	Hydroxyzine	Meperidine	Metoclopramide	Midazolam	Morphine	Nalbuphine	Pentazocine	Pentobarbital	Perphenazine	Prochlorperazine	Promazine	Promethazine	Ranitidine	Scopolamine Hbr	Secobarbital	Thiethylperazine
	C	C	C	C	C	C	C	C	C	C	C	C	C	C	C	I
	C	C	C	C	C		C	I	C	C		C		C	I	C
	C	C	C	C	C		C	I	C	C	C	C	C	C	I	
								I							I	
	I	I	I		I	I	I	I	I	I	I	I		I	I	I
	I	C	C	I	C		C	I	C	I	I	I	C	C	I	
	C	C	C	C	C		C	I	C	C	C	C	C	C	I	
	C	C	C		C	C	C	I	C	C	C	C		C	I	
	C	C	C		C		C	I	C	C	C	C	C	C	I	
	C	C			C		I	I		C	C	C	C	C	I	
		I			I		I				I					
	▓	C	C		C	C	C	I		C	C	C	I	C	I	
	C	▓	C		I		C	I	C	C	C	C	C	C	I	
	C	C	▓		C		C		C	C	C	C	C	C	I	
	C		C	▓	C	C		I	I	I	C	C	I	C		C
	C	I	C		▓		C	I	C	C	C	C	C	C	I	
	C					▓		I		C		*	C	C	I	C
	C	C	C		C		▓	I	C	C	C	C	C	C	I	
	I	I			I	I	I	▓	I	I	I	I	I	C	I	
		C	C		C		C	I	▓	C			C	C	C	I
	C	C	C		C	C	C	I	C	▓		C	C	C	C	I
	C	C	C		C		C	I		C	▓	C		C	I	
	C	C	C		C	C	C	I	C	C	C	▓	C	C	I	
		C	C	I	C	C	C			C	C		▓	C		C
	C	C	C		C	C	C	C	C	C	C	C	C	▓	I	
	I	I	I			I	I	I	I	I	I	I	I		▓	I
					C				I				C		I	▓

Parenteral compatibility occurs when two or more drugs are successfully mixed without liquefaction, deliquescence, or precipitation.

Drug Monographs New to This Edition
(See Appendix A, Selected New Drugs)

abacavir
alitretinoin
aminolevulinic acid
amprenavir
bexarotene
cilostazol
coagulation factor VIIa,
    recombinant
denileukin diftitox
dexmedetomidine
dofetilide
doxercalciferol
entacapone
epirubicin
exemestane
ganirelix
gatifloxacin
interferon alfa-n 1
    lymphoblastoid
levalbuterol
levetiracetam

levobupivacaine
lymphocyte immune globulin
    (anti-thymocyte)
modafinil
moxifloxacin
nitric oxide
octreotide
orlistat
oseltamivir
perindopril
pioglitazone
poractant alfa
rabeprazole
rapacuronium
rofecoxib
rosiglitazone
sirolimus
temozolomide
zaleplon
zanamivir

 GET CONNECTED!

Receive our free online drug updates!

Visit us at

www.mosby.com/MERLIN/nursingdrugupdates/Skidmore/

and you'll be assured of receiving the most up-to-the-minute drug information, including*:

- Updates on recently approved drugs
- Names and brief descriptions of new drugs
- Drug alerts
- Updated drug information
- Hyperlinks to drug information websites

Visit our website today to get connected!

---

*Not every update will include each of these items. Information released by the FDA and other developments will determine the contents of each update.

Mosby's

2001
Nursing
Drug
Reference

Linda Skidmore-Roth, R.N., M.S.N., N.P.

Consultant
Littleton, Colorado

Formerly, Nursing Faculty,
New Mexico State University,
Las Cruces, New Mexico;
El Paso Community College,
El Paso, Texas

 Mosby

A Harcourt Health Sciences Company

St. Louis   London   Philadelphia   Sydney   Toronto

Mosby

A Harcourt Health Sciences Company

Vice President, Nursing Editorial Director: Sally Schrefer
Executive Editor, Nursing: N. Darlene Como
Developmental Editor: Tamara Myers
Project Manager: Deborah L. Vogel
Production Editor: Ed Alderman
Designer: Bill Drone

Printed in the United States of America

Mosby, Inc.
A Harcourt Health Sciences Company
11830 Westline Industrial Drive
St. Louis, Missouri 63146

ISSN 1044-8470
ISBN 0-323-00981-6

01 02 03 04 GW/RDC 9 8 7 6 5 4 3 2

Consultants

Phyllis Baker, R.N., Ed.D.
Associate Professor,
Saint Xavier University,
School of Nursing,
Chicago, Illinois

Jean Krajicek Bartek, Ph.D.,
A.R.N.P.
Associate Professor,
University of Nebraska Medical
    Center,
Colleges of Nursing and Medicine
    (Pharmacology),
Omaha, Nebraska

Barbara A. Brunow, R.N., M.S.N.
Instructor, Providence Hospital,
School of Nursing,
Sandusky, Ohio

Marcia Buck, Pharm.D., F.C.C.P.
Clinical Pharmacy Specialist,
Clinical Associate Professor,
University of Virginia Children's
    Medical Center,
Department of Pharmacy Services,
Charlottesville, Virginia

Connie L. Bush, R.N., M.S.
Associate Professor, Nursing,
Niagara County Community
    College,
Sanborn, New York

Judy E. Davidson, R.N., M.S.,
C.C.R.N.
Clinical Nurse Specialist,
University of California San Diego
    Medical Center,
San Diego, California

Jane Doyle, R.N., B.S.N., M.S.,
M.B.A.
Nursing Faculty,
Mount Wachusett Community
    College,
Gardner, Massachusetts

Laurel A. Eisenhauer, R.N., Ph.D.
Professor of Nursing,
Boston College School of Nursing,
Chestnut Hill, Massachusetts

Tim Engelhardt, B.Sc., Pharm.D.
Manager, Pharmacy Services,
Calgary District Hospital Group,
Calgary, Alberta

Theresa M. Hulub, R.N., M.S.Ed.,
M.S.N.
Professor of Nursing Education,
Niagara County Community
    College,
Sanborn, New York

Kimberly A. Hunter, Pharm.D.
Assistant Professor of Pharmacy
    Practice,
Washington State University
    College of Pharmacy;
Geriatric Clinical Pharmacist,
Sacred Heart Medical Center,
Spokane, Washington

Jon E. Lewis, B.A., Ph.D.
Senior Research Scientist and
    Director,
Respiratory Diseases,
Marion Merrell Dow Research
    Institute,
Cincinnati, Ohio

Edwina A. McConnell, R.N., Ph.D.
Independent Nurse Consultant,
Madison, Wisconsin

Diane Moro, R.N., M.S.
Nursing Instructor,
St. Joseph's Hospital Health Center,
School of Nursing,
Syracuse, New York

Rosemary A. Pine, R.N., M.S.N.
Assistant Professor of Nursing,
Department Chair, ADN Program,
Houston Baptist University,
Houston, Texas

Norma L. Pinnell, R.N., M.S.N.
Instructor, Southern Illinois
    University,
School of Nursing,
Edwardsville, Illinois

Mary Quintas, R.N.
Miles Community College,
Department of Nursing,
Miles City, Montana

Robert T. Reilly, Pharm.D.
Associate Director of Pharmacy,
    Clinical Services,
Thomason Hospital,
El Paso, Texas

Roberta Roynayne, R.N., B.Sc.N.,
M.Sc.
Assistant Professor,
University of Ottawa,
School of Nursing,
Ottawa, Ontario

Carol Ruscin, R.N., B.S.
Level I Faculty,
Baptist Medical System,
School of Nursing,
Little Rock, Arkansas

Lori Schoonover, Pharm.D.
Assistant Professor, Pharmacy,
Washington State University,
Spokane, Washington

Roberta J. Secrest, Ph.D., Pharm.D.,
R.Ph.
Associate Scientist,
Marion Merrell Dow Research
    Institute,
Cincinnati, Ohio

John R. White, Jr., Pharm.D.
Assistant Professor,
Washington State University,
College of Pharmacy,
Spokane, Washington

Preface

Since the first publication of *Mosby's Nursing Drug Reference* in 1988, more than 100 U.S. and Canadian pharmacists and consultants have reviewed the book's content closely. Today, as we enter the new millennium, *Mosby's 2001 Nursing Drug Reference* has been more completely revised and updated than ever! The new edition features more than 1000 new drug facts—including revised nursing considerations and patient/family teaching guidelines, as well as hundreds of newly researched side effects, adverse reactions, precautions, interactions, contraindications, and IV therapy information. To keep our readers up to date, Appendix A, "Selected new drugs," also presents detailed monographs for 38 new drugs recently approved by the FDA (see the page facing the title page for a complete list). Included are monographs for zaleplon (Sonata), used for short-term treatment of insomnia; rabeprazole (Aciphex), for erosive/ulcerative gastroesophageal reflux disease (GERD); epirubicin (Ellence), used in breast cancer; and sirolimus (Rapamune), used to prevent renal organ transplant rejection. In addition, Appendix B, "Recent FDA drug approvals," provides generic/trade names and uses for 8 of the most recently approved drugs, for which complete information was not yet available at press time.

To keep pace with current consumer trends, Appendix I, "Herbal products," lists more than 80 popular herbal supplements and their uses. A special herbal product icon also appears throughout the text, highlighting more than 370 potential interactions between drugs and herbal products, 103 of which are new to this edition. To help ensure safe drug administration, Appendix H, "Look-alike/sound-alike drug names," lists nearly 200 pairs of drug names that may be easily confused. Another feature designed to help nurses identify common drugs and deliver high-quality patient care is a 16-page full-color insert containing 160 photographs of frequently prescribed tablets and capsules. The photos in this drug identification guide are arranged alphabetically by generic name, with common trade names and dosage strengths included. In addition, Appendix E, "Combination products," includes entries for 682 commonly used combination products, their components, and their uses. Appendix F, "Rarely used drugs," features 11 new monographs. The new Appendix G, "Less frequently used antihistamines," presents information on less commonly used products in a convenient tabular format that includes generic and common trade name(s), uses, dosages and routes, available forms, interactions, and contraindications. The updated Windows disk inside the back cover includes additional drug information that complements that found in the book. The 2001 edition also includes free Internet updates on the "Nursing Drug Updates" page of the Mosby website at *www.mosby.com* (this page's URL is www1.mosby.com/Mosby/nursing_drug_updates/). The information on this site is updated throughout the year to provide users with the very latest drug information.

Within the drug monographs themselves, *Mosby's 2001 Nursing Drug Reference* includes numerous useful features that make finding essential information fast and easy. For example, instructions for giving drugs by various routes (IV, IM, PO, etc.) are grouped together under the Nursing Considerations' "Administer" subsection. These route subheadings appear in boldfaced type, making this crucial information easy to retrieve in the clinical setting. All drug compatibility information is also located under this monograph subheading. In addition, the "Dosages and routes" section of each monograph also features IV, IM, PO, and other route designations in boldfaced type to make them easier to locate. To help organize closely related drug information for convenient reference, the book also features nine new detailed monographs that group all chemically similar forms of a single drug together into a single monograph. These monographs include: calcitonin, human and salmon; clindamycin hydrochloride, palmitate, and phosphate; diphtheria, tetanus toxoids, and pertussis vaccines, both acellular and whole; doxorubicin and doxorubicin liposome; fluoride, oral and topical; haemophilus b vaccines, including diphtheria CRM_{197} protein conjugate, diphtheria toxoid conjugate (PRP-D), and meningococcal protein conjugate (PRP-OMP); haloperidol, haloperidol decanoate, and haloperidol lactate; fluphenazine decanoate, enanthate, and hydrochloride; and magnesium salts, citrate, hydroxide, oxide, and sulfate. To ensure that readers can locate drug information quickly and easily, cross-references to each individual drug included in a grouped monograph appear in alphabetical order where they would normally be found in the book. Similarly, cross-references to each of the new drug monographs included in Appendix A appear throughout the body of the book.

The guiding principle behind this book is to provide easy access to drug information and nursing considerations that specifically tell the nurse what to do in terms consistent with the nursing process. Every detail—down to the paper, typeface, cover, binding, use of color, and appendixes—is carefully chosen with the user in mind.

This book is organized into three main sections. General information about the various drug categories is included after the table of contents, on blue-screened pages for quick reference. The individual drug monographs appear next, arranged in alphabetical order by generic name. The book includes monographs for more than 1300 generic and 4500 trade medications. Common trade names are given for all drugs regularly used in the United States and Canada, with drugs available only in Canada identified by an asterisk. The final section of the book consists of the appendixes, which are easily identified by the wide blue thumb tabs on their edges.

The following information is provided, whenever possible, for safe, effective administration of each drug:

Pronunciation: Pronunciations help the nursing student master the more complex generic names.

R/OTC: Prescription (R) or over-the-counter (OTC) designation is included in each drug monograph.

Functional and chemical classifications: All known broad functional and chemical classifications are given. These classifications allow the nurse to see similarities and dissimilarities among drugs in the same functional but different chemical classes.

Controlled-substance schedule: Schedules are included for the United States (I, II, III, IV, V) and Canada (F, G).

Action: Pharmacologic properties are described in concise terms. Action is discussed to the cellular level when known.

Uses: Provides drug applications.

Investigational uses: Provides drug applications for those uses that may be encountered in practice but are not yet FDA-approved.

Dosages and routes: All available and approved dosages and routes are given for adult, pediatric, and geriatric patients.

Available forms: All available forms—including tablets, capsules, extended-release, injectables (IV, IM, SC), solutions, creams, ointments, lotions, gels, shampoos, elixirs, suspensions, suppositories, sprays, aerosols, and lozenges—are provided.

Side effects/adverse reactions: Grouped by body system, common side effects are *italicized,* and life-threatening reactions are in ***bold italic type,*** allowing the nurse to quickly identify common and life-threatening reactions.

Contraindications: Contraindications are instances in which a medication absolutely should not be given. When the FDA has assigned pregnancy safety categories D or X, it appears here.

Precautions: Special precautionary steps are given here, including FDA pregnancy safety categories A, B, and C.

Pharmacokinetics: Metabolism, distribution, and elimination are provided for all dosage forms, if known.

Interactions: This section includes confirmed drug, food, and smoking interactions. The reaction is listed first, followed by the drug or nutrient causing that interaction, when applicable.

"Herb-Drug Interaction" icon: More than 370 icons (⌀) highlight potential interactions between herbal products and prescription or OTC drugs.

Lab test interferences: Known lab test interferences are provided.

Nursing considerations: Highlighted nursing considerations are organized to foster use of the nursing process: Assess, Administer, Perform/provide, Evaluate, and Teach patient/family. Nursing considerations are consistently organized under these headings to help the nurse group interventions that can be used for planning nursing care.

Compatibilities: Syringe, Y-site, and additive compatibilities and incompatibilities are listed for drugs where applicable under "Administer." If no compatibilities are listed for a drug, this denotes that the necessary compatibility testing has not been done and that compatibility information is unknown. To ensure safety, assume that the drug may not be mixed with other drugs unless specifically stated.

"Nursing Alert" icon: Certain items are highlighted with an arrow (◆) to alert the user to pay particular attention to an item that may be dangerous.

"Do Not Crush" icon: Includes more than 100 icons (⊘) denoting drugs that may not be administered in crushed form.

Treatment of overdose: Drugs and treatment for overdoses are provided for appropriate drugs.

The following appendixes are included to further enhance the usability of this reference: Selected new drugs; Recent FDA drug approvals; Ophthalmic, otic, nasal, and topical products; Commonly used antiinfectives in adults and children; Combination products; Rarely used drugs; Less frequently used antihistamines; Look-alike/sound-alike drug names; Herbal products; FDA pregnancy categories; Controlled substance chart; Abbreviations; Weights and equivalents; Formulas for drug calculations; and Nomogram for calculation of body surface area. Drug-to-drug and drug-to-solution IV compatibility charts have been printed inside the front and back covers for quick access.

I am indebted to the nursing and pharmacology consultants who reviewed the manuscript and galley pages and thank them for their criticism and encouragement. I would also like to thank Darlene Como and Dana Knighten, my editors, whose active encouragement and enthusiasm have made this book better than it might otherwise have been. I am likewise grateful to Ed Alderman, Mike McConnell, and Graphic World, Inc., for the coordination of the production process.

Linda Skidmore-Roth

Contents

Individual drugs, 67

Appendixes

Index, 1125

ALPHA-ADRENERGIC BLOCKERS

Action: Acts by binding to α-adrenergic receptors, causing dilation of peripheral blood vessels. Lowers peripheral resistance, resulting in decreased blood pressure.

Uses: Used for pheochromocytoma, prevention of tissue necrosis and sloughing associated with extravasation of IV vasopressors.

Side effects/adverse reactions: The most common side effects are hypotension, tachycardia, nasal stuffiness, nausea, vomiting, and diarrhea.

Contraindications: Hypersensitive reactions may occur, and allergies should be identified before these products are given. Patients with myocardial infarction, coronary insufficiency, angina, or other evidence of coronary artery disease should not use these products.

Pharmacokinetics: Onset, peak, and duration vary among products.

Interactions: Vasoconstrictive and hypertensive effects of epinephrine are antagonized by α-adrenergic blockers.

Possible nursing diagnoses:
- Altered tissue perfusion *[uses]*
- Risk for injury *[adverse reactions]*
- Sleep pattern disturbance *[adverse reactions]*

NURSING CONSIDERATIONS

Assess:
- Electrolytes: K, Na, Cl, CO_2
- Weight daily, I&O
- B/P lying, standing before starting treatment, q4h thereafter
- Nausea, vomiting, diarrhea
- Skin turgor, dryness of mucous membranes for hydration status

Administer:
- Starting with low dose, gradually increasing to prevent side effects
- With food or milk for GI symptoms

Evaluate:
- Therapeutic response: decreased B/P, increased peripheral pulses

Teach patient/family:
- To avoid alcoholic beverages
- To report dizziness, palpitations, fainting
- To change position slowly or fainting may occur
- To take drug exactly as prescribed
- To avoid all OTC products (cough, cold, allergy) unless directed by prescriber

---

Generic names

phenoxybenzamine   phentolamine

ANESTHETICS—GENERAL/LOCAL

Action: Anesthetics (general) act on the CNS to produce tranquilization and sleep before invasive procedures. Anesthetics (local) inhibit conduction of nerve impulses from sensory nerves.

Uses: General anesthetics are used to premedicate for surgery, induction and maintenance in general anesthesia. For local anesthetics, refer to individual product listing for indications.

Side effects/adverse reactions: The most common side effects are dystonia, akathisia, flexion of arms, fine tremors, drowsiness, restlessness, and hypotension. Also common are chills, respiratory depression, and laryngospasm.

Contraindications: Persons with CVA, increased intracranial pressure, severe hypertension, cardiac decompensation should not use these products, since severe adverse reactions can occur.

Precautions: Anesthetics (general) should be used with caution in the elderly, cardiovascular disease (hypotension, bradydysrhythmias), renal disease, liver disease, Parkinson's disease, children <2 yr. The precaution for anesthetics (local) is pregnancy.

Pharmacokinetics: Onset, peak, and duration vary widely among products. Most products are metabolized in the liver and excreted in urine.

Interactions: MAOIs, tricyclics, phenothiazines may cause severe hypotension or hypertension when used with local anesthetics. CNS depressants will potentiate general and local anesthetics.

Possible nursing diagnoses:
General:
• Risk for injury *[adverse reactions]*
• Knowledge deficit *[teaching]*
Local:
• Pain *[uses]*
• Knowledge deficit *[teaching]*

NURSING CONSIDERATIONS
Assess:
• VS q10min during IV administration, q30min after IM dose
Administer:
• Anticholinergic preoperatively to decrease secretions
• Only with crash cart, resuscitative equipment nearby
Perform/provide:
• Quiet environment for recovery to decrease psychotic symptoms
Evaluate:
• Therapeutic response: maintenance of anesthesia, decreased pain

Generic names (Injectables only)

General anesthetics
droperidol
etomidate
fentanyl
fentanyl/droperidol
fentanyl transdermal
ketamine (Appx F)
methohexital
midazolam
propofol
thiopental

Local anesthetics
chloroprocaine
etidocaine
lidocaine
procaine
ropivacaine
tetracaine

ANTACIDS

Action: Antacids are basic compounds that neutralize gastric acidity and decrease the rate of gastric emptying. Products are divided into those containing aluminum, magnesium, calcium, or a combination of these.

Uses: Hyperacidity is decreased by antacids in conditions such as peptic ulcer disease, reflux esophagitis, gastritis, and hiatal hernia.

Side effects/adverse reactions: The most common side effect caused by aluminum-containing antacids is constipation, which may lead to fecal impaction and bowel obstruction. Diarrhea occurs often when magnesium products are given. Alkalosis may occur when systemic products are used. Constipation occurs more frequently than laxation with calcium carbonate. The release of CO_2 from carbonate-containing antacids causes belching, abdominal distention, and flatulence. Sodium bicarbonate may act as a systemic antacid and produce systemic electrolyte disturbances and alkalosis. Calcium carbonate and sodium bicarbonate may cause rebound hyperacidity and milk-alkali syndrome. Alkaluria may occur when products are used on a long-term basis, particularly in persons with abnormal renal function.

Contraindications: Sensitivity to aluminum or magnesium products may cause hypersensitive reactions. Aluminum products should not be used by persons sensitive to aluminum; magnesium products should not be used by persons sensitive to magnesium. Check for sensitivity before administering.

Precautions: Magnesium products should be given cautiously to patients with renal insufficiency and during pregnancy and lactation. Sodium content of antacids may be significant; use with caution for patients with hypertension, CHF, or those on a low-sodium diet.

Pharmacokinetics: Duration is 20-40 min. If ingested 1 hr after meals, acidity is reduced for at least 3 hr.

Interactions: Drugs whose effects may be increased by some antacids: quinidine, amphetamines, pseudoephedrine, levodopa, valproic acid, dicumarol. Drugs whose effects may be decreased by some antacids: cimetadine, corticosteroids, ranitidine, iron salts, phenothiazines, phenytoin, digoxin, tetracyclines, ketoconazole, salicylates, isoniazid.

Possible nursing diagnoses:

- Pain *[uses]*
- Constipation *[adverse reactions]*
- Diarrhea *[adverse reactions]*

NURSING CONSIDERATIONS

Assess:

- Aggravating and alleviating factors of epigastric pain or hyperacidity; identify the location, duration, and characteristics of epigastric pain
- GI symptoms, including constipation, diarrhea, abdominal pain; if severe abdominal pain with fever occurs, these drugs should not be given
- Renal symptoms, including increasing urinary pH, electrolytes

Administer:

- All products with an 8-oz glass of water to ensure absorption in the stomach
- Another antacid if constipation occurs with aluminum products

Evaluate:

- The therapeutic effectiveness of the drug; absence of epigastric pain and decreased acidity should occur

Teach patient/family:

- Not to take other drugs within 1-2 hr of antacid administration, since antacids may impair absorption of other drugs

---

Generic names

aluminum hydroxide
bismuth subsalicylate
calcium carbonate
dihydroxyaluminum
   sodium carbonate

magaldrate
magnesium oxide
sodium bicarbonate

ANTIANGINALS

Action: The antianginals are divided into the nitrates, calcium channel blockers, and β-adrenergic blockers. The nitrates dilate coronary arteries, causing decreased preload, and dilate systemic arteries, causing decreased afterload. Calcium channel blockers dilate coronary arteries, decrease SA/AV node conduction. β-Adrenergic blockers decrease heart rate so that myocardial O_2 use is decreased. Dipyridamole selectively dilates coronary arteries to increase coronary blood flow.

Uses: Antianginals are used in chronic stable angina pectoris, unstable angina, vasospastic angina. Some (i.e., calcium channel blockers and β-blockers) may be used for dysrhythmias and in hypertension.

Side effects/adverse reactions: The most common side effects are postural hypotension, headache, flushing, dizziness, nausea, edema, and drowsiness. Also common are rash, dysrhythmias, and fatigue.

Contraindications: Persons with known hypersensitivity, increased intracranial pressure, or cerebral hemorrhage should not use some of these products.

Precautions: Antianginals should be used with caution in postural hypotension, pregnancy, lactation, children, renal disease, and hepatic injury.

Pharmacokinetics: Onset, peak, and duration vary widely among coronary products. Most products are metabolized in the liver and excreted in urine.

Interactions: Please check individual monographs since interactions vary widely among products.

Possible nursing diagnoses:
- Altered tissue perfusion: cardiopulmonary *[uses]*
- Pain *[uses]*
- Risk for injury *[uses]*
- Knowledge deficit *[teaching]*
- Decreased cardiac output *[adverse reactions]*

NURSING CONSIDERATIONS

Assess:
- Orthostatic B/P, pulse
- Pain: duration, time started, activity being performed, character
- Tolerance if taken over long period
- Headache, light-headedness, decreased B/P; may indicate a need for decreased dosage

Perform/provide:
- Storage protected from light, moisture; place in cool environment

Evaluate:
• Therapeutic response: decrease, prevention of anginal pain
Teach patient/family:
• To keep tabs in original container
• Not to use OTC products unless directed by prescriber
• To report bradycardia, dizziness, confusion, depression, fever
• To take pulse at home, advise when to notify prescriber
• To avoid alcohol, smoking, sodium intake
• To comply with weight control, dietary adjustments, modified exercise program
• To carry Medic Alert ID to identify drug that you are taking, allergies
• To make position changes slowly to prevent fainting

Generic names

Nitrates
amyl nitrite (Appx F)
isosorbide
nitroglycerin

β-Adrenergic blockers
atenolol
dipyridamole
metoprolol
nadolol
propranolol

Calcium channel blockers
amlodipine
bepridil
diltiazem
nicardipine
nifedipine
verapamil

ANTICHOLINERGICS

Action: Anticholinergics inhibit the muscarinic actions of acetylcholine at receptor sites in the autonomic nervous system; anticholinergics are also known as antimuscarinic drugs.

Uses: Anticholinergics are used for a variety of conditions: gastrointestinal anticholinergics are used to decrease motility (smooth muscle tone) in the GI, biliary, and urinary tracts and for their ability to decrease gastric secretions (propantheline, glycopyrrolate); decreasing involuntary movements in parkinsonism (benztropine, trihexyphenidyl); bradydysrhythmias (atropine); nausea and vomiting (scopolamine); and as cycloplegic mydriatics (atropine, hematropine, scopolamine, cyclopentolate, tropicamide).

Side effects/adverse reactions: The most common side effects are dry mouth, constipation, urinary retention, urinary hesitancy, headache, and dizziness. Also common is paralytic ileus.

Contraindications: Persons with narrow-angle glaucoma, myasthenia gravis, or GI/GU obstruction should not use some of these products.

Precautions: Anticholinergics should be used with caution in patients who are elderly, pregnant, or lactating or in those with prostatic hypertrophy, CHF, or hypertension; use with caution in presence of high environmental temp.

Pharmacokinetics: Onset, peak, and duration vary widely among products. Most products are metabolized in the liver and excreted in urine.

Interactions: Increased anticholinergic effects may occur when used with MAOIs and tricyclic antidepressants and amantadine. Anticholinergics may cause a decreased effect of phenothiazines and levodopa.

Possible nursing diagnoses:
• Decreased cardiac output *[uses]*
• Constipation *[adverse reactions]*
• Knowledge deficit *[teaching]*

NURSING CONSIDERATIONS

Assess:
• I&O ratio; retention commonly causes decreased urinary output
• Urinary hesitancy, retention; palpate bladder if retention occurs
• Constipation; increase fluids, bulk, exercise if this occurs
• For tolerance over long-term therapy, dose may need to be increased or changed
• Mental status: affect, mood, CNS depression, worsening of mental symptoms during early therapy

Administer:
• Parenteral dose with patient recumbent to prevent postural hypotension
• With or after meals to prevent GI upset; may give with fluids other than water
• Parenteral dose slowly; keep in bed for at least 1 hr after dose; monitor vital signs
• After checking dose carefully; even slight overdose can lead to toxicity

Perform/provide:
• Storage at room temp
• Hard candy, frequent drinks, sugarless gum to relieve dry mouth

Evaluate:
• Therapeutic response: decreased secretions, absence of nausea and vomiting

Teach patient/family:
• To avoid driving or other hazardous activities; drowsiness may occur

• To avoid OTC medication: cough, cold preparations with alcohol, antihistamines unless directed by prescriber

Generic names

atropine	methantheline
benztropine	propantheline
biperiden	scopolamine (Appx C)
cyclopentolate (Appx C)	scopolamine (transdermal)
dicyclomine	trihexyphenidyl
glycopyrrolate	tropicamide (Appx C)
homatropine (Appx C)	
hyoscyamine	

ANTICOAGULANTS

Action: Anticoagulants interfere with blood clotting by preventing clot formation.

Uses: Anticoagulants are used for deep-vein thrombosis, pulmonary emboli, myocardial infarction, open-heart surgery, disseminated intravascular clotting syndrome, atrial fibrillation with embolization, transfusion, and dialysis.

Side effects/adverse reactions: The most serious adverse reactions are hemorrhage, agranulocytosis, leukopenia, eosinophilia, and thrombocytopenia, depending on the specific product. The most common side effects are diarrhea, rash, and fever.

Contraindications: Persons with hemophilia, leukemia with bleeding, peptic ulcer disease, thrombocytopenic purpura, blood dyscrasias, acute nephritis, and subacute bacterial endocarditis should not use these products.

Precautions: Anticoagulants should be used with caution in alcoholism, elderly, and pregnancy.

Pharmacokinetics: Onset, peak, and duration vary widely among products. Most products are metabolized in the liver and excreted in urine.

Interactions: Salicylates, steroids, and nonsteroidal antiinflammatories will potentiate the action of anticoagulants. Anticoagulants may cause serious effects; please check individual monographs.

Possible nursing diagnoses:

• Altered tissue perfusion *[uses]*
• Risk for injury *[side effects]*
• Knowledge deficit *[teaching]*

NURSING CONSIDERATIONS

Assess:

- Blood studies (Hct, platelets, occult blood in stools) q3mo
- Partial prothrombin time, which should be 1½-2 × control PPT qd, also APTT, ACT
- B/P, watch for increasing signs of hypertension
- Bleeding gums, petechiae, ecchymosis; black, tarry stools; hematuria
- Fever, skin rash, urticaria
- Needed dosage change q1-2wk

Administer:

- At same time each day to maintain steady blood levels
- Do not massage area or aspirate when giving SC injection; give in abdomen between pelvic bone, rotate sites; do not pull back on plunger; leave in for 10 sec; apply gentle pressure for 1 min
- Without changing needles
- Avoiding all IM injections that may cause bleeding

Perform/provide:

- Storage in tight container

Evaluate:

- Therapeutic response: decrease of deep-vein thrombosis

Teach patient/family:

- To avoid OTC preparations that may cause serious drug interactions unless directed by prescriber
- That drug may be held during active bleeding (menstruation), depending on condition
- To use soft-bristle toothbrush to avoid bleeding gums, avoid contact sports, use electric razor
- To carry a Medic Alert ID identifying drug taken
- To report any signs of bleeding: gums, under skin, urine, stools

---

Generic names

ardeparin	heparin
dalteparin	lepirudin
danaparoid	warfarin
enoxaparin	

ANTICONVULSANTS

Action: Anticonvulsants are divided into the barbiturates (p. 35), benzodiazepines (p. 37), hydantoins, succinimides, and miscellaneous products. Barbiturates and benzodiazepines are discussed in separate sections. Hydantoins act by inhibiting the spread of seizure activity in the motor cortex. Succinimides act by inhibiting spike and wave formation; they also decrease amplitude, frequency, duration, and spread of discharge in seizures.

Uses: Hydantoins are used in generalized tonic-clonic seizures, status epilepticus, and psychomotor seizures. Succinimides are used for absence (petit mal) seizures. Barbiturates are used in generalized tonic-clonic and cortical focal seizures.

Side effects/adverse reactions: Bone marrow depression is the most life-threatening adverse reaction associated with hydantoins or succinimides. The most common side effects are GI symptoms. Other common side effects for hydantoins are gingival hyperplasia and CNS effects such as nystagmus, ataxia, slurred speech, and mental confusion.

Contraindications: Hypersensitive reactions may occur, and allergies should be identified before these products are given.

Precautions: Persons with renal or hepatic disease should be watched closely.

Pharmacokinetics: Onset, peak, and duration vary widely among products. Most products are metabolized in the liver and excreted in urine, bile, and feces.

Interactions: Decreased effects of estrogens, oral contraceptives (hydantoins).

Possible nursing diagnoses:
- Risk for injury *[uses]*
- Noncompliance *[teaching]*
- Sleep pattern disturbance *[adverse reactions]*

NURSING CONSIDERATIONS
Assess:
- Renal function studies, including BUN, creatinine, serum uric acid, urine creatinine clearance before and during therapy
- Blood studies: RBC, Hct, Hgb, reticulocyte counts qwk for 4 wk then qmo
- Hepatic studies: AST, ALT, bilirubin, creatinine
- Mental status, including mood, sensorium, affect, behavorial changes; if mental status changes, notify prescriber
- Eye problems, including need for ophthalmic exam before, during, and after treatment (slit lamp, fundoscopy, tonometry)

• Allergic reactions, including red, raised rash; if this occurs, drug should be discontinued

• Blood dyscrasia, including fever, sore throat, bruising, rash, jaundice

• Toxicity, including bone marrow depression, nausea, vomiting, ataxia, diplopia, cardiovascular collapse, Stevens-Johnson syndrome

Administer:

• With food, milk to decrease GI symptoms

Perform/provide:

• Good oral hygiene is important for hydantoins

Evaluate:

• Therapeutic response, including decreased seizure activity; document on patient's chart

Teach patient/family:

• To carry ID card or Medic Alert bracelet stating drugs taken, condition, prescriber's name, phone number

• To avoid driving, other activities that require alertness

Generic names

Hydantoins
fosphenytoin
phenytoin

Succinimides
ethosuximide
methsuximide (Appx F)

Miscellaneous
acetazolamide
carbamazepine
clonazepam
diazepam

felbamate
gabapentin
lamotrigine
magnesium sulfate
paraldehyde (Appx F)
paramethadione (Appx F)
phenacemide (Appx F)
phenobarbital
primidone
tiagabine
topiramate
valproate/valproic acid,
    divalproex sodium

ANTIDEPRESSANTS

Action: Antidepressants are divided into the tricyclics, MAOIs, and miscellaneous antidepressants. The tricyclics work by blocking reuptake of norepinephrine and serotonin into nerve endings and increasing action of norepinephrine and serotonin in nerve cells. MAOIs act by increasing concentrations of endogenous epinephrine, norepinephrine, serotonin, dopamine in storage sites in CNS by inhibition of MAO; increased concentration reduces depression.

Uses: Antidepressants are used for depression and, in some cases, enuresis in children.

Side effects/adverse reactions: The most serious adverse reactions are paralytic ileus, acute renal failure, hypertension, and hypertensive crisis, depending on the specific product. Common side effects are dizziness, drowsiness, diarrhea, dry mouth, retention, and orthostatic hypotension.

Contraindications: The contraindications to antidepressants are convulsive disorders, prostatic hypertrophy, severe renal, hepatic, cardiac disease depending on the type of medication.

Precautions: Antidepressants should be used cautiously in suicidal patients, severe depression, schizophrenia, hyperactivity, diabetes mellitus, pregnancy, and the elderly.

Pharmacokinetics: Onset, peak, and duration vary widely among products. Most products are metabolized in the liver and excreted in urine.

Interactions: Please check individual monographs since interactions vary widely among products.

Possible nursing diagnoses:
- Ineffective individual coping [uses]
- Risk for injury [uses/adverse reactions]
- Knowledge deficit [teaching]

NURSING CONSIDERATIONS

Assess:
- B/P (lying, standing), pulse q4h; if systolic B/P drops 20 mm Hg, hold drug, notify prescriber; take vital signs q4h in patients with cardiovascular disease
- Blood studies: CBC, leukocytes, differential, cardiac enzymes if patient is receiving long-term therapy
- Hepatic studies: AST, ALT, bilirubin, creatinine
- Weight qwk; appetite may increase with drug
- EPS, primarily in elderly: rigidity, dystonia, akathisia
- Mental status: mood, sensorium, affect, suicidal tendencies, increase in psychiatric symptoms: depression, panic
- Urinary retention, constipation; constipation is more likely to occur in children, elderly
- Withdrawal symptoms: headache, nausea, vomiting, muscle pain, weakness; do not usually occur unless drug was discontinued abruptly
- Alcohol consumption; if alcohol is consumed, hold dose until morning

Administer:
- Increased fluids, bulk in diet if urinary retention, constipation occur
- With food or milk for GI symptoms
- Gum, hard candy, or frequent sips of water for dry mouth

Perform/provide:
- Storage in tight container at room temp; do not refreeze
- Assistance with ambulation during beginning therapy, since drowsiness, dizziness occur
- Safety measures including side rails primarily in elderly
- Checking to see PO medication swallowed

Evaluate:
- Therapeutic response: decreased depression

Teach patient/family:
- That therapeutic effects may take 2-3 wk
- To use caution in driving, other activities requiring alertness because of drowsiness, dizziness, blurred vision
- To avoid alcohol ingestion, other CNS depressants
- Not to discontinue medication quickly after long-term use; may cause nausea, headache, malaise
- To wear sunscreen or wide-brimmed hat, since photosensitivity may occur

---

Generic names

Tetracyclics
mirtazapine

Tricyclics
amitriptyline
amoxapine
clomipramine
desipramine (Appx F)
doxepin
imipramine
nortriptyline
protriptyline
trimipramine

Miscellaneous
bupropion
nefazodone
trazodone
venlafaxine

MAOIs
phenelzine
tranylcypromine

SSRIs
citalopram
fluoxetine
fluvoxamine
paroxetine
sertraline

ANTIDIABETICS

Action: Antidiabetics are divided into the insulins that decrease blood sugar, phosphate, and potassium and increase blood pyruvate and lactate; and oral antidiabetics that cause functioning β-cells in the pancreas to release insulin, improve the effect of endogenous and exogenous insulin.
Uses: Insulins are used for ketoacidosis and diabetes mellitus types I (IDDM) and II (NIDDM); oral antidiabetics are used for stable adult-onset diabetes mellitus type II (NIDDM).

Side effects/adverse reactions: The most common side effect of insulin and oral antidiabetics is hypoglycemia. Other adverse reactions to oral antidiabetics include blood dyscrasias, hepatotoxicity, and rarely, cholestatic jaundice. Adverse reactions to insulin products include allergic responses and more rarely, anaphylaxis.

Contraindications: Hypersensitive reactions may occur, and allergies should be identified before these products are given. Oral antidiabetics should not be used in juvenile or brittle diabetes, diabetic ketoacidosis, severe renal disease, or severe hepatic disease.

Precautions: Oral antidiabetics should be used with caution in the elderly, in cardiac disease, pregnancy, lactation, and in the presence of alcohol.

Pharmacokinetics: Onset, peak, and duration vary widely among products. Oral antidiabetics are metabolized in the liver, with metabolites excreted in urine, bile, and feces.

Interactions: Interactions vary widely among products. Check individual monographs for specific information.

Possible nursing diagnoses:
• Altered nutrition: more than body requirements *[uses]*

NURSING CONSIDERATIONS

Assess:
• Blood, urine glucose levels during treatment to determine diabetes control (oral products)
• Fasting blood glucose, 2 hr PP (60-100 mg/dl normal fasting level) (70-130 mg/dl normal 2-hr level)
• Hypoglycemic reaction that can occur during peak time

Administer:
• Insulin after warming to room temp by rotating in palms to prevent lipodystrophy from injecting cold insulin
• Human insulin to those allergic to beef or pork
• Oral antidiabetic 30 min before meals

Perform/provide:
• Rotation of injection sites when giving insulin; use abdomen, upper back, thighs, upper arm, buttocks; rotate sites within one of these regions; keep a record of sites

Evaluate:
• Therapeutic response, including decrease in polyuria, polydipsia, polyphagia, clear sensorium, absence of dizziness, stable gait

Teach patient/family:
• To avoid alcohol and salicylates except on advice of prescriber
• Symptoms of ketoacidosis: nausea, thirst, polyuria, dry mouth, decreased B/P; dry, flushed skin; acetone breath, drowsiness, Kussmaul respiration

• Symptoms of hypoglycemia: headache, tremors, fatigue, weakness; and that candy or sugar should be carried to treat hypoglycemia
• To test urine for glucose/ketones tid if this drug is replacing insulin
• To continue weight control, dietary restrictions, exercise, hygiene

Generic names

chlorpropamide (Appx F)
glipizide
glyburide
insulin lispro
insulin, regular
insulin, regular concentrated
insulin, zinc suspension
  (Lente)
insulin, zinc suspension
  extended (Ultralente)

insulin, zinc suspension,
  prompt (Semilente)
metformin
miglitol
pioglitazone (Appx A)
repaglinide
rosiglitazone (Appx A)
tolbutamide

ANTIDIARRHEALS

Action: Antidiarrheals work by various actions, including direct action on intestinal muscles to decrease GI peristalsis; by inhibiting prostaglandin synthesis responsible for GI hypermotility; by acting on mucosal receptors responsible for peristalsis; or by decreasing water content of stools.

Uses: Antidiarrheals are used for diarrhea of undetermined causes.

Side effects/adverse reactions: The most serious adverse reactions of some products are paralytic ileus, toxic megacolon, and angioneurotic edema. The most common side effects are constipation, nausea, dry mouth, and abdominal pain.

Contraindications: Persons with severe ulcerative colitis, pseudomembranous colitis with some products.

Precautions: Antidiarrheals should be used with caution in the elderly, pregnancy, lactation, children, dehydration.

Pharmacokinetics: Onset, peak, and duration vary widely among products. Most products are metabolized in the liver and excreted in urine.

Interactions: Please check individual monographs, since interactions vary widely among products.

Possible nursing diagnoses:
• Diarrhea *[uses]*
• Constipation *[adverse reactions]*
• Fluid volume deficit *[adverse reactions]*
• Knowledge deficit *[teaching]*

NURSING CONSIDERATIONS
Assess:
• Electrolytes (K, Na, Cl) if on long-term therapy
• Bowel pattern before; for rebound constipation after termination of medication
• Response after 48 hr; if no response, drug should be discontinued
• Dehydration in children
Administer:
• For 48 hr only
Evaluate:
• Therapeutic response: decreased diarrhea
Teach patient/family:
• To avoid OTC products
• Not to exceed recommended dose

Generic names

bismuth subsalicylate
difenoxin
kaolin/pectin

loperamide
opium tincture

ANTIDYSRHYTHMICS

Action: Antidysrhythmics are divided into four classes and miscellaneous antidysrhythmics:
• Class I increases the duration of action potential and effective refractory period and reduces disparity in the refractory period between a normal and infarcted myocardium; further subclasses include Ia, Ib, Ic
• Class II decreases the rate of SA node discharge, increases recovery time, slows conduction through the AV node, and decreases heart rate, which decreases O_2 consumption in the myocardium
• Class III increases the duration of action potential and the effective refractory period
• Class IV inhibits calcium ion influx across the cell membrane during cardiac depolarization; decreases SA node discharge, decreases conduction velocity through the AV node
• Miscellaneous antidysrhythmics include those such as adenosine, which slows conduction through the AV node, and digoxin, which decreases conduction velocity and prolongs the effective refractory period in the AV node
Uses: These products are used for PVCs, tachycardia, hypertension, atrial fibrillation, angina pectoris.

Side effects/adverse reactions: Side effects and adverse reactions vary widely among products.

Contraindications: Contraindications vary widely among products.

Precautions: Precautions vary widely among products.

Pharmacokinetics: Onset, peak, and duration vary widely among products.

Interactions: Interactions vary widely among products; check individual monographs for specific information.

Possible nursing diagnoses:
- Decreased cardiac output *[uses]*
- Altered tissue perfusion: cardiopulmonary *[uses]*
- Diarrhea *[adverse reactions]*
- Impaired gas exchange *[adverse reactions]*

NURSING CONSIDERATIONS

Assess:
- ECG continuously to determine drug effectiveness, PVCs, or other dysrhythmias
- IV infusion rate to avoid causing nausea, vomiting
- For dehydration or hypovolemia
- B/P continuously for hypotension, hypertension
- I&O ratio
- Serum potassium
- Edema in feet and legs daily

Evaluate:
- Therapeutic response, including decrease in B/P in hypertension; decreased B/P, edema, moist rales in CHF

Teach patient/family:
- To comply with dosage schedule, even if patient is feeling better
- To report bradycardia, dizziness, confusion, depression, fever

Generic names

Class I	*Class II*
moricizine	acebutolol
	esmolol
Class Ia	propranolol
disopyramide	sotalol
procainamide	
quinidine	*Class III*
	amiodarone
Class Ib	bretylium
lidocaine	ibutilide
mexiletine	
phenytoin	*Class IV*
tocainide	verapamil
Class Ic	*Miscellaneous*
flecainide	adenosine
indecainide (Appx F)	atropine
propafenone	digoxin

ANTIFUNGALS (SYSTEMIC)

Action: Antifungals act by increasing cell membrane permeability in susceptible organisms by binding sterols and decreasing potassium, sodium, and nutrients in the cell.

Uses: Antifungals are used for infections of histoplasmosis, blastomycosis, coccidiomycosis, cryptococcosis, aspergillosis, phycomycosis, candidiasis, sporotrichosis causing severe meningitis, septicemia, and skin infections.

Side effects/adverse reactions: The most serious adverse reactions include renal tubular acidosis, permanent renal impairment, anuria, oliguria, hemorrhagic gastroenteritis, acute liver failure, and blood dyscrasias. Some common side effects include hypokalemia, nausea, vomiting, anorexia, headache, fever, and chills.

Contraindications: Persons with severe bone depression or hypersensitivity should not use these products.

Precautions: Antifungals should be used with caution in renal disease, pregnancy, and hepatic disease.

Pharmacokinetics: Onset, peak, and duration vary widely among products. Most products are metabolized in the liver and excreted in urine.

Interactions: Please check individual monographs since interactions vary widely among products.

Possible nursing diagnoses:
• Risk for infection *[uses]*
• Risk for injury *[adverse reactions]*
• Knowledge deficit *[teaching]*

NURSING CONSIDERATIONS
Assess:
• VS q15-30min during first infusion; note changes in pulse, B/P
• I&O ratio; watch for decreasing urinary output, change in specific gravity; discontinue drug to prevent permanent damage to renal tubules
• Blood studies: CBC, K, Na, Ca, Mg q2wk
• Weight weekly; if weight increases over 2 lb/wk, edema is present; renal damage should be considered
• For renal toxicity: increasing BUN, if >40 mg/dl or if serum creatinine >3 mg/dl; drug may be discontinued or dosage reduced
• For hepatotoxicity: increasing AST, ALT, alk phosphatase, bilirubin
• For allergic reaction: dermatitis, rash; drug should be discontinued, antihistamines (mild reaction) or epinephrine (severe reaction) administered
• For hypokalemia: anorexia, drowsiness, weakness, decreased reflexes, dizziness, increased urinary output, increased thirst, paresthesias
• For ototoxicity: tinnitus (ringing, roaring in ears), vertigo, loss of hearing (rare)
Administer:
• IV using in-line filter (mean pore diameter >1 μm) using distal veins; check for extravasation, necrosis q8h
• Drug only after C&S confirms organism, drug needed to treat condition; make sure drug is used in life-threatening infections
Perform/provide:
• Protection from light during infusion, cover with foil
• Symptomatic treatment as ordered for adverse reactions: aspirin, antihistamines, antiemetics, antispasmodics
• Storage protected from moisture and light; diluted sol is stable for 24 hr
Evaluate:
• Therapeutic response: decreased fever, malaise, rash, negative C&S for infecting organism
Teach patient/family:
• That long-term therapy may be needed to clear infection (2 wk-3 mo depending on type of infection)

Generic names

amphotericin B
fluconazole
flucytosine
griseofulvin

itraconazole
ketoconazole
miconazole
nystatin

ANTIHISTAMINES

Action: Antihistamines compete with histamines for H_1-receptor sites. They antagonize in varying degrees most of the pharmacologic effects of histamines.

Uses: Products are used to control the symptoms of allergies, rhinitis, and pruritus.

Side effects/adverse reactions: Most products cause drowsiness; however, two of the newer products, astemizole and terfenadine, produce little, if any, drowsiness. Other common side effects are headache and thickening of bronchial secretions. Serious blood dyscrasias may occur, but are rare. Urinary retention, GI effects occur with many of these products.

Contraindications: Hypersensitivity to H_1-receptor antagonists occurs rarely. Patients with acute asthma and lower respiratory tract disease should not use these products since thick secretions may result. Other contraindications include narrow-angle glaucoma, bladder neck obstruction, stenosing peptic ulcer, symptomatic prostatic hypertrophy, newborn, lactation.

Precautions: These products must be used cautiously in conjunction with intraocular pressure since they increase intraocular pressure. Caution should also be used in patients with renal and cardiac disease, hypertension, seizure disorders, pregnancy, lactation, and in the elderly.

Pharmacokinetics: Onset varies from 20-60 min, with duration lasting 4-12 hr. In general, pharmacokinetics vary widely among products.

Interactions: Barbiturates, narcotics, hypnotics, tricyclic antidepressants, or alcohol can increase CNS depression when taken with antihistamines.

Possible nursing diagnoses:
• Ineffective airway clearance *[uses]*

NURSING CONSIDERATIONS
Assess:
• I&O ratio; be alert for urinary retention, frequency, dysuria; drug should be discontinued if these occur
• CBC during long-term therapy, since hemolytic anemia, although rare, may occur

- Blood dyscrasias: thrombocytopenia, agranulocytosis (rare)
- Respiratory status, including rate, rhythm, increase in bronchial secretions, wheezing, chest tightness
- Cardiac status, including palpitations, increased pulse, hypotension

Administer:
- With food or milk to decrease GI symptoms; absorption may be decreased slightly
- Whole (sustained release tabs)

Perform/provide:
- Hard candy, gum, frequent rinsing of mouth for dryness

Evaluate:
- Therapeutic response, including absence of allergy symptoms, itching

Teach patient/family:
- To notify prescriber if confusion, sedation, hypotension occur
- To avoid driving, other hazardous activity if drowsiness occurs
- To avoid concurrent use of alcohol, other CNS depressants
- To discontinue a few days before skin testing

Generic names

acrivastine/pseudoephedrine
azatadine
azelastine
brompheniramine
budesonide
cetirizine
chlorpheniramine
clemastine
cyproheptadine

dexchlorpheniramine
diphenhydramine
fexofenadine
loratadine
promethazine
trimeprazine
tripelennamine
triprolidine

ANTIHYPERTENSIVES

Action: Antihypertensives are divided into angiotensin-converting enzyme (ACE) inhibitors, β-adrenergic blockers, calcium channel blockers, centrally acting adrenergics, diuretics, peripherally acting antiadrenergics, and vasodilators. β-Blockers, calcium channel blockers, and diuretics are discussed in separate sections. Angiotensin-converting enzyme inhibitors act by selectively suppressing renin-angiotensin I to angiotensin II; dilation of arterial and venous vessels occurs. Centrally acting adrenergics act by inhibiting the sympathetic vasomotor center in the CNS that reduces impulses in the sympathetic nervous system; blood pressure, pulse rate, and cardiac output decrease. Peripherally acting antiadrenergics inhibit sympathetic vasoconstriction by inhibiting release of norepinephrine and/or depleting norepinephrine stores in adrenergic nerve endings. Vasodilators act on arteriolar smooth muscle by producing direct relaxation or vasodilation; a reduction in blood pressure, with concomitant increases in heart rate and cardiac output, occurs.

Uses: Used for hypertension and for heart failure not responsive to conventional therapy. Some products are used in hypertensive crisis, angina, and for some cardiac dysrhythmias.

Side effects/adverse reactions: The most common side effects are marked hypotension, bradycardia, tachycardia, headache, nausea, and vomiting. Side effects and adverse reactions may vary widely between classes and specific products.

Contraindications: Hypersensitive reactions may occur, and allergies should be identified before these products are given. Antihypertensives should not be used in patients with heart block or in children.

Precautions: Antihypertensives should be used with caution in the elderly, in dialysis patients, and in the presence of hypovolemia, leukemia, and electrolyte imbalances.

Pharmacokinetics: Onset, peak, and duration vary widely among products. Most products are metabolized in the liver, with metabolites excreted in urine, bile, and feces.

Interactions: Interactions vary widely among products; check individual monographs for specific information.

Possible nursing diagnoses:
• Altered tissue perfusion *[uses]*
• Decreased cardiac output *[uses]*
• Diarrhea *[adverse reactions]*
• Impaired gas exchange *[adverse reactions]*

NURSING CONSIDERATIONS
Assess:
• Blood studies: neutrophil; decreased platelets occur with many of the products
• Renal studies: protein, BUN, creatinine; watch for increased levels that may indicate nephrotic syndrome; obtain baselines in renal and liver function studies before beginning treatment
• Edema in feet and legs daily
• Allergic reaction, including rash, fever, pruritus, urticaria: drug should be discontinued if antihistamines fail to help
• Symptoms of CHF: edema, dyspnea, wet rales, B/P
• Renal symptoms: polyuria, oliguria, frequency
Perform/provide:
• Supine or Trendelenburg position for severe hypotension

Evaluate:
• Therapeutic response, including decrease in B/P in hypotension; decreased B/P, edema, moist rales in CHF

Teach patient/family:
• To comply with dosage schedule, even if feeling better
• To rise slowly to sitting or standing position to minimize orthostatic hypotension

---

Generic names

Angiotensin-converting enzyme inhibitors
benazepril
enalapril
fosinopril
quinapril
ramipril
trandolapril

Angiotensin II receptor blocker
candesartan
irbesartan
losartan
telmisartan
valsartan

Centrally acting adrenergics
clonidine
guanabenz
guanfacine
methyldopa

Peripherally acting antiadrenergics
guanadrel
guanethidine
prazosin
reserpine
terazosin

Vasodilators
diazoxide
fenoldopam
hydralazine
minoxidil
nitroprusside

Antiadrenergic combined
α-/β-*blocker*
labetalol

ANTIINFECTIVES

Action: Antiinfectives are divided into several groups, which include but are not limited to penicillins, cephalosporins, aminoglycosides, sulfonamides, tetracyclines, monobactam, erythromycins, and quinolones. These drugs act by inhibiting the growth and replication of susceptible bacterial organisms.

Uses: Used for infections of susceptible organisms. These products are effective against bacterial, rickettsial, and spirochete infections.

Side effects/adverse reactions: The most common side effects are nausea, vomiting, and diarrhea. Adverse reactions include bone marrow depression and anaphylaxis.

Contraindications: Hypersensitivity reactions may occur, and allergies should be identified before these products are given. Cross-sensitivity can occur between products of different classes (penicillins or cephalosporins). Many persons allergic to penicillins are also allergic to cephalosporins.

Precautions: Antiinfectives should be used with caution in persons with renal and liver disease.

Pharmacokinetics: Onset, peak, and duration vary widely among products. Most products are metabolized in the liver, and metabolites are excreted in urine, bile, and feces.

Interactions: Interactions vary widely among products; check individual monographs for specific information.

Possible nursing diagnoses:
• Risk for infection *[uses]*
• Diarrhea *[adverse reactions]*

NURSING CONSIDERATIONS
Assess:
• Nephrotoxicity, including increased BUN, creatinine
• Blood studies: AST, ALT, CBC, Hct, bilirubin; test monthly if patient is on long-term therapy
• Bowel pattern qd; if severe diarrhea occurs, drug should be discontinued
• Urine output; if decreasing, notify prescriber; may indicate nephrotoxicity
• Allergic reaction, including rash, fever, pruritus, urticaria; drug should be discontinued
• Bleeding: ecchymosis, bleeding gums, hematuria, stool guaiac daily
• Overgrowth of infection: perineal itching, fever, malaise, redness, pain, swelling, drainage, rash, diarrhea, change in cough, sputum

Administer:
• For 10-14 days to ensure organism death, prevention of superinfection
• After C&S completed; drug may be taken as soon as culture is taken

Evaluate:
• Therapeutic response, including absence of fever, fatigue, malaise, draining wounds

Teach patient/family:
• To comply with dosage schedule, even if feeling better
• To report sore throat, bruising, bleeding, joint pain; may indicate blood dyscrasias (rare)

Generic names

Aminoglycosides
amikacin
azithromycin
clarithromycin
gentamicin
kanamycin
neomycin
streptomycin
tobramycin

Cephalosporins
cefaclor
cefadroxil
cefamandole
cefazolin
cefdinir
cefepime
cefixime
cefmetazole
cefonicid
cefoperazone
ceforanide
cefotaxime
cefprozil
ceftibuten
cefuroxime
cephalexin
cephalothin
cephapirin
cephradine
moxalactam

Fluoroquinolones
alatrofloxacin/trovafloxacin
ciprofloxacin
enoxacin
levofloxacin

lomefloxacin
nalidixic acid
norfloxacin
ofloxacin
sparfloxacin

Miscellaneous
meropenem

Penicillins
amoxicillin/clavulanate
ampicillin/sulbactam
cloxacillin
dicloxacillin
imipenem/cilastatin
mezlocillin
nafcillin
oxacillin
penicillin G benzathine
penicillin G potassium
penicillin G procaine
penicillin G sodium
penicillin V potassium
piperacillin
ticarcillin
ticarcillin/clavulanate

Sulfonamides
sulfasalazine
sulfisoxazole

Tetracyclines
demeclocycline
doxycycline
minocycline
tetracycline

ANTINEOPLASTICS

Action: Antineoplastics are divided into alkylating agents, antimetabolites, antibiotic agents, hormonal agents, and miscellaneous agents. Alkylating agents act by cross-linking strands of DNA. Antimetabolites act by inhibiting DNA synthesis. Antibiotic agents act by inhibiting RNA synthesis and by delaying or inhibiting mitosis. Hormones alter the effects of androgens, luteinizing hormone, follicle-stimulating hormone, and estrogen by changing the hormonal environment.

Uses: Uses vary widely among products and classes of drugs. They are used to treat leukemia, Hodgkin's disease, lymphomas, and other tumors throughout the body.

Side effects/adverse reactions: Most products cause thrombocytopenia, leukopenia, and anemia, and if these reactions occur, the drug may have to be stopped until the problem is corrected. Other side effects include nausea, vomiting, glossitis, and hair loss. Some products also cause hepatotoxicity, nephrotoxicity, and cardiotoxicity.

Contraindications: Hypersensitive reactions may occur, and allergies should be identified before these products are given. Also, persons with severe liver and kidney disease should not use these products unless the benefits outweigh the risks.

Precautions: Persons with bleeding, severe bone marrow depression, or renal or hepatic disease should be watched closely.

Pharmacokinetics: Onset, peak, and duration vary widely among products. Most products cross the placenta and are excreted in breast milk and in urine.

Interactions: Toxicity may occur when used with other antineoplastics or radiation.

Possible nursing diagnoses:
- Risk for infection *[adverse reactions]*
- Altered nutrition: less than body requirements *[adverse reactions]*
- Altered oral mucous membrane *[adverse reactions]*

NURSING CONSIDERATIONS

Assess:
- CBC, differential, platelet count weekly; withhold drug if WBC is <4000/mm^3 or platelet count is <75,000/mm^3; notify prescriber of results
- Renal function studies, including BUN, creatinine, serum uric acid, and urine creatinine clearance before and during therapy
- I&O ratio; report fall in urine output of 30 ml/hr
- Monitor temp q4h (may indicate beginning infection)
- Liver function tests before and during therapy (bilirubin, AST, ALT, LDH) as needed or monthly
- Bleeding, including hematuria, guaiac, bruising or petechiae, mucosa, or orifices q8h; obtain prescription for viscous Xylocaine (lidocaine)
- Yellowing of skin, sclera, dark urine, clay-colored stools, itchy skin, abdominal pain, fever, diarrhea
- Edema in feet, joint pain, stomach pain, shaking
- Inflammation of mucosa, breaks in skin

Administer:
- Checking IV site for irritation; phlebitis
- Epinephrine for hypersensitivity reaction
- Antibiotics for prophylaxis of infection

Perform/provide:
- Strict asepsis, protective isolation if WBC levels are low
- Comprehensive oral hygiene, using careful technique and soft-bristle brush

Evaluate:
- Therapeutic response, including decreased tumor size

Teach patient/family:
- To report signs of infection, including increased temp, sore throat, malaise
- To report signs of anemia, including fatigue, headache, faintness, shortness of breath, irritability
- To report bleeding and avoid use of razors or commercial mouthwash

---

Generic names

Alkylating agents
busulfan
carboplatin
carmustine
chlorambucil
cisplatin
cyclophosphamide
dacarbazine
lomustine
mechlorethamine
melphalan
streptozocin (Appx F)
thiotepa

Antimetabolites
capecitabine
cytarabine
doxorubicin
etoposide
fludarabine (Appx F)
fluorouracil
mercaptopurine
thioguanine (6-TG)

Antibiotic agents
bleomycin
dactinomycin
daunorubicin
epirubicin
methotrexate
mitomycin
mitoxantrone
plicamycin

Hormonal agents
aminoglutethimide
estramustine (Appx F)
flutamide
goserelin
irinotecan
leuprolide
megestrol
mitotane (Appx F)
nilutamide
tamoxifen
testolactone
topotecan

Miscellaneous
altretamine
anastrozole
asparaginase
cladribine
gemcitabine
interferon alfa-2A
interferon alfa-2B
irinotecan
pentostatin
porfimer
procarbazine
rituximab
vinblastine
vincristine
vinorelbine

ANTIPARKINSON AGENTS

Action: Antiparkinson agents are divided into cholinergics and dopamine agonists. Cholinergics work by blocking or competing at central acetylcholine receptors; dopamine agonists work by decarboxylation to dopamine or by activation of dopamine receptors; monoamine oxidase type B inhibitors work by increasing dopamine activity by inhibiting MAO type B activity.

Uses: Antiparkinson agents are used alone or in combination for patients with Parkinson's disease.

Side effects/adverse reactions: Side effects and adverse reactions vary widely among products. The most common side effects include involuntary movements, headache, numbness, insomnia, nightmares, nausea, vomiting, dry mouth, and orthostatic hypotension.

Contraindications: Persons with hypersensitivity, narrow-angle glaucoma, and undiagnosed skin lesions should not use these products.

Precautions: Antiparkinson agents should be used with caution in pregnancy, lactation, children, renal, cardiac, hepatic disease, and affective disorder.

Pharmacokinetics: Onset, peak, and duration vary widely among products. Most products are metabolized in the liver and excreted in urine.

Interactions: Please check individual monographs since interactions vary widely among products.

Possible nursing diagnoses:
• Risk for injury *[uses]*
• Risk for impaired physical mobility *[uses]*
• Knowledge deficit *[teaching]*

NURSING CONSIDERATIONS
Assess:
• B/P, respiration
• Mental status: affect, mood, behavioral changes, depression, complete suicide assessment

Administer:
• Drug up until NPO before surgery
• Adjust dosage depending on patient response
• With meals; limit protein taken with drug
• Only after MAOIs have been discontinued for 2 wk

Perform/provide:
• Assistance with ambulation, during beginning therapy
• Testing for diabetes mellitus, acromegaly if on long-term therapy

Evaluate:
• Therapeutic response: decrease in akathisia, increased mood
Teach patient/family:
• To change positions slowly to prevent orthostatic hypotension
• To report side effects: twitching, eye spasm; indicate overdose
• To use drug exactly as prescribed; if drug is discontinued abruptly, parkinsonian crisis may occur

---

Generic names

amantadine	levodopa
benztropine	pramipexole
biperiden	selegiline
bromocriptine	tolcapone
cabergoline	trihexyphenidyl
carbidopa-levodopa	

ANTIPSYCHOTICS

Action: Antipsychotics/neuroleptics are divided into several subgroups: phenothiazines, thioxanthenes, butyrophenones, dibenzoxazepines, dibenzodiazepines, and indolones and other heterocyclic compounds. Although chemically different, these subgroups share many pharmacologic and clinical properties. All antipsychotics work to block postsynaptic dopamine receptors in the brain that are responsible for psychotic behavior, including hallucinations, delusions, and paranoia.

Uses: Antipsychotic behavior is decreased in conditions such as schizophrenia, paranoia, and mania. These agents are also effective for severe anxiety, intractable hiccups, nausea, vomiting, behavioral problems in children, and for relaxation before surgery.

Side effects/adverse reactions: The most common side effects include EPS such as pseudoparkinsonism, akathisia, dystonia, and tardive dyskinesia, which may be controlled by use of antiparkinsonian agents. Serious adverse reactions such as hypotension, agranulocytosis, cardiac arrest, and laryngospasm have occurred. Other common side effects include dry mouth and photosensitivity.

Contraindications: Persons with liver damage, severe hypertension or coronary disease, cerebral arteriosclerosis, blood dyscrasias, bone marrow depression, parkinsonism, severe depression, narrow-angle glaucoma, children <12 yr, or persons withdrawing from alcohol or barbiturates should not use antipsychotics until these conditions are corrected.

Precautions: Caution must be used when antipsychotics are given to the elderly since metabolism is slowed and adverse reactions can occur rapidly. Hepatic and renal disease may cause poor metabolism and excretion of the drug. Seizure threshold is decreased with these products; increases in the dose of anticonvulsants may be required. Persons with diabetes mellitus, prostatic hypertrophy, chronic respiratory disease, and peptic ulcer disease should be monitored closely.

Pharmacokinetics: Onset, peak, and duration vary widely with different products and routes. Products are metabolized by the liver, are excreted in urine as metabolites, are highly bound to plasma proteins, cross the placenta, and enter breast milk. Half-life can be extended over 3 days.

Interactions: Because other CNS depressants can cause oversedation, these combinations should be used carefully. Anticholinergics may decrease the therapeutic actions of phenothiazines and also cause increased anticholinergic effects.

Possible nursing diagnoses:
• Altered thought processes *[uses]*
• Sensory/perceptual alterations *[uses]*

NURSING CONSIDERATIONS
Assess:
• Bilirubin, CBC, liver function studies qmo, since these drugs are metabolized in the liver and excreted in urine
• I&O ratio: palpate bladder if low urinary output occurs, since urinary retention occurs with many of these products
• Affect, orientation, LOC, reflexes, gait, coordination, sleep pattern disturbances
• Dizziness, faintness, palpitations, tachycardia on rising
• B/P lying and standing; wide fluctuations between lying and standing B/P may require dosage or product change, since orthostatic hypotension is occurring
• EPS, including akathisia, tardive dyskinesia, pseudoparkinsonism
Administer:
• Antiparkinsonian agent if EPS occur
• Liquid concentrates mixed in glass of juice or cola, since taste is unpleasant; avoid contact with skin when preparing liquid concentrate or parenteral medications
Perform/provide:
• Supervised ambulation until stabilized on medication; do not involve in strenuous exercise program because fainting is possible; patient should not stand still for long periods
• Increased fluids to prevent constipation
• Sips of water, candy, gum for dry mouth

Evaluate:
• Therapeutic response: decrease in excitement, hallucinations, delusions, paranoia, reorganization of thought patterns, speech

Teach patient/family:
• To rise from sitting or lying position gradually, since fainting may occur
• To remain lying down for at least 30 min after IM injections
• To avoid hot tubs, hot showers, or tub baths, since hypotension may occur
• To wear a sunscreen or protective clothing to prevent burns
• To take extra precautions during hot weather to stay cool; heat stroke can occur
• To avoid driving, other activities requiring alertness until response to medication is known
• That drowsiness or impaired mental/motor activity is evident the first 2 wk, but tends to decrease over time

---

Generic names

Phenothiazines
chlorpromazine
fluphenazine
mesoridazine
perphenazine
prochlorperazine
promazine
thioridazine
thiothixene
trifluoperazine

Butyrophenone
haloperidol

Miscellaneous
loxapine
molindone (Appx F)
olanzapine
quetiapine
risperidone

ANTITUBERCULARS

Action: Antituberculars act by inhibiting RNA or DNA, or interfering with lipid and protein synthesis, thereby decreasing tubercle bacilli replication.

Uses: Antituberculars are used for pulmonary tuberculosis.

Side effects/adverse reactions: They vary widely among products. Most products can cause nausea, vomiting, anorexia, and rash. Serious adverse reactions include renal failure, nephrotoxicity, ototoxicity, and hepatic necrosis.

Contraindications: Persons with severe renal disease or hypersensitivity should not use these products.

Precautions: Antituberculars should be used with caution with pregnancy, lactation, and hepatic disease.

Pharmacokinetics: Onset, peak, and duration vary widely among products. Most products are metabolized in the liver and excreted in urine.

Interactions: Please check individual monographs since interactions vary widely among products.

Possible nursing diagnoses:
- Risk for infection *[uses]*
- Risk for injury *[adverse reactions]*
- Knowledge deficit *[teaching]*
- Noncompliance *[teaching]*

NURSING CONSIDERATIONS

Assess:
- Signs of anemia: Hct, Hgb, fatigue
- Liver studies qwk: ALT, AST, bilirubin
- Renal status before, qmo: BUN, creatinine, output, specific gravity, urinalysis
- Hepatic status: decreased appetite, jaundice, dark urine, fatigue

Administer:
- For some of these agents on empty stomach, 1 hr ac (only for isoniazid and rifampin) or 2 hr pc
- Antiemetic if vomiting occurs
- After C&S is completed; qmo to detect resistance

Evaluate:
- Therapeutic response: decreased symptoms of TB, culture negative

Teach patient/family:
- That compliance with dosage schedule, duration is necessary
- That scheduled appointments must be kept; relapse may occur
- To avoid alcohol while taking drug
- To report flulike symptoms: excessive fatigue, anorexia, vomiting, sore throat; unusual bleeding, yellowish discoloration of skin/eyes

---

Generic names

cycloserine	rifabutin
ethambutol	rifampin
isoniazid	streptomycin
pyrazinamide	

ANTITUSSIVES/EXPECTORANTS

Action: Antitussives act by suppressing the cough reflex by direct action on the cough center in the medulla. Expectorants act by liquefying and reducing the viscosity of thick, tenacious secretions.

Uses: Antitussives/expectorants are used to treat cough occurring in pneumonia, bronchitis, TB, cystic fibrosis, and emphysema; as an adjunct in atelectasis (expectorants); and nonproductive cough (antitussives).

Side effects/adverse reactions: The most common side effects are drowsiness, dizziness, and nausea.

Contraindications: Some products are contraindicated in hypothyroidism, iodine sensitivity, pregnancy, and lactation.

Precautions: Some products should be used cautiously in asthmatic, elderly, and debilitated patients.

Pharmacokinetics: Onset, peak, and duration vary widely among products. Some products are metabolized in the liver and excreted in urine.

Interactions: Please check individual monographs since interactions vary widely among products.

Possible nursing diagnoses:
- Ineffective breathing pattern [uses]
- Ineffective airway clearance [uses]
- Knowledge deficit [teaching]

NURSING CONSIDERATIONS

Assess:
- Cough: type, frequency, character (including sputum)

Administer:
- Decreased dose to elderly patients; their metabolism may be slowed

Perform/provide:
- Increased fluids to liquefy secretions
- Humidification of patient's room

Evaluate:
- Therapeutic response: absence of cough

Teach patient/family:
- To avoid driving, other hazardous activities until patient is stabilized on this medication
- To avoid smoking, smoke-filled rooms, perfumes, dust, environmental pollutants, cleaners that increase cough

---

Generic names

acetylcysteine
ammonium chloride (Appx F)
benzonatate (Appx F)
codeine

dextromethorphan
guaifenesin
hydrocodone

ANTIVIRALS

Action: Antivirals act by interfering with DNA synthesis that is needed for viral replication.

Uses: Antivirals are used for mucocutaneous herpes simplex virus, herpes genitalis (HSV_1, HSV_2), advanced HIV infections, herpes simplex virus encephalitis, varicella-zoster encephalomyelitis.

Side effects/adverse reactions: Serious adverse reactions are fatal metabolic encephalopathy, blood dyscrasias, and acute renal failure. Common side effects are nausea, vomiting, anorexia, diarrhea, headache, vaginitis, and moniliasis.

Contraindications: Persons with hypersensitivity, or immunosuppressed individuals with herpes zoster should not use these products.

Precautions: Antivirals should be used with caution in renal disease, liver disease, lactation, pregnancy, and dehydration.

Pharmacokinetics: Onset, peak, and duration vary widely among products. Most products are metabolized in the liver and excreted in urine.

Interactions: Please check individual monographs since interactions vary widely among products.

Possible nursing diagnoses:
• Risk for infection *[uses]*
• Risk for injury *[adverse reactions]*
• Knowledge deficit *[teaching]*

NURSING CONSIDERATIONS
Assess:
• Signs of infection, anemia
• I&O ratio; report hematuria, oliguria, fatigue, weakness; may indicate nephrotoxicity; check for protein in urine during treatment
• Any patient with compromised renal system, since drug is excreted slowly in poor renal system function; toxicity may occur rapidly
• Liver studies: AST, ALT
• Blood studies: WBC, RBC, Hct, Hgb, bleeding time; blood dyscrasias may occur; drug should be discontinued
• Renal studies: urinalysis, protein, BUN, creatinine, CrCl
• C&S before drug therapy; drug may be taken as soon as culture is taken; repeat C&S after treatment
• Bowel pattern before, during treatment; if severe abdominal pain with bleeding occurs, drug should be discontinued
• Skin eruptions: rash, urticaria, itching
• Allergies before treatment, reaction of each medication; record allergies on chart in bright red letters

Administer:
• Increased fluids to 3 L/day to decrease crystalluria when given IV

Perform/provide:
• Storage at room temp for up to 12 hr after reconstitution
• Adequate intake of fluids (2 L) to prevent deposit in kidneys

Evaluate:
• Therapeutic response: absence or control of infection

Teach patient/family:
• That drug does not cure infection, just controls symptoms
• To report sore throat, fever, fatigue; could indicate superinfection
• That drug must be taken in equal intervals around the clock to maintain blood levels for duration of therapy
• To notify prescriber of side effects of bruising, bleeding, fatigue, malaise; may indicate blood dyscrasias

Generic names

abacavir (Appx A)
acyclovir
amantadine
cidofovir
delavirdine (Appx F)
didanosine
famciclovir
foscarnet
ganciclovir
indinavir

nelfinavir
nevirapine
rimantadine
ritonavir
saquinavir
stavudine
vidarabine
zalcitabine
zidovudine

BARBITURATES

Action: Barbiturates act by decreasing impulse transmission to the cerebral cortex.

Uses: All forms of epilepsy can be controlled, since the seizure threshold is increased. Uses also include febrile seizures in children, sedation, insomnia, hyperbilirubinemia, chronic cholestasis with some of these products. Ultra-short-acting barbiturates are used as anesthetics.

Side effects/adverse reactions: The most common side effects are drowsiness and nausea. Serious adverse reactions such as Stevens-Johnson syndrome and blood dyscrasias may occur with high doses and long-term treatment.

Contraindications: Hypersensitivity may occur, and allergies should be identified before administering. Barbiturates are identified as pregnancy category D and should not be used in pregnancy. Other contraindications include porphyria and marked impairment of liver function.

Precautions: Caution must be used when these products are given to the elderly or debilitated; usually smaller doses are needed since metabolism is slowed. Persons with renal and hepatic disease may show delayed excretion. Barbiturates may produce excitability in children.

Pharmacokinetics: Onset of action can be slow, up to 1 hr, with a peak of 8 hr and a duration of 3-10 hr. These drugs are metabolized by the liver, excreted by the kidneys, cross the placenta, and enter breast milk.

Interactions: Increased CNS depressant effect may occur with alcohol, MAOIs, sedatives, or narcotics. These products should be used together cautiously. Oral anticoagulants, corticosteroids, griseofulvin, quinidine, oral contraceptives, and theophylline may show a decreased effect when used with barbiturates.

Possible nursing diagnoses:
- Sleep pattern disturbance *[uses]*
- Risk for injury *[adverse reactions]*

NURSING CONSIDERATIONS
Assess:
- Hepatic and renal studies: AST, ALT, bilirubin, creatinine, LDH, alkaline phosphatase, BUN if patient is on long-term therapy, since these products are metabolized and excreted by the liver and kidneys
- Blood studies: CBC, hematocrit, hemoglobin, and prothrombin time if patient is on long-term therapy, since these products increase the possibility of bleeding and blood dyscrasias
- Barbiturate toxicity: hypotension, pulmonary constriction; cold, clammy skin; cyanosis of lips, insomnia, nausea, vomiting, hallucinations, delirium, weakness

Evaluate:
- Therapeutic response, including appropriate sedation or seizure control

Teach patient/family:
- That physical dependency may result when used for extended periods (45-90 days, depending on dose)
- To avoid driving, activities that require alertness since drowsiness and dizziness may occur
- To abstain from alcohol or other psychotropic medications unless directed by prescriber
- Not to discontinue medication abruptly after long-term use; withdrawal symptoms will occur

---

Generic names

pentobarbital	secobarbital
phenobarbital	thiopental

BENZODIAZEPINES

Action: Benzodiazepines potentiate the effects of γ-aminobutyric acid (GABA), including any other inhibitory transmitters in the CNS, resulting in decreased anxiety.

Uses: Anxiety is relieved in conditions such as phobic disorders. Benzodiazepines are also used for acute alcohol withdrawal to relieve the possibility of delirium tremens, and some products are used for relaxation before surgery.

Side effects/adverse reactions: The most common side effects are dizziness, drowsiness, blurred vision, and orthostatic hypotension. Most adverse effects are mediated through the CNS. There is a risk of physical dependence and abuse.

Contraindications: Hypersensitivity, acute narrow-angle glaucoma, children <6 mo, liver disease (clonazepam), lactation (diazepam).

Precautions: Caution must be used when these products are given to the elderly or debilitated; usually smaller doses are needed, since metabolism is slowed. Persons with renal and hepatic disease may show delayed excretion. Clonazepam may increase incidence of seizures.

Pharmacokinetics: Onset of action is ½-1 hr, with a peak of 1-2 hr and a duration of 4-6 hr. These drugs are metabolized by the liver, excreted by the kidneys, cross the placenta, and enter breast milk.

Interactions: Increased CNS depressant effect may occur with other CNS depressants. These products should be used together cautiously. Alcohol should not be used; fatal reactions can occur. The serum concentration and toxicity of digoxin may be increased.

Possible nursing diagnoses:

- Anxiety *[uses]*
- Risk for injury *[adverse reactions]*

NURSING CONSIDERATIONS
Assess:

- B/P (lying, standing), pulse; if systolic B/P drops 20 mm Hg, hold drug, notify prescriber; orthostatic hypotension is severe
- Hepatic and renal studies: AST, ALT, bilirubin, creatinine, LDH, alkaline phosphatase
- Physical dependency, withdrawal symptoms, including headache, nausea, vomiting, muscle pain, weakness after long-term use

Administer:

- With food or milk for GI symptoms; may give crushed if patient is unable to swallow medication whole

Evaluate:
• Therapeutic response, including relaxation or decreased anxiety

Teach patient/family:
• That drug should not be used for everyday stress or long-term; not to take more than prescribed amount since drug is habit-forming
• To avoid driving and activities that require alertness since drowsiness and dizziness occur
• To abstain from alcohol, other psychotropic medications unless directed by prescriber
• Not to discontinue medication abruptly after long-term use; withdrawal symptoms will occur

---

Generic names

alprazolam	lorazepam
chlordiazepoxide	midazolam
clonazepam	oxazepam
diazepam	temazepam
flurazepam	triazolam

BETA-ADRENERGIC BLOCKERS

Action: β-Blockers are divided into selective and nonselective blockers. Nonselective blockers produce a fall in blood pressure without reflex tachycardia or reduction in heart rate through a mixture of β-blocking effects; elevated plasma renins are reduced. Selective β-blockers competitively block stimulation of $β_1$-receptors in cardiac smooth muscle; these drugs produce chronotropic and inotropic effects.

Uses: β-Blockers are used for hypertension, ventricular dysrhythmias, and prophylaxis of angina pectoris.

Side effects/adverse reactions: The most common side effects are orthostatic hypotension, bradycardia, diarrhea, nausea, vomiting. Serious adverse reactions include blood dyscrasias, bronchospasm, and CHF.

Contraindications: Hypersensitive reactions may occur, and allergies should be identified before these products are given. β-Adrenergic blockers should not be used in heart block, CHF, or cardiogenic shock.

Precautions: β-Blockers should be used with caution in the elderly or in renal and thyroid disease, COPD, CAD, diabetes mellitus, pregnancy, or asthma.

Pharmacokinetics: Onset, peak, and duration vary widely among products. Most products are metabolized in the liver, with metabolites excreted in urine, bile, and feces.

Interactions: Interactions vary widely among products; check individual monographs for specific information.

Possible nursing diagnoses:
- Altered tissue perfusion *[uses]*
- Decreased cardiac output *[uses]*
- Diarrhea *[adverse reactions]*
- Impaired gas exchange *[adverse reactions]*

NURSING CONSIDERATIONS

Assess:
- Renal studies, including protein, BUN, creatinine; watch for increased levels that may indicate nephrotic syndrome; obtain baselines in renal and liver function studies before beginning treatment
- I&O, weight daily
- B/P during beginning treatment and periodically thereafter; pulse q4h, note rate, rhythm, quality
- Apical/radial pulse before administration; notify prescriber of significant changes
- Edema in feet and legs daily

Administer:
- PO ac, hs; tablets may be crushed or swallowed whole
- Reduced dosage in renal dysfunction

Evaluate:
- Therapeutic response, including decrease in B/P in hypertension, decreased B/P, edema, moist rales in CHF

Teach patient/family:
- To comply with dosage schedule, even if feeling better
- To rise slowly to sitting or standing position to minimize orthostatic hypotension
- To report bradycardia, dizziness, confusion, depression, fever
- To take pulse at home; advise when to notify prescriber
- To comply with weight control, dietary adjustment, modified exercise program
- To wear support hose to minimize effects of orthostatic hypotension
- Not to discontinue drug abruptly; taper over 2 wk; may precipitate angina

Generic names

Selective β₁-receptor blockers
acebutolol
atenolol
esmolol
metoprolol

Combined α₁-, β₁-, and β₂-receptor blocker
labetalol

Nonselective β₁- and β₂-blockers
carteolol
nadolol
pindolol
propranolol
timolol

BRONCHODILATORS

Action: Bronchodilators are divided into anticholinergics, α/β-adrenergic agonists, β-adrenergic agonists, and phosphodiesterase inhibitors. Anticholinergics act by inhibiting interaction of acetylcholine at receptor sites on bronchial smooth muscle; α/β-adrenergic agonists by relaxing bronchial smooth muscle and increasing diameter of nasal passages; β-adrenergic agonists by action on β₂-receptors, which relaxes bronchial smooth muscle; phosphodiesterase inhibitors by blocking phosphodiesterase increase cAMP, which mediates smooth muscle relaxation in the respiratory system.

Uses: Bronchodilators are used for bronchial asthma, bronchospasm associated with bronchitis, emphysema, or other obstructive pulmonary diseases, Cheyne-Stokes respirations, prevention of exercise-induced asthma.

Side effects/adverse reactions: The most common side effects are tremors, anxiety, nausea, vomiting, and irritation in throat. The most serious adverse reactions include bronchospasm and dyspnea.

Contraindications: Persons with hypersensitivity, narrow-angle glaucoma, tachydysrhythmias, and severe cardiac disease should not use some of these products.

Precautions: Bronchodilators should be used with caution in lactation, pregnancy, hyperthyroidism, hypertension, prostatic hypertrophy, and seizure disorders.

Pharmacokinetics: Onset, peak, and duration vary widely among products. Most products are metabolized in the liver and excreted in urine.

Interactions: Please check individual monographs since interactions vary widely among products.

Possible nursing diagnoses:
• Ineffective airway clearance [uses]
• Activity intolerance [uses]

- Risk for injury *[adverse reactions]*
- Knowledge deficit *[teaching]*

NURSING CONSIDERATIONS

Assess:
- Respiratory function: vital capacity, forced expiratory volume, ABGs, lung sounds, heart rate and rhythm

Administer:
- After shaking, exhale, place mouthpiece in mouth, inhale slowly, hold breath, remove, exhale slowly
- Gum, sips of water for dry mouth
- PO with meals to decrease gastric irritation

Perform/provide:
- Storage in light-resistant container, do not expose to temps over 86° F (30° C)

Evaluate:
- Therapeutic response: absence of dyspnea, wheezing

Teach patient/family:
- Not to use OTC medications; extra stimulation may occur
- Use of inhaler; review package insert with patient
- To avoid getting aerosol in eyes
- To wash inhaler in warm water qd and dry
- To avoid smoking, smoke-filled rooms, persons with respiratory infections

Generic names

albuterol	isoproterenol
aminophylline	levalbuterol
atropine	metaproterenol
bitolterol	oxtriphylline
dyphylline	pirbuterol
ephedrine	terbutaline
epinephrine	theophylline
ipratropium	

CALCIUM CHANNEL BLOCKERS

Action: These products act by inhibiting calcium ion influx across the cell membrane in cardiac and vascular smooth muscle. This action produces relaxation of coronary vascular smooth muscle, dilates coronary arteries, slows SA/AV node conduction, and dilates peripheral arteries.

Uses: These products are used for chronic stable angina pectoris, vaso-spastic angina, dysrhythmias, hypertension, and unstable angina.

Side effects/adverse reactions: The most common side effects are dysrhythmias and edema. Also common are headache, fatigue, drowsiness, and flushing.

Contraindications: Persons with 2nd or 3rd degree heart block, sick sinus syndrome, hypotension of <90 mm Hg systolic, Wolff-Parkinson-White syndrome, or cardiogenic shock should not use these products since worsening of those conditions may occur.

Precautions: CHF may worsen since edema may be increased. Hypotension may worsen since B/P is decreased. Patients with renal and liver disease should use these products cautiously since they are metabolized in the liver and excreted by the kidneys.

Pharmacokinetics: Onset, peak, and duration vary widely with route of administration. Drugs are metabolized by the liver and excreted in the urine primarily as metabolites.

Interactions: Increased levels of digoxin and theophylline may occur when used with these products. Increased effects of β-blockers and antihypertensives may occur with calcium channel blockers.

Possible nursing diagnoses:
• Altered tissue perfusion: cardiopulmonary [uses]
• Decreased cardiac output [adverse reactions]

NURSING CONSIDERATIONS
Assess:
• Cardiac system, including B/P, pulse, respirations, ECG intervals (PR, QRS, QT)
Administer:
• PO before meals and hs
Evaluate:
• Therapeutic response, including decreased anginal pain, decreased B/P, dysrhythmias
Teach patient/family:
• How to take pulse before taking drug; patient should record or graph pulses to identify changes
• To avoid hazardous activities until stabilized on this drug, since dizziness commonly occurs
• Need for compliance in all areas of medical regimen, including diet, exercise, stress reduction, drug therapy

Generic names

diltiazem
felodipine
nicardipine

nifedipine
verapamil

CARDIAC GLYCOSIDES

Action: Products act by inhibiting sodium and potassium ATPase and then making more calcium available to activate contracted proteins. Cardiac contractility and cardiac output are increased.

Uses: These products are used for CHF, atrial fibrillation, atrial flutter, atrial tachycardia, and rapid digitalization in these disorders.

Side effects/adverse reactions: The most common side effects are cardiac disturbances, headache, hypotension, GI symptoms. Also common are blurred vision and yellow-green halos.

Contraindications: Hypersensitive reactions may occur, and allergies should be identified before these products are given. Also, persons with ventricular tachycardia, ventricular fibrillation, and carotid sinus syndrome should not use these products.

Precautions: Persons with acute MI and those who have or may develop serum potassium, calcium, or magnesium imbalances should use these products cautiously. Also, persons with AV block, severe respiratory disease, hypothyroidism, renal and liver disease, and the elderly should exercise caution when these drugs are prescribed.

Pharmacokinetics: Onset, peak, and duration vary widely with the route of administration. Digitoxin is inactivated by the liver, and inactive metabolites are excreted in urine. Digoxin is excreted in urine mainly as the parent drug and metabolites.

Interactions: Toxicity may occur when used with diuretics, succinylcholine, quinidine, and thioamines. Increased blood levels may occur with propantheline bromide, spironolactone, quinidine, verapamil, aminoglycosides (PO), amiodarone, anticholinergics, and quinine. Diuretics may increase toxicity.

Possible nursing diagnoses:
- Altered tissue perfusion: cardiopulmonary *[uses]*
- Decreased cardiac output *[adverse reactions]*

NURSING CONSIDERATIONS
Assess:
- Cardiac system, including B/P, pulse, respirations, and increased urine output

• Apical pulse for 1 min before giving drug; if pulse <60 bpm, take again in 1 hr; if still <60 bpm, notify prescriber
• Electrolytes, including K, Na, Cl, Mg; renal function studies, including BUN and creatinine; and blood studies, including AST, ALT, bilirubin
• I&O ratio, daily weights
• Monitor therapeutic drug levels

Administer:
• K supplements if ordered for K levels <3 mg/dl

Evaluate:
• Therapeutic response, including decreased weight, edema, pulse, respiration, and increased urine output

Teach patient/family:
• How to take pulse before taking drug; patient should record or graph pulse to identify changes
• To avoid hazardous activities until stabilized on this drug, since dizziness commonly occurs
• Need for compliance in all areas of medical regimen, including diet, exercise, stress reduction, drug therapy

---

Generic names

digitoxin   digoxin

CHOLINERGICS

Action: Cholinergics act by preventing destruction of acetylcholine, which increases concentration at sites where acetylcholine is released; this exaggerates the effects of acetylcholine and facilitates transmission of impulses across the myoneural junction. Cholinergics may also act by stimulating receptors for acetylcholine.

Uses: Cholinergics are used for myasthenia gravis, as antagonists of nondepolarizing neuromuscular blockade, postoperative bladder distention and urinary distention, and postoperative ileus.

Side effects/adverse reactions: The most serious adverse reactions are respiratory depression, bronchospasm, constriction, laryngospasm, respiratory arrest, convulsions, and paralysis. The most common side effects are nausea, diarrhea, and vomiting.

Contraindications: Persons with obstruction of the intestine or renal system should not use these products.

Precautions: Caution should be used in patients with bradycardia, hypotension, seizure disorders, bronchial asthma, coronary occlusion, hyperthyroidism, lactation, and in children.

Pharmacokinetics: Onset, peak, and duration vary widely among products. Most products are metabolized in the liver and excreted in urine.

Interactions: Please check individual monographs since interactions vary widely among products.

Possible nursing diagnoses:

- Altered urinary elimination *[uses]*
- Ineffective breathing pattern *[uses]*
- Knowledge deficit *[teaching]*
- Noncompliance *[teaching]*

NURSING CONSIDERATIONS

Assess:

- VS, respiration q8h
- I&O ratio; check for urinary retention or incontinence
- Bradycardia, hypotension, bronchospasm, headache, dizziness, convulsions, respiratory depression; drug should be discontinued if toxicity occurs

Administer:

- Only with atropine sulfate available for cholinergic crisis
- Only after all other cholinergics have been discontinued
- Increased doses if tolerance occurs
- Larger doses after exercise or fatigue
- On empty stomach for better absorption

Perform/provide:

- Storage at room temp

Evaluate:

- Therapeutic response: increased muscle strength, hand grasp, improved muscle gait, absence of labored breathing (if severe)

Teach patient/family:

- That drug is not a cure; it only relieves symptoms (myasthenia gravis)
- To wear Medic Alert ID specifying myasthenia gravis, drugs taken

---

Generic names

bethanechol	physostigmine (Appxs C, F)
edrophonium	pyridostigmine
neostigmine	

CHOLINERGIC BLOCKERS

Action: Cholinergic blockers inhibit or block acetylcholine at receptor sites in the autonomic nervous system.

Uses: Many products are used to decrease secretions before surgery, to reverse neuromuscular blockade, and to decrease motility of GI, biliary, urinary tracts. Other products are used for parkinsonian symptoms, including dystonia associated with neuroleptic drugs.

Side effects/adverse reactions: The most common side effects are dryness of the mouth and constipation, which can be prevented by frequent rinsing of the mouth and by increasing water and bulk in the diet.

Contraindications: Hypersensitivity can occur, and allergies should be identified before administering these products. Persons with GI and GU obstruction should not use these products since constipation and urinary retention may occur. They are also contraindicated in angle-closure glaucoma and myasthenia gravis.

Precautions: Caution must be used when these products are given to the elderly, since metabolism is slowed. Also, persons with tachycardia or prostatic hypertrophy should use these products with caution.

Pharmacokinetics: Onset, peak, and duration vary with route.

Interactions: Increase in anticholinergic effect occurs when used with narcotics, barbiturates, antihistamines, MAOIs, phenothiazines, and amantadine.

Possible nursing diagnoses:
• Impaired physical mobility *[uses]*
• Pain *[uses]*

NURSING CONSIDERATIONS

Assess:
• I&O ratio; be alert for urinary retention, frequency, dysuria; drug should be discontinued if these occur
• Urinary hesitancy, retention; palpate bladder if retention occurs
• Constipation; increase fluids, bulk, exercise
• For tolerance over long-term therapy, dose may have to be increased or changed
• Mental status: affect, mood, CNS depression, worsening of mental symptoms during early therapy

Administer:
• With food or milk to decrease GI symptoms
• Parenteral dose with patient recumbent to prevent postural hypotension; give parenteral dose slowly, monitoring vital signs

Perform/provide:
• Hard candy, gum, frequent rinsing of mouth for dryness
Evaluate:
• Therapeutic response, including absence of cramps and EPS
Teach patient/family:
• To avoid driving, other hazardous activity if drowsiness occurs
• To avoid concurrent use of cough, cold preparations with alcohol, antihistamines unless directed by prescriber
• To use with caution in hot weather since medication may increase susceptibility to heat stroke

---

Generic names

atropine	glycopyrrolate
benztropine	scopolamine
biperiden	trihexyphenidyl

CORTICOSTEROIDS

Action: Corticosteroids are divided into glucocorticoids and mineralocorticoids. Glucocorticoids decrease inflammation by the suppression of migration of polymorphonuclear leukocytes, fibroblasts, increased capillary permeability, and lysosomal stabilization. They also have varied metabolic effects and modify the body's immune responses to many stimuli. Mineralocorticoids act by increasing resorption of sodium by increasing hydrogen and potassium excretion in the distal tubule.

Uses: Glucocorticoids are used to decrease inflammation and for immunosuppression. In addition, some products may be given for allergy, adrenal insufficiency, or cerebral edema. Mineralocorticoids are given for adrenal insufficiency or adrenogenital syndrome.

Side effects/adverse reactions: The most common side effects include change in behavior, including insomnia and euphoria; GI irritation, including peptic ulcer; metabolic reactions, including hypokalemia, hyperglycemia, and carbohydrate intolerance; and sodium and fluid retention. Most adverse reactions are dose dependent.

Contraindications: Hypersensitivity may occur and should be identified before administering. Since these products mask infection, they should not be used in systemic fungal infections or amebiasis. Mothers taking pharmacologic doses of corticosteroids should not nurse.

Precautions: Caution must be used when these products are prescribed for diabetic patients since hyperglycemia may occur. Also, patients with glaucoma, seizure disorders, peptic ulcer, impaired renal function, CHF, hypertension, ulcerative colitis, or myasthenia gravis should be monitored closely if corticosteroids are given. Use with caution in children and the elderly and during pregnancy.

Pharmacokinetics: For oral preparations, the onset of action occurs between 1 and 2 hr, and duration can be up to 2 days, with a half-life of 2-4 days. Pharmacokinetics vary widely among products. These products cross the placenta and appear in breast milk.

Interactions: Decreased corticosteroid effect may occur with barbiturates, rifampin, phenytoin; corticosteroid dose may have to be increased. There is a possibility of GI bleeding when used with salicylates, indomethacin. Steroids may reduce salicylate levels. When using with digitalis glycosides, potassium-depleting diuretics, and amphotericin, serum potassium levels should be monitored.

Possible nursing diagnoses:

• Risk for infection *[adverse reactions]*
• Body image disturbance *[adverse reactions]*
• Risk for violence: self-directed (suicide) *[adverse reactions]*

NURSING CONSIDERATIONS

Assess:

• Potassium, blood sugar, urine glucose while on long-term therapy; hypokalemia and hyperglycemia are common
• Weight daily; notify prescriber of weekly gain >5 lb, since these products alter fluid and electrolyte balance
• I&O ratio; be alert for decreasing urinary output and increasing edema
• Plasma cortisol levels during long-term therapy (normal level is 138-635 nmol/L SI U when drawn at 8 AM)
• Infection, including increased temp, WBC, even after withdrawal of medication; drug masks symptoms of infection
• Adrenal insufficiency: nausea, anorexia, fatigue, dizziness, dyspnea, weakness, joint pain
• Potassium depletion, including paresthesias, fatigue, nausea, vomiting, depression, polyuria, dysrhythmias, weakness
• Mental status, including affect, mood, behavioral changes, aggression; if severe personality changes occur, including depression, drug may have to be tapered and then discontinued

Administer:

• With food or milk to decrease GI symptoms

Evaluate:

• Therapeutic response, including decreased inflammation

Teach patient/family:
• That ID as steroid user should be carried
• Not to discontinue this medication abruptly, or adrenal crisis can result
• Teach patient all aspects of drug use, including cushingoid symptoms
• That single daily or alternate-day doses should be taken in the morning before 9 AM (for replacement therapy)
• To take with meals or a snack

Generic names

Glucocorticoids	methylprednisolone
beclomethasone	prednisolone
betamethasone	prednisone
cortisone	rimexolone (Appx C)
dexamethasone	triamcinolone
flunisolide	
hydrocortisone	*Mineralocorticoid*
hydrocortisone sodium phosphate	fludrocortisone

DIURETICS

Action: Diuretics are divided into subgroups: thiazides and thiazide-like diuretics, loop diuretics, carbonic anhydrase inhibitors, osmotic diuretics, and potassium-sparing diuretics. Each one of these subgroups has its own mechanism of action. Thiazides and thiazide-like diuretics increase excretion of water and sodium by inhibiting resorption in the early distal tubule. Loop diuretics inhibit resorption of sodium and chloride in the thick ascending limb of the loop of Henle. Carbonic anhydrase inhibitors increase sodium excretion by decreasing sodium-hydrogen ion exchange throughout the renal tubule. Carbonic anhydrase inhibitors also decrease secretion of aqueous humor in the eye and thus decrease intraocular pressure. Osmotic diuretics increase the osmotic pressure of glomerular filtrate, thus decreasing net absorption of sodium. The potassium-sparing diuretics interfere with sodium resorption at the distal tubule, thus decreasing potassium excretion.

Uses: Blood pressure is reduced in hypertension; edema is reduced in CHF; intraocular pressure is decreased in glaucoma.

Side effects/adverse reactions: Hypokalemia, hyperuricemia, and hyperglycemia occur most frequently with thiazide diuretics. Aplastic anemia, blood dyscrasias, volume depletion, and dehydration may occur when thiazide-like diuretics, loop diuretics, or carbonic anhydrase inhibitors are given. Side effects and adverse reactions vary widely for the miscellaneous products.

Contraindications: Persons with electrolyte imbalances (Na, Cl, K), dehydration, or anuria should not be given these products until the problem is corrected.

Precautions: Caution must be used when diuretics are given to the elderly, since electrolyte disturbances and dehydration can occur rapidly. Hepatic and renal disease may cause poor metabolism and excretion of the drug.

Pharmacokinetics: Onset, peak, and duration vary widely among the different subgroups of these drugs.

Interactions: Cholestyramine and colestipol will decrease the absorption of thiazide diuretics. Concurrent use of thiazides with diazoxide may increase hyperuricemia, hyperglycemia, and antihypertensive effects of thiazides. Ototoxicity may occur when loop diuretics are used with aminoglycosides. Thiazide and loop diuretics may increase therapeutic and toxic effects of lithium.

Possible nursing diagnoses:
- Fluid volume excess [uses]
- Decreased cardiac output [adverse reactions]

NURSING CONSIDERATIONS

Assess:
- Weight, I&O daily to determine fluid loss; check skin turgor for dehydration
- Electrolytes: K, Na, Cl; include BUN, blood sugar, CBC, serum creatinine, blood pH, ABGs, uric acid, Ca; electrolyte imbalances may occur quickly
- B/P lying, standing; postural hypotension may occur since fluid loss occurs first from intravascular spaces
- Signs of metabolic alkalosis, including drowsiness and restlessness
- Signs of hypokalemia with some products, including postural hypotension, malaise, fatigue, tachycardia, leg cramps, weakness

Administer:
- In AM to avoid interference with sleep if using drug as a diuretic
- K replacement if K is less than 3 mg/dl

Evaluate:
- Therapeutic response: improvement in edema of feet, legs, sacral area daily if medication is being used in CHF; improvement in B/P if medication is being used as a diuretic; improvement in intraocular pressure if medication is being used to decrease aqueous humor in the eye

Teach patient/family:
- To take drug early in the day (diuretic) to prevent nocturia

Generic names

Thiazides
chlorothiazide
hydrochlorothiazide

Thiazide-like
chlorthalidone
indapamide
metolazone

Loop
bumetanide
ethacrynate/ethacrynic
furosemide
torsemide

Carbonic anhydrase inhibitors
acetazolamide
methazolamide

Potassium-sparing
amiloride
spironolactone
triamterene

Osmotic
mannitol
urea

HISTAMINE H$_2$ ANTAGONISTS

Action: Histamine H$_2$ antagonists act by inhibiting histamine at the H$_2$-receptor site in parietal cells, which inhibits gastric acid secretion.

Uses: Histamine H$_2$ antagonists are used for short-term treatment of duodenal and gastric ulcers and maintenance therapy for duodenal ulcer; gastroesophageal reflux disease.

Side effects/adverse reactions: The most serious adverse reactions are agranulocytosis, thrombocytopenia, neutropenia, aplastic anemia, exfoliative dermatitis. The most common side effects are confusion (not with ranitidine), headache, and diarrhea.

Contraindications: Persons with hypersensitivity should not use these products.

Precautions: Caution should be used in pregnancy, lactation, child <16 yr, organic brain syndrome, hepatic disease, renal disease.

Pharmacokinetics: Onset, peak, and duration vary widely among products. Most products are metabolized in the liver and excreted in urine.

Interactions: Antacids interfere with absorption of histamine H$_2$ antagonists. Check individual monographs for other interactions.

Possible nursing diagnoses:

- Pain *[uses]*
- Risk for injury *[bleeding]*
- Knowledge deficit *[teaching]*

NURSING CONSIDERATIONS

Assess:

- Gastric pH (>5 should be maintained)
- I&O ratio, BUN, creatinine

Administer:

- With meals for prolonged drug effect
- Antacids 1 hr before or 1 hr after cimetidine
- IV slowly; bradycardia may occur; give over 30 min

Perform/provide:

- Storage of diluted sol at room temp for up to 48 hr

Evaluate:

- Therapeutic response: decreased pain in abdomen

Teach patient/family:

- That gynecomastia, impotence may occur, but are reversible
- To avoid driving, other hazardous activities until patient is stabilized on this medication
- To avoid black pepper, caffeine, alcohol, harsh spices, extremes in temp of food
- To avoid OTC preparations: aspirin, cough, cold preparations
- That drug must be continued for prescribed time to be effective
- To report bruising, fatigue, malaise; blood dyscrasias may occur

---

Generic names

cimetidine   ranitidine
famotidine

IMMUNOSUPPRESSANTS

Action: Immunosuppressants act by inhibiting lymphocytes (T).

Uses: Most products are used for organ transplants to prevent rejection.

Side effects/adverse reactions: The most serious adverse reactions are albuminuria, hematuria, proteinuria, renal failure, and hepatotoxicity. The most common side effects are overgrowth of oral *Candida,* gum hyperplasia, tremors, and headache. The most serious adverse reactions for azathioprine are hematologic (leukopenia and thrombocytopenia) and GI (nausea and vomiting). There is a risk of secondary infection.

Contraindications: Products are contraindicated in hypersensitivity.

Precautions: Caution should be used in severe renal disease, severe hepatic disease, and pregnancy.

Pharmacokinetics: Onset, peak, and duration vary widely among products. Most products are metabolized in the liver and excreted in urine.

Interactions: Please check individual monographs since interactions vary widely among products.

Possible nursing diagnoses:
• Risk for infection *[adverse reactions]*
• Risk for injury *[uses]*
• Knowledge deficit *[teaching]*

NURSING CONSIDERATIONS

Assess:
• Renal studies: BUN, creatinine at least qmo during treatment, 3 mo after treatment
• Liver function studies: alk phosphatase, AST (SGOT), ALT (SGPT), bilirubin
• Drug blood levels during treatment
• Hepatotoxicity: dark urine, jaundice, itching, light-colored stools; drug should be discontinued

Administer:
• For several days before transplant surgery
• With meals for GI upset or drug mixed with chocolate milk
• With oral antifungal for *Candida* infections

Evaluate:
• Therapeutic response: absence of rejection

Teach patient/family:
• To report fever, chills, sore throat, fatigue, since serious infections may occur
• To use contraceptive measures during treatment, for 12 wk after ending therapy

---

Generic names

azathioprine	muromonab-CD3
basiliximab	sirolimus
cyclosporine	tacrolimus

LAXATIVES

Action: Laxatives are divided into bulk products, lubricants, osmotics, saline laxative stimulants, and stool softeners. Bulk laxatives work by absorbing water and expanding to increase moisture content and bulk in the stool. Lubricants increase water retention in the stool, causing reabsorption of water in the bowel. Stimulants act by increasing peristalsis by direct effect on the intestine. Saline draws water into the intestinal lumen.

Osmotics increase distention and promote peristalsis. Stool softeners reduce surface tension of liquids of the bowel.

Uses: Laxatives are used as a preparation for bowel and rectal exam, constipation, and stool softener.

Side effects/adverse reactions: The most common side effects are nausea, abdominal cramps, and diarrhea.

Contraindications: Persons with GI obstruction, perforation, gastric retention, toxic colitis, megacolon, abdominal pain, nausea, vomiting, or fecal impaction should not use these products.

Precautions: Caution should be used in rectal bleeding, large hemorrhoids, and anal excoriation.

Pharmacokinetics: Onset, peak, and duration vary among products.

Interactions: Please check individual monographs since interactions vary widely among products.

Possible nursing diagnoses:
• Constipation *[uses]*
• Diarrhea *[adverse reactions]*
• Knowledge deficit *[teaching]*

NURSING CONSIDERATIONS
Assess:
• Blood, urine electrolytes if drug is used often by patient
• I&O ratio: to identify fluid loss
• Cause of constipation; identify whether fluids, bulk, or exercise is missing from lifestyle
• Cramping, rectal bleeding, nausea, vomiting; if these symptoms occur, drug should be discontinued

Administer:
• Alone only with water for better absorption; do not take within 1 hr of antacids, milk, or cimetidine

Evaluate:
• Therapeutic response: decrease in constipation

Teach patient/family:
• To swallow tabs whole; not to chew
• Not to use laxatives for long-term therapy; bowel tone will be lost
• That normal bowel movements do not always occur daily
• Not to use in presence of abdominal pain, nausea, vomiting
• To notify prescriber of abdominal pain, nausea, vomiting
• To notify prescriber if constipation is unrelieved or if symptoms of electrolyte imbalance: muscle cramps, pain, weakness, dizziness

Generic names

Bulk laxatives
calcium polycarbophil
methylcellulose
psyllium

Lubricants
mineral oil

Osmotic agents
glycerin
lactulose

Saline laxatives
magnesium salts
sodium biphosphate/phosphate

Stimulants
bisacodyl
cascara sagrada
senna

Stool softeners
docusate

NEUROMUSCULAR BLOCKING AGENTS

Action: Neuromuscular blocking agents are divided into depolarizing and nondepolarizing blockers. They act by inhibiting transmission of nerve impulses by binding with cholinergic receptor sites.

Uses: Neuromuscular blocking agents are used to facilitate endotracheal intubation and skeletal muscle relaxation during mechanical ventilation, surgery, or general anesthesia.

Side effects/adverse reactions: The most serious adverse reactions are prolonged apnea, bronchospasm, cyanosis, respiratory depression, and malignant hyperthermia. The most common side effects are bradycardia and decreased motility.

Contraindications: Persons who are hypersensitive should not be given this product.

Precautions: Caution should be used in pregnancy, thyroid disease, collagen disease, cardiac disease, lactation, children <2 yr, electrolyte imbalances, dehydration, neuromuscular disease (myasthenia gravis), and respiratory disease.

Pharmacokinetics: Onset, peak, and duration vary widely among products. Most products are metabolized in the liver and excreted in urine.

Interactions: Aminoglycosides potentiate neuromuscular blockade. See individual monographs.

Possible nursing diagnoses:
- Ineffective breathing pattern *[uses]*
- Risk for injury *[adverse reactions]*
- Knowledge deficit *[teaching]*

NURSING CONSIDERATIONS
Assess:
• For electrolyte imbalances (K, Mg); may lead to increased action of this drug
• Vital signs (B/P, pulse, respirations, airway) q15min until fully recovered; rate, depth, pattern of respirations, strength of hand grip
• I&O ratio; check for urinary retention, frequency, hesitancy
• Recovery: decreased paralysis of face, diaphragm, leg, arm, rest of body
• Allergic reactions: rash, fever, respiratory distress, pruritus; drug should be discontinued

Administer:
• Using nerve stimulator by anesthesiologist to determine neuromuscular blockade
• Anticholinesterase to reverse neuromuscular blockade
• IV undiluted over 1-2 min (only by qualified person, usually an anesthesiologist)

Perform/provide:
• Storage in light-resistant container, cool area
• Reassurance if communication is difficult during recovery from neuromuscular blockade

Evaluate:
• Therapeutic response: paralysis of jaw, eyelid, head, neck, rest of body

---

Generic names

atracurium	pancuronium
cisatracurium	pipecuronium
doxacurium	succinylcholine
gallamine	tubocurarine
mivacurium	vecuronium

NONSTEROIDAL ANTIINFLAMMATORIES

Action: Nonsteroidals decrease prostaglandin synthesis by inhibiting an enzyme needed for biosynthesis.

Uses: Nonsteroidal antiinflammatories are used to treat mild to moderate pain, osteoarthritis, rheumatoid arthritis, and dysmenorrhea.

Side effects/adverse reactions: The most serious adverse reactions are nephrotoxicity (dysuria, hematuria, oliguria, azotemia), blood dyscrasias, and cholestatic hepatitis. The most common side effects are nausea, abdominal pain, anorexia, dizziness, and drowsiness.

Contraindications: Persons with hypersensitivity, asthma, severe renal disease, and severe hepatic disease should not use these products.

Precautions: Caution should be used in pregnancy, lactation, children, bleeding disorders, GI disorders, cardiac disorders, hypersensitivity to other antiinflammatory agents, and the elderly.

Pharmacokinetics: Onset, peak, and duration vary widely among products. Most products are metabolized in the liver and excreted in urine.

Interactions: Please check individual monographs since interactions vary widely among products.

Possible nursing diagnoses:
- Chronic pain *[uses]*
- Impaired physical mobility *[uses]*
- Knowledge deficit *[teaching]*
- Noncompliance *[teaching]*

NURSING CONSIDERATIONS
Assess:
- Renal, liver, blood studies: BUN, creatinine, AST, ALT, Hgb, before treatment, periodically thereafter
- Audiometric, ophthalmic examination before, during, and after treatment
- For eye, ear problems: blurred vision, tinnitus; may indicate toxicity

Administer:
- With food to decrease GI symptoms; however, best to take on empty stomach to facilitate absorption

Perform/provide:
- Storage at room temp

Evaluate:
- Therapeutic response: decreased pain, stiffness in joints, decreased swelling in joints, ability to move more easily

Teach patient/family:
- To report blurred vision, ringing, roaring in ears; may indicate toxicity
- To avoid driving, other hazardous activities if dizziness, drowsiness occur, especially elderly
- To report change in urine pattern, increased weight, edema, increased pain in joints, fever, blood in urine; indicate nephrotoxicity
- That therapeutic effects may take up to 1 mo

Generic names

celecoxib
diclofenac
etodolac
fenoprofen
flurbiprofen (Appx C)
ibuprofen
indomethacin
ketoprofen

ketorolac
mefenamic acid (Appx F)
nabumetone
naproxen
piroxicam
sulindac
tolmetin

OPIOID ANALGESICS

Action: Opioid analgesics act by depressing pain impulse transmission at the spinal cord level by interacting with opioid receptors. Products are divided into opiates and nonopiates.

Uses: Most products are used to control moderate to severe pain and are used before and after surgery.

Side effects/adverse reactions: GI symptoms, including nausea, vomiting, anorexia, constipation, and cramps are the most common side effects. Other common side effects include light-headedness, dizziness, sedation. Serious adverse reactions such as respiratory depression, respiratory arrest, circulatory depression, and increased intracranial pressure may result but are less common and usually dose dependent.

Contraindications: Hypersensitive reactions occur frequently. Check for sensitivity before administering. These drugs should not be used if narcotic addiction is suspected, and they are also contraindicated in acute bronchial asthma and upper airway obstruction.

Precautions: Caution must be used when these products are given to a person with an addictive personality since the possibility of addiction is so great. Also, they may worsen intracranial pressure. Persons with severe heart disease, hepatic or renal disease, respiratory conditions, or seizure disorders should be monitored closely for worsening condition.

Pharmacokinetics: Onset of action is immediate by IV route and rapid by IM and PO routes. Peak occurs from 1-2 hr, depending on route, with a duration of 2-8 hr. These agents cross the placenta and appear in breast milk.

Interactions: Barbiturates, other narcotics, hypnotics, antipsychotics, or alcohol can increase CNS depression when taken with narcotics.

Possible nursing diagnoses:
• Pain *[uses]*
• Impaired gas exchange *[adverse reactions]*

NURSING CONSIDERATIONS

Assess:
• I&O ratio; be alert for urinary retention, frequency, dysuria; drug should be discontinued if these occur
• Respiratory dysfunction, including respiratory depression, rate, rhythm, character; notify prescriber if respirations are <12/min
• CNS changes: dizziness, drowsiness, hallucinations, euphoria, LOC, pupil reaction
• Allergic reactions: rash, urticaria
• Need for pain medication; use pain scoring

Administer:
• With antiemetic if nausea or vomiting occurs
• When pain is beginning to return; determine dosage interval by response

Perform/provide:
• Assistance with ambulation; patient should not be ambulating during drug peak

Evaluate:
• Therapeutic response, including decrease in pain

Teach patient/family:
• To report any symptoms of CNS changes, allergic reactions, or shortness of breath
• That physical dependency may result when used for extended periods
• That withdrawal symptoms may occur, including nausea, vomiting, cramps, fever, faintness, anorexia
• To avoid alcohol and other CNS depressants

Generic names

alfentanil
buprenorphine
butorphanol
codeine
dezocine
fentanyl
fentanyl transdermal
hydromorphone
levorphanol

meperidine
methadone
morphine
nalbuphine
oxycodone
oxymorphone
pentazocine
propoxyphene
remifentanil

SALICYLATES

Action: Salicylates have analgesic, antipyretic, and antiinflammatory effects. The antiinflammatory and analgesic activities may be mediated through the inhibition of prostaglandin synthesis. Antipyretic action results from inhibition of the hypothalamic heat-regulating center.

Uses: The primary uses of salicylates are relief of mild to moderate pain and fever and in inflammatory conditions such as arthritis, thromboembolic disorders, and rheumatic fever.

Side effects/adverse reactions: The most common side effects are GI symptoms and rash. Serious blood dyscrasias and hepatotoxicity may result when used for long periods at high doses. Tinnitus or impaired hearing may indicate that blood salicylate levels are reaching or exceeding the upper limit of the therapeutic range.

Contraindications: Hypersensitivity to salicylates is common. Check for sensitivity before administering. Persons with bleeding disorders, GI bleeding, and vit K deficiency should not use these products since salicylates increase prothrombin time. Children should not use these products since salicylates have been associated with Reye's syndrome.

Precautions: Caution is needed when salicylates are given to patients with anemia, hepatic or renal disease, or Hodgkin's disease. Caution should also be exercised in pregnancy and lactation.

Pharmacokinetics: Onset of action occurs in 15-30 min, with a peak of 1-2 hr and a duration up to 6 hr. These drugs are metabolized by the liver and excreted by the kidneys.

Interactions: Increased effects of anticoagulants, insulin, methotrexate, heparin, valproic acid, and oral sulfonylureas may occur when used with salicylates. Aspirin may decrease serum concentrations of nonsteroidal antiinflammatory agents.

Possible nursing diagnoses:
• Pain *[uses]*
• Impaired physical mobility *[uses]*
• Activity intolerance *[uses]*
• Sensory/perceptual alterations: auditory *[adverse reactions]*
• Ineffective thermoregulation *[uses]*

NURSING CONSIDERATIONS

Assess:
• Hepatic and renal studies: AST, ALT, bilirubin, creatinine, LDH, alk phosphatase, BUN if patient is on long-term therapy, since these products are metabolized and excreted by the liver and kidney
• Blood studies: CBC, hematocrit, hemoglobin, and prothrombin time if

patient is on long-term therapy, since these products increase the possibility of bleeding and blood dyscrasias

• Hepatotoxicity: dark urine, clay-colored stools; yellowing of skin, sclera; itching, abdominal pain, fever, diarrhea, which may occur with long-term use

• Ototoxicity: tinnitus; ringing, roaring in ears; audiometric testing is needed before and after long-term therapy

Administer:

• With food or milk to decrease gastric irritation; give 30 min before or 1 hr after meals with a full glass of water

Evaluate:

• Therapeutic response, including decreased pain, fever

Teach patient/family:

• That blood sugar levels should be monitored closely if patient is diabetic

• Not to exceed recommended dosage; acute poisoning may result

• That therapeutic response takes 2 wk in arthritis

• To avoid use of alcohol, since GI bleeding may result

• To notify prescriber of ringing in the ears or persistent GI pain

• To take with full glass of water to reduce risk of lodging in esophagus

---

Generic names

aspirin	magnesium salicylate
choline salicylate	salsalate

THROMBOLYTICS

Action: Thrombolytics act by activating conversion of plasminogen to plasmin (fibrinolysin): plasmin is able to break down clots (fibrin).

Uses: Thrombolytics are used to treat deep-vein thrombosis, pulmonary embolism, arterial thrombosis, arterial embolism, arteriovenous cannula occlusion, lysis of coronary artery thrombi after MI, and acute, evolving transmural MI.

Side effects/adverse reactions: Serious adverse reactions include GI, GU, intracranial retroperitoneal bleeding, and anaphylaxis. The most common side effects are decreased Hct, urticaria, headache, and nausea.

Contraindications: Persons with hypersensitivity, active bleeding, intraspinal surgery, neoplasms of the CNS, ulcerative colitis/enteritis, severe hypertension, renal disease, hepatic disease, hypocoagulation, COPD, subacute bacterial endocarditis, rheumatic valvular disease, cerebral embolism/thrombosis/hemorrhage, recent intraarterial diagnostic procedure or surgery (10 days), and recent major surgery should not use these products.

Precautions: Caution should be used in arterial emboli from left side of heart and pregnancy.

Pharmacokinetics: Onset, peak, and duration vary widely among products. Most products are metabolized in the liver and excreted in urine.

Interactions: Please check individual monographs since interactions vary widely among products.

Possible nursing diagnoses:

• Risk for injury *[uses]*

NURSING CONSIDERATIONS

Assess:

• VS, B/P, pulse, resp, neuro signs, temp at least q4h; temp >104° F (40° C) indicator of internal bleeding; cardiac rhythm following intracoronary administration; systolic pressure increase of >25 mm Hg should be reported to prescriber

• For neurologic changes that may indicate intracranial bleeding

• Retroperitoneal bleeding: back pain, leg weakness, diminished pulses

• Allergy: fever, rash, itching, chill; mild reaction may be treated with antihistamines

• For bleeding during 1st hr of treatment: hematuria, hematemesis, bleeding from mucous membranes, epistaxis, ecchymosis

• Blood studies (Hct, platelets, PTT, PT, TT, APTT) before starting therapy; PT or APTT must be less than ×2 control before starting therapy; TT or PT q3-4h during treatment

Administer:

• As soon as thrombi identified; not useful for thrombi over 1 wk old

• Cryoprecipitate or fresh, frozen plasma if bleeding occurs

• Loading dose at beginning of therapy; may require increased loading doses

• Heparin after fibrinogen level is over 100 mg/dl. Heparin infusion to increase PTT to 1.5-2 × baseline for 3-7 days

• About 10% of patients have high streptococcal antibody titers requiring increased loading doses

• IV therapy using 0.8 μm filter

Perform/provide:

• Storage of reconstituted drug in refrigerator; discard after 24 hr

• Bed rest during entire course of treatment

• Avoidance of venous or arterial puncture, inj, rectal temp

• Treatment of fever with acetaminophen or aspirin

• Pressure for 30 sec to minor bleeding sites; inform prescriber if this does not attain hemostasis; apply pressure dressing

Evaluate:

• Therapeutic response: resolution of thrombosis, embolism

Generic names

alteplase
anistreplase

streptokinase
urokinase

THYROID HORMONES

Action: Acts by increasing metabolic rates, resulting in increased cardiac output, O_2 consumption, body temp, blood volume, growth, development at cellular level, respiratory rate, enzyme system activity.

Uses: Products are used for thyroid replacement.

Side effects/adverse reactions: The most common side effects include insomnia, tremors, tachycardia, palpitations, angina, dysrhythmias, weight loss, and changes in appetite. Serious adverse reactions include thyroid storm.

Contraindications: Persons with adrenal insufficiency, myocardial infarction, or thyrotoxicosis should not use these products.

Precautions: The elderly and patients with angina pectoris, hypertension, ischemia, cardiac disease, or diabetes mellitus or insipidus should be watched closely when using these products. Caution should be used in pregnancy (A) and lactation.

Pharmacokinetics: Pharmacokinetics vary widely among products; check specific monographs.

Interactions:
• Impaired absorption of thyroid products may occur when administered with cholestyramine (separate by 4-5 hr)
• Increased effects of anticoagulants, sympathomimetics, tricyclic antidepressants, catecholamines may occur
• Decreased effects of digitalis, glycosides, insulin, hypoglycemics may occur
• Decreased effects of thyroid products may occur with estrogens

Possible nursing diagnoses:
• Knowledge deficit *[teaching]*
• Noncompliance *[teaching]*
• Body image disturbance *[adverse reactions]*

NURSING CONSIDERATIONS
Assess:
• B/P, pulse before each dose
• I&O ratio
• Weight qd in same clothing, using same scale, at same time of day
• Height, growth rate if given to a child

• T_3, T_4, which are decreased; radioimmunoassay of TSH, which is increased; ratio uptake, which is decreased if patient is on too low a dosage of medication
• Increased nervousness, excitability, irritability; may indicate overdosage, usually after 1-3 wk of treatment
• Cardiac status: angina, palpitation, chest pain, change in VS

Administer:
• At same time each day to maintain drug level
• Only for hormone imbalances, not to be used for obesity, male infertility, menstrual conditions, lethargy

Perform/provide:
• Removal of medication 4 wk before RAIU test

Evaluate:
• Therapeutic response: absence of depression; increased weight loss; diuresis; pulse; appetite; absence of constipation; peripheral edema; cold intolerance; pale, cool, dry skin; brittle nails; alopecia; coarse hair; menorrhagia; night blindness; paresthesias; syncope; stupor; coma; rosy cheeks

Teach patient/family:
• That hair loss will occur in child and is temporary
• To report excitability, irritability, anxiety; indicates overdose
• Not to switch brands unless directed by prescriber
• That hypothyroid child will show almost immediate behavior/personality change
• That treatment drug is not to be taken to reduce weight
• To avoid OTC preparations with iodine; read labels
• To avoid iodine in food, iodinized salt, soybeans, tofu, turnips, some seafood, some bread

---

Generic names

levothyroxine (T_4)	liotrix
liothyronine (T_3)	thyroid USP

VASODILATORS

Action: Vasodilators have various modes of action. Please check individual monographs for specific action.
Uses: Vasodilators are used to treat intermittent claudication, arteriosclerosis obliterans, vasospasm and muscular ischemia, ischemic cerebral vascular disease, hypertension, and angina.

Side effects/adverse reactions: The most common side effects are headache, nausea, hypotension or hypertension, and ECG changes.

Contraindications: Some drugs are contraindicated in acute MI, paroxysmal tachycardia, and thyrotoxicosis.

Precautions: Caution should be used in uncompensated heart disease or peptic ulcer disease.

Pharmacokinetics: Onset, peak, and duration vary widely among products. Most products are metabolized in the liver and excreted in urine.

Interactions: Please check individual monographs since interactions vary widely among products.

Possible nursing diagnoses:

- Decreased cardiac output *[uses]*
- Altered tissue perfusion: cardiopulmonary *[uses]*
- Knowledge deficit *[teaching]*

NURSING CONSIDERATIONS

Assess:

- Bleeding time in individuals with bleeding disorders
- Cardiac status: B/P, pulse, rate, rhythm, character; watch for increasing pulse

Administer:

- With meals to reduce GI symptoms

Perform/provide:

- Storage in tight container at room temp

Evaluate:

- Therapeutic response: ability to walk without pain, increased temp in extremities, increased pulse volume

Teach patient/family:

- That medication is not cure; may need to be taken continuously
- That it is necessary to quit smoking to prevent excessive vasoconstriction
- That improvement may be sudden, but usually occurs gradually over several wk
- To report headache, weakness, increased pulse, as drug may have to be decreased or discontinued
- To avoid hazardous activities until stabilized on medication; dizziness may occur

---

Generic names

amyl nitrite (Appx F)
dipyridamole
hydralazine
isoxsuprine (Appx F)

minoxidil
papaverine (Appx F)
tolazoline

VITAMINS

Action: Action varies widely among products and classes; check specific monographs.

Uses: Vitamins are used to correct and prevent vitamin deficiencies.

Side effects/adverse reactions: There are no side effects or adverse reactions with the water-soluble vitamins (C, B). However, fat-soluble vitamins (A, D, E, K) may accumulate in the body and cause adverse reactions (see specific monographs).

Contraindications: Hypersensitive reactions may occur, and allergies should be identified before these products are given.

Pharmacokinetics: Onset, peak, and duration vary widely among products; check individual monographs for specific information.

Possible nursing diagnoses:
• Altered nutrition: less than body requirements *[uses]*

NURSING CONSIDERATIONS

Administer:
• PO with food for better absorption

Perform/provide:
• Storage in tight, light-resistant container

Evaluate:
• Therapeutic response: no vitamin deficiency

Teach patient/family:
• Not to take more than prescribed amount

Generic names

Fat-soluble
phytonadione (vita-
    min K_1)
vitamin A
vitamin D
vitamin E

cyanocobalamin B_{12}/hydroxo-
    cobalamin (B_{12}a)
pyridoxine (B_6)
riboflavin (B_2)
thiamine (B_1)

Water-soluble
ascorbic acid (C)

Miscellaneous
    multivitamins

abacavir
See appendix a—selected new drugs

---

acarbose (R_x)
(ay-car'bose)
Prandese*, Precose
Func. class.: Oral antidiabetic
Chem. class.: α-Glucosidase inhibitor

Action: Delays digestion of ingested carbohydrates, results in smaller rise in blood glucose after meals; does not increase insulin production
Uses: Non–insulin-dependent diabetes mellitus (NIDDM) Type II, alone or in combination with a sulfonylurea
Dosage and routes:
• *Adult:* **PO** 25 mg tid initially, with first bite of meal; maintenance dose may be increased to 50-100 mg tid; dosage adjustment at 4-9 wk intervals
• *Adult <60 kg:* Not to exceed 50 mg PO tid
• *Available forms:* Tabs 50, 100 mg
Side effects/adverse reactions:
GI: Abdominal pain, diarrhea, flatulence, increased serum transaminase level
Contraindications: Hypersensitivity, diabetic ketoacidosis, cirrhosis, inflammatory bowel disease, colonic ulceration, partial intestinal obstruction, chronic intestinal disease, serum creatinine >2 mg/dl
Precautions: Pregnancy (B), renal disease, lactation, children, hepatic disease
Pharmacokinetics: Metabolized in GI tract, excreted as intact drug in urine, half-life 2 hr
Interactions:
• Effect of acarbose may be decreased: digestive enzymes, intestinal absorbents
• Increased hypoglycemia: sulfonylureas, insulin, calcium channel blockers, corticosteroids, estrogen, oral contraceptives, phenothiazines, phenytoin, sympathomimetics, diuretics, thyroid, isoniazid, nicotinic acid
Lab test interferences:
Decrease: Calcium, vit B_6
Increase: AST, bilirubin
NURSING CONSIDERATIONS
Assess:
• Hypoglycemia, hyperglycemia; even though drug does not cause hypoglycemia, if patient is on sulfonylureas or insulin, hypoglycemia may be additive; if hypoglycemia occurs, treat with dextrose, or if severe, IV glucose or glucagon.
• 1 hr postprandial for establishing effectiveness, then glycosylated Hgb q3mo
• Monitor AST q3mo × 1 yr and periodically thereafter
Administer:
PO
• Tid with first bite of each meal
Perform/provide:
• Storage in tight container in cool environment
Evaluate:
• Therapeutic response: decreased signs/symptoms of diabetes mellitus (polyuria, polydipsia, polyphagia, clear sensorium, absence of dizziness, stable gait)
Teach patient/family:
• The symptoms of hypo/hyperglycemia, what to do about each
• That medication must be taken as prescribed; explain consequences of discontinuing medication abruptly
• To avoid OTC medications unless approved by health-care provider
• That diabetes is lifelong illness; that this drug is not a cure

- To carry a Medic Alert ID for emergency purposes
- That diet and exercise regimen must be followed

---

acebutolol (R)
(a-se-byoo'toe-lole)
Monitan*, Sectral
Func. class.: Antihypertensive, β_1-blocker, antidysrhythmic (II)

Action: Competitively blocks stimulation of β-adrenergic receptors within vascular smooth muscle; decreases rate of SA node discharge, increases recovery time, slows conduction of AV node resulting in decreased heart rate (negative chronotropic effect), which decreases O_2 consumption in myocardium; also decreases renin-aldosterone-angiotensin system at high doses, inhibits β_2-receptors in bronchial system (high doses)

Uses: Mild to moderate hypertension, sinus tachycardia, persistent atrial extrasystoles, tachydysrhythmias

Investigational uses: Prophylaxis of MI, treatment of angina pectoris, tremor, mitral valve prolapse, thyrotoxicosis, idiopathic hypertrophic subaortic stenosis

Dosage and routes:
Hypertension
- *Adult:* **PO** 400 mg qd or in 2 divided doses; may be increased to desired response; maintenance 200-1200 mg/qd in 2 divided doses

Ventricular dysrhythmia
- *Adult:* **PO** 200 mg bid, may increase gradually, usual range 600-1200 mg daily; should be tapered over 2 wk before discontinuing
- *Geriatric:* not to exceed 800 mg qd
- *Renal dose:* CrCl 50-25 ml/min, reduce dose by 50%; if <25 ml/min reduce dose by 75%

Available forms: Caps 200, 400 mg; tabs 200, 400 mg*

Side effects/adverse reactions:
CV: **Profound hypotension, bradycardia, CHF,** cold extremities, postural hypotension, **2nd- or 3rd-degree heart block**
CNS: Insomnia, fatigue, dizziness, mental changes, memory loss, hallucinations, depression, lethargy, drowsiness, strange dreams, catatonia
GI: Nausea, diarrhea, vomiting, **mesenteric arterial thrombosis, ischemic colitis**
INTEG: Rash, fever, alopecia, dry skin
HEMA: **Agranulocytosis, thrombocytopenia, purpura**
EENT: Sore throat; dry, burning eyes
GU: **Impotence,** decreased libido, dysuria, nocturia
ENDO: Increased hypoglycemic response to insulin
RESP: **Bronchospasm,** dyspnea, wheezing, cough
MS: Joint pain, cramping

Contraindications: Hypersensitivity to β-blockers, cardiogenic shock, heart block (2nd-, 3rd-degree), sinus bradycardia, CHF, cardiac failure

Precautions: Major surgery, pregnancy (B), lactation, diabetes mellitus, renal disease, thyroid disease, COPD, asthma, well-compensated heart failure, aortic, mitral valve, hepatic disease

Pharmacokinetics:
PO: Onset 1-1½ hr, peak 2-4 hr, duration 10-12 hr, half-life 6-7 hr, excreted unchanged in urine, protein binding 5%-15%

Interactions:
- Increased hypotension, bradycardia: reserpine, hydralazine, methyldopa, prazosin, anticholinergics,

---

cardiac glycosides, diltiazem, verapamil, diuretics, other antihypertensives

• Decreased antihypertensive effects: NSAIDs

• Increased hypoglycemic effect: insulin, oral antidiabetics

• Decreased bronchodilation: theophyllines, β_2-agonists

⚕ May increase acebutolol effect: buckthorn bark/berry, aloe, rhubarb root, senna leaf/fruits, cascara sagrada bark

⚕ Dysrhythmia: Ephedra

Lab test interferences:

Positive: ANA

NURSING CONSIDERATIONS

Assess:

• B/P during beginning treatment, periodically thereafter; pulse q4h; note rate, rhythm, quality

• Apical/radial pulse before administration; notify prescriber of any significant changes (pulse <60 bpm); signs of CHF (dyspnea, crackles, weight gain, jugular vein distension)

• Baselines in renal, liver function tests before therapy begins

• Edema in feet, legs daily: monitor I&O

• Skin turgor, dryness of mucous membranes for hydration status, especially elderly

Administer:

PO

• Drug ac, hs, tablet may be crushed or swallowed whole; give with food to prevent GI upset

Perform/provide:

• Storage protected from light, moisture; place in cool environment

Evaluate:

• Therapeutic response: decreased B/P after 1-2 wk; decreased dysrhythmias

Teach patient/family:

◆Not to discontinue drug abruptly, taper over 2 wk; do not double dose;

if a dose is missed, take as soon as remembered up to 4 hr before next dose

• Not to use OTC products containing α-adrenergic stimulants (such as nasal decongestants, OTC cold preparations) unless directed by prescriber

• To report low pulse, dizziness, confusion, depression, fever

• To take pulse at home, advise when to notify prescriber

• To comply with weight control, dietary adjustments, modified exercise program

• To carry Medic Alert ID to identify drug, allergies

• To avoid hazardous activities if dizziness is present

• To report symptoms of CHF: difficult breathing, especially on exertion or when lying down, night cough, swelling of extremities

Treatment of overdose: Lavage, IV atropine for bradycardia, IV theophylline for bronchospasm, digitalis, O_2, diuretic for cardiac failure, IV glucose for hypoglycemia, IV diazepam (or phenytoin) for seizures

acetaminophen (OTC)

(a-seat-a-mee'noe-fen)
Abenol*, Acephen, Aceta, Actamin, Actimol, Aminofen, Apacet, APAP, Apo-Acetaminophen*, Aspirin Free Pain Relief, Atasol*, Banesin, Children's Feverall, Dapa, Datril, Exdol*, FemEtts, Genapap, Genebs, Halenol, Liquiprin, Mapap, Maranox, Meda, Panadol, Redutemp, Robigesic*, Rounax*, Silapap, Snaplets-FR, St. Joseph Aspirin-Free, Tapanol, Tempra, Tylenol, Uni-Ace, Valorin

Func. class.: Nonnarcotic analgesic, antipyretic

Chem. class.: Nonsalicylate, para-aminophenol derivative

Action: May block pain impulses peripherally that occur in response to inhibition of prostaglandin synthesis; does not possess antiinflammatory properties; antipyretic action results from inhibition of prostaglandins in the CNS (hypothalamic heat-regulating center)

Uses: Mild to moderate pain or fever

Dosage and routes:
• *Adult and child >12 yr:* **PO/RECT** 325-650 mg q4h prn, not to exceed 4 g/day
• *Child:* **PO** 10-15 mg/kg q4h
• *Child 6-12 yr:* **RECT** 325 mg q4-6h
• *Child 3-6 yr:* **RECT** 125 mg q4-6h
• *Child 1-3 yr:* **RECT** 80 mg q4h
• *Child 3-11 mo:* **RECT** 80 mg q6h
Available forms: Rect supp 120, 125, 325, 600, 650 mg; soft chew tabs 80, 160 mg; caps 500 mg; elix 120, 160, 325 mg/5 ml; liq 160 mg/5 ml, 500 mg/15 ml; sol 100 mg/1 ml, 120 mg/2.5 ml; granules 80 mg/ packet, 80 mg/cap; tabs 160, 325, 500, 650 mg

Side effects/adverse reactions:
SYST: **Anaphylaxis**
HEMA: **Leukopenia, neutropenia, hemolytic anemia (long-term use), thrombocytopenia, pancytopenia**
CNS: Stimulation, drowsiness
GI: Nausea, vomiting, abdominal pain, **hepatotoxicity**
INTEG: Rash, urticaria, **angioedema**
TOXICITY: **Cyanosis, anemia, neutropenia, jaundice, pancytopenia, CNS stimulation, delirium followed by vascular collapse, convulsions, coma, death**

Contraindications: Hypersensitivity, intolerance to tartrazine (yellow dye #4), alcohol, table sugar, saccharin, depending on product

Precautions: Anemia, hepatic disease, renal disease, chronic alcoholism, pregnancy (B), elderly, lactation

Pharmacokinetics: Well absorbed PO, rectal absorption varies
PO: Onset 10-30 min, peak ½-2 hr, duration 3-4 hr
RECT: Onset slow, peak 1-2 hr, duration 3-4 hr; 85%-90% metabolized by liver, excreted by kidneys; metabolites may be toxic if overdose occurs; widely distributed, crosses placenta in low concentrations, excreted in breast milk, half-life 1-4 hr

Interactions:
• Decreased effect, increased hepatotoxicity: barbiturates, alcohol, carbamazepine, hydantoins, rifampin, sulfinpyrazone
• Hypoprothrombinemia: warfarin, long-term use, high doses of acetaminophen
• Bone marrow suppression: zidovudine

Lab test interferences:
Interference: Chemstrip G, Dextrostix, Visidex II, 5-HIAA

NURSING CONSIDERATIONS
Assess:

- Liver function studies: AST, ALT, bilirubin, creatinine prior to therapy if long-term therapy is anticipated; may cause hepatic toxicity at doses >4 g/day with chronic use
- Renal function studies: BUN, urine creatinine, occult blood, albumin, if patient is on long-term therapy; presence of blood or albumin indicates nephritis
- Blood studies: CBC, pro-time if patient is on long-term therapy
- I&O ratio; decreasing output may indicate renal failure (long-term therapy)
- For fever and pain: type of pain, location, intensity, duration
- For chronic poisoning: rapid, weak pulse; dyspnea; cold, clammy extremities; report immediately to prescriber
- Hepatotoxicity: dark urine; clay-colored stools; yellowing of skin, sclera; itching, abdominal pain; fever; diarrhea if patient is on long-term therapy
- Allergic reactions: rash, urticaria; if these occur, drug may have to be discontinued

Administer:
PO

- Crushed or whole; chewable tablets may be chewed; give with full glass of water
- With food or milk to decrease gastric symptoms if needed

Perform/provide:

- Storage of suppositories <80° F (27° C)

Evaluate:

- Therapeutic response: absence of pain, fever

Teach patient/family:

- Not to exceed recommended dosage; acute poisoning with liver damage may result
- That acute toxicity includes symptoms of nausea, vomiting, abdominal pain; prescriber should be notified immediately
- To read label on other OTC drugs; many contain acetaminophen and may cause toxicity if taken concurrently
- To recognize signs of chronic overdose: bleeding, bruising, malaise, fever, sore throat
- To notify prescriber of pain or fever lasting over 3 days
- **Treatment of overdose:** Drug level, gastric lavage, activated charcoal; administer oral acetylcysteine to prevent hepatic damage (see acetylcysteine monograph), monitor for bleeding

---

acetazolamide (R)

(a-set-a-zole'a-mide)
acetazolamide, Apo-Acetazolamide*, Dazamide, Diamox, Diamox Sequels

Func. class.: Diuretic, carbonic anhydrase inhibitor, antiglaucoma agent, antiepileptic
Chem. class.: Sulfonamide derivative

Action: Inhibits carbonic anhydrase activity in proximal renal tubules to decrease reabsorption of water, sodium, potassium, bicarbonate; decreases carbonic anhydrase in CNS, increasing seizure threshold; able to decrease aqueous humor in eye, which lowers intraocular pressure
Uses: Open-angle glaucoma, narrow-angle glaucoma (preoperatively, if surgery delayed), epilepsy (petit mal, grand mal, mixed), edema in CHF, drug-induced edema, acute mountain sickness
Investigational uses: Prevention of uric acid/cystine renal stones, decrease CSF production in infants with hydrocephalus

---

Dosage and routes:

Closed-angle glaucoma
• *Adult:* **PO/IM/IV** 250 mg q4h or 250 mg bid, to be used for short-term therapy

Open-angle glaucoma
• *Adult:* **PO/IM/IV** 250 mg-1 g/day in divided doses for amounts over 250 mg or 500 mg SR bid

Edema in CHF
• *Adult:* **IM/IV** 250-375 mg/day in AM
• *Child:* **IM/IV** 5 mg/kg/day in AM

Seizures
• *Adult:* **PO/IM/IV** 4-30 mg/kg/day, in 1-4 divided doses usual range 375-1000 mg/day
• *Child:* **PO/IM/IV** 8-30 mg/kg/day in divided doses tid or qid, or 300-900 mg/m²/day, not to exceed 1 g/day

Mountain sickness
• *Adult:* **PO** 250 mg q8-12h

Renal stones
• *Adult:* **PO** 250 mg hs

Infants with hydrocephalus
• *Infant:* **IV** 5 mg/kg/dose q6h, may be increased up to 100 mg/kg/day if tolerated

Available forms: Tabs 125, 250 mg; caps sust rel 500 mg; inj 500 mg

Side effects/adverse reactions:
GU: Frequency, polyuria, **uremia,** glucosuria, hematuria, dysuria, crystalluria, renal calculi
CNS: Drowsiness, paresthesia, anxiety, depression, headache, dizziness, confusion, stimulation, fatigue, **convulsions,** sedation, nervousness
GI: Nausea, vomiting, anorexia, constipation, diarrhea, melena, weight loss, **hepatic insufficiency,** taste alterations
EENT: Myopia, tinnitus
INTEG: Rash, pruritus, urticaria, fever, **Stevens-Johnson syndrome,** photosensitivity
ENDO: Hyperglycemia
HEMA: Aplastic anemia, hemolytic anemia, leukopenia, agranulocytosis, thrombocytopenia, purpura, pancytopenia
META: Hypokalemia, hyperchloremic acidosis

Contraindications: Hypersensitivity to sulfonamides, severe renal disease, severe hepatic disease, electrolyte imbalances (hyponatremia, hypokalemia), hyperchloremic acidosis, Addison's disease, long-term use in narrow-angle glaucoma, COPD

Precautions: Hypercalciuria, pregnancy (C), lactation

Pharmacokinetics:
PO: Onset 1-1½ hr, peak 2-4 hr, duration 8-12 hr
PO-SUS REL: Onset 2 hr, peak 3-6 hr, duration 18-24 hr
IV: Onset 2 min, peak 15 min, duration 4-5 hr, 65% absorbed if fasting (oral), 75% absorbed if given with food; half-life 2½-5½ hr; excreted unchanged by kidneys (80% within 24 hr), crosses placenta

Interactions:
• Increased action of amphetamines, procainamide, quinidine, anticholinergics
• Increased excretion of lithium
• Increased toxicity: salicylates
• Toxicity: cyclosporine
• Decreased acetazolamide effect: methenamine
• Increased side effects: diflunisal
• Decreased primidone levels

Lab test interferences:
False positive: Urinary protein, 17 hydroxysteroid
Decrease: Thyroid iodine uptake

NURSING CONSIDERATIONS
Assess:
• Weight daily, I&O daily to determine fluid loss; effect of drug may be decreased if used qd; monitor the elderly for dehydration
• For cross-sensitivity between other sulfonamides and this drug

◆ = Nursing alert   ✔ = Herb-drug interaction   ⊘ = Do not crush

• B/P lying, standing; postural hypotension may occur

• Electrolytes: K, Na, chloride; also BUN, blood sugar, CBC, serum creatinine, blood pH, ABGs, liver function tests; I&O, glucose, patient may need to be on a high-K diet

Administer:

• In AM to avoid interference with sleep if using drug as diuretic

• K replacement if K level is less than 3.0 mg/dl

PO

• With food if nausea occurs; absorption may be decreased slightly

🚫 Do not break, crush, or chew sus rel caps

IV

• After diluting 500 mg in >5 ml sterile H_2O for injection; direct IV—give at 100-500 mg/min; may be diluted further in LR, D_5W, $D_{10}W$, 0.45% NaCl, 0.9% NaCl, or Ringer's sol and infused over 4-8 hr; use within 24 hr of dilution

Additive compatibilities: Cimetidine, ranitidine

Perform/provide:

• Storage in dark, cool area; use reconstituted solution within 24 hr

Evaluate:

• Therapeutic response: improvement in edema of feet, legs, sacral area daily if medication is being used in CHF; or decrease in aqueous humor if medication is being used in glaucoma

Teach patient/family:

• To take exactly as prescribed; if dose is missed, take as soon as remembered; do not double dose

• To notify prescriber if sore throat, unusual bleeding, bruising, paresthesias, tremors, flank pain, or skin rash occurs

• To use sunscreen to prevent photosensitivity; to monitor blood glucose and urine for sugar

• To avoid hazardous activities if drowsiness occurs

Treatment of overdose: Lavage if taken orally; monitor electrolytes; administer dextrose in saline; monitor hydration, CV, renal status

---

acetylcysteine (℞)

(a-se-teel-sis'tay-een)
Mucomyst*, Mucosal, Parvolex*

Func. class.: Mucolytic; antidote—acetaminophen

Chem. class.: Amino acid L-cysteine

Action: Decreases viscosity of secretions by breaking disulfide links of mucoproteins; increases hepatic glutathione, which is necessary to inactivate toxic metabolites in acetaminophen overdose

Uses: Acetaminophen toxicity; bronchitis; pneumonia; cystic fibrosis; emphysema; atelectasis; tuberculosis; complications of thoracic, cardiovascular surgery; diagnosis in bronchial lab tests

Dosage and routes:

Mucolytic

• *Adult and child:* **INSTILL** 1-2 ml (10%-20% sol) q1-4h prn or 3-5 ml (20% sol) or 6-10 ml (10% sol) tid or qid

Acetaminophen toxicity

• *Adult and child:* **PO** 140 mg/kg, then 70 mg/kg q4h × 17 doses to total of 1330 mg/kg

Available forms: Sol 10%, 20%

Side effects/adverse reactions:

CNS: Dizziness, drowsiness, headache, fever, chills

GI: Nausea, stomatitis, constipation, vomiting, anorexia, *hepatotoxicity*

EENT: Rhinorrhea, tooth damage

CV: Hypotension

INTEG: Urticaria, rash, fever, clamminess

*RESP: **Bronchospasm,** burning, **hemoptysis,*** chest tightness

Contraindications: Hypersensitivity, increased intracranial pressure, status asthmaticus

Precautions: Hypothyroidism, Addison's disease, CNS depression, brain tumor, asthma, hepatic disease, renal disease, COPD, psychosis, alcoholism, convulsive disorders, lactation, pregnancy (B)

Pharmacokinetics:

INH/INSTILL: Onset 1 min, duration 5-10 min, metabolized by liver, excreted in urine

Interactions:

• Do not use with iron, copper, rubber

• Do not mix with antibiotics: tetracycline, chlortetracycline, oxytetracycline, erythromycin lactobionate, amphotericin B, sodium ampicillin; iodized oil, chymotrypsin, trypsin, hydrogen peroxide

NURSING CONSIDERATIONS

Assess:

• Cough: type, frequency, character, including sputum

• Rate, rhythm of respirations, increased dyspnea; sputum; discontinue if bronchospasm occurs

• VS, cardiac status including checking for dysrhythmias, increased rate, palpitations

• ABGs for increased CO_2 retention in asthma patients

• Antidotal use: liver function tests, pro-time, BUN, glucose, electrolytes, acetaminophen levels; inform prescriber if dose is vomited or vomiting is persistent

• Nausea, vomiting, rash; notify prescriber if these occur

Administer:

PO

• Antidotal use: give within 24 hr; give with cola or soft drink to disguise taste; can be given with H_2O through tubes; use within 1 hr

INSTILL

• By syringe 2-3 doses of 1-2 ml of 20% or 2-4 ml of 10% solution

• Decreased dose to elderly patients; their metabolisms may be slowed

• Only if suction machine is available

• Before meals ½-1 hr for better absorption, to decrease nausea

• 20% solutions diluted with NS or water for injection; may give 10% solution undiluted

• Only after patient clears airway by deep breathing, coughing

Perform/provide:

• Storage in refrigerator; use within 96 hr of opening

• Assistance with inhaled dose: bronchodilator if bronchospasm occurs

• Mechanical suction if cough insufficient to remove excess bronchial secretions

• Gum, hard candy, frequent rinsing of mouth for dryness of oral cavity

Evaluate:

• Therapeutic response: absence of purulent secretions when coughing; absence of hepatic damage in acetaminophen toxicity

Teach patient/family:

• About mucolytic use

• That unpleasant odor will decrease after repeated use

• That discoloration of solution after bottle is opened does not impair its effectiveness

---

activated charcoal (OTC)

Actidose-Aqua, CharcoAid, CharcoAid 2000, Liqui-Char

Func. class.: Antiflatulent; antidote

Action: Binds poisons, toxins, irritants; increases adsorption in GI

---

tract; inactivates toxins and binds until excreted

Uses: Poisoning

Dosage and routes:

• Children should not get more than 1 dose of products with sorbitol

Poisoning

• *Adult and child:* **PO** 30-100 g or 1 g/kg, minimum dose 30 g/250 ml of water, may give 20-40 g q6h for 1-2 days in severe poisoning

Available forms: Powder 15, 25*, 30, 40, 120, 125, 240 g/container; oral susp 12.5 g/60 ml, 15 g/72 ml, 15 g/120 ml, 25 g/120 ml, 30 g/120 ml, 50 g/240 ml; Canada 15 g/120 ml, 25 g/125 ml, 50 g/225 ml, 50 g/250 ml

Side effects/adverse reactions:

GI: Nausea, black stools, vomiting, constipation, diarrhea

Contraindications: Hypersensitivity to this drug, unconsciousness, semiconsciousness, poisoning of cyanide, mineral acids, alkalis

Pharmacokinetics:

PO: Excreted in feces

Interactions:

• Inactivation of: ipecac, acetylcysteine

NURSING CONSIDERATIONS

Assess:

• Respiration, pulse, B/P to determine charcoal effectiveness if taken for barbiturate/narcotic poisoning

Administer:

PO

• After inducing vomiting unless vomiting contraindicated (i.e., cyanide or alkalis)

• After mixing with water or fruit juice to form thick syrup; do not use dairy products to mix charcoal

• Repeat dose if vomiting occurs soon after dose; give with a laxative to promote elimination; alone, do not administer with ipecac

• After spacing at least 1 hr before or after other drugs, or absorption will be decreased

Perform/provide:

• Container closed tightly to prevent absorption of gases

NG

• Through a nasogastric tube if patient unable to swallow

Evaluate:

• Therapeutic response: LOC-alert (poisoning)

Teach patient/family:

• That stools will be black

• How to prevent further poisonings

---

acyclovir (℞)

(ay-sye'kloe-ver)

Avirax*, Zovirax

Func. class.: Antiviral

Chem. class.: Acyclic purine nucleoside analog

Action: Interferes with DNA synthesis by conversion to acyclovir triphosphate, causing decreased viral replication, time of lesional healing

Uses: Mucocutaneous herpes simplex virus, herpes genitalis (HSV-1, HSV-2), varicella infections, herpes zoster, herpes simplex encephalitis

Investigational uses: Cytomegalovirus, HSV after transplant, mononucleosis, herpes simplex

Dosage and routes:

• Lengthen dosing interval in renal disease CrCl <50 ml/min

Herpes simplex

• *Adult and child >12 yr:* **IV INF** 5 mg/kg over 1 hr q8h × 5 days

• *Child <12 yr:* **IV INF** 250 mg/m^2 or 30 mg/kg/day divided q8h over 1 hr × 5 days

Genital herpes

• *Adult:* **PO** 200 mg q4h (5×/day while awake) for 5 days to 6 mo

---

depending on whether initial, recurrent, or chronic

Herpes simplex encephalitis
- *Adult:* IV 10 mg/kg over 1 hr q8h × 10 days
- *Child >6 mo:* IV 500 mg/m² q8h × 10-14 days

Herpes zoster
- *Adult:* PO 800 mg × 7-10 days; IV 5 mg/kg q8h

Children with immunosuppression:
- *Child >2 yr:* 20 mg/kg qid × 5 days

Varicella-zoster
- *Adult:* PO 1000 mg q6h × 5 days or 600-800 mg q4h (5×/day while awake); IV 500 mg/m² q8h or 10 mg/kg q8h × 7d
- *Child:* PO 10-20 mg/kg (max 800 mg) qid × 5 days; IV 500 mg/m² q8h or 10 mg/kg q8h × 7d

Available forms: Caps 200 mg; inj 500 mg, oral susp, tabs 400, 800 mg
Side effects/adverse reactions:
CNS: Tremors, confusion, lethargy, hallucinations, **convulsions,** dizziness, *headache,* encephalopathic changes
GI: Nausea, vomiting, diarrhea, increased ALT, AST, abdominal pain, glossitis, colitis
GU: **Oliguria, proteinuria, hematuria,** vaginitis, moniliasis, **glomerulonephritis, acute renal failure,** changes in menses, polydipsia
EENT: Gingival hyperplasia
INTEG: Rash, urticaria, pruritus, pain or phlebitis at IV site, unusual sweating, alopecia
MS: Joint pain, leg pain, muscle cramps
Contraindications: Hypersensitivity
Precautions: Lactation, hepatic disease, renal disease, electrolyte imbalance, dehydration, pregnancy (B)
Pharmacokinetics:
Distributed widely; crosses placenta, CSF concentrations are 50% plasma

IV: Onset immediate, peak immediate, duration unknown, half-life 20 min-3 hr (terminal); metabolized by liver, excreted by kidneys as unchanged drug (95%)
PO: Absorbed minimally; onset unknown, peak 1½-2 hr, terminal half-life 3½ hr
Interactions:
- Increased levels, toxicity: probenecid
- Synergistic effect: interferon
- Drowsiness side effects: zidovudine

NURSING CONSIDERATIONS
Assess:
- Signs of infection, anemia
- I&O ratio; report hematuria, oliguria, fatigue, weakness; may indicate nephrotoxicity; check for protein in urine during treatment
◆ Any patient with compromised renal system, since drug is excreted slowly in poor renal system function; toxicity may occur rapidly
- Liver studies: AST, ALT
- Blood studies: WBC, RBC, Hct, Hgb, bleeding time; blood dyscrasias may occur; drug should be discontinued
- Renal studies: urinalysis, protein, BUN, creatinine, CrCl
- C&S before drug therapy; drug may be taken as soon as culture is taken; repeat C&S after treatment; determine the presence of other sexually transmitted diseases
- Bowel pattern before, during treatment; if severe abdominal pain with bleeding occurs, drug should be discontinued
- Skin eruptions: rash, urticaria, itching
- Allergies before treatment, reaction of each medication; place allergies on chart in bright red letters

---

◆ = Nursing alert   ✐ = Herb-drug interaction   ⊘ = Do not crush

Administer:
PO
🚫 Do not break, crush, or chew caps
IV
• Increased fluids to 3 L/day to decrease crystalluria

• After reconstituting with 10 ml compatible solution/500 mg of drug, concentration of 50 mg/ml, shake, use within 12 hr (<7 mg/ml); give over at least 1 hr (constant rate) by infusion pump to prevent nephrotoxicity; do not reconstitute with sol containing benzyl alcohol in neonates

• Lower dose in acute or chronic renal failure

Additive compatibilities: Fluconazole

Solution compatibilities: D$_5$W, LR, or NaCl (D$_5$ 0.9% NaCl, 0.9% NaCl) solutions

Y-site compatibilities: Allopurinol, amikacin, ampicillin, amphotericin B, cefamandole, cefazolin, cefonicid, cefoperazone, cefotaxime, cefoxitin, ceftazidime, ceftizoxime, ceftriaxone, cefuroxime, cephapirin, chloramphenicol, cholesteryl sulfate complex, cimetidine, clindamycin, dexamethasone sodium phosphate, dimenhydrinate, diphenhydramine, doxorubicin, doxycycline, erythromycin, famotidine, filgrastim, fluconazole, gallium, gentamicin, granisetron, heparin, hydrocortisone sodium succinate, hydromorphone, imipenem/cilastatin, lorazepam, magnesium sulfate, melphalan, methylprednisolone sodium succinate, metoclopramide, metronidazole, multivitamin, nafcillin, oxacillin, paclitaxel, penicillin G potassium, pentobarbital, perphenazine, piperacillin, potassium chloride, propofol, ranitidine, remifentanil, sodium bicarbonate, tacrolimus, teniposide, theophylline, thiotepa, ticarcillin, tobramycin, trimethoprim - sulfamethoxazole, vancomycin, zidovudine

Perform/provide:
• Storage at room temperature for up to 12 hr after reconstitution; if refrigerated, sol may show a precipitate that clears at room temperature

• Adequate intake of fluids (2 L) to prevent deposit in kidneys

Evaluate:
• Therapeutic response: absence of itching, painful lesions; crusting and healed lesions

Teach patient/family:
• To take as prescribed; if dose is missed, take as soon as remembered up to 1 hr before next dose; do not double dose

• That drug may be taken orally before infection occurs; drug should be taken when itching or pain occurs, usually before eruptions

• That sexual partners need to be told that patient has herpes; they can become infected; condoms must be worn to prevent reinfections

• That drug does not cure infection, just controls symptoms and does not prevent infecting others

◆ To report sore throat, fever, fatigue (may indicate superinfection)

• That drug must be taken in equal intervals around the clock to maintain blood levels for duration of therapy

• To notify prescriber of side effects of bruising, bleeding, fatigue, malaise; may indicate blood dyscrasias

• To seek dental care during treatment to prevent gingival hyperplasia

Treatment of overdose: Discontinue drug, hemodialysis, resuscitate if needed

---

adenosine (Rx)

(a-den'oh-seen)

Adenocard

Func. class.: Antidysrhythmic

Chem. class.: Endogenous nucleoside

Action: Slows conduction through AV node, can interrupt reentry pathways through AV node, and can restore normal sinus rhythm in patients with paroxysmal supraventricular tachycardia (PSVT)

Uses: PSVT

Dosage and routes:
• *Adult:* IV BOL 6 mg; if conversion to normal sinus rhythm does not occur within 1-2 min, give 12 mg by rapid IV BOL; may repeat 12 mg dose again in 1-2 min
• *Infants and children:* 0.05 mg/kg, if not effective, increase dose by 0.05 mg/kg q2min to a max of 0.25 mg/kg or 12 mg

Available forms: Inj 3 mg/ml

Side effects/adverse reactions:
GI: Nausea, metallic taste, throat tightness, groin pressure
RESP: Dyspnea, chest pressure, hyperventilation
CNS: Lightheadedness, dizziness, arm tingling, numbness, apprehension, blurred vision, headache
CV: Chest pain, *atrial tachydysrhythmias,* sweating, palpitations, hypotension, *facial flushing*

Contraindications: Hypersensitivity, 2nd- or 3rd-degree heart block, AV block, sick sinus syndrome, atrial flutter, atrial fibrillation

Precautions: Pregnancy (C), lactation, children, asthma, elderly

Pharmacokinetics: Cleared from plasma in <30 sec, half-life 10 sec

Interactions:
• Increased effects of adenosine: dipyridamole
• Decreased activity of adenosine: theophylline or other methylxanthines (caffeine)
• Higher degree of heart block: carbamazepine
• Possible ventricular fibrillation: digoxin, verapamil

🖊 May cause increased adenosine effect: buckthorn bark/berry, cascara sagrada bark, rhubarb root, senna leaf/fruits, aloe

🖊 Decreased adenosine effect: guarana

NURSING CONSIDERATIONS
Assess:
• B/P continuously for fluctuations
• I&O ratio, electrolytes (K, Na, Cl)
• Cardiac status: B/P, pulse, respiration, ECG intervals (PR, QRS, QT)
• Respiratory status: rate, rhythm, lung fields for rales, watch for respiratory depression; lung fields, bilateral rales may occur in CHF patient; increased respiration, increased pulse, drug should be discontinued
• CNS effects: dizziness, confusion, psychosis, paresthesias, convulsions; drug should be discontinued

Administer:
IV bolus
• Undiluted; give 6 mg or less by rapid inj; if using an IV line, use port near insertion site, flush with normal saline (50 ml)

Solution compatibilities: D_5LR, D_5W, LR, 0.9% NaCl

Perform/provide:
• Storage at room temperature; sol should be clear; discard unused drug

Evaluate:
• Therapeutic response: decreased anginal pain, B/P, dysrhythmias, heart rate
• Treatment of overdose: Defibrillation, vasopressor for hypotension

---

◆ = Nursing alert   🖊 = Herb-drug interaction   🚫 = Do not crush

alatrofloxacin (R)
(ah-lat-troh-floks'ah-sin)
Trovan IV
trovafloxacin (R)
(tro-vah-floks'ah-sin)
Trovan
Func. class.: Antiinfective
Chem. class.: Fluoroquinolone

Action: Interferes with conversion of intermediate DNA fragments into high-molecular-weight DNA in bacteria; DNA gyrase inhibitor

Uses: Nosocomial pneumonia; *Escherichia coli, Proteus aeruginosa, Haemophilus influenzae, Staphylococcus aureus;* community-acquired pneumonia: *Streptococcus pneumoniae, H. influenzae, S. aureus, Klebsiella pneumoniae, Mycoplasma pneumoniae, Moraxella catarrhalis, Legionella pneumophila, Citrobacter pneumoniae;* chronic bronchitis, acute sinusitis, complicated intraabdominal infections, gyn/pelvic infections, skin/skin structure infections, UTIs, chronic bacterial prostatitis, urethral gonorrhea in males, PID, cervicitis caused by susceptible organisms

Dosage and routes:
• *Adult:* **IV/PO** 200-300 mg qd for 7-14 days, depending on infection
Available forms: Sol for inj 5 mg/ml (alatrofloxacin); tabs 100, 200 mg (trovafloxacin)

Side effects/adverse reactions:
CNS: Headache, *dizziness,* insomnia, anxiety, psychosis, *seizures*
HEMA: Anemia, **thrombocytopenia, leukopenia,** decreased Hgb; Hct, increased platelets
GI: Nausea, flatulence, vomiting, diarrhea, abdominal pain, **pseudomembranous colitis**
MS: Arthralgia, myalgia

GU: Vaginitis, crystalluria, increased BUN, creatinine
INTEG: Rash, pruritus, photosensitivity
Contraindications: Hypersensitivity to quinolones, seizure disorders, cerebral atherosclerosis, photosensitivity
Precautions: Pregnancy (C), lactation, children
Pharmacokinetics: Metabolized in liver, excreted in urine unchanged
Interactions:
• Decreased absorption: antacids with aluminum, magnesium, citric acid buffered with sodium citrate, sucralfate, iron products, IV morphine
Solution compatibilities: D_5, ½NaCl, D_5 ½NaCl, D_5/0.2% NaCl
NURSING CONSIDERATIONS
Assess:
• For previous sensitivity reaction to fluoroquinolones
• For signs and symptoms of infection: characteristics of sputum, WBC >10,000, fever; obtain baseline information before and during treatment
• For CNS disorders, since other quinolones can cause CNS stimulation, seizures
• C&S before beginning drug therapy to identify if correct treatment has been initiated
• For allergic reactions: rash, urticaria, pruritus, chills, fever, joint pain; may occur a few days after therapy begins; epinephrine and resuscitation equipment should be available for anaphylactic reaction
• Bowel pattern qd; if severe diarrhea occurs, drug should be discontinued
• For overgrowth of infection, perineal itching, fever, malaise, redness, pain, swelling, drainage, rash, diarrhea, change in cough, sputum

---

Side effects: *italics* = common; **bold italics** = life-threatening

Evaluate:

• Therapeutic response: absence of signs/symptoms of infection (WBC <10,000/mm^3, temp WNL)

Teach patient/family:

• To contact prescriber if vaginal itching, loose foul-smelling stools, or furry tongue occurs (may indicate superinfection); to report itching, rash, pruritus, urticaria, tendon pain

• To notify prescriber of diarrhea with blood or pus, may indicate pseudomembranous colitis

• To prevent sun exposure

• That drug may be taken without regard to meals; separate aluminum, magnesium, iron, or sucralfate by 2 hr

---

albumin, normal serum 5%/25% (℞)

(al-byoo′min)
Albuminar 5%, Albuminar 25%, Albutein 5%, Albutein 25%, Buminate 5%, Buminate 25%, Plasbumin 5%, Plasbumin-25%

Func. class.: Blood derivative
Chem. class.: Placental human plasma

Action: Exerts oncotic pressure, which expands volume of circulating blood and maintains cardiac output

Uses: Restores plasma volume in burns, hyperbilirubinemia, shock, hypoproteinemia, prevention of cerebral edema, cardiopulmonary bypass procedures, ARDS

Dosage and routes:

Burns

• *Adult:* **IV** dose to maintain plasma albumin at 30-50 g/L, use 5% sol initially, then 25% sol after 24 hr

Shock

• *Adult:* **IV** 500 ml of 5% sol q30 min, as needed

• *Child:* 0.5-1 g/kg/dose

Hypoproteinemia

• *Adult:* **IV** 1000-2000 ml of 5% sol qd, not to exceed 5-10 ml/min or 25-100 g of 25% sol qd, not to exceed 3 ml/min, titrated to patient response

Hyperbilirubinemia/erythroblastosis fetalis

• *Infant:* **IV** 1 g of 25% sol/kg before transfusion

Available forms: Inj 50, 250 mg/ml (5%, 25%)

Side effects/adverse reactions:

GI: Nausea, vomiting, increased salivation

INTEG: Rash, urticaria

CNS: Fever, chills, flushing, headache

RESP: Altered respirations, *pulmonary edema*

CV: Fluid overload, hypotension, erratic pulse, tachycardia

Contraindications: Hypersensitivity, CHF, severe anemia, renal insufficiency

Precautions: Decreased salt intake, decreased cardiac reserve, lack of albumin deficiency, hepatic disease, renal disease, pregnancy (C)

Pharmacokinetics: In hyponutrition states, metabolized as protein/energy source

Lab test interferences:

False increase: Alk phosphatase

NURSING CONSIDERATIONS

Assess:

• Blood studies Hct, Hgb; if serum protein declines, dyspnea, hypoxemia can result

• Decreased B/P, erratic pulse, respiration

• I&O ratio: urinary output may decrease

◆ CVP, pulmonary wedge pressure will increase if overload occurs

---

◆ = Nursing alert   ✐ = Herb-drug interaction   ⊘ = Do not crush

• Allergy: fever, rash, itching, chills, flushing, urticaria, nausea, vomiting, hypotension, requires discontinuation of infusion, use of new lot if therapy reinstituted

• CVP reading: distended neck veins indicate circulatory overload; shortness of breath, anxiety, insomnia, expiratory rales, frothy blood-tinged cough, cyanosis indicate pulmonary overload

Administer:

IV

• Slowly, to prevent fluid overload; dilute with NS for injection or D_5W; 5% may be given undiluted; 25% may be given diluted or undiluted, give over 4 hr, use infusion pump

Solution compatibilities: LR, NaCl, Ringer's, D_5W, $D_{10}W$, $D_{2\frac{1}{2}}W$, dextrose/saline, dextran$_6$ D_5, dextran$_6$ NaCl 0.9%, dextrose/Ringer's, dextrose/LR

Y-site compatibilities: Diltiazem, lorazepam

Perform/provide:

• Adequate hydration before, during administration

• Check type of albumin; some stored at room temperature, some need to be refrigerated

Evaluate:

• Therapeutic response: increased B/P, decreased edema, increased serum albumin levels, increased plasma protein

---

albuterol (R)

(al-byoo'ter-ole)

Airet, albuterol, Proventil, Proventil Repetabs, Ventolin, Ventolin Rotacaps, Volmax

Func. class.: Adrenergic β$_2$-agonist, sympathomimetic, bronchodilator

Action: Causes bronchodilation by action on β$_2$ (pulmonary) receptors by increasing levels of cAMP, which relaxes smooth muscle; produces bronchodilation, CNS, cardiac stimulation, as well as increased diuresis and gastric acid secretion; longer acting than isoproterenol

Uses: Prevention of exercise-induced asthma, bronchospasm, bronchitis, emphysema, bronchiectasis, or other pulmonary disease

Investigational uses: Hyperkalemia in dialysis patients

Dosage and routes:

To prevent exercise-induced bronchospasm

• *Adult:* **INH** 2 puffs 15 min before exercising; **NEB/IPPB** 5 mg tid-qid

Other respiratory conditions

• *Adult and child ≥12 yr:* **INH** 1-2 puffs q4h; **PO** 2-4 mg tid-qid, not to exceed 8 mg; Volmax ext rel 8 mg q12h; Repetabs 4-8 mg q12h

• *Geriatric:* 2 mg tid-qid, may increase gradually to 8 mg tid-qid

• *Child 2-12 yr:* **INH** 0.1 mg/kg tid (max 2.5 mg tid-qid)

• *Adult and child > 4 yr:* **INH CAP** 200 µg cap inhaled q4-6h using Rotahaler

Prevention of exercise-induced bronchospasm

• *Adult and child >4 yr:* 200 µg cap inhaled 15 min before exercise

Available forms: Aerosol 90 µg/actuation; tabs 2, 4 mg; syr 2 mg/5 ml; ext rel 4, 8 mg; inh sol 0.083, 0.5%; inh cap 200 µg

Side effects/adverse reactions:

CNS: Tremors, anxiety, insomnia, headache, dizziness, stimulation, *restlessness,* hallucinations, flushing, irritability

CV: Palpitations, tachycardia, hypertension, angina, hypotension, dysrhythmias

EENT: Dry nose, irritation of nose and throat

GI: Heartburn, nausea, vomiting

MISC: Flushing, sweating, anorexia, bad taste/smell changes

MS: Muscle cramps

RESP: Cough, wheezing, dyspnea, **bronchospasm,** dry throat

Contraindications: Hypersensitivity to sympathomimetics, tachydysrhythmias, severe cardiac disease, heart block

Precautions: Lactation, pregnancy (C), cardiac disorders, hyperthyroidism, diabetes mellitus, hypertension, prostatic hypertrophy, narrow-angle glaucoma, seizures, exercise-induced bronchospasm (aerosol) in children <12 years

Pharmacokinetics: Well absorbed PO, extensively metabolized in the liver and tissues, crosses placenta, breast milk, blood-brain barrier

PO: Onset ½ hr, peak 2½ hr, duration 4-6 hr, half-life 2½ hr

PO-ER: Onset ½ hour; peak 2-3 hr; duration 12 hr

INH: Onset 5 min, peak 1-1½ hr, duration 4-6 hr, half-life 4 hr

Interactions:

• Increased action of aerosol bronchodilators

• Increased action of albuterol: tricyclic antidepressants, MAOIs, other adrenergics

• May inhibit action of albuterol: other β-blockers

• Severe hypotension: oxytoxics

• Toxicity: theophylline

• ECG changes/hypokalemia: diuretics

NURSING CONSIDERATIONS

Assess:

• Respiratory function: vital capacity, forced expiratory volume, ABGs, lung sounds, heart rate and rhythm (baseline)

• That patient has not received theophylline therapy before giving dose

• Patient's ability to self-medicate

• For evidence of allergic reactions

Administer:

Inhalation

• In geriatric patients, a spacing device is advised

• After shaking, exhale, place mouthpiece in mouth, inhale slowly, hold breath, remove, exhale slowly

• Gum, sips of water for dry mouth

PO

• With meals to decrease gastric irritation

• Syrup to children (no alcohol, sugar)

Perform/provide:

• Storage in light-resistant container, do not expose to temperatures over 86° F (30° C)

Evaluate:

• Therapeutic response: absence of dyspnea, wheezing after 1 hr, improved airway exchange, improved ABGs

Teach patient/family:

• To use exactly as prescribed; take missed dose when remembered, alter dosing schedule

• Not to use OTC medications; excess stimulation may occur

• Use of inhaler; review package insert with patient; use demonstration, return demonstration

• To avoid getting aerosol in eyes; blurring of vision may result

• To wash inhaler in warm water qd and dry

• To avoid smoking, smoke-filled rooms, persons with respiratory infections

◆ That paradoxic bronchospasm may occur and to stop drug immediately

• To limit caffeine products such as chocolate, coffee, tea, and colas

Treatment of overdose: Administer a β₁-adrenergic blocker

◆ = Nursing alert   ∥ = Herb-drug interaction   ⊘ = Do not crush

aldesleukin (℞)

(al-dess-loo'ken)

Interleukin-2, IL-2, Proleukin

Func. class.: Miscellaneous antineoplastic

Chem. class.: Interleukin-2, human recombinant (cytokine)

Action: Enhancement of lymphocyte mitogenesis and stimulation of IL-2-dependent cell lines; enhancement of lymphocyte cytotoxicity; induction of killer cell activity; induction of interferon γ-production; results in activation of cellular immunity, cytokines, and inhibition of tumor growth

Uses: Metastatic renal cell carcinoma in adults, phase II for HIV in combination with zidovudine, melanoma

Investigational uses: Kaposi's sarcoma given with zidovudine, metastatic melanoma given with cyclophosphamide, non-Hodgkin's lymphoma given with lymphokine-activated killer cells, AIDS (phase I) given with zidovudine

Dosage and routes:

• *Adult:* **IV INF** 600,000 IU/kg (0.037 mg/kg) q8h over 15 min × 14 doses; off 9 days, repeat schedule for another 14 doses, for a max of 28 doses/course

Available forms: Powder for inj 22 million IU/vial

Side effects/adverse reactions:

CV: Hypotension, sinus tachycardia, dysrhythmias, bradycardia, PVCs, PACs, myocardial ischemia, *myocardial infarction, cardiac arrest, capillary leak syndrome*

RESP: Pulmonary congestion, dyspnea, *pulmonary edema, respiratory failure,* tachypnea, pleural effusion, wheezing

GI: Nausea, vomiting, diarrhea, stomatitis, anorexia, GI bleeding, dyspepsia, constipation, *intestinal perforation*/ileus, jaundice, ascites

HEMA: Anemia, *thrombocytopenia, leukopenia, coagulation disorders, leukocytosis, eosinophilia*

CNS: Mental status changes, dizziness, sensory dysfunction, syncope, motor dysfunction, fever, chills, headache

GU: *Oliguria/anuria, proteinuria, hematuria,* dysuria, *renal failure*

INTEG: Pruritus, erythema, rash, dry skin, *exfoliative dermatitis,* purpura, petechiae, urticaria

MS: Arthralgia, myalgia

SYST: Infection

Contraindications: Hypersensitivity, abnormal thallium stress test or pulmonary function tests, organ allografts

Precautions: CNS metastases, bacterial infections, renal/hepatic/cardiac/pulmonary disease, pregnancy (C), lactation, children, anemia, thrombocytopenia

Pharmacokinetics: Renal elimination half-life 85 min; onset 4 wk, duration ≤12 mo

Interactions:

• Potentiate hypotension: antihypertensives

• Reduced antitumor effectiveness: corticosteroids

• Increased toxicity: aminoglycosides, indomethacin, cytotoxic chemotherapy, methotrexate, asparaginase, doxorubicin

• Unpredictable reactions: psychotropics

Lab test interferences:

Increase: Bilirubin, BUN, serum creatinine, transaminase, alk phosphatase; hypomagnesemia, acidosis hypocalcemia, hypophosphatemia, hypokalemia, hyperuricemia, hypoalbuminemia, hypoproteinemia, hyponatremia, hyperkalemia, alkalosis (toxic effect of drug)

Side effects: *italics* = common; ***bold italics*** = life-threatening

NURSING CONSIDERATIONS

Assess:

• CBC, differential, platelet count weekly; withhold drug if WBC is <4000/mm³ or platelet count is <75,000/mm³; notify prescriber of these results

◆ Capillary leak syndrome including a drop in mean arterial pressure (2-12 hr after initiating therapy); hypotension and hypoperfusion will occur

• Renal function studies: BUN, serum uric acid, urine CrCl, electrolytes before, during therapy; I&O ratio; report fall in urine output to <30 ml/hr

• Monitor temperature q4h; fever may indicate beginning infection

• Liver function tests before, during therapy: bilirubin, AST, ALT, alk phosphatase as needed or monthly

• ECG; watch for ST-T wave changes, low QRS and T, possible dysrhythmias (sinus tachycardia, PVCs)

• Baselines in pulmonary function; document FEV >2 L or ≥75% prior to therapy; check daily VS, pulse oximetry, dyspnea, rales, ABGs

• Stress thallium study prior to therapy; document normal ejection fraction, unimpaired wall motion

• Bleeding: hematuria, guaiac, bruising or petechiae, mucosa or orifices q8h

• Buccal cavity q8h for dryness, sores, ulceration, white patches, oral pain, bleeding, dysphagia

• Local irritation, pain, burning at injection site

• GI symptoms: frequency of stools, cramping

• Acidosis, signs of dehydration: rapid respirations, poor skin turgor, decreased urine output, dry skin, restlessness, weakness

Administer:

IV

• Hydrocortisone, dexamethasone or sodium bicarbonate (1 mEq/1 ml) for extravasation, apply ice compresses

• Antiemetic 30-60 min before giving drug to prevent vomiting

• IV after diluting 22 million IU (1.3 mg)/1.2 ml sterile H₂O for inj at site of vial and swirl, do not shake; dilute dose with 50 ml D₅W and give over 15 min; use plastic bag; do not use an in-line filter, give through Y-tube or 3-way stopcock

• Dopamine 1-5 kg/min before onset of hypotension; decreased dose preserves kidney output

Y-site compatibilities: Amikacin, amphotericin B, calcium gluconate, diphenhydramine, dopamine, fluconazole, foscarnet, gentamicin, heparin, IV fat emulsion, magnesium sulfate, metoclopramide, morphine, ondansetron, piperacillin, potassium chloride, ranitidine, ticarcillin, tobramycin, TPN #145, trimethoprim/sulfamethoxazole

Perform/provide:

• Liquid diet: carbonated beverage, gelatin (Jell-O) may be added if patient is not nauseated or vomiting

• Rinsing of mouth tid-qid with water, club soda; brushing of teeth bid-tid with soft brush or cotton-tipped applicators for stomatitis; use unwaxed dental floss

• Storage in refrigerator of diluted drug; do not freeze; administer within 48 hr; bring to room temperature before infusing; discard unused portion

Evaluate:

• Therapeutic response: decreased tumor size, spread of malignancy

Teach patient/family:

• To use a nonhormonal contraceptive method during therapy

◆ = Nursing alert   ▰ = Herb-drug interaction   ⊘ = Do not crush

• To report any complaints, side effects to nurse or prescriber
• To avoid foods with citric acid, hot or rough texture
• To report any bleeding, white spots, ulcerations in mouth to prescriber; tell patient to examine mouth qd
• To avoid crowds and persons with infections when granulocyte count is low

---

alendronate (℞)

(al-en-drone'ate)

Fosamax

Func. class.: Bone-resorption inhibitor

Chem. class.: Biphosphonate

Action: Absorbs calcium phosphate crystal in bone and may directly block dissolution of hydroxyapatite crystals of bone; inhibits bone resorption, apparently without inhibiting bone formation, mineralization

Uses: Osteoporosis in postmenopausal women, Paget's disease

Dosage and routes:

Osteoporosis in postmenopausal women
• *Adult and elderly:* **PO** 10 mg qd
Paget's disease
• *Adult and elderly:* **PO** 40 mg qd × 6 mo

Available forms: Tabs 5, 10, 40 mg

Side effects/adverse reactions:

CNS: Headache

META: Anemia, hypokalemia, hypomagnesemia, hypophosphatemia

GI: Abdominal pain, anorexia, constipation, nausea, vomiting, esophageal ulceration

MS: Bone pain

CV: Hypertension

GU: UTI, fluid overload

Contraindications: Hypersensitivity to biphosphonates, hypocalcemia

Precautions: Children, lactation, pregnancy (C), CrCl <35 ml/min, esophageal disease, ulcers, gastritis

Pharmacokinetics: Rapidly cleared from circulation, taken up mainly by bones, eliminated primarily through kidneys

Interactions:
• Decreased absorption: antacids, calcium supplements
• GI reactions: NSAIDs, salicylates
• Increased alendronate effect: ranitidine
• Drug/food: decreased absorption

NURSING CONSIDERATIONS

Assess:
• Electrolytes; renal function studies; Ca, P, Mg, K; confirm osteoporosis with bone density test before use
• For hypercalcemia: paresthesia, twitching, laryngospasm, Chvostek's, Trousseau's signs
• Alk phosphatase levels of 2 × upper limit of normal are indicated for Paget's disease

Administer:

PO
• For 6 months to be effective in Paget's disease; take with 8 oz of water 30 min ac

Perform/provide:
• Storage in cool environment, out of direct sunlight

Evaluate:
• Therapeutic response: increased bone mass, absence of fractures

Teach patient/family:
• To remain upright for 30 min after dose to prevent esophageal irritation
• To take in AM before food, other meds, take with 6-8 oz of water (no mineral water)
• To take calcium, vit D if dietary intake is lacking
• To use weight-bearing exercise to increase bone density

---

alfentanil (℞)

(al-fen′ta-nil)

Alfenta, Rapifen*

Func. class.: Narcotic analgesic

Chem. class.: Opiate, synthetic

Controlled Substance Schedule II

Action: Inhibits ascending pain pathways in limbic system, thalamus, midbrain, hypothalamus

Uses: In combination with other drugs in general anesthesia, as a primary anesthetic in general surgery, monitored anesthesia care (MAC)

Dosage and routes:

Anesthesia <30 min
Combination

• *Adult:* IV 8-50 μg/kg, may increase by 3-15 μg/kg

Anesthetic induction

• *Adult:* IV 3-5 μg/kg, then 0.5-1.5 μg/kg/min; total dose is 8-40 μg/kg

Anesthesia 30-60 min
Induction

• *Adult:* IV 20-50 μg/kg

Maintenance

• *Adult:* IV 5-15 μg/kg; may give up to 75 μg/kg total dose

Continuous anesthesia >45 min
Induction

• *Adult:* IV 50-75 μg/kg

Maintenance

• *Adult:* IV 0.5-3.0 μg/kg/min; rate should be decreased by 30%-50% after 1 hr maintenance **INF;** may be increased to 4 μg/kg/min or **BOL** doses of 7 μg/kg

Induction of anesthesia >45 min

• *Adult:* IV 130-245 μg/kg, then 0.5-1.5 μg/kg/min

MAC
Induction

• *Adult:* IV duration ≤½ hr 3-8 μg/kg

Maintenance

• *Adult:* 3-5 μg/kg q5-20min to 1 μg/kg/min, total dose 3-40 μg/kg

Available forms: Inj 500 μg/ml

Side effects/adverse reactions:

CNS: Drowsiness, dizziness, confusion, headache, sedation, euphoria, delirium, agitation, anxiety

GI: Nausea, vomiting, anorexia, constipation, cramps, dry mouth

GU: Urinary retention, dysuria

INTEG: Rash, urticaria, bruising, flushing, diaphoresis, pruritus

EENT: Tinnitus, blurred vision, miosis, diplopia

CV: Palpitation, bradycardia, change in B/P, facial flushing, syncope, asystole

*RESP: **Respiratory depression, apnea***

MS: Rigidity

Contraindications: Child <12 yr, hypersensitivity

Precautions: Pregnancy (C), lactation, increased intracranial pressure, acute MI, severe heart disease, renal disease, hepatic disease, asthma, respiratory conditions, convulsive disorders, elderly

Pharmacokinetics: Half-life 1-2 hr, 90% bound to plasma proteins, duration 30 min

Interactions:

• Respiratory depression, hypotension, profound sedation: alcohol, sedative/hypnotics, or other CNS depressants, antihistamines, phenothiazines, fluconazole

• CNS toxicity: cimetidine

⚜ Increased CNS depression: kava

Lab test interferences:

Increase: Amylase, lipase

NURSING CONSIDERATIONS

Assess:

• I&O ratio, check for decreasing output; may indicate urinary retention, especially in elderly

• CNS changes: dizziness, drowsiness, hallucinations, euphoria, LOC, pupil reaction

• Allergic reactions: rash, urticaria

◆ = Nursing alert   ⚜ = Herb-drug interaction   Ⓢ = Do not crush

◆ Respiratory dysfunction: respiratory depression, character, rate, rhythm: notify prescriber if respirations are <12/min; CV status: bradycardia, syncope

Administer:

Direct IV

• Over 1½-3 min; use tuberculin syringe

Continuous IV

• By diluting 20 ml of drug in 230 ml of diluent (40 µg/ml); discontinue inf 15 min before surgery is completed

Solution compatibilities: LR, 0.9% NaCl, D₅W, D₅/0.9% NaCl

Syringe compatibilities: Atracurium

Y-site compatibilities: Cisatracurium, etomidate, propofol, remifentanil

Perform/provide:

• Storage in light-resistant container at room temperature

Evaluate:

• Therapeutic response: maintenance of anesthesia

Teach patient/family:

• That after surgery, another analgesic will be available for pain

• The reason for and expected results of this drug

Treatment of overdose: Nalaxone HCl 0.2-0.8 mg IV, O₂, IV fluids, vasopressors

---

alitretinoin
See appendix a—selected new drugs

---

allopurinol (℞)

(al-oh-pure′i-nole)

allopurinol, Apo-Allopurinol*, Lopurin*, Purimol*, Zyloprim

Func. class.: Antigout drug

Chem. class.: Xanthene oxidase inhibitor

Action: Inhibits the enzyme xanthine oxidase, reducing uric acid synthesis

Uses: Chronic gout, hyperuricemia associated with malignancies, recurrent calcium oxalate calculi, Chagas' disease, cutaneous/visceral leishmaniasis

Dosage and routes:

Gout/hyperuricemia

• *Adult:* **PO** 200-600 mg qd depending on severity, not to exceed 800 mg/day

• *Child 6-10 yr:* 300 mg qd

• *Child <6 yr:* 150 mg qd

Impaired renal function

• *Adult:* **PO** 200 mg qd when CrCl is 20 to 30 ml/min

• *Adult:* **PO** 100 mg qd (CrCl <20 ml/min)

Recurrent calculi

• *Adult:* **PO** 200-300 mg qd

Uric acid nephropathy prevention

• *Adult and child >10 yr:* **PO** 600-800 mg qd × 2-3 days

Available forms: Tabs, scored 100, 300 mg

Side effects/adverse reactions:

*HEMA: **Agranulocytosis, thrombocytopenia, aplastic anemia, pancytopenia, leukopenia, bone marrow suppression, eosinophilia***

CNS: Headache, drowsiness, neuritis, paresthesia

GI: Nausea, vomiting, anorexia, malaise, metallic taste, cramps, peptic ulcer, diarrhea, stomatitis

*MISC: Myopathy, arthralgia, hepatomegaly, **cholestatic jaundice, re-***

---

nal failure, exfoliative dermatitis
EENT: Retinopathy, cataracts, epistaxis
INTEG: Fever, chills, dermatitis, pruritus, purpura, erythema, ecchymosis, alopecia
Contraindications: Hypersensitivity
Precautions: Pregnancy (C), lactation, renal disease, hepatic disease, children
Pharmacokinetics:
PO: Peak 2-4 hr; excreted in feces, urine; half-life 2-3 hr, terminal half-life 18-30 hr
Interactions:
• Increased action of oral anticoagulants, chlorpropamide, cyclophosphamide, hydantoin, theophylline, vidarabine, ACE inhibitors, mercaptopurine, azathioprine
• Possible kidney stone formation: ammonium chloride, Vit C, potassium/sodium phosphate
• Decreased effects of probenecid
• Rash: ampicillin, amoxicillin, bacampicillin
• Increased allopurinol toxicity: thiazide diuretics
• Decreased effects of allopurinol: aluminum salts
• Increased bone marrow depression: antineoplastics
NURSING CONSIDERATIONS
Assess:
• Uric acid levels q2wk; uric acid levels should be 6 mg/dl or less
• CBC, AST, BUN, creatinine before starting treatment, monthly
• I&O ratio; increase fluids to 2 L/day to prevent stone formation
• Nutritional status: discourage organ meat, sardines, salmon, legumes, gravies (high-purine foods), alcohol
Administer:
PO
• With meals, to prevent GI symptoms

• A few days before antineoplastic therapy
Evaluate:
• Therapeutic response: decreased pain in joints, decreased stone formation in kidneys
Teach patient/family:
• That tabs may be crushed
• To take as prescribed; if dose is missed, take as soon as remembered; do not double dose
• To increase fluid intake to 2 L/day
• To report skin rash, stomatitis, malaise, fever, aching; drug should be discontinued
• To avoid hazardous activities if drowsiness or dizziness occurs
• To avoid alcohol, caffeine; will increase uric acid levels
• To avoid large doses of vitamin C; kidney stone formation may occur
• To maintain a diet enhancing urine alkalinity, e.g., dairy products
• To reduce dairy products, refined sugars, sodium, meat if taking for calcium oxalate stones

---

alprazolam (R)
(al-pray′zoe-lam)
Apo-Alpraz*, Novo-Alprazol*, Nu-Alpraz*, Xanax
Func. class.: Antianxiety
Chem. class.: Benzodiazepine

Controlled Substance Schedule IV
Action: Depresses subcortical levels of CNS, including limbic system, reticular formation
Uses: Anxiety, panic disorders, anxiety with depressive symptoms
Investigational uses: Depression, social phobia, premenstrual syndrome
Dosage and routes:
Anxiety disorder
• *Adult:* **PO** 0.25-0.5 mg tid, not to exceed 4 mg/day in divided doses

---

 = Nursing alert   = Herb-drug interaction   ⊘ = Do not crush

• *Elderly:* **PO** 0.125-0.25 mg bid; increase by 0.125 as needed
Panic disorder
• *Adult:* **PO** 0.5 mg may increase q3-4d by 1 mg/day or less
Premenstrual syndrome
• *Adult:* **PO** 0.25 mg tid
Social phobia
• *Adult:* **PO** 2-8 mg/day
Available forms: Tabs 0.25, 0.5, 1, 2 mg
Side effects/adverse reactions:
CNS: Dizziness, drowsiness, confusion, headache, anxiety, tremors, stimulation, fatigue, depression, insomnia, hallucinations
GI: Constipation, dry mouth, nausea, vomiting, anorexia, diarrhea
INTEG: Rash, dermatitis, itching
CV: Orthostatic hypotension, ***ECG changes, tachycardia,*** hypotension
EENT: Blurred vision, tinnitus, mydriasis
Contraindications: Hypersensitivity to benzodiazepines, narrow-angle glaucoma, psychosis, pregnancy (D), lactation, child <18 yr
Precautions: Elderly, debilitated, hepatic disease, renal disease
Pharmacokinetics:
PO: Onset 30 min, peak 1-2 hr, duration 4-6 hr, therapeutic response 2-3 days; metabolized by liver, excreted by kidneys; crosses placenta, breast milk; half-life 12-15 hr
Interactions:
• Increased CNS depression: anticonvulsants, alcohol, antihistamines, sedative/hypnotics
• Increased digoxin levels: digoxin
• Increased plasma levels of TCAs: tricyclic antidepressants
• Decreased alprazolam clearance: cimetidine
• Decreased action of levodopa
🗡 Increased CNS depression, coma: kava
Lab test interferences:
Increase: AST/ALT

NURSING CONSIDERATIONS
Assess:
• B/P lying, standing; pulse; if systolic B/P drops 20 mm Hg, hold drug, notify prescriber
• Hepatic studies: AST, ALT, bilirubin, creatinine, LDH, alk phosphatase
• For indications of increasing tolerance and abuse
• Mental status: mood, sensorium, affect, sleeping pattern, drowsiness, dizziness, especially in elderly
◆Physical dependency, withdrawal symptoms: anxiety, panic attacks, agitation, convulsions, headache, nausea, vomiting, muscle pain, weakness; withdrawal seizures may occur after rapid decrease in dose or abrupt discontinuation
• Suicidal tendencies
Administer:
PO
• With food or milk for GI symptoms
• Crushed if patient is unable to swallow medication whole
Perform/provide:
• Assistance with ambulation during beginning therapy; drowsiness/dizziness occurs
Evaluate:
• Therapeutic response: decreased anxiety, restlessness, sleeplessness
Teach patient/family:
• Not to double doses; take exactly as prescribed; if dose is missed, take within 1 hr as scheduled
• That drug may be taken with food
• Not to use for everyday stress or longer than 4 mo unless directed by prescriber; not to take more than prescribed amount; may be habit forming
• To avoid OTC preparations unless approved by prescriber
• To avoid driving, activities that require alertness, since drowsiness may occur

• To avoid alcohol ingestion or other psychotropic medications unless directed by prescriber
• Not to discontinue medication abruptly after long-term use
• To rise slowly or fainting may occur, especially elderly
• That drowsiness may worsen at beginning of treatment

Treatment of overdose: Lavage, VS, supportive care

---

alprostadil (℞)
(al-pros'ta-dil)
Caverject, Edex, Muse, PGEI, prostaglandin E$_1$, Prostin VR*, Prostin VR Pediatric
Func. class.: Hormone
Chem. class.: Prostaglandin E$_1$

Action: Relaxes smooth muscles of ductus arteriosus; results in increased O$_2$ content throughout body; causes erection by dilation of cavernosal arteries and relaxation of trabecular muscle, this leads to the trapping of blood

Uses: To maintain patent ductus arteriosus (temporary treatment), erectile dysfunction

Dosage and routes:
Patent ductus arteriosus
• Infants: **IV INF** 0.1 µg/kg/min, until desired response, then reduce to lowest effective amount, 0.4 µg/kg/min not likely to produce greater beneficial effects
Erectile dysfunction of vasculogenic or mixed etiology, psychogenic
• Men: **INTRACAVERNOSAL** 2.5 µg may increase by 2.5 µg; may then increase by 5-10 µg until adequate response occurs; **INTRAURETHRAL:** administer as needed to achieve erection
Available forms: Inj 500 µg/ml;

lyopholized powder for inj 6.15, 11.9, 23.2 µg; 5, 10, 20, 40 µg/single dose vial; pellet 125, 250, 500, 1000 µg

Side effects/adverse reactions:
MS: Deformities of long bones in neonates treated for prolonged periods
MISC: **Sepsis,** hypokalemia, **peritonitis,** hypoglycemia, hyperkalemia
RESP: **Apnea, bradypnea, wheezing, respiratory depression**
HEMA: **DIC** (disseminated intravascular coagulation), **thrombocytopenia,** anemia, **bleeding**
CNS: Fever, **convulsions,** lethargy, hypothermia, stiffness, hyperirritability, **cerebral bleeding**
GI: Diarrhea, regurgitation, hyperbilirubinemia
GU: Oliguria, hematuria, **anuria**
CV: **Bradycardia, tachycardia,** hypotension, **CHF, ventricular fibrillation, shock,** flushing, **cardiac arrest,** edema
Local (Caverject): Penile pain, prolonged erection, penile fibrosis, penile rash, edema, hematoma, ecchymosis
Systems (Caverject): Headache, dizziness, flu symptoms, sinusitis, nasal congestion, hypertension, back pain, prostatic disorder

Contraindications: Hypersensitivity, respiratory distress syndrome (RDS)

Precautions: Bleeding disorders

Pharmacokinetics: Up to 80% metabolized in lungs, excreted in urine (metabolites)

NURSING CONSIDERATIONS
Assess:
• ABGs, arterial pH, arterial pressure, continuous ECG; if arterial pressure decreases, reduce or stop drug
◆ Apnea and bradycardia; if these occur, be prepared to support ventilation

---

◆ = Nursing alert   ✦ = Herb-drug interaction   ⊘ = Do not crush

• Increased pH, B/P, output, decreased ratio of PA to AP (restricted systemic blood flow)

Administer:

IV infusion

• Only with emergency equipment available and by trained clinicians (patent ductus arteriosus)

• After diluting with NS or D_5W injection to a concentration of 500 μg/ml, dilute further with 0.9% NaCl, D_5W; 500 μg of drug/250 ml of dilute = 2 μg/ml; 0.1 μg/kg/min run at 0.05 ml/kg/min, use infusion pump; do not mix with diluents using benzyl alcohol, *fatal toxic syndrome may occur*

Perform/provide:

• Arterial pressure measurement during infusion

• Refrigeration for drug; discard all mixed unused portion

Evaluate:

• Therapeutic response: increased PO_2 (cyanotic heart disease); erection

Teach patient/family:

• About the diagnosis, prognosis, treatment

• The method for self-injection (erectile disorder), amount to be used, disposal of needle; refrigerate; alternate sides of the penis with each inj; do not inj >3×/wk; there is little control over erection; allow 24 hr between doses; notify healthcare provider of new penile pain, nodules, or signs of infection

Treatment of overdose: Discontinue drug, provide supportive measures

---

alteplase ($\mathbb{R}$)

(al-ti-plaze')

Activase, tissue plasminogen activator, TPA

Func. class.: Thrombolytic enzyme

Chem. class.: Tissue plasminogen activator (TPA)

Action: Produces fibrin conversion of plasminogen to plasmin; able to bind to fibrin, convert plasminogen in thrombus to plasmin, which leads to local fibrinolysis, limited systemic proteolysis

Uses: Lysis of obstructing thrombi associated with acute MI, ischemic conditions requiring thrombolysis, i.e., PE, DVT, unclotting arteriovenous shunts, acute ischemic CVA

Investigational uses: Unstable angina

Dosage and routes:

• *Adult >65 kg:* **IV** a total of 100 mg; 6-10 mg given **IV BOL** over 1-2 min, 60 mg given over first hour, 20 mg given over second hour, 20 mg given over third hour; or 1.25 mg/kg given over 3 hr for smaller patients

Accelerated INF

• *Adult:* **IV BOL** 15 mg; then 0.75 mg/kg over ½ hr; 0.5 mg/kg over 1 hr

Available forms: Powder for inj 20 mg (11.6 million IU/vial), 50 mg (29 million IU/vial), 100 mg (58 million IU/vial)

Side effects/adverse reactions:

*SYST: **GI, GU, intracranial, retroperitoneal bleeding,** surface bleeding*

*CV: **Sinus bradycardia, ventricular tachycardia, accelerated idioventricular rhythm***

INTEG: Urticaria, rash

Contraindications: Hypersensitivity, active internal bleeding, recent CVA, severe uncontrolled hypertension, intracranial/intraspinal surgery/trauma, aneurysm

Precautions: Pregnancy (C), lactation, children

Pharmacokinetics: Cleared by liver, 80% cleared within 10 min of drug termination, onset immediate, peak 45 min, duration 4 hr

Interactions:

• Increased bleeding: anticoagulants, salicylates, dipyridamole

Lab test interferences:
Increase: PT, APTT, TT

NURSING CONSIDERATIONS
Assess:

• VS, B/P, pulse, respirations, neurologic signs, temperature at least q4h; temperature >104° F (40° C) indicates internal bleeding; monitor rhythm closely; ventricular dysrhythmias may occur with hyperfusion; monitor heart, breath sounds, neuro status, peripheral pulses

 For bleeding during first hour of treatment and 24 hr after procedure: hematuria, hematemesis, bleeding from mucous membranes, epistaxis, ecchymosis; guaiac all body fluids, stools. Do not use 150 mg or more total dose; intracranial bleeding may occur

• Allergy: fever, rash, itching, chills; mild reaction may be treated with antihistamines

• Blood studies (Hct, platelets, PTT, PT, TT, APTT) before starting therapy; PT or APTT must be less than 2 × control before starting therapy TT or PT q3-4h during treatment

Administer:
Intermittent IV inf

• After reconstituting with provided diluent, add appropriate amount of sterile water for injection (no preservatives) 20 mg vial/20 ml or 50 mg vial/50 ml to make 1 mg/ml, mix by slow inversion or dilute with NaCl, D_5W to a concentration of 0.5 mg/ml; 1.5 to <0.5 mg/ml may result in precipitation of drug; use 18 G needle; flush line with NaCl after administration

• Heparin therapy after thrombolytic therapy is discontinued, TT, ACT, or APTT less than 2 × control (about 3-4 hr)

• Reconstituted IV solution within 8 hr or discard

• Within 6 hr of coronary occlusion for best results

Additive compatibilities: Lidocaine, morphine, nitroglycerin

Y-site compatibilities: Lidocaine, metoprolol, propranolol

Perform/provide:

• Avoidance of invasive procedures, injection, rectal temperature

• Pressure for 30 sec to minor bleeding sites; 30 min to sites of atrial puncture, followed by pressure dressing; inform prescriber if this does not attain hemostasis; apply pressure dressing

• Storage of powder at room temperature or refrigerate; protect from excessive light

Evaluate:

• Therapeutic response: lysis of thrombi

Teach patient/family:

• The purpose and expected results of the treatment; to report adverse reactions

A

altretamine (℞)

(al-tret′a-meen)
Hexalen, hexamethylmela-
mine, Hexastat*

Func. class.: Misc. antineoplastic

Chem. class.: S-triazine derivative (formerly known as hexa-
methylmelamine)

Action: Products of metabolism
form covalent adducts with tissue
macromolecules including DNA,
which may be responsible for cytotoxicity; activity is not cell cycle
phase specific

Uses: Palliative treatment of recurrent, persistent ovarian cancer following first-line treatment with cisplatin or alkylating agent–based
combination

Dosage and routes:
• *Adult:* **PO** 260 mg/m^2/day for 14
or 21 days in a 28-day cycle; give in
4 divided doses after meals and at hs
Available forms: Caps 50 mg

Side effects/adverse reactions:
GI: Nausea, anorexia, vomiting, increased alk phosphatase, ***hepatic
toxicity***
CNS: Peripheral sensory neuropathy, fatigue, *seizures,* mood disorders, disorders of consciousness,
ataxia, dizziness, vertigo
*HEMA: **Leukopenia, thrombocytopenia, anemia***
GU: Increased BUN, serum creatinine
INTEG: Rash, pruritus, alopecia

Contraindications: Hypersensitivity, severe bone marrow depression,
severe neurologic toxicity

Precautions: Pregnancy (D), lactation, children

Pharmacokinetics:
PO: Well absorbed orally, rapidly

metabolized in liver, metabolites excreted in urine; peak ½-3 hr

Interactions:
• Possible increased toxicity of al-
tretamine: cimetidine
• Severe orthostatic hypotension:
MAOI

NURSING CONSIDERATIONS
Assess:
• CBC, differential, platelet count
weekly, withhold drug if WBC is
<2000 or platelet count is <75,000
or granulocyte count is <1000/mm^3;
notify prescriber of results
• Renal function studies: BUN, serum uric acid, urine CrCl before,
during therapy
• I&O ratio; report fall in urine output of 30 ml/hr
• Temperature q4h; may indicate
beginning infection
• Liver function tests before, during
therapy (bilirubin, AST, ALT, LDH)
as needed or monthly

Administer:
PO
• Antacid before oral agent, give
drug after meals, at hs
• Antiemetic 30-60 min before giv-
ing drug to prevent vomiting
• Antibiotics for prophylaxis of in-
fection

Perform/provide:
• Strict medical asepsis, protective
isolation if WBC levels are low

Evaluate:
• Therapeutic response: decreased
tumor size, spread of malignancy

Teach patient/family:
• To report signs of infection: increased temperature, sore throat, flu
symptoms
• To report signs of anemia: fatigue,
headache, faintness, shortness of
breath, irritability
• To report bleeding; avoid use of
razors, commercial mouthwash
• To avoid use of aspirin products,
ibuprofen

Side effects: *italics* = common; ***bold italics*** = life-threatening

• That hair may be lost during therapy; a wig or hairpiece may make patient feel better; new hair may be different in color, texture (rare)

---

aluminum hydroxide (otc)

AlternaGEL, Alu-Cap, Alugel*, aluminum hydroxide, Alu-Tab, Amphojel, Dialume

Func. class.: Antacid, hypophosphatemic

Chem. class.: Aluminum product

Action: Neutralizes gastric acidity, binds phosphates in GI tract; these phosphates are excreted

Uses: Antacid, hyperphosphatemia in chronic renal failure

Investigational uses: Stress ulcer, GI bleeding

Dosage and routes:
• *Adult:* **SUSP** 5-10 ml 1 hr pc, hs; **PO** 600 mg 1 hr pc, hs, chewed with milk or water

Hyperphosphatemia in renal failure
• *Adult:* **SUSP** 500 mg-2 g bid-qid

GI bleeding
• *Infant:* 2-5 ml/dose q1-2h
• *Child:* **PO** 5-15 ml/dose q1-2h

Available forms: Caps 400, 500 mg; tabs 300, 500 mg; chewable tabs 600 mg; susp 450 mg/5 ml, 600 mg/5 ml; liq 320 mg/5 ml, 600 mg/5 ml, 675 mg/5 ml

Side effects/adverse reactions:
GI: Constipation, anorexia, ***obstruction,*** fecal impaction

META: Hypophosphatemia, hypercalciuria

Contraindications: Hypersensitivity to this drug or aluminum products

Precautions: Elderly, fluid restriction, decreased GI motility, GI obstruction, dehydration, renal disease, sodium-restricted diets, pregnancy (C), lactation

Pharmacokinetics:
PO: Onset 20-40 min, duration ½-1½ hr, excreted in feces

Interactions:
• Decreased effectiveness of tetracyclines, allopurinol, corticosteroids, diflunisal, H_2-antagonists, penicillamine, thyroid hormones, ticlopidine anticholinergics, phenothiazines, isoniazid, quinidine, phenytoin, digitalis, iron salts, warfarin, ketoconazole, ciprofloxacin; separate by at least 2 hr

NURSING CONSIDERATIONS
Assess:
• Phosphate levels, since drug is bound in GI system
• Hypophosphatemia: anorexia, weakness, fatigue, bone pain, hyporeflexia
• Constipation; increase bulk in diet if needed
• Urinary pH, Ca^{++}, electrolytes

Administer:
PO
• Laxatives or stool softeners if constipation occurs, especially elderly
• After shaking liquid
• With small amount of water or milk

NG
• By nasogastric tube if patient unable to swallow

Evaluate:
• Therapeutic response: absence of pain, decreased acidity

Teach patient/family:
• To increase fluids to 2 L/day unless contraindicated; measures to prevent constipation
• To avoid phosphate foods (most dairy products, eggs, fruits, carbonated beverages) during drug therapy
• Not to use for prolonged periods in patients with low serum phosphate or if on a low-sodium diet

---

◆ = Nursing alert   ✐ = Herb-drug interaction   ⊘ = Do not crush

- To add cheese, corn, pasta, plums, prunes, lentils after drug is discontinued
- That stools may appear white or speckled
- To check with prescriber after 2 wk of self-prescribed antacid use

---

amantadine (℞)

(a-man'ta-deen)
amantadine HCl, Symadine, Symmetrel
Func. class.: Antiviral, antiparkinsonian agent
Chem. class.: Tricyclic amine

Action: Prevents uncoating of nucleic acid in viral cell, preventing penetration of virus to host; causes release of dopamine from neurons

Uses: Prophylaxis or treatment of influenza type A, extrapyramidal reactions, parkinsonism, respiratory tract infections

Investigational uses: Neuroleptic malignant syndrome, cocaine dependency, enuresis

Dosage and routes:

Influenza type A

- *Adult and child >12 yr:* **PO** 200 mg/day in single dose or divided bid
- *Child 9-12 yr:* **PO** 100 mg bid
- *Child 1-9 yr:* **PO** 4.4-8.8 mg/kg/day divided bid-tid, not to exceed 200 mg/day

Extrapyramidal reaction/parkinsonism

- *Adult:* **PO** 100 mg bid, up to 400 mg/day in EPS; give for 1 wk, then 100 mg as needed up to 400 mg in parkinsonism; CrCl 40-50 ml/min 100 mg/day; CrCl 30 ml/min 200 mg 2×/wk; CrCl 20 ml/min 100 mg 3×/wk; CrCl <10 ml/min 100 mg alternating with 200 mg q7days

Available forms: Caps 100 mg; syr 50 mg/5 ml

Side effects/adverse reactions:

CNS: Headache, dizziness, drowsiness, fatigue, *anxiety*, psychosis, *depression, hallucinations*, tremors, **convulsions**, confusion, *insomnia*

CV: Orthostatic hypotension, **CHF**

INTEG: Photosensitivity, dermatitis

EENT: Blurred vision

HEMA: **Leukopenia**

GI: Nausea, vomiting, constipation, dry mouth

Contraindications: Hypersensitivity, lactation, child <1 yr, eczematic rash

Precautions: Epilepsy, CHF, orthostatic hypotension, psychiatric disorders, hepatic disease, renal disease, peripheral edema, elderly, pregnancy (C)

Pharmacokinetics:

PO: Onset 48 hr, half-life 24 hr, not metabolized, excreted in urine (90%) unchanged, crosses placenta, excreted in breast milk

Interactions:

- Increased anticholinergic response: atropine, other anticholinergics
- Increased CNS stimulation: CNS stimulants
- Decreased renal excretion of amantadine: triamterene, hydrochlorothiazide

🖉 Increased anticholinergic effect: belladonna leaf/root, henbane leaf

🖉 Increased action/side effects: pheasant's eye herb, quinine, scopolia root

NURSING CONSIDERATIONS

Assess:

- CHF, confusion, mottling of skin
- Bowel pattern before, during treatment
- Skin eruptions, photosensitivity after administration of drug
- Respiratory status: rate, character, wheezing, tightness in chest

---

Side effects: *italics* = common; ***bold italics*** = life-threatening

- Allergies before initiation of treatment, reaction of each medication
- Signs of infection

Administer:
- Before exposure to influenza; continue for 10 days after contact
- At least 4 hr before hs to prevent insomnia
- After meals for better absorption, to decrease GI symptoms

Perform/provide:
- Storage in tight, dry container

Evaluate:
- Therapeutic response: absence of fever, malaise, cough, dyspnea in infection; tremors, shuffling gait in Parkinson's disease

Teach patient/family:
- To change body position slowly to prevent orthostatic hypotension
- About aspects of drug therapy: need to report dyspnea, weight gain, dizziness, poor concentration, dysuria, behavioral changes
- To avoid hazardous activities if dizziness, blurred vision occurs
- To take drug exactly as prescribed; parkinsonian crisis may occur if drug is discontinued abruptly; do not double dose; if a dose is missed, do not take within 4 hr of next dose; caps may be opened and mixed with food
- To avoid alcohol

Treatment of overdose: Withdraw drug, maintain airway, administer epinephrine, aminophylline, O₂, IV corticosteroids, physostigmine

---

amifostine (℞)
(a-mi-foss'teen)
Ethyol

Func. class.: Cytoprotective agent for cisplatin

Action: Binds and detoxifies damaging metabolites of cisplatin by converting this drug by alkaline phosphatase in tissue to an active free thiol compound

Uses: Used to reduce renal toxicity when cisplatin is given in ovarian cancer

Dosage and routes:
- *Adult:* IV 910 mg/m² qd, within ½ hr before chemotherapy

Available forms: Powder for inj 500 mg/vial with 500 mg mannitol

Side effects/adverse reactions:
CNS: Dizziness, somnolence
EENT: Sneezing
INTEG: Flushing
CV: Hypotension
GI: Nausea, vomiting, hiccups
MISC: Hypocalcemia, rash, chills

Contraindications: Hypersensitivity to mannitol, aminothiol; hypotension, dehydration, lactation

Precautions: Elderly, CV disease, pregnancy (C), children

Pharmacokinetics: Metabolized to free thiol compound, half-life 8 min, onset 5-8 min

Interactions:
- Increased hypotension: antihypertensives

NURSING CONSIDERATIONS
Assess:
- Fluid status before administration; administer antiemetic prior to administration to prevent severe nausea and vomiting; also, dexamethasone 20 mg IV and a serotonin antagonist such as ondansetron or granisetron
- Calcium levels before and during treatment; calcium supplements may be given for low calcium levels
- B/P prior to and q5min during infusion; if severe hypotension occurs, give IV 0.9% NaCl to expand fluid volume, place in Trendelenburg position

Administer:
Intermittent IV inf
- Intermittent inf after reconstituting with 9.5 ml of sterile 0.9% NaCl,

---

further dilute with 0.9% NaCl to a concentration of 5-40 mg/ml, give at a rate over 15 min within ½ hr of chemotherapy

Y-site compatibilities: Amikacin, aminophylline, ampicillin, ampicillin/sulbactam, aztreonam, bleomycin, bumetanide, buprenorphine, butorphanol, calcium gluconate, carboplatin, carmustine, cefazolin, cefonicid, cefotaxime, cefotetan, cefoxitin, ceftazidime, ceftizoxime, ceftriaxone, cefuroxime, cimetidine, ciprofloxacin, clindamycin, cyclophosphamide, cytarabine, dacarbazine, dactinomycin, daunorubicin, dexamethasone, diphenhydramine, dobutamine, dopamine, doxorubicin, doxycycline, droperidol, enalaprilat, etoposide, famotidine, floxuridine, fluconazole, fludarabine, fluorouracil, furosemide, gallium, gentamicin, granisetron, haloperidol, heparin, hydrocortisone, hydromorphone, idarubicin, ifosfamide, imipenem-cilastatin, leucovorin, lorazepam, magnesium sulfate, mannitol, mechlorethamine, meperidine, mesna, methotrexate, methylprednisolone, metoclopramide, metronidazole, mezlocillin, mitomycin, mitoxantrone, morphine, nalbuphine, netilmicin, ondansetron, piperacillin, plicamycin, potassium chloride, promethazine, rantidine, sodium bicarbonate, streptozocin, teniposide, thiotepa, ticarcillin, ticarcillin/clavulanate, tobramycin, trimethoprim-sulfamethoxazole, trimetrexate, vancomycin, vinblastine, vincristine, zidovudine

Additive incompatibilities: Do not mix with other drugs or solutions

Teach patient/family:
• The reason for the medication and expected results
• That side effects may cause severe nausea, vomiting, decreased B/P, chills, dizziness, somnolence, hiccups, sneezing

amikacin (℞)
(am-i-kay'sin)
amikacin sulfate, Amikin
Func. class.: Antibiotic
Chem. class.: Aminoglycoside

Action: Interferes with protein synthesis in bacterial cell by binding to ribosomal subunit, which causes misreading of genetic code; inaccurate peptide sequence forms in protein chain, causing bacterial death

Uses: Severe systemic infections of CNS, respiratory, GI, urinary tract, bone, skin, soft tissues caused by *Proteus aeruginosa, Escherichia coli, Enterobacter, Acinetobacter, Providencia, Citrobacter, Staphylococcus, Serratia, Proteus, Klebsiella* pneumonia

Investigational uses: *Mycobacterium avium* complex (intrathecal or intraventricular)

Dosage and routes:
Severe systemic infections
• *Adult and child:* **IV INF** 15 mg/kg/day in 2-3 divided doses q8-12h in 100-200 ml D₅W over 30-60 min, not to exceed 1.5 g; decreased doses are needed in poor renal function as determined by blood levels, renal function studies; **IM** 15 mg/kg/day in divided doses q8-12h; qd or extended interval dosing as an alternative dosing regimen
• *Infant:* **IV INF** 10 mg/kg initially, then 7.5 mg/kg q12h in D₅W over 1-2 hr

Severe urinary tract infections
• *Adult:* **IM** 250 mg q12h
Adult with poor renal function:
5-7.5 mg/kg initially, then increased as determined by blood levels, renal function studies

Available forms: Inj 50, 250 mg/ml

Side effects/adverse reactions:

*GU: **Oliguria, hematuria, renal damage, azotemia, renal failure, nephrotoxicity***

CNS: Confusion, depression, numbness, tremors, *convulsions,* muscle twitching, *neurotoxicity,* dizziness, vertigo, tinnitus

*EENT: **Ototoxicity,** deafness,* visual disturbances

*HEMA: **Agranulocytosis, thrombocytopenia,** leukopenia,* eosinophilia, anemia

GI: Nausea, vomiting, anorexia; increased ALT, AST, bilirubin; hepatomegaly, *hepatic necrosis,* splenomegaly

CV: Hypotension or hypertension, palpitations

INTEG: Rash, burning, urticaria, dermatitis, alopecia

Contraindications: Mild to moderate infections, hypersensitivity to aminoglycosides

Precautions: Neonates, mild renal disease, pregnancy (D), myasthenia gravis, lactation, hearing deficits, Parkinson's disease, elderly

Pharmacokinetics:

IM: Onset rapid, peak 1-2 hr

IV: Onset immediate, peak 1-2 hr; plasma half-life 2-3 hr, prolonged up to 7 hr in infants; not metabolized, excreted unchanged in urine, crosses placental barrier, poor penetration into CSF

Interactions:

• Increased neuromuscular blockade, respiratory depression: anesthetics, nondepolarizing neuromuscular blockers

• Inactivation of amikacin: parenteral penicillins; cephalosporins; do not use together

• May increase serum trough and peak: indomethacin

• Mask ototoxicity: dimenhydrinate

• Nephrotoxicity: cephalosporins

NURSING CONSIDERATIONS

Assess:

• Weight before treatment; calculation of dosage is usually based on ideal body weight but may be calculated on actual body weight

• I&O ratio; urinalysis daily for proteinuria, cells, casts; report sudden change in urine output

• VS during infusion; watch for hypotension, change in pulse

• IV site for thrombophlebitis including pain, redness, swelling q30 min; change site if needed; apply warm compresses to discontinued site

• Serum peak, drawn at 30-60 min after IV infusion or 60 min after IM injection, trough level drawn just before next dose; peak 20-30 μg/ml, trough 4-8 μg/ml; adjust dosage per levels

• Urine pH if drug is used for UTI; urine should be kept alkaline

• Renal impairment by securing urine for CrCl testing, BUN, serum creatinine; lower dosage should be given in renal impairment (CrCl <80 ml/min)

◆ Deafness by audiometric testing, ringing, roaring in ears, vertigo; assess hearing before, during, after treatment

• Dehydration: high specific gravity, decrease in skin turgor, dry mucous membranes, dark urine

• Overgrowth of infection, including increased temperature, malaise, redness, pain, swelling, perineal itching, diarrhea, stomatitis, change in cough, sputum

• C&S before starting treatment to identify organism

• Vestibular dysfunction: nausea, vomiting, dizziness, headache; drug should be discontinued if severe

---

◆ = Nursing alert   ⫰ = Herb-drug interaction   🚫 = Do not crush

• Injection sites for redness, swelling, abscesses; use warm compresses at site
Administer:
IM
• Injection in large muscle mass; rotate injection sites
• Bicarbonate to alkalinize urine if ordered for UTI because drug is most active in alkaline environment
Intermittent IV inf
• Dilute 500 mg of drug/100-200 ml of IV D_5W, D_5RL, D_5NaCl, or 0.9% NaCl and give over ½-1 hr; flush after administration with D_5W or 0.9% NaCl
• In evenly spaced doses to maintain blood level
Additive compatibilities: Amobarbital, ascorbic acid inj, bleomycin, calcium chloride, calcium gluconate, cefepime, cefoxitin, chloramphenicol, chlorpheniramine, cimetidine, ciprofloxacin, clindamycin, cloxacillin, colistimethate, dimenhydrinate, diphenhydramine, epinephrine, ergonovine, fluconazole, furosemide, hyaluronidase, hydrocortisone, lincomycin, metaraminol, metronidazole, metronidazole/sodium bicarbonate, norepinephrine, pentobarbital, phenobarbital, phytonadione, polymyxin B, prochlorperazine, promethazine, ranitidine, secobarbital, sodium bicarbonate, succinylcholine, vancomycin, verapamil
Syringe compatibilities: Clindamycin, doxapram
Y-site compatibilities: Acyclovir, amifostine, amiodarone, amsacrine, aztreonam, cefepime, cisatracurium, cyclophosphamide, dexamethasone, diltiazem, enalaprilat, esmolol, filgrastim, fluconazole, fludarabine, foscarnet, furosemide, granisetron, idarubicin, IL-2, labetalol, lorazepam, magnesium sulfate, melphalan, midazolam, morphine, on-

dansetron, paclitaxel, perphenazine, remifentanil, sargramostim, teniposide, thiotepa, TPN #54, #61, #91, #203, #204, #212, vinorelbine, warfarin, zidovudine
Perform/provide:
• Adequate fluids of 2-3 L/day, unless contraindicated, to prevent irritation of tubules
• Flush of IV line with NS or D_5W after infusion
• Supervised ambulation, other safety measures with vestibular dysfunction
Evaluate:
• Therapeutic response: absence of fever, draining wounds, negative C&S after treatment
Teach patient/family:
• To report headache, dizziness, symptoms for overgrowth of infection, renal impairment
◆To report loss of hearing, ringing, roaring in ears or feeling of fullness in head
Treatment of hypersensitivity: Hemodialysis, exchange transfusion in the newborn, monitor serum levels of drug, may give ticarcillin or carbenicillin

---

amiloride (℞)
(a-mill'oh-ride)
amiloride HCl, Midamor
Func. class.: Potassium-sparing diuretic
Chem. class.: Pyrazine

Action: Acts primarily on proximal distal tubule by inhibiting reabsorption of sodium, H_2O, and increasing potassium retention
Uses: Edema in CHF in combination with other diuretics, for hypertension, adjunct with other diuretics to maintain potassium
Investigational uses: Cystic fibrosis (INH), lithium-induced polyuria

Dosage and routes:
• *Adult:* PO 5 mg qd, may be increased to 10-20 mg qd if needed
Available forms: Tabs 5 mg
Side effects/adverse reactions:
GU: Polyuria, dysuria, urinary frequency, impotence
ELECT: Hyperkalemia
RESP: Cough, dyspnea, shortness of breath
CNS: Headache, dizziness, fatigue, weakness, paresthesias, tremor, depression, anxiety
GI: Nausea, diarrhea, dry mouth, *vomiting, anorexia,* cramps, constipation, abdominal pain, jaundice, bleeding
EENT: Loss of hearing, tinnitus, blurred vision, nasal congestion, increased intraocular pressure
INTEG: Rash, pruritus, alopecia, urticaria
MS: Cramps, joint pain
CV: Orthostatic hypotension, dysrhythmias, angina
HEMA: Aplastic anemia, neutropenia

Contraindications: Anuria, hypersensitivity, hyperkalemia, impaired renal function

Precautions: Dehydration, pregnancy (B), diabetes, acidosis, lactation

Pharmacokinetics:
PO: Onset 2 hr, peak 6-10 hr, duration 24 hr; excreted in urine, feces, half-life 6-9 hr

Interactions:
• Enhanced action of antihypertensives
• Hyperkalemia: other potassium-sparing diuretics, potassium products, ACE inhibitors, salt substitutes
• Decreased effect of amiloride: NSAIDs
• Lithium toxicity: lithium

• Drug/food: possible hyperkalemia: foods high in potassium
Lab test interferences:
Interference: GTT

NURSING CONSIDERATIONS
Assess:
• Weight, I&O daily to determine fluid loss; effect of drug may be decreased if used qd
• B/P lying, standing; postural hypotension may occur
• Electrolytes: K, Na, Cl; glucose (serum), BUN, CBC, serum creatinine, blood pH, ABGs
• Improvement in CVP q8h
• Rashes, temperature elevation qd
• Confusion, especially in elderly; take safety precautions if needed
Administer:
PO
• In AM to avoid interference with sleep if using drug as a diuretic
• With food; if nausea occurs, absorption may be decreased slightly
Evaluate:
• Therapeutic response: improvement in edema of feet, legs, sacral area daily if medication is being used in CHF
Teach patient/family:
• To take as prescribed; if dose is missed, take when remembered within 1 hr of next dose
• About adverse reactions: muscle cramps, weakness, nausea, dizziness, blurred vision
• To take with food or milk for GI symptoms
• To take early in day to prevent nocturia
• To avoid potassium-rich foods: oranges, bananas; salt substitutes, dried fruits
Treatment of overdose: Lavage if taken orally, monitor electrolytes, administer sodium bicarbonate for $K^+ > 6.5$ mEq/L, monitor hydration, CV, renal status

◆ = Nursing alert   ∥ = Herb-drug interaction   ⊘ = Do not crush

amino acid injection (R)

(a-mee'noe)

FreAmine, HepatAmine

Func. class.: Nitrogen product

Action: Needed for anabolism to maintain structure, decrease catabolism, promote healing

Uses: Hepatic encephalopathy, cirrhosis, hepatitis, nutritional support in cancer

Dosage and routes:

• *Adult:* **IV** 80-120 g/day; 500 ml of amino acids/500 ml D_{50} given over 24 hr

Available forms: Inj; many strengths, types

Side effects/adverse reactions:

CNS: Dizziness, headache, confusion, *loss of consciousness*

CV: Hypertension, **CHF, pulmonary edema**

GI: Nausea, vomiting, liver fat deposits, abdominal pain

GU: Glycosuria, osmotic diuresis

ENDO: Hyperglycemia, rebound hypoglycemia, electrolyte imbalances, hyperosmolar syndrome, hyperosmolar hyperglycemic nonketotic syndrome, alkalosis, acidosis, hypophosphatemia, hyperammonemia, dehydration, hypocalcemia

INTEG: Chills, flushing, warm feeling, rash, urticaria, extravasation necrosis, phlebitis at injection site

Contraindications: Hypersensitivity, severe electrolyte imbalances, anuria, severe liver damage, maple syrup urine disease, PKU

Precautions: Renal disease, pregnancy (C), lactation, children, diabetes mellitus, CHF

NURSING CONSIDERATIONS

Assess:

• Electrolytes (K, Na, Ca, Cl, Mg), blood glucose, ammonia, phosphate, ketones

• Renal, liver function studies: BUN, creatinine, ALT, AST, bilirubin

• Injection site for extravasation: redness along vein, edema at site, necrosis, pain, hard tender area; site should be changed immediately

• Respiratory function q4h: auscultate lung fields bilaterally for crackles, respirations, quality, rate, rhythm

• Temperature q4h for increased fever, indicating infection; if infection suspected, infusion is discontinued, tubing bottle cultured

◆For impending hepatic coma: asterixis, confusion, uremic fetor, lethargy

• Hyperammonemia: nausea, vomiting, malaise, tremors, anorexia, convulsions

Administer:

Continuous IV

• Up to 40% protein and dextrose (up to 12.5%) via peripheral vein; stronger solutions require central IV administration

• TPN only mixed with dextrose to promote protein synthesis

• Immediately after mixing under strict aseptic technique, use infusion pump, in-line filter (0.22 μm) unless mixed with fat emulsion and dextrose (3 in 1)

◆Using careful monitoring technique; do not speed up infusion; pulmonary edema, glucose overload will result

Additive compatibilities: Amikacin, aminophylline, aztreonam, calcium gluconate, cefamandole, cefazolin, cefepime, cefotaxime, cefoxitin, cefsulodin, ceftazidime, ceftriaxone, cefuroxime, cimetidine, clindamycin, cyanocobalamin, cyclophosphamide, cyclosporine, cytarabine, dopamine, epoetin, erythromycin, famotidine, folic acid, fosphenytoin, furosemide, heparin, insulin (regular), isoproterenol, lidocaine, meperidine, metaraminol, methicillin, methotrexate, methyldopate, methylprednisolone, metoclopramide, morphine, nafcillin, netilmicin, nizatidine, norepinephrine, ondansetron, oxacillin, penicillin G potassium, penicillin G sodium, phytonadione, polymyxin B, sodium bicarbonate, tacrolimus, tobramycin, vancomycin

Y-site compatibilities: Amikacin, aminophylline, amoxicillin, ampicillin, ascorbic acid inj, atracurium, azlocillin, aztreonam, bumetanide, buprenorphine, calcium gluconate, carboplatin, cefamandole, cefonicid, cefoperazone, cefotaxime, cefotetan, cefoxitin, ceftazidime, ceftizoxime, ceftriaxone, cefuroxime, cephalothin, cephapirin, chloramphenicol, chlorpromazine, cimetidine, clindamycin, clonazepam, dexamethasone, diazepam, digoxin, diphenhydramine, dobutamine, dopamine, doxycycline, droperidol, enalaprilat, epinephrine, erythromycin, famotidine, fentanyl, flucloxacillin, fluconazole, folic acid, foscarnet, gentamicin, granisetron, haloperidol, heparin, hydrocortisone, hydromorphone, hydroxyzine, idarubicin, ifosfamide, IL-2, imipenem/cilastatin, insulin (regular), isoproterenol, kanamycin, lidocaine, meperidine, methicillin, metronidazole, mezlocillin, miconazole, leucovorin, levorphanol, lorazepam, magnesium sulfate, mannitol, mesna, morphine, moxalactam, multivitamins, nafcillin, netilmicin, nitroglycerin, nitroprusside, norepinephrine, octreotide, ofloxacin, ondansetron, oxacillin, paclitaxel, penicillin G, penicillin G potassium, pentobarbital, phenobarbital, piperacillin, potassium chloride, prochlorperazine, ranitidine, salbutamol, sargramostim, tacrolimus, thiotepa, ticarcillin, ticarcillin/clavulanate, tobramycin, trimethoprim-sulfamethoxazole, urokinase, vancomycin, vecuronium, zidovudine

Perform/provide:
• Storage depends on type of solution; consult manufacturer
• Changing dressing and IV tubing to prevent infection q24-48h

Evaluate:
• Therapeutic response: weight gain, decrease in jaundice in liver disorders, increased LOC

Teach patient/family:
• The reason for use of TPN
• If chills, sweating are experienced, report at once
• About infusion pump and blood glucose monitoring

---

amino acid solution (R)
Aminees, Aminosyn, Branch Amin, FreAmine III, NeprAmine, Novamine, ProcalAmine, Ren Amin, Travasol, Trophmine
Func. class.: Nitrogen product

Action: Needed for anabolism to maintain structure, decrease catabolism, promote healing

Uses: Nutritional support in cancer, trauma, intestinal obstruction, short bowel syndrome, severe malabsorption

Dosage and routes:
• *Adult:* IV 1-1.5 g/kg/day titrated to patient's needs
• *Child:* IV 2-3 g/kg/day titrated to patient's needs

Available forms: Inj, many types, strengths

Side effects/adverse reactions:
CNS: Dizziness, headache, confusion, *loss of consciousness*

◆ = Nursing alert   ∥ = Herb-drug interaction   Ⓢ = Do not crush

CV: Hypertension, ***CHF, pulmonary edema***

GI: Nausea, vomiting, liver fat deposits, abdominal pain, jaundice

GU: Glycosuria, osmotic diuresis

ENDO: Hyperglycemia, rebound hypoglycemia, electrolyte imbalances, hyperosmolar syndrome, hyperosmolar hyperglycemic nonketotic syndrome, alkalosis, acidosis, hypophosphatemia, hyperammonemia, dehydration, hypocalcemia

INTEG: Chills, flushing, warm feeling, rash, urticaria, extravasation necrosis, phlebitis at injection site

Contraindications: Hypersensitivity, severe electrolyte imbalances, anuria, severe liver damage, maple syrup urine disease, PKU

Precautions: Renal disease, pregnancy (C), lactation, children, diabetes mellitus, CHF

NURSING CONSIDERATIONS

Assess:

• Electrolytes (K, Na, Ca, Cl, Mg), blood glucose, ammonia, phosphate

• Renal, liver function studies: BUN, creatinine, ALT, AST, bilirubin

• Injection site for extravasation: redness along vein, edema at site, necrosis, pain, hard tender area; site should be changed immediately

• Monitor respiratory function q4h: auscultate lung fields bilaterally for crackles, respirations, quality, rate, rhythm

• Monitor temperature q4h for increased fever, indicating infection; if infection suspected, discontinue infusion, culture tubing, bottle

• Urine glucose q6h using Tes-Tape, Clinistix, which are not affected by infusion substances; blood glucose is preferred testing method

• Hyperammonemia: nausea, vomiting, malaise, tremors, anorexia, convulsions

Administer:

Continuous IV

• Up to 40% protein and dextrose (up to 12.5%) via peripheral vein; stronger solutions require central IV administration, use infusion pump

• TPN only mixed with dextrose to promote protein synthesis

• Immediately after mixing in pharmacy under strict aseptic technique using laminar flow hood, use infusion pump, in-line filter (0.22 μm) unless mixed with fat emulsion and dextrose (3 in 1)

◆ Using careful monitoring technique; do not speed up infusion; pulmonary edema, glucose overload will result

Y-site compatibilities: Cefamandole, cefazolin, cefoperazone, cefotaxime, cefoxitin, cephalothin, cephapirin, chloramphenicol, clindamycin, digoxin, dobutamine, dopamine, doxycycline, erythromycin lactobionate, fat emulsion, foscarnet, furosemide, gentamicin, isoproterenol, kanamycin, lidocaine, meperidine, methicillin, mezlocillin, miconazole, morphine, nafcillin, netilmicin, norepinephrine, oxacillin, penicillin G potassium, piperacillin, sargramostim, ticarcillin, tobramycin, urokinase, vancomycin

Perform/provide:

• Storage depends on type of solution; consult label

• Dressing and IV tubing change q24-48h to prevent infection

Evaluate:

• Therapeutic response: weight gain, decrease in jaundice in liver disorders, increased serum albumin

Teach patient/family:

• The reason for use of TPN

• That any chills, sweating should be reported at once

• About infusion pump and blood glucose monitoring

---

aminoglutethimide (℞)

(a-meen-oh-gloo-teth'i-mide)
Cytadren
Func. class.: Antineoplastic, adrenal steroid inhibitor
Chem. class.: Hormone

Action: Acts by inhibiting DNA, RNA, protein synthesis; is derived from *Streptomyces verticillus;* replication is decreased by binding to DNA, which causes strand splitting; phase specific in G_2 and M phases; blocks biosynthesis of all steroid hormones (cortisol, androgens, progestins)

Uses: Suppression of adrenal function in Cushing's syndrome, adrenal cancer

Dosage and routes:
• *Adult:* **PO** 250 mg qid at 6 hr intervals, may increase by 250 mg/day q1-2wk, not to exceed 2 g/day
Available forms: Tabs 250 mg

Side effects/adverse reactions:
*GI: Nausea, vomiting, anorexia, **hepatotoxicity***
*HEMA: **Agranulocytosis, thrombocytopenia, transient leukopenia***
INTEG: Rash, pruritus, hirsutism
*CV: **Hypotension,** tachycardia*
CNS: Drowsiness, morbilliform skin rash, dizziness, headache, lethargy

Contraindications: Hypersensitivity, hypothyroidism, pregnancy (D)

Precautions: Renal disease, hepatic disease, respiratory disease

Pharmacokinetics: Half-life 13 hr, metabolized in liver, excreted in urine, crosses placenta

Interactions:
• Accelerated metabolism: dexamethasone, medroxyprogesterone
• Decreased effect of: anticoagulants, theophylline
• Increased drug clearance: digoxin
• Increased aminoglutethimide effect: alcohol

Lab test interferences:
Decrease: plasma cortisol, thyroxine, urinary aldosterone
Increase: Alk phos, AST, TSH

NURSING CONSIDERATIONS
Assess:
• Renal function studies: BUN, serum uric acid, urine CrCl, electrolytes before, during therapy
• I&O ratio; report fall in urine output of 30 ml/hr
• Monitor temperature q4h; may indicate beginning infection
• Liver function tests before, during therapy (bilirubin, AST, ALT, LDH) as needed or monthly
• RBC, Hct, Hgb, since these may be decreased
• Yellowing of skin, sclera, dark urine, clay-colored stools, itchy skin, abdominal pain, fever, diarrhea
• Symptoms indicating severe allergic reaction: rash, pruritus, urticaria, purpuric skin lesions, itching, flushing

Administer:
PO
• Antacid before oral agent; give last dose of the day after evening meal before bedtime

Perform/provide:
• Liquid diet, including cola, Jell-O; dry toast or crackers as ordered may be added if patient is not nauseated or vomiting
• Nutritious diet with iron and vitamin supplements as ordered

Evaluate:
• Therapeutic response: decrease in size of tumor or decrease in Cushing's syndrome

Teach patient/family:
• To report any complaints, side effects to nurse or prescriber
• That masculinization can occur, is reversible after discontinuing treatment

---

◆ = Nursing alert   ∅ = Herb-drug interaction   ⊘ = Do not crush

- To avoid self-administration of adjuvant corticosteroids
- That drowsiness may occur and to avoid driving or operating heavy machinery

aminolevulinic acid
See appendix a—selected new drugs

aminophylline (R)
(am-in-off'i-lin)
Aminophyllin, Phyllocontin, Truphylline
Func. class.: Spasmolytic
Chem. class.: Xanthine, ethylenediamide

Action: Relaxes smooth muscle of respiratory system by blocking phosphodiesterase, which increases cyclic AMP; increased cyclic AMP alters intracellular calcium ion movements; produces bronchodilation, increased pulmonary blood flow, relaxation of respiratory tract

Uses: Bronchial asthma, bronchospasm, Cheyne-Stokes respirations

Investigational uses: Apnea in infancy for respiratory/myocardial stimulation, Cheyne-Stokes respirations as a respiratory stimulant

Dosage and routes:
- *Adult:* **PO** 500 mg, then 250-500 mg q6-8h; **CONT IV** 0.3-0.9 mg/kg/hr (maintenance); **RECT** 500 mg q6-8h
- *Child:* **PO** 7.5 mg/kg, then 3-6 mg/kg q6-8h; **IV** 7.5 mg/kg, then 3-6 mg/kg q6-8h injected over 5 min; do not exceed 25 mg/min; may give loading dose of 5.6 mg/kg over ½ hr; **CONT IV** 1 mg/kg/hr (maintenance); for children/infants use drug without preservative or alcohol
- *Neonate:* **IV/PO** 1 mg/kg initially

for plasma increases of each 2 µg/ml, then 1 mg/kg q12h

Available forms: Inj 250 mg/10 ml, 500 mg/20 ml, 100 mg/100 ml in 0.45% NaCl, 200 mg/100 ml in 0.45% NaCl; rect supp 250, 500 mg, oral liq 105 mg/5 ml; tabs 100, 200 mg, tabs con rel 225 mg

Side effects/adverse reactions:
CNS: Anxiety, restlessness, insomnia, *dizziness*, **convulsions,** headache, light-headedness, muscle twitching
CV: Palpitations, sinus tachycardia, hypotension, flushing, dysrhythmias, increased respiratory rate
GI: Nausea, vomiting, anorexia, diarrhea, bitter taste, dyspepsia, anal irritation (suppositories), epigastric pain
RESP: Tachypnea
INTEG: Flushing, urticaria, *rectal irritation* (suppositories)
GU: Urinary frequency

Contraindications: Hypersensitivity to xanthines, tachydysrhythmias
Precautions: Elderly, CHF, cor pulmonale, hepatic disease, active peptic ulcer disease, diabetes mellitus, hyperthyroidism, hypertension, children, pregnancy (C), lactation, glaucoma, prostatic hypertrophy

Pharmacokinetics: Well absorbed PO; extended rel well absorbed slowly, rectal supp is erratic, rectal sol is absorbed quickly; metabolized by liver (caffeine); excreted in urine; crosses placenta; appears in breast milk; half-life 3-12 hr; half-life increased in geriatric patients, hepatic disease, CHF
PO: Onset ¼ hr, peak 1-2 hr, duration 6-8 hr
PO-ER: Unknown, peak 4-7 hr, duration 8-12 hr
IV: Onset rapid, duration 6-8 hr
REC: Onset erratic, peak 1-2 hr, duration 6-8 hr

Interactions:
• Increased action of aminophylline: cimetidine, propranolol, erythromycin
• Dysrhythmias: halothane
• May increase effects of anticoagulants
• Cardiotoxicity: β-blockers
• Increased elimination: smoking
• Increased aminophylline levels: calcium channel blockers, cimetidine, disulfiram, interferon, macrolide antibiotics, methotrexate, oral contraceptives, quinolone antibiotics
• Decreased effects of lithium
• Decreased effects of: adenosine, beta blockers
• May increase or decrease aminophylline levels: carbamazepine, loop diuretics, isoniazid
• Synergistic toxicity: sympathomimetics
• Decreased effects of: aminophylline, rifampin, barbiturates, nicotine, phenytoin

Lab test interferences:
Increase: Plasma free fatty acids

NURSING CONSIDERATIONS
Assess:
• Theophylline blood levels (therapeutic level is 10-20 μg/ml); toxicity may occur with small increase above 20 μg/ml, especially elderly
• Monitor I&O; diuresis occurs; dehydration may occur in elderly or children
• Whether theophylline was given recently (24 hr)
• Respiratory rate, rhythm, depth; auscultate lung fields bilaterally; notify prescriber of abnormalities
• Allergic reactions: rash, urticaria; if these occur, drug should be discontinued

Administer:
• Avoid IM injection; pain and tissue damage may occur

PO
• After meals to decrease GI symptoms; absorption may be effected with a full glass of water
🚫 Do not break, crush, or chew enteric-coated or ER tabs

Rectal
• If patient is unable to take PO; retain rectal dose for ½ hr

IV
• Only clear sol; flush IV line before dose
• After diluting in 5% dextrose to decrease burning sensation at injection site; only clear solutions
• May be diluted for IV INF in 100-200 ml in D_5W, $D_{10}W$, $D_{20}W$, 0.9% NaCl, 0.45% NaCl, LR

Additive compatibilities: Amobarbital, bretylium, calcium gluconate, chloramphenicol, cibenzoline, cimetidine, dexamethasone, diphenhydramine, dopamine, erythromycin lactobionate, esmolol, floxacillin, flumazenil, furosemide, heparin, hydrocortisone, lidocaine, mephentermine, meropenem, methicillin, methyldopate, metronidazole/sodium bicarbonate, nitroglycerin, pentobarbital, phenobarbital, potassium chloride, ranitidine, secobarbital, sodium bicarbonate, terbutaline

Syringe compatibilities: Heparin, metoclopramide, pentobarbital, thiopental

Y-site compatibilities: Allopurinol, amifostine, amphotericin B, amrinone, aztreonam, ceftazidime, cholesteryl sulfate complex, cimetidine, cladribine, doxorubicin liposome, enalaprilat, esmolol, famotidine, filgrastim, fluconazole, fludarabine, foscarnet, gallium, granisetron, heparin sodium with hydrocortisone sodium succinate, labetalol, melphalan, meropenem, morphine, netilmicin, paclitaxel, pancuronium, piperacillin/tazobactam, potassium

---

◆ = Nursing alert   ▮ = Herb-drug interaction   🚫 = Do not crush chloride, propofol, ranitidine, remifentanil, sargramostim, tacrolimus, teniposide, thiotepa, tolazoline, vecuronium, vit B/C

Perform/provide:

• Storage of diluted solution for 24 hr if refrigerated

Evaluate:

• Therapeutic response: decreased dyspnea, respiratory stimulation in infancy, clear lung fields bilaterally

Teach patient/family:

• To take doses as prescribed, not to skip dose, not to double dose

• To check OTC medications, current prescription medications for ephedrine; will increase CNS stimulation; not to drink alcohol or caffeine products (tea, coffee, chocolate, colas)

• To avoid hazardous activities; dizziness may occur

• If GI upset occurs, to take drug with 8 oz water; avoid food, since absorption may be decreased

• To remain in bed 15-20 min after rectal suppository is inserted to avoid removal

◆ To notify prescriber of toxicity: insomnia, anxiety, nausea, vomiting, rapid pulse, convulsions

• To notify prescriber of change in smoking habit; a change in dose may be required

• To increase fluids to 2 L/day to decrease secretion viscosity

---

amiodarone (℞)

(a-mee-o′da-rone)
Cordarone

Func. class.: Antidysrhythmic (class III)

Chem. class.: Iodinated benzofuran derivative

Action: Prolongs duration of action potential and effective refractory period, noncompetitive α- and β-adrenergic inhibition; increases PR and QT intervals, decreases sinus rate

Uses: Severe ventricular tachycardia, supraventricular tachycardia, atrial fibrillation, ventricular fibrillation not controlled by first-line agents

Dosage and routes:

• *Adult:* **PO** loading dose 800-1600 mg/day 1-3 wk; then 600-800 mg/day 1 mo; maintenance 200-600 mg/day

• *Child:* **PO** loading dose 10-15 mg/kg/day in 1-2 divided doses for 4-14 days then 5 mg/kg/day

• *Adult:* **IV** loading dose (first rapid) 150 mg over the first 10 min then slow 360 mg over the next 6 hr; maintenance 540 mg given over the remaining 18 hr, decrease rate of the slow infusion to 0.5 mg/min

Available forms: Tabs 200 mg; inj 50 mg/ml

Side effects/adverse reactions:

CNS: Headache, dizziness, involuntary movement, tremors, peripheral neuropathy, malaise, fatigue, ataxia, paresthesias, insomnia

GI: Nausea, vomiting, diarrhea, abdominal pain, anorexia, constipation, *hepatotoxicity*

CV: Hypotension, bradycardia, sinus arrest, CHF, dysrhythmias, *SA node dysfunction*

INTEG: Rash, photosensitivity, blue-gray skin discoloration, alopecia, spontaneous ecchymosis

EENT: Blurred vision, halos, photophobia, *corneal microdeposits,* dry eyes

ENDO: Hyperthyroidism or hypothyroidism

MS: Weakness, pain in extremities

RESP: Pulmonary fibrosis, pulmonary inflammation

MISC: Flushing, abnormal taste or smell, edema, abnormal salivation, coagulation abnormalities

---

Precautions: Goiter, Hashimoto's thyroiditis, SN dysfunction, 2nd- or 3rd-degree AV block, electrolyte imbalances, pregnancy (D), bradycardia, lactation

Pharmacokinetics:

PO: Onset 1-3 wk, peak 2-10 hr; half-life 15-100 days; metabolized by liver, excreted by kidneys

Interactions:

• Bradycardia: β-blockers, calcium channel blockers

• Increased levels of digitalis, quinidine, procainamide, flecainide, disopyramide, phenytoin, theophylline

• Increased anticoagulant effects: warfarin

• Torsades de pointes: antidysrhythmics

• Increased hypotension: antihypertensives

• Bradycardia, arrest: lidocaine

✎ May increase amiodarone effect: aloe, buckthorn bark/berry, cascara sagrada bark, rhubarb root, senna leaf/fruits

Lab test interferences:

Increase: T_4

NURSING CONSIDERATIONS

Assess:

• I&O ratio; electrolytes (K, Na, Cl)

• Liver function studies: AST, ALT, bilirubin, alk phosphatase

• Chest x-ray, thyroid function tests

• ECG continuously to determine drug effectiveness, measure PR, QRS, QT intervals, check for PVCs, other dysrhythmias

• For dehydration or hypovolemia

• B/P continuously for hypotension, hypertension

• For rebound hypertension after 1-2 hr

• CNS symptoms: confusion, psychosis, numbness, depression, involuntary movements; if these occur, drug should be discontinued

• Hypothyroidism: lethargy, dizziness, constipation, enlarged thyroid gland, edema of extremities, cool, pale skin

• Hyperthyroidism: restlessness, tachycardia, eyelid puffiness, weight loss, frequent urination, menstrual irregularities, dyspnea; warm, moist skin

◆Pulmonary toxicity: dyspnea, fatigue, cough, fever, chest pain; drug should be discontinued

• Cardiac rate, respiration: rate, rhythm, character, chest pain

Administer:

PO

• Loading dose with food to decrease nausea

Intermittent IV inf

• 1000 mg/24 hr during loading/maintenance

• Initial loading: Add 3 ml (150 mg) 100 ml D_5W (1.5 mg/ml) give over 10 min

• Loading inf: Add 18 ml (900 mg) 500 ml D_5W (1.8 mg/ml) give over next 6 hr

• Maintenance inf: Give remainder of loading inf 540 mg over 18 hr (0.5 mg/min)

Continuous inf

• After 24 hr, give 1-6 mg/ml at 0.5 mg/ml, do not exceed 30 mg/min

Additive compatibilities: Dobutamine, lidocaine, potassium chloride, procainimide, verapamil

Y-site compatibilities: Amikacin, bretylium, clindamycin, dobutamine, dopamine, doxycycline, erythromycin, esmolol, gentamicin, insulin, isoproterenol, labetalol, lidocaine, metaraminol, metronidazole, midazolam, morphine, nitroglycerin, norepinephrine, penicillin G potassium, phentolamine, phenylephrine, potassium chloride, procainamide, tobramycin, vancomycin

Solution compatibility: D_5W, 0.9% NaCl

◆ = Nursing alert   ✎ = Herb-drug interaction   ⃠ = Do not crush

Evaluate:
• Therapeutic response: decrease in ventricular tachycardia, supraventricular tachycardia or fibrillation
Teach patient/family:
• To take this drug as directed; avoid missed doses
• To use sunscreen or stay out of sun to prevent burns
• To report side effects immediately
• That skin discoloration is usually reversible
• That dark glasses may be needed for photophobia
Treatment of overdose: O_2, artificial ventilation, ECG, administer dopamine for circulatory depression, administer diazepam or thiopental for convulsions, isoproterenol

---

amitriptyline (℞)

(a-mee-trip′ti-leen)
amitriptyline HCl, Apo-Amitriptyline*, Elavil, Endep, Levate*, Novo-Triptyn*
Func. class.: Antidepressant—tricyclic
Chem. class.: Tertiary amine

Action: Blocks reuptake of norepinephrine, serotonin into nerve endings, increasing action of norepinephrine, serotonin in nerve cells
Uses: Major depression
Investigational uses: Chronic pain management, prevention of cluster/migraine headaches
Dosage and routes:
Depression
• *Adult:* **PO** 50-100 mg hs, may increase to 200 mg qd, not to exceed 300 mg/day; **IM** 20-30 mg qid, or 80-120 mg hs
• *Adolescent:* **PO** 30 mg/day in divided doses, may be increased to 150 mg/day

• *Geriatric:* Generally avoided due to anticholinergic side effects; if used **PO** 10-25 mg at hs, increase by 10-25/wk as tolerated
Cluster/migraine headache
• *Adult:* **PO** 50-150 mg/day
Chronic pain
• *Adult:* **PO** 75-150 mg/day
Available forms: Tabs 10, 25, 50, 75, 100, 150 mg; inj 10 mg/ml
Side effects/adverse reactions:
HEMA: **Agranulocytosis, thrombocytopenia, eosinophilia, leukopenia**
CNS: Dizziness, drowsiness, confusion, headache, anxiety, tremors, stimulation, weakness, insomnia, nightmares, EPS (elderly), increased psychiatric symptoms, *seizures*
GI: Constipation, dry mouth, nausea, vomiting, *paralytic ileus,* increased appetite, cramps, epigastric distress, jaundice, *hepatitis,* stomatitis
GU: Retention
INTEG: Rash, urticaria, sweating, pruritus, photosensitivity
CV: Orthostatic hypotension, *ECG changes, tachycardia, hypertension,* palpitations
EENT: Blurred vision, tinnitus, mydriasis, ophthalmoplegia
Contraindications: Hypersensitivity to tricyclic antidepressants, recovery phase of myocardial infarction, narrow-angle glaucoma
Precautions: Suicidal patients, convulsive disorders, prostatic hypertrophy, schizophrenia, psychosis, severe depression, increased intraocular pressure, narrow-angle glaucoma, urinary retention, cardiac disease, hepatic disease, renal disease, hyperthyroidism, electroshock therapy, elective surgery, child <12 yr, pregnancy (C), lactation, elderly
Pharmacokinetics:
PO/IM: Onset 45 min, peak 2-12 hr, therapeutic response 4-10 days; me-

---

tabolized by liver; excreted in urine, feces; crosses placenta, excreted in breast milk, half-life 31-46 hr

Interactions:

• Increased risk of agranulocytosis: Antithyroid agents

• Increased amitriptyline levels, toxicity: cimetidine, fluoxetine, phenothiazines, oral contraceptives

• Decreased effects of: guanethidine, clonidine, indirect-acting sympathomimetics (ephedrine)

• Increased effects of: direct-acting sympathomimetics (epinephrine), alcohol, barbiturates, benzodiazepines, CNS depressants

• Hyperpyretic crisis, convulsions, hypertensive episode: MAOIs, clonidine

🍃 Increased CNS depression: kava

🍃 Increased anticholinergic effect: belladonna leaf/root, henbane leaf

🍃 Increased action of amitriptyline: scopolia root

Lab test interferences:

Increase: Serum bilirubin, blood glucose, alk phosphatase

NURSING CONSIDERATIONS
Assess:

• B/P lying, standing; pulse q4h; if systolic B/P drops 20 mm Hg, hold drug, notify prescriber; take vital signs q4h in patients with cardiovascular disease

• Blood studies: CBC, leukocytes, differential, cardiac enzymes if patient is receiving long-term therapy

• Blood level: therapeutic 100-250 ng/ml; toxic >500 ng/ml

• Hepatic studies: AST, ALT, bilirubin

• Weight qwk; appetite may increase with drug

• ECG for flattening of T wave, prolongation of QTc interval, bundle branch block, AV block, dysrhythmias in cardiac patients

• EPS primarily in elderly: rigidity, dystonia, akathisia

• Mental status: mood, sensorium, affect, suicidal tendencies; increase in psychiatric symptoms: depression, panic

• Urinary retention, constipation; constipation is most likely to occur in children and elderly

• Withdrawal symptoms: headache, nausea, vomiting, muscle pain, weakness; do not usually occur unless drug was discontinued abruptly

• Alcohol consumption; if alcohol is consumed, hold dose until morning

Administer:

PO

• Increased fluids, bulk in diet if constipation, urinary retention occur, especially elderly

• With food or milk for GI symptoms

• Crushed if patient is unable to swallow medication whole

• Dosage hs if oversedation occurs during day; may take entire dose hs; elderly may not tolerate once/day dosing

Perform/provide:

• Storage at room temperature; do not freeze

• Assistance with ambulation during beginning therapy, since drowsiness/dizziness occurs

• Gum; hard, sugarless candy; or frequent sips of water for dry mouth

Evaluate:

• Therapeutic response: decrease in depression, absence of suicidal thoughts

Teach patient/family:

• To take medication as directed; do not double dose; that therapeutic effects may take 2-3 wk

• To use caution in driving, other activities requiring alertness because of drowsiness, dizziness, blurred vision; to avoid rising quickly from

sitting to standing, especially elderly
• To avoid alcohol ingestion, other CNS depressants
• Not to discontinue medication quickly after long-term use: may cause nausea, headache, malaise
• To wear sunscreen or large hat, since photosensitivity occurs
Treatment of overdose: ECG monitoring, induce emesis, lavage, activated charcoal, administer anticonvulsant

---

amlodipine (℞)
(am-loe'di-peen)
Norvasc
Func. class.: Antianginal, calcium channel blocker
Chem. class.: Dihydropyridine

Action: Inhibits calcium ion influx across cell membrane during cardiac depolarization; produces relaxation of coronary vascular smooth muscle, peripheral vascular smooth muscle; dilates coronary vascular arteries; increases myocardial oxygen delivery in patients with vasospastic angina

Uses: Chronic stable angina pectoris, hypertension, vasospastic angina

Dosage and routes:
Angina
• *Adult:* **PO** 5-10 mg qd
Hypertension
• *Adult:* **PO** 5 mg qd initially, may increase up to 10 mg/day
Available forms: Tabs 2.5, 5, 10 mg
Side effects/adverse reactions:
CV: Dysrhythmia, edema, bradycardia, hypotension, palpitations, syncope, AV block
GI: Nausea, vomiting, diarrhea, gastric upset, constipation, abdominal cramps, flatulence, anorexia
GU: Nocturia, polyuria

INTEG: Rash, pruritus, urticaria, hair loss
CNS: Headache, fatigue, dizziness, anxiety, depression, insomnia, paresthesia, somnolence, asthenia
OTHER: Flushing, nasal congestion, sweating, shortness of breath, sexual difficulties, muscle cramps, cough, weight gain, tinnitus, epistaxis
Contraindications: Sick sinus syndrome, 2nd- or 3rd-degree heart block, hypotension less than 90 mm Hg systolic, hypersensitivity
Precautions: CHF, hypotension, hepatic injury, pregnancy (C), lactation, children, renal disease, elderly
Pharmacokinetics:
PO: Onset not determined, peak 6-12 hr, half-life 30-50 hr; metabolized by liver, excreted in urine (90% as metabolites)
Interactions:
• Increased hypotension: alcohol, fentanyl, quinidine, antihypertensives, nitrates
• Decreased antihypertensive effect: NSAIDs
⊘ May increase hypotensive effect: grapefruit
NURSING CONSIDERATIONS
Assess:
• Cardiac status: B/P, pulse, respiration, ECG; some patients have developed severe angina, acute MI after calcium channel blockers if obstructive CAD is severe
Administer:
PO
• Once a day
Evaluate:
• Therapeutic response: decreased anginal pain, decreased B/P
Teach patient/family:
• To take drug as prescribed, do not double or skip dose
• To avoid hazardous activities until stabilized on drug, dizziness is no longer a problem

---

• To avoid OTC drugs unless directed by prescriber
• To comply in all areas of medical regimen: diet, exercise, stress reduction, drug therapy
• To notify prescriber of irregular heartbeat, shortness of breath, swelling of feet and hands, pronounced dizziness, constipation, nausea, hypotension

Treatment of overdose: Defibrillation, β-agonists, IV calcium inotropic agents, diuretics, atropine for AV block, vasopressor for hypotension

---

amoxapine (℞)

(a-mox′a-peen)

amoxapine, Asendin

Func. class.: Antidepressant—tetracyclics

Chem. class.: Dibenzoxazepine derivative—secondary amine

Action: Blocks reuptake of norepinephrine, serotonin into nerve endings, increasing action of norepinephrine, serotonin in nerve cells

Uses: Depression

Dosage and routes:
• *Adult:* PO 50 mg tid, may increase to 100 mg tid on 3rd day of therapy; not to exceed 300 mg/day unless lower doses have been given for at least 2 wk, may be given daily dose hs, not to exceed 600 mg/day in hospitalized patients
• *Elderly:* PO 25 mg hs, may increase by 25 mg/wk, up to 150 mg/day in divided doses

Available forms: Tabs 25, 50, 100, 150 mg

Side effects/adverse reactions:

*HEMA: **Agranulocytosis, thrombocytopenia, eosinophilia, leukopenia***

CNS: Dizziness, drowsiness, confu-

sion, headache, anxiety, tremors, stimulation, weakness, insomnia, nightmares, EPS (elderly), increased psychiatric symptoms, paresthesia, ***neuroleptic malignant syndrome,*** impairment of sexual functioning

GI: Dry mouth, constipation, nausea, vomiting, ***paralytic ileus,*** increased appetite, cramps, epigastric distress, jaundice, ***hepatitis,*** stomatitis

*GU: Retention, **acute renal failure***

INTEG: Rash, urticaria, sweating, pruritus, photosensitivity

CV: Orthostatic hypotension, ECG changes, tachycardia, hypertension, palpitations

EENT: Blurred vision, tinnitus, mydriasis, ophthalmoplegia

Contraindications: Hypersensitivity to tricyclic antidepressants, recovery phase of myocardial infarction, convulsive disorders, prostatic hypertrophy

Precautions: Suicidal patients, severe depression, increased intraocular pressure, narrow-angle glaucoma, urinary retention, cardiac disease, hepatic disease, hyperthyroidism, electroshock therapy, elective surgery, elderly, pregnancy (C)

Pharmacokinetics:

PO: Steady state 2-7 days; metabolized by liver, excreted by kidneys, crosses placenta, half-life 8 hr

Interactions:
• Increased CNS depression: CNS depressants
• Decreased amoxapine effect: barbiturates
• Increased amoxapine level: cimetidine, fluoxetine, fluvoxamine, paroxetine, sertraline
• Increased hypertensive effect: clonidine, epinephrine, norepinephrine
• Hyperpyretic crisis, convulsions, hypertensive episode: MAOIs
⧸ Increased CNS depression: kava

⬥ = Nursing alert   ⧸ = Herb-drug interaction   ⊘ = Do not crush

🖋 May increase anticholinergic effects: belladonna leaf/root, henbane leaf

🖋 Increased action of amoxapine: scopolia root

Lab test interferences:
Increase: LFTs, blood glucose
Decrease: WBC, blood glucose

NURSING CONSIDERATIONS
Assess:
• B/P lying, standing; pulse q4h; if systolic B/P drops 20 mm Hg, hold drug, notify prescriber; take vital signs q4h in patients with cardiovascular disease
• Blood studies: CBC, leukocytes, differential, cardiac enzymes if patient is receiving long-term therapy
• Blood level: ther 20-100 ng/ml
• Hepatic studies: AST, ALT, bilirubin
• Weight qwk; appetite may increase with drug
• ECG for flattening of T wave, bundle branch block, AV block, dysrhythmias in cardiac patients
• EPS primarily in elderly: rigidity, dystonia, akathisia
• Mental status: mood, sensorium, affect, suicidal tendencies; increase in psychiatric symptoms: depression, panic; confusion (elderly)
• Urinary retention, constipation; constipation is more likely to occur in children, elderly
• Withdrawal symptoms: headache, nausea, vomiting, muscle pain, weakness; do not usually occur unless drug is discontinued abruptly
• Alcohol consumption; if alcohol is consumed, hold dose until morning

Administer:
PO
• Increased fluids, bulk in diet if constipation, urinary retention occur, especially in elderly
• Crushed if patient is unable to swallow medication whole, with food or milk for GI symptoms
• Dosage hs if oversedation occurs during day; may take entire dose hs; elderly may not tolerate once/day dosing

Perform/provide:
• Storage at room temperature; do not freeze
• Assistance with ambulation during beginning therapy, since drowsiness/dizziness occurs
• Safety measures including side rails primarily for elderly
• Check to see PO medication swallowed
• Gum, hard candy, or frequent sips of water for dry mouth

Evaluate:
• Therapeutic response: decreased depression, absence of suicidal thoughts

Teach patient/family:
• To take as directed, not to double dose
• That therapeutic effects may take 2-3 wk
• To use caution in driving or other activities requiring alertness because of drowsiness, dizziness, blurred vision
• To avoid alcohol ingestion, other CNS depressants
• Not to discontinue medication quickly after long-term use; may cause nausea, headache, malaise
• To wear sunscreen or large hat, since photosensitivity occurs

Treatment of overdose: ECG monitoring, induce emesis, lavage, activated charcoal, administer anticonvulsant

---

Side effects: *italics* = common; ***bold italics*** = life-threatening

amoxicillin (℞)

(a-mox-i-sill'in)
amoxicillin, Amoxil, Apo-moxi*, Novamoxin*, Nu-Amoxi*, Polymox, Trimox, Wymox

Func. class.: Broad-spectrum antiinfective

Chem. class.: Aminopenicillin

Action: Interferes with cell wall replication of susceptible organisms; the cell wall, rendered osmotically unstable, swells and bursts from osmotic pressure

Uses: For gram-positive cocci *(Staphylococcus aureus, Streptococcus pyogenes, Streptococcus faecalis, Streptococcus pneumoniae),* gram-negative cocci *(Neisseria gonorrhoeae, N. meningitidis),* gram-positive bacilli *(Corynebacterium diphtheriae, Listeria monocytogenes),* gram-negative bacilli *(Haemophilus influenzae, Escherichia coli, Proteus mirabilis, Salmonella);* in combination *Helicobacter pylori*

Investigational uses: Lyme disease, *Chlamydia trachomatis* in pregnancy

Dosage and routes:
Systemic infections
• *Adult:* PO 750 mg-1.5 g qd in divided doses q8h
• *Child:* PO 20-50 mg/kg/day in divided doses q8h
Renal disease
• CrCl 10-50 ml/min dose q12h; CrCl <10 ml/min dose q24h
Gonorrhea/urinary tract infections
• *Adult:* PO 3 g given with 1 g probenecid as a single dose
Chlamydia trachomatis
• *Adult:* PO 500 mg/day × 1 wk
Bacterial endocarditis prophylaxis
• *Child:* PO 50 mg/kg/hr before and 25 mg/kg 6 hr after procedure
Available forms: Caps 250, 500 mg; chew tabs 125, 250 mg; powder for oral susp 50 mg/ml, 125, 250 mg/5 ml

Side effects/adverse reactions:
HEMA: Anemia, increased bleeding time, ***bone marrow depression, granulocytopenia***
GI: Nausea, vomiting, diarrhea, increased AST, ALT, abdominal pain, glossitis, colitis, ***pseudomembranous colitis***
CNS: Headache
SYST: ***Anaphylaxis, respiratory distress,*** *serum sickness*
INTEG: Urticaria, rash

Contraindications: Hypersensitivity to penicillins

Precautions: Pregnancy (B), lactation, hypersensitivity to cephalosporins, neonates, renal disease

Pharmacokinetics:
PO: Peak 2 hr, duration 6-8 hr; half-life 1-1⅓ hr, metabolized in liver, excreted in urine, crosses placenta, enters breast milk

Interactions:
• Increased amoxicillin level: probenecid
• Decreased effectiveness of oral contraceptives
• Amoxicillin-induced skin rash: allopurinol
🌿 Delayed or reduced absorption: khat; separate by ≥2 hr

Lab test interferences:
False positive: Urine glucose, urine protein

NURSING CONSIDERATIONS
Assess:
• I&O ratio; report hematuria, oliguria, since penicillin in high doses is nephrotoxic
• Any patient with a compromised renal system, since drug is excreted slowly in poor renal system function; toxicity may occur rapidly
• Liver studies: AST, ALT
• Blood studies: WBC, RBC, Hgb and Hct, bleeding time

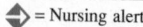

- Renal studies: urinalysis, protein, blood, BUN, creatinine
- Culture, sensitivity before drug therapy; drug may be given as soon as culture is taken
- Bowel pattern before, during treatment
- Skin eruptions after administration of penicillin to 1 wk after discontinuing drug
- Respiratory status: rate, character, wheezing, tightness in the chest
- Allergies before initiation of treatment, reaction of each medication; place allergies on chart in bright red

Administer:

PO

- After C&S completed
- Shake suspension well before each dose

Perform/provide:

- Adrenaline, suction, tracheostomy set, endotracheal intubation equipment on unit
- Adequate intake of fluids (2 L) during diarrhea episodes
- Scratch test to assess allergy after securing order from prescriber; usually done when penicillin is only drug of choice
- Storage in tight container; after reconstituting, oral suspension refrigerated for 2 wk or stored at room temperature for 1 wk

Evaluate:

- Therapeutic response: absence of fever, draining wounds

Teach patient/family:

- That caps may be opened and contents taken with fluids
- To take as prescribed, not to double dose
- All aspects of drug therapy: need to complete entire course of medication to ensure organism death (10-14 days); culture may be taken after completed course of medication

To report sore throat, fever, fatigue, diarrhea (may indicate superinfection or agranulocytopenia)
- That drug must be taken in equal intervals around the clock to maintain blood levels; take on empty stomach with a full glass of water
- To wear or carry a Medic Alert ID if allergic to penicillins

Treatment of anaphylaxis: Withdraw drug, maintain airway, administer epinephrine, aminophylline, O_2, IV corticosteroids

---

amoxicillin/clavulanate potassium (Ŗ)

(a-mox-i-sill'in)

Augmentin, Clavulin*

Func. class.: Broad-spectrum antiinfective

Chem. class.: Aminopenicillin β-lactamase inhibitor

Action: Interferes with cell wall replication of susceptible organisms; the cell wall, rendered osmotically unstable, swells and bursts from osmotic pressure; combination increases spectrum of activity against β-lactamase–resistant organisms

Uses: Sinus infections, pneumonia, otitis media, skin infection, UTI; effective for strains of *Escherichia coli, Proteus mirabilis, Haemophilus influenzae, Streptococcus faecalis, Streptococcus pneumoniae,* and some β-lactamase–producing organisms

Dosage and routes:

- *Adult:* **PO** 250-500 mg q8h or 500-875 mg q12h depending on severity of infection

Renal disease

- CrCl 10-30 ml/min dose q12h; CrCl <10 ml/min dose q24h

• *Child:* **PO** 20-40 mg/kg/day in divided doses q8h or 25-45 mg/kg/day in divided doses q12h

Available forms: Tabs 250, 500, 875 mg/125 mg clavulanate; chew tabs 125, 200, 250, 400 mg; powder for oral susp 125, 200, 250, 400 mg/5 ml

Side effects/adverse reactions:

HEMA: Anemia, ***bone marrow depression, granulocytopenia, leukopenia, eosinophilia,*** thrombocytopenic purpura

GI: Nausea, diarrhea, vomiting, increased AST, ALT, abdominal pain, glossitis, colitis, black tongue, ***pseudomembranous colitis***

GU: Oliguria, proteinuria, hematuria, *vaginitis, moniliasis,* ***glomerulonephritis***

CNS: Headache, fever

META: Hyperkalemia, hypokalemia, alkalosis, hypernatremia

INTEG: Rash, urticaria

Contraindications: Hypersensitivity to penicillins

Precautions: Pregnancy (B), lactation, hypersensitivity to cephalosporins; neonates, renal disease

Pharmacokinetics:

PO: Peak 2 hr, duration 6-8 hr; half-life 1-1⅓ hr, metabolized in liver, excreted in urine, crosses placenta, excreted in breast milk

Interactions:

• Increased amoxicillin levels: probenecid

• Decreased action of: oral contraceptives

• Amoxicillin-induced skin rash: allopurinol

🍃 Delayed/reduced absorption: khat; separate by ≥2 hr

Lab test interferences:

False positive: Urine glucose, urine protein

NURSING CONSIDERATIONS
Assess:

• I&O ratio; report hematuria, oliguria since penicillin in high doses is nephrotoxic

• Any patient with a compromised renal system since drug is excreted slowly in poor renal system function; toxicity may occur

• Liver studies: AST, ALT

• Blood studies: WBC, RBC, Hgb and Hct, bleeding time

• Renal studies: urinalysis, protein, blood, BUN, creatinine

• Culture, sensitivity before drug therapy; drug may be given as soon as culture is taken

• Bowel pattern before, during treatment

• Skin eruptions after administration of penicillin to 1 wk after discontinuing drug

• Respiratory status: rate, character, wheezing, tightness in chest

• Allergies before initiation of treatment, reaction of each medication; place allergies on chart in bright red

Administer:
PO

• After C&S completed

• Only as directed, 2 (250 mg tab) not equivalent to 1 (500 mg tab) due to strength of clavulanate

• Shake suspension well before each dose

Perform/provide:

• Adrenaline, suction, tracheostomy set, endotracheal intubation equipment on unit

• Adequate intake of fluids (2 L) during diarrhea episodes

• Scratch test to assess allergy after securing order from prescriber; usually done when penicillin is only drug of choice

• Storage refrigerated for 2 wk or room temperature for 1 wk

Evaluate:

• Therapeutic response: absence of fever, draining wounds

⬥ = Nursing alert   🍃 = Herb-drug interaction   🚫 = Do not crush

Teach patient/family:
• To take as prescribed, not to double dose
• All aspects of drug therapy: need to complete entire course of medication to ensure organism death (10-14 days); culture may be taken after completed course of medication
◆ To report sore throat, fever, fatigue (may indicate superinfection or agranulocytosis)
• That drug must be taken in equal intervals around the clock to maintain blood levels
• To wear or carry a Medic Alert ID if allergic to penicillins
• To notify nurse of diarrhea
Treatment of hypersensitivity: Withdraw drug, maintain airway, administer epinephrine, aminophylline, O_2, IV corticosteroids for anaphylaxis

---

amphetamine (℞)

(am-fet´a-meen)
amphetamine sulfate
Func. class.: Cerebral stimulant
Chem. class.: Amphetamine

Controlled Substance Schedule II
Action: Increases release of norepinephrine, dopamine in cerebral cortex to reticular activating system
Uses: Narcolepsy, exogenous obesity, attention deficit disorder
Dosage and routes:
Narcolepsy
• *Adult:* **PO** 5-60 mg qd in divided doses
• *Child >12 yr:* **PO** 10 mg qd increasing by 10 mg/day at weekly intervals
• *Child 6-12 yr:* **PO** 5 mg qd increasing by 5 mg/wk, max 60 mg/day

Attention deficit disorder
• *Child >6 yr:* **PO** 5 mg qd-bid increasing by 5 mg/day at weekly intervals
• *Child 3-6 yr:* **PO** 2.5 mg qd increasing by 2.5 mg/day at weekly intervals
Obesity
• *Adult:* **PO** 5-30 mg in divided doses 30-60 min before meals
Available forms: Tabs 5, 10 mg
Side effects/adverse reactions:
CNS: Hyperactivity, insomnia, restlessness, talkativeness, dizziness, headache, chills, stimulation, dysphoria, irritability, aggressiveness, tremor, dependence, addiction
GI: Nausea, vomiting, anorexia, dry mouth, diarrhea, constipation, weight loss, metallic taste, cramps
GU: Impotence, change in libido
CV: Palpitations, tachycardia, hypertension, dysrhythmias, decreased heart rate
INTEG: Urticaria
Contraindications: Hypersensitivity to sympathomimetic amines, hyperthyroidism, hypertension, glaucoma, severe arteriosclerosis, drug abuse, cardiovascular disease, anxiety, lactation
Precautions: Gilles de la Tourette's disorder, lactation, child <3 yr, pregnancy (C)
Pharmacokinetics:
PO: Onset 30 min, peak 1-3 hr, duration 4-20 hr, metabolized by liver, excreted by kidneys, crosses placenta, breast milk, half-life 10-30 hr
Interactions:
• Hypertensive crisis: MAOIs or within 14 days of MAOIs
• Increased effect of amphetamine: acetazolamide, antacids, caffeine
• Decreased antidiabetic requirement: insulin, oral antidiabetics
• Altered CNS effect: phenothiazines, haloperidol, tricyclics
• Decreased effect of amphetamine:

urinary acidifiers (ascorbic acid, ammonium chloride)

💊 May decrease amphetamine effect: kava

Lab test interferences:

Increase: Plasma corticosteroids

Interfere: Urinary steroid

NURSING CONSIDERATIONS

Assess:

• VS, B/P, since this drug may reverse antihypertensives; check patients with cardiac disease more often

• CBC, urinalysis, in diabetes: blood sugar, urine sugar; insulin changes may be required since eating will decrease

• Height; growth rate in children may be decreased

• Mental status: mood, sensorium, affect, stimulation, insomnia; aggressiveness may occur

• Physical dependency; should not be used for extended time; dose should be discontinued gradually

◆ Withdrawal symptoms: headache, nausea, vomiting, muscle pain, weakness

• Drug tolerance will develop after long-term use; dosage should not be increased if tolerance develops

Administer:

PO

• At least 6 hr before hs to avoid sleeplessness

• For obesity only if patient is on weight-reduction program that includes dietary changes, exercise; patient will develop tolerance, and weight loss won't occur without additional methods; give 30-60 min before meals

• Gum, hard candy, frequent sips of water for dry mouth

Evaluate:

• Therapeutic response: decreased activity in attention deficit disorder; absence of sleeping during day in narcolepsy; decrease in weight

Teach patient/family:

• Not to double dose; if dose is missed, take up to 6 hr before hs; that prescription cannot be refilled

• To decrease caffeine consumption (coffee, tea, cola, chocolate), which may increase irritability, stimulation

• To avoid OTC preparations unless approved by prescriber; to avoid alcohol ingestion

• To taper off drug over several weeks, or depression, increased sleeping, lethargy may occur

• To avoid hazardous activities until patient is stabilized on medication

• To get needed rest; patients will feel more tired at end of day

• That seizure threshold is decreased in patients with seizure disorders

Treatment of overdose: Administer fluids, hemodialysis, peritoneal dialysis, antihypertensives for increased B/P; ammonium Cl for increased excretion

---

amphotericin B deoxycholate
(am-foe-ter′i-sin)
Fungizone

amphotericin B cholesteryl
Amphotec

amphotericin B lipid complex
Abelcet

amphotericin B liposome
AmBisome

Func. class: Antifungal

Chem. class.: Amphoteric polyene

Action: Increases cell membrane permeability in susceptible organisms by binding sterols; decreases

---

◆ = Nursing alert   💊 = Herb-drug interaction   🚫 = Do not crush potassium, sodium, and nutrients in cell

Uses: Histoplasmosis, blastomycosis, coccidioidomycosis, cryptococcosis, aspergillosis, phycomycosis, candidiasis, sporotrichosis causing severe meningitis, septicemia, skin infections

Investigational uses: Candiduria (bladder irrigation)

Dosage and routes:

Deoxycholate

• *Adult:* IV Give test dose of 1 mg; then 0.25 mg/kg, increase qd slowly to 0.5 mg/kg, may give 1 mg/kg/day or 1.5 mg/kg qid

• *Child:* IV 0.25 mg/kg infused initially, increase by 0.25 mg/kg qod to max of 1 mg/kg/day

• *Adult/child:* **TOP** apply 2-4×daily

• *Adult/child:* **PO** 1 ml qid

Cholesteryl sulfate

• *Adult/child:* IV 3-4 mg/kg/day, max 6 mg/kg/day

Lipid complex

• *Adult/child:* IV 5 mg/kg/day

Liposome

• *Adult/child:* IV Fungal infections 3-5 mg/kg q24h

Visceral leishmaniasis 3-4 mg/kg q24h days 1-5, decrease dose

Available forms: Amphotericin deoxycholate inj 50 mg vial oral susp 100 mg/ml; *amphotericin B cholesteryl* powder for inj 50 mg/20 ml, 100 mg/50 ml; *amphotericin B lipid complex* susp for inj 100 mg/20 ml vial

Side effects/adverse reactions:

EENT: Tinnitus, deafness, diplopia, blurred vision

INTEG: Burning, irritation, pain, necrosis at injection site with extravasation, flushing, dermatitis, skin rash (topical route)

CNS: Headache, fever, chills, peripheral nerve pain, paresthesias, peripheral neuropathy, *convulsions,* dizziness

GU: Hypokalemia, azotemia, hyposthenuria, *renal tubular acidosis,* nephrocalcinosis, *permanent renal impairment, anuria, oliguria*

GI: Nausea, vomiting, anorexia, diarrhea, cramps, *hemorrhagic gastroenteritis, acute liver failure*

MS: Arthralgia, myalgia, generalized pain, weakness, weight loss

HEMA: Normochromic, normocytic anemia, *thrombocytopenia, agranulocytosis, leukopenia, eosinophilia,* hypokalemia, hyponatremia, hypomagnesemia

Contraindications: Hypersensitivity, severe bone marrow depression

Precautions: Renal disease, pregnancy (B), lactation

Pharmacokinetics:

IV: Peak 1-2 hr, initial half-life 24 hr, metabolized in liver, excreted in urine (metabolites), breast milk, highly bound to plasma proteins; penetrates poorly CSF, bronchial secretions, aqueous humor, muscle, bone

Interactions:

• Synergistic effect: flucytosine

• Increased nephrotoxicity: other nephrotoxic antibiotics (aminoglycosides, cisplatin, vancomycin, cyclosporine, polymyxin B)

• Increased hypokalemia: corticosteroids, digitalis, skeletal muscle relaxants, thiazides

• Antagonism: miconazole

🍇 Increased possibility of nephrotoxicity: gossypol

NURSING CONSIDERATIONS

Assess:

• VS q15-30min during first infusion; note changes in pulse, B/P

• I&O ratio; watch for decreasing urinary output, change in specific gravity; discontinue drug to prevent permanent damage to renal tubules

• Blood studies: CBC, K, Na, Ca, Mg q2wk, BUN, creatinine weekly

• Weight weekly; if weight increases over 2 lb/wk, edema is present; renal damage should be considered

◆ For renal toxicity: increasing BUN, serum creatinine; if BUN is >40 mg/dl or if serum creatinine >3 mg/dl, drug may be discontinued or dosage reduced

◆ For hepatotoxicity: increasing AST, ALT, alk phosphatase, bilirubin

• For allergic reaction: dermatitis, rash; drug should be discontinued, antihistamines (mild reaction) or epinephrine (severe reaction) administered

• For hypokalemia: anorexia, drowsiness, weakness, decreased reflexes, dizziness, increased urinary output, increased thirst, paresthesias

• For ototoxicity: tinnitus (ringing, roaring in ears) vertigo, loss of hearing (rare)

Administer:

• Do not confuse three different types

IV

• Drug only after C&S confirms organism, drug needed to treat condition; make sure drug is used in life-threatening infections

Deoxycholate

• After diluting 50 mg/10 ml sterile water (no preservatives) (5 mg-1 ml), shake, dilute with 500 ml of D_5W to concentration of 0.1 mg/ml

• Test dose of 1 mg/20 ml D_5W; give over 10-30 min

Intermittent IV inf

• IV using in-line filter (mean pore diameter >1 micron) using distal veins; check for extravasation, necrosis q8h; use an infusion pump; administer over 6 hr; rapid infusion may result in circulation collapse

Additive compatibilities: Fluconazole, heparin, hydrocortisone, sodium bicarbonate

Syringe compatibilities: Heparin

Y-site compatibilities: Aldesleukin, diltiazem, doxorubicin liposome, famotidine, remifentanil, tacrolimus, teniposide, thiotepa, zidovudine

Solution compatibilities: D_5W

Perform/provide:

• Acetaminophen and diphenhydramine 30 min prior to inf to reduce fever, chills, headache

• Storage protected from moisture and light; diluted solution is stable for 24 hr at room temperature

Evaluate:

• Therapeutic response: decreased fever, malaise, rash, negative C&S for infecting organism

Teach patient/family:

• That long-term therapy may be needed to clear infection (2 wk-3 mo depending on type of infection)

---

ampicillin (℞)

(am-pi-sill'in)

Amcill, Ampicin*, Apo-Ampi*, D-Amp*, NovoAmpicillin*, Nu- Ampi*, Omnipen, Omnipen-N, Penbriten*, Polycillin, Polycillin-N, Principen, Totacillin, Totacillin-N

Func. class.: Broad-spectrum antiinfective

Chem. class.: Aminopenicillin

Action: Interferes with cell wall replication of susceptible organisms; the cell wall, rendered osmotically unstable, swells, bursts from osmotic pressure

Uses: Effective for gram-positive cocci *(Staphylococcus aureus, Streptococcus pyogenes, Streptococcus faecalis, Streptococcus pneumoniae)*, gram-negative cocci *(Neisseria gonorrhoeae, N. meningitidis)*, gram-negative bacilli *(Haemophilus influenzae, Proteus mirabilis, Salmonella, Shigella, Lis-*

◆ = Nursing alert   ✹ = Herb-drug interaction   ⊘ = Do not crush *teria monocytogenes)*, gram-positive bacilli

Dosage and routes:

Systemic infections

• *Adult and child ≥40 kg (88 lbs):* **PO** 1-2 g qd in divided doses q6h; **IV/IM** 2-8 g qd in divided doses q4-6h

• *Child <40 kg:* **PO** 25-100 mg/kg/day in divided doses q6h; **IV/IM** 25-50 mg/kg/day in divided doses q8h

Renal disease

• CrCl 10-30 ml/min dose q6-12h; <10 ml/min dose q12h

Meningitis

• *Adult:* **IV** 8-14 g/day in divided doses q3-4h

• *Child:* **IV** 100-200 mg/kg/day in divided doses q3-4h

Gonorrhea

• *Adult and child ≥ 45 kg (99 lbs):* **PO** 3.5 g given with 1 g probenecid as a single dose

Available forms: Powder for inj 125, 250, 500 mg, 1, 2 g; IV inj 500 mg, 1, 2 g; caps 250, 500 mg; powder for oral susp 100 mg, 125, 250, 500 mg/5 ml

Side effects/adverse reactions:

INTEG: Rash, urticaria

HEMA: Anemia, increased bleeding time, ***bone marrow depression, granulocytopenia***

*GI: Nausea, vomiting, diarrhea, **pseudomembranous colitis***

GU: Oliguria, proteinuria, hematuria, *vaginitis, moniliasis, **glomerulonephritis***

CNS: Lethargy, hallucinations, anxiety, depression, twitching, ***coma, convulsions***

*MISC: **Anaphylaxis***

Contraindications: Hypersensitivity to penicillins

Precautions: Pregnancy (B), lactation; hypersensitivity to cephalosporins; neonates, renal disease

Pharmacokinetics:

PO: Peak 2 hr, duration 6-8 hr

IV: Peak 5 min

IM: Peak 1 hr

Half-life 50-110 min; metabolized in liver; excreted in urine, bile, breast milk; crosses placenta

Interactions:

• Increased ampicillin concentrations: probenecid

• Decreased effectiveness of oral contraceptives

• Increased ampicillin-induced skin rash: allopurinol

🖋 Delayed/reduced absorption: khat; separate by ≥2 hr

Lab test interferences:

False positive: Urine glucose, urine protein

NURSING CONSIDERATIONS

Assess:

• I&O ratio; report hematuria, oliguria, since penicillin in high doses is nephrotoxic

◆ Any patient with compromised renal system, since drug is excreted slowly in poor renal system function; toxicity may occur

• Liver studies: AST, ALT

• Blood studies: WBC, RBC, Hgb and Hct, bleeding time

• Renal studies: urinalysis, protein, blood, BUN, creatinine

• Culture, sensitivity before drug therapy; drug may be taken as soon as culture is taken

• Bowel pattern before, during treatment

• Skin eruptions after administration of penicillin to 1 wk after discontinuing drug

• Respiratory status: rate, character, wheezing, tightness in chest

• Allergies before initiation of treatment; reaction of each medication; place allergies on chart in bright red

Administer:

PO

• On empty stomach for best absorption (1-2 hr ac or 2-3 hr pc)

• Shake suspension well before each dose

IV

• After diluting with sterile H_2O 0.9-1.2 ml/125 mg drug, administer over 3-5 min (up to 500 mg), 10-15 min (>500 mg) by direct IV; may be diluted in 50 ml or more of D_5W, D_5 ½ NaCl to a concentration of 30 mg/ml or less; IV sol is stable for 1 hr; give at prescribed rate

• After C&S completed

Additive compatibilities: Cefotiam, clindamycin, erythromycin, floxacillin, furosemide

Syringe compatibilities: Chloramphenicol, colistimethate, diatrizoate, heparin, iohexol, iopamidol, iothalamate, ioxaglate, procaine

Y-site compatibilities: Acyclovir, allopurinol, amifostine, aztreonam, cyclophosphamide, doxorubicin liposome, enalaprilat, esmolol, famotidine, filgrastim, fludarabine, foscarnet, granisetron, heparin, insulin (regular), labetalol, magnesium sulfate, melphalan, meperidine, morphine, multivitamins, oflaxacin, perphenazine, phytonadione, potassium chloride, propofol, remifentanil, tacrolimus, teniposide, theophylline, thiotepa, tolazoline, vit B/C

Perform/provide:

• Adrenaline, suction, tracheostomy set, endotracheal intubation equipment on unit

• Adequate intake of fluids (2 L) during diarrhea episodes

• Scratch test to assess allergy after securing order from prescriber; usually done when penicillin is only drug of choice

• Storage in tight container; after reconstituting, oral suspension refrigerated for 2 wk or stored at room temperature for 1 wk

Evaluate:

• Therapeutic response: absence of temperature, draining wounds

Teach patient/family:

• That tabs may be crushed; caps may be opened and mixed with water

• To take oral ampicillin on empty stomach with full glass of water

• All aspects of drug therapy: need to complete entire course of medication to ensure organism death (10-14 days); culture may be taken after completed course of medication

◆ To report sore throat, fever, fatigue, diarrhea (may indicate superinfection); report rash or other signs of allergy

• That drug must be taken in equal intervals around the clock to maintain blood levels

• To wear or carry a Medic Alert ID if allergic to penicillins

Treatment of anaphylaxis: Withdraw drug, maintain airway, administer epinephrine, aminophylline, O_2, IV corticosteroids

---

ampicillin, sulbactam (℞)

Unasyn

Func. class.: Broad-spectrum antiinfective

Chem. class.: Aminopenicillin with β-lactamase inhibitor

Action: Interferes with cell wall replication of susceptible organisms; the cell wall, rendered osmotically unstable, swells, bursts from osmotic pressure; combination extends spectrum of activity by β-lactamase inhibition

---

◆ = Nursing alert   🌿 = Herb-drug interaction   🚫 = Do not crush

Uses: Skin infections, pneumonia (*Staphylococcus aureus, Escherichia coli, Klebsiella, Proteus mirabilis, Bacteroides fragilis, Haemophilus influenzae, Enterobacter, Acinetobacter calcoaceticus*), intraabdominal infections (*Enterobacter, Klebsiella, Bacteroides, E. coli*), gynecologic infections (*E. coli, Bacteroides*), meningitis, septicemia

Dosage and routes:
• *Adult:* IV 1 g ampicillin, 0.5 g sulbactam to 2 g ampicillin and 1 g sulbactam q6h, not to exceed 4 g/day sulbactam

Renal disease
• CrCl 15-29 ml/min dose q12h; CrCl 5-14 ml/min dose q24h
• *Child:* IV 100-200 mg/kg/day (ampicillin component) divided q6h

Available forms: Powder for inj 1.5 g (1 g ampicillin, 0.5 g sulbactam), 3 g (2 g ampicillin, 1 g sulbactam), 10 g (10 g ampicillin, 5 g sulbactam)

Side effects/adverse reactions:
HEMA: Anemia, increased bleeding time, ***bone marrow depression, granulocytopenia***
GI: *Nausea, vomiting, diarrhea,* increased AST, ALT, abdominal pain, glossitis, colitis, ***pseudomembranous colitis***
GU: Oliguria, proteinuria, hematuria, *vaginitis, moniliasis,* ***glomerulonephritis***
CNS: Lethargy, hallucinations, anxiety, depression, twitching, ***coma, convulsions***
MISC: ***Anaphylaxis***

Contraindications: Hypersensitivity to penicillins

Precautions: Pregnancy (B), lactation, hypersensitivity to cephalosporins, neonates, renal disease

Pharmacokinetics:
IV: Peak 5 min; half-life 50-110 min; little metabolized in liver, 75% to 85% of both drugs excreted in urine, diffuses to breast milk, crosses placenta

Interactions:
• Decreased oral contraceptive effect
• Increased ampicillin level: probenecid
• Ampicillin-induced skin rash: allopurinol
🍃 Delayed/reduced absorption: khat; separate by ≥2 hr

Lab test interferences:
False positive: Urine glucose, urine protein

NURSING CONSIDERATIONS
Assess:
• Bowel pattern before, during treatment
• Respiratory status: rate, character, wheezing, tightness in chest
• I&O ratio; report hematuria, oliguria, since penicillin in high doses is nephrotoxic
◆ Any patient with compromised renal system, since drug is excreted slowly in poor renal system function; toxicity may occur rapidly
• Liver studies: AST, ALT if on longterm therapy
• Blood studies: WBC, RBC, Hct, Hgb, bleeding time
• Renal studies: urinalysis, protein, blood, BUN, creatinine
• C&S before drug therapy; drug may be given as soon as culture is taken
• Skin eruptions after administration of ampicillin to 1 wk after discontinuing drug
• Allergies before initiation of treatment; reaction of each medication; report allergies on chart in bright red

Administer:

Side effects: *italics* = common; ***bold italics*** = life-threatening

IV

• After diluting 1.5 g/4 ml or more sterile H_2O for inj (375 mg/ml); allow to stand until foaming stops; dilute further in 50 ml or more of D_5W, NaCl, administer within 1 hr after reconstitution; give as an intermittent inf over 15-30 min

Additive compatibilities: Aztreonam

Y-site compatibilities: Amifostine, aztreonam, cefepime, enalaprilat, famotidine, filgrastim, fluconazole, fludarabine, gallium, granisetron, heparin, insulin (regular), meperidine, morphine, paclitaxel, remifentanil, tacrolimus, teniposide, theophylline, thiotepa

Perform/provide:

• Adrenaline, suction, tracheostomy set, endotracheal intubation equipment on unit for possible anaphylaxis

• Adequate intake of fluids (2 L) during diarrhea episodes

• Scratch test to assess allergy after securing order from prescriber; usually done when penicillin is only drug choice

• Storage in tight container, out of light

Evaluate:

• Therapeutic response: absence of fever, draining wounds, negative C&S

Teach patient/family:

• To report sore throat, fever, fatigue, persistent diarrhea (may indicate superinfection)

• To wear or carry Medic Alert ID if allergic to penicillin products

Treatment of anaphylaxis: Withdraw drug, maintain airway, administer epinephrine, aminophylline, O_2, IV corticosteroids

---

amprenavir

See appendix a—selected new drugs

---

amrinone (℞)

(am′ri-none)

Inocor

Func. class.: Cardiac inotropic agent

Chem. class.: Bipyrimidine derivative

Action: Positive inotropic agent with vasodilator properties; reduces preload and afterload by direct relaxation of vascular smooth muscle, increases cardiac output

Uses: Short-term management of CHF that has not responded to other medication; can be used with digitalis

Dosage and routes:

• *Adult and child:* **IV BOL** 0.75 mg/kg given over 2-3 min; start inf of 5-10 µg/kg/min; may give another bol 30 min after start of therapy, not to exceed 10 mg/kg total daily dose

Available forms: Inj 5 mg/ml

Side effects/adverse reactions:

HEMA: Thrombocytopenia

CV: Dysrhythmias, hypotension, headache, chest pain

GI: Nausea, vomiting, anorexia, abdominal pain, *hepatotoxicity (rare), ascites,* jaundice, hiccups

INTEG: Allergic reactions, burning at injection site

HEMA: Thrombocytopenia

RESP: Pleuritis, *pulmonary densities, hypoxemia*

Contraindications: Hypersensitivity to this drug or bisulfites, severe aortic disease, severe pulmonic valvular disease, acute MI

Precautions: Lactation, pregnancy

◆ = Nursing alert　　🖉 = Herb-drug interaction　　🚫 = Do not crush

(C), children, renal disease, hepatic disease, atrial flutter/fibrillation, elderly

Pharmacokinetics:

IV: Onset 2-5 min, peak 10 min, duration variable; half-life 4-6 hr, metabolized in liver, excreted in urine as drug and metabolites 60%-90%

Interactions:

• Excessive hypotension: antihypertensives, disopyramide

• Additive effect: cardiac glycosides

🖉 Possible increased action of amrinone: cascara sagrada bark, aloe, buckthorn bark/berry, ephedra, senna pod/leaf

Lab test interferences:

Decrease: Serum K

Increase: Hepatic enzymes

NURSING CONSIDERATIONS

Assess:

• B/P and pulse q5min during infusion; if B/P drops 30 mm Hg, stop infusion and call prescriber

• Electrolytes: K, S, Cl, Ca; renal function studies: BUN, creatinine; blood studies: platelet count; monitor fluid status (CVP) in elderly

• ALT, AST, bilirubin daily

• I&O ratio and weight qd; diuresis should increase with continuing therapy

◆ If platelets are <150,000/mm^3, drug is usually discontinued and another drug started

• Extravasation; change site q48h

Administer:

• Do not mix directly with glucose solutions; chemical reaction occurs over 24 hr; precipitate forms if amrinone and furosemide come in contact

• Into running dextrose infusion through Y-connector or directly into tubing; may give undiluted over 2-3 min or dilute with NS to 1-3 mg/ml, run at prescribed rate

• By infusion pump for doses other than bolus

• Potassium supplements if ordered for potassium levels <3.0

Syringe compatibilities: Propranolol, verapamil

Y-site compatibilities: Aminophylline, atropine, bretylium, calcium chloride, cimetidine, cisatracurium, digoxin, dobutamine, dopamine, epinephrine, famotidine, hydrocortisone, isoproterenol, lidocaine, metaraminol, methylprednisolone, nitroglycerin, nitroprusside, norepinephrine, phenylephrine, potassium chloride, propofol, propranolol, remifentanil, verapamil

Evaluate:

• Therapeutic response: increased cardiac output, decreased PCWP, adequate CVP, decreased dyspnea, fatigue, edema, ECG

Teach patient/family:

• That burning may occur at IV site

• To report adverse reactions promptly

Treatment of overdose: Discontinue drug, support circulation

---

anagrelide (℞)

(a-na′gre-lide)

Agrylin

Func. class.: Antiplatelet

Chem. class.: Imidazo-quinazolinone

Action: Reduces platelet count and prevents early platelet shape changes in response to aggregating agents thus inhibiting platelet aggregation

Uses: Essential thrombocythemia, polycythemia vera, chronic myelogenous leukemia

Dosage and routes:
• *Adult:* **PO** 0.5 mg qid or 1 mg bid, may be adjusted after 1 wk, max 10 mg/day or 2.5 mg single dose
Available forms: Caps 0.5, 1.0 mg
Side effects/adverse reactions:
CV: Postural hypotension, tachycardia, palpitations, ***CHF, MI, cardiomyopathy, cardiomegaly, complete heart block, atrial fibrillation,*** dysrhythmia
CNS: Headache, dizziness, *seizures*
INTEG: Rash
*HEMA: **Anemia, thrombocytopenia, ecchymosis, lymphadenoma***
Contraindications: Hypersensitivity, hypotension
Precautions: Pregnancy (C), lactation
Pharmacokinetics:
PO: Peak 1 hr, duration >24 hr: metabolized in liver: excreted in feces/urine
Interactions:
• Decreased absorption: sucralfate
• Drug/food: decreased bioavailability
NURSING CONSIDERATIONS
Assess:
• B/P, pulse during treatment until stable; take B/P lying, standing; orthostatic hypotension is common
• Cardiac status: chest pain, what aggravates or ameliorates condition
Administer:
• On an empty stomach: 1 hr before meals or 2 hr after; give with 8 oz water for better absorption
Perform/provide:
• Storage at room temperature
Evaluate:
• Therapeutic response: increased platelet count
Teach patient/family:
• That medication is not a cure: may have to be taken continuously in evenly spaced doses only as directed
• That it is necessary to quit smoking to prevent excessive vasoconstriction
• To avoid hazardous activities until stabilized on medication; dizziness may occur
• To rise slowly from sitting or lying to prevent orthostatic hypotension
• Not to use alcohol or OTC medications unless approved by prescriber
• To report cardiac reactions, increased bruising, bleeding
• To use contraception (female, child-bearing age)

---

anastrozole
(an-a-stroh′zole)
Arimidex
Func. class.: Antineoplastic
Chem. class.: Aromatase inhibitor

Action: Lowers serum estradiol concentrations; many breast cancers have strong estrogen receptors
Uses: Advanced breast carcinoma not responsive to other therapy in estrogen-receptor-positive patients (usually postmenopausal)
Dosage and routes:
• *Adult:* **PO** 1 mg qd
Available forms: Tabs 1 mg
Side effects/adverse reactions:
*HEMA: **Leukopenia***
GI: Nausea, vomiting, altered taste (anorexia), diarrhea, constipation, abdominal pain, dry mouth
GU: Vaginal bleeding, pruritus vulvae, UTI
INTEG: Rash, alopecia
CV: Chest pain, hypertension, thrombophlebitis
CNS: Hot flashes, headache, lightheadedness, depression, dizziness, confusion, insomnia, anxiety
RESP: Cough, sinusitis
MS: Bone pain, myalgia

⬥ = Nursing alert   🌿 = Herb-drug interaction   ⊘ = Do not crush

Contraindications: Hypersensitivity, pregnancy (D)

Precautions: Leukopenia, thrombocytopenia, lactation, children, elderly, liver disease, renal disease

Pharmacokinetics:

PO: Peak 4-7 hr, half-life 50 hr, excreted in feces, urine

Lab test interferences:

Increase: GGT, AST, ALT, alk phosphatase, cholesterol, LDL

NURSING CONSIDERATIONS

Assess:

• CBC, differential, platelet count qwk; withhold drug if WBC is <3500/mm³ or platelet count is <100,000/mm³; notify prescriber

• Bleeding: hematuria, guaiac, bruising, petechiae, mucosa or orifices q8h

• Effects of alopecia on body image; discuss feelings about body changes

• Symptoms indicating severe allergic reactions: rash, pruritus, urticaria, purpuric skin lesions, itching, flushing

Administer:

PO

• Antiemetic 30-60 min before giving drug to prevent vomiting

Perform/provide:

• Storage in light-resistant container at room temp

Evaluate:

• Therapeutic response: decreased tumor size, spread of malignancy

Teach patient/family:

• To report any complaints, side effects to prescriber

• That vaginal bleeding, pruritus, hot flashes are reversible after discontinuing treatment

• To report vaginal bleeding immediately

• That tumor flare—increase in size of tumor, increased bone pain—may occur and will subside rapidly; may take analgesics for pain

• That hair may be lost during treatment; a wig or hairpiece may make patient feel better; new hair may be different in color, texture

---

anistreplase (℞)

(ah-nis'tre-place)

anisoylated plasminogen, APSAC, Eminase

Func. class.: Thrombolytic enzyme

Chem. class.: Anisoylated plasminogen streptokinase activator complex

---

Action: Promotes thrombolysis by promoting conversion of plasminogen to plasmin

Uses: Acute MI for lysis of coronary artery thrombi

Dosage and routes:

• *Adult:* **IV INJ** 30 U over 2-5 min as soon as possible after onset of symptoms

Available forms: Powder, lyophilized 30 U/vial

Side effects/adverse reactions:

HEMA: Decreased Hct; *GI, GU, intracranial, retroperitoneal,* surface bleeding; *thrombocytopenia*

INTEG: Rash, urticaria, phlebitis at inj site, itching, flushing

CNS: Headache, fever, sweating, agitation, dizziness, paresthesia, tremor, vertigo

GI: Nausea, vomiting

RESP: Altered respirations, dyspnea, *bronchospasm, lung edema*

MS: Low back pain, arthralgia

CV: Hypotension, *dysrhythmias,* conduction disorders

SYST: *Anaphylaxis (rare)*

Contraindications: Hypersensitivity, active internal bleeding, intraspinal or intracranial surgery, neoplasms of CNS, severe hypertension, cerebral embolism/thrombosis/

---

hemorrhage, hypersensitivity to this drug or streptokinase

Precautions: Arterial emboli from left side of heart, pregnancy (C), ulcerative colitis/enteritis, renal disease, hepatic disease, hypocoagulation, COPD, subacute bacterial endocarditis, rheumatic valvular disease, intraarterial diagnostic procedure or surgery (10 days), recent major surgery, lactation

Pharmacokinetics: Half-life 105 min

Interactions:

• Increased bleeding potential: aspirin, indomethacin, phenylbutazone, anticoagulants, dipyridamole

🌿 Increased risk of bleeding: bromelain

Lab test interferences:

Increase: PT, APTT, TT

Decrease: Fibrinogen, plasminogen

NURSING CONSIDERATIONS

Assess:

• VS, B/P, pulse, respirations, neurologic signs, temperature at least q4h, temp >104° F (40° C) or indicators of internal bleeding, cardiac rhythm after intracoronary administration; monitor ECG, treat bradycardia, ventricular changes

• Allergy: fever, rash, itching, chills; mild reaction may be treated with antihistamines

◆ Bleeding during first hr of treatment (hematuria, hematemesis, bleeding from mucous membranes, epistaxis, ecchymosis), continue to monitor for 24 hr after treatment

• Blood studies (Hct, platelets, PTT, PT, TT, APTT) before starting therapy; PT or APTT must be less than 2 × control before starting therapy; TT or PT q3-4h during treatment

Administer:

IV, direct

• Reconstitute single-dose vial/5 ml sterile water for injection (not bac-

teriostatic water), and roll (not shake) to enhance reconstitution; give over 2-5 min by direct IV, give within ½ hr of reconstitution or discard, do not add other meds to vial or syringe; give within 6 hr of thrombi identification for best results

• Cryoprecipitate or fresh frozen plasma if bleeding occurs

• Heparin therapy after thrombolytic therapy is discontinued, TT or APTT less than 2 × control (about 3-4 hr)

• About 10% of patients have high streptococcal antibody titers, requiring increased loading doses

Perform/provide:

• Bed rest during entire course of treatment; handle patient as little as possible during therapy

• Storage of powder in refrigerator; use within 30 min after reconstitution

• Avoid invasive procedures: inj, rectal temperature

• Treat fever with acetaminophen

• Pressure of 30 sec to minor bleeding sites, 30 min to sites of arterial puncture followed by dressing; inform prescriber if hemostasis not attained; apply pressure dressing

Evaluate:

• Therapeutic response: absence of thrombi formation in MI, improved ventricular function

---

◆ = Nursing alert   *🌿* = Herb-drug interaction   ⊘ = Do not crush

antihemophilic factor (AHF) (℞)

(an-tee-hee-moe-fill'ik)
antihemophilic factor,
Alphanate, Helixate, Hemofil M, Humate-P, Koate H.P., Kogenate, Monoclate-P, Recombinate

Func. class.: Hemostatic
Chem. class.: Factor VIII

Action: Necessary for clotting; activates factor X in conjunction with activated factor IX; transforms prothrombin to thrombin

Uses: Hemophilia A, patients with acquired circulating factor VIII inhibitors, factor VIII deficiency

Dosage and routes:
Massive hemorrhage
• *Adult and child:* **IV** 40-50 U/kg, then 20-25 U/kg q8-12h

Overt bleeding
• *Adult and child:* **IV** 15-25 U/kg, then 8-15 U/kg q8-12h × 4 days

Hemorrhage near vital organs
• *Adult and child:* **IV** 15 U/kg, then 8 U/kg q8h × 2 days, then 4 U/kg q8h × 2 days

Minor hemorrhage
• *Adult and child:* **IV** 8-10 U/kg/q24h × 2-3 days or 8 U/kg q12h × 2 days, then q24h × 2 days

Joint bleeding
• *Adult and child:* **IV** 5-10 U/kg q8-12h × 1-2 days

Available forms: Inj 250, 500, 1000, 1500 U/vial (number of units noted on label)

Side effects/adverse reactions:
GI: Nausea, vomiting, abdominal cramps, jaundice, ***viral hepatitis***
INTEG: Rash, flushing, *urticaria,* stinging at injection site
CNS: Headache, *lethargy, chills, fever, flushing*
HEMA: ***Thrombosis, hemolysis, risk of hepatitis B, HIV***
CV: Hypotension, tachycardia
RESP: ***Bronchospasm***
MISC: ***Anaphylaxis***

Contraindications: Hypersensitivity, monoclonal antibody-derived factor VIII

Precautions: Neonates/infants, hepatic disease; blood types A, B, AB; pregnancy (C), factor VIII inhibitor

Pharmacokinetics:
IV: Half-life 4 hr, terminal 15 hr

Interactions:
• Do not admix with other drugs

NURSING CONSIDERATIONS
Assess:
• Blood studies (coagulation factors assay by % normal: 5% prevents spontaneous hemorrhage, 30%-50% for surgery, 80%-100% for severe hemorrhage)
• I&O, urine color; notify prescriber if urine becomes orange, red
• Pulse: discontinue infusion if significant increase
• Hct, Coombs' test with blood types A, B, AB
• Test for factor VIII inhibitors before starting treatment, may require concomitant antiinhibitor coagulant complex therapy
• Allergy: fever, rash, itching, jaundice; give diphenhydramine HCl (Benadryl), continue therapy if reaction is mild
• Blood group of patient, donors (if applicable; most factor VIII not from specific blood group donors)
◆ Bleeding: ankles, knees, elbows, other joints

Administer:
IV
• After rotating gently to mix
• Using plastic syringe to reconstitute, and administer; adheres to glass; use another needle as a vent when reconstituting

• After dilution with warm NS, D₅W, LR, give within 3 hr

IV infusion

• Give at ≤2 ml/min if concentration exceeds 34 U/ml or over 3 min if concentration is less than 34 U/ml

Perform/provide:

• Storage in refrigerator; do not freeze; after reconstitution, do not refrigerate; give within 3 hr

Evaluate:

• Therapeutic response: absence of bleeding

Teach patient/family:

• To report any signs of bleeding: gums, under skin, urine, stools, emesis; review methods to prevent bleeding

• To avoid salicylates (increase bleeding tendencies)

• To prepare, administer factor VIII concentrates at first sign of danger

• To advise health professionals of treatment for hemophilia

• The signs of viral hepatitis, AIDS

• That immunization for hepatitis B may be given first

• To report hives, urticaria, chest tightness, hypotension; may be monoclonal antibody-derived factor VIII

• To be checked q2-3mo for HIV screen

• To carry ID describing disease process

---

antithrombin III, human (℞)

(an'tee-throm-bin)
ATnativ, Thrombate III
Func. class.: Antithrombin
Chem. class.: Pooled human plasma

Action: Inactivates thrombin and the activated forms of factors IX, X, XI, XII, resulting in inhibition of coagulation

Uses: Hereditary antithrombin III deficiency in connection with surgical or obstetric procedures or for thromboembolism

Dosage and routes: Dosage is individualized; after first dose, antithrombin III level should increase to about 120% of normal; thereafter maintain at levels >80%; this is usually achieved by administering maintenance doses q24h

Available forms: Lyophilized powder, 50 ml infusion bottles containing 500 IU antithrombin III with 10 ml sterile water for injection

Side effects/adverse reactions:

*SYST: **Bleeding,** surface bleeding, **anaphylaxis,** vasodilatory effects*

Precautions: Pregnancy (C), lactation, children

Pharmacokinetics: Unknown

Interactions:

• Increased anticoagulant effect: heparin, aspirin

• Do not administer with other drugs in syringe or solutions

NURSING CONSIDERATIONS

Assess:

• AT-III levels bid until stabilized, then qd before dose

• VS, B/P, pulse, respirations, neurologic signs, temperature at least q4h, temperature 104° F (40° C) or indicators of internal bleeding, cardiac rhythm

◆ For child born of parents with hereditary AT-III deficiency, obtain AT-III levels immediately after birth

◆ For neurologic changes that may indicate intracranial bleeding

◆ Retroperitoneal bleeding: back pain, leg weakness, diminished pulses

Administer:

• Heparin after fibrinogen level is over 100 mg/dl; heparin infusion to

---

◆ = Nursing alert   ✍ = Herb-drug interaction   ⊘ = Do not crush increase PTT to 1.5-2 × baseline for 3-7 days

IV

• After reconstituting 500 IU/10 ml of NS or D₅W; do not shake; rotate to dissolve; allow to warm to room temperature; use within 3 hr of reconstitution; give 50 IU or less/min; do not exceed 100 IU/min using 0.22 or 0.45 microfilter

Perform/provide:

• Bed rest during entire course of treatment

• Avoidance of venous or arterial puncture, inj, rectal temperature

• Treatment of fever with acetaminophen or aspirin

Evaluate:

• Therapeutic response: absence of thrombi formation

Teach patient/family:

• About drug use and expected results; to report adverse reactions

---

anti-thymocyte

See lymphocyte immune globulin in appendix a—selected new drugs

---

ardeparin (R)

(are-de-pear'in)

Normiflo

Func. class.: Anticoagulant

Chem. class.: Low-molecular-weight heparin

Action: Prevents conversion of fibrinogen to fibrin and prothrombin to thrombin by enhancing inhibitory effects of antithrombin III

Uses: Prevention of deep vein thrombosis after knee replacement surgery

Dosage and routes:

• *Adult:* **SC** 50 antifactor XaU/kg q12h the evening of the day of knee replacement surgery or the follow-

ing AM continued until patient is fully ambulatory or 2 wk, whichever is first

Available forms: Inj 5,000, 10,000 anti XaU/0.5 ml

Side effects/adverse reactions:

CNS: **Intracranial bleeding,** fever

SYST: Hypersensitivity, **hemorrhage, anaphylaxis** possible

HEMA: **Thrombocytopenia,** anemia

INTEG: Pruritus, superficial wound infection, ecchymosis, rash

Contraindications: Hypersensitivity to this drug, pork products, heparin, or other anticoagulants; hemophilia, leukemia with bleeding, thrombocytopenic purpura, cerebrovascular hemorrhage, cerebral aneurysm, severe hypertension, other severe cardiac disease

Precautions: Elderly, pregnancy (C), hepatic disease, severe renal disease, blood dyscrasias, subacute bacterial endocarditis, acute nephritis, lactation, child, recent childbirth, peptic ulcer disease, pericarditis, pericardial effusion, recent lumbar puncture, vasculitis, other diseases where bleeding is possible

Pharmacokinetics: Unknown

Interactions:

• Increased risk of bleeding: aspiration, oral anticoagulants, platelet inhibitors, NSAIDs

🖋 May increase risk of bleeding: bromelain, cinchona bark

NURSING CONSIDERATIONS

Assess:

• For blood studies (Hct, occult blood in stools, CBC, platelets, urinalysis) during treatment since bleeding can occur

◆For bleeding gums, petechiae, ecchymosis, black tarry stools, hematuria, epistaxis, decrease in Hct, B/P; may indicate bleeding, possible hemorrhage; notify prescriber immediately, drug should be discontinued, protamine should be = to dose of

---

Side effects: *italics* = common; **bold italics** = life-threatening

drug given; 1 mg protamine = 100 anti-Xa U of drug

• For hypersensitivity: fever, skin rash, urticaria; notify prescriber immediately

Administer:

• By SC only; have patient sit or lie down; SC inj may be around the navel in a ∪-shape, upper outer side of thigh or upper outer quadrangle of the buttocks; rotate inj sites

• Changing needles is not recommended

Evaluate:

• Therapeutic response: absence of deep-vein thrombosis

Teach patient/family:

• To avoid OTC preparations that may cause serious drug interactions unless directed by prescriber; may contain aspirin; other anticoagulants, NSAIDs

• To use soft-bristle toothbrush to avoid bleeding gums, avoid contact sports, use electric razor, avoid IM injection

• To report any signs of bleeding: gums, under skin, urine, stools; unusual bruising, hematoma at inj site

Treatment of overdose: Protamine sulfate 1% given IV

---

ascorbic acid
(vit C) (OTC, ℞)
(a-skor′bic)

ascorbic acid, Ascorbicap, Cebid, Cecon, Cenolate, Cetane, Cevalin, Cevi-Bid, Ce-Vi-Sol, C-Span, Dull-C, Flavorcee, Mega-C/A Plus, Ortho/CS, Redoxon*, Vita-C

Func. class.: Vit C—water-soluble vitamin

Action: Needed for wound healing, collagen synthesis, antioxidant, carbohydrate metabolism

Uses: Vit C deficiency, scurvy, delayed wound and bone healing, chronic disease, urine acidification, before gastrectomy

Investigational uses: Acidification of urine, common cold prevention

Dosage and routes:

RDA

Neonates and up to 6 mo: 30 mg

Infants 6 mo-1 yr: 35 mg

Child 1-3 yr: 40 mg

Child 4-10 yr: 45 mg

Child 11-14 yr: 50 mg

Adult and child ≥ 15 yr: 60 mg

Pregnancy: 70 mg

Lactation: 90 mg

Scurvy

• *Adult:* **PO/SC/IM/IV** 100 mg-500 mg qd, then 50 mg or more qd

• *Child:* **PO/SC/IM/IV** 100-300 mg qd, then 35 mg or more qd

Wound healing/chronic disease/ fracture

• *Adult:* **SC/IM/IV/PO** 200-500 mg qd

• *Child:* **SC/IM/IV/PO** 100-200 mg added doses

Urine acidification

• *Adult:* 4-12 g qd in divided doses

• *Child:* 500 mg q6-8h

Available forms: Tabs 25, 50, 100, 250, 500, 1000, 1500 mg; tabs effervescent 1000 mg; tabs chewable 100, 250, 500 mg; tabs timed release 500, 750, 1000, 1500 mg; caps timed release 500 mg; crys 4 g/tsp; powd 4 g/tsp; liq 35 mg/0.6 ml; sol 100 mg/ml; syr 20 mg/ml, 500 mg/5 ml; inj SC, IM, IV 100, 250, 500 mg/ml

Side effects/adverse reactions:

CNS: Headache, insomnia, dizziness, fatigue, flushing

GI: Nausea, vomiting, diarrhea, anorexia, heartburn, cramps

GU: Polyuria, urine acidification, oxalate or urate renal stones

HEMA: **Hemolytic anemia in patients with G6PD**

Contraindications: None significant

Precautions: Gout, pregnancy (C); diabetes, renal calculi (large doses)

Pharmacokinetics:

PO, INJ: Metabolized in liver, unused amounts excreted in urine (unchanged) and metabolites, crosses placenta, breast milk

Interactions:

• Increased effects of salicylates, oral contraceptives, estrogens, oral iron
• Increased side effects of PAS, digitalis, sulfonamides
• Decreased effects of heparin, warfarin (massive doses)

Lab test interferences:

False positive: Negatives in glucose tests

False negative: Occult blood

NURSING CONSIDERATIONS

Assess:

• I&O ratio
• Ascorbic acid levels throughout treatment if continued deficiency is suspected
• Nutritional status: citrus fruits, vegetables
• Injection sites for inflammation

Administer:

IV, direct

• Undiluted by direct IV 100 mg over at least 1 min, rapid inf may cause fainting

Intermittent IV inf

• Diluted with D₅W, D₅NaCl, NS, LR, Ringer's, sodium lactate and given over 15 min

Additive compatibilities: Amikacin, calcium chloride, calcium gluceptate, calcium gluconate, cephalothin, chloramphenicol, chlorpromazine, colistimethate, cyanocobalamin, diphenhydramine, heparin, kanamycin, methicillin, methyldopa, penicillin G potassium, polymyxin B, prednisolone, procaine, prochlorperazine, promethazine, verapamil

Syringe compatibilities: Metoclopramide

Y-site compatibilities: Warfarin

Evaluate:

• Therapeutic response: absence of anorexia, irritability, pallor, joint pain, hyperkeratosis, petechiae, poor wound healing

Teach patient/family:

🚫 Do not break, crush, or chew ext rel tab

• That caps may be opened and contents mixed with jelly
• The necessary foods in diet
• That if oral contraceptives are taken, increased levels of vit C are needed
• That smoking decreases vit C levels, not to exceed prescribed dose; increases will be excreted in urine, except time release

---

asparaginase (℞)

(a-spare′a-gi-nase)

Elspar, Kidrolase*

Func. class.: Antineoplastic

Chem. class.: E. coli enzyme

Action: Indirectly inhibits protein synthesis in tumor cells; without amino acid, DNA, RNA synthesis is halted; asparagine, protein synthesis is halted; G₁ phase of cell cycle specific; a nonvesicant

Uses: Acute lymphocytic leukemia in combination with other antineoplastics

Investigational uses: Lymphosarcoma, other leukemias

Dosage and routes:

In combination

• *Adult:* IV 1000 IU/kg/day × 10 days given over 30 min; **IM** 6000 IU/m²/day

Sole induction

• *Adult:* IV 200 IU/kg/day × 28 days

Available forms: Inj 10,000 IU

Side effects/adverse reactions:

SYST: **Anaphylaxis, hypersensitivity**

HEMA: **Thrombocytopenia, leukopenia, myelosuppression, anemia, decreased clotting factors**

GI: Nausea, vomiting, anorexia, cramps, stomatitis, **hepatotoxicity, pancreatitis**

GU: Urinary retention, **renal failure,** glycosuria, polyuria, azotemia, uric acid neuropathy

INTEG: Rash, urticaria, chills, fever

ENDO: Hyperglycemia

RESP: **Fibrosis, pulmonary infiltrate**

CV: Chest pain

CNS: Neuritis, dizziness, headache, **coma,** depression, fatigue, confusion, hallucinations

Contraindications: Hypersensitivity, infants, pregnancy (C), lactation, pancreatitis

Precautions: Renal disease, hepatic disease

Pharmacokinetics: Half-life 4-9 hr, terminal 1.4-1.8 hr

Interactions:

• Decreased action of methotrexate

• Increased toxicity: vincristine, prednisone

Lab test interferences:

Decrease: Thyroid function tests

NURSING CONSIDERATIONS

Assess:

• For signs and symptoms of pancreatitis (nausea, vomiting, severe abdominal pain), anaphylaxis (bronchospasm, dyspnea), cyanosis

• CBC, differential, platelet count weekly; withhold drug if WBC is <4000 or platelet count is <75,000; notify prescriber of these results

• Pulmonary function tests, chest x-ray studies before, during therapy; chest x-ray film should be obtained q2wk during treatment

• Renal function studies: BUN, serum uric acid, ammonia urine CrCl, electrolytes before, during therapy

• I&O ratio; report fall in urine output of 30 ml/hr

• Monitor temperature q4h; may indicate beginning infection

• Liver function tests before, during therapy (bilirubin, AST, ALT, LDH) as needed or monthly

• RBC, Hct, Hgb, since these may be decreased

• Serum, urine glucose levels

• Bleeding: hematuria, guaiac, bruising or petechiae, mucosa or orifices q8h

Dyspnea, rales, nonproductive cough, chest pain, tachypnea, fatigue, increased pulse, pallor, lethargy, swelling around eyes or lips; anaphylaxis may occur; risk of hypersensitivity increases with repeated dose

• Jaundice of skin and sclera, dark urine, clay-colored stools, itchy skin, abdominal pain, fever, diarrhea

• Local irritation, pain, burning, discoloration at injection site

• Symptoms indicating severe allergic reaction: rash, pruritus, urticaria, purpuric skin lesions, itching, flushing, dyspnea

• Frequency of stools, characteristics: cramping, acidosis; signs of dehydration: rapid respirations, poor skin turgor, decreased urine output, dry skin, restlessness, weakness

Administer:

IM

• Reconstitute with 2 ml NaCl/10,000 U/vial, refrigerate, use within 8 hr

IV, direct

• After intradermal skin testing and desensitization, give 0.1 ml (2 IU) intradermally after reconstituting with 5 ml sterile H_2O or 0.9% NaCl for injection; then add 0.1 ml of reconstituted drug to 9.9 ml diluent (20 IU/ml); observe for 1 hr, check for wheal

• Allopurinol or sodium bicarbonate to reduce uric acid levels, alkalinization of urine

Intermittent IV inf

• Using 21G, 23G, 25G needle; administer by slow IV infusion via Y-tube or 3-way stopcock of flowing D_5W or NS infusion over 30 min diluting 10,000 IU/5 ml of sterile H_2O or 0.9% NaCl (no preservatives) (2000 IU/ml); use of filter may be necessary if fibers are present

Y-site compatibilities: Methotrexate, sodium bicarbonate

Perform/provide:

• Deep-breathing exercises with patient 3-4 ×/day; place in semi-Fowler's position

• Increase fluid intake to 2-3 L/day to prevent urate deposits, calculi formation

• Diet low in purines: absence of organ meats (kidney, liver), dried beans, peas to maintain alkaline urine

• Rinsing of mouth 3-4 ×/day with water, club soda

• Brushing of teeth 2-3 ×/day with soft brush or cotton-tipped applicators for stomatitis; use unwaxed dental floss

• Warm compresses at injection site for inflammation

• Nutritious diet with iron, vitamin supplements

• HOB raised to facilitate breathing

Evaluate:

• Therapeutic response: decreased exacerbations in ALL

Teach patient/family:

• To report any complaints or side effects to nurse or prescriber

• To report any changes in breathing or coughing

Treatment of anaphylaxis: Administer epinephrine, diphenhydramine, IV corticosteroids

A

---

aspirin (OTC)

(as´pir-in)

acetylsalicylic acid, Acuprin, Apo-ASA*, Apo-Asen*, Arthrinol*, Arthrisin*, Artria S.R., A.S.A., Aspergum, Aspirin*, Aspir-Low, Aspirtab, Astrin*, Bayer, Easprin, Ecotrin, 8-Hour Bayer Timed Release, Empirin, Entrophen*, Halfprin, Norwich Extra-Strength, Novasen*, PMS-ASA*, Sloprin, St. Joseph Children's, Supasa*, Therapy Bayer, ZORprin

Func. class.: Nonnarcotic analgesic, nonsteroidal antiinflammatory, antipyretic, antiplatelet

Chem. class.: Salicylate

Action: Blocks pain impulses in CNS, inhibition of prostaglandin synthesis; antipyretic action results from vasodilation of peripheral vessels; decreases platelet aggregation

Uses: Mild to moderate pain or fever including rheumatoid arthritis, osteoarthritis, thromboembolic disorders; transient ischemic attacks, rheumatic fever, postmyocardial infarction, prophylaxis of MI, ischemic stroke, angina

Investigational uses: Prevention of cataracts (long-term use), prevention of pregnancy loss in women with clotting disorders

Dosage and routes:

Arthritis

• *Adult:* **PO** 2.6-5.2 g/day in divided doses q4-6h

• *Child:* **PO** 90-130 mg/kg/day in divided doses q4-6h

Pain/fever

• *Adult:* **PO/RECT** 325-650 mg q4h prn, not to exceed 4 g/day

---

• *Child:* **PO/RECT** 40-100 mg/kg/day in divided doses q4-6h prn
Kawasaki disease
• *Child:* **PO** 80-120 mg/kg/day in 4 divided doses, maintenance 3-8 mg/kg/day as a single dose × 8 wk
Thromboembolic disorders
• *Adult:* **PO** 325-650 mg/day or bid
Transient ischemic attacks
• *Adult:* **PO** 650 mg qid or 325 mg qid
MI, stroke prophylaxis
• *Adult:* **PO** 81-650 mg/day
Available forms: Tabs 325, 500, 650, 975 mg; chewable tabs 81 mg; tabs controlled-release 800 mg; tabs time-release 650 mg; supp 120, 200, 300, 600 mg, 1.2 g; cream; gum 227.5 mg

Side effects/adverse reactions:
HEMA: ***Thrombocytopenia, agranulocytosis, leukopenia, neutropenia, hemolytic anemia,*** increased pro-time, APTT, bleeding time
CNS: Stimulation, drowsiness, dizziness, confusion, ***convulsion,*** headache, flushing, hallucinations, ***coma***
GI: Nausea, vomiting, ***GI bleeding,*** diarrhea, heartburn, anorexia, ***hepatitis***
INTEG: Rash, urticaria, bruising
EENT: Tinnitus, hearing loss
CV: Rapid pulse, pulmonary edema
RESP: Wheezing, hyperpnea
ENDO: Hypoglycemia, hyponatremia, hypokalemia
SYST: ***Reye's syndrome (children)***

Contraindications: Hypersensitivity to salicylates, tartrazine (FDC yellow dye #5), GI bleeding, bleeding disorders, children <12 yr, children with flulike symptoms, pregnancy (D) 3rd trimester, lactation, vit K deficiency, peptic ulcer

Precautions: Anemia, hepatic disease, renal disease, Hodgkin's disease, pre/postoperatively, gastritis, asthmatic patients with nasal polyps or aspirin sensitivity, pregnancy (C)

Pharmacokinetics: Well absorbed PO; enteric and rectal products may be erratic
PO: Onset 15-30 min, peak 1-2 hr, duration 4-6 hr
REC: Onset slow, duration 4-6 hr; metabolized by liver, inactive metabolites excreted by kidneys, crosses placenta, excreted in breast milk; half-life 1-3½ hr, up to 30 hr in large doses

Interactions:
• Decreased effects of aspirin: antacids (high doses), steroids, urinary alkalizers, corticosteroids
• Increased bleeding: alcohol, heparin, plicamycin, cefamandole
• Increased effects of warfarin, insulin, methotrexate, thrombolytic agents, penicillins, phenytoin, valproic acid, oral hypoglycemics, sulfonamides
• Increased salicylate levels: urinary acidifiers, ammonium chloride, nizatidine
• Decreased effects of probenecid, spironolactone, sulfinpyrazone, sulfonylamides, NSAIDs, beta blockers
• Gastric ulcer: steroids, antiinflammatories, NSAIDs
�herb Increased risk of bleeding: horse chestnut, kelpware

Lab test interferences:
Increase: Coagulation studies, liver function studies, serum uric acid, amylase, CO_2, urinary protein
Decrease: Serum K, PBI, cholesterol
Interference: Urine catecholamines, pregnancy test, urine glucose tests (Clinistix, Tes-Tape)

NURSING CONSIDERATIONS
Assess:
• Liver function studies: AST, ALT, bilirubin, creatinine if patient is on long-term therapy

---

◆ = Nursing alert   🌒 = Herb-drug interaction   🚫 = Do not crush

• Renal function studies: BUN, urine creatinine if patient is on long-term therapy
• Blood studies: CBC, Hct, Hgb, pro-time if patient is on long-term therapy
• I&O ratio; decreasing output may indicate renal failure (long-term therapy)
◆ Hepatotoxicity: dark urine, clay-colored stools, yellowing of skin, sclera, itching, abdominal pain, fever, diarrhea if patient is on long-term therapy
• Allergic reactions: rash, urticaria; if these occur, drug may have to be discontinued
• Renal dysfunction: decreased urine output
• Ototoxicity: tinnitus, ringing, roaring in ears; audiometric testing needed before, after long-term therapy
• Visual changes: blurring, halos; corneal, retinal damage
• Edema in feet, ankles, legs
• Drug history; many drug interactions
• Pain: location, duration, type, intensity, prior to dose and 1 hr after
• Musculoskeletal status: ROM prior to dose
• Fever; length of time and related symptoms

Administer:
PO
• Crushed or whole; chewable tablets may be chewed
🚫 Do not crush enteric product
• With food or milk to decrease gastric symptoms; give 30 min before or 2 hr after meals

Evaluate:
• Therapeutic response: decreased pain, inflammation, fever

Teach patient/family:
• To report any symptoms of hepatotoxicity, renal toxicity, visual changes, ototoxicity, allergic reactions, bleeding (long-term therapy)
• To take with 8 oz H_2O and sit upright for ½ hr after dose
• Not to exceed recommended dosage; acute poisoning may result
• To read label on other OTC drugs; many contain aspirin
• That the therapeutic response takes 2 wk (arthritis)
• To report tinnitus, confusion, diarrhea, sweating, hyperventilation
• To avoid alcohol ingestion; GI bleeding may occur
• That patients who have allergies may develop allergic reactions
• To avoid buffered or effervescent products
• That medication is not to be given to children or teens with flulike symptoms or chickenpox; Reye's syndrome may develop

Treatment of overdose: Lavage, activated charcoal, monitor electrolytes, VS

---

atenolol (℞)

(a-ten'oh-lole)
Apo-Atenol*, atenolol*, Nu-Atenol, Tenormin
Func. class.: Antihypertensive, antianginal
Chem. class.: β-Blocker, β-1, β-2-blocker (high doses)

Action: Competitively blocks stimulation of β-adrenergic receptor within vascular smooth muscle; produces negative chronotropic activity, negative inotropic activity (decreases rate of SA node discharge, increases recovery time), slows conduction of AV node, decreases heart rate, decreases O_2 consumption in myocardium; also decreases renin-aldosterone-angiotensin system at high doses, inhibits β-2 receptors in bronchial system at higher doses

---

Uses: Mild to moderate hypertension, prophylaxis of angina pectoris, suspected or known myocardial infarction

Investigational uses: Dysrhythmia, mitral valve prolapse, pheochromocytoma, hypertrophic cardiomyopathy, vascular headaches, thyrotoxicosis, tremors, alcohol withdrawal

Dosage and routes:
• *Adult:* **IV** 5 mg, repeat in 10 min if initial dose is well tolerated, then start **PO** dose 10 min after last **IV** dose
• *Adult:* **PO** 50 mg qd, increasing q1-2wk to 100 mg qd; may increase to 200 mg qd for angina
• *Elderly:* **PO** 25 mg/day initially

Renal disease
• CrCl 15-35 ml/min, max 50 mg/day; CrCl <15 ml/min max dose 50 mg qod; hemodialysis 25-50 mg after dialysis

Available forms: Tabs 25, 50, 100 mg; inj 5 mg/10 ml

Side effects/adverse reactions:
CV: ***Profound hypotension, bradycardia, CHF,*** *cold extremities, postural hypotension, 2nd- or 3rd-degree heart block*
CNS: Insomnia, fatigue, dizziness, mental changes, memory loss, hallucinations, depression, lethargy, drowsiness, strange dreams, catatonia
GI: Nausea, diarrhea, vomiting, ***mesenteric arterial thrombosis, ischemic colitis***
INTEG: Rash, fever, alopecia
HEMA: ***Agranulocytosis, thrombocytopenia, purpura***
EENT: Sore throat, dry burning eyes
GU: Impotence
ENDO: Increased hypoglycemic response to insulin
RESP: ***Bronchospasm,*** dyspnea, wheezing

Contraindications: Hypersensitivity to β-blockers, cardiogenic shock, 2nd- or 3rd-degree heart block, sinus bradycardia, cardiac failure, pregnancy (D)

Precautions: Major surgery, lactation, diabetes mellitus, renal disease, thyroid disease, CHF, COPD, asthma, well-compensated heart failure

Pharmacokinetics:
PO: Peak 2-4 hr; half-life 6-7 hr, excreted unchanged in urine, protein binding 5%-15%

Interactions:
• Increased hypotension, bradycardia: reserpine, hydralazine, methyldopa, prazosin, anticholinergics, digoxin, diltiazem, verapamil, cardiac glycosides, antihypertensives
• Increased hypoglycemic effect: insulin, oral antidiabetics
• Mutual inhibition: sympathomimetics (cough, cold preparations)

Lab test interferences:
Interference: Glucose/insulin tolerance tests

NURSING CONSIDERATIONS
Assess:
• I&O, weight daily
• B/P, pulse q4h; note rate, rhythm, quality
• Apical/radial pulse before administration; notify prescriber of any significant changes (<50 bpm)
• Baselines in renal, liver function tests before therapy begins
• Edema in feet, legs daily
• Skin turgor, dryness of mucous membranes for hydration status

Administer:
PO
• Drug ac, hs, tablet may be crushed or swallowed whole
• Reduced dosage in renal dysfunction

IV, direct
• Undiluted over 5 min

IV infusion
• Diluted in 10-50 ml of D_5W, D_5/NaCl, or NS and give as an infusion at prescribed rate

---

◆ = Nursing alert   ∥ = Herb-drug interaction   ⊘ = Do not crush

Y-site compatibilities: Meperidine, meropenem, morphine

Perform/provide:
• Storage protected from light, moisture; place in cool environment

Evaluate:
• Therapeutic response: decreased B/P after 1-2 wk

Teach patient/family:
◆Not to discontinue drug abruptly, taper over 2 wk
• Not to use OTC products unless directed by prescriber
• To report bradycardia, dizziness, confusion, depression, fever
• To take pulse at home; advise when to notify prescriber
• To limit alcohol, smoking, sodium intake
• To comply with weight control, dietary adjustments, modified exercise program
• To carry Medic Alert ID to identify drug that you are taking, allergies
• To avoid hazardous activities if dizziness is present
• That drug may mask symptoms of hypoglycemia in diabetic patients

Treatment of overdose: Lavage, IV atropine for bradycardia, IV theophylline for bronchospasm, digitalis, O₂, diuretic for cardiac failure, hemodialysis

---

atorvastatin (R)
(at-or′va-sta-tin)
Lipitor
Func. class.: Antilipidemic
Chem. class.: Synthetically derived fermentation product

Action: Inhibits HMG-CoA reductase enzyme, which reduces cholesterol synthesis

Uses: As an adjunct in primary hypercholesterolemia (types Ia, Ib), dysbetalipoproteinemia, elevated triglyceride levels

Dosage and routes:
• *Adult:* **PO** 10 mg qd, usual range 10-80, dosage adjustments may be made in 2-4 wk intervals

Available forms: Tabs 10, 20, 40 mg

Side effects/adverse reactions:
INTEG: Rash, pruritus, alopecia
GI: Dyspepsia, flatus, *liver dysfunction,* pancreatitis
EENT: Lens opacities
MS: Myalgia
CNS: Headache

Contraindications: Hypersensitivity, pregnancy (X), lactation, active liver disease

Precautions: Past liver disease, alcoholism, severe acute infections, trauma, hypotension, uncontrolled seizure disorders, severe metabolic disorders, electrolyte imbalance

Pharmacokinetics: Metabolized in liver, highly protein bound, excreted primarily in urine, half-life 14 hr; protein binding 98%

Interactions:
• Possible rhabdomyolysis: azole antifungals, cyclosporine, erythromycin, niacin
• Increased serum level of digoxin
• Increased levels of oral contraceptives
• Increased levels of atorvastatin: erythromycin, itraconazole

NURSING CONSIDERATIONS

Assess:
• Cholesterol levels periodically during treatment
• Liver function studies q1-2mo during the first 1½ yr of treatment; AST, ALT, liver function tests may be increased
• Renal studies in patients with compromised renal system: BUN, I&O ratio, creatinine
• Eyes with slit lamp before, 1 mo after treatment begins, annually; lens opacities may occur

---

Administer:
PO
• Total daily dose any time of day
Perform/provide:
• Storage in cool environment in tight container protected from light
Evaluate:
• Therapeutic response: decrease in cholesterol to desired level after 8 wk
Teach patient/family:
• That blood work and eye exam will be necessary during treatment
• To report blurred vision, severe GI symptoms, headache
• That previously prescribed regimen will continue: low-cholesterol diet, exercise program
• Not to take drug if pregnant

---

atovaquone (℞)
(a-toe'va-kwon)
Mepron
Func. class.: Antiprotozoal
Chem. class.: Aromatic diamide derivative, analog of ubiquinone

---

Action: Interferes with DNA/RNA synthesis in protozoa
Uses: *Pneumocystis carinii* infections in patients intolerant of trimethoprim/sulfamethoxazole
Dosage and routes:
• *Adult and adolescents 13-16 yr:* **PO** 750 mg/food bid for 21 days
Prevention of Pneumocystis carinii pneumonia (PCP)
• *Adults and adolescents 13-16 yr:* **PO** 1500 mg qd with food
Available forms: 750 mg/5 ml, susp
Side effects/adverse reactions:
CV: Hypotension
HEMA: Anemia, leukopenia
INTEG: Pruritus, urticaria, *rash*, oral monilia
GI: Nausea, vomiting, diarrhea, anorexia, increased AST and ALT, acute pancreatitis, constipation, abdominal pain
CNS: Dizziness, headache, anxiety
META: Hyperkalemia, hyperglycemia, hyponatremia
Contraindications: Hypersensitivity or history of developing life-threatening allergic reactions to any component of the formulation
Precautions: Blood dyscrasias, hepatic disease, diabetes mellitus, pregnancy (C), lactation, children, elderly
Pharmacokinetics: Excreted unchanged in feces (94%), highly protein bound (99%)
Interactions:
• Use caution when administering concurrently with other highly plasma protein-bound drugs with narrow therapeutic indices
• Decreased effect of atovaquone: rifampin, rifabutin
NURSING CONSIDERATIONS
Assess:
• Signs of infection, anemia
• Bowel pattern before, during treatment
• Respiratory status: rate, character, wheezing, dyspnea
• Allergies before treatment, reaction of each medication
Administer:
PO
• With food because of increased absorption of the drug and higher plasma concentrations
Evaluate:
• Therapeutic response: decreased temperature, ability to breathe
Teach patient/family:
• To take with food to increase plasma concentrations

---

atracurium (℞)
(a-tra-kyoor'ee-um)
Tracrium
Func. class.: Neuromuscular blocker (nondepolarizing)
Chem. class.: Biquaternary ammonium ester

Action: Inhibits transmission of nerve impulses by binding with cholinergic receptor sites, antagonizing action of acetylcholine

Uses: Facilitation of endotracheal intubation, skeletal muscle relaxation during mechanical ventilation, surgery, or general anesthesia

Dosage and routes:
• *Adult and child >2 yr:* **IV BOL** 0.3-0.5 mg/kg, then 0.08-0.10 mg/kg 20-45 min after first dose if needed for prolonged procedures
• *Child, 1 mo-2 yr:* **IV BOL** 0.3-0.4 mg/kg

Available forms: Inj 10 mg/ml

Side effects/adverse reactions:
CV: Bradycardia, tachycardia; increased, decreased B/P
RESP: ***Prolonged apnea, bronchospasm, cyanosis, respiratory depression***
EENT: Increased secretions
INTEG: Rash, flushing, pruritus, urticaria
MS: Inadequate or prolonged block

Contraindications: Hypersensitivity

Precautions: Pregnancy (C), cardiac disease, lactation, children <2 yr, electrolyte imbalances, dehydration, neuromuscular disease, respiratory disease

Pharmacokinetics:
IV: Onset 2 min, duration 20-60 min; half-life 2 min, terminal 29 min, excreted in urine, feces (metabolites), crosses placenta

Interactions:
• Increased neuromuscular blockade: aminoglycosides, clindamycin, enflurane, isoflurane, lincomycin, lithium, magnesium salts, opioid analgesics, polymyxin antibiotics, procainamide, quinidine, thiazides, trimethaphan, verapamil
• Decreased neuromuscular blockade: edrophonium, neostigmine, phenytoin, pyridostigmine, theophylline

NURSING CONSIDERATIONS
Assess:
• For electrolyte imbalances (K, Mg); may lead to increased action of this drug
• Vital signs (B/P, pulse, respirations, airway) until fully recovered; rate, depth, pattern of respirations, strength of hand grip
• I&O ratio; check for urinary retention, frequency, hesitancy
• Recovery: decreased paralysis of face, diaphragm, leg, arm, rest of body
• Allergic reactions: rash, fever, respiratory distress, pruritus; drug should be discontinued

Administer:
• Do not administer IM
IV
• Using nerve stimulator by anesthesiologist to determine neuromuscular blockade
• Anticholinesterase to reverse neuromuscular blockade
• IV undiluted by direct IV over 5 min, or diluted in 10-50 ml of D_5W, ½ NaCl or NS and give as an infusion at prescribed rate
• By slow IV over 1-2 min (only by qualified person)

Additive compatibilities: Bretylium, cimetidine, dobutamine, dopamine, esmolol, gentamicin, isoproterenol, lidocaine, morphine, potassium chloride, procainamide, vancomycin

---

Syringe compatibilities: Afatanil, fentanyl, midazolam, sufentanil

Y-site compatibilities: Cefazolin, cefuroxime, cimetidine, dobutamine, dopamine, epinephrine, esmolol, etomidate, fentanyl, gentamicin, heparin, hydrocortisone, isoproterenol, lorazepam, midazolam, morphine, nitroglycerine, ranitidine, sodium nitroprusside, trimethoprim/sulfamethoxazole, vancomycin

Perform/provide:
• Storage in light-resistant area
• Reassurance if communication is difficult during recovery from neuromuscular blockade

Evaluate:
• Therapeutic response: paralysis of jaw, eyelid, head, neck, rest of body

Treatment of overdose: Edrophonium or neostigmine, atropine, monitor VS; mechanical ventilation

---

atropine (Ŗ)
(a'troe-peen)
Atropair, Atro-Pen, Atropisol, Isopto-Atropine, I-Tropina, Minims Atopine*, Ocu-Tropine

Func. class.: Antidysrhythmic, anticholinergic parasympatholytic

Chem. class.: Belladonna alkaloid

Action: Blocks acetylcholine at parasympathetic neuroeffector sites; increases cardiac output, heart rate by blocking vagal stimulation in heart; dries secretions by blocking vagus

Uses: Bradycardia, bradydysrhythmia, reversal of anticholinesterase agents, insecticide poisoning, blocking cardiac vagal reflexes, decreasing secretions before surgery, antispasmodic with GU, biliary surgery, bronchodilator

Dosage and routes:
Bradycardia/bradydysrhythmia
• *Adult:* IV BOL 0.5-1 mg given q3-5min, not to exceed 2 mg
• *Child:* IV BOL 0.01-0.03 mg/kg up to 0.4 mg or 0.3 mg/m^2; may repeat q4-6h; min dose 0.1 mg to avoid paradoxical reaction

Insecticide poisoning
• *Adult and child:* IM/IV 2 mg qh until muscarinic symptoms disappear, may need 6 mg qh

Presurgery
• *Adult:* SC/IM/IV 0.4-0.6 mg before anesthesia
• *Child:* SC 0.1-0.4 mg 30 min before surgery

Available forms: Inj 0.05, 0.1, 0.3, 0.4, 0.5, 0.8, 1 mg/ml; tabs 0.4, 0.6 mg

Side effects/adverse reactions:
GU: Retention, hesitancy, impotence, dysuria

CNS: Headache, dizziness, involuntary movement, confusion, psychosis, anxiety, coma, flushing, drowsiness, insomnia, weakness; delirium (elderly)

GI: Dry mouth, nausea, vomiting, abdominal pain, anorexia, constipation, *paralytic ileus,* abdominal distention, altered taste

CV: Hypotension, paradoxical bradycardia, angina, PVCs, hypertension, *tachycardia,* ectopic ventricular beats

INTEG: Rash, urticaria, contact dermatitis, dry skin, flushing

EENT: Blurred vision, photophobia, glaucoma, eye pain, pupil dilation, nasal congestion

MISC: Suppression of lactation, decreased sweating

Contraindications: Hypersensitivity to belladonna alkaloids, angle-closure glaucoma, GI obstructions, myasthenia gravis, thyrotoxicosis, ulcerative colitis, prostatic hypertrophy, tachycardia/tachydysrhyth-

---

◆ = Nursing alert   ∥ = Herb-drug interaction   ⊘ = Do not crush

mias, asthma, acute hemorrhage, hepatic disease, myocardial ischemia

Precautions: Pregnancy (C), renal disease, lactation, CHF, tachydysrhythmia, hyperthyroidism, COPD, hepatic disease, child <6 yr, hypertension, elderly, intraabdominal infection, Down syndrome, spastic paralysis, gastric ulcer

Pharmacokinetics: Well absorbed PO, IM, SC; half-life 13-40 hr, excreted by kidneys unchanged (70%-90% in 24 hr); metabolized in liver, 40%-50% crosses placenta, excreted in breast milk

IV: Peak 2-4 min, duration 4-6 hr

IM/SC: Onset 15-50 min; peak 30 min, duration 4-6 hr

PO: Onset ½ hr; peak ½-1 hr; duration 4-6 hr

Interactions:

• Decreased effect of atropine: antacids

• Mucosal lesions: potassium chloride wax-matrix tab

• Decreased absorption: ketoconazole, levodopa

• EPS: methotrimeprazine

• Increased anticholinergic effects, tricylic antidepressants, amantadine, MAOIs, quinidine, phenothiazines, meperidine, glutethimide, antiparkinson agents, antidysrhythmics, amantadine

⚕ Possible increased action of atropine: chronic use/abuse of cascara sagrada bark, buckthorn bark/berry, rhubarb root, senna leaf/fruits, aloe

NURSING CONSIDERATIONS
Assess:

• I&O ratio; check for urinary retention, daily output

• ECG for ectopic ventricular beats, PVC, tachycardia, in cardiac patients

• For bowel sounds; check for constipation

• Respiratory status: rate, rhythm, cyanosis, wheezing, dyspnea, engorged neck veins

• Increased intraocular pressure: eye pain, nausea, vomiting, blurred vision, increased tearing

• Cardiac rate: rhythm, character, B/P continuously

• Allergic reaction: rash, urticaria

Administer:

PO

• Increased bulk, water in diet if constipation occurs

• ½ hr ac

IM

• Atropine flush may occur in children and is not harmful

IV

• Undiluted or diluted with 10 ml sterile H_2O, give at 0.6 mg/min, give through Y-tube or 3-way stopcock; do not add to IV sol; may cause paradoxical bradycardia lasting 2 min

Additive compatibilities: Dobutamine, furosemide, meropenem, netilmicin, sodium bicarbonate, verapamil

Syringe compatibilities: Benzquinamide, butorphanol, chlorpromazine, cimetidine, dimenhydrinate, diphenhydramine, droperidol, fentanyl, glycopyrrolate, heparin, hydromorphone, hydroxyzine, meperidine, metoclopramide, midazolam, milrinone, morphine, nalbuphine, pentazocine, perphenazine, prochlorperazine, promazine, promethazine, propiomazine, ranitidine, scopolamine, sufentanil

Y-site compatibilities: Amrinone, etomidate, famotidine, heparin, hydrocortisone, meropenem, nafcillin, potassium chloride, sufentanil, vit B/C

Perform/provide:

• Sugarless hard candy, gum, frequent rinsing of mouth for dryness

Evaluate:

• Therapeutic response: decreased dysrhythmias, increased heart rate, secretions; GI, GU spasms; bronchodilation

Teach patient/family:

• To report blurred vision, chest pain, allergic reactions

• Not to perform strenuous activity in high temperatures; heat stroke may result

• To take as prescribed; not to skip doses

• Not to operate machinery if drowsiness occurs

• Not to take OTC products without approval of prescriber

Treatment of overdose: O_2, artificial ventilation, ECG; administer dopamine for circulatory depression; administer diazepam or thiopental for convulsions; assess need for antidysrhythmics

---

auranofin (℞)

(au-rane'oh-fin)
Ridaura
Func. class.: Antiinflammatory
Chem. class.: Active gold compound (29%)

Action: Antiinflammatory action unknown; may decrease phagocytosis, lysosomal activity, or prostaglandin synthesis; decreases concentration of rheumatoid factor, immunoglobulins

Uses: Rheumatoid arthritis

Investigational uses: SLE, psoriatic arthritis, pemphigus

Dosage and routes:

• *Adult:* PO 6 mg qd or 3 mg bid; may increase to 9 mg/day after 3 mo

Available forms: Caps 3 mg

Side effects/adverse reactions:

*HEMA: **Thrombocytopenia, agranulocytosis, aplastic anemia, leukopenia, eosinophilia, neutropenia***

INTEG: Rash, pruritus, dermatitis, **exfoliative dermatitis**, urticaria, alopecia, photosensitivity

CNS: Dizziness, confusion, hallucinations, **seizures,** EEG abnormalities

GI: Diarrhea, abdominal cramping, stomatitis, nausea, vomiting, enterocolitis, anorexia, flatulence, metallic taste, dyspepsia, jaundice, increased AST, ALT, glossitis, gingivitis, melena, constipation

*GU: **Proteinuria, hematuria,*** increased BUN, creatinine, vaginitis

MISC: Iritis, corneal ulcers, gold deposits in ocular tissues

*RESP: **Interstitial pneumonitis, fibrosis,*** cough, dyspnea

Contraindications: Hypersensitivity to gold, necrotizing enterocolitis, bone marrow aplasia, child <6 yr, lactation, pulmonary fibrosis, exfoliative dermatitis, blood dyscrasias, recent radiation therapy, renal/hepatic disease, marked hypertension, uncontrolled CHF

Precautions: Elderly, CHF, diabetes mellitus, allergic conditions, ulcerative colitis, renal disease, liver disease, pregnancy (C)

Pharmacokinetics:

PO: Absorbed by GI tract, peak 2 hr, steady state 8-16 wk, excreted in urine, feces

Interactions:

• May increase levels of phenytoin

Lab test interferences:

False positive: TB test

NURSING CONSIDERATIONS

Assess:

• Respiratory status: dyspnea, wheezing; if respiratory problems occur, drug should be discontinued

• I&O ratio

• Urine: hematuria, proteinuria; increased BUN, creatinine; may require decrease in dosage

---

⬥ = Nursing alert   ⧄ = Herb-drug interaction   ⊘ = Do not crush

• Platelet counts qmo; drug should be discontinued if <100,000/mm³
• Hepatic test: ALT, AST, alk phosphatase
• Diarrhea stools; if severe, drug should be discontinued
• Allergy: rash, dermatitis, pruritus; drug should be discontinued if any of these occur
◆ Gold toxicity: decreased Hgb, WBC <4000/mm³, granulocytes <1500/mm³, platelets <100,000/mm³, severe diarrhea, stomatitis, hematuria, rash, itching, proteinuria

Administer:

PO
• Bid or may give as single dose qAM with food or drink

Evaluate:
• Therapeutic response: ability to move joints with less pain

Teach patient/family:
• That drug must be taken as prescribed to be useful, to obtain lab work monthly
🚫 Not to break, crush, or chew caps
• That diarrhea is common, but if blood appears in stools or urine, notify prescriber at once; that patient should check for bruising, petechiae, bleeding gums
• To report abnormal skin conditions, stomatitis, fatigue, jaundice; may indicate blood dyscrasias
• To avoid exposure to sunlight or ultraviolet light; to use sunscreen to prevent burns
• That therapeutic effect may take 3-4 mo
• To use diluted hydrogen peroxide for mild stomatitis, avoid hot spicy foods, food with high acidic content; use soft toothbrush, rinse more frequently, floss daily
• That contraception should be used during treatment

---

aurothioglucose/gold sodium thiomalate (℞)

(aur-oh-thye-oh-gloo'kose)
Solganal/Aurolate
Func. class.: Antiinflammatory
Chem. class.: Active gold compound (50%)

Action: Antiinflammatory action unknown; may decrease phagocytosis, lysosomal activity, prostaglandin synthesis

Uses: Rheumatoid arthritis, psoriatic arthritis

Dosage and routes:
• *Adult:* **IM** 10 mg, then 25 mg qwk × 2-3 wk, then 50 mg/wk until total of 1 g is administered, then 25-50 mg q3-4wk if there is improvement without toxicity (aurothioglucose) total of 800 mg-1 g
• *Adult:* **IM** 10 mg, then 25 mg after 1 wk, then 50 mg qwk for total of 14-20 doses, then 50 mg q2wk × 4, then 50 mg q3wk × 4, then 50 mg qmo for maintenance (gold sodium thiomalate)
• *Child 6-12 yr:* **IM** 1 mg/kg/wk × 20 wk, or ¼ of adult dose (aurothioglucose)
• *Child:* **IM** 1 mg/kg/wk × 20 wk, then q3-4wk if improvement without toxicity (gold sodium thiomalate) not to exceed 2.5 mg

Available forms: Inj 50 mg/ml

Side effects/adverse reactions:
EENT: Iritis, corneal ulcers
HEMA: ***Thrombocytopenia, agranulocytosis, aplastic anemia, leukopenia, eosinophilia, neutropenia***
INTEG: Rash, pruritus, dermatitis, urticaria, alopecia, photosensitivity, ***exfoliative dermatitis, angioedema***
GI: Stomatitis, nausea, vomiting, metallic taste, jaundice, ***hepatitis,*** diarrhea, cramping, flatulence

---

Side effects: *italics* = common; ***bold italics*** = life-threatening

GU: Proteinuria, hematuria, ***nephrosis, tubular necrosis***
RESP: Interstitial pneumonitis, pharyngitis, ***pulmonary fibrosis***
CNS: Dizziness, EEG abnormalities, ***encephalitis,*** confusion, hallucinations
CV: Bradycardia, rapid pulse
SYST: ***Anaphylaxis***

Contraindications: Hypersensitivity to gold, systemic lupus erythematosus, uncontrolled diabetes mellitus, marked hypertension, recent radiation therapy, CHF, lactation, renal disease, liver disease

Precautions: Decreased tolerance in elderly, children, blood dyscrasias, pregnancy (C)

Pharmacokinetics:
IM: Peak 4-6 hr; half-life 3-27 days; excreted in urine, feces; half-life increases up to 168 days with 11th dose

Interactions:
• Photosensitivity: ultraviolet light
Lab test interferences:
False reading: Protein-bound iodine test

NURSING CONSIDERATIONS
Assess:
• Respiratory status: dyspnea, wheezing; if respiratory problems occur, drug should be discontinued
• I&O ratio
• For pregnancy before administration; do not give in pregnancy
• Urine: hematuria, proteinuria; increased BUN, creatinine; may require decrease in dosage
• Platelet counts qmo; drug should be discontinued if <100,000/mm^3
• Hepatic test: ALT, AST, alk phosphatase
• Diarrhea stools; if severe, drug should be discontinued
• Allergy: rash, dermatitis, pruritus; drug should be discontinued if any of these occur

◆ Gold toxicity: decreased Hgb, WBC <4000/mm^3, granulocytes <1500/mm^3, platelets <100,000/mm^3, severe diarrhea, stomatitis, hematuria, rash, itching, proteinuria, use dimercaprol for acute toxicity
Administer:
IM
• Bid or may give as single dose qAM
• Deep IM, never IV
• Slowly, keep patient recumbent for 10 min after injection, monitor for transient reaction
Evaluate:
• Therapeutic response: ability to move joints with less pain
Teach patient/family:
• That drug must be taken as prescribed to be useful
• To obtain lab work monthly
• That diarrhea is common, but if blood appears in stools or urine, notify prescriber at once; that patient should check for bruising, petechiae, bleeding gums
• To report skin conditions, stomatitis, fatigue, jaundice, which may indicate blood dyscrasias; report fever, chills, which may indicate infection
• That therapeutic effect may take 3-4 mo
• To use dilute hydrogen peroxide for mild stomatitis; avoid hot, spicy foods and food with high acidic content; use soft toothbrush, rinse more frequently
• That contraception should be used during treatment
• To use sunscreen to prevent burns

◆ = Nursing alert   ∥ = Herb-drug interaction   ⊘ = Do not crush

---

azathioprine (R)

(ay-za-thye′oh-preen)

Imuran

Func. class.: Immunosuppressant

Chem. class.: Purine analog

Action: Produces immunosuppression by inhibiting purine synthesis in cells

Uses: Renal transplants to prevent graft rejection, refractory rheumatoid arthritis, refractory ITP, glomerulonephritis, nephrotic syndrome, bone marrow transplant

Investigational uses: Myasthenia gravis, chronic ulcerative colitis, Crohn's disease, Behçet's disease

Dosage and routes:

Prevention of rejection

• *Adult and child:* **PO, IV** 3-5 mg/kg/day, then maintenance (PO) of at least 1-2 mg/kg/day

Refractory rheumatoid arthritis

• *Adult:* **PO** 1/mg/kg/day, may increase dose after 2 mo by 0.5 mg/kg/day, not to exceed 2.5 mg/kg/day

Renal disease

• CrCl 10-50 ml/min 75% of dose; CrCl <10 ml/min 50% of dose

Available forms: Tabs 50 mg; inj 100 mg

Side effects/adverse reactions:

GI: Nausea, vomiting, stomatitis, esophagitis, *pancreatitis, hepatotoxicity, jaundice*

HEMA: **Leukopenia, thrombocytopenia, anemia, pancytopenia**

INTEG: Rash

MS: Arthralgia, muscle wasting

Contraindications: Hypersensitivity, pregnancy (D), lactation

Precautions: Severe renal disease, severe hepatic disease, elderly

Pharmacokinetics: Metabolized in liver, excreted in urine (active metabolite), crosses placenta

Lab test interferences:

Interfere: CBC, diff count

Decrease: Uric acid

Increase: LFTs

Interactions:

• Leukopenia: ACE inhibitors; cotrimoxazole, myelopoiesis

• Decreased immune response: vaccines

• Decreased action of warfarin: warfarin

• Increased action of azathioprine: allopurinol

• Do not admix with other drugs

NURSING CONSIDERATIONS

Assess:

• Blood studies: Hgb, WBC, platelets during treatment monthly; if leukocytes are <3000/mm³, drug should be discontinued

• Liver function studies: alk phosphatase, AST, ALT, bilirubin

◆Hepatotoxicity: dark urine, jaundice, itching, light-colored stools, increased LFTs; drug should be discontinued

Administer:

• All medications PO if possible, avoiding IM injections, since bleeding may occur

PO

• With meals to reduce GI upset

IV

• After diluting 100 mg/10 ml of sterile H₂O for inj; rotate to dissolve; may further dilute with 50 ml or more saline or glucose in saline

• For several days before transplant surgery

Solution compatibilities: D₅W, NaCl 0.9%, NaCl 0.45%

Evaluate:

• Therapeutic response: absence of graft rejection, immunosuppression in autoimmune disorders

Teach patient/family:

• That therapeutic response may take 3-4 mo in rheumatoid arthritis

• To report fever, rash, severe diarrhea, chills, sore throat, fatigue, since serious infections may occur

• To use contraceptive measures during treatment, for 12 wk after ending therapy; to avoid vaccinations

• To avoid crowds to reduce risk of infection

• To use soft-bristled toothbrush to prevent bleeding

---

azelastine (R)

(ay′ze-lass-teen)

Astelin

Func. class.: Antihistamine; leukotriene synthesis inhibitor

Chem. class.: Phthalazinone derivative

Action: Inhibits synthesis and release of leukotrienes; antagonizes action of acetylcholine, histamine, serotonin

Uses: Seasonal allergic rhinitis

Dosages and routes:

• *Adult and child ≥12 yr:* **Nasal** 2 sprays/nostril bid

Available forms: Spray 137 μg/actuation

Side effects/adverse reactions:

CNS: Sedation (more common with increased doses), increased drowsiness

MISC: Weight increases, myalgia

Contraindications: Hypersensitivity, acute asthma attacks, lower respiratory tract disease

Precautions: Pregnancy (C), increased intraocular pressure, bronchial asthma

Pharmacokinetics: Peak 2-3 hr, half-life 22 hr; metabolized in liver, excreted in urine

Interactions:

• Additive CNS depressant effects: alcohol, other CNS depressants

NURSING CONSIDERATIONS

Administer:

• By nasal spray: remove cap/safety clip from spray pump

• Prime pump if using for 1st time by pushing 4 times quickly, away from face, blow nose, then place tip of pump into one nostril, while holding other nostril closed, tilt head forward and spray into nostril; repeat in other nostril; put cover/safety clip back on

Perform/provide:

• Storage in tight container at room temperature

Evaluate:

• Therapeutic response: absence of running or congested nose

Teach patient/family:

• To avoid driving, other hazardous activities if drowsiness occurs

---

azithromycin (R)

(ay-zi-thro-my′sin)

Zithromax

Func. class.: Antiinfective

Chem. class.: Macrolide (azalide)

Action: Binds to 50S ribosomal subunits of susceptible bacteria and suppresses protein synthesis; much greater spectrum of activity than erythromycin

Uses: Mild to moderate infections of the upper respiratory tract, lower respiratory tract, uncomplicated skin and skin structure infections caused by *Moraxella catarrhalis, Streptococcus pneumoniae, Streptococcus pyogenes, Staphylococcus aureus, Streptococcus agalactiae, Mycoplasma pneumoniae, Haemophilus influenzae, Clostridium, Legionella pneumophila;* nongonococcal ure-

---

◆ = Nursing alert   ⫽ = Herb-drug interaction   Ⓝ = Do not crush thritis or cervicitis due to *Chlamydia trachomatis*; in children: acute otitis media (*H. influenzae, M. catarrhalis, S. pneumoniae*) PO; community-acquired pneumonia *(Citrobacter pneumoniae, H. influenzae, M. pneumoniae, S. pneumoniae)* PO; pharyngitis/tonsillitis *(S. pyogenes);* prophylaxis of disseminated *Mycobacterium avium* complex (MAC)

Dosage and routes:
• *Adult:* PO 500 mg on day 1, then 250 mg qd on days 2-5 for a total dose of 1.5 g; may give a one-time dose of 1 g for chlamydial infections; 1200 mg qwk for MAC prophylaxis IV 500 mg qd ≥2 days, then 500 mg qd to complete 7-10 day therapy for community-acquired pneumonia
• *Adult:* IV 500 mg qd × 2 days, then 250 mg qd to complete 7 day therapy for pelvic inflammatory disease (PID)
• *Child ≥2 yr:* 12 mg/kg qd for 5 days
• *Child <6 mo:* 10 mg/kg on day 1, then 5 mg/kg qd
Available forms: Caps 250; tabs 250, 600 mg; powder for inj 500 mg; powder for oral susp 100 mg/5 ml, 200 mg/5 ml, 1 g/packet

Side effects/adverse reactions:
INTEG: Rash, urticaria, pruritus, photosensitivity
CV: Palpitations, chest pain
CNS: Dizziness, headache, vertigo, somnolence
GI: Nausea, vomiting, diarrhea, **hepatotoxicity,** abdominal pain, stomatitis, heartburn, dyspepsia, flatulence, melena, *cholestatic jaundice*
GU: Vaginitis, moniliasis, nephritis
Contraindications: Hypersensitivity to azithromycin or erythromycin
Precautions: Pregnancy (B), lacta-

tion; hepatic, renal, cardiac disease; elderly, <6 mo for otitis media, <2 yr for pharyngitis, tonsillitis
Pharmacokinetics: Peak 2-4 hr, duration 24 hr, half-life 11-57 hr, excreted in bile, feces, urine primarily as unchanged drug
Interactions:
• Toxicity; ergotamine
• Increased effects of oral anticoagulants, digoxin, theophylline, methylprednisolone, cyclosporine, bromocriptine, disopyramide, triazolam, carbamazepine, phenytoin
• Decreased clearance of: triazolam
• Dysrhythmias: astemizole, pimozide
• Decreased absorption of azithromycin: food, aluminium, magnesium antacids
NURSING CONSIDERATIONS
Assess:
• I&O ratio; report hematuria, oliguria in renal disease
• Liver studies: AST, ALT; CBC with differential
• Renal studies: urinalysis, protein, blood
• C&S before drug therapy; drug may be taken as soon as culture is taken; C&S may be repeated after treatment
• For superinfection: sore throat, fever, fatigue
• Bowel pattern before, during treatment
• Respiratory status: rate, character, wheezing, tightness in chest; discontinue drug if these occur
Administer:
• Caps/susp 1 hr ac or 2 hr pc; tabs may be taken without regard to food Reconstitute 1 g packet for susp with 60 ml water, mix, rinse glass with more water and have patient drink to consume all medication
IV
• Reconstitute 500 mg of drug/4.8 ml sterile water for inj (100 mg/ml);

shake, dilute with ≥250 ml 0.9% NaCl, 0.45% NaCl, or LR to 1-2 mg/ml
• Give 500 mg/hr or more, never give IM or as a bolus

Perform/provide:
• Storage at room temperature

Evaluate:
• Therapeutic response: C&S negative for infection; decreased signs of infection

Teach patient/family:
• To report sore throat, fever, fatigue (may indicate superinfection)
• Not to take aluminum/magnesium-containing antacids simultaneously with this drug (PO)
• To notify nurse of diarrhea stools, dark urine, pale stools, yellow discoloration of eyes or skin, severe abdominal pain
• To take at evenly spaced intervals; complete dosage regimen

Treatment of hypersensitivity: Withdraw drug, maintain airway, administer epinephrine, aminophylline, O_2, IV corticosteroids

---

aztreonam (R)

(az-tree'oh nam)
Azactam
Func. class.: Miscellaneous antibiotic
Chem. class.: Monobactam

Action: Inhibits organisms by inhibiting bacterial cell wall synthesis, which causes death of organism (bactericidal)

Uses: Urinary tract infection; septicemia; skin, muscle, bone infection; and other infections caused by gram-negative organisms

Investigational uses: May be used instead of spectinomycin for acute uncomplicated gonorrhea in patients with penicillin-resistant gonococci

Dosage and routes:
Urinary tract infections
• *Adult:* **IV/IM** 500 mg-1 g q8-12h
Systemic infections
• *Adult:* **IV/IM** 1-2 g q8-12h
• *Child:* **IV/IM** 90-120 mg/kg/day divided q6-8h
Severe systemic infections
• *Adult:* **IV/IM** 2 g q6-8h; do not exceed 8 g/day
Continue treatment for 48 hr after negative culture or until patient is asymptomatic

Available forms: Powder for inj 500 mg, 1, 2 g

Side effects/adverse reactions:
HEMA: Anemia, increased bleeding time, **bone marrow depression, granulocytopenia**
GI: Nausea, vomiting, diarrhea, increased AST, ALT, abdominal pain, glossitis, colitis, **pseudomembranous colitis**
CNS: Lethargy, hallucinations, anxiety, depression, twitching, **coma, convulsions,** malaise, fever (pediatric)
EENT: Tinnitus, diplopia, nasal congestion
GU: Vaginal candidiasis, vaginitis, breast tenderness, increased BUN, creatinine
INTEG: Rash (pediatric)

Contraindications: Hypersensitivity to this drug, penicillins, cephalosporins

Precautions: Pregnancy (B), lactation, children, impaired renal, hepatic function, elderly

Pharmacokinetics:
IV: Peak immediate, trough 8 hr
IM: Peak 1 hr
Half-life: 1.7 hr; half-life prolonged in renal disease; protein binding 56%; metabolized by liver; excreted in urine 60%-70%; small amounts appear in breast milk, placenta

---

⬥ = Nursing alert   ⫽ = Herb-drug interaction   ⊘ = Do not crush

Interactions:
• Synergistic effect: other anti-infectives, β-lactamase antibiotics, aminoglycosides
• Antagonist effect: Cefoxitin, imipenem
• Increased aztreonam level: Probenecid
• Incompatible with nafcillin, metronidazole, cephradine

Lab test interferences:
Interfere: Urine glucose using Clinitest/Benedict's reagent
Positive: Coombs' test

NURSING CONSIDERATIONS
Assess:
• Signs of bruising, bleeding, anemia
• Bowel pattern before, during treatment
• I&O ratio; report hematuria, oliguria, since this drug in high doses is nephrotoxic
◆ Any patient with compromised renal system, since drug is excreted slowly in poor renal system function; toxicity may occur rapidly
• Liver studies: AST, ALT
• Blood studies: WBC, RBC, Hgb, Hct, bleeding time
• Renal studies: urinalysis, protein, blood, serum creatinine, BUN
• Skin eruptions after administration of drug to 1 wk after discontinuing drug
• Allergies before initiation of treatment, reaction of medication; highlight allergies on chart

Administer:
IM
• Dilute each g with at least 3 ml of 0.9% NaCl; give into large muscle
• Give drug after C&S completed
IV, direct
• After diluting with 6-10 ml sterile H_2O/15-30 ml drug; give over 3-5 min

IV inf
• After diluting with 3 ml or more sterile H_2O/1 g drug; then dilute with 50-100 ml of D_5W, 0.9% NaCl, LR, D_5, D_{10} solution; give over ½-1 hr, by Y-tube or 3-way stopcock; flush tubing before and after administration

Additive compatibilities: Ampicillin/sulbactam, cefazolin, ciprofloxacin, clindamycin, gentamicin, tobramycin

Syringe compatibilities: Clindamycin

Y-site compatibilities: Allopurinol, amifostine, amikacin, aminophylline, ampicillin, ampicillin/sulbactam, bleomycin, bumetanide, buprenorphine, butorphanol, calcium gluconate, carboplatin, carmustine, cefazolin, cefepime, cefonicid, cefoperazone, cefotaxime, cefotetan, cefoxitin, ceftazidime, ceftizoxime, ceftriaxone, cefuroxime, cimetidine, ciprofloxacin, cisatracurium, cisplatin, clindamycin, cyclophosphamide, cytarabine, dacarbazine, dactinomycin, dexamethasone, diltiazem, diphenhydramine, dobutamine, dopamine, doxorubicin, doxorubicin liposome, doxycycline, droperidol, enalaprilat, etoposide, famotidine, filgrastim, floxuridine, fluconazole, fludarabine, fluorouracil, foscarnet, furosemide, gallium, gentamicin, granisetron, haloperidol, heparin, hydrocortisone, hydromorphone, hydroxyzine, idarubicin, ifosfamide, imipenem-cilastatin, insulin (regular), leucovorin, magnesium sulfate, mannitol, mechlorethamine, melphalan, meperidine, mesna, methotrexate, methylprednisolone, metoclopramide, mezlocillin, minocycline, morphine, nalbuphine, netilmicin, ondansetron, piperacillin, piperacillin/tazobactam, plicamycin, potassium chloride, promethazine, propofol, ranitidine, remifentanil, sargramostim, sodium bicarbonate, teniposide, theophylline, thiotepa, ticarcillin, ticarcillin/clavulanate, tobramycin, trimethoprim-sulfamethoxazole, vinblastine, vincristine, vinorelbine, zidovudine

Perform/provide:
• Adequate fluid intake (2 L) during diarrhea episodes
• Storage in refrigerator

Evaluate:
• Therapeutic response: absence of fever, purulent drainage, redness, inflammation, temp

Teach patient/family:
• That culture may be taken after completed course of medication
• To report sore throat, fever, fatigue (may indicate superinfection)

---

bacitracin (℞)

(bass-i-tray′sin)
BACI-IM, Baciquent, Bacitin*
Func. class.: Antiinfective, misc.
Chem. class.: *Bacillus subtilis* derivative (polypeptide)

Action: Inhibits bacterial cell wall synthesis, interfering with osmotic pressure within cell

Uses:
Staphylococcal pneumonia, empyema

Dosage and routes:
• *Infant >2.5 kg:* **IM** 1000 U/kg/day in divided doses q8-12h
• *Infant ≤2.5 kg:* **IM** 900 U/kg/day in divided doses q8-12h
Available forms: Inj 50,000 U

Side effects/adverse reactions:
EENT: Ototoxicity
CV: Hypotension
INTEG: Rash, pain at injection site
GI: Nausea, vomiting, diarrhea
GU: **Proteinuria, casts, azotemia,** *oliguria, anuria, increased BUN, creatinine, tubular/glomerular necrosis*

Contraindications: Hypersensitivity, severe renal disease (IM use)
Precautions: Pregnancy (C), lactation, renal disease
Pharmacokinetics: Peak 1-2 hr, duration > 12 hr, metabolized in liver, excreted in urine

Interactions:
• Increased nephrotoxicity: aminoglycosides, polymyxin
• Increased neuromuscular blockade: nondepolarizing skeletal muscle relaxants, inhalation anesthetics

NURSING CONSIDERATIONS

Assess:
• Any patient with compromised renal system; drug is excreted slowly in poor renal system function; toxicity may occur rapidly
• Renal studies: urinalysis, protein, blood, BUN, creatinine, urine pH (keep above 6.0); I&O ratio; report oliguria, change in urinary output; high doses are nephrotoxic
• C&S before drug therapy; drug may be taken as soon as culture is taken; repeat C&S after treatment
• Bowel pattern before, during treatment; if severe diarrhea occurs, drug should be discontinued
• Allergies before treatment, reaction of each medication; report allergies on chart in bright red; notify all people giving drugs; skin eruptions, itching; rash, urticaria, erythema

Administer:
IM
• After reconstituting with NS
• IM in deep muscle mass; rotate injection site; do not give IV/SC

Perform/provide:
• Storage in refrigerator; protect from direct sunlight

 = Nursing alert   = Herb-drug interaction   ⊘ = Do not crush

Evaluate:
• Therapeutic response: absence of fever, cough, dyspnea, malaise, temp, negative C&S
Teach patient/family:
• To report sore throat, fever, fatigue (may indicate superinfection); reduced frequency of urination

---

baclofen (℞)

(bak'loe-fen)
Lioresal, Lioresal Intrathecal
Func. class.: Skeletal muscle relaxant, central acting
Chem. class.: GABA chlorophenyl derivative

Action: Inhibits synaptic responses in CNS by decreasing GABA, which decreases neurotransmitter function; decreases frequency, severity of muscle spasms
Uses: Spasticity in spinal cord injury, multiple sclerosis
Dosage and routes:
• *Adult:* **PO** 5 mg tid × 3 days, then 10 mg tid × 3 days, then 15 mg tid × 3 days, then 20 mg tid × 3 days, then titrated to response, not to exceed 80 mg/day
• *Child >2 yr:* **PO** 10-15 mg/kg/day divided q8h titrate to max 40 mg/day
• *Child ≥8 yr:* as above, max 60 mg/day
• **INTRATHECAL:** Use implantable intrathecal **INF** pump; use screening trial of 3 separate **BOL** doses if needed (50 µg/ml, 75 µg/1.5 ml, 100 µg/2 ml). Initial: double screening dose that produced result and give over 24 hr: increase by 10%-30% q24h only. Maintenance: 1200-1500 µg/day
Available forms: Tabs 10, 20 mg; intrathecal inj 10 mg/20 ml (500 µg/ml), 10 mg/5 ml (2000 µg/ml)

Side effects/adverse reactions:
CNS: Dizziness, weakness, fatigue, drowsiness, headache, *disorientation,* insomnia, paresthesias, tremors, **seizures**
EENT: Nasal congestion, blurred vision, mydriasis, tinnitus
CV: Hypotension, chest pain, palpitations, edema
GI: Nausea, constipation, *vomiting,* increased AST, alk phosphatase, abdominal pain, dry mouth, anorexia
GU: Urinary frequency
INTEG: Rash, pruritus
Contraindications: Hypersensitivity
Precautions: Peptic ulcer disease, renal disease, hepatic disease, stroke, seizure disorder, diabetes mellitus, pregnancy (C), lactation, elderly
Pharmacokinetics:
PO: Peak 2-3 hr, duration >8 hr, half-life 2½-4 hr, partially metabolized in liver, excreted in urine (unchanged)
INTRATHECAL: CSF levels with plasma levels 100 times oral route
Interactions:
• Increased CNS depression: alcohol, tricyclic antidepressants, opiates, barbiturates, sedatives, hypnotics
🍵 May increase CNS depression: kava
Lab test interferences:
Increase: AST, alk phosphatase, blood glucose
NURSING CONSIDERATIONS
Assess:
• B/P, weight, blood sugar, and hepatic function periodically
◆ For increased seizure activity in epilepsy patient; this drug decreases seizure threshold
• I&O ratio; check for urinary frequency
• EEG in epileptic patients; poor seizure control has occurred in patients taking this drug

---

• Allergic reactions: rash, fever, respiratory distress
• Severe weakness, numbness in extremities
• Tolerance: increased need for medication, more frequent requests for medication, increased pain
• CNS depression: dizziness, drowsiness, psychiatric symptoms
• Dosage, as individual titration is required

Administer:
PO
• With meals for GI symptoms
IT
• Do not use IT inj IV, IM, SC, epidural
Additive compatibilities: Morphine
Perform/provide:
• Storage in tight container at room temperature
• Assistance with ambulation if dizziness or drowsiness occurs
Evaluate:
• Therapeutic response: decreased pain, spasticity
Teach patient/family:
• Not to discontinue medication quickly; hallucinations, spasticity, tachycardia will occur; drug should be tapered off over 1-2 wk
• Not to take with alcohol, other CNS depressants
• To avoid hazardous activities if drowsiness or dizziness occurs
• To avoid using OTC medication: cough preparations, antihistamines, unless directed by prescriber
Treatment of overdose: Induce emesis of conscious patient, lavage, dialysis

basiliximab (℞)
(bas-ih-liks'ih-mab)
Simulect
Func. class.: Immunosuppressive
Chem. class.: Murine/human monoclonal antibody (Interleukin-2) receptor antagonist

Action: Binds to and blocks the IL-2 receptor, which is selectively expressed on the surface of activated T-lymphocytes; impairs the immune system to antigenic challenges
Uses: Acute allograft rejection in renal transplant patients when used with cyclosporine and corticosteroids
Dosage and routes:
• *Adult:* IV 20 mg × 2 doses; 1st dose within 2 hr before transplant surgery; 2nd dose given 4 days after transplantation
• *Child 2-15 yr:* 12 mg/m^2 × 2 doses; 1st dose within 2 hr before transplant surgery; 2nd dose given 4 days after transplantation
Available forms: Powder for inj 20 mg
Side effects/adverse reactions:
CNS: Pyrexia, chills, tremors, headache, insomnia
*RESP: Dyspnea, wheezing, **pulmonary edema***
CV: Chest pain, angina, ***cardiac failure***, hypotension
MS: Arthralgia, myalgia
GI: Vomiting, nausea, diarrhea, constipation, abdominal pain
MISC: Infection, moniliasis
Contraindications: Hypersensitivity
Precautions: Pregnancy (B), infections, elderly, lactation, children
NURSING CONSIDERATIONS
Assess:
• Blood studies: Hgb, WBC, plate-

lets during treatment qmo; if leukocytes are <3000/mm^3, drug should be discontinued
• Liver function studies: alk phosphatase, AST, ALT, bilirubin
• Hepatotoxicity: dark urine, jaundice, itching, light-colored stools; drug should be discontinued

Administer:
• All medications PO if possible; avoid IM injection, since infection may occur

IV
• After adding 5 ml sterile water for inj, shake gently to dissolve, reconstitute to a vol of 50 ml with 0.9% NaCl or D$_5$, gently invert bag, do not shake

Evaluate:
• Therapeutic response: absence of graft rejection

Teach patient/family:
• To report fever, chills, sore throat, fatigue, since serious infection may occur

---

beclomethasone (℞)

(be-kloe-meth'a-sone)
Beclodisk*, Becloforte Inhaler*, Beclovent, Beclovent Rotocaps*, Vanceril
Func. class.: Corticosteroid, synthetic
Chem. class.: Glucocorticoid

Action: Prevents inflammation by depression of migration of polymorphonuclear leukocytes, fibroblasts, reversal of increased capillary permeability and lysosomal stabilization; does not suppress hypothalamus and pituitary function
Uses: Chronic asthma, rhinitis
Dosage and routes:
• *Adult:* INH 2-4 puffs tid-qid, not to exceed 20 inhalations/day
• *Child: 6-12 yr:* INH 1-2 puffs tid-qid, not to exceed 10 inhalations/day
Available forms: Aerosol 42 µg/actuation

Side effects/adverse reactions:
RESP: **Bronchospasm,** wheezing, cough
GI: Dry mouth
EENT: Hoarseness, candidal infections of oral cavity, sore throat
MISC: **Angioedema, adrenal insufficiency,** facial edema
Contraindications: Hypersensitivity, status asthmaticus (primary treatment), nonasthmatic bronchial disease; bacterial, fungal, viral infections of mouth, throat, lungs; children <3 yr
Precautions: Nasal disease/surgery, pregnancy (C), lactation
Pharmacokinetics:
INH: Onset 10 min, excreted in feces (metabolites), half-life 3-15 hr, crosses placenta, metabolized in lungs, liver, GI system
NURSING CONSIDERATIONS
Assess:
• For fungal infection in mucous membranes
• Adrenal function periodically for HPA axis suppression during prolonged therapy, monitor growth/development
Administer:
• INH with water to decrease possibility of fungal infections
• Titrated dose, use lowest effective dose
• PO, using a spacer device for proper dose
Perform/provide:
• Gum, rinsing of mouth for dry mouth
Evaluate:
• Therapeutic response: decreased dyspnea, wheezing, dry rales on auscultation

---

Teach patient/family:
• To carry or wear ID as steroid user
• To gargle/rinse mouth after each use to prevent oral fungal infections
• That in times of stress, systemic corticosteroids may be needed to prevent adrenal insufficiency; do not discontinue oral drug abruptly, taper slowly
• To notify prescriber if therapeutic response decreases; dosage adjustment may be needed
• Proper administration technique
• To wash inhaler with warm water and dry after each use
• All aspects of drug usage, including cushingoid symptoms
• The symptoms of adrenal insufficiency: nausea, anorexia, fatigue, dizziness, dyspnea, weakness, joint pain, depression

---

benazepril (℞)
(ben-aze'uh-pril)
Lotensin
Func. class.: Antihypertensive
Chem. class.: Angiotensin-converting enzyme (ACE) inhibitor

Action: Selectively suppresses renin-angiotensin-aldosterone system; inhibits ACE, preventing conversion of angiotensin I to angiotensin II; results in dilation of arterial, venous vessels
Uses: Hypertension, alone or in combination with thiazide diuretics
Dosage and routes:
• *Adult:* **PO** 10 mg qd initially, then 20-40 mg/day divided bid or qd (without a diuretic); 5 mg **PO** qd (with a diuretic)
• *Renal dose:* CrCl <30 ml/min 5 mg **PO** qd, max 40 mg/day
• *Geriatric:* **PO** 5-10 mg/day initially

Available forms: Tabs 5, 10, 20, 40 mg
Side effects/adverse reactions:
CV: Hypotension, postural hypotension, syncope, palpitations, angina
GU: Increased BUN, creatinine, decreased libido, impotence, urinary tract infection
HEMA: Neutropenia, agranulocytosis
INTEG: Rash, flushing, sweating
RESP: Cough, asthma, bronchitis, dyspnea, sinusitis
META: Hyperkalemia, hyponatremia
GI: Nausea, constipation, vomiting, gastritis, melena
CNS: Anxiety, hypertonia, insomnia, paresthesia, headache, dizziness, fatigue
MS: Arthralgia, arthritis, myalgia
MISC: Angioedema
Contraindications: Hypersensitivity to ACE inhibitors, pregnancy (D) 2nd/3rd trimester, lactation, children
Precautions: Impaired renal, liver function, dialysis patients, hypovolemia, blood dyscrasias, CHF, COPD, asthma, elderly, bilateral renal artery stenosis, pregnancy (C) 1st trimester
Pharmacokinetics:
PO: Peak ½-1 hr, serum protein binding 97%, half-life 10-11 hr, metabolized by liver (metabolites), excreted in urine
Interactions:
• Increased hypotension: diuretics, other antihypertensives
• Increased hyperkalemia: potassium-sparing diuretics, potassium supplements
• Increased serum levels of lithium
Lab test interferences:
Increase: BUN, creatinine, LFTs, bilirubin, uric acid, blood glucose

---

◆ = Nursing alert   🦋 = Herb-drug interaction   ⊘ = Do not crush

NURSING CONSIDERATIONS
Assess:

• Blood studies: neutrophils, decreased platelets

• B/P at peak/trough level of drug, orthostatic hypotension, syncope when used with diuretic

• Renal studies: protein, BUN, creatinine; increased levels may indicate nephrotic syndrome; monitor urine for protein

• Potassium levels, although hyperkalemia rarely occurs

• Allergic reactions: rash, fever, pruritus, urticaria; drug should be discontinued if antihistamines fail to help

• Renal symptoms: polyuria, oliguria, frequency, dysuria

Perform/provide:

• Storage in tight container at 86° F (30° C) or less

Evaluate:

• Therapeutic response: decrease in B/P

Teach patient/family:

• Not to discontinue drug abruptly

• Not to use OTC products (cough, cold, allergy) unless directed by prescriber; do not use salt substitutes containing potassium without consulting prescriber

• The importance of complying with dosage schedule, even if feeling better

• To notify prescriber of pregnancy, drug will need to be discontinued

• To rise slowly to sitting or standing position to minimize orthostatic hypotension

• To notify prescriber of mouth sores, sore throat, fever, swelling of hands or feet, irregular heartbeat, chest pain

• To report excessive perspiration, dehydration, vomiting, diarrhea; may lead to fall in B/P

• That drug may cause dizziness, fainting, light-headedness; may occur during first few days of therapy

• That drug may cause skin rash or impaired perspiration

• How to take B/P, and normal readings for age group

Treatment of overdose: 0.9% NaCl IV INF, hemodialysis

---

benztropine ($\textbf{R}$)

(benz'troe-peen)

Apo-Benztropin*, benztropine mesylate, Bensylate*, Cogentin, PMS-Benztropine*

Func. class.: Cholinergic blocker
Chem. class.: Tertiary amine

Action: Blockade of central acetylcholine receptors

Uses: Parkinson symptoms, EPS associated with neuroleptic drugs

Dosage and routes:
Drug-induced EPS

• *Adult:* **IM/IV** 1-4 mg qd-bid; give **PO** dose as soon as possible; **PO** 1-2 mg bid/tid, increase by 0.5 mg q5-6 days

• *Child:* **IM/IV** 0.02-0.05 mg/kg/dose 1-2 ×/day

• *Geriatric:* **PO** 0.5 mg qd-bid, increase by 0.5 mg q5-6d

Parkinson symptoms

• *Adult:* **PO** 0.5-6 mg qd, increase 0.5 mg q5-6d titrated to patient response, max 6 mg qd

Acute dystonic reactions

• *Adult:* **IM/IV** 1-2 mg, may increase to 1-2 mg bid (PO)

Available forms: Tabs 0.5, 1, 2 mg; inj 1 mg/ml

Side effects/adverse reactions:
MS: Muscular weakness, cramping
INTEG: Rash, urticaria, dermatoses
MISC: Increased temperature, flushing, decreased sweating, hyperthermia, heat stroke, numbness of fingers

---

CNS: Anxiety, restlessness, irritability, delusions, hallucinations, headache, sedation, depression, incoherence, dizziness, memory loss; confusion, delirium (elderly)

EENT: Blurred vision, photophobia, dilated pupils, difficulty swallowing, dry eyes, mydriasis, increased intraocular tension, angle-closure glaucoma

CV: Palpitations, tachycardia, hypotension, bradycardia

GI: Dryness of mouth, constipation, nausea, vomiting, abdominal distress, ***paralytic ileus,*** epigastric distress

GU: Hesitancy, retention, dysuria

Contraindications: Hypersensitivity, narrow-angle glaucoma, myasthenia gravis, GI/GU obstruction, child <3 yr, peptic ulcer, megacolon, prostate hypertrophy

Precautions: Pregnancy (C), elderly, lactation, tachycardia, liver, kidney disease, drug abuse history, dysrhythmias, hypotension, hypertension, psychiatric patients, children

Pharmacokinetics:
IM/IV: Onset 15 min, duration 6-10 hr
PO: Onset 1 hr, duration 6-10 hr

Interactions:
• Increased anticholinergic effect: antihistamines, phenothiazines, tricyclics, disopyramide, quinidine
• Decreased absorption: antidiarrheals

NURSING CONSIDERATIONS
Assess:
• I&O ratio; commonly causes decreased urinary output; urinary hesitancy, retention; palpate bladder if retention occurs
• Parkinsonism, EPS: shuffling gait, muscle rigidity, involuntary movements
• Constipation; increase fluids, bulk, exercise if this occurs

• Mental status: affect, mood, CNS depression, worsening of mental symptoms during early therapy
• Use caution in hot weather; drug may increase susceptibility to stroke by decreasing sweating
• For benztropine "buzz" or "high," patients may imitate EPS

Administer:
PO
• With or after meals to prevent GI upset; may give with fluids other than water
• At hs to avoid daytime drowsiness in patient with parkinsonism
IV
• Undiluted IV (1 mg = 1 ml) dose at ≤1 mg/>1 min; keep in bed for at least 1 hr after dose

Syringe compatibilities: Chlorpromazine, fluphenazine, metoclopramide, perphenazine, thiothixene

Y-site compatibilities: Fluconazole, tacrolimus

Perform/provide:
• Storage at room temperature
• Hard candy, gum, frequent drinks, to relieve dry mouth

Evaluate:
• Therapeutic response: absence of involuntary movements

Teach patient/family:
• That tabs may be crushed and mixed with food
• Not to discontinue this drug abruptly; to taper off over 1 wk
• To avoid driving, other hazardous activities; drowsiness may occur
• To avoid OTC medication: cough, cold preparations with alcohol, antihistamines unless directed by prescriber

---

◆ = Nursing alert   ⬮ = Herb-drug interaction   🚫 = Do not crush

bepridil (R)
(be'pri-dil)
Bepadin, Vascor
Func. class.: Calcium channel blocker, antianginal

Action: Inhibits calcium ion influx across cell membrane during cardiac depolarization; produces relaxation of coronary vascular smooth muscle, dilates coronary arteries, decreases SA/AV node conduction, dilates peripheral arteries

Uses: Chronic stable angina, used alone or in combination with propranolol

Dosage and routes:

Angina
• *Adult:* PO 200 mg qd, after 10 days may increase dose if needed, max dose 400 mg/day
Available forms: Tabs, film-coated, 200, 300, 400 mg

Side effects/adverse reactions:
CV: Dysrhythmia, edema, CHF, bradycardia, hypotension, palpitations, AV block, *torsades de pointes*
GI: Nausea, vomiting, diarrhea, gastric upset, constipation, increased liver function studies
GU: Nocturia, polyuria
CNS: Headache, fatigue, drowsiness, dizziness, anxiety, depression, weakness, insomnia, confusion, light-headedness, nervousness
HEMA: Agranulocytosis

Contraindications: Sick sinus syndrome, 2nd- or 3rd-degree heart block, Wolff-Parkinson-White syndrome, hypotension less than 90 mm Hg systolic, cardiogenic shock, history of serious ventricular dysrhythmias

Precautions: CHF, hypotension, hepatic injury, pregnancy (C), lactation, children, renal disease, idiopathic hypertropic subaortic stenosis (IHSS), concomitant β-blocker therapy

Pharmacokinetics: Onset 1 hr, peak 2-3 hr, duration 24 hr, 99% plasma protein bound, half-life 42 hr; completely metabolized in the liver and excreted in urine and feces

Interactions:
• Increased prolongation of QT, depression of AV node: cardiac glycosides, antidysrhythmics
• Increased hypotension: fentanyl
• Increased levels of digoxin
🥄 Increased antianginal effect: cat's claw, chicory
🥄 Increased hypotensive effects: grapefruit

Lab test interferences:
Increase: Liver function tests, aminotransferase, CPK, LDH

NURSING CONSIDERATIONS
Assess:
• Cardiac status: B/P, pulse, respiration, ECG intervals (PR, QRS, QT), dysrhythmias
Administer:
PO
• Before meals, hs; adjust no more frequently than q10 days
Evaluate:
• Therapeutic response: decreased anginal pain
Teach patient/family:
• How to take pulse before taking drug; record or graph should be kept; use demonstration, return demonstration
• To avoid hazardous activities until stabilized on drug, dizziness no longer a problem
• To limit caffeine consumption
🚫 Not to break, crush, or chew tabs
• To avoid OTC drugs unless directed by a prescriber
• The importance of compliance with all areas of medical regimen: diet, exercise, stress reduction, drug therapy

Treatment of overdose: Defibrillation, atropine for AV block, vasopressor for hypotension

---

betamethasone (℞)
(bay-ta-meth'a-sone)
Betnelan*, Celestone
betamethasone acetate/ betamethasone sodium phosphate (℞)
Celestone Soluspan
betamethasone sodium phosphate (℞)
Celestone Phosphate, Selestoject
Func. class.: Corticosteroid, synthetic
Chem. class.: Glucocorticoid, long-acting

Action: Decreases inflammation by suppressing migration of polymorphonuclear leukocytes, fibroblasts, reversal of increased capillary permeability and lysosomal stabilization

Uses: Immunosuppression, severe inflammation, prevention of neonatal respiratory distress syndrome (by administration to mother)

Dosage and routes:
• *Adult:* **PO** 0.6-7.2 mg qd; **IM/IV** 0.6-7.2 mg qd in joint or soft tissue (sodium phosphate)
• *Child:* **PO** 17.5 µg/kg/day in 3 divided doses; **IM** 17.5 µg/kg/day in 3 divided doses every 3rd day or 5.8-8.75 µg/kg/day as a single dose (adrenal insufficiency)
• *Child:* **PO** 62.5-250 µg/kg/day in 3 divided doses; **IM** 20.8-125 µg/ kg/day of the base q12-24h (other uses)

Available forms: Betamethasone:

tabs 500; 600 µg, tabs, effervescent 500 µg*, syrup 600 µg/5 ml; betamethasone acetate/betamethasone sodium phosphate: inj susp acetate 3 mg/sodium phosphate (= to 3 mg base); betamethasone sodium phosphate: inj 4 mg (= to 3 mg base)/ml

Side effects/adverse reactions:
INTEG: Acne, poor wound healing, ecchymosis, bruising, petechiae
CNS: Depression, flushing, sweating, headache, ecchymosis, bruising, mood changes
CV: Hypertension, **circulatory collapse, thrombophlebitis, embolism,** tachycardia, **necrotizing angiitis, CHF**
HEMA: **Thrombocytopenia**
MS: Fractures, osteoporosis, weakness
GI: Diarrhea, nausea, abdominal distention, **GI hemorrhage,** increased appetite, **pancreatitis**
EENT: Fungal infections, increased intraocular pressure, blurred vision

Contraindications: Psychosis, hypersensitivity, idiopathic thrombocytopenia, acute glomerulonephritis, amebiasis, fungal infections, nonasthmatic bronchial disease, child <2 yr, AIDS, TB

Precautions: Pregnancy (C), lactation, diabetes mellitus, glaucoma, osteoporosis, seizure disorders, ulcerative colitis, CHF, myasthenia gravis, renal disease, esophagitis, peptic ulcer

Pharmacokinetics:
PO: Onset 1-2 hr, peak 1 hr, duration 3 days
IM/IV: Onset 10 min, peak 4-8 hr, duration 1-1½ days
Metabolized in liver, excreted in urine as steroids, crosses placenta

Interactions:
• Decreased action of betamethasone: barbiturates, rifampin, phenytoin

---

◆ = Nursing alert   ∥ = Herb-drug interaction   ⊘ = Do not crush

• Decreased effects of anticoagulants, antidiabetics, insulin, isoniazid, toxoids, vaccines, salicylates

• GI bleeding: NSAIDs, alcohol, salicylates, indomethacin

🖋 Potassium deficiency: chronic use/abuse of cascara sagrada bark, buckthorn bark/berry, rhubarb root, senna leaf/fruits, aloe

🖋 Increased action/side effects: squill, lily of the valley, pheasant's eye

Lab test interferences:

Increase: Cholesterol, sodium, blood glucose, uric acid, calcium, urine glucose

Decrease: Calcium, potassium, T_4, T_3, thyroid ^{131}I uptake test, urine 17-OHCS, 17-KS, PBI

False negative: Skin allergy tests

NURSING CONSIDERATIONS

Assess:

• Potassium, blood sugar, urine glucose while on long-term therapy; hypokalemia and hyperglycemia

• Weight daily; notify prescriber of weekly gain >5 lb

• B/P q4h, pulse; notify prescriber if chest pain occurs

• I&O ratio; be alert for decreasing urinary output and increasing edema

• Plasma cortisol levels during long-term therapy (normal level: 138-635 nmol/L SI units when drawn at 8 AM)

Administer:

PO

• With food or milk to decrease GI symptoms

IM

• Inject deeply in large muscle mass, rotate sites, avoid deltoid, use 21G needle

• In one dose in AM to prevent adrenal suppression, avoid SC administration; may damage tissue

IV

• Only sodium phosphate product;

give >1 min; may be given by IV INF in compatible sol

• After shaking suspension (parenteral)

• Titrated dose; use lowest effective dose

Y-site compatibilities: Heparin, hydrocortisone, potassium chloride, vit B/C

Perform/provide:

• Assistance with ambulation in patient with bone tissue disease to prevent fractures

Evaluate:

• Therapeutic response: ease of respirations, decreased inflammation

• Infection: increased temperature, WBC even after withdrawal of medication; drug masks infection symptoms

• Potassium depletion: paresthesias, fatigue, nausea, vomiting, depression, polyuria, dysrhythmias, weakness

• Edema, hypertension, cardiac symptoms

• Mental status: affect, mood, behavioral changes, aggression

Teach patient/family:

• That ID as steroid user should be carried

• To notify prescriber if therapeutic response decreases; dosage adjustment may be needed

◆ Not to discontinue abruptly; adrenal crisis can result

• To avoid OTC products: salicylates, alcohol in cough products, cold preparations unless directed by prescriber

• All aspects of drug usage including cushingoid symptoms

• The symptoms of adrenal insufficiency: nausea, anorexia, fatigue, dizziness, dyspnea, weakness, joint pain

bethanechol (℞)

(be-than'e-kole)
bethanechol chloride,
Duvoid, Myotonachol,
Urebeth, Urecholine

Func. class.: Cholinergic stimulant

Chem. class.: Synthetic choline ester

Action: Stimulates muscarinic ACh receptors directly; mimics effects of parasympathetic nervous system stimulation; stimulates gastric motility, stimulates micturition

Uses: Urinary retention (postoperative, postpartum), neurogenic atony of bladder with retention

Dosage and routes:
• *Adult:* **PO** 10-50 mg bid-qid; **SC** 2.5-10 mg tid-qid prn
• *Child:* **PO** 0.6 mg/kg/day divided in 3-4 doses/day

Test dose
• *Adult:* **SC** 2.5 mg repeated 15-30 min intervals × 4 doses to determine effective dose

Available forms: Tabs 5, 10, 25, 50 mg; inj 5 mg/ml

Side effects/adverse reactions:
INTEG: Rash, urticaria, flushing, increased sweating
CNS: Dizziness
GI: Nausea, bloody diarrhea, belching, vomiting, cramps, fecal incontinence
CV: Hypotension, bradycardia, orthostatic hypotension, reflex tachycardia, *cardiac arrest, circulatory collapse*
GU: Urgency
RESP: Acute asthma, dyspnea, bronchoconstriction
EENT: Miosis, increased salivation, lacrimation, blurred vision

Contraindications: Hypersensitivity, severe bradycardia, asthma, severe hypotension, hyperthyroidism, peptic ulcer, parkinsonism, seizure disorders, CAD, COPD, coronary occlusion, mechanical obstruction, peritonitis, recent urinary or GI surgery

Precautions: Hypertension, pregnancy (C), lactation, child <8 yr

Pharmacokinetics:
PO: Onset 30-90 min, duration 1-6 hr
SC: Onset 5-15 min, duration 2 hr, excreted by kidneys

Interactions:
• Increased action or toxicity: cholinergic agonists, anticholinesterase
• Severe hypotension: ganglionic blockers

Lab test interferences:
Increase: AST, lipase/amylase, bilirubin, BSP

NURSING CONSIDERATIONS
Assess:
• B/P, pulse; observe after parenteral dose for 1 hr
• I&O ratio; check for urinary retention or urge incontinence
• Bradycardia, hypotension, bronchospasm, headache, dizziness, convulsions, respiratory depression; drug should be discontinued if toxicity occurs

Administer:
• To avoid nausea and vomiting, take on an empty stomach
SC
◆ Parenteral dose by SC route; use of IM, IV may result in cardiac arrest
◆ Only with atropine sulfate available for cholinergic crisis
• Only after all other cholinergics have been discontinued
• Increased doses if tolerance occurs

Perform/provide:
• Storage at room temperature
• Bedpan/urinal if given for urinary retention

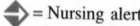

◆ = Nursing alert   🖋 = Herb-drug interaction   🚫 = Do not crush

• Use of rectal tube if ordered, to increase passage of gas when used for abdominal distention
Evaluate:
• Therapeutic response: absence of urinary retention, abdominal distention
Teach patient/family:
• To take drug exactly as prescribed; 1 hr ac or 2 hr pc
• To make position changes slowly; orthostatic hypotension may occur
Treatment of overdose: Administer atropine 0.6-1.2 mg IV or IM (adult)

---

bexarotene
See appendix a—selected new drugs

---

bicalutamide (℞)
(bye-kal-u′ta-mide)
Casodex
Func. class.: Antineoplastic hormone
Chem. class.: Nonsteroidal antiandrogen

Action: Binds to cytosol androgen in target tissue, which competitively inhibits the action to androgens
Uses: Prostate cancer in combination with luteinizing hormone–releasing hormone (LHRH) analog
Dosage and routes:
• *Adult:* PO 50 mg qd with LHRH
Available forms: Tabs 50 mg
Side effects/adverse reactions:
GI: Diarrhea, constipation, nausea, vomiting, increased liver enzyme test
CV: Hot flashes, hypertension
CNS: Dizziness, paresthesia, insomnia
INTEG: Rash, sweating
GU: Nocturia, hematuria, UTI, impotence, gynecomastia, urinary incontinence

MISC: Infection, anemia, dyspnea, bone pain, headache, asthenia, back pain, flu syndrome
Contraindications: Hypersensitivity, pregnancy (X)
Precautions: Renal, hepatic disease, elderly, lactation
Pharmacokinetics: Well absorbed, metabolized by liver, excreted in urine, feces
Interactions:
• May displace anticoagulants from their binding sites
Lab test interferences:
Increase: AST, ALT, bilirubin, BUN, creatinine
Decrease: Hgb, WBC
NURSING CONSIDERATIONS
Assess:
• For diarrhea, constipation, nausea, vomiting
• For hot flashes, gynecomastia (assure patient that these are common side effects)
• Prostate specific antigen (PSA), liver function studies
Administer:
PO
• At same time each day, either AM or PM, with/without food
• With LHRH treatment; start at same time for both drugs
Evaluate:
• Therapeutic response: decreased tumor size, decreased spread of malignancy
Teach patient/family:
• To recognize, report signs of anemia, hepatoxicity, renal toxicity

---

biperiden (℞)
(bye-per′i-den)
Akineton
Func. class.: Cholinergic blocker

Action: Centrally acting competitive anticholinergic
Uses: Parkinson symptoms, EPS

Side effects: *italics* = common; ***bold italics*** = life-threatening

secondary to neuroleptic drug therapy

Dosage and routes:
Extrapyramidal symptoms
• *Adult:* **PO** 2 mg qd-tid; **IM/IV** 2 mg q30min, if needed, not to exceed 8 mg/24 hr
Parkinson symptoms
• *Adult:* **PO** 2 mg tid-qid; max 16 mg/24 hr
Available forms: Tabs 2 mg; inj 5 mg/ml (lactate)

Side effects/adverse reactions:
CNS: Confusion, anxiety, restlessness, irritability, delusions, hallucinations, headache, sedation, depression, incoherence, dizziness, euphoria, tremors, memory loss
EENT: Blurred vision, photophobia, dilated pupils, difficulty swallowing, mydriasis, increased intraocular tension, angle-closure glaucoma
CV: Palpitations, tachycardia, postural hypotension, bradycardia
GI: Dryness of mouth, constipation, nausea, vomiting, abdominal distress, *paralytic ileus*
GU: Hesitancy, retention, dysuria
INTEG: Rash, urticaria, dermatoses
MISC: Increased temperature, flushing, decreased sweating, hyperthermia, *heat stroke,* numbness of fingers, weakness, cramping

Contraindications: Hypersensitivity, narrow-angle glaucoma, myasthenia gravis, GI/GU obstruction, megacolon, stenosing peptic ulcers, prostatic hypertrophy

Precautions: Pregnancy (C), elderly, lactation, tachycardia, dysrhythmias, liver or kidney disease, drug abuse, hypotension, hypertension, psychiatric patients, children

Pharmacokinetics:
IM/IV: Onset 15 min, duration 6-10 hr
PO: Onset 1 hr, duration 6-10 hr

Interactions:
• Increased levels of digoxin, levodopa

• Increased schizophrenic symptoms: haloperidol
• Increased anticholinergic effect: antihistamines, phenothiazines, amantadine, tricyclics
• Decreased biperiden absorption: antacids
• Increased sedation: alcohol

NURSING CONSIDERATIONS
Assess:
• I&O ratio; retention commonly causes decreased urinary output
• Parkinsonism, EPS: shuffling gait, muscle rigidity, involuntary movements
• Patient response if anticholinergics are given
• Urinary hesitancy, retention; palpate bladder if retention occurs
• Constipation; increase fluids, bulk, exercise if this occurs
• For tolerance over long-term therapy; dose may have to be increased or changed
• Mental status: affect, mood, CNS depression, worsening of mental symptoms during early therapy
Administer:
PO
• With or after meals to prevent GI upset; may give with fluids other than water
• At hs to avoid daytime drowsiness in patients with parkinsonism
IM/IV
• With patient recumbent to prevent postural hypotension, give undiluted 2 mg or less over 1 min or more
Perform/provide:
• Storage at room temperature
• Hard candy, gum, frequent drinks to relieve dry mouth
Evaluate:
• Therapeutic response: absence of involuntary movements
Teach patient/family:
• To use caution in hot weather; drug

---

may increase susceptibility to heat stroke, decreases sweating
• Not to discontinue this drug abruptly; to taper off over 1 wk
• To avoid driving, other hazardous activities; drowsiness may occur
• To avoid OTC medication: cough, cold preparations with alcohol, antihistamines unless directed by prescriber

---

bisacodyl (℞, OTC)

(bis-a-koe′dill)
Bisacolax*, Bisc-Evac, Bisco-Lax, Carter's Little Pills, Dacodyl, Deficol, Dulcagen, Dulcolax, Fleet Bisacodyl, Fleet Laxative, Laxit*, Therelax
Func. class.: Laxative, stimulant
Chem. class.: Diphenylmethane

Action: Acts directly on intestine by increasing motor activity; thought to irritate colonic intramural plexus
Uses: Short-term treatment of constipation, bowel or rectal preparation for surgery, examination
Dosage and routes:
• *Adult ≥12 yr:* PO 5-15 mg in PM or AM; may use up to 30 mg for bowel or rectal preparation; **RECT** 10 mg
• *Child >3 yr:* PO 5-10 mg as a single dose
• *Child >2 yr-11 yr:* RECT 10 mg as a single dose
• *Child <2 yr:* RECT 5 mg as a single dose
Available forms: Enteric-coated tabs 5 mg; rect supp 5, 10 mg; rect sol: 10 mg/37 ml; enema 0.33 mg/ml, 10 mg/5 ml; powder for rectal sol/ 1.5 mg bisacodyl/2.5 g tannic acid
Side effects/adverse reactions:
CNS: Muscle weakness
GI: Nausea, vomiting, anorexia, *cramps,* diarrhea, rectal burning (suppositories)
META: Protein-losing enteropathy, alkalosis, hypokalemia, ***tetany,*** electrolyte, fluid imbalances
Contraindications: Hypersensitivity, rectal fissures, abdominal pain, nausea, vomiting, appendicitis, acute surgical abdomen, ulcerated hemorrhoids, acute hepatitis, fecal impaction, intestinal/biliary tract obstruction
Precautions: Pregnancy (C), lactation
Pharmacokinetics:
PO: Onset 6-10 hr
RECT: Onset 15-60 min
Metabolized by liver; excreted in urine, bile, feces, breast milk
Interactions:
• Gastric irritation: antacids, milk, H₂-blockers
• Increased action/side effects: lily of the valley, pheasant's eye, squill
NURSING CONSIDERATIONS
Assess:
• Blood, urine electrolytes if drug is used often by patient
• I&O ratio to identify fluid loss
• Cause of constipation; identify whether fluids, bulk, or exercise missing from lifestyle
• Cramping, rectal bleeding, nausea, vomiting; if these symptoms occur, drug should be discontinued
Administer:
PO
• Alone only with water for better absorption; do not take within 1 hr of other drugs or within 1 hr of antacids, milk, or cimetidine
• In AM or PM
Evaluate:
• Therapeutic response: decrease in constipation
Teach patient/family:
🚫 To swallow tabs whole; do not break, crush, or chew tabs

• Not to use laxatives for long-term therapy; bowel tone will be lost

• That normal bowel movements do not always occur daily

• Not to use in presence of abdominal pain, nausea, vomiting

• To notify prescriber if constipation is unrelieved or if symptoms of electrolyte imbalance occur: muscle cramps, pain, weakness, dizziness

---

bismuth subsalicylate (OTC)

(bis'muth sub-sal-iss'uh-late)
Bismatrol, Bismatrol Extra Strength, Bismed, Pepto-Bismol, Pepto-Bismol Maximum Strength, Pink Bismuth, PMS-Bismuth Subsalicylate

Func. class.: Antidiarrheal
Chem. class.: Salicylate

Action: Inhibits prostaglandin synthesis responsible for GI hypermotility; stimulates absorption of fluid and electrolytes

Uses: Diarrhea (cause undetermined), prevention of diarrhea when traveling; may be included to treat *Helicobacter pylori*

Dosage and routes:

• *Adult:* **PO** 30 ml or 2 tabs q30-60min, not to exceed 8 doses per day for >2 days

• *Child 10-14 yr:* **PO** 15 ml

• *Child 6-9 yr:* **PO** 10 ml

• *Child 3-6 yr:* **PO** 5 ml

Available forms: Chewable tabs 262 mg; susp 262 mg/15 ml, 524 mg/15 ml

Side effects/adverse reactions:

HEMA: Increased bleeding time
GI: Increased fecal impaction (high doses), dark stools
CNS: Confusion, twitching

EENT: Hearing loss, tinnitus, metallic taste, blue gums, black tongue (chew tabs)

Contraindications: Child <3 yr, history of GI bleeding, renal disease

Precautions: Anticoagulant therapy, immobility

Pharmacokinetics:

PO: Onset 1 hr, peak 2 hr, duration 4 hr

Interactions:

• Possible salicylate toxicity: salicylates

• Increased effects of oral anticoagulants, oral antidiabetics

• Decreased absorption of: tetracycline

🌢 Increased absorption of bismuth: sarsaparilla root

Lab test interferences:

Interference: Radiographic studies of GI system

NURSING CONSIDERATIONS
Assess:

• Electrolytes (K, Na, Cl) if diarrhea is severe or continues long term; assess skin turgor

• Bowel pattern before drug therapy, after treatment

Administer:

PO

• Increased fluids to rehydrate the patient

Evaluate:

• Therapeutic response: decreased diarrhea or absence of diarrhea when traveling

Teach patient/family:

• To chew or dissolve in mouth; do not swallow whole; shake liquid before using

• To avoid other salicylates unless directed by prescriber; not to give to children, possibility of Reye's syndrome

• That stools may turn black; tongue may darken; impaction may occur in debilitated patients

---

◆ = Nursing alert 🌢 = Herb-drug interaction 🚫 = Do not crush

• To stop use if symptoms do not improve within 2 days or become worse, or if diarrhea is accompanied by high fever

---

bisoprolol (R)
(bis-oh'pro-lole)
Zebeta
Func. class.: Antihypertensive
Chem. class.: β₁-blocker

Action: Preferentially and competitively blocks stimulation of β₁-adrenergic receptors within cardiac muscle (decreases rate of SA node discharge, increases recovery time), slows conduction of AV node, decreases heart rate, which decreases O₂ consumption in myocardium; decreases renin-aldosterone-angiotensin system; inhibits β₂-receptors in bronchial and vascular smooth muscle at high doses

Uses: Mild to moderate hypertension

Investigational uses: Angina pectoris, supraventricular tachycardia

Dosage and routes:
• *Adult:* PO 2.5-5 mg qd; may increase if necessary to 20 mg qd
Renal/hepatic dose: 2.5 mg PO, titrate upward
Available forms: Tabs 5, 10 mg

Side effects/adverse reactions:
MS: Joint pain, arthralgia
MISC: Facial swelling, weight gain, decreased exercise tolerance
CV: ***Ventricular dysrhythmias, profound hypotension, bradycardia, CHF,*** cold extremities, postural hypotension, ***2nd- or 3rd-degree heart block***
CNS: Vertigo, headache, insomnia, fatigue, dizziness, mental changes, memory loss, hallucinations, depression, lethargy, drowsiness, strange dreams, catatonia, peripheral neuropathy
GI: Nausea, diarrhea, vomiting, ***mesenteric arterial thrombosis,*** ischemic colitis, flatulence, gastritis, gastric pain
INTEG: Rash, fever, alopecia, pruritus, sweating
HEMA: ***Agranulocytosis, thrombocytopenia,*** purpura, eosinophilia
EENT: Sore throat; dry, burning eyes
GU: Impotence, decreased libido
ENDO: Increased hypoglycemic response to insulin
RESP: ***Bronchospasm,*** dyspnea, wheezing, cough, nasal stuffiness

Contraindications: Hypersensitivity to β-blockers, cardiogenic shock, heart block (2nd, 3rd degree), sinus bradycardia, CHF, cardiac failure

Precautions: Major surgery, pregnancy (C), lactation, children, diabetes mellitus, renal or hepatic disease, thyroid disease, COPD, asthma, well-compensated heart failure, aortic or mitral valve disease, peripheral vascular disease, myasthenia gravis

Pharmacokinetics:
PO: Peak 2-4 hr; half-life 9-12 hr, 50% excreted unchanged in urine, protein binding 30%; metabolized in liver to inactive metabolites

Interactions:
• Decreased antihypertensive effect: NSAIDs
• Hypotension: reserpine, guanethidine
• Myocardial depression: calcium channel blockers

Lab test interferences:
Increase: AST and ALT
Interference: Glucose/insulin tolerance tests

NURSING CONSIDERATIONS
Assess:
• B/P during beginning treatment, periodically thereafter; pulse q4h: note rate, rhythm, quality

---

• Apical/radial pulse before administration; notify prescriber of any significant changes (pulse <50 bpm)
• Baselines in renal, liver function tests before therapy begins
• Edema in feet, legs daily
• Skin turgor, dryness of mucous membranes for hydration status, especially elderly
Administer:
PO
• Drug ac, hs, tablet may be crushed or swallowed whole
• Reduced dosage in renal and hepatic dysfunction
Perform/provide:
• Storage protected from light, moisture; place in cool environment
Evaluate:
• Therapeutic response: decreased B/P after 1-2 wk
Teach patient/family:
• Not to discontinue drug abruptly, may cause precipitate angina
• Not to use OTC products containing α-adrenergic stimulants (such as nasal decongestants, OTC cold preparations) unless directed by prescriber
• To report bradycardia, dizziness, confusion, depression, fever
• To take pulse at home; advise when to notify prescriber
• To avoid alcohol, smoking, sodium intake
• To comply with weight control, dietary adjustments, modified exercise program
• To carry Medic Alert ID to identify drug taking, allergies
• To avoid hazardous activities if dizziness is present
◆To report symptoms of CHF: difficulty breathing, especially on exertion or when lying down, night cough, swelling of extremities
Treatment of overdose: Lavage, IV atropine for bradycardia, IV theophylline for bronchospasm; digitalis, O_2, diuretic for cardiac failure; hemodialysis, IV glucose for hypoglycemia; IV diazepam (or phenytoin) for seizures

---

bitolterol (℞)
(bye-tole′ter-ole)
Tornalate
Func. class.: Bronchodilator, adrenergic β₂-agonist
Chem. class.: Acid ester of colterol

Action: Causes bronchodilation by action on β₂-receptors with increased synthesis of cAMP; relaxes bronchial smooth muscle; inhibits mast cell degranulation; stimulates cilia to remove secretions with very little effect on heart rate
Uses: Asthma, bronchospasm
Dosage and routes:
Inhaler
• *Adult and child >12 yr:* **INH** 2 puffs, wait 1-3 min before 3rd puff if needed, not to exceed 3 **INH** q6h or 2 **INH** q4h
Nebulization
• *Adult and child >12 yr:* **INH** 0.5 ml (1 mg) tid by intermittent flow or 1.25 mg tid by continuous flow, max 8 mg (intermittent), 14 mg (continuous)
Available forms: Aerosol 0.37 mg/actuation, 0.2% neb sol
Side effects/adverse reactions:
CNS: Tremors, anxiety, insomnia, headache, dizziness, stimulation, restlessness, hallucinations
EENT: Dry nose, irritation of nose and throat
CV: Palpitations, tachycardia, hypertension, angina, hypotension
GI: Heartburn, nausea, vomiting, anorexia
MS: Muscle cramps
*RESP: **Bronchospasm,*** dyspnea

◆ = Nursing alert   ∥ = Herb-drug interaction   ⊘ = Do not crush

Contraindications: Hypersensitivity to sympathomimetics

Precautions: Lactation, pregnancy (C), cardiac disorders, hyperthyroidism, diabetes mellitus

Pharmacokinetics:
INH: Onset 3 min, peak ½-1 hr, duration 5-8 hr

Interactions:
• Increased action of aerosol bronchodilators
• Increased action of bitolterol: tricyclic antidepressants, MAOIs
• May inhibit action when used with other β-blockers

NURSING CONSIDERATIONS
Assess:
• Respiratory function: vital capacity, forced expiratory volume, ABGs

Administer:
Inhalation
• After shaking, exhale, place mouthpiece in mouth, inhale slowly, hold breath, remove, exhale slowly

Perform/provide:
• Storage in light-resistant container, do not expose to temperatures over 86° F (30° C)
• Gum, sips of water for dry mouth

Evaluate:
• Therapeutic response: absence of dyspnea, wheezing over 1 hr

Teach patient/family:
• Not to use OTC medications; excess stimulation may occur
• To use inhaler; review package insert with patient, provide demonstration, return demonstration
• To avoid getting aerosol in eyes
• To wash inhaler in warm water and dry qd
• All aspects of drug; to avoid smoking, smoke-filled rooms, persons with respiratory infections

Treatment for overdose: Administer a β₂-adrenergic blocker

---

bleomycin (℞)
(blee-oh-mye'sin)
Blenoxane
Func. class.: Antineoplastic, antibiotic
Chem. class.: Glycopeptide

Action: Inhibits synthesis of DNA, RNA, protein; derived from *Streptomyces verticillus;* replication is decreased by binding to DNA, which causes strand splitting; phase specific in the G_2 and M phases; a nonvesicant

Uses: Cancer of head, neck, penis, cervix, vulva of squamous cell origin, Hodgkin's disease, lymphosarcoma, reticulum cell sarcoma, testicular carcinoma, malignant pleural effusion

Dosage and routes:
• *Adult and child:* **SC/IV/IM** 0.25-0.5 U/kg 1-2 times/wk or 10-20 U/m², then 1 U/day or 5 U/wk; may also be given by **CONT INF;** do not exceed total dose, 400 U in lifetime

Malignant pleural effusion
• *Adult:* 60 U as a single bolus intrapleural inj; 0.9% NaCl given through a thoracostomy tube following drainage of excess pleural fluid and complete lung expansion, remove after 4 hr

Available forms: Powder for inj, 15, 30 U

Side effects/adverse reactions:
*SYST: **Anaphylaxis***
GI: Nausea, vomiting, anorexia, stomatitis, weight loss
INTEG: Rash, hyperkeratosis, nail changes, alopecia, fever and chills
*RESP: **Fibrosis,** pneumonitis, wheezing, **pulmonary toxicity***
CNS: Fever, chills
IDIOSYNCRATIC REACTION: Hypo-

tension, confusion, fever, chills, wheezing

Contraindications: Hypersensitivity, pregnancy (D)

Precautions: Renal, hepatic, respiratory disease

Pharmacokinetics: Half-life 2 hr; when CrCl >35 ml/min, half-life is increased in lower clearance; metabolized in liver, 50% excreted in urine (unchanged)

Interactions:
• Increased toxicity: other antineoplastics, radiation therapy
• Decreased serum digoxin levels: digoxin

Lab test interferences:
Increase: Uric acid
• Decreased serum phenytoin levels: phenytoin

NURSING CONSIDERATIONS
Assess:
• IM test dose
• Pulmonary function tests: chest x-ray film before and during therapy; should be obtained q2wk during treatment
• Temperature q4h; fever may indicate beginning infection
• Serum creatinine
• Dyspnea, rales, unproductive cough, chest pain, tachypnea, fatigue, increased pulse, pallor, lethargy
• Effects of alopecia and skin color on body image; discuss feelings about body changes
• Buccal cavity q8h for dryness, sores, ulceration, white patches, oral pain, bleeding, dysphagia
• Local irritation, pain, burning, discoloration at injection site
◆ Symptoms indicating severe allergic reaction: rash, pruritus, urticaria, purpuric skin lesions, itching, flushing

Administer:
• Antiemetic 30-60 min before giving drug to prevent vomiting, con-

tinue antiemetics 6-10 hr after treatment
• Topical or systemic analgesics for pain of stomatitis as ordered; antihistamines and antipyretics for fever and chills

IM/SC
• After reconstituting 5 U/1-5 ml sterile H_2O, D_5W, 0.9% NaCl, or bacteriostatic water for inj; do not use products containing benzyl alcohol when giving to neonates

Direct IV
• After reconstituting 15 U or less/5 ml or more of D_5W or 0.9% NaCl; after further diluting with 50-100 ml D_5W or 0.9% NaCl, give 15 U or less/10 min through Y-tube or 3-way stopcock
• Two test doses 2-5 U before initial dose; monitor for anaphylaxis

Intrapleural
• 60 U/50-100 ml of 0.9% NaCl

Additive compatibilities: Amikacin, cephapirin, dexamethasone, diphenhydramine, fluorouracil, gentamicin, heparin, hydrocortisone, phenytoin, streptomycin, tobramycin, vinblastine, vincristine

Solution compatibilities: 0.9% NaCl

Syringe compatibilities: Cisplatin, cyclophosphamide, doxorubicin, droperidol, fluorouracil, furosemide, heparin, leucovorin, methotrexate, metoclopramide, mitomycin, vinblastine, vincristine

Y-site compatibilities: Allopurinol, amifostine, aztreonam, cefepime, cisplatin, cyclophosphamide, doxorubicin, doxorubicin liposome, droperidol, filgrastim, fludarabine, fluorouracil, granisetron, heparin, leucovorin, melphalan, methotrexate, metoclopramide, mitomycin, ondansetron, paclitaxel, piperacillin/tazobactam, sargramostim, teniposide, thiotepa, vinblastine, vincristine, vinorelbine

---

◆ = Nursing alert   ⫽ = Herb-drug interaction   ⃠ = Do not crush

Perform/provide:

• Storage for 2 wk after reconstituting at room temperature; discard unused portions

• Deep-breathing exercises with patient tid-qid; place in semi-Fowler's position

• Liquid diet: carbonated beverage; gelatin may be added if patient is not nauseated or vomiting

• Rinsing of mouth tid-qid with water, club soda; brushing of teeth with baking soda bid-tid with soft brush or cotton-tipped applicators for stomatitis; use unwaxed dental floss

• HOB raised to facilitate breathing

Evaluate:

• Therapeutic response: decrease in size of tumor

Teach patient/family:

• To report any complaints, side effects to nurse or prescriber

• To report any changes in breathing, coughing, fever

• That hair may be lost during treatment, and wig or hairpiece may make patient feel better; that new hair may be different in color, texture

• To avoid foods with citric acid, hot or rough texture

• To report any bleeding, white spots, ulcerations in mouth; to examine mouth qd and report symptoms

---

bretylium (R)

(bre-til'ee-um)

Bretylate*, bretylium tosylate, Bretylol

Func. class.: Antidysrhythmic (Class III)

Chem. class.: Quaternary ammonium compound

Action: After a transient release of norepinephrine, inhibits further release by postganglionic nerve endings; prolongs duration of action potential and effective refractory period

Uses: Serious ventricular tachycardia, cardioversion, ventricular fibrillation; for short-term use only

Dosage and routes:

Severe ventricular fibrillation

• *Adult:* **IV BOL** 5 mg/kg, over 15-30 sec; increase to 10 mg/kg repeated q15min, up to 30 mg/kg; **IV INF** 1-2 mg/min or give 5-10 mg/kg over 10 min q6h (maintenance)

Ventricular tachycardia

• *Adult:* **IV INF** 500 mg diluted in 50 ml D$_5$W or NS, infuse over 10-30 min, may repeat in 1 hr, maintain with 1-2 mg/min or 5-10 mg/kg over 10-30 min q6h; **IM** 5-10 mg/kg undiluted; repeat in 1-2 hr if needed; maintain with same dose q6-8h

• *Child:* 2-5 mg/kg/dose

Renal disease

• CrCl 10-50 ml/min 25%-50% dose; CrCl <10 ml/min avoid use

Available forms: Inj 50 mg/ml; 1, 2, 4 mg/ml prefilled syringes

Side effects/adverse reactions:

CNS: Syncope, dizziness, confusion, psychosis, anxiety

GI: Nausea, vomiting

CV: Hypotension, postural hypotension, bradycardia, angina, PVCs, substernal pressure, transient hypertension, precipitation of angina

RESP: ***Respiratory depression***

Contraindications: Hypersensitivity, digitalis toxicity, aortic stenosis, pulmonary hypertension

Precautions: Renal disease, pregnancy (C), lactation, children

Pharmacokinetics: Well absorbed by IM/IV routes

IV: Onset 5 min, duration 6-24 hr

IM: Onset ½-2 hr, duration 6-24 hr Half-life 4-17 hr, excreted unchanged by kidneys (70%-80% in 24 hr), not metabolized

Interactions:

• Increased or decreased effects of bretylium: quinidine, procainamide, propranolol, other antidysrhythmics

• Hypotension: antihypertensives

• Increased effects of: sympathomimetics

🌿 Increased action of bretylium: chronic use/abuse of cascara sagrada bark, aloe, buckthorn bark/berry, rhubarb root, senna leaf/fruits

NURSING CONSIDERATIONS
Assess:

• ECG continuously to determine drug effectiveness, PVCs, other dysrhythmias

• IV INF rate to avoid causing nausea, vomiting

• For dehydration or hypovolemia

• B/P continuously for hypotension, hypertension; orthostatic hypotension; keep supine until hypotension subsides

• I&O ratio

• If systolic B/P <75 mm Hg, notify prescriber

• For rebound hypertension after 1-2 hr

• Cardiac status: rate, rhythm, character, continuously

Administer:
IM

• Inj, rotate sites, inject <5 ml in any one site to prevent tissue necrosis, may repeat 1-2 hr

IV, direct

• Undiluted over 15-30 sec (ventricular fibrillation); may repeat in 15-30 min, not to exceed 30 mg/kg/24 hr

Intermittent IV inf

• Dilute 500 mg of drug/50 ml or more D$_5$W, 0.9% NaCl, D$_5$/0.45%, D$_5$/0.9% NaCl, D$_5$/LR, give over 15-30 min

Continuous IV inf

• Dilute further; give at 1-2 mg diluted sol/min via infusion pump

• Reduced dosage slowly with ECG monitoring, discontinue over 3-5 days, maintain on oral dysrhythmic

Additive compatibilities: Aminophylline, atracurium, calcium chloride, calcium gluconate, digoxin, dopamine, esmolol, insulin (regular), lidocaine, potassium chloride, quinadine, verapamil

Y-site compatibilities: Amiodarone, amrinone, cisatracurium, diltiazem, dobutamine, famotidine, isoproterenol, ranitidine, remifentanil

Perform/provide:

• Place patient in supine position unless otherwise ordered; assist with ambulation

• Have suction equipment available

Evaluate:

• Therapeutic response: absence of ventricular tachycardia, fibrillation

Teach patient/family:

• To make position changes slowly; orthostatic hypotension may occur

Treatment of overdose: O$_2$, artificial ventilation, ECG; administer dopamine for circulatory depression; administer diazepam or thiopental for convulsions

---

bromocriptine (℞)
(broe-moe-krip'teen)
Parlodel
Func. class.: Dopamine receptor agonist, ovulation stimulant
Chem. class.: Ergot alkaloid derivative

Action: Inhibits prolactin release by activating postsynaptic dopamine receptors; activation of striatal dopamine receptors may be reason for improvement in Parkinson's disease

Uses: Female infertility, Parkinson's disease, prevention of postpartum

---

◆ = Nursing alert   🌿 = Herb-drug interaction   🚫 = Do not crush

lactation, amenorrhea caused by hyperprolactinemia, acromegaly

Dosage and routes:

Hyperprolactinemic indications/ female infertility
• *Adult:* **PO** 1.25-2.5 mg with meals; may increase by 2.5 mg q3-7d, usual 5-7.5 mg

Acromegaly
• *Adult:* **PO** 1.25-2.5 mg × 3 days hs; may increase by 1.25-2.5 mg q3-7d; usual range 20-30 mg/day, max 100 mg/day

Postpartum lactation
• *Adult:* **PO** 2.5 mg qd-tid with meal × 14 or 21 days

Parkinson's disease
• *Adult:* **PO** 1.25 mg bid with meals, may increase q2-4wk by 2.5 mg/day, not to exceed 100 mg qd

Available forms: Caps 5 mg; tabs 2.5 mg

Side effects/adverse reactions:

EENT: Blurred vision, diplopia, burning eyes, nasal congestion

CNS: Headache, depression, restlessness, anxiety, nervousness, confusion, *convulsions,* hallucinations, dizziness, fatigue, drowsiness, abnormal involuntary movements, psychosis

GU: Frequency, retention, incontinence, diuresis

GI: Nausea, vomiting, anorexia, cramps, constipation, diarrhea, dry mouth, GI hemorrhage

INTEG: Rash on face, arms, alopecia

CV: Orthostatic hypotension, decreased B/P, palpitation, extra systole, *shock,* dysrhythmias, bradycardia

Contraindications: Hypersensitivity to ergot, severe ischemic disease, severe peripheral vascular disease

Precautions: Lactation, hepatic disease, renal disease, children, pituitary tumors, pregnancy (B)

Pharmacokinetics:

PO: Peak 1-3 hr, duration 4-8 hr, 90%-96% protein bound, half-life 3 hr, metabolized by liver (inactive metabolites), 85%-98% of dose excreted in feces

Interactions:

• Decreased action of bromocriptine: phenothiazines, oral contraceptives, progestins, estrogens, haloperidol, loxapine, methyldopa, metoclopramide, MAOIs, reserpine
• Increased action of antihypertensives, levodopa
• Disulfiram-like reaction: alcohol
⬥ Decreased effect of bromocriptine: chaste tree fruit

Lab test interferences:

Increase: Growth hormone, AST, ALT, CK, BUN, uric acid, alk phosphatase

NURSING CONSIDERATIONS

Assess:

• B/P; establish baseline, compare with other reading; this drug decreases B/P

Administer:

PO
• With meal to prevent GI symptoms
• At hs so dizziness, orthostatic hypotension do not occur

Perform/provide:
• Storage at room temperature in tight container

Evaluate:
• Therapeutic response (Parkinson's disease): decreased dyskinesia, decreased slow movements, decreased drooling

Teach patient/family:
• That tabs may be crushed and mixed with food
• To change position slowly to prevent orthostatic hypotension
• To use contraceptives during treatment with this drug; pregnancy may occur; to use methods other than oral contraceptives

• That therapeutic effect for Parkinson's disease may take 2 mo: galactorrhea, amenorrhea
• To avoid hazardous activity if dizziness occurs

---

brompheniramine (℞)

(brome-fen-ir'a-meen)
Bromphen, brompheniramine, Chlorphed, Codimal-A, Conjec-B, Cophene-B, Dehist, Dimetane, Dimetane Extentabs, Dimetapp Allergy Liqui-Gels, Histaject Modified, Nasahist-B, ND Stat Revised, Oraminic II, Veltane

Func. class.: Antihistamine
Chem. class.: Alkylamine, H_1-receptor antagonist

Action: Acts on blood vessels, GI, respiratory system by competing with histamine for H_1-receptor site; decreases allergic response by blocking histamine

Uses: Allergy symptoms, rhinitis

Dosage and routes:
• *Adult:* **PO** 4-8 mg tid-qid, not to exceed 36 mg/day; time rel 8-12 mg bid-tid, not to exceed 36 mg/day; **IM/IV/SC** 10 mg q6-12h, not to exceed 40 mg/day
• *Child >6 yr:* **PO** 2 mg tid-qid, not to exceed 12 mg/day; **IM/IV/SC** 0.125 mg/kg
• *Child <6 yr:* Only as directed by prescriber

Available forms: Tabs 4, 8, 12 mg; tabs, ext rel 8, 12 mg; elix 2 mg/5 ml; inj 10 mg/ml

Side effects/adverse reactions:
CNS: Dizziness, drowsiness, poor coordination, fatigue, anxiety, euphoria, confusion, paresthesia, neuritis
CV: Hypotension, palpitations, tachycardia

RESP: Increased thick secretions, wheezing, chest tightness
*HEMA: **Thrombocytopenia, agranulocytosis, hemolytic anemia***
GI: Dry mouth, nausea, vomiting, anorexia, constipation, diarrhea
INTEG: Photosensitivity
GU: Retention, dysuria, frequency, impotence
EENT: Blurred vision, dilated pupils, tinnitus, nasal stuffiness, dry nose, throat, mouth

Contraindications: Hypersensitivity to H_1-receptor antagonists, acute asthma attack, lower respiratory tract disease, child <6 yr

Precautions: Increased intraocular pressure, renal disease, cardiac disease, hypertension, bronchial asthma, seizure disorder, stenosed peptic ulcers, hyperthyroidism, prostatic hypertrophy, bladder neck obstruction, pregnancy (C), lactation

Pharmacokinetics:
PO: Peak 2-5 hr, duration to 48 hr; metabolized in liver, excreted by kidneys, excreted in breast milk, half-life 12-34 hr

Interactions:
• Increased CNS depression: barbiturates, opiates, hypnotics, tricyclic antidepressants, alcohol
• Increased anticholinergic effect: MAOIs
• Incompatible with aminophylline, insulins, pentobarbital
 Increased CNS depression: kava
 Increased anticholinergic effect: henbane leaf

Lab test interferences:
Interfere: Skin allergy tests

NURSING CONSIDERATIONS
Assess:
• Be alert for urinary retention, frequency, dysuria; drug should be discontinued if these occur
• CBC during long-term therapy
• Blood dyscrasias: thrombocytope-

 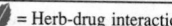

nia, agranulocytosis (rare) during long-term therapy

• Respiratory status: rate, rhythm, increase in bronchial secretions, wheezing, chest tightness

Administer:

PO

• With meals if GI symptoms occur; absorption may slightly decrease

IV, direct

• Undiluted or diluted with 10 ml 0.9% NaCl, given over 1 min or more

IV inf

• Dilute in D_5W, 0.9% NaCl given at prescribed rate

Perform/provide:

• Hard candy, gum, frequent rinsing of mouth for dryness

• Storage in tight container at room temperature

Evaluate:

• Therapeutic response: absence of running or congested nose or rashes

Teach patient/family:

🚫 Not to break, crush, or chew sustained release forms

• All aspects of drug use; to notify prescriber if confusion/sedation/hypotension occurs

• To avoid driving, other hazardous activities if drowsiness occurs

• To avoid use of alcohol, other CNS depressants while taking drug

Treatment of overdose: Administer ipecac syrup or lavage, diazepam, vasopressors, barbiturates (short-acting)

---

budesonide (℞)

(byoo-des′oh-nide)

Pulmicort Turbuhaler

Func. class.: Glucocorticoid

Chem. class.: Nonhalogenated

Action: Prevents inflamma~~tion~~ depression of migration of

phonuclear leukocytes, fibroblasts, reversal of increased capillary permeability and lysosomal stabilization; does not suppress hypothalamus and pituitary function

Uses: Rhinitis, asthma; Crohn's disease

Dosage and routes:

• *Adult and child >12 yr:* **INH** 400-600 µg/day; **NASAL:** 200-400 µg/day

Available forms: Nasal aerosol 50 µg; dry powder for INH 200 µg/metered dose

Side effects/adverse reactions:

CNS: Headache, insomnia, hypertonia, syncope

EENT: Sinusitis, pharyngitis, rhinitis, oral candidiasis

GI: Dry mouth, dyspepsia, nausea, vomiting, abdominal pain

MISC: Ecchymosis, fever, *hypersensitivity,* flulike symptoms

MS: Back pain, myalgias, fractures

RESP: Nasal irritation, cough, nasal bleeding, *respiratory infections,* **bronchospasm**

Contraindications: Hypersensitivity, status asthmaticus

Precautions: Pregnancy (C), lactation, children, *TB,* fungal, bacterial, systemic viral infections, ocular herpes simplex, nasal septal ulcers

Pharmacokinetics: Unknown

Interactions:

• Decreased budesonide metabolism: ketoconazole

NURSING CONSIDERATIONS

Assess:

• Respiratory status: rate, rhythm, increase in bronchial ~~thick~~ wheezing, chest ~~tightness~~ fluids, corticosteroids, infections

• For increased intraocular pressure, discontinue use if increase occurs

Administer:
Inhalation
• Use scissors to open pouch
• Use Turbuhaler upright to load, prime when using first time, turn grip to the right, then left to click in place; to provide dose turn to right, then to the left, click in place. Place mouthpiece between lips, inhale forcefully, do not exhale through Turbuhaler, rinse after use

Perform/provide:
• Storage at 59°-86° F (15°-30° C); keep away from heat, open flame

Evaluate:
• Therapeutic response: absence of asthma, rhinitis

Teach patient/family:
• To notify prescriber of pharyngitis, nasal bleeding
• Not to exceed recommended dose; adrenal suppression may occur
• To carry medical ID identifying steroid use
• To read and follow package directions
• To prevent exposure to infections, especially viral

alone or as adjunct with antihypertensives such as spironolactone, triamterene

Dosage and routes:
• *Adult:* **PO** 0.5-2.0 mg qd; may give 2nd or 3rd dose at 4-5 hr intervals, not to exceed 10 mg/day; may be given on alternate days or intermittently; **IV/IM** 0.5-1.0 mg; may give 2nd or 3rd dose at 2-3 hr intervals, not to exceed 10 mg/day
• *Child:* **PO/IM/IV** 0.02-0.1 mg/kg q12h, max 10 mg/day

Available forms: Tabs 0.5, 1, 2 mg; inj 0.25 mg/ml

Side effects/adverse reactions:
GU: Polyuria, **renal failure,** glycosuria
ELECT: Hypokalemia, hypochloremic alkalosis, hypomagnesemia, hyperuricemia, hypocalcemia, hyponatremia
CNS: Headache, fatigue, weakness, vertigo
GI: Nausea, diarrhea, dry mouth, vomiting, anorexia, cramps, upset stomach, abdominal pain, ***acute pancreatitis, jaundice***
EENT: **Loss of hearing,** ear pain, tinnitus, blurred vision
INTEG: Rash, pruritus, purpura, ***Stevens-Johnson syndrome,*** sweating, photosensitivity
MS: Muscular cramps, arthritis, stiffness, tenderness
ENDO: Hyperglycemia
HEMA: **Thrombocytopenia**
CV: **Chest pain,** hypotension, ***circulatory collapse,*** ECG changes, dehydration

Contraindications: Hypersensitivity to sulfonamides, anuria, hepatic coma

Precautions: Dehydration, ascites, renal disease, pregnancy (C), cirrhosis, lactation

---

bumetanide (Ŗ)
(byoo-met'a-nīd)
Bume...
...*unc. cl...,* Lo...
Cl...m. cla...: Sul...diuretic
...*...ide de-*
...ative

Acts on ascendin...
...hibiting reabsor...
Use...
renal...
pulm...CHF, liver dis...coma
syndr...otic syndrom...*cautions:* Dehydration, ascites,
Invest...ites (nephrotic...renal disease, pregnancy (C),
= Nurs...n, anasarca...irrhosis, lactation
...ye be used...inetics:
Herb-drug inter...hr, peak 1-2 hr, du-

⊘ = Do not crush

IM: Onset 40 min, duration 4 hr

IV: Onset 5 min, peak 15-30 min, duration 2-3 hr, excreted by kidneys, crosses placenta, excreted in breast milk

Interactions:

- Decreased diuretic effect: indomethacin, NSAIDs, probenecid
- Ototoxicity: aminoglycosides
- Increased toxicity: lithium, digitalis
- Increased diuresis, electrolyte loss: metolazone
- Hypokalemia: potassium-wasting drugs, corticosteroids
- Decreased effects of antidiabetics

NURSING CONSIDERATIONS

Assess:

- Hearing with high IV doses
- Weight, I&O daily to determine fluid loss; if urinary output decreases or azotemia occurs, drug should be discontinued; the safest dosage schedule is on alternate days
- B/P lying, standing; postural hypotension may occur
- Electrolytes: K, Na, Cl; include BUN, blood sugar, CBC, serum creatinine, blood pH, ABGs, uric acid, Ca, Mg
- Blood glucose if patient is diabetic; blood uric acid levels in those with gout
- Improvement in edema of feet, legs, sacral area daily if medication is being used in CHF
- Signs of metabolic alkalosis: drowsiness, restlessness
- Signs of hypokalemia: postural hypotension, malaise, fatigue, tachycardia, leg cramps, weakness
- Rashes, temperature elevation qd
- Confusion, especially in elderly; take safety precautions if needed
- For digitalis toxicity in patients taking digitalis products; lithium toxicity in those taking lithium

Administer:

- In AM to avoid interference with sleep if using drug as a diuretic
- Potassium replacement if potassium is less than 3.0

PO

- With food if nausea occurs; absorption may be decreased slightly

IV, direct

- Direct IV undiluted over at least 1 min through Y-tube or 3-way stopcock or heplock

Intermittent IV

- Dilute in LR, D_5W, 0.9% NaCl (rarely given by this method)

Additive compatibilities: Floxacillin, furosemide

Syringe compatibilities: Doxapram

Y-site compatibilities: Allopurinol, amifostine, aztreonam, cefepime, cisatracurium, cladribine, diltiazem, filgrastim, granisetron, lorazepam, melphalan, meperidine, morphine, piperacillin/tazobactam, propofol, remifentanil, teniposide, thiotepa, vinorelbine

Evaluate:

- Therapeutic response: decreased edema, B/P

Teach patient/family:

- To increase fluid intake to 2-3 L/day unless contraindicated, to take K supplement, to rise slowly from lying or sitting position
- To recognize adverse reactions: muscle cramps, weakness, nausea, dizziness
- To take with food or milk for GI symptoms
- To take early in day to prevent nocturia
- To use sunscreen to prevent photosensitivity

Treatment of overdose: Lavage if taken orally; monitor electrolytes; administer dextrose in saline; r itor hydration, CV, renal stat

buprenorphine (R)

(byoo-pre-nor'feen)
Buprenex

Func. class.: Opioid analgesic
Chem. class.: Thebaine derivative

Controlled Substance Schedule V
Action: Depresses pain impulse transmission at the spinal cord level by interacting with opioid receptors
Uses: Moderate to severe pain
Dosage and routes:
• *Adult:* **IM/IV** 0.3-0.6 mg q6h prn, reduce dosage in elderly
• *Child 2-12 yr:* **IM/IV** 2-6 μg/kg q4-6h
• *Geriatric:* **PO** 0.15 mg q6h prn
Available forms: Inj 0.3 mg/ml (1 ml vials)
Side effects/adverse reactions:
CNS: Drowsiness, dizziness, confusion, headache, sedation, euphoria, **increased intracranial pressure**
GI: Nausea, vomiting, anorexia, constipation, cramps
GU: Increased urinary output, dysuria
INTEG: Rash, urticaria, bruising, flushing, diaphoresis, pruritus
EENT: Tinnitus, blurred vision, *miosis,* diplopia
CV: Palpitations, bradycardia, change in B/P, tachycardia
RESP: **Respiratory depression,** dyspnea, hypoventilation
Contraindications: Hypersensitivity, addiction (narcotic)
Precautions: Addictive personality, pregnancy (C), lactation, increased intracranial pressure, MI (acute), severe heart disease, respiratory depression, hepatic disease, renal disease
Pharmacokinetics:
IM: Onset 10-30 min, peak ½ hr, duration 3-4 hr

IV: Onset 1 min, peak 5 min, duration 2-5 hr
Metabolized by liver; excreted by kidneys; crosses placenta; excreted in breast milk; half-life 2½-3½ hr; 96% bound to plasma proteins
Interactions:
• Effects may be increased with other CNS depressants: alcohol, opioids, sedative/hypnotics, antipsychotics, skeletal muscle relaxants, MAOIs
🍃 Increased CNS depression: kava
NURSING CONSIDERATIONS
Assess:
• I&O ratio; check for decreasing output; may indicate urinary retention
• CNS changes, dizziness, drowsiness, hallucinations, euphoria, LOC, pupil reaction; withdrawal in narcotic-dependent persons; if dependence occurs, within 2 wk of discontinuing drug withdrawal symptoms will occur
• Allergic reactions: rash, urticaria
• Respiratory dysfunction: respiratory depression, character, rate, rhythm; notify prescriber if respirations are <12/min
• Need for pain medication, tolerance
Administer:
IV, direct
• Undiluted over 3-5 min, titrate to patient response
• With antiemetic if nausea, vomiting occur
• When pain is beginning to return; determine dosage interval by patient response
Additive compatibilities: Atropine, bupivacaine, diphenhydramine, droperidol, glycopyrrolate, haloperidol, hydroxyzine, promethazine, scopolamine
Syringe compatibilities: Midazolam
Y-site compatibilities: Allopurinol, amifostine, aztreonam, cefepime, cisatracurium, cladribine,

filgrastim, granisetron, melphalan, piperacillin/tazobactam, propofol, remifentanil, teniposide, thiotepa, vinorelbine

Perform/provide:
• Assistance with ambulation if needed

Evaluate:
• Therapeutic response: decrease in pain, absence of grimacing

Teach patient/family:
• To report any symptoms of CNS changes, allergic reactions
• That tolerance may result when used for extended periods

Treatment of overdose: Naloxone HCl (Narcan) 0.2-0.8 mg IV, O_2, IV fluids, vasopressors

---

bupropion (R̸)
(byoo-proe′pee-on)
Wellbutrin, Wellbutrin SR, Zyban
Func. class.: Misc. antidepressant, smoking deterrent
Chem. class.: Aminoketone

Action: Inhibits reuptake of dopamine, serotonin, norepinephrine
Uses: Depression, smoking cessation

Dosage and routes:
Depression
• *Adult:* PO 100 mg bid initially, then increase after 3 days to 100 mg tid if needed; may increase after 1 mo to 150 mg tid
• *Geriatric:* PO 50-100 mg/day, may increase by 50-100 mg q3-4 day

Smoking cessation
• *Adult:* PO 150 mg bid, begin with 150 mg qd × 3 days, then 300 mg/day; continue for 7-12 wk
Available forms: Tabs 75, 100 mg; tab sust rel 150 mg

Side effects/adverse reactions:
*CNS: Headache, agitation, confusion, **seizures,** delusions, insomnia,* sedation, tremors
CV: Dysrhythmias, hypertension, palpitations, tachycardia, hypotension, ***complete AV block***
GI: Nausea, vomiting, dry mouth, increased appetite, constipation
GU: Impotence, urinary frequency, retention
INTEG: Rash, pruritus, sweating
EENT: Blurred vision, auditory disturbance

Contraindications: Hypersensitivity, seizure disorder, eating disorders

Precautions: Renal and hepatic disease, recent MI, cranial trauma, pregnancy (B), lactation, children

Pharmacokinetics: Onset 2-4 wk, half-life 8-24 hr; metabolized by liver, steady state 1½-5 wk

Interactions:
• Increased adverse reactions, seizures: levodopa, MAOIs, phenothiazines, tricyclic antidepressants, benzodiazepines, alcohol, antidepressants, theophylline, systemic steroids
• Increased bupropion toxicity: ritonavir
• Decreased bupropion effect: carbamazepine, phenobarbital, phenytoin
• Increased bupropion level: cimetidine
🌢 Increased CNS depression: kava
🌢 May increase anticholinergic effect: belladonna leaf/root

NURSING CONSIDERATIONS
Assess:
• For increased risk of seizures; if patient has excessively used CNS depressants and OTC stimulants, dosage of bupropion should not be exceeded
• For smoking cessation after 7 wk; if progress has not been made, drug should be discontinued

---

• Mental status: mood, sensorium, affect, suicidal tendencies, increase in psychiatric symptoms
• Withdrawal symptoms: headache, nausea, vomiting, muscle pain, weakness if drug is discontinued abruptly

Administer:

PO

• Increased fluids, bulk in diet if constipation occurs
• With food or milk for GI symptoms
• Gum, hard candy, or frequent sips of water for dry mouth

Perform/provide:

• Assistance with ambulation during beginning therapy, since sedation occurs
• Safety measures, primarily in elderly

Evaluate:

• Therapeutic response: decreased depression, ability to function in daily activities, ability to sleep throughout the night

Teach patient/family:

• That therapeutic effects may take 2-4 wk; not to increase dose without prescriber's approval; that treatment for smoking cessation lasts 7-12 wk
• To use caution in driving, other activities requiring alertness; sedation, blurred vision may occur
• To avoid alcohol ingestion, other CNS depressants
• Not to discontinue medication quickly after long-term use; may cause nausea, headache, malaise
• Not to use with nicotine patches unless directed by prescriber, may increase B/P
• That risk of seizures is increased when dose is exceeded, or if patient has seizure disorder
• To notify prescriber, if pregnant

Treatment of overdose: ECG monitoring; induce emesis, lavage, activated charcoal; administer anticonvulsant

---

buspirone (℞)

(byoo-spye′rone)

BuSpar

Func. class.: Antianxiety agent

Chem. class.: Azaspirodecanedione

Action: Acts by inhibiting the action of serotonin (5-HT)

Uses: Management and short-term relief of anxiety disorders

Dosage and routes:

• *Adult:* **PO** 5 mg tid; may increase by 5 mg/day q2-3d, not to exceed 60 mg/day

Available forms: Tabs 5, 10, 15 mg

Side effects/adverse reactions:

CNS: Dizziness, headache, depression, stimulation, insomnia, nervousness, light-headedness, numbness, paresthesia, incoordination, tremors, excitement, involuntary movements, confusion, akathisia

GI: Nausea, dry mouth, diarrhea, constipation, flatulence, increased appetite, rectal bleeding

CV: Tachycardia, palpitations, hypotension, hypertension, ***CVA, CHF, MI***

EENT: Sore throat, tinnitus, blurred vision, nasal congestion; red, itching eyes; change in taste, smell

GU: Frequency, hesitancy, menstrual irregularity, change in libido

MS: Pain, weakness, muscle cramps, spasms

RESP: Hyperventilation, chest congestion, shortness of breath

INTEG: Rash, edema, pruritus, alopecia, dry skin

MISC: Sweating, fatigue, weight gain, fever

Contraindications: Hypersensitivity, child <18 yr

◆ = Nursing alert   🌿 = Herb-drug interaction   ⊘ = Do not crush

Precautions: Pregnancy (B), lactation, elderly, impaired hepatic/renal function

Pharmacokinetics: Half-life 2-3 hr rapidly absorbed, metabolized by liver, excreted in feces

Interactions:
• Decreased buspirone effects: rifampin
• Increased B/P: MAOIs; do not use together
• Increased CNS depression: psychotropic drugs, alcohol (avoid use)
  / Increased CNS depression: kava
  / Increased peak concentration of buspirone: grapefruit

NURSING CONSIDERATIONS
Assess:
• B/P (lying, standing), pulse; if systolic B/P drops 20 mm Hg, hold drug, notify prescriber
• CNS reactions since some reactions may be unpredictable
• Mental status: mood, sensorium, affect, sleeping pattern, drowsiness, dizziness

Administer:
PO
• With food or milk for GI symptoms
• Crushed if patient unable to swallow medication whole
• Sugarless gum, hard candy, frequent sips of water for dry mouth

Perform/provide:
• Assistance with ambulation during beginning therapy; drowsiness, dizziness occur
• Safety measures if drowsiness occurs
• Check to see PO medication swallowed

Evaluate:
• Therapeutic response: decreased anxiety, restlessness, sleeplessness

Teach patient/family:
• That drug may be taken with food
• To avoid OTC preparations unless approved by prescriber

• To avoid activities requiring alertness since drowsiness may occur
• To avoid alcohol ingestion, other psychotropic medications, unless directed by prescriber
• Not to discontinue medication abruptly after long-term use
• To rise slowly because fainting may occur, especially elderly
• That drowsiness may worsen at beginning of treatment
• That 1-2 wk of therapy may be required before therapeutic effects occur

Treatment of overdose: Gastric lavage, VS, supportive care

---

busulfan (Ŗ)
(byoo-sul'fan)
Myleran
Func. class.: Antineoplastic alkylating agent
Chem. class.: Nitrosurea

Action: Changes essential cellular ions to covalent bonding with resultant alkylation; this interferes with normal biologic function of DNA; activity is not phase specific; action is due to myelosuppression

Uses: Chronic myelocytic leukemia

Dosage and routes:
• *Adult:* **PO** 4-12 mg/day initially until WBC levels fall to 10,000/mm^3, then drug is stopped until WBC levels raise over 50,000/mm^3, then 1-3 mg/day
• *Child:* **PO** 0.06-0.12 mg/kg or 1.8-4.6 mg/m^2 day; dose is titrated to maintain WBC levels at 20,000/mm^3

Available forms: Tabs 2 mg

Side effects/adverse reactions:
*HEMA: **Thrombocytopenia, leukopenia, pancytopenia, severe bone marrow depression***

GI: Nausea, vomiting, *diarrhea, weight loss*

GU: Impotence, sterility, amenorrhea, gynecomastia, *renal toxicity,* hyperuremia, adrenal insufficiency-like syndrome

INTEG: Dermatitis, hyperpigmentation, alopecia

*RESP: **Irreversible pulmonary fibrosis,** pneumonitis*

*OTHER: **Chromosomal aberrations***

Contraindications: Radiation, chemotherapy, lactation, pregnancy (3rd trimester) (D), blastic phase of chronic myelocytic leukemia, hypersensitivity

Precautions: Childbearing age women and men, leukopenia, thrombocytopenia, anemia, hepatotoxicity, renal toxicity

Pharmacokinetics: Well absorbed orally; excreted in urine; crosses placenta; excreted in breast milk

Interactions:

• Increased toxicity: other antineoplastics or radiation

• Increased risk of bleeding: anticoagulants, aspirin

NURSING CONSIDERATIONS
Assess:

• CBC, differential, platelet count weekly; withhold drug if WBC is <4000/mm^3 or platelet count is <75,000/mm^3; notify prescriber of results

• Pulmonary function tests, chest x-ray films before, during therapy; chest film should be obtained q2wk during treatment; pulmonary fibrosis may occur up to 10 yr after treatment with busulfan

• Renal function studies: BUN, serum uric acid, urine CrCl before, during therapy

• I&O ratio; report fall in urine output <30 ml/hr

• Monitor for cold, fever, sore throat (may indicate beginning infection)

• For decreased hyperuricemia

• Bleeding: hematuria, guaiac, bruising or petechiae, mucosa or orifices q8h, no rectal temps

• Dyspnea, rales, nonproductive cough, chest pain, tachypnea

• Food preferences; list likes, dislikes

• Edema in feet, joint, stomach pain, shaking

• Inflammation of mucosa, breaks in skin; use viscous xylocaine for oral pain

Administer:
PO

• Antacid before oral agent, give drug after evening meal, before bedtime, antiemetic 30-60 min before giving drug to prevent vomiting

• Allopurinol or sodium bicarbonate to maintain uric acid levels, alkalinization of urine

Perform/provide:

• Comprehensive oral hygiene

• Strict medical asepsis, protective isolation if WBC levels are low

• Deep breathing exercises with patient tid-qid; place in semi-Fowler's position for pulmonary reactions

• Increase fluid intake to 2-3 L/day to prevent urate deposits, calculi formation

• Diet low in purines: organ meats (kidney, liver), dried beans, peas to maintain alkaline urine

• Storage in tight container

Evaluate:

• Therapeutic response: decreased exacerbations of chronic myelocytic leukemia

Teach patient/family:

• About protective isolation precautions

• To avoid use of products containing aspirin or ibuprofen, razors, commercial mouthwash

• To report signs of anemia (fatigue, headache, irritability, faintness, shortness of breath)

◆ = Nursing alert   ⫽ = Herb-drug interaction   ⊘ = Do not crush

B

• To report symptoms of bleeding (hematuria, tarry stools)
• That impotence or amenorrhea can occur, are reversible after discontinuing treatment
• To report any changes in breathing or coughing even several months after treatment

---

butorphanol (R)

(byoo-tor′fa-nole)
Stadol, Stadol NS
Func. class.: Narcotic analgesic
Chem. class.: Opiate

Controlled Substance Schedule IV
Action: Depresses pain impulse transmission at the spinal cord level by interacting with opioid receptors
Uses: Moderate to severe pain
Investigational uses: Migraine headache, pain
Dosage and routes:
• *Adult:* **IM** 1-4 mg q3-4h prn; **IV** 0.5-2 mg q3-4h prn; **INTRANASAL,** 1 spray in one nostril q3-4h; may give another dose 1-1½ hr later; repeat if needed q3-4h
Geriatric: ½ adult dose at 2× the interval
Renal disease
• CrCl 10-50 ml/min 75% dose; CrCl <10 ml/min 50% dose
Available forms: Inj 1, 2 mg/ml; nasal spray 10 mg/ml
Side effects/adverse reactions:
CNS: Drowsiness, dizziness, confusion, headache, sedation, euphoria, weakness, hallucinations
GI: Nausea, vomiting, anorexia, constipation, cramps
GU: Increased urinary output, dysuria, urinary retention
INTEG: Rash, urticaria, bruising, flushing, diaphoresis, pruritus

EENT: Tinnitus, blurred vision, miosis, diplopia
CV: Palpitations, bradycardia, change in B/P
*RESP: **Respiratory depression,** pulmonary hypertension*
Contraindications: Hypersensitivity, addiction (narcotic), CHF, myocardial infarction
Precautions: Addictive personality, pregnancy (C), lactation, increased intracranial pressure, respiratory depression, hepatic disease, renal disease, child <18 yr
Pharmacokinetics:
IM: Onset 10-30 min, peak ½ hr, duration 3-4 hr
IV: Onset 1 min, peak 5 min, duration 2-4 hr
INTRANASAL: Onset within 15 min, peak 1-2 hr, duration 4-5 hr
Metabolized by liver; excreted by kidneys; crosses placenta; excreted in breast milk; half-life 2½-3½ hr
Interactions:
• Increased CNS effects: alcohol, opioids, sedative/hypnotics, antipsychotics, skeletal muscle relaxants
🌢 Increased CNS depression: kava
NURSING CONSIDERATIONS
Assess:
• For decreasing output; may indicate urinary retention
◆ For withdrawal symptoms in opioid-dependent patients: pulmonary embolus, vascular occlusion, abscesses, ulcerations
• CNS changes: dizziness, drowsiness, hallucinations, euphoria, LOC, pupil reaction
• Allergic reactions: rash, urticaria
• Respiratory dysfunction: respiratory depression, character, rate, rhythm; notify prescriber if respirations are <10/min
• Need for pain medication, physical dependence

Administer:
• With antiemetic if nausea, vomiting occur
• When pain is beginning to return; determine dosage interval by patient response

IM
• Deeply in large muscle mass

IV
• Undiluted at a rate of <2 mg/>3-5 min, titrate to patient response

Syringe compatibilities: Atropine, chlorpromazine, cimetidine, diphenhydramine, droperidol, fentanyl, hydroxyzine, meperidine, methotrimerprazine, metoclopramide, midazolam, morphine, pentazocine, perphenazine, prochlorperazine, promethazine, scopolamine, thiethylperazine

Y-site compatibilities: Allopurinol, amifostine, aztreonam, cefepime, cisatracurium, cladribine, doxorubicin liposome, enalaprilat, esmolol, filgrastim, fludarabine, granisetron, labetalol, melphalan, paclitaxel, piperacillin/tazobactam, propofol, remifentanil, sargramostim, tenoposide, thiotepa, vinorelbine

Perform/provide:
• Storage in light-resistant container at room temperature
• Assistance with ambulation
• Safety measures: night-light, call bell within easy reach, especially elderly

Evaluate:
• Therapeutic response: decrease in pain

Teach patient/family:
• To report any symptoms of CNS changes, allergic reactions
• That physical dependency may result when used for extended periods
• That withdrawal symptoms may occur: nausea, vomiting, cramps, fever, faintness, anorexia

Treatment of overdose: Naloxone HCl (Narcan) 0.2-0.8 mg IV, O_2, IV fluids, vasopressors

---

calcifediol (℞)
(kal-si-fe-dye'ole)
Calderol
Func. class.: Vit D analog, 25-hydroxyvitamin D_3
Chem. class.: Sterol

Action: Increases intestinal absorption of calcium for bones; increases renal tubular absorption of phosphate; increases mobilization of calcium from bones, bone resorption
Uses: Metabolic bone disease with chronic renal failure, osteopenia, osteomalacia, hypocalcemia
Dosage and routes:
• *Adult:* **PO** 300-350 µg qwk divided into qd or qod doses; may increase q4wk
• *Supplement Elderly:* **PO** 20 µg qd
Available forms: Caps 20, 50 µg
Side effects/adverse reactions:
EENT: Tinnitus, conjunctivitis, photophobia, rhinorrhea
CNS: Drowsiness, headache, vertigo, fever, lethargy
GI: Nausea, diarrhea, vomiting, jaundice, anorexia, dry mouth, constipation, cramps, metallic taste
MS: Myalgia, arthralgia, decreased bone development
GU: Polyuria, hypercalciuria, hyperphosphatemia, hematuria
CV: Dysrhythmias
Contraindications: Hypersensitivity, hyperphosphatemia, hypercalcemia, vit D toxicity
Precautions: Pregnancy (C), renal calculi, lactation, CV disease, elderly
Pharmacokinetics:
PO: Peak 4 hr, duration 15-20 days; half-life 12-22 days

◆ = Nursing alert   ∥ = Herb-drug interaction   ⊘ = Do not crush

Interactions:

• Decreased absorption of calcifediol: cholestyramine, colestipol, mineral oil, fat-soluble vitamins

• Hypercalcemia: thiazide diuretics, calcium supplements

• Cardiac dysrhythmias: cardiac glycosides

• Decreased effect of this drug: corticosteroids

• Hypermagnesemia: magnesium antacids

• Increased metabolism of vit D: phenytoin

• Toxicity: other vit D products

Lab test interferences:

False increase: Cholesterol

Interfere: Alk phosphatase, electrolytes

NURSING CONSIDERATIONS

Assess:

• BUN, urinary calcium, AST, ALT, cholesterol, creatinine, uric acid, chloride, magnesium, electrolytes, urine pH, phosphate; may increase; calcium should be kept at 9-10 mg/dl, vit D 50-135 IU/dl, phosphate 70 mg/dl

• Alk phosphatase; may be decreased

• For increased blood level, since toxic reactions may occur rapidly

• For dry mouth, metallic taste, polyuria, bone pain, muscle weakness, headache, fatigue, tinnitus, change in LOC, irregular pulse, dysrhythmias, increased respirations, anorexia, nausea, vomiting, cramps, diarrhea, constipation; may indicate hypercalcemia

• Renal status: decreased urinary output (oliguria, anuria), edema in extremities, weight gain 5 lb, periorbital edema

• Nutritional status, diet for sources of vit D (milk, some seafood), calcium (dairy products, dark green vegetables), phosphates (dairy products)

Administer:

PO

🚫 Do not break, crush, or chew caps

• May be increased q4wk depending on blood level

Perform/provide:

• Storage in tight, light-resistant container at room temperature

• Restriction of sodium, potassium if required; ensure adequate calcium intake

• Restriction of fluids if required for chronic renal failure

Evaluate:

• Therapeutic response: calcium levels 9-10 mg/dl, decreasing symptoms of bone disease

Teach patient/family:

• The symptoms of hypercalcemia

• About foods rich in calcium

---

calcitonin (human) (℞)

(kal-sih-toh'nin)

Cibacalcin

calcitonin (salmon) (℞)

Calcimir, Miacalcin, Miacalcin Nasal Spray, Osteocalcin, Salmonine

Func. class.: Parathyroid agents (calcium regulator)

Chem. class.: Polypeptide hormone

Action: Decreases bone resorption, blood calcium levels; increases deposits of calcium in bones

Uses: Paget's disease

Dosage and routes:

Human

Paget's disease

• *Adult:* SC 0.5 mg/day initially; may require 0.5 mg bid × 6 mo, then decrease until symptoms reappear

---

Side effects: *italics* = common; ***bold italics*** = life-threatening

Salmon
Postmenopausal osteoporosis
• *Adult:* **SC/IM** 100 IU/day; **NA-SAL** 200 IU qd alternating nostrils qd, activate pump before 1st dose
Paget's disease
• *Adult:* **SC/IM** 100 IU qd, maintenance 50-100 IU qd or qod
Hypercalcemia
• *Adult:* **SC/IM** 4 IU/kg q12h, increase to 8 IU/kg q12h if response is unsatisfactory
Available forms: Human: Inj (SC) 500 mg vial; Salmon: Inj 100 IU, 200 IU/ml, nasal spray 200 IU/actuation
Side effects/adverse reactions:
INTEG: Rash, flushing, pruritus of earlobes, edema of feet
CNS: Headache, tetany, chills, weakness, dizziness
GU: Diuresis
GI: Nausea, diarrhea, vomiting, anorexia, abdominal pain, salty taste, epigastric pain
MS: Swelling, tingling of hands
CV: Chest pressure
RESP: Dyspnea
Contraindications: Hypersensitivity
Precautions: Renal disease, children, lactation, osteogenic sarcoma, pregnancy (C)
Pharmacokinetics:
IM/SC: Onset 15 min, peak 4 hr, duration 8-24 hr; metabolized by kidneys, excreted as inactive metabolites
NURSING CONSIDERATIONS
Assess:
• GI symptoms, polyuria, flushing, head swelling, tingling, headache; may indicate hypercalcemia
• Nutritional status; diet for sources of vit D (milk, some seafood), calcium (dairy products, dark green vegetables), phosphates
• BUN, creatinine, uric acid, chloride, electrolytes, urine pH, urinary calcium, magnesium, phosphate, urinalysis (calcium should be kept at 9-10 mg/dl, vit D 50-135 IU/dl), alk phosphatase baseline, q3-6mo
• Increased drug level, since toxic reactions occur rapidly; have calcium chloride on hand if calcium level drops too low; check for tetany
• Urine for sediment
Administer:
Human
SC
• By SC route only; rotate injection sites; use within 6 hr of reconstitution; give hs to minimize nausea, vomiting
Salmon
IM
• After test dose of 10 IU/ml, 0.1 ml intradermally; watch 15 min; give only with epinephrine and emergency meds available
• IM injection slowly in deep muscle mass; rotate sites
Perform/provide:
• Storage at <77° F (25° C); protect from light
Evaluate:
• Therapeutic response: calcium levels 9-10 mg/dl, decreasing symptoms of Paget's disease
Teach patient/family:
• The method of injection if patient will be responsible for self-medication
• To report difficulty swallowing or any change in side effects to prescriber immediately

---

◆ = Nursing alert   ⫻ = Herb-drug interaction   ⊘ = Do not crush

calcitriol (℞)

(kal-sih-try'ole)
Calcijex, Rocaltrol, (1,25-dihydroxycholecalciferol)
Func. class.: Parathyroid agent (calcium regulator)
Chem. class.: Vit D hormone

Action: Increases intestinal absorption of calcium, provides calcium for bones, increases renal tubular resorption of phosphate

Uses: Hypocalcemia in chronic renal disease, hypoparathyroidism, pseudohypoparathyroidism

Dosage and routes:
Hypocalcemia
• *Adult:* **PO** 0.25 μg qd, may increase by 0.25 μg/day q4-8wk; maintenance 0.25 μg qod-1 μg qd

Hypoparathyroidism/pseudohypoparathyroidism
• *Adult and child >1 yr:* **PO** 0.25 μg qd, may be increased q2-4wk; maintenance 0.25-2 μg qd

Available forms: Caps 0.25, 0.5 μg; inj 1 μg, 2 μg/ml

Side effects/adverse reactions:
CNS: Drowsiness, headache, vertigo, fever, lethargy
GI: Nausea, diarrhea, vomiting, jaundice, anorexia, dry mouth, constipation, cramps, metallic taste
MS: Myalgia, arthralgia, decreased bone development
GU: Polyuria, hypercalciuria, hyperphosphatemia, hematuria

Contraindications: Hypersensitivity, hyperphosphatemia, hypercalcemia, vit D toxicity

Precautions: Pregnancy (C), renal calculi, lactation, CV disease

Pharmacokinetics:
PO: Peak 4 hr, duration 15-20 days, half-life 3-6 hr

Interactions:
• Decreased absorption of calcitriol: cholestyramine, mineral oil, fat-soluble vitamins
• Hypercalcemia: thiazide diuretics, calcium supplements
• Cardiac dysrhythmias: cardiac glycosides, verapamil
• Hypermagnesemia: magnesium antacids
• Increased metabolism of vit D: phenytoin
• Toxicity: other vit D products

Lab test interferences:
False increase: Cholesterol
Interfere: Alk phosphatase, electrolytes

NURSING CONSIDERATIONS
Assess:
• BUN, urinary calcium, AST, ALT, cholesterol, creatinine, albumin, uric acid, chloride, magnesium, electrolytes, urine pH, phosphate; may increase calcium, should be kept at 9-10 mg/dl, vit D 50-135 IU/dl, phosphate 70 mg/dl
• Alk phosphatase; may be decreased
• For increased drug level, since toxic reactions may occur rapidly
• For dry mouth, metallic taste, polyuria, bone pain, muscle weakness, headache, fatigue, change in LOC, dysrhythmias, increased respirations, anorexia, nausea, vomiting, cramps, diarrhea, constipation; may indicate hypercalcemia
• Renal status: decreased urinary output (oliguria, anuria), edema in extremities, weight gain 5-7 lb, periorbital edema
• Nutritional status, diet for sources of vit D (milk, some seafood); calcium (dairy products, dark green vegetables), phosphates (dairy products) must be avoided

Perform/provide:
• Storage protected from light, heat, moisture
• Restriction of sodium, potassium if required

Side effects: *italics* = common; ***bold italics*** = life-threatening

• Restriction of fluids if required for chronic renal failure

Evaluate:

• Therapeutic response: calcium 9-10 mg/dl, decreasing symptoms of hypocalcemia, hypoparathyroidism

Teach patient/family:

• The symptoms of hypercalcemia

• About foods rich in calcium

• To avoid products with sodium: cured meats, dairy products, cold cuts, olives, beets, pickles, soups, meat tenderizers in chronic renal failure

• To avoid products with potassium: oranges, bananas, dried fruit, peas, dark green leafy vegetables, milk, melons, beans in chronic renal failure

• To avoid OTC products containing calcium, potassium, or sodium in chronic renal failure

• To avoid all preparations containing vit D

• To monitor weight weekly

Ⓢ Not to break, crush, or chew caps

---

calcium carbonate
(PO-OTC, IV-℞)

Alka-Mints, Amitone, Apo-Cal*, BioCal, Calcarb, Calci-Chew, Calci-Mix, Calcilac, Calcite*, Calglycine*, Cal-Plus, Calsan*, Caltrate 600, Caltrate Jr., Chooz, Dicarbosil, Equilet, Gencalc, Liquid-Cal, Liquid-Cal-600, Maalox Antacid Caplets, Mallamint, Mylanta Lozenges*, Nephro-Calci, Nu-Cal*, Os-Cal 500, Oysco 500, Oystercal 500, Oyst-Cal 500, Rolaids Calcium Rich, Titralac, Tums, Tums E-X Extra Strength

Func. class.: Antacid, calcium supplement

Chem. class.: Calcium product

Action: Neutralizes gastric acidity

Uses: Antacid, calcium supplement; not suitable for chronic therapy

Dosage and routes:

• *Adult:* **PO** 350 mg-1.5 g or 2 pieces of gum 1 hr pc and hs

Available forms: Chewable tabs 350, 420, 500, 750, 850, 1000, 1250 mg; tabs 500, 600, 650, 1000, 1250 mg; gum 500 mg; susp 1250 mg/5 ml; lozenges 600 mg

Side effects/adverse reactions:

GI: Constipation, anorexia, nausea, vomiting, flatulence, diarrhea, rebound hyperacidity, eructation

Contraindications: Hypersensitivity, hypercalcemia, hyperparathyroidism, bone tumors

Precautions: Elderly, fluid restriction, decreased GI motility, GI obstruction, dehydration, renal disease, pregnancy (C), lactation

---

Pharmacokinetics:
PO: Onset 20 min, duration 20-180 min, excreted in feces

Interactions:
• Increased plasma levels of quinidine, amphetamines
• Decreased levels of salicylates, calcium channel blockers, ketoconazole, tetracyclines, iron salts
/ Increased action/side effects: lily of the valley, pheasant's eye, squill

NURSING CONSIDERATIONS
Assess:
• Ca^+ (serum, urine), Ca^+ should be 8.5-10.5 mg/dl, urine Ca^+ should be 150 mg/day, monitor weekly
◆ Milk-alkali syndrome: nausea, vomiting, disorientation, headache
• Constipation; increase bulk in the diet if needed
• Hypercalcemia: headache, nausea, vomiting, confusion

Administer:
PO
• As antacid 1 hr pc and hs
• As supplement 1½ hr pc and hs
• Only with regular tablets or capsules; do not give with enteric-coated tablets
• Laxatives or stool softeners if constipation occurs

Evaluate:
• Therapeutic response: absence of pain, decreased acidity

Teach patient/family:
• To increase fluids to 2 L unless contraindicated, to add bulk to diet for constipation
• Not to switch antacids unless directed by prescriber
• That therapeutic dose recommendations are figured as elemental calcium

---

**calcium chloride/
calcium gluceptate/
calcium gluconate/
calcium lactate (℞)**
Func. class.: Electrolyte replacement—calcium product

C

Action: Cation needed for maintenance of nervous, muscular, skeletal, enzyme reactions, normal cardiac contractility, coagulation of blood; affects secretory activity of endocrine, exocrine glands

Uses: Prevention and treatment of hypocalcemia, hypermagnesemia, hypoparathyroidism, neonatal tetany, cardiac toxicity caused by hyperkalemia, lead colic, hyperphosphatemia, vit D deficiency

Dosage and routes:
Calcium chloride
• *Adult:* IV 500 mg-1 g q1-3d as indicated by serum calcium levels, give at <1 ml/min; IV 200-800 mg injected in ventricle of heart
• *Child:* IV 25 mg/kg over several min

Calcium gluceptate
• *Adult:* IV 5-20 ml; IM 2-5 ml
• *Newborn:* 0.5 ml/100 ml of blood transfused

Calcium gluconate
• *Adult:* PO 0.5-2 g bid-qid; IV 0.5-2 g at 0.5 ml/min (10% solution)
• *Child:* PO/IV 500 mg/kg/day in divided doses

Calcium lactate
• *Adult:* PO 325 mg-1.3 g tid with meals
• *Child:* PO 500 mg/kg/day in divided doses

Available forms: Many; check product listings

Side effects/adverse reactions:
INTEG: Pain, burning at IV site, severe venous thrombosis, necrosis, extravasation

---

HYPERCALCEMIA: Drowsiness, lethargy, muscle weakness, headache, constipation, *coma,* anorexia, nausea, vomiting, polyuria, thirst

CV: Shortened QT, heart block, hypotension, bradycardia, dysrhythmias, *cardiac arrest*

GI: Vomiting, nausea, constipation

Contraindications: Hypercalcemia, digitalis toxicity, ventricular fibrillation, renal calculi

Precautions: Pregnancy (C), lactation, children, renal disease, respiratory disease, cor pulmonale, digitalized patient, respiratory failure

Interactions:
• Increased dysrhythmias: digitalis glycosides

• *Calcium chloride*

🌿 Increased action/side effects: lily of the valley, pheasant's eye, squill

Lab test interferences:
Increase: 11-OCHS
False decrease: Magnesium
Decrease: 17-OHCS

NURSING CONSIDERATIONS
Assess:
• ECG for decreased QT and T wave inversion: hypercalcemia, drug should be reduced or discontinued, consider cardiac monitoring
• Calcium levels during treatment (8.5-11.5 g/dl is normal level)
• Cardiac status: rate, rhythm, CVP, (PWP, PAWP if being monitored directly)

Administer:
PO
• With or following meals to enhance absorption
IM
• IM injection may cause severe burning, necrosis, tissue sloughing; warm sol to body temp before administering only gluconate/gluceptate

IV
• Undiluted or diluted with equal amounts of NS to a 5% sol for inj, give 0.5-1 ml/min
• Through small-bore needle into large vein; if extravasation occurs, necrosis will result (IV)

• *Calcium chloride*

Additive compatibilities: Amikacin, ascorbic acid, bretylium, cephapirin, chloramphenicol, dopamine, hydrocortisone, isoproterenol, lidocaine, methicillin, norepinephrine, penicillin G potassium, penicillin G sodium, pentobarbital, phenobarbital, sodium bicarbonate, verapamil, vit B/C

Syringe compatibilities: Milrinone
Y-site compatibilities: Amrinone, dobutamine, epinephrine, esmolol, morphine, paclitaxel

• *Calcium gluceptate*

Additive compatibilities: Ascorbic acid injection, isoproterenol, lidocaine, norepinephrine, phytonadione, sodium bicarbonate

• *Calcium gluconate*

Additive compatibilities: Amikacin, aminophylline, ascorbic acid injection, bretylium, cephapirin, chloramphenicol, cisatracurium, corticotropin, dimenhydrinate, doxorubicin liposome, erythromycin, furosemide, heparin, hydrocortisone, lidocaine, magnesium sulfate, methicillin, norepinephrine, penicillin G potassium, penicillin G sodium, phenobarbital, potassium chloride, remifentanil, tobramycin, vancomycin, verapamil, vit B/C

Syringe compatibilities: Aldesleukin, allopurinol, amifostine, aztreonam, cefazolin, cefepime, ciprofloxacin, cladribine, dobutamine, enalaprilat, epinephrine, famotidine, filgrastim, granisetron, heparin/hydrocortisone, labetalol, melphalan, midazolam, netilmicin, piperacillin/tazobactam, potassium chloride, prochlorperazine, propofol, sargramostim, tacrolimus, teniposide, thiotepa, tolazoline, vinorelbine, vit B/C

Perform/provide:

• Seizure precautions: padded side rails, decreased stimuli (noise, light); place airway suction equipment, padded mouth gag if Ca levels are low

• Store at room temperature

Evaluate:

• Therapeutic response: decreased twitching, paresthesias, muscle spasms, absence of tremors, convulsions, dysrhythmias, dyspnea, laryngospasm, negative Chvostek's sign, negative Trousseau's sign

Teach patient/family:

• To remain recumbent ½ hr after IV dose

• To add foods high in vit D

• To add calcium-rich foods to diet: dairy products, shellfish, dark green leafy vegetables; decrease oxalate-rich and zinc-rich foods: nuts, legumes, chocolate, spinach, soy

• To prevent injuries, avoid immobilization

---

calcium polycarbophil (OTC)

(pol-ee-kar'boe-fil)

Equalactin, Fiberall, FiberCon, Fiber-Lax, Mitrolan

Func. class.: Laxative

Chem. class.: Bulk-forming

Action: Attracts water, expands in intestine to increase peristalsis; also absorbs excess water in stool; decreases diarrhea

Uses: Constipation, irritable bowel syndrome (diarrhea), acute, nonspecific diarrhea

Dosage and routes:

• *Adult:* **PO** 1 g qd-qid prn, not to exceed 6 g/24 hr

• *Child 6-12 yr:* **PO** 500 mg bid prn, not to exceed 3 g/24 hr

• *Child 3-6 yr:* **PO** 500 mg bid prn, not to exceed 1.5 g/24 hr

Available forms: Chew tabs 500, 625, 1250 mg; tabs 500, 625 mg

Side effects/adverse reactions:

*GI: **Obstruction,*** abdominal distention, flatus, laxative dependence

Contraindications: Hypersensitivity, GI obstruction

Precautions: Pregnancy (C), lactation

Pharmacokinetics:

PO: Onset 12-24 min, peak 1-3 days

Interactions:

⚠ Increased action/side effects: lily of the valley, pheasant's eye, squill

NURSING CONSIDERATIONS

Assess:

• Cause of constipation; identify whether fluids, bulk, or exercise is missing from lifestyle

• Cramping, rectal bleeding, nausea, vomiting; if these symptoms occur, drug should be discontinued

Administer:

PO

• Alone for better absorption; do not take within 1 hr of other drugs

• In morning or evening (oral dose)

Evaluate:

• Therapeutic response: decreased constipation

Teach patient/family:

• Not to use laxatives for long-term therapy; laxative dependence will result

• That normal bowel movements do not always occur daily

• Not to use in presence of abdominal pain, nausea, vomiting

• To notify prescriber if constipation is unrelieved or if symptoms of

---

electrolyte imbalance occur: muscle cramps, pain, weakness, dizziness

• To chew thoroughly (chew tab) and follow with water

---

calfactant (R)

(cal-fak′tant)
Infasurf
Func. class.: Natural lung surfactant extract

Action: Replenishes surfactant and restores surface activity to the lungs in premature infants

Uses: Prevention and treatment (rescue) of respiratory distress syndrome in premature infants

Dosage and routes:
• Newborn: **INTRATRACHEAL INSTILL:** 3 ml/kg of birth wt, given as 2 doses of 1.5 ml/kg, repeat doses of 3 ml/kg of birth wt until up to 3 doses 12 hr apart have been given

Available forms: Susp 35 mg phospholipids/ml in 0.9% NaCl with 0.65 mg proteins in single-use vials containing 6 ml susp

Side effects/adverse reactions:
Concurrent illnesses that have occurred during treatment are in bold
RESP: Pulmonary air leaks, pulmonary interstitial emphysema, apnea, pulmonary hemorrhage
SYST: Patent ductus arteriosus, intracranial hemorrhage, severe intracranial hemorrhage, necrotizing enterocolitis, posttreatment sepsis, posttreatment infection, bradycardia, oxygen desaturation, pallor, vasoconstriction, hypotension, hypertension

Precautions: Bradycardia, rales, infections

Pharmacokinetics: Becomes lung associated within hours of administration

NURSING CONSIDERATIONS
Assess:
• Respiratory rate, rhythm, character, chest expansion, color, transcutaneous saturation, ABGs
• Endotracheal tube placement before dosing; for apnea after endotracheal administration
• Reflux of drug into the endotracheal tube during administration; stop drug if this occurs, and if needed, increase peak inspiratory pressure on the ventilator by 4-5 cm H_2O until tube is cleared
• Infant for repeat dosing using radiographic confirmation of RDS; repeat doses should be given as above; ventilator settings for repeat doses FIo_2 were decreased by 0.2 or amount to prevent cyanosis; ventilator rate of 30/min; inspiratory time <1 sec; if infant's pretreatment rate was >30, it was left unchanged during dosing; resume usual ventilator management after dosing

Administer:
• After suctioning
• By endotracheal administration only by persons trained in neonatal intubation and ventilation
• After using a No. 5 Fr end-hole catheter inserted into the endotracheal tube with the tip protruding just beyond the end of the endotracheal tube; shorten the catheter before insertion; do not insert the drug into the mainstem bronchus
• Divide doses and administer with infant in different positions
• Determine dosing by weight of infant; slowly withdraw contents into plastic syringe through 20G needle; do not filter or shake; attach premeasured No. 5 Fr catheter to syringe; fill with drug and discard excess through catheter so only dose to be given remains in syringe
• For prevention dosing, stabilize, weigh, and intubate infant; give drug

---

within 15 min of birth if possible; position infant and inject first dose through catheter over 2-3 sec; remove catheter and manually ventilate with O_2 to prevent cyanosis (60 bpm) and sufficient positive pressure to promote adequate air exchange and chest wall excursion

• For rescue dosing, give dosing as soon as infant is placed on ventilator after birth; immediately before administering dose, change ventilator settings to 60/min, inspiratory time 0.5 sec, FIo_2 1; position infant and inject first dose through catheter over 2-3 sec; remove catheter; return to mechanical ventilator

• Ventilate infant for >30 sec or until stable after prevention or rescue strategy; reposition for next dose; same procedure for subsequent dosing; do not suction for at least 1 hr after dosing unless airway obstruction is evident; resume ventilator therapy after dosing

Perform/provide:

• Reduction in peak ventilator inspiratory pressures immediately if chest expansion improves substantially after dose

• Reduction in FIo_2 in small, repeated steps when infant becomes pink and transcutaneous oxygen saturation is in excess of 95%; oxygen saturation should remain between 90% and 95%

• Suctioning of all infants before administration to prevent mucus plugging; if endotracheal tube obstruction is suspected, remove obstruction and replace tube immediately

• Storage in refrigerator; protect from light; warm to room temperature for >20 min or warm in hand >8 min before giving; do not use artificial warming methods; enter a vial only once; unopened, unused vials that have been warmed to room temperature may be rerefrigerated within 8 hr of warming; do not warm and return to refrigerator more than once

Evaluate:

• Therapeutic response: significant improvement in respiratory status

---

candesartan (Ŗ)

(can-deh-sar′tan)
Atacand
Func. class.: Antihypertensive
Chem. class.: Angiotensin II receptor (Type AT_1)

Action: Blocks the vasoconstrictor and aldosterone-secreting effects of angiotensin II; selectively blocks the binding of angiotensin II to the AT_1 receptor found in tissues

Uses: Hypertension, alone or in combination

Dosage and routes:
• *Adult:* **PO** 16 mg qd initially in patients who are not volume depleted, range 8-32 mg/day; may be given with a diuretic
Available forms: Tabs 4, 8, 16, 32 mg

Side effects/adverse reactions:
CNS: Dizziness, fatigue, headache
GI: Diarrhea, nausea, abdominal pain, vomiting
MS: Arthralgia, pain
RESP: Cough, upper respiratory infection
*SYST: **Angioedema***
CV: Chest pain, peripheral edema
EENT: Sinusitis, rhinitis, pharyngitis

Contraindications: Hypersensitivity

Precautions: Hypersensitivity to ACE inhibitors; pregnancy (C) 1st trimester, (D) 2nd and 3rd trimesters; lactation; children; elderly

---

Side effects: *italics* = common; ***bold italics*** = life-threatening

Pharmacokinetics: Extensively metabolized, excreted in urine and feces

NURSING CONSIDERATIONS
Assess:
• For pregnancy, this drug can cause fetal death when given in pregnancy
• Response and adverse reactions especially in renal disease
• For severe hypotension, place supine, give 0.9% NaCl IV
• B/P, pulse q4h; note rate, rhythm, quality; electrolytes: K, Na, Cl; baselines in renal, liver function tests before therapy begins
• Skin turgor, dryness of mucous membranes for hydration status; for angioedema
Administer:
• Without regard to meals
Evaluate:
• Therapeutic response: decreased B/P
Teach patient/family:
• To comply with dosage schedule, even if feeling better
• To notify prescriber of mouth sores, fever, swelling of hands or feet, irregular heartbeat, chest pain
• That excessive perspiration, dehydration, vomiting, diarrhea may lead to fall in blood pressure; to consult prescriber if these occur
• That drug may cause dizziness, fainting; light-headedness may occur
• To rise slowly to sitting or standing position to minimize orthostatic hypotension
• To notify prescriber immediately if pregnant; not to use during lactation

capecitabine (℞)
(cap-eh-sit′ah-bean)
Xeloda
Func. class.: Antineoplastic, antimetabolite
Chem. class.: Fluoropyrimidine carbamate

Action: Competes with physiologic substrate of DNA synthesis, thus interfering with cell replication in the S phase of cell cycle (before mitosis); drug is converted to 5-FU
Uses: Metastatic breast cancer
Dosage and routes:
• *Adult:* **PO** 2500 mg/m^2/day in 2 divided doses q12h at end of meal × 2 wk, then 1 wk rest period; given in 3 wk cycles
Available forms: Tabs 150, 500 mg
Side effects/adverse reactions:
HEMA: **Neutropenia, lymphopenia, thrombocytopenia, myelosuppression,** anemia
GI: Nausea, vomiting, anorexia, diarrhea, stomatitis, abdominal pain, constipation, anorexia, dyspepsia, **intestinal obstruction**
OTHER: Hyperbilirubinemia, eye irritation, pyrexia, edema, myalgia, limb pain, *pyrexia,* dehydration
INTEG: Hand and foot syndrome, dermatitis, nail disorder
CNS: Dizziness, headache, *paresthesia, fatigue,* insomnia
Contraindications: Hypersensitivity to 5-FU, infants, pregnancy (D)
Precautions: Renal disease, hepatic disease, lactation, children, elderly
Pharmacokinetics: Readily absorbed, peak 1½ hr; food decreases absorption; extensively metabolized in the liver; elimination half-life 45 min
Interactions:
• Increased toxicity: leucovorin

 = Nursing alert   = Herb-drug interaction   ⃠ = Do not crush

• Increased capecitabine levels: ant-acid

NURSING CONSIDERATIONS

Assess:

• CBC (RBC, Hct, Hgb), differential, platelet count weekly; withhold drug if WBC is <4000/mm^3, platelet count is <75,000/mm^3, or RBC, Hct, Hgb low; notify prescriber of these results

• Renal function studies: BUN, serum uric acid, urine creatinine clearance, electrolytes before and during therapy

• Monitor temperature q4h; fever may indicate beginning infection; no rectal temperatures

• Liver function tests before and during therapy: bilirubin, ALT, AST, alk phosphatase, as needed or monthly

• Bleeding: hematuria, heme-positive stools, bruising or petechiae, mucosa or orifices q8h

• Dyspnea, rales, unproductive cough, chest pain, tachypnea, fatigue, increased pulse, pallor, lethargy; personality changes, with high doses

• Edema in feet, joint pain, stomach pain, shaking

• For hand and foot syndrome: paresthesia, tingling, painful/painless swelling, blistering, erythema with severe pain of hands or feet

• For toxicity: severe diarrhea, nausea, vomiting, stomatitis

• Buccal cavity q8h for dryness, sores or ulceration, white patches, oral pain, bleeding, dysphagia

• GI symptoms: frequency of stools, cramping, if severe diarrhea occurs, fluid and electrolytes may need to be given

Administer:

• Antiemetic 30-60 min before giving drug and prn

Perform/provide:

• Rinsing of mouth tid-qid with water, club soda; brushing of teeth bid-tid with soft brush or cotton-tipped applicators for stomatitis; use unwaxed dental floss

Evaluate:

• Therapeutic response: decreased tumor size, spread of malignancy

Teach patient/family:

• To avoid foods with citric acid, hot or rough texture if stomatitis is present; to take drug with water ½ hr pc 5AM, PM

• To avoid pregnancy while on this drug; to avoid using while lactating

• Not to double dose, if dose is missed

• To immediately report severe diarrhea, vomiting, stomatitis, fever over 100° F (37.8° C), hand and foot syndrome, anorexia

• To report signs of infection: increased temperature, sore throat, flu symptoms

• To report signs of anemia: fatigue, headache, faintness, shortness of breath, irritability

• To report bleeding; to avoid use of razors, commercial mouthwash

---

captopril (℞)

(kap'toe-pril)

Capoten, Novo-Captoril*

Func. class.: Antihypertensive

Chem. class.: Angiotensin-converting enzyme inhibitor (ACE)

Action: Selectively suppresses renin-angiotensin-aldosterone system; inhibits ACE; preventing conversion of angiotensin I to angiotensin II; results in dilation of arterial, venous vessels

Uses: Hypertension, CHF, left ventricular dysfunction after MI, diabetic nephropathy

---

Dosage and routes:
Malignant hypertension
• *Adult:* PO 25 mg increasing q2h until desired response, not to exceed 450 mg/day
Hypertension
• *Adult:* PO initial dose: 25 mg bid-tid; may increase to 50 mg bid-tid at 1-2 wk intervals; usual range: 25-150 mg bid-tid; max 450 mg
• *Child:* PO 0.3-0.5 mg/kg/dose, titrate up to 6 mg/kg/day in 2-4 divided doses
CHF
• *Adult:* PO 12.5 mg bid-tid; may increase to 50 mg bid-tid; after 14 days, may increase to 150 mg tid if needed
LVD after MI
• *Adult:* PO 50 mg tid, may begin treatment 3 days after MI; give 6.25 mg as a single dose, then 12.5 mg tid, increase to 25 mg tid for several days, then to 50 mg tid
Diabetic nephropathy
• *Adult:* PO 25 mg tid
Available forms: Tabs 12.5, 25, 50, 100 mg
Side effects/adverse reactions:
CV: Hypotension, postural hypotension, *tachycardia,* angina
GU: Impotence, dysuria, nocturia, proteinuria, ***nephrotic syndrome, acute reversible renal failure,*** polyuria, oliguria, urinary frequency
*HEMA: **Neutropenia, agranulocytosis, pancytopenia, thrombocytopenia,*** anemia
INT: Rash, *angioedema*
*RESP: **Bronchospasm,*** *dyspnea, cough*
GI: Loss of taste, increased LFTs
CNS: Fever, chills
*MISC: **Angioedema,*** hyperkalemia
Contraindications: Hypersensitivity, lactation, heart block, children, K-sparing diuretics, bilateral renal artery stenosis
Precautions: Dialysis patients, hypovolemia, leukemia, scleroderma, lupus erythematosus, blood dyscrasias, CHF, diabetes mellitus, renal disease, thyroid disease, COPD, asthma, pregnancy (C)
Pharmacokinetics:
PO: Peak 1 hr; duration 6-12 hr; half-life 6-7 hr; metabolized by liver (metabolites), excreted in urine; crosses placenta; excreted in breast milk
Interactions:
• Increased hypotension: diuretics, other antihypertensives
• Decreased captopril effect: antacids, NSAIDs
• Possible toxicity: lithium
• Hypoglycemia: insulin, oral antidiabetics
• Increased digoxin level: digoxin
• Do not use with potassium-sparing diuretics, sympathomimetics, potassium supplements
Lab test interferences:
False positive: Urine acetone
NURSING CONSIDERATIONS
Assess:
• Blood studies: neutrophils, decreased platelets
• B/P, pulse rates baseline, frequently
• Renal studies: protein, BUN, creatinine; watch for increased levels that may indicate nephrotic syndrome
• Baselines in renal, liver function tests before therapy begins
• Edema in feet, legs daily
• Allergic reaction: rash, fever, pruritus, urticaria; drug should be discontinued if antihistamines fail to help
• Symptoms of CHF: edema, dyspnea, wet rales, B/P
Administer:
• 1 hr ac or 1½ hr pc
Perform/provide:
• Storage in tight container at 86° F (30° C) or less

◆ = Nursing alert　　🥢 = Herb-drug interaction　　🚫 = Do not crush

Evaluate:
• Therapeutic response: decrease in B/P in hypertension, edema, moist rales (CHF)

Teach patient/family:
• That tabs may be crushed and mixed with food
• To take 1 hr before meals or 1½ hr pc
• Not to discontinue drug abruptly
• Not to use OTC products (cough, cold, or allergy) unless directed by prescriber
• To avoid sunlight or wear sunscreen if in sunlight; photosensitivity may occur
• To comply with dosage schedule, even if feeling better
• To rise slowly to sitting or standing position to minimize orthostatic hypotension
• To notify prescriber of mouth sores, sore throat, fever, swelling of hands or feet, irregular heartbeat, chest pain, signs of angioedema
• That excessive perspiration, dehydration, vomiting; diarrhea may lead to fall in blood pressure; consult prescriber if these occur
• That dizziness, fainting, lightheadedness may occur during first few days of therapy
• That skin rash or impaired perspiration may occur
• How to take B/P
• To report if pregnancy is suspected

Treatment of overdose: 0.9% NaCl IV/INF; hemodialysis

carbamazepine (R)
(kar-ba-maz'e-peen)
Apo-Carbamazepine*, Atretol, Carbatrol, Epitol, Mazepine*, Novo-Carbamaz*, PMS-Carbamazepine*, Tegretol, Tegretol CR*, Tegretol-XR
Func. class.: Anticonvulsant
Chem. class.: Iminostilbene derivative

Action: Inhibits nerve impulses by limiting influx of sodium ions across cell membrane in motor cortex

Uses: Tonic-clonic, complex-partial, mixed seizures; trigeminal neuralgia, diabetic neuropathy

Investigational uses: Diabetes insipidus, bipolar disorder, neurogenic pain, schizophrenia, psychotic behavior with dementia

Dosage and routes:
Seizures
• *Adult and child >12 yr:* **PO** 200 mg bid, may be increased by 200 mg/day in divided doses q6-8h; maintenance 800-1200 mg/day maximum 1200 mg/day; adjustment is needed to minimum dose to control seizures; ext rel give bid
• *Child <12 yr:* **PO** 10-20 mg/kg/day in 3-4 divided doses
Trigeminal neuralgia
• *Adult:* **PO** 100 mg bid with meals; may increase 100 mg q12h until pain subsides, not to exceed 1.2 g/day; maintenance is 200-400 mg bid

Available forms: Tabs, chewable 100 mg; tabs 200 mg; ext-rel tabs 100*, 200*, 400* mg; oral susp 100 mg/5 ml; caps, ext rel 200, 300 mg

Side effects/adverse reactions:
*HEMA: **Thrombocytopenia, agranulocytosis, leukocytosis, neutropenia, aplastic anemia, eosinophilia,*** increased pro-time
ENDO: SIADH (elderly)

*CNS: Drowsiness, dizziness, confusion, fatigue, **paralysis**, headache, hallucinations, **worsening of seizures***

GI: Nausea, constipation, diarrhea, anorexia, vomiting, abdominal pain, stomatitis, glossitis, increased liver enzymes, **hepatitis**

INTEG: Rash, Stevens-Johnson syndrome, urticaria

EENT: Tinnitus, dry mouth, blurred vision, diplopia, nystagmus, conjunctivitis

*CV: **Hypertension, CHF, dysrhythmias, AV block,*** hypotension, aggravation of cardiac artery disease

RESP: Pulmonary hypersensitivity (fever, dyspnea, pneumonitis)

GU: Frequency, retention, albuminuria, glycosuria, impotence, increased BUN

Contraindications: Hypersensitivity to carbamazepine or tricyclic antidepressants, bone marrow depression, concomitant use of MAOIs

Precautions: Glaucoma, hepatic disease, renal disease, cardiac disease, psychosis, pregnancy (C), lactation, child <6 yr

Pharmacokinetics:

PO: Onset slow, peak 4-8 hr; metabolized by liver; excreted in urine, feces; crosses placenta, blood-brain barrier; excreted in breast milk; half-life 14-16 hr

Interactions:

• CNS toxicity: lithium

• Increased carbamazepine levels: cimetidine, clarithromycin, danazol, diltiazem, erythromycin, fluoxetine, fluvoxamine, isoniazid, propoxyphene, valproic acid, verapamil

• Decreased effects of benzodiazepines, doxycycline, felbamate, haloperidol, oral contraceptives, phenobarbital, phenytoin, primidone, theophylline, thyroid hormones, warfarin

• Increased effects of desmopressin, lithium, lypressin, vasopressin

◆ Fatal reaction: MAOIs

🍷 Increased peak concentration of carbamazepine: grapefuit

🍷 Decreased carbamazepine metabolism, increased levels: quinine

NURSING CONSIDERATIONS
Assess:

• Renal studies: urinalysis, BUN, urine creatinine q3mo

• Blood studies: RBC, Hct, Hgb, reticulocyte counts qwk for 4 wk then qmo; if myelosuppression occurs, drug should be discontinued

• Hepatic studies: ALT, AST, bilirubin

• Drug levels during initial treatment or when changing dose; should remain at 4-12 µg/ml; anorexia may indicate increased blood levels

• Description of seizures

• Mental status: mood, sensorium, affect, behavioral changes; if mental status changes, notify prescriber

• Eye problems: need for ophthalmic examinations before, during, after treatment (slit lamp, fundoscopy, tonometry)

• Allergic reaction: purpura, red, raised rash; if these occur, drug should be discontinued

• Blood dyscrasias: fever, sore throat, bruising, rash, jaundice

◆ Toxicity: bone marrow depression, nausea, vomiting, ataxia, diplopia, cardiovascular collapse, Stevens-Johnson syndrome

Administer:

PO

• With food, milk to decrease GI symptoms

• Chewable tablets; tell patient to chew tablet, not swallow it whole

• Shake oral susp before use

• Mix an equal amount of water, D_5W, 0.9% NaCl when giving by NG tube, flush tube with 100 ml of above sol

---

◆ = Nursing alert   🍷 = Herb-drug interaction   🚫 = Do not crush

Perform/provide:
• Storage at room temperature
• Hard candy, gum, frequent rinsing for dry mouth
• Assistance with ambulation during early part of treatment; dizziness occurs
Evaluate:
• Therapeutic response: decreased seizure activity, document on patient's chart
Teach patient/family:
• To carry Medic Alert ID stating patient's name, drugs taken, condition, prescriber's name, phone number
• To avoid driving, other activities that require alertness usually the first 3 days of treatment
• Not to discontinue medication quickly after long-term use
• That urine may turn pink to brown
Treatment of overdose: Lavage, VS

---

carbidopa-levodopa
(℞)
(kar-bi-doe'pa) (lee-voe-doe'pa)
carbidopa/levodopa
Sinemet, Sinemet CR
Func. class.: Antiparkinson agent
Chem. class.: Catecholamine

Action: Decarboxylation of levodopa to periphery is inhibited by carbidopa; more levodopa is made available for transport to brain and conversion to dopamine in the brain
Uses: Parkinson's disease, parkinsonism resulting from carbon monoxide, chronic manganese intoxication, cerebral arteriosclerosis, restless leg syndrome
Dosage and routes:
• *Adult:* **PO** 3-6 tabs of 25 mg carbidopa/250 mg levodopa qd in divided doses, not to exceed 8 tabs/

day; **SUST REL** 1 tablet bid at intervals of not less than 6 hr usual: 2-8 tabs/day at intervals of 4-8 hr
Available forms: Tabs 10/100, 25/100, 25 mg carbidopa/250 mg levodopa; sust rel tab: 50 mg/200 mg carbidopa/levodopa (Sinemet CR)
Side effects/adverse reactions:
HEMA: **Hemolytic anemia, leukopenia, agranulocytosis**
CNS: Involuntary choreiform movements, hand tremors, fatigue, headache, anxiety, twitching, numbness, weakness, confusion, agitation, insomnia, nightmares, psychosis, hallucination, hypomania, severe depression, dizziness
GI: Nausea, vomiting, anorexia, abdominal distress, dry mouth, flatulence, dysphagia, bitter taste, diarrhea, constipation
INTEG: Rash, sweating, alopecia
CV: Orthostatic hypotension, tachycardia, hypertension, palpitation
EENT: Blurred vision, diplopia, dilated pupils
MISC: Urinary retention, incontinence, weight change, dark urine
Contraindications: Hypersensitivity, narrow-angle glaucoma, undiagnosed skin lesions
Precautions: Renal disease, cardiac disease, hepatic disease, respiratory disease, MI with dysrhythmias, convulsions, peptic ulcer, pregnancy (C), lactation
Pharmacokinetics:
PO: Peak 1-3 hr, excreted in urine (metabolites)
Interactions:
• Hypertensive crisis: MAOIs
• Decreased effects of levodopa: anticholinergics, hydantoins, papaverine, pyridoxine, benzodiazepines
• Increased effects of levodopa: antacids, metoclopramide
• Drug/food: increased pyridoxine will decrease levodopa effect

---

- Decreased absorption of levodopa: protein

Decreased action, increased EPS: Indian snakeroot

Increased Parkinson symptoms: kava

Lab test interferences:

False positive: Urine ketones, Coombs' test

False negative: Urine glucose

False increase: Uric acid, urine protein

Decrease: VMA, BUN, creatinine

NURSING CONSIDERATIONS

Assess:

- B/P, respiration; orthostatic B/P
- Mental status: affect, mood, behavioral changes, depression, complete suicide assessment
- Muscle twitching, blepharospasm that may indicate toxicity
- Renal, liver, hematopoietic tests, also for diabetes, acromegaly if on long-term therapy

Administer:

PO

- Drug until NPO before surgery
- Adjust dosage to response
- With meals; limit protein taken with drug
- Only after MAOIs have been discontinued for 2 wk; if previously on levodopa, discontinue for at least 8 hr before change to carbidopa-levodopa

Perform/provide:

- Assistance with ambulation during beginning therapy

Evaluate:

- Therapeutic response: decrease in akathisia, improved mood

Teach patient/family:

🚫 Not to crush or chew cont rel tabs; may be broken in half

- To change positions slowly to prevent orthostatic hypotension
- To report side effects: twitching, eye spasms; indicate overdose
- To use drug exactly as prescribed; if discontinued abruptly, parkinsonian crisis may occur; prescriber may recommend drug-free holidays
- That urine, sweat may darken
- To use physical activities to maintain mobility, lessen spasms
- That improvement may not occur for 3-4 mo

---

carboplatin (℞)

(kar-boe-pla'-tin)

Paraplatin, Paraplatin-AQ*

Func. class.: Antineoplastic alkylating agent

Chem. class.: Platinum coordination compound

Action: Produces interstrand DNA cross-links and, to a lesser extent, DNA-protein cross-links; activity is not cell cycle phase specific

Uses: Palliative treatment of ovarian carcinoma recurrent after treatment with other antineoplastic agents

Dosage and routes (single agent):

- *Adult:* **IV INF** 360 mg/m^2 given over >15 min on day 1 q4wk; do not repeat single intermittent courses until neutrophil count is >2,000/mm^3 and platelet count is >100,000/mm^3

Renal dose

CrCl 41-59 ml/min 250 mg/m^2, CrCl 16-40 ml/min 200 mg/m^2

Available forms: Inj 50, 150, 450 mg/vial

Side effects/adverse reactions:

EENT: Tinnitus, hearing loss, *vestibular toxicity*

HEMA: Thrombocytopenia, leukopenia, pancytopenia, neutropenia, anemia, bleeding

CV: Cardiac abnormalities

GI: Severe nausea, vomiting, diarrhea, weight loss

GU: Renal tubular damage, renal insufficiency, impotence, sterility, amenorrhea, gynecomastia

---

⬥ = Nursing alert   🍟 = Herb-drug interaction   🚫 = Do not crush

INTEG: Alopecia, dermatitis, rash, erythema, pruritus, urticaria
CNS: **Convulsions, central neurotoxicity,** peripheral neuropathy
RESP: Mucositis
META: Hypomagnesemia, hypocalcemia, hypokalemia, hyponatremia, hyperuremia

Contraindications: Hypersensitivity to this drug, platinum products, mannitol; severe bone marrow depression, significant bleeding, pregnancy (D)

Precautions: Radiation therapy within 1 mo, chemotherapy within 1 mo, lactation, liver disease

Pharmacokinetics: Initial half-life 1-2 hr, postdistribution half-life 2 ½-6 hr, not bound to plasma proteins, excreted by the kidneys

Interactions:
• Increased nephrotoxicity or ototoxicity: aminoglycosides
• Increased risk of bleeding: aspirin
• Increased toxicity: radiation, bone marrow suppressants
• Increased myelosuppression: myelosuppressives

Lab test interferences:
Increase: AST, BUN, alk phosphatase, bilirubin, creatinine

NURSING CONSIDERATIONS
Assess:
• CBC, differential, platelet count weekly; withhold drug if WBC count is <4000/mm^3 or platelet count is <100,000/mm^3; notify prescriber of results
• Renal function studies: BUN, creatinine, serum uric acid, urine CrCL before and during therapy
• I&O ratio; report fall in urine output to <30 ml/hr
• Monitor temperature q4h (may indicate beginning of infection)
• Liver function tests before and during therapy (bilirubin, AST, ALT, LDH) as needed or monthly

• Bleeding; hematuria, stool guaiac, bruising or petechiae, mucosa or orifices q8h
• Dyspnea, rales, unproductive cough, chest pain, tachypnea
• Effects of alopecia on body image; discuss feelings about body changes
• Jaundice of skin, sclera, dark urine, clay-colored stools, itchy skin, abdominal pain, fever, diarrhea
• Edema in feet, joint pain, stomach pain, shaking

Administer:
• Antiemetic 30-60 min before giving drug and prn for vomiting
IV
• After diluting 10 mg/ml of sterile water for inj, D$_5$W, NS (10 mg/ml); then further dilute with the same sol 1-4 mg/ml; give over 15 min or more (INT INF)
• IV INF over 5-6 hr; do not use needles or IV administration sets containing aluminum; may cause precipitate
• Diuretic (furosemide 40 mg IV) after infusion

Additive compatibilities: Cisplatin, etoposide, floxuridine, ifosfamide, ifosfamide/etoposide, paclitaxel

Solution compatibilities: D$_5$/0.2% NaCl, D$_5$/0.45% NaCl, D$_5$/0.9% NaCl, 0.9% NaCl, D$_5$W, sterile water for inj

Y-site compatibilities: Allopurinol, amifostine, aztreonam, cefepime, cladribine, doxorubicin liposome, filgrastim, fludarabine, granisetron, melphalan, ondansetron, paclitaxel, piperacillin/tazobactam, propofol, sargramostim, teniposide, thiotepa, vinorelbine

Perform/provide:
• Storage protected from light at room temperature; reconstituted sol stable for 8 hr at room temp

---

Side effects: *italics* = common; ***bold italics*** = life-threatening

Evaluate:

• Therapeutic response: decreasing size of tumor, spread of malignancy

Teach patient/family:

• That impotence or amenorrhea can occur; reversible after treatment is discontinued, to notify prescriber if pregnancy is suspected

• Not to breastfeed during treatment

• To avoid OTC drugs with aspirin

• To notify prescriber of fever, fatigue, sore throat, and bleeding, bruising

• That hair may be lost during treatment; a wig or hairpiece may make patient feel better; new hair may be different in color, texture

---

carboprost (℞)

(kar′boe-prost)

Hemabate, Prostin/15M*

Func. class.: Oxytocic, abortifacient

Chem. class.: Prostaglandin

Action: Stimulates uterine contractions, causing complete abortion in approximately 16 hr

Uses: Abortion at 13-20 wk gestation, postpartum hemorrhage caused by uterine atony not controlled by other methods

Dosage and routes:

To induce abortion

• *Adult:* **IM** 250 µg, then 250 µg q1½- 3½ h, may increase to 500 µg if no response, not to exceed 12 mg total dose

Postpartum hemorrhage

• *Adult:* **IM** 250 µg, repeat at 15-90 min intervals; max total dosage 2 mg

Available forms: Inj 250 µg/ml

Side effects/adverse reactions:

CNS: Fever, chills, headache

GI: Nausea, vomiting, diarrhea

Contraindications: Hypersensitivity, severe hepatic disease, severe renal disease, PID, respiratory disease, cardiac disease

Precautions: Asthma, anemia, jaundice, diabetes mellitus, convulsive disorders, past uterine surgery, pregnancy (C)

Pharmacokinetics: Onset 15 min, peak 2 hr; metabolized in lungs, liver; excreted in urine (metabolites)

Interactions:

• Increased action: other oxytocics

🌿 Hypertension: ephedra

NURSING CONSIDERATIONS

Assess:

• B/P, pulse; watch for change that may indicate hemorrhage

• Respiratory rate, rhythm, depth; notify prescriber of abnormalities

• For length, duration of contraction; notify prescriber of contractions lasting over 1 min or absence of contractions

• For incomplete abortion, pregnancy must be terminated by another method; drug is teratogenic

Administer:

IM

• In deep muscle mass; rotate injection sites if additional doses are given

Perform/provide:

• Emotional support before and after the abortion

Evaluate:

• Therapeutic response: expulsion of fetus, control of bleeding

Teach patient/family:

• To report increased blood loss, abdominal cramps, increased temperature, foul-smelling lochia

• Some methods of comfort control and pain control

---

carisoprodol (℞)

(kar-eye-soe-proe'dole)

carisoprodol, Soma, Vanadom

Func. class.: Skeletal muscle relaxant, central acting

Chem. class.: Meprobamate congener

Action: Depresses CNS by blocking interneuronal activity in descending reticular formation, spinal cord, producing sedation

Uses: Relieving pain, stiffness in musculoskeletal disorders

Dosage and routes:

• *Adult and child >12 yr:* **PO** 350 mg tid and hs

Available forms: Tabs 350 mg

Side effects/adverse reactions:

CNS: Dizziness, weakness, drowsiness, headache, tremor, depression, insomnia, ataxia, irritability

EENT: Diplopia, temporary loss of vision

HEMA: Eosinophilia

RESP: Asthmatic attacks

CV: Postural hypotension, tachycardia

GI: Nausea, vomiting, hiccups, epigastric discomfort

INTEG: Rash, pruritus, fever, facial flushing, ***erythema multiforme***

*SYST: **Angioedema, anaphylaxis***

Contraindications: Hypersensitivity, child <12 yr, intermittent porphyria

Precautions: Renal disease, hepatic disease, addictive personality, pregnancy (C), elderly, lactation

Pharmacokinetics:

PO: Onset ½ hr, peak 4 hr, duration 4-6 hr; metabolized by liver; excreted in urine; crosses placenta; excreted in breast milk (large amounts); half-life 8 hr

Interactions:

• Increased CNS depression: alcohol, tricyclic antidepressants, narcotics, barbiturates, sedatives, hypnotics

⚘ May increase CNS depression: kava

NURSING CONSIDERATIONS

Assess:

• Blood studies: CBC, WBC, differential; blood dyscrasias may occur

• Liver function studies: AST, ALT, alk phosphatase; hepatitis may occur

• ECG in epileptic patients; poor seizure control has occurred with patients taking this drug

• Idiosyncratic reaction, anaphylaxis within a few min or hr of 1st to 4th dose

• Allergic reactions: rash, fever, respiratory distress

• Severe weakness, numbness in extremities

• Psychologic dependency: increased need for medication, more frequent requests for medication, increased pain

• CNS depression: dizziness, drowsiness, psychiatric symptoms

Administer:

PO

• With meals for GI symptoms

Perform/provide:

• Storage in tight container at room temperature

• Assistance with ambulation if dizziness, drowsiness occurs, especially elderly

Evaluate:

• Therapeutic response: decreased pain, spasticity

Teach patient/family:

• Not to discontinue medication quickly after long-term use; insomnia, nausea, headache, spasticity, tachycardia may occur; taper over 1-2 wk

• Not to take with alcohol, other CNS depressants

• To avoid hazardous activities if drowsiness, dizziness occur
• To avoid using OTC medication: cough preparations, antihistamines, unless directed by prescriber

Treatment of overdose: Induce emesis of conscious patient, lavage, dialysis

---

carmustine (R)
(kar-mus'teen)
BiCNU, BCNU, Gliadel
Func. class.: Antineoplastic alkylating agent
Chem. class.: Nitrosourea

Action: Alkylates DNA, RNA; is able to inhibit enzymes that allow synthesis of amino acids in proteins; activity is not cell cycle phase specific

Uses: Brain tumors such as glioblastoma, medulloblastoma, astrocytoma; multiple myeloma, Hodgkin's disease, other lymphomas; GI, breast, bronchogenic, renal carcinomas

Dosage and routes:
• *Adult:* **IV** 75-100 mg/m² over 1-2 hr × 2 days or 200 mg/m² × 1 dose q6-8wk; if WBC is 3000-3999/mm³ give 50% of dose; if WBC is 2000-2999/mm³ and platelets are 25,000-75,000/mm³ give 25% of dose; withhold dose if WBC is <2000/mm³ and platelets are <25,000/mm³
• *Adult:* **INTRACAVITARY** wafer: 8 inserted into resection cavity
Available forms: Powder for inj 100 mg; wafer 7.7 mg (intracavitary)

Side effects/adverse reactions:
HEMA: Thrombocytopenia, leukopenia, myelosuppression, anemia
GI: Nausea, vomiting, anorexia, stomatitis, *hepatotoxicity*
GU: Azotemia, *renal failure*

INTEG: Burning, hyperpigmentation at injection site
RESP: Fibrosis, pulmonary infiltrate

Contraindications: Hypersensitivity, leukopenia, thrombocytopenia
Precautions: Pregnancy (D), lactation
Pharmacokinetics: Degraded within 15 min; crosses blood-brain barrier; 70% excreted in urine within 96 hr; 10% excreted as CO_2; fate of 20% is unknown

Interactions:
• Increased toxicity: other antineoplastics, radiation, cimetidine
• Risk of bleeding: aspirin, anticoagulants
• Myelosuppression: myelosuppressive agents

NURSING CONSIDERATIONS
Assess:
• CBC, differential, platelet count weekly; withhold drug if WBC is <2000 or platelet count is <25,000; notify prescriber of results
• Liver function tests: AST, ALT, bilirubin
• Pulmonary function tests, chest x-ray films before, during therapy; chest film should be obtained q2wk during treatment
• Renal function studies: BUN, serum uric acid, urine CrCl before, during therapy
• I&O ratio; report fall in urine output of 30 ml/hr
• Monitor for cold, cough, fever (may indicate beginning infection)
• Bleeding: hematuria, guaiac, bruising, petechiae, mucosa, orifices q8h
• Dyspnea, rales, unproductive cough, chest pain, tachypnea

Administer:
• Blood transfusions or RBC colony-stimulating factors to counter anemia
• Antiemetic 30-60 min before giving drug to prevent vomiting

---

◆ = Nursing alert   ∅ = Herb-drug interaction   🚫 = Do not crush

• Antibiotics for prophylaxis of infection
• All medications PO, if possible, avoid IM inj if platelets are <100,000/mm³

Wafer
• Foil pouches may be kept at room temp for 6 hr if unopened
🚫 If wafers are broken in several pieces, they should not be used

IV
• After diluting 100 mg drug/3 ml ethyl alcohol (provided); then further dilute 27 ml sterile H₂O for inj; then dilute with 100-500 ml 0.9% NaCl or D₅W, give over 1 hr or more, reduce rate if discomfort is felt; use only glass containers

Y-site compatibilities: Amifostine, aztreonam, cefepime, filgrastim, fludarabine, granisetron, melphalan, ondansetron, piperacillin/tazobactam, sargramostim, teniposide, thiotepa, vinorelbine

Perform/provide:
• Storage of reconstituted sol in refrigerator for 24 hr, or room temp for 8 hr
• Increase fluid intake to 2-3 L/day to prevent urate deposits, calculi formation
• Rinsing of mouth tid-qid with water or club soda; brushing of teeth bid-tid with soft brush or cotton-tipped applicators for stomatitis; use unwaxed dental floss, use viscous lidocaine (Xylocaine)
• Warm compresses at injection site for inflammation; reduce flow rate if patient complains of burning at infusion site

Evaluate:
• Therapeutic response: decreasing size of tumor, spread of malignancy

Teach patient/family:
• To report any changes in breathing or coughing
• To avoid foods with citric acid, hot or rough texture if stomatitis is present
• To report any bleeding, white spots, ulceration in mouth to prescriber; tell patient to examine mouth qd
• To avoid use of aspirin, ibuprofen, razors, commercial mouthwash
• To report signs of anemia (fatigue, irritability, shortness of breath, faintness)
• To report signs of infection (sore throat, fever)

carteolol (℞)
(kar-tee'oh-lole)
Cartrol, Ocupress
Func. class.: Antihypertensive
Chem. class.: Nonselective β-blocker

Action: Produces fall in B/P without reflex tachycardia or significant reduction in heart rate through mixture of α-blocking, β-blocking effects and intrinsic sympathomimetic activity; elevated plasma renins are reduced

Uses: Mild to moderate hypertension, ophthalmic, intraocular, open-angle glaucoma

Dosage and routes:
• *Adult:* **PO** 2.5 mg qd initially, may gradually increase to desired response, max 10 mg/day; **OPHTH** 1 gtt bid

Renal disease
• CrCl >60 ml/min give dose q24h; CrCl 20-60 ml/min give dose q48h; CrCl <20 ml/min give dose q72h
• *Available forms:* Tabs 2.5, 5 mg; ophth sol 1%

Side effects/adverse reactions:
CV: Orthostatic hypotension, ***bradycardia, CHF, chest pain, ventricular dysrhythmias, AV block, peripheral vascular insufficiency,*** palpitations

CNS: Dizziness, mental changes, drowsiness, fatigue, headache, catatonia, depression, anxiety, nightmares, paresthesia, lethargy, insomnia, decreased concentration

GI: Nausea, vomiting, diarrhea, dry mouth, flatulence, constipation, anorexia

INTEG: Rash, alopecia, urticaria, pruritus, fever

*HEMA: **Agranulocytosis, thrombocytopenic purpura (rare)***

EENT: Tinnitus, visual changes, sore throat, double vision, dry, burning eyes

GU: Impotence, dysuria, ejaculatory failure, urinary retention

*RESP: **Bronchospasm,** dyspnea,* wheezing, nasal stuffiness, pharyngitis

MS: Joint pain, arthralgia, muscle cramps, pain

OTHER: Facial swelling, decreased exercise tolerance, weight change, Raynaud's disease

Contraindications: Hypersensitivity to β-blockers, cardiogenic shock, heart block (2nd or 3rd degree), sinus bradycardia, bronchial asthma

Precautions: Major surgery, pregnancy (C), lactation, CHF, diabetes mellitus, renal disease, thyroid disease, COPD, well-compensated heart failure, nonallergic bronchospasm

Pharmacokinetics:

PO: Onset 1-2 hr, peak 2-4 hr, duration 8-12 hr, half-life 6-8 hr; metabolized by liver (metabolites inactive); excreted in urine, bile; crosses placenta; excreted in breast milk

Interactions:

• Decreased carteolol effect: thyroid

• Increased myocardial depression: phenytoin (IV), verapamil

• Increased hypertension: MAOIs, amphetamines

• Decreased CV effect: dopamine, dobutamine

• Decreased antihypertensive effect: NSAIDs

• Increased hypotension: other antihypertensives, clonidine, nitrates, general anesthetics, alcohol (large amts)

• Increased hypoglycemic effect: insulin, oral antidiabetics

• Decreased bronchodilating effects of theophylline, β-agonists

NURSING CONSIDERATIONS

Assess:

• I&O, weight daily; edema in feet, legs daily

• B/P, pulse q4h; note rate, rhythm, quality; apical/radial pulse before administration; notify prescriber of any significant changes

• Baselines in renal, liver function tests before therapy begins

• Skin turgor, dryness of mucous membranes for hydration status

• Blood glucose in those taking insulin/oral antidiabetics

Administer:

PO

• Drug ac, hs; tablet may be crushed or swallowed whole

Ophthalmic

• Bid, 1 gtt in each eye

Perform/provide:

• Storage in dry area at room temperature; do not freeze

Evaluate:

• Therapeutic response: decreased B/P after 1-2 wk

Teach patient/family:

• Not to discontinue drug abruptly; taper over 2 wk or may precipitate angina

• Not to use OTC products containing α-adrenergic stimulants (nasal decongestants, OTC cold preparations) unless directed by prescriber

---

⬥ = Nursing alert   ⫻ = Herb-drug interaction   🚫 = Do not crush

• To report bradycardia, dizziness, confusion, depression, fever

• To take pulse at home, advise when to notify prescriber

• To avoid alcohol, smoking, sodium intake

• To comply with weight control, dietary adjustments, modified exercise program

• To carry Medic Alert ID to identify drug being taken, allergies

• To avoid hazardous activities if dizziness is present

• To report symptoms of CHF: difficulty breathing, especially on exertion or when lying down, night cough, swelling of extremities

• To take medication hs to minimize orthostatic hypotension

• The method of instillation if using ophthalmic

Treatment of overdose: Lavage, IV atropine for bradycardia, IV theophylline for bronchospasm, digitalis, O_2, diuretic for cardiac failure; administer vasopressor (norepinephrine) for hypotension, isoproterenol for heart block

---

carvedilol (℞)

(kar-ved′i-lole)

Coreg

Func. class.: α/β-adrenergic blocker

Action: A mixture of nonselective α/β-adrenergic blocking activity; decreases cardiac output, exercise-induced tachycardia, reflex orthostatic tachycardia; causes vasodilation, reduction in peripheral vascular resistance

Uses: Essential hypertension alone or in combination with other antihypertensives, CHF

Investigational uses: Angina pectoris, idiopathic cardiomyopathy

Dosage and routes:
Essential hypertension
• *Adult:* **PO** 6.25 mg bid × 7-14 days; if tolerated well, then increase to 12.5 mg bid × 7-14 days; if tolerated well, may be increased (if needed) to 25 mg bid; not to exceed 50 mg qd

Congestive heart failure
• *Adult:* **PO** 3.125 mg bid × 2 wk; if tolerated well, give 6.25 mg bid × 2 wk, then double q2wk to max dose

Angina pectoris
• *Adult:* **PO** 25-50 mg bid

Idiopathic cardiomyopathy
• *Adult:* **PO** 6.25-25 mg bid

Available forms: Tabs 3.125, 6.25, 12.5, 25 mg

Side effects/adverse reactions:
CNS: Dizziness, somnolence, insomnia, ataxia, hyperesthesia, paresthesia, vertigo, depression

GI: Diarrhea, abdominal pain, increased alk phosphatase, ALT/AST

CV: Bradycardia, postural hypotension, dependent edema, peripheral edema, *AV block,* extrasystoles, hypertension, hypotension, palpitations, peripheral ischemia

RESP: Rhinitis, pharyngitis, dyspnea

MISC: Fatigue, injury, back pain, UTI, viral infection, hypertriglyceridemia, *thrombocytopenia*

Contraindications: Hypersensitivity, bronchial asthma, class IV decompensated cardiac failure, 2nd or 3rd-degree heart block, cardiogenic shock, severe bradycardia

Precautions: Cardiac failure, hepatic injury, peripheral vascular disease, anesthesia, major surgery, diabetes mellitus, thyrotoxicosis, elderly, pregnancy (C), lactation, children, emphysema, chronic bronchitis, renal disease

---

Side effects: *italics* = common; ***bold italics*** = life-threatening

Pharmacokinetics: Readily and extensively absorbed PO, >98% bound to plasma proteins, extensively metabolized by liver, excreted through bile into feces, terminal half-life 5-9 hr with increases in elderly, hepatic disease

Interactions:

• Increased hypoglycemia: antidiabetic agents

• Decreased heart rate, B/P: clonidine

• Increased concentrations of digoxin

• Increased levels of carvedilol: cimetidine

• Decreased levels of carvedilol: rifampin

• Conduction disturbances: calcium channel blockers

• Bradycardia, hypotension: MAOIs, reserpine

NURSING CONSIDERATIONS
Assess:

◆ Renal studies, including protein, BUN, creatinine; watch for increased levels that may indicate nephrotic syndrome; obtain baselines in renal, liver function studies before beginning treatment

• Liver function studies, jaundice; if LFTs are elevated, drug should be discontinued

• I&O, weight daily

• B/P during beginning treatment, periodically thereafter; pulse q4h, note rate, rhythm, quality

• Apical/radial pulse before administration; notify prescriber of significant changes

• Edema in feet, legs daily

Administer:
PO

• Drug ac, hs; tablets may be crushed or swallowed whole

• Reduced dosage in renal dysfunction; give with food to decrease orthostatic hypotension

Evaluate:

• Therapeutic response: decreased B/P in hypertension

Teach patient/family:

• To comply with dosage schedule, even if feeling better, that improvement may take several wk

• To rise slowly to sitting or standing position to minimize orthostatic hypotension

• To report bradycardia, dizziness, confusion, depression, fever; weight gain, SOB

• To take pulse at home; advise when to notify prescriber

• Not to discontinue drug abruptly, taper over 1-2 wk

• To avoid hazardous activities until stabilized on medication; dizziness may occur

---

**cascara sagrada/
cascara sagrada
aromatic fluid extract/
cascara sagrada fluid
extract** (OTC)
(kas-kar′a)

Func. class.: Laxative
Chem. class.: Anthraquinone

Action: Direct chemical irritation in colon; increases propulsion of stool

Uses: Constipation; bowel or rectal preparation for surgery or examination

Dosage and routes:

• *Adult:* PO 325 mg hs; **FLUID** 1 ml qd; **AROMATIC FLUID** 5 ml qd

• *Child 2-12 yr:* **PO/FLUID/ AROMATIC FLUID** ½ adult dose

• *Child <2 yr:* **PO/FLUID/AROMATIC FLUID** ¼ adult dose

Available forms: Tabs 325 mg; fluid extract 1 g/ml; aromatic fluid extract 1 g/ml

---

◆ = Nursing alert   ▮ = Herb-drug interaction   ⊘ = Do not crush

Side effects/adverse reactions:
GI: Nausea, vomiting, anorexia, cramps, diarrhea
META: Hypocalcemia, enteropathy, alkalosis, hypokalemia, ***tetany***
Contraindications: Hypersensitivity, GI bleeding, obstruction, CHF, lactation, abdominal pain, nausea/vomiting, appendicitis, acute surgical abdomen, alcoholics (aromatic form)
Precautions: Pregnancy (C)
Pharmacokinetics:
PO: Peak 6-12 hr; metabolized by liver; excreted by kidneys, in feces
Interactions:
• Decreased absorption of these drugs: antibiotics, digitalis, nitrofurantoin, salicylates, tetracyclines, oral anticoagulants

◢ Increased action/side effects: lily of the valley, pheasant's eye, squill
NURSING CONSIDERATIONS
Assess:
• Monitor blood, urine electrolytes if drug is used often by patient; check I&O ratio to identify fluid loss
• Cause of constipation; identify whether fluids, bulk, or exercise missing from lifestyle
• Cramping, rectal bleeding, nausea, vomiting; if these symptoms occur, drug should be discontinued
Administer:
• Alone for better absorption; do not take within 1 hr of other drugs or within 1 hr of antacids, milk
• In morning or evening (oral dose)
Evaluate:
• Therapeutic response: decrease in constipation
Teach patient/family:
🚫 To swallow tabs whole; do not break, crush, or chew
• Not to use laxatives for long-term therapy; bowel tone will be lost
• That normal bowel movements do not always occur daily
• Not to use in presence of abdominal pain, nausea, vomiting

• To notify prescriber if constipation unrelieved or of symptoms of electrolyte imbalance: muscle cramps, pain, weakness, dizziness

---

celecoxib (℞)
(sel-eh-cox′ib)
Celebrex
Func. class.: Nonsteroidal antiinflammatory

Action: Inhibits prostaglandin synthesis by decreasing enzyme needed for biosynthesis; analgesic, antiinflammatory, antipyretic properties
Uses: Acute, chronic rheumatoid arthritis, osteoarthritis
Dosage and routes:
Osteoarthritis
• *Adult:* **PO** 200 mg/day as a single dose
Rheumatoid arthritis
• *Adult:* **PO** 100-200 mg bid
Available forms: Caps 100, 200 mg
Side effects/adverse reactions:
CNS: Fatigue, anxiety, depression, nervousness, paresthesia
*CV: **Tachycardia,** angina, **MI,** palpitations, dysrhythmias, hypertension, fluid retention*
EENT: Tinnitus, hearing loss, blurred vision, glaucoma, cataract, conjunctivitis, eye pain
*GI: Nausea, anorexia, vomiting, constipation, dry mouth, diverticulitis, gastritis, gastroenteritis, hemorrhoids, hiatal hernia, stomatitis, **GI bleeding***
*GU: **Nephrotoxicity:** dysuria, **hematuria, oliguria, azotemia,** cystitis, UTI*
*HEMA: **Blood dyscrasias,** epistaxis, bruising, anemia*
INTEG: Purpura, rash, pruritus, sweating, erythema, petechiae, photosensitivity, alopecia
RESP: Pharyngitis, shortness of breath, pneumonia, coughing

Contraindications: Hypersensitivity to aspirin, iodides, other NSAIDs, asthma

Precautions: Pregnancy (C), lactation, children, bleeding disorders, GI disorders, cardiac disorders, hypersensitivity to other antiinflammatory agents

Pharmacokinetics: Well absorbed, crosses placenta, bound to plasma proteins, metabolized in liver, excreted by kidneys, peak 3 hr

Interactions:
• Increased effect of: anticoagulants
• Decreased effect of: aspirin, ACE inhibitors, diuretics
• Increased adverse reactions: glucocorticoids, NSAIDs, aspirin
• Increased toxicity: lithium, antineoplastics

NURSING CONSIDERATIONS
Assess:
• For pain of rheumatoid arthritis, osteoarthritis; check ROM, inflammation of joints, characteristics of pain
• Blood counts during therapy; watch for decreasing platelets; if low, therapy may need to be discontinued, restarted after hematologic recovery
◆ For blood dyscrasias (thrombocytopenia): bruising, fatigue, bleeding, poor healing

Administer:
PO
• With food or milk to decrease gastric symptoms
🚫 Do not crush, dissolve, or chew caps

Evaluate:
Therapeutic response: decreased pain in arthritic conditions; decreased inflammation in arthritic conditions

Teach patient/family:
• That drug must be continued for prescribed time to be effective; to avoid other NSAIDs, aspirin

• To report bleeding, bruising, fatigue, malaise since blood dyscrasias do occur
🚫 To take with a full glass of water to enhance absorption; do not crush, break, or chew

---

◆ = Nursing alert   🖋 = Herb-drug interaction   🚫 = Do not crush

CEPHALOSPORINS—1ST GENERATION

cefadroxil (℞)
(sef-a-drox′ill)
cefadroxil, Duricef, Ultracef

cefazolin (℞)
(sef-a′zoe-lin)
Ancef, cefazolin, Kefzol

cephalexin (℞)
(sef-a-lex′in)
Apo-Cephalex*, Cefanex, C-Lexin, cephalexin, Keflex, Keftab, Novo-Lexin*, Nu-Cephalex*

cephalothin (℞)
(sef-a-loe′thin)
cephalothin, Keflin

cephapirin (℞)
(sef-a-pye′rin)
Cefadyl, cephapirin

cephradine (℞)
(sef′ra-deen)
cephradine, Velosef
Func. class.: Antiinfective
Chem. class.: Cephalosporin (1st generation)

Action: Inhibits bacterial cell wall synthesis, rendering cell wall osmotically unstable, leading to cell death by binding to cell wall membrane

Uses:

cefadroxil: gram-negative bacilli: *Escherichia coli, Proteus mirabilis, Klebsiella* (UTI only); gram-positive organisms: *Streptococcus pneumoniae, S. pyogenes, Staphylococcus aureus;* upper, lower respiratory tract, urinary tract, skin infections, otitis media; tonsillitis; and UTIs

cefazolin: gram-negative bacilli: *Haemophilus influenzae, Escherichia coli, Proteus mirabilis, Klebsiella;* gram-positive organisms: *Staphylococcus aureus;* upper, lower

---

* = Canada only   Side effects: *italics* = common; ***bold italics*** = life-threatening

respiratory tract, urinary tract, skin infections, bone, joint, biliary, genital infections, endocarditis, surgical prophylaxis, septicemia

cephalexin: gram-negative bacilli: *Haemophilus influenzae, Escherichia coli, Proteus mirabilis, Klebsiella;* gram-positive organisms: *Streptococcus pneumoniae, S. pyogenes, Staphylococcus aureus;* upper, lower respiratory tract, urinary tract, skin, bone infections, otitis media

cephalothin: gram-negative bacilli: *Haemophilus influenzae, Escherichia coli, Proteus mirabilis, Klebsiella, Salmonella, Shigella;* gram-positive organisms: *Streptococcus pneumoniae, S. pyogenes, Staphylococcus aureus;* upper, lower respiratory tract, skin infections, bone infections, endocarditis, septicemia, bacterial peritonitis

cephapirin: gram-negative bacilli: *Haemophilus influenzae, Escherichia coli, Proteus mirabilis, Klebsiella;* gram-positive organisms: *Streptococcus pneumoniae, S. viridans, Staphylococcus aureus;* lower respiratory tract, skin infections, endocarditis, bacterial peritonitis

cephradine: gram-negative bacilli: *Haemophilus influenzae, Escherichia coli, Proteus mirabilis, Klebsiella;* gram-positive organisms: *Streptococcus pneumoniae, S. pyogenes, Staphylococcus aureus;* serious respiratory tract, skin infections, urinary tract infections, otitis media

Dosage and routes:

cefadroxil
• *Adult:* PO 1-2 g qd or q12h in divided doses, give a loading dose of 1 g initially
• *Child:* PO 30/kg/day in divided doses

Renal dose: CrCl 25-50 ml/min 1 gm, then 500 mg q12h; CrCl 10-24 ml/min 500 mg q24h; CrCl <10 ml/min 500 mg q36h

Available forms: Caps 500 mg; tabs 1 g; oral susp 125, 250, 500 mg/5 ml

cefazolin

Life-threatening infections
• *Adult:* IM/IV 1-2 g q6h
• *Child >1 mo:* IM/IV 100 mg/kg in 3-4 divided doses

Mild/moderate infections
• *Adult:* IM/IV 250 mg-1 g q8h
• *Child >1 mo:* IM/IV 25-50 mg/kg in 3-4 equal doses

Renal dose: CrCl 35-54 ml/min: 250-1000 mg q12h; CrCl 10-34 ml/min: 50% of dose q12h; CrCl <10 ml/min: 50% of dose q18-24h

Available forms: Inj 500 mg, 1 g; infusion 500 mg, 1 g/50 ml vial

cephalexin

Renal dose: CrCl <40 ml/min give q8-12h; CrCl 5-10 ml/min give q12h; CrCl <5 ml/min give q24h

Moderate infections
• *Adult:* PO 250-500 mg q6h
• *Child:* PO 25-50 mg/kg/day in 4 equal doses

Moderate skin infections
• *Adult:* PO 500 mg q12h

Severe infections
• *Adult:* PO 500 mg-1 g q6h
• *Child:* PO 50-100 mg/kg/day in 4 equal doses

Available forms: Caps 250, 500 mg; tabs 250, 500 mg, 1 g; oral susp 125, 250 mg/5ml

cephalothin

Renal dose: CrCl 26-50 ml/min 1.5 g q6h; CrCl 10-25 ml/min 1 g q6h; CrCl <10 ml/min 500 mg q6h

Moderate infections
• *Adult:* IM/IV 500 mg-1 g q4-6h
• *Child:* IM/IV 14-27 mg/kg q4h or 20-40 mg/kg q6h

Uncomplicated gonorrhea
• *Adult:* IM 2 g as a single dose

Severe infections
• *Adult:* IM/IV 1-2 g q4h

◆ = Nursing alert   ∥ = Herb-drug interaction   ⊘ = Do not crush

• *Child:* **IM/IV** 80-160 mg/kg/day in divided doses q4h
Available forms: Powder for inj 1, 2, 20 g

cephapirin
• *Adult:* **IM/IV** 500 mg-1 g q4-6h
• *Child:* **IM/IV** 40-80 mg/kg/day in divided doses q6h or 10-20 mg/kg q6h
Renal dose: CrCl <10 ml/min give q12h
Available forms: Powder for inj 500 mg, 1, 2, 20 g; IV only 1, 2, 4 g

cephradine
• *Adult:* **PO** 250 mg-1 g q6-12h
• *Child >1 yr:* **PO** 6-12 mg/kg q6h
Renal dose: CrCl > 20 ml/min 500 mg q6h; CrCl 5-20 ml/min 250 mg q6h
Available forms: Caps 250, 500 mg; oral susp 125, 250 mg/5ml

Side effects/adverse reactions:
CNS: Headache, dizziness, weakness, paresthesia, fever, chills
GI: Nausea, vomiting, *diarrhea, anorexia,* pain, glossitis, bleeding; increased AST, ALT, bilirubin, LDH, alk phosphatase; abdominal pain, *pseudomembranous colitis*
GU: Proteinuria, vaginitis, pruritus, candidiasis, increased BUN, *nephrotoxicity, renal failure*
HEMA: Leukopenia, thrombocytopenia, agranulocytosis, anemia, *neutropenia, lymphocytosis, eosinophilia, pancytopenia, hemolytic anemia*
INTEG: Rash, urticaria, dermatitis, *anaphylaxis*
RESP: Dyspnea

Contraindications: Hypersensitivity to cephalosporins, infants <1 mo
Precautions: Hypersensitivity to penicillins, pregnancy (B), lactation, renal disease
Pharmacokinetics:
cefadroxil: Peak 1-1½ hr, half-life 1-2 hr; 20% bound by plasma proteins; crosses placenta; excreted in breast milk

cefazolin
IM: Peak ½-2 hr, half-life 1½-2¼ hr
IV: Peak 10 min; eliminated unchanged in urine; 70% to 86% protein bound
cephalexin: Peak 1 hr, duration 6-8 hr, half-life 30-72 min; 5%-15% bound by plasma proteins; 90%-100% eliminated unchanged in urine; crosses placenta; excreted in breast milk

cephalothin
IV: Peak 15 min
IM: Peak 30 min
Half-life ½-1 hr, 65%-80% bound by plasma proteins, 50%-75% eliminated unchanged in urine in 8 hr; crosses placenta, excreted in breast milk, deacetylated in kidneys, liver

cephapirin
IV: Peak 5 min
IM: Peak 30 min
Half-life 21-47 min; 44%-50% bound by plasma proteins; 40%-70% eliminated unchanged in urine; crosses placenta; excreted in breast milk; metabolized in liver
cephradine: Peak 1 hr, half-life 0.75-1.5 hr; 20% bound by plasma proteins; 80%-90% eliminated unchanged in urine; crosses placenta; excreted in breast milk

Interactions:
• Increased toxicity: aminoglycosides, furosemide, probenecid
Lab test interferences:
False increase: Creatinine (serum urine), urinary 17-KS
False positive: Urinary protein, direct Coombs' test, urine glucose
Interference: Cross-matching
NURSING CONSIDERATIONS
Assess:
• Sensitivity to penicillin and other cephalosporins

• Nephrotoxicity: increased BUN, creatinine

• I&O daily

• Blood studies: AST, ALT, CBC, Hct, bilirubin, LDH, alk phosphatase, Coombs' test monthly if patient is on long-term therapy

• Electrolytes: K, Na, Cl monthly if patient is on long-term therapy

• Bowel pattern qd; if severe diarrhea occurs, drug should be discontinued; may indicate pseudomembranous colitis

• Urine output: if decreasing, notify prescriber; may indicate nephrotoxicity

• Allergic reactions: rash, urticaria, pruritus, chills, fever, joint pain; angioedema; may occur few days after therapy begins

• Bleeding: ecchymosis, bleeding gums, hematuria, stool guaiac daily

• Overgrowth of infection: perineal itching, fever, malaise, redness, pain, swelling, drainage, rash, diarrhea, change in cough, sputum

Administer:

cefadroxil

• For 10-14 days to ensure organism death, prevent superinfection

• With food if needed for GI symptoms

• Shake susp, refrigerate, discard after 2 wk

• After C&S completed

cefazolin

• IV; check for irritation, extravasation often; dilute in 10 ml sterile H_2O for inj and run over 3-5 min; may be further diluted with 50-100 ml of NS, D_5W sol and run over ½-1 hr by Y-tube or 3-way stopcock

• For 10-14 days to ensure organism death, prevent superinfection

• After C&S completed

Additive compatibilities: Aztreonam, clindamycin, famotidine, fluconazole, metronidazole, verapamil

Syringe compatibilities: Heparin, vit B

Y-site compatibilities: Acyclovir, allopurinol, amifostine, atracurium, aztreonam, calcium gluconate, cyclophosphamide, diltiazem, doxorubicin liposome, enalaprilat, esmolol, famotidine, filgrastim, fluconazole, fludarabine, foscarnet, heparin, hydromorphone, insulin (regular), labetalol, lidocaine, magnesium sulfate, melphalan, meperidine, midazolam, morphine, multivitamins, ondansetron, perphenazine, pancuronium, remifentanil, sargramostim, tacrolimus, teniposide, theophylline, thiotepa, vecuronium, vit B/C, warfarin

cephalexin

• Shake susp, refrigerate, discard after 2 wk

• For 10-14 days to ensure organism death, prevent superinfection

• With food if needed for GI symptoms

• After C&S

cephalothin

• Clear solution; do not give cloudy sol

• IV after diluting 1 g or less/10 ml or more of sterile H_2O for inj; give over 3-5 min; may be further diluted with 50 ml D_5W, NS by Y-tube or 3-way stopcock; run over 15-30 min; discontinue primary IV during administration; may also be given by continuous infusion

• Store 96 hr refrigerated, 24 hr room temp

• IM after reconstituting with 4 ml sterile H_2O for inj/1 g vial

• For 10-14 days to ensure organism death, prevent superinfection

• After C&S

• Insert IM in deep muscle mass, massage

Additive compatibilities: Ascorbic acid, chloramphenicol, clindamycin, fluorouracil, hydrocortisone,

---

◆ = Nursing alert   ⫸ = Herb-drug interaction   ⊘ = Do not crush

isoproterenol, magnesium sulfate, metaraminol, methicillin, methotrexate, potassium chloride, prednisolone, procaine, sodium bicarbonate, vit B/C

Syringe compatibilities: Cimetidine

Y-site compatibilities: Cyclophosphamide, famotidine, heparin, hydromorphone, magnesium sulfate, meperidine, morphine, multivitamins, perphenazine, potassium chloride, vit B/C

cephapirin
• IV after diluting 1 g or less/10 ml or more NS, D_5W, or bacteriostatic H_2O for inj; give 1 g or less/5 min or more; may be further diluted in 50-100 ml of D_5W, NS; run over 15 min; discontinue primary IV during administration; may also be given by continuous infusion, store refrigerated 96 hr, room temp 24 hr
• For 10-14 days to ensure organism death, prevent superinfection
• After C&S

Additive compatibilities: Bleomycin, calcium chloride, calcium gluconate, chloramphenicol, diphenhydramine, ergonovine, heparin, hydrocortisone, metaraminol, oxacillin, penicillin G potassium, pentobarbital, phenobarbital, phytonadione, potassium chloride, sodium bicarbonate, succinylcholine, verapamil, vit B, warfarin

Y-site compatibilities: Acyclovir, cyclophosphamide, famotidine, heparin, hydrocortisone, hydromorphone, magnesium sulfate, meperidine, morphine, multivitamins, perphenazine, potassium chloride, vit B/C

cephradine
• Shake suspension well before each dose
• For 10-14 days to ensure organism death, prevent superinfection

• With food if needed for GI symptoms
• After C&S

Evaluate:
• Therapeutic response: decreased symptoms of infection, negative C&S

Teach patient/family:
• If diabetic, to use Clinistix or Ketodiastix to check blood glucose level
• Not to drink alcohol or use meds with alcohol: reaction may occur
• To use yogurt or buttermilk to maintain intestinal flora, decrease diarrhea
• To take all medication prescribed for length of time ordered
• To report sore throat, bruising, bleeding, joint pain (may indicate blood dyscrasias [rare])

Treatment of anaphylaxis: Epinephrine, antihistamines; resuscitate if needed

CEPHALOSPORINS—2ND GENERATION

cefaclor (R̥)
(sef'a-klor)
Ceclor
cefamandole (R̥)
(sef-a-man'dole)
Mandol
cefmetazole (R̥)
(sef-met'a-zole)
Zefazone
cefonicid (R̥)
(se-fon'i-sid)
Monocid
cefotetan (R̥)
(sef'oh-tee-tan)
Cefotan
cefoxitin (R̥)
(se-fox'i-tin)
Mefoxin
cefprozil (R̥)
(sef-proe'zill)
Cefzil
cefuroxime (R̥)
(sef-yoor-ox'eem)
Ceftin, Kefurox, Zinacef
loracarbef (R̥)
(lor-a-kar'beff)
Lorabid
Func. class.: Antiinfective
Chem. class.: Cephalosporin
(2nd generation)

Action: Inhibits bacterial cell wall synthesis, rendering cell wall osmotically unstable, leading to cell death by binding to cell wall membrane
Uses:
cefaclor: Gram-negative bacilli: *Haemophilus influenzae, Escherichia coli, Proteus mirabilis, Klebsiella;* gram-positive organisms: *Streptococcus pneumoniae, S. pyo-genes, Staphylococcus aureus;* respiratory tract, urinary tract, skin, bone, joint infections, otitis media
cefamandole: Gram-negative bacilli: *Haemophilus influenzae, Escherichia coli, Proteus mirabilis, Klebsiella;* gram-positive organisms: *Streptococcus pneumoniae, S. pyo-genes, Staphylococcus aureus;* upper, lower respiratory tract, urinary tract, skin infections, peritonitis, septicemia, surgical prophylaxis
cefmetazole: Gram-negative bacilli: *Haemophilus influenzae, Escherichia coli, Proteus, Klebsiella, Bacteroides fragilis;* gram-positive organisms: *Streptococcus pneumoniae, S. pyogenes, Staphylococcus aureus;* anaerobes, including *Clostridium;* infections of lower respiratory tract, urinary tract, skin, bone, intraabdominal infections
cefonicid: Gram-negative bacilli: *Haemophilus influenzae, Escherichia coli, Proteus mirabilis, Klebsiella;* gram-positive organisms: *Streptococcus pneumoniae, S. pyo-genes, Staphylococcus aureus;* lower respiratory tract, urinary tract, skin infections, otitis media, peritonitis, septicemia
cefotetan: Gram-negative organisms: *Haemophilus influenzae, Escherichia coli, E. aerogenes, Proteus mirabilis, Klebsiella, Citrobacter, Enterobacter, Salmonella, Shigella, Acinetobacter, Bacteroides fragilis, Neisseria, Serratia;* gram-positive organisms: *Streptococcus pneumoniae, S. pyogenes, Staphylococcus aureus;* upper, lower, serious respiratory tract, urinary tract, skin, bone, joint, gynecologic, gonococcal, intraabdominal infections
cefoxitin: Gram-negative bacilli: *Haemophilus influenzae, Escherichia coli, Proteus, Klebsiella, Bacteroides fragilis, Neisseria gonorrhoeae;* gram-positive organisms:

Streptococcus pneumoniae, S. pyogenes, Staphylococcus aureus; anaerobes including *Clostridium,* lower respiratory tract, urinary tract, skin, bone, gynecologic, gonococcal infections, septicemia, peritonitis

cefprozil: Pharyngitis/tonsillitis, otitis media, secondary bacterial infection of acute bronchitis, and acute bacterial exacerbation of chronic bronchitis and uncomplicated skin and skin structure infections; acute sinusitis

cefuroxime: Gram-negative bacilli: *Haemophilus influenzae, Escherichia coli, Neisseria, Proteus mirabilis, Klebsiella;* gram-positive organisms: *Streptococcus pneumoniae, S. pyogenes, Staphylococcus aureus;* serious lower respiratory tract, urinary tract, skin, bone, joint, gonococcal infections, septicemia, meningitis

loracarbef: Gram-negative bacilli: *Haemophilus influenzae, Escherichia coli, Proteus mirabilis, Klebsiella;* gram-positive organisms: *Streptococcus pneumoniae, S. pyogenes, Staphylococcus aureus;* upper and lower respiratory tract, urinary tract, skin infections, otitis media, pharyngitis, tonsillitis

Dosage and routes:

cefaclor
• *Adult:* **PO** 250-500 mg q8h, not to exceed 4 g/day or 375-500 mg (ext rel) q12h × 7-10 days
• *Child >1 mo:* **PO** 20-40 mg/kg qd in divided doses q8h, or total daily dose may be divided and given q12h, not to exceed 1 g/day

Acute bacterial exacerbations of chronic bronchitis or acute bronchitis
• *Adult:* 500 mg/12 hr × 1 wk (ext rel)

Pharyngitis/tonsillitis
• *Adult:* 375 mg/12 hr × 10 days (ext rel)

Available forms: Caps 250, 500 mg; oral susp 125, 187, 250, 375 mg/5 ml; tabs, ext rel 375, 500 mg

cefamandole
• *Adult:* **IM/IV** 500 mg-1 g q4-8h; may give up to 2 g q4h for severe infections
• *Child >1 mo:* **IM/IV** 8.3-16.7 mg/kg q4h, not to exceed adult dose
• Dosage reduction indicated in renal impairment (CrCl <50 ml/min)

Available forms: Inj 1, 2, 10 g

cefmetazole
Renal dose: CrCl <50 ml/min 1-2 g q12h; CrCl 10-29 ml/min 1-2 g q24h; CrCl <10 ml/min 1-2 g q48h
• *Adult:* **IV** 2 g divided q6-12h × 5-14 days

Available forms: Powder for inj 1, 2 g/vial

cefonicid
Life-threatening infections
• *Adult:* **IM/IV BOL** or **INF** 0.5-2 g/24 hr; divide in two doses if giving 2 g
• Dosage reduction indicated in renal impairment

Available forms: Inj 500 mg, 1, 10 g

cefotetan
Renal dose: CrCl 10-30 ml/min give q24h; CrCl <10 ml/min give q48h
• *Adult:* **IV/IM** 1-2 g q12h × 5-10 days

Perioperative prophylaxis
• *Adult:* **IV** 1-2 g ½-1 hr before surgery

Available forms: Inj 1, 2, 10 g

cefoxitin
Renal dose: CrCl <50 ml/min give q8-12h; CrCl 10-29 ml/min give q24h; CrCl <10 ml/min give q24-48h
• *Adult:* **IM/IV** 1-2 g q6-8h
• Dosage reduction indicated in renal impairment (CrCl <50 ml/min)

Uncomplicated gonorrhea: 2 g IM as single dose with 1 g **PO** probenecid at same time

Severe infections
• *Adult:* **IM/IV** 2 g q4h
• *Child ≥3 mo:* **IM/IV** 80-160 mg/kg/day divided q4-6h; max 12 g/day

Available forms: Powder for inj 1, 2, 10 g

cefprozil
Renal dose: CrCl <30 ml/min 50% of dose

Upper respiratory infections
• *Adult:* **PO** 500 mg q24h × 10 days

Otitis media
• *Child 6 mo-12 yr:* **PO** 15 mg/kg q12h × 10 days

Lower respiratory infections
• *Adult:* **PO** 500 mg q12h × 10 days

Skin/skin structure infections
• *Adult:* **PO** 250-500 mg q12h × 10 days

Available forms: Tabs 250, 500 mg; susp 125, 250 mg/5 ml

cefuroxime
• *Adult and child:* **PO** 250 mg q12h; may increase to 500 mg q12h in serious infections
• *Adult:* **IM/IV** 750 mg-1.5 g q8h for 5-10 days

Urinary tract infections
• *Adult:* **PO** 125 mg q12h; may increase to 250 mg q12h if needed

Otitis media
• *Child <2 yr:* **PO** 125 mg bid
• *Child >2 yr:* **PO** 250 mg bid

Surgical prophylaxis
• *Adult:* **IV** 1.5 g ½-1 hr preop

Severe infections
• *Adult:* **IM/IV** 1.5 g q6h; may give up to 3 g q8h for bacterial meningitis
• *Child >3 mo:* **IM/IV** 50-100 mg/kg/day; may give up to 200-240 mg/kg/day **IV** in divided doses for bacterial meningitis (not recommended)
• Dosage reduction indicated in severe renal impairment (CrCl <20 ml/min)

Uncomplicated gonorrhea
• *Adult:* 1.5 g **IM** as single dose with oral probenecid in 2 separate sites

Available forms: Tabs 125, 250, 500 mg; inj 150, 750 mg, 1.5, 7.5 g; inj 750 mg; 1.5 g powder

loracarbef
Renal dose: CrCl 10-49 ml/min 50% of dose; CrCl <10 ml/min q3-5 days
• *Adult and child >13:* **PO** 200-400 mg q12h
• *Child <12 yr:* **PO** 15-30 mg/kg/day in 2 divided doses q12h

Available forms: Caps 200, 400 mg; 100, 200 mg/5 ml oral susp

Side effects/adverse reactions:
CNS: Dizziness, headache, fatigue, paresthesia, fever, chills, confusion
GI: Diarrhea, nausea, vomiting, anorexia, dysgeusia, glossitis, bleeding; increased AST, ALT, bilirubin, LDH, alk phosphatase; abdominal pain, loose stools, flatulence, heartburn, stomach cramps, colitis, jaundice
INTEG: Rash, urticaria, dermatitis, **Stevens-Johnson syndrome**
GU: Vaginitis, pruritus, candidiasis, increased BUN, **nephrotoxicity, renal failure,** pyuria, dysuria, reversible interstitial nephritis
HEMA: **Leukopenia, thrombocytopenia, agranulocytosis,** anemia, **neutropenia, lymphocytosis, eosinophilia, pancytopenia, hemolytic anemia, leukocytosis, granulocytopenia**
RESP: Dyspnea
SYST: **Anaphylaxis, serum sickness**
Contraindications: Hypersensitivity to cephalosporins or related antibiotics, seizures
Precautions: Pregnancy (B), lactation, children, renal disease
Pharmacokinetics:
cefaclor:
PO: Peak ½-1 hr, ext rel peak 1½-2½ hr, half-life 36-54 min; 25%

 = Nursing alert   ✦ = Herb-drug interaction   ⊘ = Do not crush

bound by plasma proteins; 60%-85% eliminated unchanged in urine in 8 hr; crosses placenta; excreted in breast milk (low concentrations)

cefamandole: Peak 1-1½ hr, half-life ½-1 hr; 60%-75% bound by plasma proteins; crosses placenta; excreted in breast milk; poor penetration into CSF

cefmetazole
IM: Peak 30-45 min; 68% bound by plasma proteins, excreted by kidneys; half-life 1-3 hr

cefonicid
IV: Onset 5 min

IM: Peak 1 hr

Half-life 4½ hr; excreted in breast milk (small amounts); 98% protein bound; poor penetration in CSF

cefotetan
IV/IM: Peak 1½-3 hr; half-life 3-5 hr, 70%-90% bound by plasma proteins, 50%-80% eliminated unchanged in urine, crosses placenta, excreted in breast milk

cefoxitin
IV: Peak 3 min

IM: Peak 15-60 min

Half-life 1 hr, 55%-75% bound by plasma proteins, 90%-100% eliminated unchanged in urine; crosses placenta, blood-brain barrier; eliminated in breast milk, not metabolized

cefprozil
PO: Peak 6-10 hr; plasma protein binding 99%; elimination half-life 25 hr; extensively metabolized to an active metabolite

cefuroxime: 65% excreted unchanged in urine, half-life 1-2 hr in normal renal function

loracarbef
PO: Peak 1 hr, half-life 1 hr; excreted in urine as unchanged drug

Interactions:

• Increased effect/toxicity: aminoglycosides, furosemide, probenecid

• Disulfiram-like reaction: alcohol

• Antagonist effect: chloramphenicol, do not use together

Lab test interferences:

False increase: Creatinine (serum urine), urinary 17-KS

False positive: Urinary protein, direct Coombs' test, urine glucose testing (Clinitest)

Interference: Cross-matching

NURSING CONSIDERATIONS
Assess:

◆ Nephrotoxicity: increased BUN, creatinine

• I&O ratio

• Blood studies: AST, ALT, CBC, Hct, bilirubin, LDH, alk phosphatase, Coombs' test qmo if patient is on long-term therapy

• Electrolytes: K, Na, Cl qmo if patient is on long-term therapy

• Bowel pattern qd; if severe diarrhea occurs, drug should be discontinued; may indicate pseudomembranous colitis

• Urine output; if decreasing, notify prescriber (may indicate nephrotoxicity)

• Allergic reactions: rash, flushing, urticaria, pruritus

• Bleeding: ecchymosis, bleeding gums, hematuria, stool guaiac daily

• Overgrowth of infection: perineal itching, fever, malaise, redness, pain, swelling, drainage, rash, diarrhea, change in cough, sputum

Administer:

cefaclor
• Shake susp, refrigerate, discard after 2 wk

• For 10-14 days to ensure organism death, prevent superinfection

• With food if needed for GI symptoms

• After C&S completed

🚫 Do not break, crush, or chew ext rel tabs

cefamandole
• IV; check often for irritation, ex-

travasation; dilute 1 g or less of drug/10 ml or more normal saline or sterile H_2O for inj; run over 3-5 min; may be further diluted with 100 ml of compatible sol and run over 15-30 min via Y-tube or 3-way stopcock; may also be diluted in 1 L compatible sol, run over prescribed rate

• For 10-14 days to ensure organism death, prevent superinfection

• After C&S completed

Additive compatibilities: Clindamycin, floxacillin, furosemide, metronidazole, verapamil

Syringe compatibilities: Heparin

Y-site compatibilities: Acyclovir, cyclophosphamide, hydromorphone, magnesium sulfate, meperidine, morphine, perphenazine

cefmetazole

• For 10-14 days to ensure organism death, prevent superinfection

• After C&S completed

Solution compatibilities: D_5W, 0.9% NaCl

Additive compatibilities: Clindamycin, famotidine, KCl

• IV after diluting 3.7 or 10 ml sterile H_2O for inj, 2 g/7 or 15 ml, shake, let stand until clear, run over 3-5 min; may be further diluted in 50-100 ml of D_5W, NS, LR to 1-20 mg/ml and run over ½-1 hr by Y-tube or 3-way stopcock

cefonicid

• IV direct dilute 0.5 g/2 ml or 1 g/2.5 ml sterile H_2O for inj and give by Y-tube or 3-way stopcock over 3-5 min

• IV INT INF may be further diluted in 50-100 ml D_5W, NS and given over 30 min; slight yellowing of sol does not affect potency

• IV; check for irritation, extravasation often

Additive compatibilities: Clindamycin

Y-site compatibilities: Acyclovir, amifostine, aztreonam, teniposide, thiotepa

cefotetan

• IV direct after diluting 1 g/10 ml sterile H_2O for inj and give over 3-5 min; may be diluted further with 50-100 ml of normal saline or D_5W, shake; run over ½-1 hr by Y-tube or 3-way stopcock; discontinue primary inf during administration

• May be stored 96 hr refrigerated or 24 hr room temp

Y-site compatibilities: Allopurinol, amifostine, aztreonam, diltiazem, famotidine, filgrastim, fluconazole, fludarabine, heparin, insulin (regular), melphalan, meperidine, morphine, paclitaxel, remifentanil, sargramostim, tacrolimus, teniposide, theophylline, thiotepa

cefoxitin

• IV after diluting 1 g or less/10 ml or more D_5W, NS and give over 3-5 min; may be diluted further with 50-100 ml of normal saline or D_5W; run over ½-1 hr by Y-tube or 3-way stopcock; discontinue primary inf during administration; by cont inf at prescribed rate; may store 96 hr refrigerated or 24 hr room temp

• For 10-14 days to ensure organism death, prevent superinfection

• After C&S completed

Additive compatibilities: Amikacin, cimetidine, clindamycin, gentamicin, kanamycin, multivitamins, sodium bicarbonate, tobramycin, verapamil, vit B/C

Syringe compatibilities: Heparin, insulin

Y-site compatibilities: Acyclovir, amifostine, amphotericin B cholesteryl sulfate complex, aztreonam, cyclophosphamide, diltiazem, doxorubicin liposome, famotidine, fluconazole, foscarnet, hydromorphone, magnesium sulfate, meperidine, morphine, ondansetron, perphenazine, remifentanil, teniposide, thiotepa

cefprozil

• For 10-14 days to ensure organism death, prevent superinfection
• After C&S
• Refrigerate/shake susp prior to use

cefuroxime

• For 10-14 days to ensure organism death, prevent superinfection
• With food if needed for GI symptoms
• After C&S

Additive compatibilities: Clindamycin, floxacillin, furosemide, metronidazole, netilmicin

Y-site compatibilities: Acyclovir, allopurinol, amifostine, atracurium, aztreonam, cyclophosphamide, diltiazem, famotidine, fludarabine, foscarnet, hydromorphone, melphalan, meperidine, morphine, ondansetron, pancuronium, perphenazine, remifentanil, sargramostim, tacrolimus, teniposide, thiotepa, vecuronium

loracarbef

• Oral susp should be shaken before giving; store for 2 wk at room temp, discard after 2 wk
• 1 hr before or 2 hr after a meal
• After C&S is completed
• For 7 days to ensure organism death, prevent superinfection

Evaluate:

• Therapeutic response: negative C&S

Teach patient/family:

• If diabetic, to use blood glucose testing
• Not to drink alcohol or take meds with alcohol or reaction may occur
• To complete full course of drug therapy, to report persistent diarrhea
• To take on an empty stomach 1 hr before or 2 hr after a meal

🚫 Not to break, crush, or chew caps
• To notify prescriber if breastfeeding or of any side effects

Treatment of overdose: Epinephrine, antihistamines; resuscitate if needed (anaphylaxis)

C

---

* = Canada only   Side effects: *italics* = common; ***bold italics*** = life-threatening

CEPHALOSPORINS—3RD/4TH GENERATIONS

cefdinir (℞)
(sef'dih-ner)
Omnicef
cefepime (℞)
(sef'e-peem)
Maxipime
cefixime (℞)
(sef-icks'ime)
Suprax
cefoperazone (℞)
(sef-oh-per'a-zone)
Cefobid
cefotaxime (℞)
(sef-oh-taks'eem)
Claforan
cefpodoxime (℞)
(sef-poe-docks'eem)
Vantin
ceftazidime (℞)
(sef'tay-zi-deem)
Ceptaz, Fortaz, Magnacef*,
Pentacef, Tazicef, Tazidime
ceftibuten (℞)
(sef-ti-byoo'tin)
Cedax
ceftizoxime (℞)
(sef-ti-zox'eem)
Cefizox
ceftriaxone (℞)
(sef-try-ax'one)
Rocephin
moxalactam (℞)
(mox'a-lak-tam)
Moxam

Func. class.: Broad-spectrum antibiotic
Chem. class.: Cephalosporin (3rd and 4th generation)

Action: Inhibits bacterial cell wall synthesis, rendering cell wall osmotically unstable, leading to cell death

Uses:
cefdinir: Gram-negative bacilli: *Haemophilus influenzae, H. parainfluenzae, M. catarrhalis;* gram-positive organisms: *Streptococcus pneumoniae, S. pyogenes, Staphylococcus aureus*
cefepime: Gram-negative bacilli: *Escherichia coli, Proteus, Klebsiella;* gram-positive organisms: *Streptococcus pneumoniae, S. pyogenes, Staphylococcus aureus;* lower respiratory tract, urinary tract, skin, bone infections
cefixime: Uncomplicated UTI *(Escherichia coli, Proteus mirabilis),* pharyngitis and tonsillitis *(Streptococcus pyogenes),* otitis media *(Haemophilus influenzae), Moraxella catarrhalis,* acute bronchitis, and acute exacerbations of chronic bronchitis *(Streptococcus pneumoniae, H. influenzae)*
cefoperazone: Gram-negative bacilli: *Haemophilus influenzae, Escherichia coli, Proteus mirabilis, Klebsiella, Enterobacter, Serratia, Citrobacter, Providencia, Proteus aeruginosa;* lower respiratory tract, urinary tract, skin, bone infections, bacterial septicemia, peritonitis, PID
cefotaxime: Gram-negative organisms: *Haemophilus influenzae, Escherichia coli, Neisseria gonorrhoeae, N. meningitidis, Proteus mirabilis, Klebsiella, Citrobacter, Serratia, Salmonella, Shigella;* gram-positive organisms: *Streptococcus pneumoniae, S. pyogenes, Staphylococcus aureus;* serious lower respiratory tract, urinary tract, skin, bone, gonococcal infections; bacteremia, septicemia, meningitis
cefpodoxime: Gram-negative bacilli: *Neisseria gonorrhoeae, Haemophilus influenzae, Escherichia coli, Proteus mirabilis, Klebsiella;* gram-positive organisms: *Streptococcus pneumoniae, S. pyogenes,*

Staphylococcus aureus; upper and lower respiratory tract, urinary tract, skin infections; otitis media, sexually transmitted diseases

ceftazidime: Gram-negative organisms: *Haemophilus influenzae, Escherichia coli, E. aerogenes, Proteus aeruginosa, P. mirabilis, Klebsiella, Citrobacter, Enterobacter, Salmonella, Shigella, Acinetobacter, Bacteroides fragilis, Neisseria, Serratia;* gram-positive organisms: *Streptococcus pneumoniae, S. pyogenes, Staphylococcus aureus;* serious upper, lower respiratory tract, urinary tract, skin, gynecologic, bone, joint, intraabdominal infections; septicemia, meningitis

ceftibuten: Pharyngitis/tonsillitis, otitis media, secondary bacterial infection of acute bronchitis

ceftizoxime: Gram-negative bacilli: *Haemophilus influenzae, Escherichia coli, E. aerogenes, Proteus mirabilis, Klebsiella, Enterobacter;* gram-positive organisms: *Streptococcus pneumoniae, S. pyogenes, Staphylococcus aureus;* serious lower respiratory tract, urinary tract, skin, intraabdominal infections, septicemia, meningitis, bone and joint infections, PID caused by *Neisseria gonorrhoeae*

ceftriaxone: Gram-negative bacilli: *Haemophilus influenzae, Escherichia coli, E. aerogenes, Proteus mirabilis, Klebsiella, Citrobacter, Enterobacter, Salmonella, Shigella, Acinetobacter, Bacteroides fragilis, Neisseria, Serratia;* gram-positive organisms: *Streptococcus pneumoniae, S. pyogenes, Staphylococcus aureus;* serious lower respiratory tract, urinary tract, skin, gonococcal, intraabdominal infections, septicemia, meningitis, bone, joint infections

moxalactam: Gram-negative bacilli: *Haemophilus influenzae, Esche-*

richia coli, Proteus mirabilis, Klebsiella, Citrobacter, Salmonella, Shigella, Serratia; gram-positive organisms: *Streptococcus pneumoniae, S. pyogenes, Staphylococcus aureus;* serious lower respiratory tract, urinary tract, skin, bone infections; septicemia, meningitis, intraabdominal infections

Dosage and routes:

cefdinir

Uncomplicated skin and skin structure infections/community-acquired pneumonia

• *Adult and child ≥ 13 yr:* **PO** 300 mg q12h × 10 days

• *Child 6 mo-12 yr:* **PO** 7 mg/kg q12h or 14 mg/kg q24h × 10 days, max 60 mg qd

Acute exacerbations of chronic bronchitis/acute maxillary sinusitis

• *Adult and child ≥ 13 yr:* **PO** 300 mg q12h or 600 mg q24h × 10 days

Pharyngitis/tonsillitis

• *Adult and child ≥ 13 yr:* **PO** 300 mg q12h or 600 mg q24h × 10 days

• *Child 6 mo-12 yr:* **PO** 7 mg/kg q12h × 5-10 days or 14 mg/kg q24h × 10 days

Renal dose

• CrCl <30 ml/min 300 mg qd (adult); 7 mg/kg qd (child)

cefepime

Urinary tract infections (mild to moderate)

• *Adult:* **IV/IM** 0.5-1 g q12h × 7-10 days

Urinary tract infections (severe)

• *Adult:* **IV** 2 g q12h × 10 days

Pneumonia (moderate to severe)

• *Adult:* **IV** 1-2 g q12h × 10 days

• Dosage reduction indicated in renal impairment (CrCl <50 ml/min)

Uncomplicated gonorrhea

• **IM** 2 g as a single dose with 1 g **PO** probenecid at the same time

Available forms: Powder for inj 500 mg, 1, 2 g

cefixime

Renal dose: CrCl 21-60 ml/min give 75% of dose; CrCl <20 ml/min give 50% of dose

• *Adult:* **PO** 400 mg qd as a single dose or 200 mg q12h

• *Child >50 kg or >12 yr:* **PO** use adult dosage

• *Child <50 kg or <12 yr:* **PO** 8 mg/kg/day as a single dose or 4 mg/kg q12h

Available forms: Tabs 200, 400 mg; powder for oral susp 100 mg/5 ml

cefoperazone

Hepatic dose: give 50% of dose

Mild/Moderate infections

• *Adult:* **IM/IV** 1-2 g q12h

Severe infections

• *Adult:* **IM/IV** 6-12 g/day divided in 2-4 equal doses

Available forms: Inj 1, 2 g

cefotaxime

• *Adult:* **IM/IV** 1-2 g q12h as a single dose

• *Child 1 mo-12 yr:* **IM/IV** 50-180 mg/kg/day divided q6h

Severe infections

• *Adult:* **IM/IV** 2 g q4h, not to exceed 12 g/day

• *Child 1 mo-12 yr:* **IM/IV** 50 mg/kg q6h

Uncomplicated gonorrhea

• *Adult:* **IM** 1 g

Dosage reduction indicated for severe renal impairment (CrCl <30 ml/min)

Available forms: Powder for inj 1, 2, 10 g; frozen inj 20, 40 mg/ml

cefpodoxime

• Reduce dose in renal disease

• *Adult >13 yr: Pneumonia:* 200 mg q12h for 14 days; *uncomplicated gonorrhea:* 200 mg single dose; *skin and skin structure:* 400 mg q12h for 7-14 days; *pharyngitis and tonsillitis:* 100 mg q12h for 10 days; *uncomplicated UTI:* 100 mg q12h for

7 days; dosing interval increased in presence of severe renal impairment

• *Child 5 mo-12 yr: acute otitis media:* 5 mg/kg q12h for 10 days; *pharyngitis/tonsillitis:* 5 mg/kg q12h (max 100 mg/dose or 200 mg/day) × 5-10 days

Available forms: Tabs 100, 200 mg/ granules for susp 50, 100 mg/5 ml

ceftazidime

Renal dose: CrCl <50 ml/min give q12h; CrCl 10-30 ml/min give q24h; CrCl <10 ml/min give q48h

• *Adult:* **IV/IM** 1-2 g q8-12h × 5-10 days

• *Child:* **IV** 30-50 mg/kg q8h not to exceed 6 g/day

• *Neonate:* **IV** 30-50 mg/kg q12h

Available forms: Inj 500 mg, 1, 2, 6 g

ceftibuten

Renal dose: CrCl <50 ml/min give 200 mg q24h; CrCl 5-20 ml/min give 100 mg q24h

• *Adult:* **PO** 400 mg qd × 10 days

• *Child 6 mo-12 yr:* **PO** 9 mg/kg qd × 10 days

Available forms: Caps 400 mg; 90, 180 mg/5 ml

ceftizoxime

Renal dose: CrCl <80 ml/min give 500-1500 mg q8h; CrCl 10-49 ml/min give 250-1000 mg q12h

• *Adult:* **IM/IV** 1-2 g q8-12h, may give up to 4 g q8h in life-threatening infections

• *Child <6 mo:* **IM/IV** 50 mg/kg q6-8h

PID

• *Adult:* **IV** 2 g q8h, may increase to 4 g q8h in severe infections

Available forms: Powder for inj 500 mg, 1, 2, 10 g; premixed 1 g, 2 g/50 ml

ceftriaxone

• *Adult:* **IM/IV** 1-2 g qd, max 2 g q12h

• *Child:* **IM/IV** 50-75 mg/kg/day in equal doses q12h

◆ = Nursing alert   🖉 = Herb-drug interaction   🚫 = Do not crush

C

Uncomplicated gonorrhea
• *Adult:* 250 mg **IM** as single dose
• Reduce dosage in severe renal impairment (CrCl <10 ml/min)
Meningitis
• *Adult and child:* **IM/IV** 100 mg/kg/day in equal doses q12h, max 4 g/day
Surgical prophylaxis
• *Adult:* **IV** 1 g ½-2 hr preop
Available forms: Inj 500 mg, 1, 2, 10 g
moxalactam
• *Adult:* **IM/IV** 2-4 g q8-12h
Mild infections
• *Adult:* **IM/IV** 250-500 mg q8-12h
Severe infections
• *Adult:* **IM/IV** 2-6 g q8h
• *Child:* **IM/IV** 50 mg/kg q6-8h
• Dosage reduction indicated even for mild renal impairment (CrCl <80 ml/min)
Available forms: Powder for inj 1, 2, 10 g
Side effects/adverse reactions:
CNS: Headache, dizziness, weakness, paresthesia, fever, chills, seizures
GI: Nausea, vomiting, diarrhea, anorexia, pain, glossitis, **bleeding;** increased AST, ALT, bilirubin, LDH, alk phosphatase; abdominal pain, *pseudomembranous colitis*
GU: Proteinuria, vaginitis, pruritus, candidiasis, increased BUN, *nephrotoxicity, renal failure*
HEMA: Leukopenia, thrombocytopenia, agranulocytosis, anemia, *neutropenia, lymphocytosis, eosinophilia, pancytopenia, hemolytic anemia*
INTEG: Rash, urticaria, dermatitis
RESP: Dyspnea
SYST: Anaphylaxis, serum sickness
Contraindications: Hypersensitivity to cephalosporins, infants <1 mo
Precautions: Hypersensitivity to penicillins, pregnancy (B), lactation, renal disease, children

Pharmacokinetics:
cefdinir
Unchanged in urine; crosses placenta, blood-brain barrier; eliminated in breast milk; not metabolized
cefepime
Peak 79 min, half-life 2 hr, 20% bound by plasma proteins, 90% excreted unchanged in urine; crosses placenta, blood-brain barrier; excreted in breast milk; not metabolized
cefixime
PO: Peak 1-2 hr, half-life 3-4 hr, 65% bound by plasma proteins, 50% eliminated unchanged in urine; crosses placenta; excreted in breast milk
cefoperazone
IV: Onset 5 min, peak 5-20 min, duration 6-8 hr
IM: Peak 1-2 hr, duration 6-8 hr
Half-life 2 hr; 70%-75% is eliminated unchanged in bile; 20%-30% unchanged in urine; excreted in breast milk (small amounts)
cefotaxime
IV: Onset 5 min
IM: Onset 30 min
Half-life 1 hr; 35%-65% is bound by plasma proteins; 40%-65% is eliminated unchanged in urine in 24 hr; 25% metabolized to active metabolites; excreted in breast milk (small amounts)
cefpodoxime
Half-life 2-3 hr; 25% bound by plasma proteins; 30% eliminated unchanged in urine in 8 hr; crosses placenta; excreted in breast milk
ceftazidime
IV/IM: Peak 1 hr, half-life ½-1 hr, 90% bound by plasma proteins, 80% eliminated unchanged in urine, crosses placenta, excreted in breast milk
ceftibuten
PO: Peak 6-10 hr; plasma protein

binding 99%; elimination half-life 25 hr; extensively metabolized to an active metabolite

ceftizoxime
IV: Onset 5 min
IM: Peak 1 hr
Half-life 5-8 hr; 90% bound by plasma proteins; 36%-60% eliminated unchanged in urine; crosses placenta; excreted in breast milk

ceftriaxone
IV: Onset 5 min
IM: Peak 1 hr
Half-life 5-8 hr, 90% bound by plasma proteins; 35%-60% eliminated unchanged in urine; crosses placenta; excreted in breast milk

moxalactam
IV: Peak 5 min
IM: Peak ½-2 hr
Half-life 1½-2½ hr, 25% bound by plasma proteins; 60%-97% eliminated unchanged in urine in 24 hr; crosses placenta, blood-brain barrier; excreted in breast milk; not metabolized

Interactions:
• Increased toxicity: aminoglycosides, furosemide, probenecid

Lab test interferences:
False increase: Urinary 17-KS
False positive: Urinary protein, direct Coombs' test, urine glucose
Interference: Cross-matching

NURSING CONSIDERATIONS
Assess:
• Sensitivity to penicillin, other cephalosporins
• Nephrotoxicity: increased BUN, creatinine
• Blood studies: AST, ALT, CBC, Hct, bilirubin, LDH, alk phosphatase, Coombs' test monthly if patient is on long-term therapy
• Electrolytes: K, Na, Cl monthly if patient is on long-term therapy
• Bowel pattern qd; if severe diarrhea occurs, drug should be discontinued; may indicate pseudomembranous colitis
• IV site for extravasation, phlebitis; change site q72h
◆ Urine output: if decreasing, notify prescriber; may indicate nephrotoxicity
• Allergic reactions: rash, urticaria, pruritus, chills, fever, joint pain, angioedema; may occur few days after therapy begins
• Bleeding: ecchymosis, bleeding gums, hematuria, stool guaiac
• Overgrowth of infection: perineal itching, fever, malaise, redness, pain, swelling, drainage, rash, diarrhea, change in cough, sputum

Administer:
cefdinir
• Oral susp after adding 39 ml water to the 60 ml bottle; 65 ml water to the 120 ml bottle; discard unused portion after 10 days
• After C&S completed
cefepime
• IV after diluting in 50-100 ml or more D_5, NS and give over 30 min
• For 7-10 days to ensure organism death, prevent superinfection
Solution compatibilities: 0.9% NaCl, D_5, D_5W, 0.5%, 10% lidocaine, bacteriostatic water for inj with parabens/benzyl alcohol
Y-site compatibilities: Doxorubicin liposome
cefixime
• For 10-14 days to ensure organism death, prevent superinfection
cefoperazone
• IV after diluting 1 g/ml sterile H_2O for inj, or 0.9% NaCl; shake, give over 3-5 min; each g may be further diluted with 20-40 ml D_5W, NS given over 30 min or as a cont inf over 6-24 hr to a concentration no greater than 25 mg/ml

• IM for concentration >250 mg/ml, dilute in sterile water, then lidocaine, inject deeply
• For 10-14 days to ensure organism death, prevent superinfection
Additive compatibilities: Cimetidine, clindamycin, furosemide
Syringe compatibilities: Heparin
Y-site compatibilities: Acyclovir, allopurinol, aztreonam, cyclophosphamide, enalaprilat, esmolol, famotidine, foscarnet, fludarabine, hydromorphone, magnesium sulfate, melphalan, morphine, teniposide, thiotepa

cefotaxime
• IV after diluting 1 g/10 ml D_5W, NS, sterile H_2O for inj and give over 3-5 min by Y-tube or 3-way stopcock; may be diluted further with 50-100 ml of normal saline or D_5W; run over ½-1 hr; discontinue primary inf during administration; or may be diluted in larger vol of sol and given as a cont inf over 6-24 hr
• For 10-14 days to ensure organism death, prevent superinfection
Additive compatibilities: Clindamycin, metronidazole, verapamil
Syringe compatibilities: Heparin, ofloxacin
Y-site compatibilities: Acyclovir, amifostine, aztreonam, cyclophosphamide, diltiazem, famotidine, fludarabine, hydromorphone, lorazepam, magnesium sulfate, melphalan, meperidine, midazolam, morphine, ondansetron, perphenazine, sargramostim, teniposide, thiotepa, tolazoline, vinorelbine

cefpodoxime
• For 10-14 days to ensure organism death, prevent superinfection
• With food to enhance absorption
Y-site compatibilities: Famotidine, fluconazole, fludarabine, insulin (regular), meperidine, morphine, sargramostim

ceftazidime
• IV after diluting 1 g/10 ml sterile H_2O for inj, shake, invert needle, push plunger, insert needle through stopper and keep in sol, expel bubbles and give over 3-5 min; may be diluted further with 50-100 ml of normal saline or D_5W; run over ½-1 hr, give through Y-tube or 3-way stopcock, discontinue primary inf during administration; store for 96 hr refrigerated, 24 hr room temp
• For 5-10 days to ensure organism death, prevent superinfection
Syringe compatibilities: Hydromorphone
Additive compatibilities: Ciprofloxacin, clindamycin, fluconazole, metronidazole, ofloxacin
Y-site compatibilities: Acyclovir, allopurinol, amifostine, aztreonam, ciprofloxacin, diltiazem, enalaprilat, esmolol, famotidine, filgrastim, fludarabine, foscarnet, granisetron, heparin, hydromorphone, labetalol, meperidine, melphalan, morphine, ondansetron, paclitaxel, ranitidine, remifentanil, tacrolimus, teniposide, theophylline, thiotepa, vinorelbine, zidovudine

ceftibuten
• For 10 days to ensure organism death, prevent superinfection

ceftizoxime
• IV after diluting 1 g/10 ml sterile water, shake and give over 3-5 min; may be diluted further with 50-100 ml NS or D_5W give through Y-tube or 3-way stopcock; run over ½-1 hr
• For 10-14 days to ensure organism death, prevent superinfection
Additive compatibilities: Clindamycin
Y-site compatibilities: Acyclovir, allopurinol, amphotericin B cholesteryl sulfate complex, aztreonam, doxorubicin liposome, enalaprilat, esmolol, famotidine, fludarabine, foscarnet, hydromorphone, labetalol,

melphalan, meperidine, morphine, ondansetron, remifentanil, sargramostim, teniposide, vinorelbine
ceftriaxone
• For 10-14 days to ensure organism death, prevent superinfection
• IV after diluting 250 mg/2.4 ml D_5W, H_2O for inj, 0.9% NaCl; may be further diluted with 50-100 ml NS, D_5W, $D_{10}W$, shake; run over ½-1 hr

Additive compatibilities: Amino acids or sodium bicarbonate, metronidazole

Y-site compatibilities: Acyclovir, allopurinol, aztreonam, cisatracurium, diltiazem, doxorubicin liposome, fludarabine, foscarnet, heparin, melphalan, meperidine, methotrexate, morphine, paclitaxel, remifentanil, sargramostim, tacrolimus, teniposide, theophylline, vinorelbine, warfarin, zidovudine
moxalactam
• For 10-14 days to ensure organism death, prevent superinfection
• IV after diluting 1 g/10 ml sterile H_2O, D_5, 0.9% NaCl; give through Y-tube over 3-5 min; may be further diluted 1 g/20 ml in D_5, 0.9% NaCl, give over ½ hr; may be added to 500-1000 ml, give over 6-24 hr
• Vit K for bleeding (10 mg/wk)

Additive compatibilities: Metronidazole, ranitidine, verapamil

Syringe compatibilities: Heparin

Y-site compatibilities: Cyclophosphamide, hydromorphone, magnesium sulfate, meperidine, morphine, perphenazine

Evaluate:
• Therapeutic response: decreased symptoms of infection; negative C&S

Teach patient/family:
• If diabetic, to check blood glucose
• To report sore throat, bruising, bleeding, joint pain; may indicate blood dyscrasias (rare)

• To report persistent diarrhea
Treatment of anaphylaxis: Epinephrine, antihistamines; resuscitate if needed

---

cerivastatin (℞)

(ser-iv′i-sta-tin)
Baycol
Func. class.: Antihyperlipidemic
Chem. class.: HMG-CoA reductase inhibitor

Action: Inhibits HMG-CoA reductase enzyme, which reduces cholesterol synthesis

Uses: As an adjunct in primary hypercholesterolemia (types IIa, IIb), mixed hyperlipidemia

Dosage and routes:
(Patient should first be placed on a cholesterol-lowering diet)
• *Adult:* **PO** 0.3 mg qd PM, may be given with a bile-acid-binding resin

Available forms: Tabs 0.2, 0.3, 0.4 mg

Side effects/adverse reactions:
GI: Flatus, nausea, constipation, diarrhea, dyspepsia, abdominal pain, heartburn, liver dysfunction
MS: Muscle cramps, myalgia, myositis, rhabdomyolysis
CNS: Dizziness, headache, tremor
INTEG: Rash, pruritus
EENT: Blurred vision, dysgeusia, lens opacities

Contraindications: Hypersensitivity, pregnancy (X), lactation, active liver disease

Precautions: Past liver disease, alcoholism, severe acute infections, trauma, hypotension, uncontrolled seizure disorders, severe metabolic disorders, electrolyte imbalances, visual disorder, children

Pharmacokinetics:
PO: Unknown

Interactions:
• Decreased absorption, decreased peak levels: cholestyramine
• Increased myalgia, myositis: cyclosporine, azole antifungals, niacin

Lab test interferences:
Interfere: Thyroid function tests
Increase: CPK, liver function tests, bilirubin

NURSING CONSIDERATIONS
Assess:
• Cholesterol levels periodically during treatment
• Liver function studies q1-2mo during the first 1½ yr of treatment; AST, ALT, liver function tests may increase
• Renal function in patients with compromised renal system: BUN, creatinine, I&O ratio

Administer:
• In evening with meal; if dose is increased, take with breakfast and evening meal

Perform/provide:
• Storage in cool environment in airtight, light-resistant container

Evaluate:
• Therapeutic response: cholesterol at desired level after 8 wk

Teach patient/family:
• That blood work and eye exam will be necessary during treatment
• To report muscle pain, fever, malaise, weakness
• That previously prescribed regimen will continue: low-cholesterol diet, exercise program
• That effect may take up to 1 mo
• Not to use if breastfeeding
• Not to use if pregnancy is being considered

---

cetirizine (℞)

(se-teer′i-zeen)
Zyrtec
Func. class.: Antihistamine
Chem. class.: Piperazine, H₁-histamine antagonist

C

Action: Acts on blood vessels, GI, respiratory system by competing with histamine for H₁-receptor site; decreases allergic response by blocking pharmacologic effects of histamine

Uses: Rhinitis, allergy symptoms

Dosage and routes:
• *Adult and child ≥6 yr:* **PO** 5-10 mg qd
• *Geriatric:* **PO** 5 mg qd, may increase to 10 mg/day

Renal/hepatic dose: CrCl 11-31 ml/min 5 mg qd

Available forms: Tabs 5, 10 mg; syrup 5 mg/5 ml

Side effects/adverse reactions:
GU: Frequency, dysuria, urinary retention, impotence
HEMA: **Hemolytic anemia, thrombocytopenia, leukopenia, agranulocytosis, pancytopenia**
RESP: Thickening of bronchial secretions, dry nose, throat
GI: Nausea, diarrhea, abdominal pain, vomiting, constipation, appetite increase, dry mouth
CNS: Headache, stimulation, drowsiness, sedation, fatigue, confusion, blurred vision, tinnitus, restlessness, tremors, paradoxical excitation in children or elderly
INTEG: Rash, eczema, photosensitivity, urticaria
CV: Hypotension, palpitations, bradycardia, tachycardia, **dysrhythmias** (rare)

Contraindications: Hypersensitivity, newborn or premature infants, lactation, severe hepatic disease

---

Side effects: *italics* = common; **bold italics** = life-threatening

Precautions: Pregnancy (B), elderly, children, respiratory disease, narrow-angle glaucoma, prostatic hypertrophy, bladder neck obstruction, asthma, elderly

Pharmacokinetics:

Peak 1-2 hr, onset rapid, protein binding 93%, half-life 8.3 hr

Interactions:

• Increased CNS depression: alcohol, other CNS depressants

• Increased anticholinergic effects: MAOIs

• May decrease cetirizine clearance: theophylline

⬗ Increased CNS depression: kava

Lab test interferences:

False negative: Skin allergy tests

NURSING CONSIDERATIONS

Assess:

• I&O ratio: be alert for urinary retention, frequency, dysuria, especially elderly; drug should be discontinued if these occur

• CBC during long-term therapy; blood dyscrasias may occur but are rare

• Respiratory status: rate, rhythm, increase in bronchial secretions, wheezing, chest tightness

Administer:

• On empty stomach 1 hr before or 2 hr after meals

Perform/provide:

• Hard candy, gum, frequent rinsing of mouth for dryness

• Storage in tight, light-resistant container

Evaluate:

• Therapeutic response: absence of running or congested nose or rashes

Teach patient/family:

• All aspects of drug use; to notify prescriber if confusion, sedation, hypotension occur

• To avoid driving, other hazardous activity if drowsiness occurs

• To avoid alcohol, other CNS depressants

• Not to exceed recommended dose; dysrhythmias may occur

• That drug is not recommended during lactation

Treatment of overdose: Administer ipecac syrup or lavage, diazepam, vasopressors, barbiturates (short-acting)

---

chloral hydrate (R)
(klor-al hye′drate)
Aquachloral, chloral hydrate, Noctec, Novochlorhydrate*, PMS-chloral hydrate*
Func. class.: Sedative/hypnotic
Chem. class.: Chloral derivative

Controlled Substance Schedule IV (USA), Schedule F (Canada)

Action: Reduction product trichloroethanol produces mild cerebral depression, which causes sleep

Uses: Sedation, insomnia

Dosage and routes:

Sedation

• *Adult:* **PO/RECT** 250 mg tid pc

• *Child:* **PO** 25-50 mg/kg tid, not to exceed 500 mg tid

Insomnia

• *Adult:* **PO/RECT** 500 mg-1 g ½ hr before hs

• *Child:* **PO/RECT** 50-75 mg/kg (one dose)

Procedure sedation

• *Child:* **PO/RECT** 25-50 mg/kg, not to exceed 100 mg/kg or 2 g

Renal disease

• CrCl <50 ml/min avoid use

Available forms: Caps 250, 500 mg; syr 250, 500 mg/5 ml; supp 325, 500, 650 mg

Side effects/adverse reactions:

HEMA: **Eosinophilia, leukopenia**

CNS: *Drowsiness,* dizziness, stimulation, nightmares, ataxia, hang-

---

◆ = Nursing alert ⬗ = Herb-drug interaction 🚫 = Do not crush over (rare), light-headedness, headache, paranoia

GI: Nausea, vomiting, flatulence, diarrhea, unpleasant taste, **gastric necrosis**

INTEG: Rash, urticaria, **angioedema,** fever, purpura, eczema

CV: Hypotension, **dysrhythmias**

RESP: Depression

Contraindications: Hypersensitivity to this drug or triclofos, severe renal disease, severe hepatic disease, GI disorders (oral forms), gastritis

Precautions: Severe cardiac disease, depression, suicidal individuals, asthma, intermittent porphyria, pregnancy (C), lactation, elderly

Pharmacokinetics:

PO: Onset 30 min-1 hr, duration 4-8 hr

RECT: Onset slow, duration 4-8 hr; metabolized by liver; excreted by kidneys (inactive metabolite) and feces; crosses placenta; excreted in breast milk; metabolite is highly protein bound

Interactions:

• Increased action: oral anticoagulants, furosemide

• Increased action of both drugs: alcohol, CNS depressants

• Decreased levels of: phenytoin

🌿 Increased CNS depression: kava

Lab test interferences:

Interference: Urine catecholamines, urinary 17-OHCS

False positive: Urine glucose (copper sulfate test), phentolamine test

NURSING CONSIDERATIONS

Assess:

• Blood studies: Hct, Hgb, RBCs, serum folate (if on long-term therapy), pro-time in patients receiving anticoagulants

• Mental status: mood, sensorium, affect, memory (long-, short-term)

• Physical dependency: more frequent requests for medication, tremors, anxiety, pinpoint pupils

• Respiratory dysfunction: respiratory depression, character, rate, rhythm; hold drug if respirations <10/min or if pupils dilated (rare)

• Blood dyscrasias: fever, sore throat, bruising, rash, jaundice, epistaxis (rare)

• History of substance abuse, cardiac disease, gastritis

Administer:

• After trying conservative measures for insomnia

• ½-1 hr before hs for sleeplessness

🚫 On empty stomach with full glass of water or juice for best absorption and to decrease corrosion (do not break, crush, or chew); after meals to decrease GI symptoms if using for sedation

Perform/provide:

• Assistance with ambulation after receiving dose, especially elderly

• Safety measure: night-light, call bell within easy reach

• Checking to see PO medication swallowed

• Check dose of syrup carefully, fatal overdoses have occurred in patients who are depressed

• Storage in dark container, suppositories in refrigerator

Evaluate:

• Therapeutic response: ability to sleep at night, decreased amount of early morning awakening if taking drug for insomnia

Teach patient/family:

• To avoid driving, other activities requiring alertness

• To avoid alcohol ingestion, CNS depressants; serious CNS depression may result

• Not to discontinue medication quickly after long-term use; drug should be tapered over 1-2 wk

• That effects may take 2 nights for benefits to be noticed

🚫 Not to break, crush, or chew caps

• Alternative measures to improve sleep (reading, exercise several hours before hs, warm bath, warm milk, TV, self-hypnosis, deep breathing)

Treatment of overdose: Lavage, activated charcoal; monitor electrolytes, vital signs

---

chlorambucil (℞)

(klor-am'byoo-sil)
Leukeran
Func. class.: Antineoplastic alkylating agent
Chem. class.: Nitrogen mustard

Action: Alkylates DNA, RNA; inhibits enzymes that allow synthesis of amino acids in proteins; activity is not cell cycle phase specific

Uses: Chronic lymphocytic leukemia, Hodgkin's disease, other lymphomas, macroglobulinemia, nephrotic syndrome, breast carcinoma, choreocarcinoma, ovarian carcinoma

Dosage and routes:

• *Adult:* **PO** 0.1-0.2 mg/kg/day for 3-6 wk initially, then 2-6 mg/day; maintenance 0.2 mg/kg for 2-4 wk; course may be repeated at 2-4 wk intervals

• *Child:* **PO** 0.1-0.2 mg/kg/day in divided doses or 4.5 mg/m^2/day as 1 dose or in divided doses

Available forms: Tabs 2 mg

Side effects/adverse reactions:

CNS: **Convulsions**

HEMA: **Thrombocytopenia, leukopenia, pancytopenia** (prolonged use), **permanent bone marrow depression**

*GI: Nausea, vomiting, diarrhea, weight loss, **hepatoxicity,** jaundice*

GU: Hyperuremia

INTEG: Alopecia (rare), dermatitis, rash, ***Stevens-Johnson syndrome***

RESP: **Fibrosis, pneumonitis**

Contraindications: Radiation therapy within 1 mo, chemotherapy within 1 mo, thrombocytopenia, smallpox vaccination, pregnancy (D), lactation

Precautions: *Pneumococcus* vaccination

Pharmacokinetics: Well absorbed orally; metabolized in liver; excreted in urine; half-life 2 hr

Interactions:

• Increased toxicity: other antineoplastics, radiation

• Increased risk of bleeding: anticoagulants, salicylates

NURSING CONSIDERATIONS

Assess:

• Bleeding: hematuria, guaiac, bruising or petechiae, mucosa or orifices q8h

• Jaundice of skin, sclera, dark urine, clay-colored stools, itchy skin, abdominal pain, fever, diarrhea

• Dyspnea, rales, unproductive cough, chest pain, tachypnea

• Effects of alopecia on body image; discuss feelings about body changes (rare)

• CBC, differential, platelet count weekly; withhold drug if WBC is <2000 or granulocyte count is <1000/mm^3; notify prescriber of results

• Pulmonary function tests, chest x-ray films before, during therapy; chest film should be obtained q2wk during treatment

• Renal function studies: BUN, serum uric acid, urine CrCl before, during therapy

• I&O ratio; report urine output of <30 ml/hr

• Monitor temperature q4h (may indicate beginning infection)

◆ = Nursing alert   🖋 = Herb-drug interaction   🚫 = Do not crush

• Liver function tests before, during therapy (bilirubin, AST, ALT, LDH) as needed or monthly

Administer:

PO

• All drugs PO if possible, avoid IM inj when platelets <100,000/mm³
• Antacid before oral agent; give drug 2 hr after evening meal, before bedtime
• Antiemetic 30-60 min before giving drug to prevent vomiting
• Allopurinol or sodium bicarbonate to maintain uric acid levels, alkalinization of urine

Perform/provide:

• Storage in tight container
• Increase fluid intake to 2-3 L/day to prevent urate deposits, calculi formation

Evaluate:

• Therapeutic response: decreased size of tumor, spread of malignancy

Teach patient/family:

• To report signs of infection: increased temperature, sore throat, flu symptoms
• To report signs of anemia: fatigue, headache, faintness, shortness of breath, irritability
• To report bleeding; avoid use of razors, commercial mouthwash
• To avoid use of aspirin products, ibuprofen
• To avoid vaccinations during treatment
• To use contraception during and several months after completion of therapy
• To report any changes in breathing or coughing

chloramphenicol (℞)

(klor-am-fen′i-kole)

chloramphenicol, Chloromycetin, Pentamycetin*

Func. class.: Antiinfective, misc

Chem. class.: Dichloroacetic acid derivative

Action: Binds to 50S ribosomal subunit, which interferes with or inhibits protein synthesis

Uses: Infections caused by *Haemophilus influenzae, Salmonella typhi, Rickettsia, Neisseria,* mycoplasma

Dosage and routes:

• *Adult and child:* **PO/IV** 50-75 mg/kg/day in divided doses q6h, 100 mg/kg/day (for meningitis only) max 4 g/day
• *Premature infants and neonates:* **IV/PO** 25 mg/kg/day in divided doses q12-24h

Available forms: Inj 1 g; caps 250 mg

Side effects/adverse reactions:

HEMA: ***Anemia, thrombocytopenia, aplastic anemia, granulocytopenia, leukopenia*** (rare)

EENT: Optic neuritis, blindness

GI: *Nausea, vomiting, diarrhea,* abdominal pain, xerostomia, glossitis, colitis, pruritus ani

INTEG: Itching, urticaria, contact dermatitis, rash

CV: ***Gray syndrome in newborns: failure to feed, pallor, cyanosis, abdominal distention, irregular respiration, vasomotor collapse***

CNS: Headache, *depression,* confusion

Contraindications: Hypersensitivity, severe renal disease, severe hepatic disease, minor infections

Precautions: Hepatic disease, renal disease, infants, children, bone marrow depression (drug-induced), pregnancy (C), lactation

Pharmacokinetics:

PO/IV: Peak 1-2 hr, duration 8 hr, half-life 1½-4 hr; conjugated in liver; excreted in urine (up to 15% as free drug, up to 80% in neonates), excreted in breast milk, feces; crosses placenta

Interactions:

• Increased action of: barbiturates, anticoagulants, hydantoins, sulfonylurea, iron products

• Decreased action of: vit B_{12}, folic acid, penicillins, rifampin

NURSING CONSIDERATIONS

Assess:

• Signs of infection, anemia

◆ Any patient with compromised renal system; drug is excreted slowly in poor renal system function; toxicity may occur rapidly

• Liver studies: AST, ALT

• Blood studies: WBC, RBC, Hct, Hgb, platelets, serum iron, reticulocytes; drug should be discontinued if bone marrow is depressed

• Renal studies: urinalysis, protein, blood, BUN, creatinine

• C&S before drug therapy; may be given as soon as culture is taken

• Drug level in impaired hepatic, renal systems; peak 15-20 mg/ml 3 hr after dose, trough 5-10 mg/ml prior to next dose

• Bowel pattern before, during treatment

• Skin eruptions, itching, dermatitis after administration

• Allergies before treatment, reaction of each medication; place allergies on chart in bright red letters; notify all people giving drugs

◆ Neonates for beginning Gray syndrome: cyanosis, abdominal distention, irregular respiration, failure to feed; drug should be discontinued immediately

Administer:

• Oral form on empty stomach with full glass of water

• IM route not recommended

IV

• After diluting 1 g/10 ml of sterile H_2O for inj or D_5W (10% sol); give >1 min; may be further diluted in 50-100 ml of D_5W; give through Y-tube, 3-way stopcock, or additive inf set; run over ½-1 hr

Additive compatibilities: Amikacin, aminophylline, ascorbic acid, calcium chloride or gluconate, cephalothin, cephapirin, colistimethate, corticotropin, cyanocobalamin, dimenhydrinate, dopamine, ephedrine, heparin, hydrocortisone, kanamycin, lidocaine, magnesium sulfate, metaraminol, methicillin, methyldopate, methylprednisolone, metronidazole, nafcillin, oxacillin, oxytocin, penicillin G potassium, penicillin G sodium, pentobarbital, phenylephrine, phytonadione, plasma protein fraction, potassium chloride, promazine, ranitidine, sodium bicarbonate, thiopental, verapamil, vit B/C

Syringe compatibilities: Ampicillin, cloxacillin, heparin, methicillin, penicillin G sodium

Y-site compatibilities: Acyclovir, cyclophosphamide, enalaprilat, esmolol, foscarnet, hydromorphone, labetalol, magnesium sulfate, meperidine, morphine, perphenazine, tacrolimus

Perform/provide:

• Storage of capsules in tight container at room temperature, reconstituted sol at room temp 30 days

Evaluate:

• Therapeutic response: decreased symptoms of infection

Teach patient/family:

• All aspects of drug therapy: the need to complete entire course to ensure organism death (10-14 days);

◆ = Nursing alert   🖊 = Herb-drug interaction   🚫 = Do not crush

culture may be taken after complete course of medication

🚫 Not to break, crush, or chew caps

• To report sore throat, fever, fatigue, unusual bleeding, bruising; could indicate bone marrow depression (may occur weeks or months after termination of drug)

• That drug must be taken in equal intervals around clock to maintain blood levels

Treatment of hypersensitivity: Withdraw drug, maintain airway, administer epinephrine, aminophylline, O_2, IV corticosteroids

---

chlordiazepoxide (℞)

(klor-dye-az-e-pox′ide)
Apo-Chlordiazepoxide*, chlordiazepoxide HCl*, Libritabs, Librium, Novopoxide*, Solium*

Func. class.: Antianxiety
Chem. class.: Benzodiazepine

Controlled Substance Schedule IV
Action: Potentiates the actions of GABA, especially in the limbic system, reticular formation
Uses: Short-term management of anxiety, acute alcohol withdrawal, preoperatively for relaxation
Dosage and routes:
Mild anxiety
• *Adult:* **PO** 5-10 mg tid-qid
• *Child >6 yr:* 5 mg bid-qid, not to exceed 10 mg bid-tid
Severe anxiety
• *Adult:* **PO** 20-25 mg tid-qid
Preoperatively
• *Adult:* **PO** 5-10 mg tid-qid on day before surgery; **IM** 50-100 mg 1 hr before surgery
Alcohol withdrawal
• *Adult:* **PO/IM/IV** 50-100 mg, not to exceed 300 mg/day

Available forms: Caps 5, 10, 25 mg; tabs 5, 10, 25 mg; powder for inj 100 mg ampule
Side effects/adverse reactions:
CNS: Dizziness, drowsiness, confusion, headache, anxiety, tremors, stimulation, fatigue, depression, insomnia, hallucinations
GI: Constipation, dry mouth, nausea, vomiting, anorexia, diarrhea
INTEG: Rash, dermatitis, itching
*CV: Orthostatic hypotension, **ECG changes, tachycardia,*** hypotension
EENT: Blurred vision, tinnitus, mydriasis
Contraindications: Hypersensitivity to benzodiazepines, narrow-angle glaucoma, psychosis, pregnancy (D), lactation, child <18 yr
Precautions: Elderly, debilitated, hepatic disease, renal disease
Pharmacokinetics:
PO: Onset 30 min, peak ½ hr, duration 4-6 hr; metabolized by liver, excreted by kidneys; crosses placenta, excreted in breast milk; half-life 5-30 hr (increased in elderly)
Interactions:
• Increased CNS depression: CNS depressants, alcohol, cimetidine
• Increased digoxin levels: digoxin
🍃 Increased CNS depression: kava
Lab test interferences:
False increase: 17-OHCS
False positive: Pregnancy test (some methods)
NURSING CONSIDERATIONS
Assess:
• B/P (lying, standing), pulse; if systolic B/P drops 20 mm Hg, hold drug, notify prescriber
• Blood studies: CBC during long-term therapy; blood dyscrasias have occurred rarely
• Hepatic studies: AST, ALT, bilirubin, creatinine, LDH, alk phosphatase during long-term therapy
• I&O; may indicate renal dysfunction

• For ataxia, oversedation in elderly, debilitated patients

• Mental status: mood, sensorium, affect, sleeping pattern, drowsiness, dizziness

• Physical dependency, withdrawal symptoms: headache, nausea, vomiting, muscle pain, weakness after long-term use

• Suicidal tendencies, paradoxic reactions such as excitement, stimulation, acute rage

• For pregnancy; drug should be avoided during pregnancy

Administer:

• With food or milk for GI symptoms

• Crushed if patient is unable to swallow medication whole

IV

• 5 ml NS/100 mg powder; agitate ampule gently; give through Y-tube or 3-way stopcock; give 100 mg or less ≥1 min; do not use IM diluent for IV use

• Keep powder from light; refrigerate, mix when ready to use

Solution compatibilities: D_5W, 0.9% NaCl

Y-site compatibilities: Heparin, hydrocortisone, potassium chloride, vit B/C

IM

• Add 2 ml diluent to powder, rotate until clear, use immediately

• Preferred route is IM

Perform/provide:

• Assistance with ambulation during beginning therapy, since drowsiness/dizziness occurs

• Check to see PO medication has been swallowed if patient is depressed, suicidal

• Sugarless gum, hard candy, frequent sips of water for dry mouth

Evaluate:

• Therapeutic response: decreased anxiety, restlessness, sleeplessness

Teach patient/family:

• That drug may be taken with food

• Not to use drug for everyday stress or use longer than 4 mo, unless directed by prescriber

• Not to take more than prescribed amount; may be habit forming

• To avoid OTC preparations unless approved by prescriber

• To avoid driving, activities that require alertness; drowsiness may occur

• To avoid alcohol ingestion, other psychotropic medications, unless directed by prescriber

• Not to discontinue medication abruptly after long-term use; may precipitate convulsions

• To rise slowly or fainting may occur, especially elderly

• That drowsiness may be worse at beginning of treatment

Treatment of overdose: Lavage, VS, supportive care, give flumazenil

---

chloroprocaine (℞)

(klor'-oh-pro-kane)

Nesacaine, Nesacaine-MPF

Func. class.: Local anesthetic

Chem. class.: Ester

Action: Competes with calcium for sites in nerve membrane that control sodium transport across cell membrane; decreases rise of depolarization phase of action potential

Uses: Epidural anesthesia, peripheral nerve block, caudal anesthesia, infiltration block

Dosage and routes:

• Varies by route of anesthesia

Available forms: Inj 1%, 2%, 3%

Side effects/adverse reactions:

CNS: Anxiety, restlessness, *convulsions, loss of consciousness,* drowsiness, disorientation, tremors, shivering

---

◆ = Nursing alert   ∥ = Herb-drug interaction   ⊘ = Do not crush

CV: **Myocardial depression, cardiac arrest, dysrhythmias,** bradycardia, hypotension, hypertension, fetal bradycardia

GI: Nausea, vomiting

EENT: Blurred vision, tinnitus, pupil constriction

INTEG: Rash, urticaria, allergic reactions, edema, burning, skin discoloration at injection site, tissue necrosis

RESP: **Status asthmaticus, respiratory arrest, anaphylaxis**

Contraindications: Hypersensitivity, child <12 yr, severe liver disease

Precautions: Elderly, severe drug allergies, pregnancy (C), lactation

Pharmacokinetics: Duration ½-1 hr; metabolized by liver; excreted in urine (metabolites)

Interactions:
• Dysrhythmias: epinephrine, halothane, enflurane
• Hypertension: MAOIs, tricyclic antidepressants, phenothiazines

NURSING CONSIDERATIONS
Assess:
• B/P, pulse, respiration during treatment
• Fetal heart tones if used during labor
• Allergic reactions: rash, urticaria, itching
• Cardiac status: ECG for dysrhythmias, pulse, B/P during anesthesia

Administer:
• Only with crash cart, resuscitative equipment nearby
• Only drugs without preservatives for epidural or caudal anesthesia

Perform/provide:
• Use of new solution; discard unused portions

Evaluate
• Therapeutic response: anesthesia necessary for procedure

Treatment of overdose: Airway, O_2, vasopressor, IV fluids, anticonvulsants for seizures

---

chloroquine (℞)

(klor'oh-kwin)
Aralen HCl, Aralen Phosphate, chloroquine phosphate
Func. class.: Antimalarial
Chem. class.: Synthetic 4-aminoquinoline derivative

Action: Inhibits parasite replications, transcription of DNA to RNA by forming complexes with DNA of parasite

Uses: Malaria of *Plasmodium vivax, P. malariae, P. ovale, P. falciparum* (some strains), amebiasis

Dosage and routes:
Malaria suppression
• *Adult and child:* **PO** 5 mg base/kg/wk on same day of week, not to exceed 300 mg base; treatment should begin 1-2 wk before exposure and for 8 wk after; if treatment begins after exposure, 600 mg base for adult and 10 mg base/kg for children in 2 divided doses 6 hr apart

Extraintestinal amebiasis
• *Adult:* **IM** 160-200 mg base qd × 10-12 days or **PO** (HCl) 600 mg base qd × 2 days, then 300 mg base qd × 2-3 wk (phosphate)
• *Child:* **IM/PO** 10 mg/kg qd (HCl) × 2-3 wk, not to exceed 300 mg/day

Available forms: Tabs 250 mg (150 mg base), 500 mg (300 mg base) phosphate; inj 50 mg (40 mg base)/ml HCl; inj 5 mg (200 mg base) phosphate

Side effects/adverse reactions:
CV: Hypotension, **heart block, asystole with syncope,** ECG changes

INTEG: Pruritus, pigmentary changes, skin eruptions, lichen planus–like eruptions, eczema, **exfoliative dermatitis**

CNS: Headache, stimulation, fatigue, *convulsion,* psychosis

EENT: Blurred vision, corneal changes, retinal changes, difficulty focusing, tinnitus, vertigo, deafness, photophobia, corneal edema

GI: Nausea, vomiting, anorexia, diarrhea, cramps

HEMA: Thrombocytopenia, agranulocytosis, hemolytic anemia, leukopenia

Contraindications: Hypersensitivity, retinal field changes

Precautions: Pregnancy (C), children, blood dyscrasias, severe GI disease, neurologic disease, alcoholism, hepatic disease, G6PD deficiency, psoriasis, eczema, lactation, porphyria

Pharmacokinetics: Metabolized in liver; excreted in urine, feces, breast milk; crosses placenta

PO: Peak 1-3 hr, half-life 3-5 days
IM: Peak 30 min

Interactions:

• Decreased action of chloroquine: magnesium, aluminum compounds, kaolin

• Reduced oral clearance and metabolism of chloroquine: cimetidine

NURSING CONSIDERATIONS
Assess:

• Ophthalmic test if long-term treatment or dosage >150 mg/day

• Liver studies qwk: AST, ALT, bilirubin

• Blood studies: CBC, since blood dyscrasias occur

• ECG during therapy; watch for depression of T waves, widening of QRS complex

• Allergic reactions: pruritus, rash, urticaria

• Blood dyscrasias: malaise, fever, bruising, bleeding (rare)

• For ototoxicity (tinnitus, vertigo, change in hearing); audiometric testing should be done before, after treatment

◆For toxicity: blurring vision; difficulty focusing; headache; dizziness; decreased knee, ankle reflexes, seizures, CV collapse; drug should be discontinued immediately

Administer:

• IM after aspirating to avoid injection into blood system, which may cause hypotension, asystole, heart block; rotate injection sites

PO

• Before or after meals at same time each day to maintain drug level

Additive compatibilities: Promethazine

Perform/provide:

• Storage in tight, light-resistant container at room temp; keep injection in cool environment

Evaluate:

• Therapeutic response: decreased symptoms of infection

Teach patient/family:

• To use sunglasses in bright sunlight to decrease photophobia

• That urine may turn rust or brown color

• To report hearing, visual problems, fever, fatigue, bruising, bleeding, which may indicate blood dyscrasias

Treatment of overdose: Induce vomiting, gastric lavage, administer barbiturate (ultrashort-acting), vasopressor; tracheostomy may be necessary

---

chlorothiazide (℞)
(klor-oh-thye′a-zide)
Diuril
Func. class.: Diuretic
Chem. class.: Thiazide; sulfonamide derivative

Action: Acts on distal tubule and thick ascending limb of the loop of Henle by increasing excretion of wa-

◆ = Nursing alert   ⫸ = Herb-drug interaction   ⊘ = Do not crush

ter, sodium, chloride, potassium, magnesium

Uses: Edema, hypertension, diuresis

Dosage and routes:

Edema, hypertension

• *Adult:* **PO/IV** 500 mg-2 g qd in 2 divided doses

Diuresis

• *Adult:* **IV** 250 mg q6-12h

• *Child >6 mo:* **PO** 20 mg/kg/day in 2 divided doses

• *Child <6 mo:* **PO** up to 40 mg/kg/day in 2 doses

Available forms: Tabs 250, 500 mg; inj 500 mg

Side effects/adverse reactions:

CNS: Paresthesia, anxiety, depression, headache, *dizziness, fatigue, weakness,* insomnia

CV: Irregular pulse, orthostatic hypotension, palpitations, volume depletion

EENT: Blurred vision

ELECT: Hypokalemia, hypercalcemia, hyponatremia, hypochloremia, hypophosphatemia, hypomagnesemia

GI: Nausea, vomiting, anorexia, constipation, diarrhea, cramps, pancreatitis, GI irritation, **hepatitis**

GU: Urinary frequency, polyuria, **uremia,** glucosuria, hematuria

HEMA: **Aplastic anemia, hemolytic anemia, leukopenia, agranulocytosis, thrombocytopenia, neutropenia**

INTEG: Rash, urticaria, purpura, photosensitivity, fever, alopecia

META: Hyperglycemia, *hyperuricemia,* increased creatinine, BUN

Contraindications: Hypersensitivity to thiazides or sulfonamides, hepatic coma, anuria, renal decompensation, pregnancy (B), lactation

Precautions: Hypokalemia, renal disease, hepatic disease, gout, COPD, lupus erythematosus, diabetes mellitus, elderly, hyperlipidemia

Pharmacokinetics: Not well absorbed PO

PO: Onset 2 hr, peak 4 hr, duration 6-12 hr; crosses placenta, excreted in breast milk, excreted unchanged by kidneys; half-life 2 hr

Interactions:

• Increased toxicity: lithium, nondepolarizing skeletal muscle relaxants, digitalis, allopurinol

• Increased hypotension: other antihypertensives, alcohol

• Decreased effects of: antidiabetics, sulfonylureas, anticoagulants

• Decreased absorption of thiazides: cholestyramine, colestipol

• Decreased hypotensive response: indomethacin, other NSAIDs

• Hypokalemia: ticarcillin, glucocorticoids, amphotericin, mezlocillin, piperacillin

• Hyperglycemia, hypotension: diazoxide

🖉 Potassium deficiency: chronic use/abuse cascara sagrada bark, aloe, buckthorn bark/berry, licorice root, senna pod/leaf

Lab test interferences:

False negative: Phentolamine and tyramine tests

Interference: Urine steroid tests

Increase: BSP retention, Ca, amylase, parathyroid test

Decrease: PBI, PSP

NURSING CONSIDERATIONS

Assess:

• Weight, I&O daily to determine fluid loss; effect of drug may be decreased if used qd

• Rate, depth, rhythm of respirations; effect of exertion

• B/P lying, standing; postural hypotension may occur, especially in elderly

• Electrolytes: K, Na, Cl; include

BUN, blood glucose, CBC, serum creatinine, blood pH, ABGs, uric acid, Ca, Mg
• Glucose in urine if patient is diabetic
• Improvement in CVP q8h
• Signs of metabolic alkalosis: drowsiness, restlessness
• Rashes, temp elevation qd
• Confusion, especially in elderly; take safety precautions if needed

Administer:
• In AM to avoid interference with sleep if using drug as a diuretic
• K replacement if K less than 3 mg/dl
• With food if nausea occurs; absorption may be decreased slightly; tablets may be crushed
• After shaking suspension

IV
• After diluting 0.5 g/18 ml or more of sterile water for inj; may be diluted further with 0.9% NaCl, D_5W, check for extravasation; give over 5 min (0.5 g/5 min)

Additive compatibilities: Cimetidine, lidocaine, nafcillin, ranitidine, sodium bicarbonate

Evaluate:
• Therapeutic response: improvement in edema of feet, legs, sacral area daily if medication is being used for CHF

Teach patient/family:
• To rise slowly from lying or sitting position; orthostatic hypotension may occur
• To notify prescriber of muscle weakness, cramps, nausea, dizziness
• That drug may be taken with food or milk; to take at same time each day; not to double dose; dehydration may occur
• That blood sugar may be increased in diabetics
• To take early in day to avoid nocturia

• To use sunscreen (not with PABA); use protective clothing to prevent photosensitivity
• To weigh weekly and notify prescriber of change of >3 lb
• To eat diet high in K
• Not to take OTC medications without consulting prescriber

Treatment of overdose: Lavage if taken orally; monitor electrolytes; administer dextrose in saline; monitor hydration, CV, renal status

---

chlorpheniramine
(OTC, ℞)

(klor-fen-ir'a-meen)
Aller-Chlor, Chlo-Amine, Chlorate, Chlor-100, Chlor-Niramine, chlorpheniramine maleate, Chlor-Pro, Chlor-Span, Chlortab, Chlor-Trimeton, Chlor-Tripolon*, GenAllerate, Novo-Pheniram*, Pedia Care Allergy Formula, Pfeiffer's Allergy, Phenetron, Telachlor, Teldrin, Trymegen

Func. class.: Antihistamine
Chem. class.: Alkylamine, H_1-receptor antagonist

Action: Acts on blood vessels, GI system, respiratory system, by competing with histamine for H_1-receptor site; decreases allergic response by blocking histamine

Uses: Allergy symptoms, rhinitis

Dosage and routes:
• *Adult:* **PO** 2-4 mg tid-qid, not to exceed 36 mg/day; **TIME-REL** 8-12 mg bid-tid, not to exceed 24 mg/day; **IM/IV/SC** 5-40 mg/day
• *Child 6-12 yr:* **PO** 2 mg q4-6h, not to exceed 12 mg/day; **SUS REL** 8 mg hs or qd, **SUS REL** not recommended for child <6 yr
• *Child 2-5 yr:* **PO** 1 mg q4-6h, not to exceed 4 mg/day

◆ = Nursing alert   ∥ = Herb-drug interaction   ⊘ = Do not crush

Available forms: Tabs, chewable 2 mg; tabs 4, 8, 12 mg; tabs, time-rel 8, 12 mg; caps, time-rel 6, 8, 12 mg; syr 2 mg/5 ml; inj 10, 100 mg/ml

Side effects/adverse reactions:

CNS: Dizziness, drowsiness, poor coordination, fatigue, anxiety, euphoria, confusion, paresthesia, neuritis

RESP: Increased thick secretions, wheezing, chest tightness

*HEMA: **Thrombocytopenia, agranulocytosis, hemolytic anemia***

GI: Dry mouth, nausea, anorexia, diarrhea

INTEG: Photosensitivity

GU: Retention, dysuria, urinary frequency

EENT: Blurred vision, dilated pupils, tinnitus, nasal stuffiness, dry nose, throat, mouth

Contraindications: Hypersensitivity to H_1-receptor antagonists, acute asthma attack, lower respiratory tract disease

Precautions: Increased intraocular pressure, renal disease, cardiac disease, hypertension, bronchial asthma, seizure disorder, stenosed peptic ulcers, hyperthyroidism, prostatic hypertrophy, bladder neck obstruction, pregnancy (B), lactation, elderly

Pharmacokinetics:

PO: Onset 20-60 min, duration 8-12 hr; detoxified in liver; excreted by kidneys (metabolites/free drug); half-life 20-24 hr

Interactions:

• Increased CNS depression: barbiturates, narcotics, hypnotics, tricyclic antidepressants, alcohol

• Increased effect of chlorpheniramine: MAOIs

🝙 Increased CNS depression: kava

🝙 Increased anticholinergic effect: henbane leaf

Lab test interferences:

False negative: Skin allergy tests

NURSING CONSIDERATIONS

Assess:

• Be alert for urinary retention, frequency, dysuria; drug should be discontinued

• Respiratory status: rate, rhythm, increase in bronchial secretions, wheezing, chest tightness

Administer:

• With meals for GI symptoms; absorption may slightly decrease

IV

• Undiluted at ≥10 mg/1 min

• The 100 mg/ml form is not to be used IV; for IM/SC use

Additive compatibilities: Amikacin

Perform/provide:

• Hard candy, gum, frequent rinsing of mouth for dryness

• Storage in tight container at room temp

Evaluate:

• Therapeutic response: absence of running, congested nose, rashes

Teach patient/family:

🚫 Not to break, crush, or chew sustained-release forms

• All aspects of drug use; to notify prescriber of confusion/sedation/hypotension, difficulty voiding

• To avoid driving, other hazardous activity if drowsiness occurs, especially elderly

• To avoid concurrent use of alcohol, other CNS depressants

Treatment of overdose: Administer ipecac syrup or lavage, diazepam, vasopressors, barbiturates (short-acting)

chlorpromazine (R)

(klor-proe'ma-zeen)
Chlorpromanyl*,
chlorpromazine HCl,
Largactil*, Novo-
Chlorpromazine*, Ormazine,
Thorazine, Thor-Prom
Func. class.: Antipsychotic/neuroleptic/antiemetic
Chem. class.: Phenothiazine-aliphatic

Action: Depresses cerebral cortex, hypothalamus, limbic system, which control activity aggression; blocks neurotransmission produced by dopamine at synapse; exhibits a strong α-adrenergic, anticholinergic blocking action; mechanism for antipsychotic effects is unclear

Uses: Psychotic disorders, mania, schizophrenia, anxiety, intractable hiccups, nausea, vomiting; preoperatively for relaxation; acute intermittent porphyria, behavioral problems in children, nonpsychotic, demented patients

Dosage and routes:

Psychiatry
• *Adult:* **PO** 10-50 mg q1-4h initially, then increase up to 2 g/day if necessary; **IM** 10-50 mg q1-4h
• *Geriatric:* Use lowest effective dose
• *Child:* **PO** 0.5 mg/kg q4-6h; **IM** 0.5 mg/kg q6-8h; **RECT** 1 mg/kg q6-8h

Nausea and vomiting
• *Adult:* **PO** 10-25 mg q4-6h prn; **IM** 25-50 mg q3h prn; **RECT** 50-100 mg q6-8h prn, not to exceed 400 mg/day; **IV** 25-50 mg qd-qid
• *Child ≥ 6 mo:* **PO** 0.55 mg/kg q4-6h; **IM** q6-8h; **RECT** 1.1 mg/kg q6-8h; max **IM** ≤ 5 yr or ≤ 22.7 kg 40 mg; max **IM** 5-10 yr or 22.7-45.5 kg, 75 mg

Intractable hiccups
• *Adult:* **PO** 25-50 mg tid-qid; **IM** 25-50 mg (only if PO dose does not work); **IV** 25-50 mg in 500-1000 ml **NS** (only for severe hiccups)

Available forms: Tabs 10, 25, 50, 100, 200 mg; ext-rel caps 30, 75, 150, 200, 300 mg; syr 10 mg/5ml; conc 30, 100 mg/ml; supp 25, 100 mg; inj 25 mg/ml

Side effects/adverse reactions:

CV: *Orthostatic hypotension,* hypertension, *cardiac arrest,* ECG changes, *tachycardia*

EENT: Blurred vision, glaucoma, dry eyes

GI: *Dry mouth, nausea, vomiting, anorexia, constipation,* diarrhea, jaundice, weight gain

GU: Urinary retention, enuresis, impotence, amenorrhea, gynecomastia, breast engorgement

HEMA: Anemia, *leukopenia, leukocytosis, agranulocytosis*

INTEG: Rash, photosensitivity, dermatitis

RESP: *Laryngospasm,* dyspnea, *respiratory depression*

CNS: **EPS:** *pseudoparkinsonism,* akathisia, dystonia, tardive dyskinesia, seizures, *headache, neuroleptic malignant syndrome (rare)*

Contraindications: Hypersensitivity, circulatory collapse, liver damage, cerebral arteriosclerosis, coronary disease, severe hypertension/hypotension, blood dyscrasias, coma, child <2 yr, brain damage, bone marrow depression, alcohol and barbiturate withdrawal

Precautions: Pregnancy (C), lactation, seizure disorders, hypertension, hepatic disease, cardiac disease, elderly

Pharmacokinetics:

PO: Absorption variable, widely distributed; onset erratic 30-60 min, duration 4-6 hr

◆ = Nursing alert   ⬭ = Herb-drug interaction   ⊘ = Do not crush

IM: Well absorbed; peak 15-20 min, duration 4 to 8 hr

IV: Onset 5 min, peak 10 min, duration unknown

PO-ER: Onset 30-60 min, peak unknown, duration 10-12 hr

REC: Onset erratic, duration 3 hr; metabolized by liver, excreted in urine (metabolites), crosses placenta, enters breast milk; 95% bound to plasma proteins; elimination half-life 10-30 hr

Interactions:

• Lowered seizure threshold: anticonvulsants

• Oversedation: other CNS depressants, alcohol, barbiturate anesthetics, antihistamines, sedatives/hypnotics, antidepressants

• Toxicity: epinephrine

• Decreased absorption: aluminum hydroxide, magnesium hydroxide antacids

• Decreased antiparkinson activity: levodopa, bromocriptine

• Decreased serum chlorpromazine: lithium, barbiturates

• Decreased anticoagulant effect: warfarin

• Increased effects of both drugs: β-adrenergic blockers, alcohol

• Increased anticholinergic effects: anticholinergics, antidepressants, antiparkinsonian agents

• Agranulocystosis: antithyroid agents

🍵 Increased CNS depression: kava

🍵 Increased anticholinergic effect: henbane leaf

Lab test interferences:

Increase: Liver function tests, cardiac enzymes, cholesterol, blood glucose, prolactin, bilirubin, PBI, cholinesterase,^{131}I, alk phosphatase, leukocytes, granulocytes, platelets

Decrease: Hormones (blood and urine)

False positive: Pregnancy tests, PKU

False negative: Urinary steroids, 17-OHCS

NURSING CONSIDERATIONS

Assess:

• Mental status: orientation, mood, behavior, presence and type of hallucinations before initial administration and monthly

• Any potentially reversible causes of behavior problems in the elderly before and during therapy

• Swallowing of PO medication; check for hoarding or giving of medication to other patients

• I&O ratio; palpate bladder if low urinary output occurs, especially in elderly

• Bilirubin, CBC, liver function studies monthly

• Urinalysis recommended before, during prolonged therapy

• Affect, orientation, LOC, reflexes, gait, coordination, sleep pattern disturbances

• B/P sitting, standing, lying; take pulse and respirations q4h during initial treatment; establish baseline before starting treatment; report drops of 30 mm Hg; obtain baseline ECG, Q-wave and T-wave changes

• Dizziness, faintness, palpitations, tachycardia on rising

🔶 For neuroleptic malignant syndrome: hyperpyrexia, muscle rigidity, increased CPK, altered mental status, for acute dystonia (check chewing, swallowing, eyes, pin rolling)

• EPS including akathisia (inability to sit still, no pattern to movements), tardive dyskinesia (bizarre movements of the jaw, mouth, tongue, extremities), pseudoparkinsonism (rigidity, tremors, pill rolling, shuffling gait)

• Skin turgor daily

• Constipation, urinary retention daily; increase bulk, H_2O in diet

---

Administer:
• IM, inject in deep muscle mass, do not give SC
• Rectal after placing in refrigerator for ½ hr if too soft to insert
• Antiparkinsonian agent for EPS
PO
• With full glass of water, milk; or with food to decrease GI upset
• Drug in liquid form mixed in glass of juice or cola if hoarding is suspected
• Periodically attempt dosage reduction in behavioral problems
IV
• After diluting 1 mg/1 ml with NS, give 1 mg or less/2 min or more; may be further diluted in 500-1000 ml of NS
Additive compatibilities: Ascorbic acid, ethacrynate, netilmicin, theophylline, vit B/C
Syringe compatibilities: Atropine, benztropine, butorphanol, diphenhydramine, doxapram, droperidol, fentanyl, glycopyrrolate, hydromorphone, hydroxyzine, meperidine, metoclopramide, midazolam, morphine, pentazocine, perphenazine, prochlorperazine, promazine, promethazine, scopolamine
Y-site compatibilities: Amsacrine, cisatracurium, cisplatin, cladribine, cyclophosphamide, cytarabine, doxorubicin, doxorubicin liposome, famotidine, filgrastim, fluconazole, granisetron, heparin, hydrocortisone, ondansetron, potassium chloride, propofol, teniposide, thiotepa, vinorelbine, vit B/C
Perform/provide:
• Decreased stimuli by dimming lights, avoiding loud noises
• Supervised ambulation until stabilized on medication; do not involve in strenuous exercise program because fainting is possible; patient should not stand still for long periods

• Increased fluids to prevent constipation
• Candy, gum, sips of water for dry mouth
• Storage in tight, light-resistant container, oral sol in amber bottle
Evaluate:
• Therapeutic response: decrease in emotional excitement, hallucinations, delusions, paranoia, reorganization of patterns of thought, speech, increase in target behaviors
Teach patient/family:
• To use good oral hygiene; frequent rinsing of mouth, sugarless gum for dry mouth
• To avoid hazardous activities until drug response is determined
🚫 Not to break, crush, or chew time-rel caps
• That orthostatic hypotension occurs often and to rise gradually from sitting or lying position
• To remain lying down for at least 30 min after IM injection
• To avoid hot tubs, hot showers, tub baths, since hypotension may occur
• To avoid abrupt withdrawal of this drug or EPS may result; drug should be withdrawn slowly
• To avoid OTC preparations (cough, hay fever, cold) unless approved by prescriber, since serious drug interactions may occur; avoid use with alcohol, CNS depressants; increased drowsiness may occur
• To use a sunscreen and sunglasses to prevent burns
• About EPS and necessity of meticulous oral hygiene, since oral candidiasis may occur
• To take antacids 2 hr before or after this drug
• To report sore throat, malaise, fever, bleeding, mouth sores; CBC should be drawn and drug discontinued
• That in hot weather, heat stroke

may occur; take extra precautions to stay cool
• Contraceptive measures
• That urine may turn pink or red
Treatment of overdose: Lavage if orally ingested; provide airway; *do not induce vomiting or use epinephrine*

---

chlorthalidone (℞)

(klor-thal'i-done)
Apo-Chlorthalidone*, chlorthalidone, Hygroton, Novo-Thalidone*, Thalitone, Uridon*
Func. class.: Diuretic
Chem. class.: Thiazide-like phthalimidine derivative

Action: Acts on distal tubule and thick ascending limb of the loop of Henle by increasing excretion of water, sodium, chloride, potassium, magnesium, bicarbonate
Uses: Edema, hypertension, diuresis, CHF, nephrotic syndrome
Dosage and routes:
• *Adult:* **PO** 25-200 mg/day or 100 mg every other day
• *Geriatric:* **PO** 12.5 mg qd, initially
• *Child:* **PO** 2 mg/kg or 60 mg/m^2 3 ×/wk
Available forms: Tabs 15, 25, 50, 100 mg
Side effects/adverse reactions:
GU: Urinary frequency, polyuria, **uremia,** glucosuria, impotence
CNS: Paresthesia, headache, *dizziness, fatigue, weakness*
GI: Nausea, vomiting, anorexia, constipation, diarrhea, cramps, pancreatitis, GI irritation, **hepatitis**
EENT: Blurred vision
INTEG: Rash, urticaria, purpura, photosensitivity, fever
META: Hyperglycemia, hyperuremia, increased creatinine, BUN, gout

*HEMA: **Aplastic anemia, hemolytic anemia, leukopenia, agranulocytosis, thrombocytopenia, neutropenia***
CV: Irregular pulse, orthostatic hypotension, palpitations, volume depletion
ELECT: Hypokalemia, hypomagnesemia, hypercalcemia, hyponatremia, hypochloremia
Contraindications: Hypersensitivity to thiazides or sulfonamides, anuria, renal decompensation, lactation
Precautions: Hypokalemia, renal disease, pregnancy (B), lactation, hepatic disease, gout, diabetes mellitus, elderly, hyperlipidemia
Pharmacokinetics:
PO: Onset 2 hr, peak 6 hr, duration 24-72 hr; excreted unchanged by kidneys; crosses placenta; enters breast milk; half-life 40 hr
Interactions:
• Increased toxicity of: lithium, nondepolarizing skeletal muscle relaxants, allopurinol
• Decreased effects of antidiabetics
• Decreased absorption of thiazides: cholestyramine, colestipol
• Hyperglycemia, hypotension: diazoxide
• Increased hypotensive effect: alcohol
• Hypokalemia: glucocorticoids, amphotericin B
� Potassium deficiency: chronic use/abuse of aloe, buckthorn bark/berry, cascara sagrada bark, licorice root, senna pod/leaf
Lab test interferences:
Increase: BSP retention, Ca, cholesterol, triglycerides, amylase
Decrease: PBI, PSP, parathyroid test
NURSING CONSIDERATIONS
Assess:
• Weight, I&O daily to determine fluid loss; effect of drug may be decreased if used qd

---

• Rate, depth, rhythm of respiration, effect of exertion
• B/P lying, standing; postural hypotension may occur
• Electrolytes: K, Mg, Na, Cl; include BUN, blood sugar, CBC, serum creatinine, blood pH, ABGs, uric acid, Ca
• Blood glucose levels if patient is diabetic
• Signs of metabolic alkalosis: drowsiness, restlessness
• Signs of hypokalemia: postural hypotension, malaise, fatigue, tachycardia, leg cramps, weakness
• Rashes, temp elevation qd
• Confusion, especially in elderly; take safety precautions if needed

Administer:
• In AM to avoid interference with sleep if using drug as a diuretic
• K replacement if K less than 3 mg/dl
• With food if nausea occurs; absorption may be decreased slightly
• Brand names Thalitone/Hygroton should not be used interchangeably

Evaluate:
• Therapeutic response: improvement in edema of feet, legs, sacral area daily if medication used in CHF

Teach patient/family:
• To rise slowly from lying or sitting position
• To notify prescriber of muscle weakness, cramps, nausea, dizziness
• That drug may be taken with food or milk
• That blood sugar may be increased in diabetics
• To use sunscreen to protect against photosensitivity
• To take early in day to avoid nocturia

Treatment of overdose: Lavage if taken orally, monitor electrolytes, administer dextrose in NS, monitor hydration, CV, renal status

---

chlorzoxazone (Ŗ)
(klor-zox'a-zone)
chlorzoxazone, Paraflex, Parafon Forte DSC, Remular-S
Func. class.: Skeletal muscle relaxant
Chem. class.: Benzoxazole derivative

Action: Inhibits multisynaptic reflex arcs
Uses: Relieving pain, spasm in musculoskeletal conditions
Dosage and routes:
• *Adult:* **PO** 250-750 mg tid-qid
• *Child:* **PO** 20 mg/kg/day in divided doses bid-tid
Available forms: Tabs 250, 500 mg; caplets 250, 500 mg
Side effects/adverse reactions:
GU: Urine discoloration
HEMA: **Granulocytopenia, anemia**
CNS: Dizziness, drowsiness, headache, insomnia, stimulation, malaise
GI: Nausea, vomiting, anorexia, diarrhea, constipation, **hepatotoxicity, jaundice**
INTEG: Rash, pruritus, petechiae, ecchymoses, **angioedema**
SYST: **Anaphylaxis**
Contraindications: Hypersensitivity, impaired hepatic function
Precautions: Pregnancy (C), lactation, hepatic disease, elderly
Pharmacokinetics:
PO: Onset 1 hr, peak 3-4 hr, duration 6 hr, half-life 1 hr; metabolized in liver; excreted in urine (metabolites)
Interactions:
• Increased CNS depression: alcohol, tricyclic antidepressants, opiates, barbiturates, sedatives, hypnotics
🍃 May increase CNS depression: kava

◆ = Nursing alert   🍃 = Herb-drug interaction   🚫 = Do not crush

NURSING CONSIDERATIONS
Assess:
• Blood studies: CBC, WBC, differential for blood dyscrasias if on long-term therapy
• Liver function studies: AST, ALT, alk phosphatase; notify prescriber of signs of hepatotoxicity
• EEG in epileptic patients; poor seizure control has occurred
• Allergic reactions: rash, fever, respiratory distress
• Severe weakness, numbness in extremities
• CNS depression: dizziness, drowsiness, psychiatric symptoms
Administer:
• With meals for GI symptoms
Perform/provide:
• Storage in tight container at room temperature
• Assistance with ambulation if dizziness or drowsiness occurs, especially elderly
Evaluate:
• Therapeutic response: decreased pain, spasticity
Teach patient/family:
• Not to discontinue abruptly; insomnia, nausea, headache, spasticity, tachycardia will occur; drug should be tapered over 1-2 wk
• Not to take with alcohol, other CNS depressants; take with food
• To avoid hazardous activities if drowsiness, dizziness occurs
• To avoid using OTC medication: cough preparations, antihistamines, unless directed by prescriber
• That urine may be orange or purple
Treatment of overdose: Gastric lavage or induce emesis, then administer activated charcoal; use other supportive treatment as necessary; monitor cardiac function

cholestyramine (R)
(koe-less-tir'a-meen)
Cholybar, LoCholest, Prevalite, Questran, Questran Light
Func. class.: Antilipemic
Chem. class.: Bile acid sequestrant

Action: Absorbs, combines with bile acids to form insoluble complex that is excreted through feces; loss of bile acids lowers cholesterol levels
Uses: Primary hypercholesterolemia, pruritus associated with biliary obstruction, diarrhea caused by excess bile acid, xanthomas
Dosage and routes:
• *Adult:* **PO** 4 g ac, and hs, not to exceed 32 g/day
• *Child:* **PO** 240 mg/kg/day in 3 divided doses with food or drink
Available forms: Pwd 9 g/4 g cholestyramine; tab 1 g
Side effects/adverse reactions:
CNS: Headache, dizziness, drowsiness, vertigo, tinnitus
MS: Muscle, joint pain
GI: Constipation, abdominal pain, nausea, fecal impaction, hemorrhoids, flatulence, vomiting, steatorrhea, peptic ulcer
INTEG: Rash, irritation of perianal area, tongue, skin
HEMA: Decreased vit A, D, K, red cell folate content; ***hyperchloremic acidosis, bleeding,*** decreased protime
Contraindications: Hypersensitivity, biliary obstruction
Precautions: Pregnancy (C), lactation, children
Pharmacokinetics:
PO: Excreted in feces, maximum effect in 2 wk

Interactions:
• Decreased absorption of: warfarin, thiazides, cardiac glycosides; acetaminophen, beta-blockers, corticosteroids, iron, thyroid hormones, fat-soluble vitamins

Lab test interferences:
Interfere: cholecystography

NURSING CONSIDERATIONS
Assess:
• Cardiac glycoside level, if both drugs are being administered
• For signs of vit A, D, K deficiency
• Fasting LDL, HDL, total cholesterol, triglyceride levels, electrolytes if on extended therapy
• Bowel pattern daily; increase bulk, H_2O in diet for constipation

Administer:
• Drug ac, hs; give all other medications 1 hr before cholestyramine or 4 hr after cholestyramine to avoid poor absorption
• Drug mixed with applesauce or stirred into beverage (2-6 oz), let stand for 2 min; do not take dry, avoid inhaling powder
• Supplemental doses of vit A, D, K, if levels are low

Evaluate:
• Therapeutic response: decreased cholesterol level (hyperlipidemia); diarrhea, pruritus (excess bile acids)

Teach patient/family:
◆ The symptoms of hypoprothrombinemia: bleeding mucous membranes, dark tarry stools, hematuria, petechiae; report immediately
• The importance of compliance; toxicity may result if doses missed
• That risk factors should be decreased: high-fat diet, smoking, alcohol consumption, absence of exercise
• Not to discontinue abruptly

---

choline salicylate (℞)
(koe′leen sa-liss′ih-late)
Arthropan
Func. class.: Nonnarcotic analgesic
Chem. class.: Salicylate

Action: Blocks pain impulses in CNS that occur in response to inhibition of prostaglandin synthesis; antipyretic action results from inhibition of hypothalamic heat-regulating center to produce vasodilation to allow heat dissipation

Uses: Mild to moderate pain or fever including arthritis, juvenile rheumatoid arthritis

Dosage and routes:
• *Adult and child >12 yr:* **PO** 870-1740 mg qid; max 6 ×/day

Pain/fever
• *Adult:* **PO** 870 mg q3-4h prn
Available forms: Liq 870 mg/5 ml

Side effects/adverse reactions:
HEMA: ***Thrombocytopenia, agranulocytosis, leukopenia, neutropenia, hemolytic anemia,*** increased pro-time
CNS: Stimulation, drowsiness, dizziness, confusion, ***convulsion,*** headache, flushing, hallucinations, ***coma***
GI: Nausea, vomiting, GI bleeding, diarrhea, heartburn, anorexia, ***hepatitis***
INTEG: Rash, urticaria, bruising
EENT: Tinnitus, hearing loss
CV: Rapid pulse, pulmonary edema
RESP: Wheezing, hyperpnea
ENDO: Hypoglycemia, hyponatremia, hypokalemia

Contraindications: Hypersensitivity to salicylates, GI bleeding, bleeding disorders, children <3 yr, vit K deficiency, children with flulike symptoms

Precautions: Anemia, hepatic dis-

◆ = Nursing alert   ▮ = Herb-drug interaction   Ⓢ = Do not crush ease, renal disease, Hodgkin's disease, renal disease, pregnancy (C), lactation

Pharmacokinetics:

PO: Onset 15-30 min; metabolized by liver; crosses placenta; excreted in breast milk, by kidneys, half-life 2-3 hr, large doses 15-30 hr

Interactions:

• Decreased effects of aspirin: antacids (high doses), steroids, urinary alkalizers, coricosteroids

• Increased bleeding: alcohol, heparin, plicamycin, cefamandole

• Increased effects of warfarin, insulin, methotrexate, thrombolytic agents, penicillins, phenytoin, valproic acid, oral hypoglycemics, sulfonamides

• Increased salicylate levels: urinary acidifiers, ammonium chloride, nizatidine

• Decreased effects of probenecid, spironolactone, sulfinpyrazone, sulfonylamides, NSAIDs, beta-blockers

• Gastric ulcer: steroids, antiinflammatories, NSAIDs

🍵 Increased risk of bleeding: horse chestnut, kelpware

Lab test interferences:

Increase: Coagulation studies, liver function studies, serum uric acid, amylase, CO_2, urinary protein

Decrease: Serum K, PBI, cholesterol

Interference: Urine catecholamines, pregnancy test

NURSING CONSIDERATIONS

Assess:

• Liver function studies: AST, ALT, bilirubin, creatinine (long-term therapy)

• Renal function studies: BUN, urine creatinine (long-term therapy)

• Blood studies: CBC, Hct, Hgb, pro-time (long-term therapy)

• I&O ratio; decreasing output may indicate renal failure (long-term therapy)

◆ Hepatotoxicity: dark urine; clay-colored stools; yellowing of skin, sclera; itching; abdominal pain; fever; diarrhea (long-term therapy)

• Allergic reactions: rash, urticaria; drug may have to be discontinued

• Renal dysfunction: decreased urine output

• Ototoxicity: tinnitus, ringing, roaring in ears; audiometric testing needed before, after long-term therapy

• Visual changes: blurring, halos, corneal, retinal damage

• Edema in feet, ankles, legs

• Drug history; many interactions

Administer:

• Mixed with fruit juice, carbonated beverage, water

Evaluate:

• Therapeutic response: decreased pain, fever, stiffness of joints

Teach patient/family:

• To report any symptoms of hepatotoxicity, renal toxicity, visual changes, ototoxicity, allergic reactions, bleeding (long-term therapy)

• Not to exceed recommended dosage; acute poisoning may result

• To read label on other OTC drugs; many contain aspirin

• That therapeutic response takes 2 wk (arthritis)

• To avoid alcohol ingestion; GI bleeding may occur

• That if anticoagulants are given with this drug, this drug should be decreased 2 wk before surgery

Treatment of overdose: Lavage, activated charcoal, monitor electrolytes, VS

chymopapain (R)
(kye′moe-pa-pane)
Chymodiactin
Func. class.: Enzyme
Chem. class.: Proteolytic

Action: Hydrolyzes noncollagenous polypeptides that maintain structure of chondromucoprotein; activity decreases pressure on disk

Uses: Herniated lumbar intervertebral disk

Dosage and routes:
• *Adult:* **INJ** 2-4 mKat U/disk injected intradiskally, not to exceed 10 mKat U in a multiple herniation

Available forms: Powder for inj 4000 U/vial

Side effects/adverse reactions:
CNS: **Paraplegia, cerebral hemorrhage, seizures,** headache, dizziness, paresthesia, numbness of extremities
INTEG: Rash, urticaria, itching
GI: Nausea, paralytic ileus
MS: *Back pain, stiffness, spasm, acute transverse myelitis,* weakness, leg pain
SYST: **Anaphylaxis, angioedema**
GU: Urinary retention

Contraindications: Hypersensitivity to this drug, papaya, meat tenderizer; severe spondylolisthesis; severe progressing paralysis; spinal cord tumor; cauda equina lesion, previous use

Precautions: Pregnancy (C), lactation, children

Pharmacokinetics: Onset 30 min, duration 24 hr

Interactions:
• Possible adverse reactions: radiographic contrast media

NURSING CONSIDERATIONS
Assess:
• RBCs, ESR before treatment
• Respiratory rate, rhythm, depth; notify prescriber of abnormalities
• Anaphylaxis for several days after injection
• Neuro status after surgery; elimination status for paralytic ileus
• For allergies: iodine, papaya, meat tenderizer; if allergies are identified, drug should not be used

Administer:
• Only with epinephrine available for anaphylaxis
• Only in lumbar spine by prescriber
• After diluting with sterile water for inj, use within 1 hr
• After completing allergy test (ChymoFAST)

Evaluate:
• Therapeutic response: absence of back pain, increased mobility

Teach patient/family:
• To report allergic reactions up to 2 wk after inj
• To be aware of possible infection: redness, swelling, pain

cidofovir (R)
(si-doh-foh′veer)
Vistide
Func. class.: Antiviral
Chem. class.: Nucleotide analog

Action: Suppresses cytomegalovirus (CMV) replication by selective inhibition of viral DNA synthesis

Uses: CMV retinitis in patients with AIDS

Dosage and routes:
• Dilute in 100 ml 0.9% saline sol before administration; probenecid must be given **PO** 2 g 3 hr prior to the cidofovir infusion and 1 g at 2 and 8 hr after ending the cidofovir infusion; give 1 L of 0.9% saline sol **IV** with each **INF** of cidofovir, give saline **INF** over 1-2 hr period immediately prior to cidofovir; patient

◆ = Nursing alert   ✔ = Herb-drug interaction   ⊘ = Do not crush

should be given a 2nd L if the patient can tolerate the fluid load (2nd L given at time of cidofovir or immediately afterward and should be given over a 1-3 hr period).

Renal dose
• CrCl <50 ml/min reduce dose

Induction
• *Adult:* **IV INF** 5 mg/kg given over 1 hr at a constant rate qwk × 2 consecutive wk

Maintenance
• *Adult:* **IV INF** 5 mg/kg given over 1 hr q2wk

Available forms: Inj 75 mg/ml

Side effects/adverse reactions:

CNS: Fever, chills, **coma,** confusion, abnormal thought, *dizziness,* bizarre dreams, *headache,* psychosis, tremors, somnolence, paresthesia, *amnesia, anxiety, insomnia,* **seizures**

CV: Dysrhythmias, hypertension/hypotension

EENT: Retinal detachment in CMV retinitis

GI: Abnormal LFTs, *nausea, vomiting, anorexia, diarrhea,* abdominal pain, **hemorrhage**

GU: **Hematuria,** increased creatinine, BUN, **nephrotoxicity**

HEMA: **Granulocytopenia, thrombocytopenia, irreversible neutropenia, anemia, eosinophilia**

INTEG: Rash, alopecia, pruritus, acne, urticaria, pain at inj site, phlebitis

RESP: Dyspnea

Contraindications: Hypersensitivity to this drug or probenecid, sulfa drugs

Precautions: Preexisting cytopenias, renal function impairment, pregnancy (C), lactation, children <6 mo, elderly, platelet count <25,000/mm^3

Pharmacokinetics: Unknown

Interactions:
• Nephrotoxicity: amphotericin B, foscarnet, aminoglycosides, pentamidine IV

NURSING CONSIDERATIONS
Assess:
• Culture before treatment is initiated; cultures of blood, urine, and throat may all be taken; CMV is not confirmed by this method; the diagnosis is made by an ophth exam
• Kidney, liver function, increased hemopoietic studies and BUN; serum creatinine, AST, ALT, creatinine, creatinine clearance, A-G ratio, baseline and drip treatment, blood counts should be done q2wk; watch for decreasing granulocytes, Hgb; if low, therapy may have to be discontinued and restarted after hematologic recovery; blood transfusions may be required
• For GI symptoms: severe nausea, vomiting, diarrhea; severe symptoms may necessitate discontinuing drug
• Electrolytes and minerals: calcium, phosphorus, magnesium, sodium, potassium; watch closely for tetany during first administration
• For symptoms of blood dyscrasias (anemia, granulocytopenia); bruising, fatigue, bleeding, poor healing
• Allergic reactions: flushing, rash, urticaria, pruritus
• For leukopenia, neutropenia, thrombocytopenia: WBCs, platelets q2d during 2×/day dosing and qwk thereafter; check for leukopenias, with qd WBC count in patients with prior leukopenia, with other nucleoside analogs, or for whom leukopenia counts are <1000 cells/mm^3 at start of treatment
• Monitor serum creatinine or creatinine clearance at least q2wk; give only to those with creatinine levels ≤1.5 mg/dl, creatinine clearance > 55 ml/min, urine protein <100 mg/dl

Administer:
IV
• Mix under strict aseptic conditions using gloves, gown, and mask, and using precautions for antineoplastic
• After diluting in 100 ml 0.9% NaCl
• Slowly; do not give by bolus IV, SC inj
• Use diluted sol within 12 hr, do not refrigerate or freeze; do not use sol with particulate matter or discoloration
Evaluate:
• Therapeutic response: Decreased symptoms of CMV
Teach patient/family:
• To notify prescriber if sore throat, swollen lymph nodes, malaise, fever occur; may indicate other infections
• To report perioral tingling, numbness in extremities, and paresthesias
• That serious drug interactions may occur if OTC products are ingested; check first with prescriber
• That drug is not a cure, but will control symptoms
• That regular ophth exams must be continued
• That major toxicities may necessitate discontinuing drug
• To use contraception during treatment and that infertility may occur; men should use barrier contraception for 90 days after treatment
Treatment of overdose: Discontinue drug; use hemodialysis, and increase hydration

---

cilostazol
See appendix a—selected new drugs

---

cimetidine (OTC, ℞)
(sye-met′i-deen)
cimetadine, Tagamet, Tagamet HBL, Tagamet HCl, Tagamet Tiltab
Func. class.: H_2-histamine receptor antagonist
Chem. class.: Imidazole derivative

Action: Inhibits histamine at H_2-receptor site in the gastric parietal cells, which inhibits gastric acid secretion

Uses: Short-term treatment of duodenal and gastric ulcers and maintenance; management of GERD and Zollinger-Ellison syndrome

Investigational uses: Prevention of aspiration pneumonitis, stress ulcers, upper GI bleeding, herpes infection, hirsutism

Dosage and routes:
Treatment of active ulcers
• *Adult:* PO 300 mg qid with meals, hs × 8 wk or 400 mg bid, 800 mg hs; after 8 wk give hs dose only; **IV BOL** 300 mg/20 ml 0.9% NaCl over 1-2 min q6h; **IV INF** 300 mg/50 ml D_5W over 15-20 min; **IM** 300 mg q6h, not to exceed 2400 mg/day
• *Child:* 20-40 mg/kg/day
Prophylaxis of duodenal ulcer
• *Adult and child >16 yr:* 400 mg hs
GERD
• *Adult:* PO 800-1600 mg/day in divided doses
Hypersecretory conditions (Zollinger-Ellison syndrome)
• *Adult:* **PO/IM/IV** 300-600 mg q6h; may increase to 12 g/day if needed
Upper GI bleeding prophylaxis
• *Adult:* IV 50 mg/hr; lowered in renal disease
Aspiration pneumonitis prophylaxis
• *Adult:* **IM/IV** 300 mg IM 1 hr

◆ = Nursing alert   ✎ = Herb-drug interaction   ⊘ = Do not crush

before anesthesia, then 300 mg **IV** q4h until patient is alert

Renal disease

• CrCl 20-40 ml/min 300 mg q8h; CrCl <20 ml/min 300 mg q12h

Available forms: Tabs 100, 200, 300, 400, 800 mg; liq 300 mg/5 ml; inj 300 mg/2 ml, 300 mg/50 ml 0.9% NaCl

Side effects/adverse reactions:

CNS: Confusion, headache, depression, dizziness, anxiety, weakness, psychosis, tremors, ***convulsions***

CV: Bradycardia, tachycardia

GI: Diarrhea, abdominal cramps, ***paralytic ileus, jaundice***

GU: Gynecomastia, galactorrhea, impotence, increase in BUN, creatinine

*HEMA: **Agranulocytosis, thrombocytopenia, neutropenia, aplastic anemia,** increase in pro-time*

INTEG: Urticaria, rash, alopecia, sweating, flushing, ***exfoliative dermatitis***

Contraindications: Hypersensitivity

Precautions: Pregnancy (B), lactation, child <16 yr, organic brain syndrome, hepatic disease, renal disease, elderly

Pharmacokinetics: Well absorbed (PO, IM)

IM/IV: Onset 10 min, peak ½ hr, duration 4-5 hr

PO: Peak 1-1½ hr, half-life 1½-2 hr; 30%-40% metabolized by liver, excreted in urine unchanged, crosses placenta, enters breast milk

Interactions:

• Increased toxicity: oral anticoagulants, benzodiazepines, betablockers, phenytoin, quinidine, theophylline, tricyclic antidepressants, lidocaine, warfarin

• Decreased absorption of cimetidine: antacids, sucralfate

• Decreased absorption: ketoconazole

Lab test interferences:

Increase: Alk phosphatase, AST, creatinine, prolactin

False positive: Gastroccult, hemoccult

False negative: Skin tests

NURSING CONSIDERATIONS

Assess:

• Gastric pH (5 or more should be maintained), also epigastric pain and duration, intensity; aggravating, ameliorating factors

• I&O ratio, BUN, creatinine, CBC with differential monthly

Administer:

• With meals for prolonged drug effect; antacids 1 hr before or 1 hr after cimetidine

IV

• After diluting 300 mg/20 ml of NS for inj; give ≥2 min; may be diluted 300 mg/50 ml of D$_5$W; run over 15-20 min; or total daily dose (900 mg) diluted in 100-1000 ml D$_5$W given over 24 hr

Additive compatibilities: Acetazolamide, amikacin, aminophylline, atracurium, cefoperazone, cefoxitin, chlorothiazide, clindamycin, colistimethate, dexamethasone, digoxin, epinephrine, erythromycin, ethacrynate, floxacillin, flumazenil, furosemide, gentamicin, insulin (regular), isoproterenol, lidocaine, lincomycin, meropenem, metaraminol, methylprednisolone, norepinephrine, nitroprusside, penicillin G potassium, phytonadione, polymyxin B, potassium chloride, protamine, quinidine, tacrolimus, vancomycin, verapamil, vit B/C

Syringe compatibilities: Atropine, butorphanol, cephalothin, diazepam, diphenhydramine, doxapram, droperidol, fentanyl, glycopyrrolate, heparin, hydromorphone, hydroxyzine, lorazepam, meperidine, midazolam, morphine, nafcillin, nalbuphine, penicillin G sodium, pentazocine, perphenazine, prochlorperazine, promazine, promethazine, scopolamine

Y-site compatibilities: Acyclovir, amifostine, aminophylline, amrinone, atracurium, aztreonam, cisatracarium, cisplatin, cladribine, cyclophosphamide, cytarabine, diltiazem, doxorubicin, doxorubicin liposome, enalaprilat, esmolol, filgrastim, fluconazole, fludarabine, foscarnet, gallium, granisetron, haloperidol, heparin, hetastarch, idarubicin, labetalol, melphalan, meropenem, methotrexate, midazolam, ondansetron, paclitaxel, pancuronium, piperacillin/tazobactam, propofol, remifentanil, sargramostim, tacrolimus, teniposide, theophylline, thiotepa, tolazoline, vecuronium, vinorelbine, zidovudine

Perform/provide:
• Storage of diluted sol at room temp up to 48 hr

Evaluate:
• Therapeutic response: decreased pain in abdomen; healing of ulcers, absence of gastroesophageal reflux, gastric pH 5

Teach patient/family:
• That gynecomastia, impotence may occur, are reversible
• To avoid driving, other hazardous activities until patient is stabilized on this medication; drowsiness or dizziness may occur
• To avoid black pepper, caffeine, alcohol, harsh spices, extremes in temp of food
• To avoid OTC preparations: aspirin, cough, cold preparations; condition may worsen
• That smoking decreases the effectiveness of the drug
• That drug must be taken exactly as prescribed and continued for prescribed time to be effective; doses not to be doubled

• To report bruising, fatigue, malaise; blood dyscrasias may occur
• To report to prescriber diarrhea, black tarry stools, sore throat, rash

---

ciprofloxacin (℞)
(sip-ro-floks'a-sin)
Cipro, Cipro IV
Func. class.: Broad-spectrum antiinfective
Chem. class.: Fluoroquinolone antibacterial

Action: Interferes with conversion of intermediate DNA fragments into high-molecular-weight DNA in bacteria; DNA gyrase inhibitor

Uses: Infection caused by susceptible *Escherichia coli, Enterobacter cloacae, Proteus mirabilis, Klebsiella pneumoniae, Proteus vulgaris, Citrobacter freundii, Serratia marcescens, Proteus aeruginosa, Staphylococcus aureus, Staphylococcus epidermidis, Enterobacter, Campylobacter jejuni, Salmonella;* chronic bacterial prostatitis, acute sinusitis

Dosage and routes:
Uncomplicated urinary tract infections
• *Adult:* **PO** 250 mg q12h; **IV** 200 mg q12h
Complicated/severe urinary tract infections
• *Adult:* **PO** 500 mg q12h; **IV** 400 mg q12h
Respiratory, bone, skin, joint infections
• *Adult:* **PO** 500-750 mg q12h; **IV** 400 mg q12h
Renal disease
• CrCl <50 ml/min **PO** 250-500 mg q12h; CrCl 5-29 ml/min **PO** 250-500 mg q18h; **IV** 200-400 mg q18-24h
Available forms: Tabs 250, 500, 750

---

mg; inj 200 mg/100 ml D₅, 400 mg/200 ml D₅; 200, 400 mg vial

Side effects/adverse reactions:
CNS: Headache, dizziness, fatigue, insomnia, depression, *restlessness*, seizures, confusion
GI: Nausea, diarrhea, increased ALT, AST, flatulence, heartburn, *vomiting*, oral candidiasis, dysphagia
INTEG: Rash, pruritus, urticaria, photosensitivity, flushing, fever, chills
MS: Tremor, arthralgia, tendon rupture

Contraindications: Hypersensitivity to quinolones

Precautions: Pregnancy (C), lactation, children, renal disease, epilepsy

Pharmacokinetics:
PO: Peak 1 hr, half-life 3-4 hr; excreted in urine as active drug, metabolites

Interactions:
• Decreased absorption of ciproflaxin: antacids containing magnesium, aluminum; zinc, iron, sucralfate
• Increased serum levels of ciprofloxacin: probenecid; monitor for toxicity
• Increased levels of: theophylline, monitor blood levels
⚠ Possible toxicity: yerba maté
• Drug/food: increased effect of: caffeine; decreased absorption: dairy products, food

NURSING CONSIDERATIONS
Assess:
• CNS symptoms: headache, dizziness, fatigue, insomnia, depression
• Kidney, liver function studies: BUN, creatinine, AST, ALT
• I&O ratio, urine pH <5.5 is ideal
• Allergic reactions: fever, flushing, rash, urticaria, pruritus

Administer:
• 2 hr before or 2 hr after antacids, zinc, iron, calcium

IV
• Over 1 hr as an INF, comes in premixed plastic INF container or diluted 20 or 40 ml vial to a final conc of 0.5-2 mg/ml of NS or D₅W; give through Y-tube or 3-way stopcock
• After clean-catch urine for C&S

Additive compatibilities: Amikacin, aztreonam, ceftazidime, cyclosporine, gentamicin, metronidazole, netilmicin, piperacillin, potassium acetate, potassium chloride, potassium phosphates, prednisolone, promethazine, propofol, ranitidine, Ringer's, sodium chloride, tobramycin, vit B/C

Y-site compatibilities: Amifostine, amino acids, aztreonam, calcium gluconate, ceftazidime, cisatracurium, digoxin, diltiazem, diphenhydramine, dobutamine, dopamine, doxorubicin liposome, gallium, gentamicin, granisetron, hydroxyzine, lidocaine, lorazepam, metoclopramide, midazolam, midodrine, piperacillin, potassium acetate, potassium chloride, potassium phosphates, prednisolone, promethazine, propofol, ranitidine, remifentanil, Ringer's, sodium chloride, tacrolimus, teniposide, thiotepa, tobramycin, verapamil

Perform/provide:
• Limited intake of alkaline foods, drugs: milk, dairy products, alkaline antacids, sodium bicarbonate

Evaluate:
• Therapeutic response: decreased pain, frequency, urgency, C&S; absence of infection

Teach patient/family:
• Not to take any products containing magnesium or calcium (such as antacids), iron, or aluminum with this drug or within 2 hr of drug
• That photosensitivity may occur; patient should avoid sunlight or use sunscreen to prevent burns

• That fluids must be increased to 3 L/day to avoid crystallization in kidneys

• If dizziness occurs, to ambulate, perform activities with assistance

• To complete full course of drug therapy

• To contact prescriber if adverse reaction occurs or if inflammation or pain in tendon occurs

---

cisatracurium
(sis-a-tra-kyoor′ee-um)
Nimbex

Func. class.: Neuromuscular blocker (nondepolarizing)

Action: Inhibits transmission of nerve impulses by binding with cholinergic receptor sites, antagonizing action of acetylcholine

Uses: Facilitation of endotracheal intubation, skeletal muscle relaxation during mechanical ventilation, surgery, or general anesthesia

Dosage and routes:

• *Adult:* **IV** 0.15-0.2 mg/kg depending on desired time to intubate and length of surgery; use peripheral nerve stimulation to evaluate dosage

• *Child 2-12 yr:* **IV** 0.1 mg/kg over 5-10 sec with halothane or opioid anesthesia

Available forms: Inj 2 mg/ml, 10 mg/ml

Side effects/adverse reactions:

CV: Bradycardia, tachycardia; increased, decreased B/P

RESP: **Prolonged apnea, bronchospasm, cyanosis, respiratory depression**

EENT: Increased secretions

INTEG: Rash, flushing, pruritus, urticaria

Contraindications: Hypersensitivity

Precautions: Pregnancy (B), cardiac disease, lactation, children <2 yr, electrolyte imbalances, dehydration, neuromuscular disease, respiratory disease

Pharmacokinetics: Onset 1-3 min, peak 2-5 min, duration 30-40 min

Interactions:

• Increased neuromuscular blockade: aminoglycosides, clindamycin, lincomycin, quinidine, local anesthetics, polymyxins, lithium, opioids, thiazides, enflurane, isoflurane, bacitracin, tetracyclines, magnesium salts

• Decreased duration of neuromuscular blockade: carbamazepine, phenytoin

• Shorter onset of neuromuscular blockade: succinylcholine

NURSING CONSIDERATIONS
Assess:

• For electrolyte imbalances (K, Mg); may lead to increased action of this drug

• Vital signs (B/P, pulse, respirations, airway) until fully recovered; rate, depth, pattern of respirations; strength of hand grip

• I&O ratio; check for urinary retention, frequency, hesitancy

• Recovery: decreased paralysis of face, diaphragm, leg, arm, rest of body

• Allergic reactions: rash, fever, respiratory distress, pruritus; drug should be discontinued

Administer:

• Using nerve stimulator by anesthesiologist to determine neuromuscular blockade

• Anticholinesterase to reverse neuromuscular blockade

• By slow IV only by qualified person, do not administer IM

Perform/provide:

• Storage in light-resistant container

• Reassurance if communication is

---

difficult during recovery from neuromuscular blockade

Evaluate:

• Therapeutic response: paralysis of jaw, eyelid, head, neck, rest of body

Treatment of overdose: Edrophonium or neostigmine, atropine, monitor VS; mechanical ventilation

---

cisplatin (Ŗ)
(sis'pla-tin)
Platinol-AQ

Func. class.: Antineoplastic alkylating agent
Chem. class.: Inorganic heavy metal

Action: Alkylates DNA, RNA; inhibits enzymes that allow synthesis of amino acids in proteins; activity is not cell cycle phase specific

Uses: Advanced bladder cancer, adjunctive in metastatic testicular cancer, adjunctive in metastatic ovarian cancer, head, neck cancer, esophagus, prostate, lung and cervical cancer, lymphoma

Dosage and routes:
Testicular cancer
• *Adult:* IV 20 mg/m^2 qd × 5 days, repeat q3wk for 3 cycles or more, depending on response
Bladder cancer
• *Adult:* IV 50-70 mg/m^2 q3-4wk
Ovarian cancer
• *Adult:* IV 100 mg/m^2 q4wk or 50 mg/m^2 q3wk with cyclophosphamide; mix with 2 L NaCl and 37.5 g mannitol over 6 hr

Available forms: Inj 0.5*, 1 mg/ml

Side effects/adverse reactions:
EENT: Tinnitus, hearing loss, vestibular toxicity
*HEMA: **Thrombocytopenia, leukopenia, pancytopenia***
CV: Cardiac abnormalities

GI: Severe nausea, vomiting, diarrhea, weight loss
*GU: **Renal tubular damage,** renal insufficiency, impotence, sterility, amenorrhea, gynecomastia, hyperuremia*
INTEG: Alopecia, dermatitis
*CNS: **Convulsions,** peripheral neuropathy*
*RESP: **Fibrosis***
META: Hypomagnesemia, hypocalcemia, hypokalemia, hypophosphatemia
*SYST: **Hypersensitivity reaction***

Contraindications: Radiation therapy or chemotherapy within 1 mo, thrombocytopenia, smallpox vaccination, pregnancy (D)

Precautions: Pneumococcus vaccination, lactation

Pharmacokinetics: Well absorbed orally, metabolized in liver, excreted in urine; half-life 2 hr

Interactions:
• Risk of bleeding: aspirin
• Ototoxicity: bumetanide, ethacrynic acid, furosemide
• Increased myelosuppression: myelosuppressive agents
• Increased nephrotoxicity: aminoglycosides
• Decreased effects of: phenytoin

Lab test interferences:
Increase: Uric acid, BUN, creatinine
Decrease: Creatinine clearance, calcium, phosphate, potassium, magnesium

NURSING CONSIDERATIONS
Assess:
• CBC, differential, platelet count weekly; withhold drug if WBC is <4000 or platelet count is <100,000; notify prescriber of results
• Renal function studies: BUN, creatinine, serum uric acid, urine CrCl before, electrolytes during therapy; dose should not be given if BUN <25 mg/dl; creatinine <1.5 mg/dl

---

Side effects: *italics* = common; ***bold italics*** = life-threatening

• I&O ratio; report fall in urine output of <30 ml/hr
• Monitor temp q4h (may indicate beginning infection)
• Liver function tests before, during therapy (bilirubin, AST, ALT, LDH) as needed or monthly
• Bleeding: hematuria, guaiac, bruising or petechiae, mucosa or orifices q8h; obtain prescription for viscous lidocaine (Xylocaine)
• Effects of alopecia on body image; discuss feelings about body changes
• Jaundice of skin, sclera; dark urine; clay-colored stools; itchy skin; abdominal pain; fever; diarrhea
• Edema in feet, joint pain, stomach pain, shaking

Administer:
IV
• After diluting 10 mg/10 ml or 50 mg/50 ml sterile H_2O for inj; withdraw prescribed dose, dilute ½ dose with 1000 ml D_5 0.2 NaCl or D_5 0.45 NaCl with 37.5 g mannitol; IV INF is given over 3-4 hr; use a 0.45 μm filter; total dose 2 L over 6-8 hr; check site for irritation, phlebitis; do not use equipment containing aluminum
• Hydrate patient with 0.9% NaCl over 8-12 hr before treatment
• Epinephrine, antihistamines, corticosteroids for hypersensitivity reaction
• Antiemetic 30-60 min before giving drug and prn
• Allopurinol or sodium bicarbonate to maintain uric acid levels, alkalinization of urine
• Diuretic (furosemide 40 mg IV) or mannitol after infusion

Additive compatibilities: Carboplatin, cyclophosphamide with etoposide, etoposide, etoposide with floxuridine, floxuridine, floxuridine with leucovorin, hydroxyzine, ifosfamide, ifosfamide with etoposide, leucovorin, magnesium sulfate, mannitol, ondansetron

Solution compatibilities: D_5/0.225% NaCl, D_5/0.45% NaCl, D_5/0.9% NaCl, D_5/0.45% NaCl with mannitol 1.875%, D_5/0.33% NaCl with KCl 20 mEq and mannitol 1.875%, 0.9% NaCl, 0.45% NaCl, 0.3% NaCl, 0.225% NaCl

Syringe compatibilities: Bleomycin, cyclophosphamide, doxapram, doxorubicin, droperidol, fluorouracil, furosemide, heparin, leucovorin, methotrexate, metoclopramide, mitomycin, vinblastine, vincristine

Y-site compatibilities: Allopurinol, aztreonam, bleomycin, chlorpromazine, cimetidine, cladribine, cyclophosphamide, dexamethasone, diphenhydramine, doxorubicin, doxorubicin liposome, droperidol, famotidine, filgrastim, fludarabine, fluorouracil, furosemide, ganciclovir, granisetron, heparin, hydromorphone, leucovorin, lorazepam, melphalan, methotrexate, methylprednisolone, metoclopramide, mitomycin, morphine, ondansetron, paclitaxel, prochlorperazine, promethazine, propofol, ranitidine, sargramostim, teniposide, vinblastine, vincristine, vinorelbine

Perform/provide:
• Comprehensive oral hygiene
• Storage protected from light in refrigerator (dry powder)
• All medications PO, if possible, avoid IM inj when platelets <100,000/mm³
• Increase fluid intake to 2-3 L/day to prevent urate deposits, calculi formation; elimination of drug

Evaluate:
• Therapeutic response: decreased tumor size, spread of malignancy

Teach patient/family:
• To report signs of infection: increased temperature, sore throat, flu symptoms

---

◆ = Nursing alert   ∥ = Herb-drug interaction   Ⓝ = Do not crush

- To report signs of anemia: fatigue, headache, faintness, shortness of breath, irritability
- To report bleeding: avoid use of razors, commercial mouthwash
- To avoid aspirin, ibuprofen
- To report any complaints or side effects to nurse or prescriber
- That impotence or amenorrhea can occur; reversible after discontinuing treatment
- To report any changes in breathing, coughing
- That hair may be lost during treatment; a wig or hairpiece may make patient feel better; new hair may be different in color, texture

---

citalopram (℞)

(sigh-tal'oh-pram)
Celexa
Func. class.: Antidepressant
Chem. class.: Selective serotonin reuptake inhibitor (SSRI)

Action: Inhibits CNS neuron uptake of serotonin but not of norepinephrine
Uses:
Major depressive disorder
Dosage and routes:
- *Adult:* **PO** 20 mg qd AM or PM, may increase if needed to 40 mg/day after 1 wk; maintenance: after 6-8 wk of initial treatment, continue for 24 wk (32 wk total), reevaluate long-term usefulness
Hepatic dose
20 mg/day, may increase to 40 mg/day if no response
Available forms: Tabs 20, 40 mg
Side effects/adverse reactions:
*CNS: Headache, nervousness, insomnia, drowsiness, anxiety, tremor, dizziness, fatigue, sedation, poor concentration, abnormal dreams, agitation, **convulsions,** apathy, eu-* phoria, hallucinations, delusions, psychosis, **suicidal attempts**
GI: Nausea, diarrhea, dry mouth, anorexia, dyspepsia, constipation, cramps, vomiting, taste changes, flatulence, decreased appetite
INTEG: Sweating, rash, pruritus, acne, alopecia, urticaria
RESP: Infection, pharyngitis, nasal congestion, sinus headache, sinusitis, cough, dyspnea, bronchitis, asthma, hyperventilation, pneumonia
*CV: Hot flashes, palpitations, angina pectoris, **hemorrhage,** hypertension, tachycardia, first-degree AV block, bradycardia, MI, thrombophlebitis*
MS: Pain, arthritis, twitching
GU: Dysmenorrhea, decreased libido, urinary frequency, UTI, amenorrhea, cystitis, impotence, urine retention
EENT: Visual changes, ear/eye pain, photophobia, tinnitus
SYST: Asthenia, viral infection, fever, allergy, chills
Contraindications: Hypersensitivity
Precautions: Pregnancy (B), lactation, children, elderly, diabetes mellitus
Pharmacokinetics:
PO: Metabolized in liver; excreted in urine; steady state 28-35 days; peak 2-4 hr; half-life 35 hr
Interactions:
- Increased effect of tricyclics
- Increased CNS effects: CNS depressants
- Increased prothrombin time: warfarin
- Do not use with MAOIs
- Increased citalopram levels: macrolides, azole antifungals
- Increased plasma levels of: β-blockers
- Decreased citalopram levels; carbamazepine

Side effects: *italics* = common; **bold italics** = life-threatening

• Increased serotonergic effects: lithium

⫸ Avoid use with St. John's wort

Lab test interferences:

• *Increase:* Serum bilirubin, blood glucose, alk phosphatase

• *Decrease:* VMA, 5-HIAA

• *False increase:* Urinary catecholamines

NURSING CONSIDERATIONS

Assess:

• Mental status: mood, sensorium, affect, suicidal tendencies, increase in psychiatric symptoms, depression, panic

• B/P (lying/standing), pulse q4h; if systolic B/P drops 20 mm Hg, hold drug, notify prescriber; take vital signs q4h in patients with cardiovascular disease

• Weight qwk; appetite may decrease or increase with drug

• ECG for flattening of T wave, bundle branch, AV block, dysrhythmias in cardiac patients

• Alcohol consumption; if alcohol is consumed, hold dose until AM

Administer:

• With food or milk for GI symptoms

• Crushed if patient is unable to swallow medication whole

• Dosages hs if oversedation occurs during the day; may take entire dose hs

Perform/provide:

• Storage at room temp; do not freeze

• Assistance with ambulation during therapy, since drowsiness, dizziness occur

• Safety measures primarily in elderly

• Check to see if PO medication swallowed

• Gum, hard candy, frequent sips of water for dry mouth

Evaluate:

• Therapeutic response: decreased depression

Teach patient/family:

• That therapeutic effect may take 2-3 wk

• To use caution in driving, other activities requiring alertness because of drowsiness, dizziness, blurred vision

• To use birth control while on this drug; to notify prescriber if pregnancy is suspected

• To avoid alcohol ingestion, other CNS depressants

• To notify prescriber if pregnant or plan to become pregnant or breastfeed

---

cladribine (CdA) ℞
(kla'dri-been)
Leustatin
Func. class.: Antineoplastic antibiotic
Chem. class.: Purine nucleoside analog

Action: Phosphylated while passively crossing the cell membrane, causing cell death by not properly repairing single-strand DNA

Uses: Treatment of active hairy cell leukemia; may be useful in chronic lymphocytic leukemia, non-Hodgkin's lymphomas, acute myeloid leukemia, autoimmune hemolytic anemia

Dosage and routes:

• *Adult:* **IV** 7 days × 0.09 mg/kg diluted with 0.9% NaCl qs to 100 ml; pass through 0.22 μm microfilter

Available forms: Inj 1 mg/ml

Side effects/adverse reactions:

CNS: Headache, dizziness, insomnia

CV: Edema, tachycardia

GI: Nausea, vomiting, anorexia, diarrhea, constipation, abdominal pain

HEMA: **Neutropenia, anemia, thrombocytopenia, bone marrow**

⬥ = Nursing alert   *⫸* = Herb-drug interaction   *⊘* = Do not crush

hypocellularity, purpura, epistaxis, petechiae

INTEG: Rash, inj site reactions, pruritus

MS: Myalgia, arthralgia

RESP: Cough, upper respiratory infection, dyspnea, shortness of breath, abnormal chest sounds, pneumonia

SYST: Fever, infection, fatigue, pain, allergic reaction, chills, ***death, sepsis***

Contraindications: Hypersensitivity

Precautions: Renal disease, pregnancy (D), lactation, children, bone marrow depression, hepatic disease, neurologic disease

Pharmacokinetics:

IV: Terminal half-life 5.4 hr

NURSING CONSIDERATIONS

Assess:

• CBC, differential, platelet count weekly; withhold drug if WBC <4000/mm^3 or platelet count <75,000/mm^3; notify prescriber

• Renal function studies: BUN, serum uric acid, urine CrCl, electrolytes before, during therapy

• I&O ratio; report urine output <30 ml/hr

• Monitor temp q4h; fever may indicate beginning infection

• Liver function tests before, during therapy: bilirubin, AST, ALT, alk phosphatase as needed or monthly

• Local irritation, pain, burning at injection site

◆ Symptoms indicating severe allergic reaction: rash, pruritus, urticaria, purpuric skin lesions, itching, flushing

• GI symptoms: frequency of stools, cramping

Administer:

IV

• Antiemetic 30-60 min before giving drug to prevent vomiting

• Use gloves, gown to mix IV sol

• Use bacteriostatic (0.9% NaCl,

0.9% benzyl alcohol preserved) to prepare 7-day inf; pass both cladribine and diluent through sterile 0.22 μm hydrophilic syr filter as each sol is introduced into inf reservoir; add dose of cladribine to inf reservoir using filter, then bacteriostatic 0.9% NaCl to bring sol total to 100 ml; after preparation, clamp line, disconnect filter, discard; aspirate air bubbles (reservoir) using syr, dry filter or sterile vat filter assembly; reclamp line, discard filter and syr; infuse continuously × 7 days

• Add dose for single daily dose to inf bag (500 ml 0.9% NaCl); infuse continuously over 24 hr; repeat daily dose × 7 days

Y-site compatibilities: Aminophylline, bumetanide, buprenorphine, butorphanol, calcium gluconate, carboplatin, chlorpromazine, cimetidine, cisplatin, cyclophosphamide, cytarabine, dexamethasone, diphenhydramine, dobutamine, dopamine, doxorubicin, droperidol, enalaprilat, etoposide, famotidine, furosemide, gallium, granisetron, haloperidol, heparin, hydrocortisone, hydrocortisone sodium phosphate, hydromorphone, hydroxyzine, idarubicin, imipramine, leucovorin, lorazepam, mannitol, meperidine, mesna, methylprednisolone, metoclopramide, mitoxantrone, morphine, nalbuphine, ondansetron, paclitaxel, potassium chloride, prochlorperazine, promethazine, ranitidine, sodium bicarbonate, teniposide, vincristine

Perform/provide:

• Storage in refrigerator; protect from light; reconstituted or diluted sol may be stored at room temp no longer than 8 hr; discard single-use vials of unused sol

---

Evaluate:
• Therapeutic response: decrease in symptoms of hairy cell leukemia
Teach patient/family:
• To report any complaints, side effects to nurse or prescriber

---

clarithromycin (Ŗ)
(klare-ith'row-my-sin)
Biaxin
Func. class.: antiinfective
Chem. class.: Macrolide

Action: Binds to 50S ribosomal subunits of susceptible bacteria and suppresses protein synthesis
Uses: Mild to moderate infections of the upper respiratory tract, lower respiratory tract, uncomplicated skin and skin structure infections caused by *Streptococcus pneumoniae, Mycoplasma pneumoniae, Legionella pneumophila, Moraxella catarrhalis, Neisseria gonorrhoeae, corynebacterium diphtheriae, Listeria monocytogenes, Haemophilus influenzae, Streptococcus pyogenes, Staphlococcus aureus, Mycobacterium avium (MAC)* complex infection in AIDS patients, *Mycobacterium intracellulare, Helicobacter pylori* in combination with omeprazole
Dosage and routes:
• *Adult:* **PO** 250-500 mg bid for 7-14 days; 500 mg bid continues for *M. avium* complex (MAC)
• *Child:* **PO** 15 mg/kg/day (max 1000 mg) divided q12h × 10 days
H. pylori *infection*
• *Adult:* **PO** 500 mg qd plus omeprazole 2 × 20 mg q AM (day 1-14), then omeprazole 20 mg q AM (days 15-28)
Available forms: Tabs 250, 500 mg; granules for oral susp 125 mg/5 ml, 250 mg/5 ml

Side effects/adverse reactions:
INTEG: Rash, urticaria, pruritus, **Stevens-Johnson syndrome**
CV: **Ventricular dysrhythmias**
HEMA: Leukopenia, thrombocytopenia, increased INR
GI: Nausea, vomiting, diarrhea, **hepatotoxicity,** abdominal pain, stomatitis, heartburn, anorexia, *abnormal taste,* **pseudomembranous colitis**
GU: Vaginitis, moniliasis
MISC: Headache
Contraindications: Hypersensitivity to this drug or macrolide antibiotics
Precautions: Pregnancy (C), lactation, hepatic, renal disease, elderly
Pharmacokinetics: Peak 2 hr, duration 12 hr, half-life 4-6 hr; metabolized by liver; excreted in bile, feces
Interactions:
• Dysrhythmias: astemizole, cisapride, pimozide
• Increased clarithromycin levels: fluconazole
• Increased effects of oral anticoagulants, digoxin, theophylline, carbamazepine
• Decreased action: clindamycin, rifampin, zidovudine
Lab test interferences:
False increase: 17-OHCS/17-KS, AST, ALT, BUN, creatinine, LDH, total bilirubin
Decrease: Folate assay, WBC
NURSING CONSIDERATIONS
Assess:
• LFTs, renal studies; report hematuria, oliguria
• C&S before drug therapy; drug may be given as soon as culture is taken; C&S may be repeated after treatment
• Bowel pattern before, during treatment
• Skin eruptions, itching

◆ = Nursing alert   ▮ = Herb-drug interaction   ⊘ = Do not crush

• Respiratory status: rate, character, wheezing, tightness in chest; discontinue drug
• Allergies before treatment, reaction of each medication

Administer:
• Adequate intake of fluids (2 L) during diarrhea episodes
• q12h to maintain serum level

Perform/provide:
• Storage at room temp

Evaluate:
• Therapeutic response: C&S negative for infection

Teach patient/family:
• To take with full glass H_2O; may give with food to decrease GI symptoms
• To report sore throat, fever, fatigue; may indicate superinfection
• To notify nurse of diarrhea, dark urine, pale stools, yellow discoloration of eyes or skin, severe abdominal pain
• To take at evenly spaced intervals; complete dosage regimen

Treatment of hypersensitivity: Withdraw drug, maintain airway, administer epinephrine, aminophylline, O_2, IV corticosteroids

---

clemastine (R)
(klem′as-teen)
Contac Allergy 12 Hour, Tavist, Antihist-1
Func. class.: Antihistamine
Chem. class.: Ethanolamine derivative, H_1-receptor antagonist

Action: Acts on blood vessels, GI, respiratory system by competing with histamine for H_1-receptor site; decreases allergic response by blocking histamine

Uses: Allergy symptoms, rhinitis, angioedema, urticaria, common cold

Dosage and routes:
• *Adult and child >12 yr:* **PO** 1.34-2.68 mg bid-tid, not to exceed 8.04 mg/day

Available forms: Tabs 1.34, 2.68 mg; syr 0.67 mg/ml

Side effects/adverse reactions:
CNS: Dizziness, drowsiness, poor coordination, fatigue, anxiety, euphoria, confusion, paresthesia, neuritis
CV: Hypotension, palpitations, tachycardia
RESP: Increased thick secretions, wheezing, chest tightness
*HEMA: **Thrombocytopenia, agranulocytosis, hemolytic anemia***
GI: Constipation, dry mouth, nausea, vomiting, anorexia, diarrhea
INTEG: Rash, urticaria, photosensitivity
GU: Urinary retention, dysuria, frequency
EENT: Blurred vision, dilated pupils, tinnitus, nasal stuffiness, dry nose, throat, mouth

Contraindications: Hypersensitivity to H_1-receptor antagonists, acute asthma attack, lower respiratory tract disease

Precautions: Increased intraocular pressure, renal disease, cardiac disease, hypertension, bronchial asthma, seizure disorder, stenosed peptic ulcers, hyperthyroidism, prostatic hypertrophy, bladder neck obstruction, pregnancy (B), lactation, elderly

Pharmacokinetics:
PO: Onset 15-60 min, peak 5-7 hr, duration 10-12 hr or more; metabolized in liver, excreted by kidneys

Interactions:
• Increased CNS depression: barbiturates, opioids, hypnotics, tricyclic antidepressants, alcohol
• Increased effect of clemastine: MAOIs

Increased CNS depression: kava

Increased anticholinergic effect: henbane leaf

Lab test interferences:

False negative: Skin allergy tests

NURSING CONSIDERATIONS

Assess:

• I&O ratio; be alert for urinary retention, frequency, dysuria; drug should be discontinued

• CBC during long-term therapy

• Blood dyscrasias: thrombocytopenia, agranulocytosis (rare)

• Respiratory status: rate, rhythm, increase in bronchial secretions, wheezing, chest tightness

• Cardiac status: palpitations, increased pulse, hypotension

Administer:

• With meals for GI symptoms; absorption may slightly decrease

Perform/provide:

• Hard candy, gum, frequent rinsing of mouth for dryness

• Storage in tight container at room temp

Evaluate:

• Therapeutic response: absence of running or congested nose or rashes

Teach patient/family:

• All aspects of drug use; to notify prescriber of confusion, sedation, hypotension

• To avoid driving, other hazardous activity if drowsiness occurs

• To avoid concurrent use of alcohol, other CNS depressants

• That drug decreases anticoagulant (oral) effect

• To change position slowly since drug may cause dizziness, hypotension (elderly)

Treatment of overdose: Administer ipecac syrup or lavage, diazepam, vasopressors, barbiturates (short-acting)

clindamycin HCl (R)
(klin-da-my′sin)
Cleocin HCl,
clindamycin palmitate (R)
Cleocin Pediatric, Dalacin C Palmitate
clindamycin phosphate (R)
Cleocin Phosphate, Dalacin C, Dalacin C Phosphate
Func. class.: Antiinfective, misc
Chem. class.: Lincomycin derivative

Action: Binds to 50S subunit of bacterial ribosomes, suppresses protein synthesis

Uses: Infections caused by staphylococci, streptococci, *Rickettsia, Fusobacterium, Actinomyces, Peptococcus, Bacteroides, Pneumocystis carinii*

Dosage and routes:

• *Adult:* **PO** 150-450 mg q6h; **IM/IV** 1.2-1.8 g/day in 2-4 divided doses, not to exceed 4800 mg/day

• *Child >1 mo:* **PO** 8-25 mg/kg/day in divided doses q6-8h; **IM/IV** 20-40 mg/kg/day in divided doses q6-8h (3-4 equal doses)

• *Child <1 mo:* 15-20 mg/kg/day divided q6-8h

• *PID: Adult:* **IV** 600 mg qid plus gentamicin

Available forms:

Phosphate: inj 150, 300, 600 mg base/4 ml; 900 mg base/ml; inj INF in D_5 300 mg, 600 mg, 900 mg; HCl: caps 75, 150, 300 mg; palmitate: oral sol 75 mg/ml

Side effects/adverse reactions:

*HEMA: **Leukopenia, eosinophilia, agranulocytosis, thrombocytopenia, polyarthritis***

◆ = Nursing alert   *▨* = Herb-drug interaction   ◎ = Do not crush

GI: Nausea, vomiting, abdominal pain, diarrhea, **pseudomembranous colitis,** anorexia, weight loss, increased AST, ALT, bilirubin, alk phosphatase; jaundice

GU: Vaginitis, urinary frequency

EENT: Rash, urticaria, pruritus, erythema, pain, abscess at injection site

Contraindications: Hypersensitivity to this drug or lincomycin, ulcerative colitis/enteritis

Precautions: Renal disease, liver disease, GI disease, elderly, pregnancy (B), lactation, tartrazine sensitivity

Pharmacokinetics:

PO: Peak 45 min, duration 6 hr

IM: Peak 3 hr, duration 8-12 hr; half-life 2½ hr; metabolized in liver; excreted in urine, bile, feces as inactive metabolites; crosses placenta; excreted in breast milk

Interactions:

• Decreased absorption: kaolin

• May block clindamycin effect: erythromycin

• Increased neuromuscular blockade: neuromuscular blockers

Lab test interferences:

Increase: Alk phosphatase, bilirubin, CPK, AST, ALT

NURSING CONSIDERATIONS
Assess:

• Liver studies: AST, ALT if on long-term therapy

• Blood studies: WBC, RBC, Hct, Hgb, platelets, serum iron, reticulocytes; drug should be discontinued if bone marrow depression occurs

• C&S before drug therapy; drug may be given as soon as culture is taken

• B/P, pulse in patient receiving drug parenterally

• Bowel pattern before, during treatment; if severe diarrhea occurs, drug should be discontinued; may indicate pseudomembranous colitis

• Skin eruptions, itching, dermatitis after administration

• Respiratory status: rate, character, wheezing, tightness in chest

• Allergies before treatment, reaction of each medication

Administer:

• IM deep injection; rotate sites

• Orally with at least 8 oz H_2O

IV

• By infusion only; do not administer bolus dose; dilute 300 mg or less/50 ml or more of D_5W, NS; may be further diluted in greater amounts of D_5W, NS and given as a cont inf in acute PID; give first dose 10 mg/min over ½ hr, then 0.75 mg/min; increased rates may be used to keep serum blood levels higher; run >10 min; no more than 1200 mg in a single 1-hr inf

Additive compatibilities: Amikacin, ampicillin, aztreonam, cefamandole, cefazolin, cefepime, cefonicid, cefoperazone, cefotaxime, cefoxitin, ceftazidime, ceftizoxime, cefuroxime, cephalothin, cimetidine, fluconazole, heparin, hydrocortisone, kanamycin, methylprednisolone, metoclopramide, metronidazole, netilmicin, ofloxacin, penicillin G, piperacillin, potassium chloride, sodium bicarbonate, tobramycin, verapamil, vit B/C

Syringe compatibilities: Amikacin, aztreonam, gentamicin, heparin

Y-site compatibilities: Amifostine, amiodarone, amphotericin B cholesteryl, amsacrine, aztreonam, cefpirome, cisatracurium, cyclophosphamide, diltiazem, doxorubicin liposome, enalaprilat, esmolol, fludarabine, foscarnet, granisetron, heparin, hydromorphone, labetalol, magnesium sulfate, melphalan, meperidine, midazolam, morphine, multivitamins, ondansetron, perphenazine, piperacillin/tazobactam, propofol, remifentanil, sargramostim, tacrolimus, teniposide, theophylline, thiotepa, vinorelbine, vit B/C, zidovudine

Perform/provide:
• Storage at room temp (caps) up to 2 wk (reconstituted)
• Epinephrine, suction, tracheostomy set, endotracheal intubation equipment on unit
• Adequate intake of fluids (2 L) during diarrhea episodes

Evaluate:
• Therapeutic response: decreased temperature, negative C&S

Teach patient/family:
• To take oral drug with full glass H₂O; may give with food to reduce GI symptoms; antiperistaltic drugs may worsen diarrhea
• All aspects of drug therapy: need to complete entire course of medication to ensure organism death (10-14 days); culture may be taken after medication course completed
◆ To report sore throat, fever, fatigue; may indicate superinfection
🚫 Not to break, crush, or chew caps
• That drug must be taken in equal intervals around clock to maintain blood levels
• To notify nurse or prescriber of diarrhea

Treatment of hypersensitivity:
Withdraw drug; maintain airway; administer epinephrine, aminophylline, O₂, IV corticosteroids

---

clofazimine (℞)
(kloe-fa′zi-meen)
Lamprene
Func. class.: Leprostatic

Action: Inhibits mycobacterial growth, binds to mycobacterial DNA; exerts antiinflammatory properties in controlling leprosy reactions

Uses: Lepromatous leprosy, dapsone-resistant leprosy, lepromatous leprosy complicated by erythema nodosum leprosum

Dosage and routes:
Erythema nodosum leprosum
• *Adult:* **PO:** 100-200 mg qd × 3 mo, then taper dosage to 100 mg when disease is controlled; do not exceed 200 mg/day

Dapsone-resistant leprosy
• *Adult:* **PO:** 100 mg/day in combination with at least one other antileprosy drug × 3 yr, then 100 mg qd clofazimine (only)

Available forms: Caps 50 mg

Side effects/adverse reactions:
GI: Diarrhea, nausea, vomiting, abdominal pain, intolerance, **GI bleeding, obstruction,** anorexia, constipation, **hepatitis,** jaundice
EENT: Pigmentation of cornea, conjunctiva, drying, burning, itching, irritation of eyes
INTEG: Pink or brown discoloration, dryness, pruritus, rash, photosensitivity, acne, monilial cheilosis
CNS: Dizziness, headache, fatigue, drowsiness
MISC: Discolored urine, feces, sputum, sweat

Contraindications: Hypersensitivity to this drug

Precautions: Pregnancy (C), lactation, children, abdominal pain, diarrhea, depression

Pharmacokinetics: Deposited in fatty tissue, reticuloendothelial system; half-life 70 days; small amount excreted in feces, sputum, sweat

Lab test interferences:
Increase: Albumin, bilirubin, AST, eosinophilia, hypokalemia, glucose, ESR

◆= Nursing alert　　　▮= Herb-drug interaction　　　🚫= Do not crush

NURSING CONSIDERATIONS

Assess:

• Liver studies qwk: ALT, AST, bilirubin

• Renal studies: BUN, creatinine, I&O, specific gravity, urinalysis before, qmo

• Blood level of drug

• Mental status often: affect, mood, behavioral changes; psychosis may occur

• Hepatic status: decreased appetite, jaundice, dark urine, fatigue

Administer:

• With meals to decrease GI symptoms

• Antiemetic if vomiting occurs

• After C&S is completed; qmo to detect resistance

Perform/provide:

• Infants to be kept with mother infected with leprosy; breastfeeding during drug therapy is encouraged

Evaluate:

• Therapeutic response: decreased symptoms of infection

Teach patient/family:

🚫 Not to break, crush, or chew caps

• That therapeutic effects may occur after 3-6 mo of drug therapy

• That compliance with dosage schedule, length is necessary

• That scheduled appointments must be kept or relapse may occur

• That drug must be taken with meals

• That skin, sweat, sputum, urine, feces discoloration, although reversible, may take several months or years to disappear

---

clomiphene (Ŗ)

(kloe'mi-feen)

Clomid, clomiphene citrate, Milophene, Serophene

Func. class.: Ovulation stimulant

Chem. class.: Nonsteroidal antiestrogenic

Action: Increases LH, FSH release from the pituitary, which increases maturation of ovarian follicle, ovulation, development of corpus luteum

Uses: Female infertility (ovulatory failure)

Dosage and routes:

• *Adult:* **PO** 50-100 mg qd × 5 days or 50-100 mg qd beginning on day 5 of cycle; may be repeated until conception occurs or 3 cycles of therapy have been completed

Available forms: Tabs 50 mg

Side effects/adverse reactions:

CV: Vasomotor flushing, phlebitis, ***deep-vein thrombosis***

EENT: Blurred vision, diplopia, photophobia

CNS: Headache, depression, restlessness, anxiety, nervousness, fatigue, insomnia, dizziness, flushing

GI: Nausea, vomiting, constipation, abdominal pain, bloating

INTEG: Rash, dermatitis, urticaria, alopecia

GU: Polyuria, urinary frequency, birth defects, spontaneous abortions, multiple ovulation, breast pain, oliguria, abnormal uterine bleeding

Contraindications: Hypersensitivity, pregnancy (X), hepatic disease, undiagnosed uterine bleeding, uncontrolled thyroid or adrenal dysfunction, intracranial lesion, ovarian cysts

Precautions: Hypertension, depression, convulsions, diabetes mellitus

---

Pharmacokinetics: Metabolized in liver, excreted in feces

Lab test interferences:
Increase: FSH/LH, BSP, thyroxine, TBG

NURSING CONSIDERATIONS
Administer:
• After discontinuing estrogen therapy
• At same time qd to maintain drug level

Evaluate:
• Therapeutic response: fertility

Teach patient/family:
• That multiple births are common
• To notify prescriber immediately if low abdominal pain occurs; may indicate ovarian cyst, cyst rupture
• To notify prescriber of photophobia, blurred vision, diplopia
• That if dose is missed, to double at next time; if more than one dose is missed, to call prescriber
• That response usually occurs 4-10 days after last day of treatment
• The method for taking, recording basal body temp to determine whether ovulation has occurred
• If ovulation can be determined (there is a slight decrease in temp, then a sharp increase for ovulation), to attempt coitus 3 days before and qod until after ovulation
• If pregnancy is suspected, to notify prescriber immediately

---

clomipramine (℞)
(kloe-mip'ra-meen)
Anafranil
Func. class.: Antidepressant, tricyclic
Chem. class.: Tertiary amine

Action: Not known; potent inhibitor of serotonin uptake; also increases dopamine metabolism; moderate anticholinergic effect

Uses: Depression, dysphoria, phobias, anxiety, agoraphobia, obsessive-compulsive disorder

Dosage and routes:
Obsessive-compulsive disorder
• *Adult:* **PO** 25 mg hs and increase gradually over 4 wk to 75-300 mg/day in divided doses
• *Child 10-18 yr:* **PO** 25-50 mg/day gradually increased; or 3 mg/kg/day, whichever is smaller, not to exceed 200 mg/day
Depression
• *Adult:* **PO** 50-150 mg/day in a single or divided dose
Anxiety/agoraphobia
• *Adult:* **PO** 25-75 mg/day
Available forms: Caps 25, 50, 75 mg

Side effects/adverse reactions:
HEMA: **Agranulocytosis, neutropenia, pancytopenia**
CV: Hypotension, tachycardia, **cardiac arrest**
CNS: Dizziness, tremors, mania, **seizures,** aggressiveness, EPS
ENDO: Galactorrhea, hyperprolactinemia
META: Hyponatremia
GI: Constipation, dry mouth, nausea, dyspepsia
GU: Delayed ejaculation, anorgasmy, urinary retention
INTEG: Diaphoresis, photosensitivity

Contraindications: Hypersensitivity

Precautions: Seizures, suicidal patients, elderly, pregnancy (C), lactation

Pharmacokinetics: Onset ≥ 2 wk, peak 2-6 hr; extensively bound to tissue and plasma proteins; demethylated in liver; active metabolites excreted in urine; half-life: 19-37 hr; steady state 1-2 wk

Interactions:
• Decreased clomipramine levels: barbiturates
• Increased clomipramine levels: ci-

---

metidine, fluoxetine, fluvoxamine, sertraline

• Increased hypertensive effect: clonidine, epinephrine, norepinephrine
• Increased CNS depression: alcohol, CNS depressants
• Hypertensive crisis, convulsions, hypertensive episode: MAOIs

🔹 Increased CNS depression: kava
🔹 Increased anticholinergic effect: belladonna leaf/root, henbane leaf
🔹 Increased action of clomipramine: scopolia root

Lab test interferences:
Increase: Prolactin, TBG
Decrease: Serum thyroid hormone

NURSING CONSIDERATIONS
Assess:
• B/P (lying, standing), pulse q4h; if systolic B/P drops 20 mm Hg, withhold drug, notify prescriber; take vital signs q4h in patients with cardiovascular disease
• ECG for flattening of T wave, QTc prolongation, bundle branch block, AV block, dysrhythmias in cardiac patients
• Blood studies: CBC, leukocytes, differential, cardiac enzymes if patient is receiving long-term therapy
• Hepatic studies: AST, ALT, bilirubin
• Mental status: mood, sensorium, affect, suicidal tendencies; increase in psychiatric symptoms: depression, panic
• Urinary retention, constipation; constipation more likely in children
• Withdrawal symptoms: headache, nausea, vomiting, muscle pain, weakness; not usual unless drug discontinued abruptly
• Alcohol consumption; if alcohol consumed, withhold dose until AM

Administer:
• Increased fluids, bulk in diet for constipation, especially elderly
• With food or milk for GI symptoms

Perform/provide:
• Storage in tight container at room temp; do not freeze
• Assistance with ambulation during beginning therapy, since drowsiness/dizziness occurs
• Safety measures, primarily in elderly
• Checking to see PO medication swallowed
• Gum, hard candy, or frequent sips of water for dry mouth

Evaluate:
• Therapeutic response: decreased anxiety, depression

Teach patient/family:
🚫 Not to break, crush, or chew caps
• That the effects may take 2-3 wk
• To use caution in driving, other activities requiring alertness because of drowsiness, dizziness, blurred vision
• To avoid alcohol ingestion, other CNS depressants
• Not to discontinue medication quickly after long-term use; may cause nausea, headache, malaise
• To wear sunscreen, protective clothing to prevent photosensitivity

Treatment of overdose: ECG monitoring; induce emesis; lavage, activated charcoal; anticonvulsant

---

clonazepam (℞)
(kloe-na′zi-pam)
Klonopin, Syn-Clonazepam*, Rivotril*

Func. class.: Anticonvulsant
Chem. class.: Benzodiazepine derivative

Controlled Substance Schedule IV
Action: Inhibits spike, wave formation in absence seizures (petit mal), decreases amplitude, frequency, duration, spread of discharge in minor motor seizures

---

Uses: Absence, atypical absence, akinetic, myoclonic seizures, Lennox-Gastaut syndrome

Investigational uses: Parkinsonian dysarthrosis, acute manic episodes, adjunction schizophrenia, neuralgias, multifocal tic disorders, restless leg syndrome

Dosage and routes:
• *Adult:* PO not to exceed 1.5 mg/day in 3 divided doses; may be increased 0.5-1 mg q3d until desired response, not to exceed 20 mg/day
• *Child <10 yr or <30 kg:* PO 0.01-0.03 mg/kg/day in divided doses q8h, not to exceed 0.05 mg/kg/day; may be increased 0.25-0.5 mg q3d until desired response, not to exceed 0.1-0.2 mg/kg/day

Available forms: Tabs 0.5, 1, 2 mg

Side effects/adverse reactions:
*HEMA: **Thrombocytopenia, leukocytosis, eosinophilia***
CNS: Drowsiness, dizziness, confusion, behavioral changes, tremors, insomnia, headache, suicidal tendencies, slurred speech
GI: Nausea, constipation, polyphagia, anorexia, xerostomia, diarrhea, gastritis, sore gums
INTEG: Rash, alopecia, hirsutism
EENT: Increased salivation, nystagmus, diplopia, abnormal eye movements
*RESP: **Respiratory depression,*** dyspnea, congestion
CV: Palpitations, bradycardia
GU: Dysuria, enuresis, nocturia, retention

Contraindications: Hypersensitivity to benzodiazepines, acute narrow-angle glaucoma, pregnancy (D)

Precautions: Open-angle glaucoma, chronic respiratory disease, lactation, renal, hepatic disease, elderly

Pharmacokinetics:
PO: Peak 1-2 hr; metabolized by liver; excreted in urine; half-life 18-50 hr

Interactions:
• Increased CNS depression: alcohol, barbiturates, opiates, antidepressants, other anticonvulsants, general anesthetics, hypnotics, sedatives
• Decreased clonazepam effect: carbamazepine, phenobarbital, phenytoin

⚗ Increased CNS depression: kava

Lab test interferences:
Increase: AST, alk phosphatase

NURSING CONSIDERATIONS
Assess:
• Blood level: ther level 20-80 ng/ml
• Renal studies: urinalysis, BUN, urine creatinine
• Blood studies: RBC, Hct, Hgb, reticulocyte counts qwk for 4 wk, then qmo
• Hepatic studies: ALT, AST, bilirubin, creatinine
• Drug levels during initial treatment (therapeutic 20-80 ng/ml)
• Signs of physical withdrawal if medication suddenly discontinued
• Mental status: mood, sensorium, affect, oversedation, behavioral changes; if mental status changes, notify prescriber
• Eye problems: need for ophthalmic exam before, during, after treatment (slit lamp, fundoscopy, tonometry)
• Allergic reaction: red, raised rash; drug should be discontinued
◆ Blood dyscrasias: fever, sore throat, bruising, rash, jaundice
• Toxicity: bone marrow depression, nausea, vomiting, ataxia, diplopia, cardiovascular collapse

Administer:
• With food, milk for GI symptoms

Perform/provide:
• Storage at room temperature
• Assistance with ambulation during early part of treatment; dizziness occurs, especially elderly

---

◆ = Nursing alert   ⚗ = Herb-drug interaction   ⊘ = Do not crush

Evaluate:

• Therapeutic response: decreased seizure activity, document on patient's chart

Teach patient/family:

• To carry ID card or Medic Alert bracelet stating name, drugs taken, condition, prescriber's name, phone number

• To avoid driving, other activities that require alertness

• To avoid alcohol ingestion, CNS depressants; increased sedation may occur

• Not to discontinue medication quickly after long-term use; taper off over several wk

Treatment of overdose: Lavage, activated charcoal, monitor electrolytes, VS, administer vasopressors

---

clonidine (℞)

(klon'i-deen)
Catapres, Catapres-TTS, clonidine HCl, Dixarit*, Duraclon

Func. class.: Antihypertensive, analgesic

Chem. class.: Central α-adrenergic agonist

Action: Inhibits sympathetic vasomotor center in CNS, which reduces impulses in sympathetic nervous system; blood pressure, pulse rate, cardiac output decrease

Uses: Mild to moderate hypertension, used alone or in combination; severe pain in cancer patients

Investigational uses: Opioid withdrawal, prevention of vascular headaches, treatment of menopausal symptoms, dysmenorrhea, attention deficit disorder

Dosage and routes:

Hypertension

• *Adult:* **PO/TRANS** 0.1 mg bid, then increase by 0.1 mg/day or 0.2 mg/day until desired response; range 0.2-0.8 mg/day in divided doses

• *Geriatric:* **PO** 0.1 mg hs, may increase gradually

• *Child:* 5-10 µg/kg/day in divided doses q8-12h, max 0.9 mg/day

Opioid withdrawal

• *Adult:* **PO** 0.3-1.2 mg/day; decreased dosage given over several days

Severe pain

• *Adult:* **CONT EPIDURAL INF** 30 µg/hr

ADHD

• *Child:* 0.05 mg/day titrate up to max 0.4 mg/day

Available forms: Tabs 0.025*, 0.1, 0.2, 0.3 mg; TRANS 2.5, 5, 7.5 mg delivering 0.1, 0.2, 0.3 mg/24 hr, respectively

Side effects/adverse reactions:

CNS: Drowsiness, sedation, headache, fatigue, nightmares, insomnia, mental changes, anxiety, depression, hallucinations, delirium

CV: Orthostatic hypotension, palpitations, **CHF,** ECG abnormalities

EENT: Taste change, parotid pain

ENDO: Hyperglycemia

GI: Nausea, vomiting, malaise, constipation, dry mouth

GU: Impotence, dysuria, *nocturia,* gynecomastia

INTEG: Rash, alopecia, facial pallor, pruritus, hives, edema, burning papules, excoriation (transdermal patches)

MS: Muscle, joint pain; leg cramps

Contraindications: Hypersensitivity

Precautions: MI (recent), diabetes mellitus, chronic renal failure, Raynaud's disease, thyroid disease, depression, COPD, child <12 yr (patches), asthma, pregnancy (C), lactation, elderly, noncompliant patients

Pharmacokinetics: Absorbed well

PO: Onset ½ to 1 hr, peak 2-4 hr, duration 8 hr; half-life 12-16 hr
TOP: Onset 3 days, duration 1 wk; metabolized by liver (metabolites), excreted in urine (30% unchanged, inactive metabolites), feces; crosses blood-brain barrier, excreted in breast milk

Interactions:
• Increased CNS depression: opiates, sedatives, hypnotics, anesthetics, alcohol
• Decreased hypotensive effects: tricyclic antidepressants, MAOIs, appetite suppressants, amphetamines
• Increased hypotensive effects: diuretics, other antihypertensive nitrates
• Increased bradycardia: β-blockers, cardiac glycosides
• AV block: verapamil
• Decreased effect of: levodopa

Lab test interferences:
Increase: Blood glucose
Decrease: VMA, catecholamines, aldosterone

NURSING CONSIDERATIONS
Assess:
• Blood studies: neutrophils, decreased platelets
• Renal studies: protein, BUN, creatinine; increased levels may indicate nephrotic syndrome
• Baselines in renal, liver function tests before therapy begins; K levels, although hyperkalemia rare
• B/P, pulse if used for hypertension
• For opiate withdrawal including fever, diarrhea, nausea, vomiting, cramps, insomnia, shivering, dilated pupils
• Edema in feet, legs daily; monitor I&O; check for falling output
• Allergic reaction: rash, fever, pruritus, urticaria; drug should be discontinued if antihistamines fail to help

• Allergic reaction from patches: rash, urticaria, angioedema; should not continue to use
• Symptoms of CHF: edema, dyspnea, wet rales, B/P
• Renal symptoms: polyuria, oliguria, frequency

Administer:
• SL if patient is unable to swallow
• PO: give last dose at hs
• Topical patch qwk; apply to site without hair; best absorption over chest or upper arm; rotate sites with each application; clean site before application; apply firmly, especially around edges
• Infusion of 0.9% NaCl (as ordered) to expand fluid volume if severe hypotension occurs

Perform/provide:
• Storage of patches in cool environment, tablets in tight container

Evaluate:
• Therapeutic response: decrease in B/P in hypertension, decrease in withdrawal symptoms (opioid), decrease in pain

Teach patient/family:
• To avoid hazardous activities, since drug may cause drowsiness
• To administer 1 hr before meals (PO)
• Not to discontinue drug abruptly or withdrawal symptoms may occur: anxiety, increased B/P, headache, insomnia, increased pulse, tremors, nausea, sweating
• Not to use OTC (cough, cold, or allergy) products unless directed by prescriber
• To avoid sunlight, wear sunscreen; photosensitivity may occur
• To comply with dosage schedule even if feeling better
• To rise slowly to sitting or standing position to minimize orthostatic hypotension, especially elderly
• To notify prescriber of mouth sores, sore throat, fever, swelling of

◆ = Nursing alert   ⫼ = Herb-drug interaction   ⊘ = Do not crush hands, feet, irregular heartbeat, chest pain, signs of angioedema

• About excessive perspiration, dehydration, vomiting; diarrhea may lead to fall in blood pressure; consult prescriber if these occur

• That drug may cause dizziness, fainting; light-headedness may occur during first few days of therapy

• That drug may cause dry mouth; use hard candy, saliva product, or frequent rinsing of mouth

• That compliance is necessary; not to skip or stop drug unless directed by prescriber

• That drug may cause skin rash or impaired perspiration

• To use patch; patch comes in two parts: drug patch and overlay to keep patch in place

• That response may take 2-3 days if drug is given transdermally; instruct on administration of patch

Treatment of overdose: Supportive treatment; administer tolazoline, atropine, dopamine prn

---

clopidogrel (℞)

(klo-pid′oh-grel)
Plavix
Func. class.: Platelet aggregation inhibitor
Chem. class.: Thienopyridine derivative

Action: Inhibits first and second phases of ADP-induced effects in platelet aggregation

Uses: Reducing the risk of stroke in high-risk patients

Dosage and routes:

• *Adult:* **PO** 75 mg qd with or without food

Available forms: Tabs 75 mg

Side effects/adverse reactions:

INTEG: Rash, pruritus

GI: Nausea, vomiting, diarrhea, GI discomfort

HEMA: Epistaxis, purpura

CV: Edema, hypertension

CNS: Headache, dizziness

MS: Arthralgia, back pain

RESP: Upper respiratory tract infection, dyspnea, rhinitis, bronchitis, cough

MISC: UTI, depression, hypercholesterolemia, chest pain, fatigue, ***intracranial hemorrhage***

Contraindications: Hypersensitivity, active bleeding

Precautions: Past liver disease, pregnancy (B), lactation, children, increased bleeding risk, neutropenia, agranulocytosis

Pharmacokinetics: Peak 1-3 hr, metabolized by liver, excreted in urine, feces

Interactions:

• Increased bleeding tendencies: anticoagulants, aspirin, NSAIDs

NURSING CONSIDERATIONS

Assess:

• Liver function studies: AST, ALT, bilirubin, creatinine (long-term therapy)

• Blood studies: CBC, Hct, Hgb, pro-time (long-term therapy)

Administer:

• With food to decrease gastric symptoms

Evaluate:

• Therapeutic response: absence of stroke

Teach patient/family:

• That blood work will be necessary during treatment

• To report any unusual bruising, bleeding to prescriber

• To take with food or just after eating to minimize GI discomfort

• To report side effects such as diarrhea, skin rashes, subcutaneous bleeding

---

clorazepate (℞)

(klor-az′e-pate)
Apo-clorazepate*, clorazepate dipotassium, Gen-XENE, NovoClopate*, Tranxene, Tranxene-SD, Tranxene T-TAB
Func. class.: Antianxiety, anticonvulsant
Chem. class.: Benzodiazepine

Controlled Substance Schedule IV
Action: Potentiates the actions of GABA, especially in limbic system, reticular formation
Uses: Anxiety, acute alcohol withdrawal, adjunct in seizure disorders
Dosage and routes:
Anxiety
• *Adult:* **PO** 15-60 mg/day
• *Geriatric:* **PO** 7.5 mg qd-bid
Alcohol withdrawal
• *Adult:* **PO** 30 mg then 30-60 mg in divided doses; day 2, 45-90 mg in divided doses; day 3, 22.5-45 mg in divided doses; day 4, 15-30 mg in divided doses; then reduce daily dose to 7.5-15 mg
Seizure disorders
• *Adult and child >12 yr:* **PO** 7.5 mg tid; may increase by 7.5 mg/wk or less, not to exceed 90 mg/day
• *Child 9-12 yr:* **PO** 7.5 mg bid; may increase by 7.5 mg/wk or less, not to exceed 60 mg/day
Available forms: Caps 3.75, 7.5, 15 mg; tabs 3.75, 7.5, 15 mg; single-dose tab 11.25, 22.5 mg
Side effects/adverse reactions:
CNS: Dizziness, drowsiness, confusion, headache, anxiety, tremors, stimulation, fatigue, depression, insomnia, hallucinations, lethargy
GI: Constipation, dry mouth, nausea, vomiting, anorexia, diarrhea
INTEG: Rash, dermatitis, itching
*CV: Orthostatic hypotension, **ECG changes, tachycardia,** hypotension

EENT: Blurred vision, tinnitus, mydriasis
Contraindications: Hypersensitivity to benzodiazepines, narrow-angle glaucoma, psychosis, pregnancy (D), lactation, child <18 yr
Precautions: Elderly, debilitated, hepatic disease, renal disease
Pharmacokinetics:
PO: Onset 15 min, peak 1-2 hr, duration 4-6 hr; metabolized by liver, excreted by kidneys; crosses placenta, breast milk; half-life 30-100 hr
Interactions:
• Increased effects of clorazepate: CNS depressants, alcohol, valproic acid, antidepressants, MAOIs, cimetidine
🌿 Increased CNS depression: kava
Lab test interferences:
Increase: AST, ALT
NURSING CONSIDERATIONS
Assess:
• B/P (lying, standing), pulse; if systolic B/P drops 20 mm Hg, hold drug, notify prescriber
• Blood studies: CBC during long-term therapy; blood dyscrasias have occurred rarely
• Hepatic studies: AST, ALT, bilirubin, creatinine, LDH, alk phosphatase
• I&O; may indicate renal dysfunction
• Mental status: mood, sensorium, affect, sleeping pattern, drowsiness, dizziness
• Physical dependency, withdrawal symptoms: headache, nausea, vomiting, muscle pain, weakness after long-term use
• Suicidal tendencies
Administer:
• With food, milk for GI symptoms
• Crushed if patient cannot swallow whole (tab only)

◆ = Nursing alert　　🌿 = Herb-drug interaction　　🚫 = Do not crush

Perform/provide:
• Assistance with ambulation during beginning therapy because of drowsiness/dizziness, especially elderly
• Safety measures, including side rails
• Check to see PO medication has been swallowed
• Sugarless gum, hard candy, frequent sips of water for dry mouth
Evaluate:
• Therapeutic response: decreased anxiety, restlessness, insomnia
Teach patient/family:
• That drug may be taken with food
• That drug is not to be used for everyday stress or used longer than 4 mo unless directed by prescriber; not to take more than prescribed amount; may be habit forming
🚫 Not to break, crush, or chew caps
• To avoid OTC preparations unless approved by prescriber
• To avoid driving, activities that require alertness; drowsiness may occur, especially in elderly
• To avoid alcohol ingestion, other psychotropic medications, unless directed by prescriber
• Not to discontinue medication abruptly after long-term use
• To rise slowly because fainting may occur
• That drowsiness may worsen at beginning of treatment
Treatment of overdose: Lavage, VS, supportive care, flumazenil

cloxacillin (℞)
(klox-a-sill'in)
Apo-Cloxi*, cloxacillin sodium, Cloxapen, Novo-Cloxin*, Nu-Clox*, Orbenin*
Func. class.: Broad-spectrum antiinfective
Chem. class.: Penicillinase-resistant penicillin

Action: Interferes with cell wall replication of susceptible organisms; the cell wall, rendered osmotically unstable, swells, bursts from osmotic pressure
Uses: Gram-positive cocci *(Staphylococcus aureus, Streptococcus pyogenes, Streptococcus pneumoniae),* penicillinase-producing staphylococci
Dosage and routes:
• *Adult:* **PO** 1-4 g/day in divided doses q6h
• *Child:* **PO** 50-100 mg/kg in divided doses q6h, max 4 g/day
Available forms: Caps 250, 500 mg; powder for oral susp 125 mg/5 ml
Side effects/adverse reactions:
HEMA: Anemia, increased bleeding time, ***bone marrow depression, granulocytopenia***
GI: Nausea, vomiting, diarrhea, increased AST, ALT, abdominal pain, glossitis, colitis
GU: ***Oliguria, proteinuria,*** hematuria, *vaginitis, moniliasis, **glomerulonephritis***
CNS: Lethargy, hallucinations, anxiety, depression, twitching, ***coma, convulsions***
Contraindications: Hypersensitivity to penicillins; neonates, severe renal, hepatic disease
Precautions: Pregnancy (B), lactation, hypersensitivity to cephalosporins

Pharmacokinetics:

PO: Peak 1 hr, duration 6 hr; half-life 30-60 min; metabolized in liver; excreted in urine, bile, breast milk; crosses placenta, poor penetration in CSF

Interactions:

• Increased cloxacillin concentrations: aspirin, probenecid, disulfiram

• Increased action of anticoagulants

• Decreased action of oral contraceptives

/ Delayed/reduced absorption: khat

Lab test interferences:

False positive: Urine glucose, urine protein

Decrease: Uric acid

NURSING CONSIDERATIONS
Assess:

• I&O ratio; report hematuria, oliguria, since penicillin in high doses is nephrotoxic

◆ Any patient with compromised renal system, since drug is excreted slowly in poor renal system function; toxicity may occur rapidly

• Liver studies: AST, ALT

• Blood studies: WBC, RBC, H&H, bleeding time

• Renal studies: urinalysis, protein, blood

• C&S before drug therapy; drug may be taken as soon as culture is taken

• Bowel pattern before, during treatment

• Skin eruptions after administration of penicillin to 1 wk after discontinuing drug

• Respiratory status: rate, character, wheezing, tightness in chest

• Allergies before initiation of treatment; reaction of each medication; place allergies on chart in bright red

Administer:

• After C&S completed

• Shake suspension well before each dose

Perform/provide:

• Adrenaline, suction, tracheostomy set, endotracheal intubation equipment on unit

• Adequate intake of fluids (2 L) during diarrhea episodes

• Scratch test to assess allergy after securing order from prescriber; usually done when penicillin is only drug of choice

• Storage in tight container; after reconstituting, store in refrigerator for 2 wk, room temp 1 wk

Evaluate:

• Therapeutic response: absence of fever, draining wounds

Teach patient/family:

🚫 Not to break, crush, or chew caps

• All aspects of drug therapy, including need to complete entire course of medication to ensure organism death (10-14 days); culture may be taken after course of medication completed

• To report sore throat, fever, fatigue (may indicate superinfection)

• To wear or carry a Medic Alert ID if allergic to penicillins

• To notify nurse of diarrhea

• To take on an empty stomach with a full glass of water

Treatment of overdose: Withdraw drug; maintain airway; administer epinephrine, aminophylline, O_2, IV corticosteroids for anaphylaxis

---

clozapine (℞)

(kloz'a-peen)
clozapine, Clozaril
Func. class.: Antipsychotic
Chem. class.: Tricyclic dibenzodiazepine derivative

Action: Interferes with dopamine receptor binding with lack of extra-

---

◆ = Nursing alert   / = Herb-drug interaction   🚫 = Do not crush pyramidal symptoms; also acts as an adrenergic, cholinergic, histaminergic, serotonergic antagonist

Uses: Management of psychotic symptoms in schizophrenic patients for whom other antipsychotics have failed

Dosage and routes:

• *Adult:* **PO** 25 mg qd or bid; may increase by 25-50 mg/day; normal range 300-450 mg/day after 2 wk; do not increase dose more than 2 × per wk; do not exceed 900 mg/day; use lowest dose to control symptoms

Available forms: Tabs 25, 100 mg

Side effects/adverse reactions:

CNS: Sedation, salivation, dizziness, headache, tremors, sleep problems, akinesia, fever, **seizures,** *sweating, akathisia, confusion, fatigue, insomnia,* depression, slurred speech, anxiety

GI: Drooling or excessive salivation, constipation, nausea, abdominal discomfort, vomiting, diarrhea, anorexia

MS: Weakness; pain in back, neck, legs; spasm

CV: Tachycardia, hypotension, hypertension, chest pain, ECG changes

GU: Urinary abnormalities, incontinence, ejaculation dysfunction, frequency, urgency, retention

RESP: Dyspnea, nasal congestion, throat discomfort

HEMA: **Leukopenia, neutropenia, agranulocytosis, eosinophilia**

Contraindications: Hypersensitivity, myeloproliferative disorders, severe granulocytopenia, CNS depression, coma, narrow-angle glaucoma

Precautions: Pregnancy (B); lactation; children <16; hepatic, renal, cardiac disease; seizures; prostatic enlargement; elderly

Pharmacokinetics: Steady state 2.5 hr; 95% protein bound; completely metabolized by liver; excreted in urine and feces (metabolites); half-life 8-12 hr

Interactions:

• Increased anticholinergic effects: anticholinergics

• Increased hypotension: antihypertensives

• Increased CNS depression: CNS depressants, psychoactives, alcohol

• Increased bone marrow suppression: antineoplastics, other drugs suppressing bone marrow

• Increased plasma concentrations: warfarin, digoxin, other highly protein-bound drugs

🥦 Increased CNS depression: kava

• Drug/food: decreased clozapine level: caffeine

Lab test interferences:

Increase: Liver function tests, cardiac enzymes, cholesterol, blood glucose, bilirubin, PBI, cholinesterase,[131]I

False positive: Pregnancy tests, PKU

False negative: Urinary steroids, 17-OHCS

NURSING CONSIDERATIONS

Assess:

• Swallowing of PO medication; check for hoarding or giving of medication to other patients

• I&O ratio; obtain baseline before treatment begins; palpate bladder if low urinary output occurs

• Bilirubin, CBC, liver function studies monthly; discontinue treatment if WBC <3000/mm^3 or agranulocyte <1500/mm^3 test qwk

• Urinalysis is recommended before, during prolonged therapy

• Affect, orientation, LOC, reflexes, gait, coordination, sleep pattern disturbances

• B/P standing and lying; take pulse and respirations q4h during initial treatment; establish baseline before starting treatment; report drops of 30 mm Hg

---

Side effects: *italics* = common; **bold italics** = life-threatening

• Dizziness, faintness, palpitations, tachycardia on rising
• EPS including akathisia (inability to sit still, no pattern to movements), tardive dyskinesia (bizarre movements of the jaw, mouth, tongue, extremities), pseudoparkinsonism (rigidity, tremors, pill rolling, shuffling gait)
• Skin turgor daily
• Constipation, urinary retention daily; if these occur, increase bulk, water in diet, especially elderly
Administer:
• Antiparkinsonian agent for EPS
Perform/provide:
• Decreased sensory input by dimming lights, avoiding loud noises
• Supervised ambulation until stabilized on medication; do not involve in strenuous exercise program because fainting is possible; patient should not stand still for long periods
• Increased fluids to prevent constipation
• Storage in tight, light-resistant container
Evaluate:
• Therapeutic response: decrease in emotional excitement, hallucinations, delusions, paranoia, reorganization of patterns of thought, speech
Teach patient/family:
• About symptoms of agranulocytosis and need for blood tests qwk; report flulike symptoms
• That orthostatic hypotension often occurs, and to rise gradually from sitting or lying position
• To avoid hot tubs, hot showers, tub baths; hypotension may occur
• To avoid abrupt withdrawal of this drug because EPS may result; drug should be withdrawn slowly
• To avoid OTC preparations (cough, hay fever, cold) unless approved by prescriber, since serious drug interactions may occur; avoid use with alcohol or CNS depressants, increased drowsiness may occur
• About compliance with drug regimen
• About EPS and necessity for meticulous oral hygiene, since oral candidiasis may occur
• To report sore throat, malaise, fever, bleeding, mouth sores; if these occur, CBC should be drawn and drug discontinued
• That heat stroke may occur in hot weather; take extra precautions to stay cool
• To avoid driving, other hazardous activities; seizures may occur
• To notify prescriber if pregnant or if pregnancy is intended
• **Treatment of overdose:** Lavage, activated charcoal; provide an airway; do not induce vomiting

coagulation factor VIIa, recombinant
See appendix a—selected new drugs

codeine (℞)
(koe'deen)
Paveral*
Func. class.: Opiate analgesic, antitussive
Chem. class.: Opiate, phenathrene derivative

Controlled Substance Schedule II, III, IV, V (depends on route)
Action: Depresses pain impulse transmission at the spinal cord level by interacting with opioid receptors, decreases cough reflex, GI motility
Uses: Moderate to severe pain, nonproductive cough
Investigational uses: Diarrhea

◆ = Nursing alert   ⫽ = Herb-drug interaction   ⃠ = Do not crush

Dosage and routes:
Pain
• *Adult:* **PO** 15-60 mg q4h prn; **IM/SC** 15-60 mg q4h prn
• *Child:* **PO** 3 mg/kg/day in divided doses q4h prn
Cough
• *Adult:* **PO** 10-20 mg q4-6h, not to exceed 120 mg/day
• *Child:* **PO** 1-1.5 mg/kg/day in 4 divided doses, not to exceed 60 mg/day
Diarrhea
• *Adult:* **PO** 30 mg; may repeat qid prn
Renal disease
• CrCl 10-50 ml/min 75% of dose; CrCl <10 ml/min 50% of dose
Available forms: Inj 15, 30, 60 mg/ml; tabs 15, 30, 60 mg; oral sol 10 mg/5 ml*, 15 mg/5 ml
Side effects/adverse reactions:
CNS: Drowsiness, sedation, dizziness, agitation, dependency, lethargy, restlessness
GI: Nausea, vomiting, anorexia, constipation
RESP: ***Respiratory depression, respiratory paralysis***
CV: Bradycardia, palpitations, orthostatic hypotension, tachycardia
GU: Urinary retention
INTEG: Flushing, rash, urticaria
Contraindications: Hypersensitivity to opiates, respiratory depression, increased intracranial pressure, seizure disorders, severe respiratory disorders
Precautions: Elderly, cardiac dysrhythmias, pregnancy (C), lactation
Pharmacokinetics: Onset 10-30 min, peak ½-1 hr, duration 4-6 hr; metabolized by liver; excreted by kidneys, in breast milk; crosses placenta; half-life 3 hr
Interactions:
• Increased CNS depression: alcohol, opiates, sedative/hypnotics, antipsychotics, skeletal muscle relaxants
🍃 Increased CNS depression: kava
NURSING CONSIDERATIONS
Assess:
• I&O ratio; check for decreasing output; may indicate urinary retention, especially elderly
• By using pain-scoring method
• For productive cough
• Cough: type, duration, ability to raise secretion
• CNS changes, dizziness, drowsiness, hallucinations, euphoria, LOC, pupil reaction
• Allergic reactions: rash, urticaria
• Respiratory dysfunction: respiratory depression, character, rate, rhythm; notify prescriber if respirations are <10/min, shallow
• Need for pain medication, tolerance
Administer:
IV
• Give slowly by direct inj
• With antiemetic for nausea, vomiting
• When pain is beginning to return; determine dosage interval by patient response
Syringe compatibilities: Glycopyrrolate, hydroxyzine
Y-site compatibilities: Cefmetazole
Perform/provide:
• Storage in light-resistant container at room temp
• Assistance with ambulation if needed
• Safety measures: top side rails, night-light, call bell
Evaluate:
• Therapeutic response: decrease in pain, absence of grimacing, decreased cough
Teach patient/family:
• To report any symptoms of CNS changes, allergic reactions

• That physical dependency may result after extended periods
• To change position slowly; orthostatic hypotension may occur
• To avoid hazardous activities if drowsiness, dizziness occurs
• To avoid alcohol, other CNS depressants unless directed by prescriber

---

colchicine (℞)

(kol'chi-seen)

Func. class.: Antigout agent
Chem. class.: Colchicum autumnale alkaloid

Action: Inhibits microtubule formation of lactic acid in leukocytes, which decreases phagocytosis and inflammation in joints

Uses: Gout, gouty arthritis (prevention, treatment); to arrest progression of neurologic disability in multiple sclerosis

Investigational uses: Hepatic cirrhosis, familial Mediterranean fever

Dosage and routes:

Prevention

• *Adult:* **PO** 0.5-1.8 mg qd depending on severity; **IV** 0.5-1 mg 1-2 × day

Treatment

• *Adult:* **PO** 0.5-1.2 mg, then 0.5-1.2 mg q1h, until pain decreases or side effects occur

Available forms: Tabs 0.5, 0.6 mg; inj 1 mg/2 ml

Side effects/adverse reactions:

MISC: Myopathy, alopecia, reversible azoospermia, peripheral neuritis

GU: Hematuria, *oliguria, renal damage*

HEMA: Agranulocytosis, thrombocytopenia, aplastic anemia, pancytopenia

GI: Nausea, vomiting, anorexia, malaise, metallic taste, cramps, peptic ulcer, diarrhea

INTEG: Chills, dermatitis, pruritus, purpura, erythema

Contraindications: Hypersensitivity; serious GI, renal, hepatic, cardiac disorders; pregnancy (D) IV

Precautions: Blood dyscrasias, pregnancy (C) PO, hepatic disease, elderly, lactation, children

Pharmacokinetics:

PO: Peak ½-2 hr, half-life 20 min; deacetylates in liver; excreted in feces (metabolites/active drug)

Interactions:

• Increased GI effects: NSAIDs
• Increased bone marrow depression: radiation, bone marrow depressants, cyclosporine
• Decreased action of vit B_{12}, may cause reversible malabsorption
• Increased colchicine effect: erythromycin
• Increased blood dyscrasias: phenylbutazone
• Decreased colchicine effect: loop diuretics

Lab test interferences:

Increase: Alk phosphatase, AST, ALT

False positive: RBC, Hgb

NURSING CONSIDERATIONS

Assess:

• I&O ratio; observe for decrease in urinary output
• CBC, platelets, reticulocytes before, during therapy (q3mo)
• Coombs' test for Coombs' negative hemolytic anemia
• For toxicity: weakness, abdominal pain, nausea, vomiting, diarrhea

Administer:

PO

• On empty stomach only, to facilitate absorption

IV

• Do not give IM or SC

• Give over 2-5 min
• Wait ≥1 wk after giving a full course of IV colchicine before giving subsequent doses
Evaluate:
• Therapeutic response: decreased stone formation on x-ray, decreased pain in kidney region, absence of hematuria, decreased pain in joints
Teach patient/family:
• To increase fluid intake to 3-4 L/day
• To avoid alcohol, OTC preparations that contain alcohol; skin rashes have occurred
• To report any pain, redness, or hard area, usually in legs
• The importance of complying with medical regimen; the possibility of bone marrow depression occurring
Treatment of overdose: D/C medication, may need opioids to treat diarrhea

---

colestipol (℞)

(koe-les'ti-pole)
Colestid
Func. class.: Antilipemic
Chem. class.: Bile sequestrant, resin exchange agent

Action: Absorbs, combines with bile acids to form insoluble complex excreted through feces; loss of bile acids lowers cholesterol levels
Uses: Primary hypercholesterolemia, xanthomas, digitalis toxicity, pruritus due to biliary obstruction, diarrhea due to bile acids
Dosage and routes:
• *Adult:* PO 15-30 g/day in 2-4 divided doses; 2-8 tabs/day
Available forms: Granules 300 g, 500 g bottles, 5 g packets; tabs 1 g
Side effects/adverse reactions:
GI: Constipation, abdominal pain, nausea, fecal impaction, hemor-

rhoids, flatulence, vomiting, steatorrhea, peptic ulcer
INTEG: Rash, irritation of perianal area, tongue, skin
HEMA: Decreased vit A, D, K, red folate content; ***hyperchloremic acidosis, bleeding, decreased pro-time***
Contraindications: Hypersensitivity, biliary obstruction
Precautions: Pregnancy (B), lactation, children, bleeding disorders
Pharmacokinetics:
PO: Excreted in feces
Interactions:
• May reduce action of thiazide, digitalis, warfarin, penicillin G, folic acid, phenylbutazone, tetracycline, corticosteroids, iron, thyroid agents, clindamycin, trimethoprim, chenodiol, fat-soluble vitamins, cephalexin, phenobarbital
• Antagonize colestipol: oral antidiabetics
Lab test interferences:
Increase: Liver function studies, chloride, PO_4
NURSING CONSIDERATIONS
Assess:
• Cardiac glycoside levels, if both drugs are being administered
• For signs of vit A, D, K deficiency
• Serum cholesterol, triglyceride levels, electrolytes (extended therapy)
• Bowel pattern daily; increase bulk, water in diet if constipation develops
Administer:
• Drug ac, hs; give all other medications 1 hr before colestipol or 4 hr after colestipol to avoid poor absorption
• Drug mixed in applesauce or stirred into beverage (2-6 oz); do not take dry; let stand for 2 min
🚫 Tabs should be swallowed whole; do not break, crush, or chew
• Supplemental doses of vit A, D, K if levels are low

Side effects: *italics* = common; ***bold italics*** = life-threatening

Evaluate:
• Therapeutic response: decreased triglycerides, diarrhea, pruritus (excess bile acids)

Teach patient/family:
◆ The symptoms of hypoprothrombinemia: bleeding mucous membranes; dark, tarry stools; hematuria, petechiae; report immediately
• That compliance is needed; toxicity may result if doses are missed
• That risk factors should be decreased: high-fat diet, smoking, alcohol consumption, absence of exercise

---

corticotropin (ACTH) (R)
(kor-ti-koe-troe'pin)
ACTH, Acthar, corticotropin, H.P. Acthar Gel
Func. class.: Pituitary hormone
Chem. class.: Adrenocorticotropic hormone

Action: Stimulates adrenal cortex to produce, secrete corticosterone, cortisol

Uses: Testing adrenocortical function, treatment of adrenal insufficiency caused by administration of corticosteroids (long term), multiple sclerosis, infantile spasms

Dosage and routes:
Testing of adrenocortical function
• *Adult:* IM/SC up to 80 U in divided doses; IV 10-25 U in 500 ml D_5W given over 8 hr
Inflammation
• *Adult:* SC/IM 40 U in 4 divided doses (aqueous) or 40 U q12-24h (gel/repository form)
Infantile spasms
• *Infant:* IM Gel 20 U/day × 2 wks, increase if needed
Available forms: Inj 25, 40 U/vial; repository inj 40, 80/ml

Side effects/adverse reactions:
INTEG: Impaired wound healing, rash, urticaria, hirsutism, petechiae, ecchymoses, sweating, acne, hyperpigmentation
*CNS: **Convulsions,*** dizziness, euphoria, insomnia, headache, mood swings, behavioral changes, depression, psychosis, ***increased intracranial pressure, papilledema***
GI: Nausea, vomiting, ***peptic ulcer perforation,*** pancreatitis, distention, ulcerative esophagitis
*CV: **Necrotizing angiitis, shock, heart failure,*** hypertension
GU: Water, sodium retention, hypokalemia
EENT: Cataracts, glaucoma
MS: Weakness, osteoporosis, compression fractures, muscle atrophy, steroid myopathy, myalgia, arthralgia
ENDO: Cushingoid symptoms, diabetes mellitus, antibody formation, growth retardation in children, menstrual irregularities

Contraindications: Hypersensitivity, scleroderma, osteoporosis, CHF, peptic ulcer disease, hypertension, systemic fungal infections, smallpox vaccination, recent surgery, ocular herpes simplex, primary adrenocortical insufficiency/hyperfunction

Precautions: Pregnancy (C), lactation, latent TB, hepatic disease, hypothyroiditis, childbearing age, psychiatric diagnosis, myasthenia gravis, acute gouty arthritis, thromboembolic disorders

Pharmacokinetics:
IV/IM/SC: Onset <6 hr, duration 2-4 hr, repository duration up to 3 days, half-life <20 min, excreted in urine

Interactions:
• Possible ulceration: salicylates, alcohol, NSAIDs
• Hypokalemia: diuretics (K-depleting), amphotericin B

◆ = Nursing alert   ⫸ = Herb-drug interaction   ⊘ = Do not crush

• Increased need for: insulin, oral hypoglycemic agents
• Decreased corticotropin effect: barbiturates, anticonvulsants, rifampin
• Increased corticotropin effect: estrogen
• Altered prothrombin time: oral anticoagulants
• Do not use with vaccines

NURSING CONSIDERATIONS
Assess:
• Baseline ECG, B/P, chest x-ray, GTT
• Pulse, B/P
• I&O ratio; weight qwk, report gain over 5 lb/wk
• 2 hr postprandial, chest x-ray, serum K, 17 KS, 17-OHCS, cortisol, during long-term treatment
• Dependent edema, moon face, pulmonary edema, cerebral edema
• Infection; drug may mask
• Increased stress in patient's life that may require increased corticosteroids
• Mental status: affect, mood, increased aggressiveness, irritability; change may require decreased steroids
• Growth rate of child
• Hypoadrenalism in neonates if drug was given during pregnancy
• Allergic reaction: rash, urticaria, fever, nausea, vomiting, dyspnea; drug should be discontinued immediately, administer epinephrine 1:1000
Administer:
• Test for hypersensitivity for individuals allergic to pork products
• Decreased Na, increase K for dependent edema
• Increased protein diet for N loss
• Gel at room temp, give deep IM using 21G needle
IV
Give over 2 min; dilute 25 U/1 ml sterile H_2O or NS or 40 U/2 ml; may dilute 10-25 U/500 ml compatible sol; give over 8 hr
Additive compatibilities: Calcium gluconate, chloramphenicol, cytarabine, dimenhydrinate, erythromycin, heparin, hydrocortisone, methicillin, norepinephrine, oxytetracycline, penicillin G potassium, potassium chloride, vancomycin, vit B/C
Perform/provide:
• Storage in refrigerator of unused portion; use within 24 hr
Evaluate:
• Therapeutic response: absence of inflammation, pain, increased muscle strength in myasthenia gravis
Teach patient/family:
• To avoid vaccinations during drug treatment
• To maintain hydration up to 2 L/day unless contraindicated
• To avoid OTC products: salicylates, products with alcohol
• Not to discontinue medication abruptly; adrenal crisis may occur; should be tapered over several wk
• To wear Medic Alert ID specifying steroid therapy
• That drug does not cure condition, only decreases symptoms
• To notify prescriber of infection: fever, sore throat, muscular pain
• To tell patient to notify anyone involved in dental or medical care that this drug is being taken

---

cortisone (R)

(kor′ti-sone)
Cortone Acetate
Func. class.: Corticosteroid, synthetic
Chem. class.: Glucocorticoid, short-acting

Action: Decreases inflammation by suppression of migration of polymorphonuclear leukocytes, fibroblasts, reversal of increased capillary permeability and lysosomal stabilization

Uses: Inflammation, severe allergy, adrenal insufficiency, collagen disorders, respiratory, dermatologic disorders

Dosage and routes:
• *Adult:* **PO/IM** 25-300 mg qd or q2d, titrated to response
• *Child:* **PO** 2.5-10 mg/kg/day; **IM** 1-5 mg/kg/day

Available forms: Tabs 5, 10, 25 mg; inj 50 mg/ml

Side effects/adverse reactions:
INTEG: Acne, poor wound healing, ecchymosis, bruising, petechiae
CNS: Depression, flushing, sweating, headache, mood changes
*CV: Hypertension, **circulatory collapse**, **thrombophlebitis**, **embolism,** tachycardia, **necrotizing angiitis, CHF,** edema
*HEMA: **Thrombocytopenia***
MS: Fractures, osteoporosis, weakness
*GI: Diarrhea, nausea, abdominal distention, **GI hemorrhage,** increased appetite, **pancreatitis***
EENT: Fungal infections, increased intraocular pressure, blurred vision

Contraindications: Psychosis, hypersensitivity, idiopathic thrombocytopenia, acute glomerulonephritis, amebiasis, fungal infections, nonasthmatic bronchial disease, child <2 yr, AIDS, TB

Precautions: Pregnancy (C), lactation, diabetes mellitus, glaucoma, osteoporosis, seizure disorders, ulcerative colitis, CHF, myasthenia gravis, renal disease, esophagitis, peptic ulcer

Pharmacokinetics:
PO: Peak 2 hr, duration 1½ days
IM: Peak 20-48 hr, duration 1½ days

Interactions:
• Decreased action of cortisone: barbiturates, rifampin, phenytoin, rifampin, theophylline
• Increased GI symptoms: salicylates, indomethacin, NSAIDs
• Decreased effects of anticoagulants, antidiabetics, toxoids, vaccines, salicylates
• Increased side effects: alcohol, salicylates, indomethacin, potassium-wasting diuretics
• Increased action of cortisone: salicylates, estrogens, indomethacin, oral contraceptives, ketoconazole, macrolide antibiotics

Potassium deficiency: chronic use/abuse cascara sagrada bark, aloe, buckthorn bark/berry, rhubarb root, senna leaf/fruits

Lab test interferences:
Increase: Cholesterol, Na, blood glucose, uric acid, Ca, urine glucose
Decrease: Ca, K, T_4, T_3, thyroid ^{131}I uptake test, urine 17-OHCS, 17-KS, PBI skin allergy tests

NURSING CONSIDERATIONS
Assess:
• K, blood sugar, urine glucose while on long-term therapy; hypokalemia and hyperglycemia
• Weight daily; notify prescriber of weekly gain >5 lb
• B/P q4h, pulse; notify prescriber if chest pain occurs
• I&O ratio; be alert for decreasing urinary output and increasing edema
• Plasma cortisol levels during long-term therapy (normal level: 138-635 nmol/L SI units if drawn at 8 AM)
• Infection: fever, WBC even after withdrawal of medication; drug masks infection
• K depletion: paresthesias, fatigue, nausea, vomiting, depression, polyuria, dysrhythmias, weakness
• Edema, hypertension, cardiac symptoms
• Mental status: affect, mood, behavioral changes, aggression

Administer:

• After shaking suspension (parenteral)

• Titrated dose; use lowest effective dose

• IM inj deeply in large mass; rotate sites; avoid deltoid; use a 21G needle

• In one dose in AM to prevent adrenal suppression; avoid SC administration; tissue may be damaged

• With food or milk to decrease GI symptoms

Perform/provide:

• Assistance with ambulation in patient with bone tissue disease to prevent fractures

Evaluate:

• Therapeutic response: ease of respirations, decreased inflammation

Teach patient/family:

• That medical ID as steroid user should be carried at all times

• To notify prescriber if therapeutic response decreases; dosage adjustment may be needed

◆ Not to discontinue abruptly or adrenal crisis can result

• To avoid OTC products: salicylates, alcohol in cough products, cold preparations unless directed by prescriber

• All aspects of drug usage, including cushingoid symptoms

• The symptoms of adrenal insufficiency: nausea, anorexia, fatigue, dizziness, dyspnea, weakness, joint pain

---

cromolyn (OTC, ℞)

(kroe'moe-lin)

Crolom, Gastrocrom, Intal, Intal Nebulizer Solution, Intal Spray Aerosol, Nasalcrom, Rynacrom*

Func. class.: Antiasthmatic

Chem. class.: Mast cell stabilizer

Action: Stabilizes the membrane of the sensitized mast cell, preventing release of chemical mediators after an antigen-IgE interaction

Uses: Allergic rhinitis, severe perennial bronchial asthma, prevention of exercise-induced bronchospasm, acute bronchospasm induced by environmental pollutants, mastocytosis

Dosage and routes:

Allergic rhinitis

• *Adult and child >6 yr:* **NASAL SOL** 1 spray in each nostril tid-qid, not to exceed 6 doses/day

Bronchospasm

• *Adult and child >6 yr:* **INH** 20 mg <1 hr before exercise

Bronchial asthma

• *Adult and child >6 yr:* **INH** 20 mg qid; **NEB** 20 mg qid by nebulization

Systemic mastocytosis

• *Adult and child >12 yr:* **PO** 200 mg qid ac and hs

• *Child 2-12 yr:* **PO** 100 mg qid ½ ac and hs

Available forms: Nasal sol 5.2 mg/ metered spray (40 mg/ml); ophth sol 4%, caps for inh, 20 mg; caps for oral sol 100 mg; neb sol 20 mg/2 ml; aerosol 800 μg/actuation

Side effects/adverse reactions:

EENT: Throat irritation, cough, nasal congestion, burning eyes

CNS: Headache, dizziness, neuritis

GU: Urinary frequency, dysuria

GI: Nausea, vomiting, anorexia, dry mouth, bitter taste

INTEG: Rash, urticaria, angioedema

MS: Joint pain/swelling

Contraindications: Hypersensitivity to this drug or lactose, status asthmaticus

Precautions: Pregnancy (B), lactation, renal disease, hepatic disease, child <5 yr

Pharmacokinetics:

INH: Peak 15 min, duration 4-6 hr; excreted unchanged in feces; half-life 80 min

ORAL: Unknown

NURSING CONSIDERATIONS
Assess:

• Eosinophil count during treatment

• Respiratory status: rate, rhythm, characteristics, cough, wheezing, dyspnea

Administer:

• For oral dose, dissolve powder in caps mixed with hot water; further dilute in cold water

• By inhalation/nebulizer only

Perform/provide:

• Gargle, sip of water to decrease irritation in throat

Evaluate:

• Therapeutic response: decrease in asthmatic symptoms; congested, runny nose

Teach patient/family:

• To clear mucus before using

• Proper inhalation technique: exhale; using inhaler, inhale deeply with head tipped back to open airway; remove; hold breath; exhale; repeat until all of drug is inhaled, use demonstration; return demonstration

• That therapeutic effect may take up to 4 wk

• Not to swallow capsule

• That drug is preventive only, not restorative

---

cyanocobalamin (vit B$_{12}$)/hydroxocobalamin (vit B$_{12}$a) (OTC, R)

(sye-an-oh-koe-bal'a-min)

Bedoz*, B$_{12}$Resin, Cobex, Crystamine, Crysti-12, Cyanabin*, Cyanoject, Cyomin, Ener-B, Pernavite, Redisol, Rubesol-1000, Rubion*, Rubramin PC, Sytobex, Vitamin B$_{12}$

Func. class.: Vit B$_{12}$, water-soluble vitamin

Action: Needed for adequate nerve functioning, protein and carbohydrate metabolism, normal growth, RBC development, cell reproduction

Uses: Vit B$_{12}$ deficiency, pernicious anemia, vit B$_{12}$ malabsorption syndrome, Schilling test, increased requirements with pregnancy, thyrotoxicosis, hemolytic anemia, hemorrhage, renal and hepatic disease

Dosage and routes:

• *Adult:* **PO** 25 µg qd × 5-10 days, maintenance 100-200 mg **IM** qmo; **IM/SC** 30-100 µg qd × 5-10 days, maintenance 100-200 µg **IM** qmo

• *Child:* **PO** 30-50 µg qd × 14 days, maintenance 100 µg **IM** qmo or more; **IM/SC** 30-50 µg qd × 14 days, maintenance 100 µg **IM** qmo or more

Pernicious anemia/malabsorption syndrome

• *Adult:* **IM** 100-1000 µg qd × 2 wk, then 100-1000 µg **IM** qmo

• *Child:* **IM** 100-500 µg over 2 wk or more given in 100-500 µg doses, then 60 µg **IM/SC** monthly

Schilling test

• *Adult and child:* **IM** 1000 µg in one dose

Available forms: Tabs 25, 50, 100,

$\Diamondsuit$ = Nursing alert $\blacksquare$ = Herb-drug interaction $\bigcirc$ = Do not crush

250, 500, 1000 μg; inj 100, 120, 1000 μg/ml

Side effects/adverse reactions:

CNS: Flushing, optic nerve atrophy

GI: Diarrhea

CV: **CHF**, peripheral vascular thrombosis, ***pulmonary edema***

INTEG: Itching, rash, pain at inj site

META: Hypokalemia

SYST: **Anaphylactic shock**

Contraindications: Hypersensitivity, optic nerve atrophy

Precautions: Pregnancy (A), lactation, children

Pharmacokinetics: Gastric intrinsic factor must be present for absorption to occur; stored in liver, kidneys, stomach; 50%-90% excreted in urine; crosses placenta, excreted in breast milk

Interactions:

• Decreased absorption: aminoglycosides, anticonvulsants, colchicine, chloramphenicol, aminosalicylic acid, K preparation, cimetidine

• Increased absorption: prednisone

Lab test interferences:

False positive: Intrinsic factor

NURSING CONSIDERATIONS

Assess:

• GI function: diarrhea, constipation

• K levels during beginning treatment

• CBC for increase in reticulocyte count during first week of therapy, then increase in RBC and hemoglobin

• Nutritional status: egg yolks, fish, organ meats, dairy products, clams, oysters: good sources of vit B_{12}

• For pulmonary edema, worsening of CHF in cardiac patients

Administer:

• With fruit juice to disguise taste; immediately after mixing

• With meals if possible for better absorption

• By IM inj for pernicious anemia for life unless contraindicated

• IV route not recommended but may be admixed in TPN solution

Additive compatibilities: Ascorbic acid, chloramphenicol, metaraminol, vit B/C

Solution compatibilities: Dextrose/Ringer's or lactated Ringer's combinations, dextrose/saline combinations, D_5W, $D_{10}W$, 0.45% NaCl, Ringer's or lactated Ringer's sol

Y-site compatibilities: Heparin, hydrocortisone, potassium chloride, vit B/C

Perform/provide:

• Protection from light and heat

Evaluate:

• Therapeutic response: decreased anorexia, dyspnea on exertion, palpitations, paresthesias, psychosis, visual disturbances

Teach patient/family:

• That treatment must continue for life for pernicious anemia

• To eat well-balanced diet

• To avoid contact with persons with infection; infections common

Treatment of overdose: Discontinue drug

---

cyclobenzaprine (℞)

(sye-kloe-ben'za-preen)

cyclobenzaprine HCl, Flexeril

Func. class.: Skeletal muscle relaxant, central acting

Chem. class.: Tricyclic amine salt

Action: Unknown; may be related to antidepressant effects

Uses: Adjunct for relief of muscle spasm and pain in musculoskeletal conditions

Dosage and routes:

• *Adult:* **PO** 10 mg tid × 1 wk, not to exceed 60 mg/day × 3 wk

---

• *Child:* 20-40 mg/kg/day in 2-4 divided doses
• *Available forms:* Tabs 10 mg
Side effects/adverse reactions:
CNS: Dizziness, weakness, drowsiness, headache, tremor, depression, insomnia, confusion, paresthesia
EENT: Diplopia, temporary loss of vision
CV: Postural hypotension, tachycardia, *dysrhythmias*
GI: Nausea, vomiting, hiccups, dry mouth, constipation
INTEG: Rash, pruritus, fever, facial flushing, sweating
GU: Urinary retention, frequency, change in libido
Contraindications: Acute recovery phase of myocardial infarction, dysrhythmias, heart block, CHF, hypersensitivity, child <12 yr, intermittent porphyria, thyroid disease
Precautions: Renal disease, hepatic disease, addictive personality, pregnancy (B), lactation, elderly
Pharmacokinetics:
PO: Onset 1 hr, peak 3-8 hr, duration 12-24 hr, half-life 1-3 days; metabolized by liver; excreted in urine; crosses placenta; excreted in breast milk
Interactions:
• Increased CNS depression: alcohol, tricyclic antidepressants, opiates, barbiturates, sedatives, hypnotics
• Do not use within 14 days of MAOI
⬤ Increased CNS depression: kava
NURSING CONSIDERATIONS
Assess:
• Blood studies: CBC, WBC, differential for blood dyscrasias
• Liver function studies: AST, ALT, alk phosphatase; hepatitis may occur
• ECG in epileptic patients; poor seizure control has occurred

• Allergic reactions: rash, fever, respiratory distress
• Severe weakness, numbness in extremities
• Psychologic dependency: increased need for medication, more frequent requests for medication, increased pain
• CNS depression: dizziness, drowsiness, psychiatric symptoms
Administer:
• With meals for GI symptoms
Perform/provide:
• Storage in tight container at room temp
• Assistance with ambulation if dizziness, drowsiness occur, especially elderly
Evaluate:
• Therapeutic response: decreased pain, spasticity; muscle spasms of acute, painful musculoskeletal conditions generally short term; long-term therapy seldom warranted
Teach patient/family:
• Not to discontinue medication abruptly; insomnia, nausea, headache, spasticity, tachycardia will occur; drug should be tapered off over 1-2 wk
• Not to take with alcohol, other CNS depressants
• To avoid hazardous activities if drowsiness/dizziness occurs
• To avoid using OTC medication: cough preparations, antihistamines, unless directed by prescriber
• To use gum, frequent sips of water for dry mouth
Treatment of overdose: Empty stomach with emesis, gastric lavage, then administer activated charcoal; use anticonvulsants if indicated; monitor cardiac function

---

◆ = Nursing alert   ▮ = Herb-drug interaction   ⊘ = Do not crush

cyclophosphamide (R)

(sye-kloe-foss'fa-mide)

Cytoxan, Neosar, Procytox*

Func. class.: Antineoplastic alkylating agent

Chem. class.: Nitrogen mustard

Action: Alkylates DNA, RNA; inhibits enzymes that allow synthesis of amino acids in proteins; is also responsible for cross-linking DNA strands; activity is not cell cycle phase specific

Uses: Hodgkin's disease; lymphomas; leukemia; cancer of female reproductive tract, lung, prostate; multiple myeloma; neuroblastoma; retinoblastoma; Ewing's sarcoma

Dosage and routes:
• *Adult:* **PO** initially 1-5 mg/kg over 2-5 days, maintenance is 1-5 mg/kg; **IV** initially 40-50 mg/kg in divided doses over 2-5 days, maintenance 10-15 mg/kg q7-10d, or 3-5 mg/kg q3d
• *Child:* **PO/IV** 2-8 mg/kg or 60-250 mg/m^2 in divided doses for 6 or more days; maintenance 10-15 mg/kg q7-10d or 30 mg/kg q3-4wk; dose should be reduced by half when bone marrow depression occurs

Renal disease
• CrCl 25-50 ml/min 50% of dose; CrCl <25 ml/min avoid use
Available forms: Inj 100, 200, 500 mg, 1, 2 g; tabs 25, 50 mg

Side effects/adverse reactions:
CV: **Cardiotoxicity** (high doses)
HEMA: **Thrombocytopenia, leukopenia, pancytopenia; myelosuppression**
GI: Nausea, vomiting, diarrhea, weight loss, colitis, **hepatotoxicity**
GU: **Hemorrhagic cystitis,** hematuria, neoplasms, amenorrhea, azoospermia, sterility, ovarian fibrosis

INTEG: *Alopecia,* dermatitis
RESP: **Fibrosis**
ENDO: Syndrome of inappropriate antidiuretic hormone (SIADH)
CNS: Headache, dizziness
Contraindications: Lactation, pregnancy (D)
Precautions: Radiation therapy
Pharmacokinetics: Metabolized by liver; excreted in urine; half-life 4-6½ hr; 50% bound to plasma proteins
Interactions:
• Increased toxicity: aminoglycosides
• Increased metabolism of cyclophosphamide: barbiturates
• Potentiation of cyclophosphamide: succinylcholine
• Increased bone marrow depression: allopurinol, thiazides
• Decreased digoxin levels: digoxin
• Decreased cyclophosphamide effect: chloramphenicol, corticosteroids
• Risk of bleeding: salicylates
Lab test interferences:
Increase: Uric acid
False positive: Pap test
False negative: PPD, mumps, trichophytin, Candida
Decrease: Pseudocholinesterase
NURSING CONSIDERATIONS
Assess:
• CBC, differential, platelet count weekly; withhold drug if WBC is <4000 or platelet count is <75,000; notify prescriber of results
• Pulmonary function tests, chest x-ray films before, during therapy; chest film should be obtained q2wk during treatment
• Renal function studies: BUN, serum uric acid, urine CrCl before, during therapy
• I&O ratio; report fall in urine output of <30 ml/hr
• Monitor temp q4h (may indicate beginning infection)

• Liver function tests before, during therapy (bilirubin, AST, ALT, LDH) as needed or monthly
• Bleeding: hematuria, guaiac, bruising or petechiae, mucosa or orifices q8h
• Dyspnea, rales, unproductive cough, chest pain, tachypnea
• Food preferences; list likes, dislikes
• Effects of alopecia on body image, discuss feelings about body changes
• Jaundice of skin, sclera; dark urine; clay-colored stools; itchy skin; abdominal pain; fever; diarrhea
• Edema in feet, joint pain, stomach pain, shaking
• Inflammation of mucosa, breaks in skin
• Buccal cavity q8h for dryness, sores or ulceration, white patches, oral pain, bleeding, dysphagia; obtain prescription for viscous lidocaine (Xylocaine)
◆ Symptoms indicating severe allergic reaction: rash, pruritus, urticaria, purpuric skin lesions, itching, flushing

Administer:
• In AM so drug can be eliminated before hs
• Fluids IV or PO before chemotherapy to hydrate patient
• Antacid before oral agent, give after evening meal, before bedtime
• Antiemetic 30-60 min before giving drug and prn
• Allopurinol or sodium bicarbonate to maintain uric acid levels, alkalinization of urine
IV
• IV after diluting 100 mg/5 ml of sterile H_2O or bacteriostatic H_2O; shake; let stand until clear; may be further diluted in up to 250 ml D_5 or NS; give 100 mg or less/min through 3-way stopcock of glucose or saline inf

• Using 21, 23, 25G needle; check site for irritation, phlebitis

Additive compatibilities: Cisplatin with etoposide, fluorouracil, hydroxyzine, methotrexate, methotrexate/fluorouracil, mitoxantrone, ondansetron

Solution compatibilities: Amino acids 4.25%/D_{25}, D_5/0.9% NaCl, D_5W, 0.9% NaCl

Syringe compatibilities: Bleomycin, cisplatin, doxapram, doxorubicin, droperidol, fluorouracil, furosemide, heparin, leucovorin, methotrexate, metoclopramide, mitomycin, vinblastine, vincristine

Y-site compatibilities: Allopurinol, amifostine, amikacin, ampicillin, azlocillin, aztreonam, bleomycin, cefamandole, cefazolin, cefepime, cefoperazone, cefotaxime, cefoxitin, cefuroxime, cephalothin, cephapirin, chloramphenicol, chlorpromazine, cimetidine, cisplatin, cladribine, clindamycin, dexamethasone, diphenhydramine, doxorubicin, doxorubicin liposome, doxycycline, droperidol, erythromycin, famotidine, filgrastim, fludarabine, fluorouracil, furosemide, gallium, ganciclovir, gentamicin, granisetron, heparin, hydromorphone, idarubicin, kanamycin, leucovorin, lorazepam, melphalan, methotrexate, methylprednisolone, metoclopramide, metronidazole, mezlocillin, minocycline, mitomycin, morphine, moxalactam, nafcillin, ondansetron, oxacillin, paclitaxel, penicillin G potassium, piperacillin, piperacillin/tazobactam, prochlorperazine, promethazine, propofol, ranitidine, sargramostim, sodium bicarbonate, teniposide, thiotepa, ticarcillin, ticarcillin-clavulanate, tobramycin, trimethoprim - sulfamethoxazole, vancomycin, vinblastine, vincristine, vinorelbine

---

◆ = Nursing alert   🍃 = Herb-drug interaction   🚫 = Do not crush

Perform/provide:

• Storage in tight container at room temperature

• Strict medical asepsis, protective isolation if WBC levels are low

• Increase fluid intake to 2-3 L/day to prevent urate deposits, calculi formation, reduce incidence of hemorrhagic cystitis

• Diet low in purines: organ meats (kidney, liver), dried beans, peas to maintain alkaline urine

• Rinsing of mouth tid-qid with water, club soda; brushing of teeth bid-tid with soft brush or cotton-tipped applicators for stomatitis; use unwaxed dental floss

• Warm compresses at injection site for inflammation

Evaluate:

• Therapeutic response: decreased tumor size, spread of malignancy

Teach patient/family:

• About protective isolation

• That amenorrhea can occur; reversible after stopping treatment

• To report any changes in breathing or coughing

• That hair may be lost during treatment; a wig or hairpiece may make patient feel better; new hair may be different in color, texture

• To avoid foods with citric acid, hot or rough texture

• To report any bleeding, white spots, ulcerations in mouth to prescriber; tell patient to examine mouth qd

• To report signs of infection: increased temperature, sore throat, flu symptoms

• To report signs of anemia: fatigue, headache, faintness, shortness of breath, irritability

• To report bleeding: avoid use of razors, commercial mouthwash

• To avoid use of aspirin products, ibuprofen

cycloserine (R)

(sye-kloe-ser′een)

Seromycin

Func. class.: Antitubercular

Chem. class.: Streptomyces orchidaceus, antibiotic

Action: Inhibits cell wall synthesis, analog of D-alanine

Uses: Pulmonary tuberculosis, extrapulmonary as adjunctive

Dosage and routes:

• *Adult:* **PO** 250 mg q12h × 14 days, then 250 mg q8h × 2 wk if no signs of toxicity, then 250 mg q6h if no signs of toxicity, not to exceed 1 g/day

• *Child:* **PO** 10-20 mg/kg/day (max 0.75-1 g) in 2 divided doses

Available forms: Caps 250 mg

Side effects/adverse reactions:

INTEG: Dermatitis, photosensitivity

CV: **CHF,** dysrhythmias

CNS: Headache, anxiety, drowsiness, tremors, **convulsions,** lethargy, depression, confusion, psychosis, aggression

HEMA: **Megaloblastic anemia,** vit B$_{12}$, folic acid deficiency, leukocytosis

Contraindications: Hypersensitivity

Precautions: Pregnancy (C), children, seizure disorders, renal disease, alcoholism (chronic), depression, severe anxiety, lactation, anemia

Pharmacokinetics:

PO: Peak 3-8 hr; excreted unchanged in urine; crosses placenta; excreted in breast milk

Interactions:

• Seizures: alcohol

• May increase CNS toxicity: isoniazid, ethionamide

Lab test interferences:

Increase: AST/ALT

NURSING CONSIDERATIONS
Assess:
• Liver studies qwk: ALT, AST, bilirubin
• CBC
• Renal studies: BUN, creatinine, I&O
• Hepatic status: fatigue, jaundice, dark urine, decreased appetite
• Blood levels of drug; keep <30 μg/ml or toxicity may occur
• Mental status often: affect, mood, behavioral changes, psychosis may occur

Administer:
• Using pipette provided; use glass container to prevent adherence to sides
• After C&S is completed, qmo to detect resistance
• Pyridoxine (200-300 mg/day) if ordered to prevent neurotoxicity

Perform/provide:
• Storage in airtight container at room temp

Evaluate:
• Therapeutic response: decreased symptoms of TB

Teach patient/family:
🚫 Not to break, crush, or chew caps
• To avoid alcohol while taking drug
• That compliance with dosage schedule, length is necessary
◆ To report neurotoxicity: confusion, headache, drowsiness, tremors, paresthesias, mental changes
• To avoid hazardous activities if drowsiness or dizziness occurs

Treatment of overdose: Administer vit B$_6$, anticonvulsants, lavage, O$_2$, assisted respiration

cyclosporine (℞)
(sye'kloe-spor-een)
Neoral, Sandimmune, Sang-Cya
Func. class.: Immunosuppressant
Chem. class.: Fungus-derived peptide

Action: Produces immunosuppression by inhibiting lymphocytes (T)
Uses: Organ transplants to prevent rejection, rheumatoid arthritis, psoriasis
Investigational uses: Pancreas, bone marrow, heart/lung transplantation
Dosage and routes:
• *Adult and child:* **PO** 15 mg/kg several hr before surgery, daily for 2 wk, reduce dosage by 2.5 mg/kg/wk to 5-10 mg/kg/day; **IV** 5-6 mg/kg several hr before surgery, daily, switch to PO form as soon as possible
Available forms: Oral sol 100 mg/ml; inj 50 mg/ml; soft gelatin caps 25, 50, 100 mg
Side effects/adverse reactions:
GI: Nausea, vomiting, diarrhea, *oral Candida, gum hyperplasia, **hepatotoxicity,*** pancreatitis
INTEG: Rash, acne, *hirsutism*
CNS: Tremors, headache
*GU: **Albuminuria, hematuria, proteinuria, renal failure***
Contraindications: Hypersensitivity
Precautions: Severe renal disease, severe hepatic disease, pregnancy (C)
Pharmacokinetics: Peak 4 hr, highly protein bound, half-life (biphasic) 1.2 hr, 25 hr; metabolized in liver; excreted in feces; crosses placenta; excreted in breast milk

---

◆ = Nursing alert   🌿 = Herb-drug interaction   🚫 = Do not crush

Interactions:
• Increased levels of: digoxin, etoposide
• Increased action of cyclosporine: amiodarone, amphotericin B, androgens, azole antifungals, calcium channel blockers, carvedilol, cimetidine, colchicine, corticosteroids, foscarnet, imipenem-cilastatin, ketoconazole, macrolides, metoclopramide, oral contraceptives
• Decreased action of cyclosporine: carbamazepine, phenobarbital, phenytoin, probucol, rifamycins, sulfamethoxazole/trimethoprim, terbinafine
• Drug/food: Slowed metabolism of drug: grapefruit

NURSING CONSIDERATIONS
Assess:
• Renal studies: BUN, creatinine at least monthly during treatment, 3 mo after treatment
• Liver function studies: alk phosphatase, AST, ALT, bilirubin
• Drug blood level during treatment
• Hepatotoxicity: dark urine, jaundice, itching, light-colored stools; drug should be discontinued
• For nephrotoxicity: 6 wk post op, acute tubular necrosis, CyA trough level >200 ng/ml, gradual rise in Cr (0.15 mg/dl/day), Cr plateau <25% above baseline, intracapsular pressure <40 mm Hg
Administer:
• For several days before transplant surgery
• With corticosteroids
• With meals for GI upset or in chocolate milk
• With oral antifungal for *Candida* infections
IV
• After diluting each 50 mg/20-100 ml of NS or D_5W; run over 2-6 hr; use an infusion pump, glass inf bottles only

Additive compatibilities: Ciprofloxacin
Solution compatibilities: D_5W, NaCl 0.9%
Y-site compatibilities: Cefmetazole, propofol, sargramostim
Evaluate:
• Therapeutic response: absence of rejection
Teach patient/family:
• To report fever, chills, sore throat, fatigue, since serious infections may occur
• To use contraceptive measures during treatment, for 12 wk after ending therapy
🚫 Not to break, crush, or chew caps

---

cyproheptadine (℞)
(si-proe-hep'ta-deen)
cyproheptadine HCl,
Periactin
Func. class.: Antihistamine, H_1-receptor antagonist
Chem. class.: Piperidine

Action: Acts on blood vessels, GI, respiratory system by competing with histamine for H_1-receptor site; decreases allergic response by blocking histamine
Uses: Allergy symptoms, rhinitis, pruritus, cold, urticaria
Investigational uses: Appetite stimulant, management of vascular headache
Dosage and routes:
• *Adult:* **PO** 4 mg tid-qid, not to exceed 0.5 mg/kg/day
• *Child 7-14 yr:* **PO** 4 mg bid-tid, not to exceed 16 mg/day
• *Child 2-6 yr:* **PO** 2 mg bid-tid, not to exceed 12 mg/day
Available forms: Tabs 4 mg; syr 2 mg/5 ml

Side effects/adverse reactions:
HEMA: **Hemolytic anemia, leukopenia, thrombocytosis, agranulocytosis**
SYST: **Anaphylactic shock**
CNS: Dizziness, drowsiness, poor coordination, fatigue, anxiety, euphoria, confusion, paresthesia, neuritis
CV: Hypotension, palpitations, tachycardia
RESP: Increased thick secretions, wheezing, chest tightness
GI: Constipation, dry mouth, nausea, vomiting, anorexia, diarrhea, weight gain
INTEG: Rash, urticaria, photosensitivity
GU: Retention, dysuria, frequency, increased appetite
EENT: Blurred vision, dilated pupils; tinnitus; nasal stuffiness; dry nose, throat, mouth

Contraindications: Hypersensitivity to H_1-receptor antagonist, acute asthma attack, lower respiratory tract disease

Precautions: Increased intraocular pressure, renal disease, cardiac disease, hypertension, bronchial asthma, seizure disorder, stenosed peptic ulcers, hyperthyroidism, prostatic hypertrophy, bladder neck obstruction, pregnancy (B), lactation, elderly

Pharmacokinetics:
PO: Duration 4-6 hr; metabolized in liver; excreted by kidneys; excreted in breast milk

Interactions:
• Increased CNS depression: barbiturates, opiates, hypnotics, tricyclic antidepressants, alcohol
• Increased effect of cyproheptadine: MAOIs
🌿 Increased CNS depression: kava
🌿 Increased anticholinergic effect: henbane leaf

Lab test interferences:
False negative: Skin allergy tests

NURSING CONSIDERATIONS
Assess:
• I&O ratio; be alert for urinary retention, frequency, dysuria; drug should be discontinued
• CBC during long-term therapy
• Respiratory status: rate, rhythm, increase in bronchial secretions, wheezing, chest tightness
• Cardiac status: palpitations, increased pulse, hypotension
Administer:
• With meals for GI symptoms; absorption may slightly decrease
Perform/provide:
• Hard candy, gum, frequent rinsing of mouth for dryness
• Storage in airtight container at room temp
Evaluate:
• Therapeutic response: absence of running or congested nose, rashes
Teach patient/family:
• All aspects of drug use; to notify prescriber of confusion, sedation, hypotension
• That this drug decreases anticoagulant (oral) effect
• To avoid driving, other hazardous activity if drowsiness occurs, especially elderly
• To avoid concurrent use of alcohol, other CNS depressants
Treatment of overdose: Ipecac syrup or lavage, diazepam, vasopressors, barbiturates (short-acting)

◆ = Nursing alert   🌿 = Herb-drug interaction   🚫 = Do not crush

cytarabine (Rx)

(sye-tare′a-been)
Ara-C, Cytosar*, Cytosar-U,
cytosine arabinoside,
DepoCyt, Tarabine PFS

Func. class.: Antineoplastic, antimetabolite

Chem. class.: Pyrimidine nucleoside

Action: Competes with physiologic substrate of DNA synthesis, thus interfering with cell replication in the S phase of the cell cycle (before mitosis)

Uses: Acute myelocytic leukemia, acute lymphocytic leukemia, chronic myelocytic leukemia, lymphomatous meningitis, and in combination for non-Hodgkin's lymphomas in children

Dosage and routes:
Acute myelocytic leukemia
• *Adult:* **IV INF** 200 mg/m^2/day × 5 days; **INTRATHECAL** 5-50 mg/m^2/day × 3 days/wk or 30 mg/m^2/day q4d

Lymphomatous meningitis
Liposomal (DepoCyt): Adult intrathecally: 50 mg q14day × 2 doses (wk 1, 3) then 50 mg q14day × 3 doses (wk 5, 7, 9) followed by 1 dose wk 13; then 50 mg q28day × 4 doses (wk 17, 21, 25, 29); if neurotoxicity occurs, reduce dose to 25 mg, if it persists, discontinue use

In combination
• *Child:* **IV INF** 100 mg/m^2/day × 5-10 days

Available forms: Inj, intrathecal 100, 500 mg, 1, 2 g; inj 20 mg/ml; liposomal 10 mg/ml

Side effects/adverse reactions:
HEMA: Thrombophlebitis, bleeding, **thrombocytopenia, leukopenia, myelosuppression, anemia**
GI: Nausea, vomiting, anorexia, diarrhea, stomatitis, **hepatotoxicity,** abdominal pain, hematemesis, **GI hemorrhage**
EENT: Sore throat, conjunctivitis
GU: Urinary retention, **renal failure, hyperuricemia**
INTEG: Rash, fever, freckling, cellulitis
RESP: **Pneumonia,** dyspnea
CV: Chest pain, **cardiopathy**
CNS: Neuritis, dizziness, headache, personality changes, ataxia, mechanical dysphasia, **coma**
CYTARABINE SYNDROME: Fever, myalgia, bone pain, chest pain, *rash,* conjunctivitis, malaise (6-12 hr after administration)

Contraindications: Hypersensitivity, infants, pregnancy (D)
Precautions: Renal disease, hepatic disease, lactation
Pharmacokinetics:
INTRATHECAL: Half-life 2 hr; metabolized in liver; excreted in urine (primarily inactive metabolite); crosses blood-brain barrier, placenta
IV: Distribution half-life 10 min, elimination half-life 1-3 hr
Interactions:
• Increased toxicity: radiation or other antineoplastics
• Decreased effects of oral digoxin

NURSING CONSIDERATIONS
Assess:
• CBC (RBC, Hct, Hgb), differential, platelet count weekly; withhold drug if WBC is <4000/mm^3, platelet count is <75,000/mm^3, or RBC, Hct, Hgb low; notify prescriber of these results
• Renal function studies: BUN, serum uric acid, urine creatinine clearance, electrolytes before and during therapy
• I&O ratio; report fall in urine output to <30 ml/hr
• Monitor temp q4h; fever may indicate beginning infection; no rectal temperatures

• Liver function tests before and during therapy: bilirubin, ALT, AST, alk phosphatase, as needed or monthly; check for jaundice of skin, sclera; dark urine; clay-colored stools; itchy skin; abdominal pain; fever; diarrhea

• Blood uric acid during therapy

◆ Cytarabine syndrome 6-12hr after inf: fever, myalgia, bone pain, chest pain, rash, conjunctivitis, malaise; corticosteroids may be ordered

• Bleeding: hematuria, heme-positive stools, bruising or petechiae, mucosa or orifices q8h

• Dyspnea, rales, unproductive cough, chest pain, tachypnea, fatigue, increased pulse, pallor, lethargy; personality changes, with high doses

• Edema in feet, joint pain, stomach pain, shaking

• Buccal cavity q8h for dryness, sores or ulceration, white patches, oral pain, bleeding, dysphagia

• Local irritation, pain, burning, discoloration at injection site

• GI symptoms: frequency of stools, cramping

• Acidosis, signs of dehydration: rapid respirations, poor skin turgor, decreased urine output, dry skin, restlessness, weakness

Administer:

• Antiemetic 30-60 min before giving drug and prn

• Allopurinol or sodium bicarbonate to maintain uric acid levels and alkalinization of the urine

• Topical or systemic analgesics for pain

• Transfusion for anemia

• Antispasmodic for GI symptoms

• Liposomal: withdraw drug immediately before use; use within 4 hr, do not save unused portions, or use in-line filter; give directly into CSF by intraventricular reservoir or by direct inj into lumbar site

• Give slowly over 1-5 min, follow with lumbar puncture, instruct patient to lie flat, give dexamethasone 4 mg bid PO or IV × 5 days beginning on day of liposomal inj

IV

• After diluting 100 mg/5 ml of sterile H_2O for inj; given by direct IV over 1-3 min through free-flowing tubing (IV); may be further diluted in 50-100 ml NS or D_5W, given over 30 min to 24 hr depending on dose

Additive compatibilities: Corticotropin, daunorubicin with etoposide, etoposide, hydroxyzine, lincomycin, mitoxantrone, ondansetron, potassium chloride, prednisolone, sodium bicarbonate, vincristine

Solution compatibilities: Amino acids, D_5/LR, D_5/0.2% NaCl, D_5/0.9% NaCl, D_{10}/0.9% NaCl, D_5W, invert sugar 10% in electrolyte #1, Ringer's LR, 0.9% NaCl, sodium lactate ⅙ mol/L, TPN #57

Syringe compatibilities: Metoclopramide

Y-site compatibilities: Amifostine, amsacrine, aztreonam, cefepime, chlorpromazine, cimetidine, cladribine, dexamethasone, diphenhydramine, doxorubicin liposome, droperidol, famitidine, filgrastim, fludarabine, gentamicin, granisetron, heparin, hydrocortisone, hydromorphone, idarubicin, lorazepam, melphalan, methotrexate, methylprednisolone, metoclopramide, morphine, ondansetron, paclitaxel, piperacillin/tazobactam, prochlorperazine, promethazine, propofol, ranitidine, sargramostim, sodium bicarbonate, teniposide, thiotepa, vinorelbine

Perform/provide:

• Strict medical asepsis and protective isolation if WBC levels are low

---

◆ = Nursing alert   ⧄ = Herb-drug interaction   ⃠ = Do not crush

• Increase fluid intake to 2-3 L/day to prevent urate deposits and calculi formation, unless contraindicated

• Diet low in purines: absence of organ meats (kidney, liver), dried beans, peas to prevent increased urate deposits

• Rinsing of mouth tid-qid with water, club soda; brushing of teeth bid-tid with soft brush or cotton-tipped applicators for stomatitis; use unwaxed dental floss

Evaluate:

• Therapeutic response: decreased tumor size, spread of malignancy

Teach patient/family:

• To report any coughing, chest pain, changes in breathing; may indicate beginning pneumonia

• To avoid foods with citric acid, hot or rough texture if stomatitis is present

• To report stomatitis: any bleeding, white spots, ulcerations in mouth; tell patient to examine mouth qd, report any symptoms; neurotoxicity

• To report signs of infection: increased temperature, sore throat, flu symptoms; neurotoxicity

• To report signs of anemia: fatigue, headache, faintness, shortness of breath, irritability

• To report bleeding; avoid use of razors, commercial mouthwash

• To avoid use of aspirin products or ibuprofen

---

dacarbazine (℞)

(da-kar′ba-zeen)

dacarbazine, DTIC*, DTIC-Dome

Func. class.: Antineoplastic alkylating agent

Chem. class.: Cytotoxic triazine

Action: Alkylates DNA, RNA; inhibits enzymes that allow synthesis of amino acids in proteins; also responsible for cross-linking DNA strands; activity is not cell cycle phase specific

Uses: Hodgkin's disease, sarcomas, neuroblastoma, malignant melanoma

Dosage and routes:

Malignant melanoma

• *Adult:* IV 2-4.5 mg/kg or 250 mg/m^2 qd × 5 days; repeat q3wk depending on response

Hodgkin's disease

• *Adult:* IV 150 mg/m^2 qd × 5 days with other agents, repeat q4wk; or 375 mg/m^2 on day 1 when given in combination, repeat q15day

• *Available forms:* Inj 100, 200 mg

Side effects/adverse reactions:

HEMA: ***Thrombocytopenia, leukopenia,*** anemia

GI: Nausea, anorexia, vomiting, ***hepatotoxicity*** (rare)

CNS: Facial paresthesia, flushing, fever, malaise

INTEG: Alopecia, dermatitis, pain at injection site

Contraindications: Lactation

Precautions: Radiation therapy, pregnancy (1st trimester) (C)

Pharmacokinetics: Metabolized by liver; excreted in urine; half-life 35 min, terminal 5 hr, 5% protein bound

Interactions:

• Decreased effectiveness of dacarbazine: phenytoin, phenobarbital

• Toxicity: bone marrow suppressants

• Bleeding: salicylates, anticoagulants

NURSING CONSIDERATIONS

Assess:

• CBC, differential, platelet count weekly; withhold drug if WBC <4000 or platelet count <75,000; notify prescriber of results

• Monitor temp q4h (may indicate beginning infection)

• Liver function tests before, during therapy (bilirubin, AST, ALT, LDH) as needed or monthly

• Bleeding: hematuria, guaiac, bruising or petechiae, mucosa or orifices q8h

• Effects of alopecia on body image, discuss feelings about body changes

• Jaundice of skin, sclera; dark urine; clay-colored stools; itchy skin; abdominal pain; fever; diarrhea

• Inflammation of mucosa, breaks in skin

Administer:

• Antiemetic 30-60 min before giving drug to prevent vomiting

• Antibiotics for prophylaxis of infection

IV

• After diluting 100 mg/9.9 ml of sterile H_2O for inj (10 mg/ml), give by direct IV over 1 min through Y-tube or 3-way stopcock; may be further diluted in 50-250 ml D_5W or NS for inj, given as an inf over ½ hr

• Watch for extravasation; give Na thiosulfate 10% 4 ml plus sterile H_2O 5 ml, 3-5 ml SC if needed

Additive compatibilities: Bleomycin, carmustine, cyclophosphamide, cytarabine, dactinomycin, doxorubicin, fluorouracil, mercaptopurine, methotrexate, ondansetron, vinblastine

Additive incompatibilities: Hydrocortisone sodium succinate, cysteine

Y-site compatibilities: Amifostine, aztreonam, filgrastim, fludarabine, granisetron, melphalan, ondansetron, paclitaxel, sargramostim, teniposide, thiotepa, vinorelbine

Perform/provide:

• Storage in light-resistant container, dry area

• Strict medical asepsis, protective isolation if WBC levels are low

• Increase fluid intake to 2-3 L/day to prevent urate deposits, calculi formation

• Warm compresses at infusion site for inflammation

Evaluate:

• Therapeutic response: decreased tumor size, spread of malignancy

Teach patient/family:

• That patient should avoid prolonged exposure to sun

• That hair may be lost during treatment; a wig or hairpiece may make the patient feel better; new hair may be different in color, texture

• To report signs of infection: fever, sore throat, flu symptoms

• To report signs of anemia: fatigue, headache, faintness, shortness of breath, irritability

• To report bleeding; avoid use of razors, commercial mouthwash

• To avoid use of aspirin products or ibuprofen

---

daclizumab (℞)

(dah-kliz'uh-mab)

Zenapax

Func. class.: Immunosuppressive

Chem. class.: Humanized IgG1 monoclonal antibody

Action: Binds to the IL-2 (interleukin-2) receptor antagonist

Uses: Acute allograft rejection in renal transplant patients

Dosage and routes:

• *Adult:* IV 1 mg/kg as part of a regimen that includes cyclosporine and corticosteroids, mix calculated vol with 50 ml of 0.9% NaCl and give via peripheral/central vein over 15 min

Available forms: Inj 25 mg/ml

◆ = Nursing alert   🍃 = Herb-drug interaction   🚫 = Do not crush

Side effects/adverse reactions:
CNS: Chills, tremors, headache, prickly sensation
*RESP: Dyspnea, wheezing, **pulmonary edema,*** coughing, atelectasis, congestion, hypoxia
GI: Vomiting, nausea, diarrhea, constipation, abdominal pain, pyrosis
CV: Hypertension, ***tachycardia, thrombosis,*** bleeding
GU: Oliguria, dysuria, ***renal tubular necrosis,*** renal damage, ***hydronephrosis***
INTEG: Impaired wound healing
Contraindications: Hypersensitivity
Precautions: Pregnancy (C), child <2 yr, lactation, elderly
NURSING CONSIDERATIONS
Assess:
• Blood studies: Hgb, WBC, platelets during treatment qmo; if leukocytes are <3000/mm³, drug should be discontinued
• Liver function studies: alk phosphatase, AST, ALT, bilirubin
• Hepatotoxicity: dark urine, jaundice, itching, light-colored stools; drug should be discontinued
• For anaphylaxis, have corticosteroids, epinephrine available
Administer:
• All other medications PO if possible
• Avoid IM injection, since infection may occur
• Protect undiluted sol from direct light; should be used with drugs for immunosuppression
Solution compatibilities: 0.9% NaCl
Evaluate:
• Therapeutic response: absence of graft rejection
Teach patient/family:
• To report fever, chills, sore throat, fatigue, since serious infection may occur

• To use contraception (women) before, during, and for 4 mo after treatment
• To avoid vaccinations during treatment
• To increase fluid intake during treatment

---

dactinomycin (Rx)
(dak-ti-noe-mye′sin)
Cosmegen
Func. class.: Antineoplastic, antibiotic

Action: Inhibits DNA, RNA, protein synthesis; derived from *Streptomyces parvullus;* replication is decreased by binding to DNA, which causes strand splitting; cell cycle nonspecific; a vesicant
Uses: Sarcomas, melanomas, trophoblastic tumors in women, testicular cancer, Wilms' tumor, rhabdomyosarcoma
Dosage and routes:
• *Adult:* **IV** 500 µg/m²/day × 5 days; stop drug for 2-4 wk; then repeat cycle
• *Child:* **IV** 15 µg/kg/day × 5 days, not to exceed 500 µg/day; stop drug until bone marrow recovery, then repeat cycle
Available forms: Inj 0.5 mg/vial
Side effects/adverse reactions:
*HEMA: **Thrombocytopenia, leukopenia, aplastic anemia***
GI: Nausea, vomiting, anorexia, stomatitis, ***hepatotoxicity,*** abdominal pain, diarrhea
INTEG: Rash, alopecia, pain at injection site, folliculitis, acne, desquamation, ***extravasation***
EENT: Chelitis, dysphagia, esophagitis
CNS: Malaise, fatigue, lethargy, fever
MS: Myalgia
Contraindications: Hypersensitivity, herpes infection, child <6 mo

Precautions: Renal disease, hepatic disease, pregnancy (C), lactation, bone marrow depression

Pharmacokinetics: Half-life 36 hr; IV onset 2-5 min; concentrates in kidneys, liver, spleen; does not cross blood-brain barrier; excreted in feces and urine

Interactions:
• Increased toxicity: other antineoplastics, radiation

Lab test interferences:
Increase: Uric acid

NURSING CONSIDERATIONS
Assess:
• CBC, differential, platelet count weekly; withhold drug if WBC is <4000/mm^3 or platelet count is <75,000/mm^3; notify prescriber
• Renal function studies: BUN, serum uric acid, urine CrCl, electrolytes before, during therapy
• I&O ratio; report fall in urine output to <30 ml/hr
• Monitor temp q4h; fever may indicate beginning infection
• Liver function tests before, during therapy: bilirubin, AST, ALT, alk phosphatase, as needed or monthly; check for jaundice of skin, sclera; dark urine; clay-colored stools; itchy skin; abdominal pain; fever; diarrhea
• Bleeding: hematuria, guaiac stools, bruising, petechiae, mucosa or orifices q8h
• Food preferences; list likes, dislikes
• Effects of alopecia on body image; discuss feelings about body changes
• Inflammation of mucosa, breaks in skin
• Buccal cavity q8h for dryness, sores, ulceration, white patches, oral pain, bleeding, dysphagia
◆ Symptoms indicating severe allergic reaction: rash, pruritus, urticaria, purpuric skin lesions, itching, flushing

• GI symptoms: frequency of stools, cramping, nausea, vomiting, anorexia
• Acidosis, signs of dehydration: rapid respirations, poor skin turgor, decreased urine output, dry skin, restlessness, weakness, sunken eyeball in children

Administer:
• Antiemetic 30-60 min before giving drug to prevent vomiting
IV
• After diluting 0.5 mg/1.1 ml of sterile H$_2$O for inj without preservative; use 2.2 ml (0.25 mg/ml), give by direct IV at 0.5 mg or less/min through Y-tube or 3-way stopcock if inf in progress; may be further diluted if required in 50 ml D$_5$W or NS for infusion; run over 10-15 min; change needles between reconstitution and direct IV administration
• Hydrocortisone, sodium thiosulfate to infiltration area, and ice compress after stopping infusion

Y-site compatibilities: Allopurinol, amifostine, aztreonam, cefepime, fludarabine, granisetron, melphalan, ondansetron, sargramostim, teniposide, thiotepa, vinorelbine

Perform/provide:
• Strict hand-washing technique, gloves and protective covering
• Liquid diet: carbonated beverages; gelatin may be added if patient is not nauseated or vomiting
• Rinsing of mouth tid-qid with water, club soda; brushing of teeth bid-qid with soft brush or cotton-tipped applicators for stomatitis; use unwaxed dental floss to prevent injury
• Storage in cool, dark environment; do not expose to bright light or freeze

Evaluate:
• Therapeutic response: decreased tumor size, spread of malignancy

Teach patient/family:
• That contraception is needed dur-

ing treatment and for 4-6 mo after discontinuing therapy

• To avoid vaccinations without order by prescriber

• That hair may be lost during treatment after 1-2 wk and that wig or hairpiece may make patient feel better; that new hair may be different in color, texture

• To avoid foods with citric acid, hot or rough texture when stomatitis is present

• To report any bleeding, white spots, ulcerations in mouth to prescriber; tell patient to examine mouth qd

• To avoid crowds, persons with known infection when granulocyte count is low

---

dalteparin (R)
(dahl'ta-pear-in)
Fragmin
Func. class.: Anticoagulant
Chem. class.: Low molecular weight heparin

Action: Prevents conversion of fibrinogen to fibrin and prothrombin to thrombin by enhancing inhibitory effects of antithrombin III

Uses: Unstable angina/non-Q-wave MI; prevention of deep vein thrombosis in abdominal surgery patients

Investigational uses: Systemic anticoagulation in venous/arterial thromboembolic complications

Dosage and routes:
• *Adult:* SC 2500 IU each day starting 1-2 hr prior to surgery and repeat qd × 5-10 days postoperatively; to be used SC only

Unstable angina/non-Q-wave MI
• *Adult:* SC 120 IU/kg, do not exceed 10,000 IU q12h with concurrent aspirin, continue until stable

Systemic anticoagulation
• *Adult:* SC 200 IU/kg qd or 100 IU/kg bid

Available forms: Prefilled syringes, 2500, 5000 IU/0.2 ml; 10,000 IU multidose vials

Side effects/adverse reactions:
CNS: ***Intracranial bleeding***
SYST: Hypersensitivity, ***hemorrhage, anaphylaxis*** possible
HEMA: ***Thrombocytopenia***
INTEG: Pruritus, superficial wound infection

Contraindications: Hypersensitivity to this drug, heparin, or other anticoagulants; hemophilia, leukemia with bleeding, thrombocytopenic purpura, cerebrovascular hemorrhage, cerebral aneurysm, severe hypertension, other severe cardiac disease

Precautions: Elderly, pregnancy (B), hepatic disease, severe renal disease, blood dyscrasias, subacute bacterial endocarditis, acute nephritis, lactation, children, recent childbirth, peptic ulcer disease, pericarditis, pericardial effusion, recent lumbar puncture, vasculitis, other diseases where bleeding is possible

Pharmacokinetics: Excreted by kidneys, half-life 2 hr, peak 4 hr, onset and duration unknown

Interactions:
• Increased risk of bleeding: aspirin, oral anticoagulants, platelet inhibitors

⚫ Possible increased risk of bleeding: bromelain, cinchona bark

NURSING CONSIDERATIONS
Assess:
• For blood studies (Hct, occult blood in stools) during treatment since bleeding can occur

◆ For bleeding gums, petechiae, ecchymosis, black tarry stools, hematuria, epistaxis, decrease in Hct, B/P; may indicate bleeding, possible hemorrhage; notify prescriber immediately, drug should be discontinued

• For hypersensitivity: fever, skin

---

rash, urticaria; notify prescriber immediately

• For needed dosage change q1-2wk; dose may need to be decreased if bleeding occurs

Administer:

• Do not give IM or IV drug route; approved is SC only; do not mix with other inj or sol

• By SC only; have patient sit or lie down; SC inj may be 2 in from umbilicus in a U-shape, upper outer side of thigh or upper outer quadrangle of the buttocks; rotate inj sites

• Changing needles is not recommended

Evaluate:

• Therapeutic response: absence of deep-vein thrombosis

Teach patient/family:

• To avoid OTC preparations that contain aspirin; other anticoagulants, serious drug interaction may occur

• To use soft-bristle toothbrush to avoid bleeding gums, avoid contact sports, use electric razor, avoid IM injection

• To report any signs of bleeding: gums, under skin, urine, stools; unusual bruising

Treatment of overdose: Protamine sulfate 1% given IV; 1 mg protamine/100 anti-Xa IU of dalteparin given

---

danaparoid (℞)

(dan-a-pair′oid)

Orgaran

Func. class.: Anticoagulant

Chem. class.: Low molecular weight heparin

Action: Prevents conversion of fibrinogen to fibrin and prothrombin to thrombin by enhancing inhibitory effects of antithrombin III

Uses: Prevention of vein thrombosis in hemodialysis, stroke, elective surgery for malignancy or total hip replacement, hip fracture surgery

Dosage and routes:

Prevention of venous thrombosis

• *Adult:* **SC** 750 anti-Xa units bid × 7-10 days

Hemodialysis

• *Adult:* **SC** 2400-4800 anti-Xa units given predialysis

Available forms: Inj 750 anti-Xa units/0.6 ml

Side effects/adverse reactions:

SYST: Hypersensitivity, ***hemorrhage***

HEMA: ***Thrombocytopenia***

INTEG: Rash

CV: ***Hemorrhage***

Contraindications: Hypersensitivity to this drug, sulfites, pork; hemophilia, leukemia with bleeding, thrombocytopenia, purpura, cerebrovascular hemorrhage, cerebral aneurysm, severe hypertension, other severe cardiac disease

Precautions: Hypersensitivity to heparin, elderly, pregnancy (B), hepatic disease, severe renal disease, blood dyscrasias, subacute bacterial endocarditis, acute nephritis, lactation, children, recent childbirth, peptic ulcer disease, pericarditis, pericardial effusion, recent lumbar puncture, vasculitis, other diseases where bleeding is possible

Pharmacokinetics: Excreted by kidneys, half-life 2-3 hr, peak 4 hr

Interactions:

• Increased risk of bleeding: aspirin, oral anticoagulants, platelet inhibitors

🌿 Increased risk of bleeding: bromelain, cinchona bark

NURSING CONSIDERATIONS

Assess:

• For blood studies (Hct, occult blood in stools) during treatment since bleeding can occur; aPTT, ACT, antifactor Xa test, platelets

---

◆ = Nursing alert   🌿 = Herb-drug interaction   🚫 = Do not crush

• For bleeding gums, petechiae, ecchymosis, black tarry stools, hematuria, epistaxis, decrease in Hct, B/P; may indicate bleeding, possible hemorrhage; notify prescriber immediately, drug should be discontinued

• For hypersensitivity: fever, skin, rash, urticaria; notify prescriber immediately

• For needed dosage change q1-2wk; dose may need to be decreased if bleeding occurs

Administer:

• By SC, have patient sit or lie down; SC inj may be around the navel in a U-shape, upper outer side of thigh or upper outer quadrangle of the buttocks; rotate inj sites

• Changing needles is not recommended

Evaluate:

• Therapeutic response: absence of deep-vein thrombosis

Teach patient/family:

• To avoid OTC preparations that may cause serious drug interactions unless directed by prescriber; may contain aspirin, other anticoagulants

• To use soft-bristle toothbrush to avoid bleeding gums, avoid contact sports, use electric razor, avoid IM injection

• To report any signs of bleeding: gums, under skin, urine, stools; unusual bruising

Treatment of overdose: Protamine sulfate 1% given IV; 1 mg protamine/100 anti-Xa IU of danaparoid given

---

danazol (R)

(da′na-zole)

Cyclomen*, danazol, Danocrine

Func. class.: Androgen

Chem. class.: α-Ethinyl testosterone derivative

D

Action: Atrophy of endometrial tissue; decreases FSH, LH, which are controlled by pituitary; this leads to amenorrhea/anovulation

Uses: Endometriosis, prevention of hereditary angioedema, fibrocystic breast disease

Dosage and routes:

Endometriosis

• *Adult:* **PO** 100-500 mg bid uninterrupted for 3-9 mo

Fibrocystic breast disease

• *Adult:* **PO** 100-400 mg qd in 2 divided doses × 2-6 mo

Hereditary angioedema prevention

• *Adult:* **PO** 200 mg bid-tid until desired response, then decrease dose to 100 mg at 1-3 mo intervals

Available forms: Caps 50, 100, 200 mg

Side effects/adverse reactions:

INTEG: Rash, acneiform lesions, oily hair, skin, flushing, sweating, acne vulgaris, alopecia, hirsutism, pruritis

CNS: Dizziness, headache, fatigue, tremors, paresthesias, flushing, sweating, anxiety, lability, insomnia, carpal tunnel syndrome

MS: Cramps, spasms

CV: Increased B/P

GU: Hematuria, amenorrhea, atrophic vaginitis, decreased libido, decreased breast size, clitoral hypertrophy, testicular atrophy

GI: Nausea, vomiting, constipation, weight gain, ***cholestatic jaundice***

EENT: Conjunctival edema, nasal congestion

ENDO: Abnormal GTT

Contraindications: Severe renal, severe cardiac, severe hepatic disease, hypersensitivity, genital bleeding (abnormal), pregnancy (X)

Precautions: Migraine headaches, seizure disorders

Interactions:

• Increased prothrombin time: anticoagulants

• Increased carbamazepine level

• Nephrotoxicity: cyclosporine

Lab test interferences:

Increase: Cholesterol

Decrease: Cholesterol, T_4, T_3, thyroid ^{131}I uptake test, 17-KS, PBI

Interference: GTT

NURSING CONSIDERATIONS
Assess:

• K, blood sugar, urine glucose while on long-term therapy

• Weight daily; notify prescriber if weekly weight gain is >5 lb; drug should be decreased or discontinued

• I&O ratio; be alert for decreasing urinary output, increasing edema

• Edema, hypertension, cardiac symptoms, jaundice

• Mental status: affect, mood, behavioral changes, aggression, sleep disorders, depression, anxiety, lability

• Signs of virilization: deepening of voice, decreased libido, facial hair that may not be reversible

• Hypercalcemia: GI symptoms, polydipsia, polyuria, increased calcium levels above 11 mg/dl, loss of muscle tone

Administer:

• With food or milk to decrease GI symptoms (i.e., nausea, vomiting, anorexia, dyspepsia)

Perform/provide:

• Storage in airtight container at room temp; do not freeze

• ROM exercise for patients who are immobile to relieve cramps and spasms

Evaluate:

• Therapeutic response: decreased pain in endometriosis; decreased size, pain in fibrocystic breast disease

Teach patient/family:

🚫 Not to break, crush, or chew caps

• To notify prescriber if therapeutic response decreases

• Not to discontinue medication abruptly; to taper over several wk

• To report menstrual irregularities; that amenorrhea usually occurs but menstruation resumes 2-3 mo after termination of therapy without medical intervention

• About routine breast self-exam and to report any increase in nodule size

• That drug should induce anovulation; reversible within 60-90 days after drug is discontinued and treatment will need to be resumed

• That endometriosis tends to recur after drug is discontinued

• To use nonhormonal contraception

• That virilization may occur, to notify prescriber

---

dantrolene (℞)

(dan′troe-leen)

Dantrium, Dantrium Intravenous

Func. class.: Skeletal muscle relaxant, direct acting

Chem. class.: Hydantoin

Action: Interferes with intracellular release of calcium from the sarcoplasmic reticulum necessary to initiate contraction; slows catabolism in malignant hyperthermia

Uses: Spasticity in multiple sclero-

---

sis, stroke, spinal cord injury, cerebral palsy, malignant hyperthermia

Dosage and routes:

Spasticity

• *Adult:* **PO** 25 mg/day; may increase by 25-100 mg bid-qid, not to exceed 400 mg/day × 1 wk

• *Child:* **PO** 1 mg/kg/day given in divided doses bid-tid; dosage may increase gradually, not to exceed 100 mg qid

Prevention of malignant hyperthermia

• *Adult and child:* **PO** 4-8 mg/kg/day in 3-4 divided doses × 1-2 days prior to procedures, give last dose 4 hr preop; **IV** 2.5 mg/kg prior to anesthesia

Malignant hyperthermia

• *Adult and child:* **IV** 1 mg/kg, may repeat to total dose of 10 mg/kg; **PO** 4-8 mg/kg/day in 4 divided doses × 3 days to prevent further hyperthermia; post-crisis follow-up 4-8 mg/kg/day for 1-3 days

Available forms: Caps 25, 50, 100 mg; powder for inj 20 mg/vial

Side effects/adverse reactions:

CNS: Dizziness, weakness, fatigue, drowsiness, headache, disorientation, insomnia, paresthesias, tremors, *seizures*

EENT: Nasal congestion, blurred vision, mydriasis

HEMA: Eosinophilia

CV: Hypotension, chest pain, palpitations

GI: Hepatic injury, nausea, constipation, vomiting, increased AST, alk phosphatase, abdominal pain, dry mouth, anorexia, hepatitis, dyspepsia

GU: Urinary frequency, nocturia, impotence, crystalluria

INTEG: Rash, pruritus, photosensitivity

Contraindications: Hypersensitivity, compromised pulmonary function, active hepatic disease, impaired myocardial function

Precautions: Peptic ulcer disease, renal disease, hepatic disease, stroke, seizure disorder, diabetes mellitus, pregnancy (C), lactation, elderly

Pharmacokinetics:

PO: Peak 5 hr; highly protein bound; half-life 8 hr; metabolized in liver; excreted in urine (metabolites)

Interactions:

• Dysrhythmias: verapamil IV

• Increased CNS depression: alcohol, tricyclic antidepressants, opiates, barbiturates, sedatives, hypnotics, antihistamines

• Increased action: warfarin, clofibrate

• Hepatotoxicity: estrogens

• Considered incompatible in sol or syringe; compatibility unknown

NURSING CONSIDERATIONS

Assess:

• For increased seizure activity, ECG in epilepsy patient; poor seizure control has occurred

• I&O ratio; check for urinary retention, frequency, hesitancy, especially elderly

• Hepatic function by frequent determination of AST, ALT; renal function studies, BUN, creatinine, CBC

• Allergic reactions: rash, fever, respiratory distress

• Severe weakness, numbness in extremities; prescriber should be notified and drug discontinued

• Tolerance: increased need for medication, more frequent requests for medication, increased pain

• CNS depression: dizziness, drowsiness, insomnia, psychiatric symptoms

◆ Signs of hepatotoxicity: jaundice, yellow sclera, pain in abdomen, nausea, fever; prescriber should be notified, drug should be discontinued

Administer:

• With meals for GI symptoms, caps may be opened and mixed with food/liquid

• IV after diluting 20 mg/60 ml sterile H₂O for inj without bacteriostatic agent (333 µg/ml); shake until clear; give by rapid IV push through Y-tube or 3-way stopcock; follow by prescribed doses immediately

Perform/provide:

• Storage in tight container at room temp; protect diluted sol from light, use within 6 hr

• Gum, frequent sips of water for dry mouth

• Assistance with ambulation if dizziness/drowsiness occurs

Evaluate:

• Therapeutic response: decreased pain, spasticity

Teach patient/family:

• Not to discontinue medication quickly; hallucinations, spasticity, tachycardia will occur; drug should be tapered off over 1-2 wk; notify prescriber of abdominal pain, jaundiced sclera, clay-colored stools, change in color of urine

• Not to take with alcohol, other CNS depressants

• That if improvement does not occur within 6 wk, prescriber may discontinue

• To avoid hazardous activities if drowsiness, dizziness occurs

• To avoid using OTC medication: cough preparations, antihistamines, unless directed by prescriber

Ⓢ Not to break, crush, or chew caps

Treatment of overdose: Induce emesis of conscious patient; lavage, dialysis

---

dapsone (DDS) (℞)
(dap'sone)
Avlosulfon*, Dapsone
Func. class.: Leprostatic
Chem. class.: Sulfone

Action: Bactericidal and bacteriostatic against *Mycobacterium leprae*

Uses: Hansen's disease, PCP (*Pneumocystis carinii* pneumonia), malaria, dermatitis herpetiformis

Dosage and routes:

Hansen's disease

• *Adult:* **PO** 100 mg qd with rifampin 600 mg qd × 6 mo, then dapsone alone for 3-10 yr

• *Child:* **PO** 1-2 mg/kg/day

PCP

• *Adult:* **PO** 50-100 mg/day usually given with trimethoprim 20 mg/kg/day in 4 divided doses for 3 wk

• *Child:* **PO** 2 mg/kg/day

Available forms: Tabs 25, 100 mg

Side effects/adverse reactions:

INTEG: ***Exfoliative dermatitis,*** photosensitivity, ***erythema nodosum, toxic erythema, toxic epidermal necrolysis***

CNS: Peripheral neuropathy, headache, anxiety, drowsiness, tremors, ***convulsions,*** lethargy, depression, confusion, psychosis, aggression

GI: Nausea, vomiting, abdominal pain, anorexia

GU: ***Proteinuria, nephrotic syndrome,*** renal papillary necrosis

EENT: Blurred vision, optic neuritis, photophobia

HEMA: ***Megaloblastic anemia***

Contraindications: Hypersensitivity to sulfones, severe anemia

Precautions: Renal disease, hepatic disease, G6PD deficiency, pregnancy (C), lactation

Pharmacokinetics: Rapid complete absorption; half-life 25-31 hr; highly

---

bound to plasma protein; metabolized in liver; excreted in urine
Interactions:
• Increased side effects: hemolytic agents
• Increased action of dapsone: probenecid, folic acid antagonists
• Decreased blood levels of dapsone: rifampin, didanosine
• Decreased bactericidal action: PABA
• Decreased GI absorption of dapsone: activated charcoal
NURSING CONSIDERATIONS
Assess:
• Temp; if >101° F (38.3° C), drug should be reduced
• Liver studies qwk: ALT, AST, bilirubin
• Renal status: BUN, creatinine, output, specific gravity, urinalysis before; qmo
• Blood levels of drug
• For anemia: Hct, Hgb, fatigue; for peripheral neuritis; or exfoliative dermatitis
• Mental status often: affect, mood, behavioral changes; psychosis may occur
• Hepatic status: decreased appetite, jaundice, dark urine, fatigue
Administer:
• With meals for GI symptoms
• Antiemetic if vomiting occurs
• After C&S is completed; qmo to detect resistance
Perform/provide:
• Infants kept with mothers infected with leprosy; breastfeeding during drug therapy encouraged; notify prescriber immediately of infant cyanosis
Evaluate:
• Therapeutic response: decreased symptoms of Hansen's disease
Teach patient/family:
• That therapeutic effects may occur after 3-6 mo of drug therapy
• That compliance with dosage schedule, duration is necessary
• To avoid hazardous machinery if drowsiness occurs; to avoid the sun, photosensitivity may occur

D

---

daunorubicin (℞)
(daw-noe-roo'bi-sin)
Cerubidine
Func. class.: Antineoplastic, antibiotic
Chem. class.: Anthracycline glycoside

Action: Inhibits DNA synthesis, primarily; derived from *Streptomyces coerulorubidus;* replication is decreased by binding to DNA, which causes strand splitting; cell cycle specific (S phase); a vesicant
Uses: Myelogenous, monocytic leukemia, acute nonlymphocytic leukemia, Ewing's sarcoma, Wilms' tumor, neuroblastoma, rhabdomyosarcoma
Dosage and routes:
Single agent
• *Adult:* **IV** 60 mg/m^2/day × 3-5 days q4wk
In combination
• *Adult:* **IV** 45 mg/m^2/day × 3 days, then 2 days of subsequent courses in combination
• *Child:* **IV** 25-60 mg/m^2 depending on cycle
Available forms: Inj 20 mg pwd/vial
Side effects/adverse reactions:
*HEMA: **Thrombocytopenia, leukopenia, anemia***
*GI: Nausea, vomiting, anorexia, mucositis, **hepatotoxicity***
GU: Impotence, sterility, amenorrhea, gynecomastia, hyperuricemia
*INTEG: Rash, **extravasation,** dermatitis, reversible alopecia, cellulitis, thrombophlebitis at injection site

---

Side effects: *italics* = common; ***bold italics*** = life-threatening

CV: **Dysrhythmias, CHF, pericarditis, myocarditis,** peripheral edema
CNS: Fever, chills
SYST: **Anaphylaxis**

Contraindications: Hypersensitivity, pregnancy (D), lactation, systemic infections, cardiac disease

Precautions: Renal, hepatic disease; gout; bone marrow depression

Pharmacokinetics: Half-life 18½ hr; metabolized by liver; crosses placenta; excreted in breast milk, urine, bile

Interactions:

• Increased toxicity: other antineoplastics, radiation

• Incompatible with dexamethasone, heparin

Lab test interferences:

Increase: Uric acid

NURSING CONSIDERATIONS
Assess:

• CBC, differential, platelet count weekly; withhold drug if WBC is <4000/mm³ or platelet count is <75,000/mm³; notify prescriber

• Blood, urine uric acid levels

• Renal function studies: BUN, serum uric acid, urine CrCl, electrolytes before, during therapy

• I&O ratio; report fall in urine output to <30 ml/hr

• Monitor temp q4h; fever may indicate beginning infection

• Liver function tests before, during therapy: bilirubin, AST, ALT, alk phosphatase as needed or monthly; check for jaundice of skin, sclera; dark urine; clay-colored stools; itchy skin; abdominal pain; fever; diarrhea

• ECG; watch for ST-T wave changes, low QRS and T, possible dysrhythmias (sinus tachycardia, heart block, PVCs)

• Bleeding: hematuria, guaiac stools, bruising or petechiae, mucosa or orifices q8h

• Food preferences; list likes, dislikes

• Effects of alopecia on body image; discuss feelings about body changes

• Inflammation of mucosa, breaks in skin

• Buccal cavity q8h for dryness, sores or ulceration, white patches, oral pain, bleeding, dysphagia

• Local irritation, pain, burning at injection site

• GI symptoms: frequency of stools, cramping

• Acidosis, signs of dehydration: rapid respirations, poor skin turgor, decreased urine output, dry skin, restlessness, weakness

• Cardiac status: B/P, pulse, character, rhythm, rate

Administer:

• Antiemetic 30-60 min before giving drug and 6-10 hr after treatment to prevent vomiting

• Allopurinol or sodium bicarbonate to reduce uric acid levels, alkalinization of urine

IV

• After diluting 20 mg/4 ml sterile H_2O for inj (5 mg/ml), rotate, further dilute in 10-15 ml NS; give over 3-5 min by direct IV through Y-tube or 3-way stopcock of inf of D_5 or NS; or dilute in 50 ml 0.9% NaCl and give over 10-15 min; or dilute in 100 ml and give over 30 min

• Hydrocortisone for extravasation; apply ice compress after stopping infusion

Additive compatibilities: Cytarabine/etoposide, hydrocortisone; not recommended for admixing

Solution compatibilities: $D_{3.3}$/0.3% NaCl, D_5W, Normosol R, Ringer's, 0.9% NaCl

Y-site compatibilities: Amifostine, filgrastim, granisetron, melphalan, methotrexate, ondansetron, sodium

---

⬦ = Nursing alert   ▰ = Herb-drug interaction   ⃠ = Do not crush bicarbonate, teniposide, thiotepa, vinorelbine

Perform/provide:

• Strict hand-washing technique, gloves, protective clothing

• Liquid diet: carbonated beverages, gelatin may be added if patient is not nauseated or vomiting

• Increased fluid intake to 2-3 L/day to prevent urate and calculi formation

• Diet low in purines: absence of organ meats (kidney, liver), dried beans, peas to reduce uric acid level

• Rinsing of mouth tid-qid with water, club soda; brushing of teeth bid-qid with soft brush or cotton-tipped applicators for stomatitis; use unwaxed dental floss

• Storage at room temp 24 hr after reconstituting or 48 hr refrigerated

Evaluate:

• Therapeutic response: decreased tumor size, spread of malignancy

Teach patient/family:

• To report signs of infection, bleeding, bruising

• That hair may be lost during treatment and wig or hairpiece may make patient feel better; tell patient that new hair may be different in color, texture

• To avoid pregnancy while on this drug

• To avoid foods with citric acid, hot or rough texture

• To report any bleeding, white spots, ulcerations in mouth; tell patient to examine mouth qd

• That urine and other body fluids may be red-orange for 48 hr

delavirdine (R)
(de-la-veer′din)
Rescriptor
Func. class.: Nonnucleoside reverse transcriptase inhibitor (NNRTI)

Action: Binds directly to reverse transcriptase and blocks RNA, DNA causing a disruption of the enzyme's site

Uses: HIV-1 in combination with zidovudine or didanosine

Dosage and routes:

• *Adult and child ≥ 16 yr:* 400 mg tid

Available forms: Tabs 100 mg

Side effects/adverse reactions:

CNS: Headache, fatigue

GI: Diarrhea, abdominal pain, nausea, vomiting, dyspepsia, *hepatotoxicity*

GU: **Nephrotoxicity**

HEMA: **Neutropenia, leukopenia, thrombocytopenia, anemia, granulocytopenia**

INTEG: Rash

MS: Pain myalgia

Contraindications: Hypersensitivity to this drug or atevirdine

Precautions: Liver disease, pregnancy (C), lactation, children, renal disease, myleosuppression

Pharmacokinetics:

Highly protein bound, half-life 6 hr

Interactions:

• Increased levels of: alprazolam, clarithromycin, dapsone, *ergots,* felodipine, midazolam, nifedipine, indinavir

• Decreased delavirdine levels: antacids, anticonvulsants, rifamycins, protease inhibitors

• Decreased action of: oral contraceptives

• Increased delavirdine levels: fluoxetine, ketoconazole

• Increased levels of both drugs: quinidine, warfarin

 Serious life-threatening adverse reaction: amphetamines, ergots, benzodiazipines, calcium channel blockers

NURSING CONSIDERATIONS
Assess:
• For signs of infection, anemia
• Liver studies: ALT, AST; renal studies
• C&S before drug therapy; drug may be taken as soon as culture is taken; repeat C&S after treatment; determine the presence of other sexually transmitted disease
• Bowel pattern before, during treatment; if severe abdominal pain with bleeding occurs, drug should be discontinued; monitor hydration
• For skin eruptions; rash, urticaria, itching
• For allergies before treatment, reaction to each medication; place allergies on chart
• Plasma delavirdine concentrations (trough 10 micromolar)
• CBC, blood chemistry, plasma HIV RNA, absolute CD4+/CD8+/cell counts/%, serum β-2 microglobulin, serum ICD+24 antigen levels
• For signs of delavirdine toxicity: severe nausea/vomiting, maculopapular rash
Evaluate:
• Therapeutic response: improvement of HIV-1 infection
Teach patient/family:
• To take as prescribed; if dose is missed, take as soon as remembered up to 1 hr before next dose; do not double dose
• That drug must be taken in equal intervals around the clock to maintain blood levels for duration of therapy
• That tabs may be dissolved in ½ cup of water, stir, when dissolved,

drink right away, rinse cup with water, and drink that to get all medication
• To make sure health care provider knows of all the medications being taken
• That if severe rash, mouth sores, swelling, aching muscles/joints, or eye redness occur, stop taking and notify health care provider
• Not to breastfeed if taking this drug

---

demeclocycline (Ᵽ)
(dem-e-kloe-sye′kleen)
Declomycin
Func. class.: Antiinfective
Chem. class.: Tetracycline

Action: Inhibits protein synthesis, phosphorylation in microorganisms by binding to 30S ribosomal subunits, reversibly binding to 50S ribosomal subunits; bacteriostatic

Uses: Uncommon gram-positive/gram-negative bacteria, protozoa, *Rickettsia, Mycoplasma, Haemophilus ducreyi, Yersinia pestis, Campylobacter fetus, Chlamydia trachomatis,* psittacosis, granuloma inguinale

Dosage and routes:
• *Adult:* **PO** 150 mg q6h or 300 mg q12h
• *Child >8 yr:* **PO** 6-12 mg/kg/day in divided doses q6-12h
Gonorrhea
• *Adult:* **PO** 600 mg, then 300 mg q12h × 4 days, total 3 g
Available forms: Tabs 150, 300 mg; caps 150 mg

Side effects/adverse reactions:
CNS: Fever, headache, paresthesia
HEMA: Eosinophilia, neutropenia, thrombocytopenia, leukocytosis, hemolytic anemia
EENT: Dysphagia, glossitis, de-

---

creased calcification of deciduous teeth, abdominal pain, oral candidiasis

GI: Nausea, vomiting, diarrhea, anorexia, enterocolitis, ***hepatotoxicity,*** flatulence, abdominal cramps, epigastric burning, stomatitis, ***pseudomembranous colitis***

CV: Pericarditis

GU: Increased BUN, polyuria, polydipsia, ***renal failure, nephrotoxicity***

*INTEG: Rash, urticaria, photosensitivity, increased pigmentation, **exfoliative dermatitis,*** pruritus, angioedema

Contraindications: Hypersensitivity to tetracyclines, children <8 yr, pregnancy (D)

Precautions: Renal disease, hepatic disease, lactation, nephrogenic diabetes insipidus

Pharmacokinetics:

PO: Peak 3-6 hr, duration 48-72 hr, half-life 10-17 hr; excreted in urine; crosses placenta; excreted in breast milk; 41%-50% bound to serum protein

Interactions:

• Decreased effect of demeclocycline: antacids, NaHCO$_3$, dairy, alkali products, iron, kaolin/pectin

• Increased effect: oral anticoagulants

• Decreased effect: penicillins, oral contraceptives

• Nephrotoxicity: methoxyflurane

🍃 Increased action: bromelain

Lab test interferences:

False negative: Urine glucose with Clinistix or Tes-Tape

False increase: Urinary catecholamines, AST, ALT, BUN

NURSING CONSIDERATIONS

Assess:

• I&O ratio

• Blood studies: PT, CBC, AST, ALT, BUN, creatinine

• Urine specific gravity, Na

• Signs of infection

• Allergic reactions: rash, itching, pruritus, angioedema

• Nausea, vomiting, diarrhea; administer antiemetic, antacids as ordered

• Overgrowth of infection: increased temp, malaise, redness, pain, swelling, drainage, perineal itching, diarrhea, changes in cough, sputum

Administer:

• On empty stomach 1 hr ac or 2 hr pc with 8 oz H$_2$O

• After C&S

• 2 hr before or after laxative or ferrous products; 3 hr after antacid or kaolin-pectin products

Perform/provide:

• Storage in tight, light-resistant container at room temp

Evaluate:

• Therapeutic response: decreased temp, absence of lesions, negative C&S

Teach patient/family:

• To avoid sun exposure; sunscreen does not seem to decrease photosensitivity

• If diabetic, to avoid use of Clinistix, Diastix, or Tes-Tape for urine glucose testing

🚫 Not to break, crush, or chew caps

• To take all prescribed medication to prevent superinfection; to discard when expires, may be toxic

• To avoid milk products; take with full glass of water

denileukin diftitox
See appendix a—selected new drugs

desmopressin (R)
(des-moe-press'in)
DDAVP, Stimate
Func. class.: Pituitary hormone
Chem. class.: Synthetic antidiuretic hormone

Action: Promotes reabsorption of water by action on renal tubular epithelium; causes smooth muscle constriction, increase in plasma factor VIII levels, which increases platelet aggregation resulting in vasopressor effect, similar to vasopressin

Uses: Hemophilia A, von Willebrand's disease type 1, nonnephrogenic diabetes insipidus, symptoms of polyuria/polydipsia caused by pituitary dysfunction, nocturnal enuresis

Dosage and routes:
Primary nocturnal enuresis
• *Child ≥6 yr:* INTRANASAL 20 µg (10 µg in each nostril) hs, may increase to 40 µg; PO 0.2 mg hs, may be increased to max 0.6 mg hs
Diabetes insipidus
• *Adult:* INTRANASAL 0.1-0.4 ml qd in divided doses (1-4 sprays with pump); IV/SC 0.5-1 ml qd in divided doses
• *Child 3 mo to 12 yr:* INTRANASAL 0.05-0.3 ml qd in divided doses
Hemophilia/von Willebrand's disease
• *Adult and child >3 mo:* IV 0.3 µg/kg in NaCl over 15-30 min; may repeat if needed

Available forms: Intranasal pipets 0.01 mg/ml, inj 4 µg/ml, Rhihal Tube del 2.5 mg/vial; tabs 0.1, 0.2 mg

Side effects/adverse reactions:
EENT: Nasal irritation, congestion, rhinitis
CNS: Drowsiness, headache, lethargy, flushing

GU: Vulval pain
GI: Nausea, heartburn, cramps
CV: Increased B/P
*SYST: **Anaphylaxis (IV)***

Contraindications: Hypersensitivity, nephrogenic diabetes insipidus
Precautions: Pregnancy (B), CAD, lactation, hypertension
Pharmacokinetics:
NASAL: Onset 1 hr, peak 1-2 hr, duration 8-20 hr, half-life 8 min, 76 min (terminal)
Interactions:
• Increased response: carbamazepine, chlorpropamide, clofibrate
• Increased adverse reactions: lithium, alcohol, demeclocycline, heparin, large doses of epinephrine
• Compatibility not known

NURSING CONSIDERATIONS
Assess:
• Pulse, B/P when giving IV or SC
• I&O ratio, weight daily; check for edema in extremities; if water retention is severe, diuretic may be prescribed
• Water intoxication: lethargy, behavioral changes, disorientation, neuromuscular excitability
• Intranasal use: nausea, congestion, cramps, headache; usually decreased with decreased dose
 For severe allergic reaction including anaphylaxis (IV route)
• For nasal mucosa changes: congestion, edema, discharge, scarring (nasal route)
• Urine vol/osmolality and plasma osmolality (diabetes insipidus)
• Factor VIII coagulant activity before using for hemostasis
Administer:
• Undiluted over 1 min in diabetes insipidus
• Diluted, one single dose/50 ml of NS (adult & child >10 kg), a single dose/10 ml as an IV INF over 15-30 min in von Willebrand's disease or hemophilia A

Perform/provide:

• Storage in refrigerator or cool environment

Evaluate:

• Therapeutic response: absence of severe thirst, decreased urine output, osmolality

Teach patient/family:

• The proper technique for nasal instillation: to insert tube into nostril to instill drug

• To avoid OTC products: cough, hay fever products, since these preparations may contain epinephrine, decrease drug response; do not use with alcohol

• To wear Medic Alert ID specifying therapy

• That if dose is missed, take when remembered up to 1 hr before next dose; do not double dose

---

dexamethasone (℞)

(dex-ah-meth′a-sone)
Decadron, Deronil*
Dexasone*, Dexon, Hexadrol, Mymethasone
dexamethasone acetate (℞)

Dalalone DP, Dalalone LA,
Decadron-LA, Decaject-LA,
Dexacen LA-8, Dexasone-LA,
Dexone LA, Solurex-LA,
dexamethasone sodium phosphate (℞)

Dalalone, Decadron Phosphate, Decaject, Dexacen-4,
Dexone, Hexadrol Phosphate, Solurex
Func. class.: Corticosteroid
Chem. class.: Glucocorticoid, long-acting

Action: Decreases inflammation by suppression of migration of polymorphonuclear leukocytes, fibroblasts, reversal of increased capillary permeability and lysosomal stabilization

Uses: Inflammation, allergies, neoplasms, cerebral edema, septic shock, collagen disorders

Dosage and routes:

Inflammation

• *Adult:* **PO** 0.75-9 mg/day or phosphate **IM** 0.5-9 mg/day; or acetate **IM** 4-16 mg into joint of tissue q1-3wk

• *Child:* **PO** 0.08-0.3 mg/kg/day in divided doses q6-12h

Shock (Phosphate)

• *Adult:* **IV** single dose 1-6 mg/kg or **IV** 40 mg q2-6h as needed up to 72h

Cerebral edema (Phosphate)

• *Adult:* **IV** 10 mg, then 4-6 mg **IM** q6h × 2-4 days, then taper over 1 wk

• *Child:* **PO** 0.2 mg/kg/day in divided doses

Adrenocortical insufficiency

• *Child:* 23.3 µg/kg/day in 3 divided doses

Available forms: dexamethasone: Tabs 0.25, 0.5, 0.75, 1, 1.5, 2, 4, 6 mg; elix 0.5 mg/5 ml; oral sol 0.5 mg/5 ml, 0.5 mg/1 ml; inj acetate 8, 16 mg/ml; inj phosphate 4, 10, 20, 24 mg/ml

Side effects/adverse reactions:

INTEG: Acne, poor wound healing, ecchymosis, petechiae

CNS: Depression, flushing, sweating, headache, mood changes, euphoria, psychosis, *seizures*

*CV: Hypertension, **circulatory collapse, thrombophlebitis, embolism,** tachycardia, edema*

*HEMA: **Thrombocytopenia***

MS: Fractures, osteoporosis, weakness

*GI: Diarrhea, nausea, abdominal distention, **GI hemorrhage,** increased appetite, **pancreatitis***

EENT: Fungal infections, increased intraocular pressure, blurred vision
ENDO: HPA suppression
META: Hypokalemia

Contraindications: Psychosis, hypersensitivity, idiopathic thrombocytopenia, acute glomerulonephritis, amebiasis, fungal infections, nonasthmatic bronchial disease, child <2 yr, AIDS, TB

Precautions: Pregnancy (C), lactation, diabetes mellitus, glaucoma, osteoporosis, seizure disorders, ulcerative colitis, CHF, myasthenia gravis, renal disease, peptic ulcer, esophagitis

Pharmacokinetics:
PO: Onset 1 hr, peak 1-2 hr, duration 2½ days
IM: (acetate) Peak 8 hr, duration 6 days
Half-life 3-4½ hr

Interactions:
• Decreased action of dexamethasone: cholestyramine, colestipol, barbiturates, rifampin, ephedrine, phenytoin, theophylline, antacids
• Decreased effects of anticoagulants, anticonvulsants, antidiabetics, ambenonium, neostigmine, isoniazid, toxoids, vaccines, anticholinesterases, salicylates, somatrem
• Increased side effects: alcohol, salicylates, indomethacin, amphotericin B, digitalis, cyclosporine, diuretics
• Increased action of dexamethasone: salicylates, estrogens, indomethacin, oral contraceptives, ketoconazole, macrolide antibiotics

🌿 Potassium deficiency: aloe, buckthorn bark/berry, cascara sagrada bark, ephedra, senna pod/leaf

Lab test interferences:
Increase: Cholesterol, Na, blood glucose, uric acid, Ca, urine glucose
Decrease: Ca, K, T_4, T_3, thyroid ^{131}I uptake test, urine 17-OHCS, 17-KS, PBI skin allergy tests

NURSING CONSIDERATIONS
Assess:
• K, blood sugar, urine glucose while on long-term therapy; hypokalemia and hyperglycemia
• Weight daily; notify prescriber of weekly gain >5 lb
• B/P q4h, pulse; notify prescriber of chest pain
• I&O ratio; be alert for decreasing urinary output, increasing edema
• Plasma cortisol levels during long-term therapy (normal: 138-635 nmol/L SI units when drawn at 8 AM)
• Infection: fever, WBC even after withdrawal of medication; drug masks infection
• Potassium depletion: paresthesias, fatigue, nausea, vomiting, depression, polyuria, dysrhythmias, weakness
• Edema, hypertension, cardiac symptoms
• Mental status: affect, mood, behavioral changes, aggression

Administer:
• Titrated dose; use lowest effective dose
• IM inj deeply in large muscle mass; rotate sites; avoid deltoid; use 21G needle
• In one dose in AM to prevent adrenal suppression; avoid SC administration, may damage tissue
• With food or milk to decrease GI symptoms

IV
• Undiluted direct over 1 min or less or diluted with NS or D_5W and give as an IV INF at prescribed rate
• After shaking suspension (parenteral); do not give suspension IV

Additive compatibilities: Aminophylline, bleomycin, cimetidine, floxacillin, furosemide, granisetron, lidocaine, meropenem, mitomycin, nafcillin, netilmicin, ondansetron, prochlorperazine, ranitidine, verapamil

---

◆ = Nursing alert   🌿 = Herb-drug interaction   🚫 = Do not crush

Syringe compatibilities: Granisetron, metoclopramide, ranitidine, sufentanil

Y-site compatibilities: Acyclovir, allopurinol, amifostine, amikacin, amphotericin B cholesteryl, amsacrine, aztreonam, cefepime, cefpirome, cisatracurium, cisplatin, cladribine, cyclophosphamide, cytarabine, doxorubicin, doxorubicin liposome, famotidine, filgrastim, fluconazole, fludarabine, foscarnet, granisetron, heparin, lorazepam, melphalan, meperidine, meropenem, morphine, ondansetron, paclitaxel, piperacillin/tazobactam, potassium chloride, propofol, remifentanil, sargramostim, sodium bicarbonate, sufentanil, tacrolimus, teniposide, theophylline, thiotepa, vinorelbine, vit B/C, zidovudine

Perform/provide:

• Assistance with ambulation in patient with bone tissue disease to prevent fractures

Evaluate:

• Therapeutic response: ease of respirations, decreased inflammation

Teach patient/family:

• That ID as steroid user should be carried

• To notify prescriber if therapeutic response decreases; dosage adjustment may be needed

◆ Not to discontinue abruptly or adrenal crisis can result

• Symptoms of adrenal insufficiency: nausea, anorexia, fatigue, dizziness, dyspnea, weakness, joint pain

• To avoid OTC products: salicylates, alcohol in cough products, cold preparations unless directed by prescriber

• To teach patient all aspects of drug usage, including cushingoid symptoms; to notify health-care provider of infection

dexmedetomidine
See appendix a—selected new drugs

D

dextran 40 (℞)
(deks′tran)
Dextran 40, Gentran 40, LMD 10%, Rheomacrodex
Func. class.: Plasma volume expander
Chem. class.: Low molecular weight polysaccharide

Action: Similar to human albumin, which expands plasma volume by drawing fluid from interstitial space to intravascular space

Uses: Expand plasma volume, prophylaxis of embolism, thrombosis

Dosage and routes:

Shock

• *Adult:* **IV INF** 500 ml over 15-30 min, total dose in 24 hr not to exceed 20 ml/kg; subsequent doses given slowly; if given >24 hr, not to exceed 10 ml/kg/day; not to exceed therapy >5 days

Thrombosis/embolism

• *Adult:* **IV INF** 500-1000 ml, then 500 ml/day × 3 days, then 500 ml q2-3 days × 2 wk if needed

Available forms: 10% dextran 40/ D_5W, 10% dextran 40/0.9% NaCl

Side effects/adverse reactions:

HEMA: Decreased hematocrit, platelet function; *increased bleeding/ coagulation times*

INTEG: Rash, urticaria, pruritus, *angioedema,* chills, fever, flushing

RESP: Wheezing, dyspnea, *bronchospasm, pulmonary edema*

CV: Hypotension, *cardiac arrest*

GU: Osmotic nephrosis, renal failure, stasis, hyponatremia

GI: Nausea, vomiting, increased AST, ALT

SYST: ***Anaphylaxis***

Contraindications: Hypersensitivity, renal failure, CHF (severe), extreme dehydration

Precautions: Active hemorrhage, pregnancy (C)

Pharmacokinetics:

IV: Expands blood vol 1-2 × amount infused; excreted in urine and feces

Interactions:

• Incompatible with chlortetracycline, phytonadione, promethazine

Lab test interferences:

False increase: Blood glucose, urinary protein, bilirubin, total protein

Interference: Rh test, blood typing/crossmatching

NURSING CONSIDERATIONS

Assess:

• VS q5min × 30 min; Hgb/Hct, if falling by 30%, notify prescriber

• CVP during infusion (5-10 cm H_2O—normal range)

• Urine output q1h; watch for increase in urinary output (common); if output does not increase, decrease or discontinue infusion

• I&O ratio and specific gravity, urine osmolarity; if specific gravity is very low, renal clearance is low; drug should be discontinued

• Allergy: rash, urticaria, pruritus, wheezing, dyspnea, bronchospasm, drug should be discontinued immediately

◆ Circulatory overload: increased pulse, respirations, SOB, wheezing, chest tightness, chest pain

• Dehydration after infusion: decreased output, decreased specific gravity of urine, increased temp, poor skin turgor, increased specific gravity, dry skin

Administer:

IV

• After prescribed dilution; may give inital 500 mg at 15-30 min; distribute remainder of daily dose over 8-24 hr

• After crossmatch is drawn, if blood is to be given also

• D_5W sol in heart failure patients as ordered

Additive compatibilities: Cloxacillin

Y-site compatibilities: Enalaprilat, famotidine

Perform/provide:

• Storage at constant temp 15°-30° C (59°-86° F); discard unused portions, protect from freezing

Evaluate:

• Therapeutic response: increased plasma volume

---

dextran 70/75 (℞)

(deks'tran)

Dextran 75, Gentran 70, Gentran 75, Macrodex

Func. class.: Plasma volume expander

Chem. class.: High molecular weight polysaccharide

Action: Similar to human albumin, which expands plasma volume by drawing fluid from interstitial spaces to intravascular space

Uses: Expand plasma volume in hypovolemic shock or impending shock

Dosage and routes:

• *Adult:* **IV INF** 500-1000 ml not to exceed 20-40 ml/min, not to exceed 10 ml/kg/24 hr if therapy >24 hr

Available forms: 70/75 dextran in 0.9% NaCl, D_5%

Side effects/adverse reactions:

HEMA: Decreased hematocrit, platelet function; ***increased bleeding/coagulation times***

INTEG: Rash, urticaria, pruritus, ***angioedema,*** chills, fever, flushing

RESP: Wheezing, dyspnea, ***bronchospasm, pulmonary edema***

◆ = Nursing alert   ▨ = Herb-drug interaction   ⊘ = Do not crush

CV: Hypotension, ***cardiac arrest***

GU: ***Osmotic nephrosis, renal failure, stasis,*** hypernatremia

GI: Nausea, vomiting, increased AST, ALT

SYST: ***Anaphylaxis***

Contraindications: Hypersensitivity, renal failure, CHF (severe), extreme dehydration

Precautions: Active hemorrhage, pregnancy (C)

Pharmacokinetics:

IV: Expands blood vol 1-2 × amount infused; excreted in urine, feces

Lab test interferences:

False increase: Blood glucose, urinary protein, bilirubin, total protein

Interference: Rh test, blood typing/crossmatching

NURSING CONSIDERATIONS

Assess:

• VS q5min × 30 min; Hgb/Hct, if falling by 30%, notify prescriber

• CVP during infusion (5-10 cm H_2O—normal range)

• Urine output q1h; watch for increase in urinary output (common); if output does not increase, decrease or discontinue infusion

• I&O ratio and specific gravity, urine osmolarity; if specific gravity is very low, renal clearance is low; drug should be discontinued

• Allergy: rash, urticaria, pruritus, wheezing, dyspnea, bronchospasm; drug should be discontinued immediately

◆ Circulatory overload: increased pulse, respirations, SOB, wheezing, chest tightness, chest pain

• Dehydration after infusion: decreased output, increased temp, poor skin turgor, increased specific gravity, dry skin

Administer:

• After prescribed dilution, may give inital 500 mg at 20-40 ml/min, reduce flow to lowest rate

• After crossmatch is drawn, if blood is to be given also

• D_5W sol in heart failure patients as ordered

Perform/provide:

• Storage at constant temp <25° C (77° F); discard unused portions; do not use unless clear

Evaluate:

• Therapeutic response: increased plasma volume

---

dextroamphetamine (℞)

(dex-troe-am-fet'a-meen)
Dexedrine, Dexedrine Spansules, dextroamphetamine, Ferndex

Func. class.: Cerebral stimulant
Chem. class.: Amphetamine

Controlled Substance Schedule II

Action: Increases release of norepinephrine, dopamine in cerebral cortex to reticular activating system

Uses: Narcolepsy, attention deficit disorder with hyperactivity

Dosage and routes:

Narcolepsy

• *Adult:* **PO** 5-60 mg qd in divided doses

• *Child >12 yr:* **PO** 10 mg qd increasing by 10 mg/day at weekly intervals

• *Child 6-12 yr:* **PO** 5 mg qd increasing by 5 mg/wk (max 60 mg/day)

Attention deficit disorder with hyperactivity

• *Child >6 yr:* **PO** 5 mg qd-bid increasing by 5 mg/day at weekly intervals

• *Child 3-6 yr:* **PO** 2.5 mg qd increasing by 2.5 mg/day at weekly intervals

---

Available forms: Tabs 5, 10 mg; caps sus rel 5, 10, 15 mg

Side effects/adverse reactions:

CNS: Hyperactivity, insomnia, restlessness, talkativeness, dizziness, headache, chills, stimulation, dysphoria, irritability, aggressiveness, tremor, dependence, addiction

GI: Anorexia, dry mouth, diarrhea, constipation, weight loss, metallic taste

GU: Impotence, change in libido

CV: Palpitations, tachycardia, hypertension, decrease in heart rate, *dysrhythmias*

INTEG: Urticaria

Contraindications: Hypersensitivity to sympathomimetic amines, hyperthyroidism, hypertension, glaucoma, severe arteriosclerosis, drug abuse, cardiovascular disease, anxiety

Precautions: Gilles de la Tourette's disorder, pregnancy (C), lactation, child <3 yr

Pharmacokinetics:

PO: Onset 30 min, peak 1-3 hr, duration 4-20 hr; metabolized by liver; urine excretion pH dependent; crosses placenta, breast milk; half-life 10-30 hr

Interactions:

◆ Hypertensive crisis: MAOIs or within 14 days of MAOIs

• Delayed absorption of: barbiturates, phenytoin

• Increased effect of dextroamphetamine: acetazolamide, antacids, sodium bicarbonate

• Increased CNS effect: haloperidol, tricyclics, phenothiazines

• Decreased effect of dextroamphetamine: ascorbic acid, ammonium chloride

• Decreased effect of: adrenergic blockers, antidiabetics

• Drug/food: increased amine effect: caffeine

NURSING CONSIDERATIONS

Assess:

• VS, B/P; this drug may reverse antihypertensives; check patients with cardiac disease often

• CBC, urinalysis; in diabetes: blood sugar, urine sugar; insulin changes may be required, since eating will decrease

• Height, growth rate in children; growth rate may be decreased

• Mental status: mood, sensorium, affect, stimulation, insomnia, irritability

• Tolerance or dependency: an increased amount may be used to get same effect; will develop after long-term use

• Overdose: pain, fever, dehydration, insomnia, hyperactivity

Administer:

• At least 6 hr before hs to avoid sleeplessness

Perform/Provide:

• Gum, hard candy, frequent sips of water for dry mouth

Evaluate:

• Therapeutic response: increased CNS stimulation, decreased drowsiness

Teach patient/family:

🚫 Not to break, crush, or chew sus rel forms

• To decrease caffeine consumption (coffee, tea, cola, chocolate); may increase irritability, stimulation

• To avoid OTC preparations unless approved by prescriber

• To taper drug over several wk; depression, increased sleeping, lethargy

• To avoid alcohol ingestion

• To avoid hazardous activities until stabilized on medication

• To get needed rest; patient will feel more tired at end of day

Treatment of overdose: Administer fluids, hemodialysis or peritoneal dialysis; antihypertensive for

---

◆ = Nursing alert   🍃 = Herb-drug interaction   🚫 = Do not crush

increased B/P, ammonium Cl for increased excretion

dextromethorphan
(OTC)

(dex-troe-meth-or'fan)
Balminil DM*, Benylin DM*, Broncho-Grippol-DM*, Children's Hold, Delsym, Dextromethorphan, Hold DM, Koffex*, Neo-DM*, Orex DM*, Pertussin, Pertussin ES, Robidex*, Robitussin Cough Calmers, Robitussin Pediatric, Sedatuss*, St. Joseph Cough Suppressant, Sucrets Cough Control, Suppress, Trocal, Vicks Formula 44

Func. class.: Antitussive, nonnarcotic
Chem. class.: Levorphanol derivative

Action: Depresses cough center in medulla by direct effect
Uses: Nonproductive cough
Dosage and routes:
• *Adult:* **PO** 10-20 mg q4h, or 30 mg q6-8h, not to exceed 120 mg/day; **SUS-REL LIQ** 60 mg bid, not to exceed 120 mg/day
• *Child 6-12 yr:* **PO** 5-10 mg q4h; **SUS-REL LIQ** 30 mg bid, not to exceed 60 mg/day
• *Child 2-6 yr:* **PO** 2.5-5 mg q4h, or 7.5 mg q6-8h, not to exceed 30 mg/day
Available forms: Loz 5, 7.5 mg; sol 3.5, 5, 7.5, 10, 15 mg/5 ml; syrup 15 mg/15 ml, 12.5 mg/5 ml; sus-action liq 30 mg/5 ml
Side effects/adverse reactions:
CNS: Dizziness
GI: Nausea
Contraindications: Hypersensitivity, asthma/emphysema, productive cough

Precautions: Nausea/vomiting, fever, persistent headache, pregnancy (C)
Pharmacokinetics:
PO: Onset 15-30 min, duration 3-6 hr
SUS: Duration 12 hr
Interactions:
• Do not give with MAOIs or within 2 wk of MAOIs
• Confusion, coma: selegiline
NURSING CONSIDERATIONS
Assess:
• Cough: type, frequency, character, including sputum
Administer:
• Decreased dose to elderly patients; metabolism may be slowed
Perform/provide:
• Increased fluids to liquefy secretions
• Humidification of patient's room
Evaluate:
• Therapeutic response: absence of cough
Teach patient/family:
• To avoid driving, other hazardous activities until patient is stabilized on this medication
• To avoid smoking, smoke-filled rooms, perfumes, dust, environmental pollutants, cleaners that increase cough
• To avoid alcohol, other CNS depressants
• To notify prescriber if cough persists over a few days

dextrose
(D-glucose) (R)
Glucose, Glutose, Insta-Glucose, Insulin Reaction
Func. class.: Caloric

Action: Needed for adequate utilization of amino acids; decreases protein, nitrogen loss; prevents ketosis
Uses: Increases intake of calories;

increases fluids in patients unable to take adequate fluids, calories orally

Dosage and routes:

• *Adult and child:* **IV** depends on individual requirements

Available forms: Inj 2.5%, 5%, 10%, 20%, 40%, 50%, 60%, 70%; oral gel 40%; chew tab 5 g

Side effects/adverse reactions:

CNS: Confusion, *loss of consciousness,* dizziness

CV: Hypertension, *CHF, pulmonary edema*

GU: Glycosuria, osmotic diuresis

ENDO: Hyperglycemia, rebound hypoglycemia, hyperosmolar syndrome, hyperglycemic nonketotic syndrome

INTEG: Chills, flushing, warm feeling, rash, urticaria, extravasation necrosis

Contraindications: Hyperglycemia, delirium tremens, hemorrhage (cranial/spinal), CHF

Precautions: Renal, liver, cardiac disease, diabetes mellitus

Interactions:

• Increased fluid retention/electrolyte excretion: coricosteroids

NURSING CONSIDERATIONS

Assess:

• Electrolytes (K, Na, Ca, Cl, Mg), blood glucose, ammonia, phosphate

• Injection site for extravasation: redness along vein, edema at site, necrosis, pain; hard, tender area; site should be changed immediately

• Monitor temp q4h for increased fever, indicating infection; if infection suspected, infusion is discontinued, tubing, bottle, catheter tip cultured

• Serum glucose in patients receiving hypotonic glucose 50% and over

• Nutritional status: calorie count by dietitian

Administer:

• Only (4%) protein and dextrose

(up to 12.5%) via peripheral vein; stronger sol: central IV administration

• May be given undiluted via prepared sol; give 10% sol, 5 ml/15 sec; 10% sol, 1000 ml/3 hr or more; 20% sol, 500 ml/½-1 hr; 50% sol, 10 ml/min; control rate, rapid infusions may cause fluid shifts

• Oral glucose preparations (gel, chew tabs) are to be used in conscious patients only; check serum blood glucose after first dose

• After changing IV catheter, dressing q24h with aseptic technique

Evaluate:

• Therapeutic response: increased weight

Teach patient/family:

• The reason for dextrose infusion

• To review hypoglycemia/hyperglycemia symptoms

• To review blood glucose monitoring procedure

---

dezocine (℞)

(dez'oh-seen)

Dalgan

Func. class.: Narcotic agonist-antagonist analgesic

Chem. class.: Opioid, synthetic

Action: Depresses pain impulse transmission at the spinal cord level by interacting with opioid receptors

Uses: Severe pain

Dosage and routes:

• *Adult:* **IM** 5-20 mg q3-6h, not to exceed 120 mg/day; **IV** 2.5-10 mg q2-4h

Available forms: Inj 5, 10, 15 mg/ml single-dose vials, multiple dose 10 mg/ml

Side effects/adverse reactions:

CV: Hypotension, pulse irregularity, hypertension, chest pain, pallor, edema, thrombophlebitis

---

◆ = Nursing alert   🖋 = Herb-drug interaction   ⊘ = Do not crush

CNS: Drowsiness, dizziness, confusion, sedation, anxiety, headache, depression, delirium, sleep disturbances, dependency

GI: Nausea, vomiting, anorexia, constipation, cramps, abdominal pain, dry mouth, diarrhea

INTEG: Injection site reactions, pruritus, rash, sweating, chills

RESP: **Respiratory depression,** hiccups

GU: Urinary frequency, hesitancy, retention

EENT: Blurred vision, slurred speech, diplopia

Contraindications: Hypersensitivity

Precautions: Addictive personality, pregnancy (C), lactation, increased intracranial pressure, respiratory depression, hepatic disease, renal disease, children <18 yr, elderly, biliary surgery, COPD, sulfite sensitivity

Pharmacokinetics:
IM: Onset 30 min, peak 50-90 min, duration 2-4 hr
IV: Onset 10 min, peak 30 min, duration 2-4 hr
Metabolized by liver; excreted by kidneys; may cross placenta

Interactions:
• Incompatibility: not known
• Increased CNS depression: alcohol, narcotics, sedative/hypnotics, antipsychotics, skeletal muscle relaxants, general anesthetics, tranquilizers

NURSING CONSIDERATIONS
Assess:
• I&O ratio; decreasing output may indicate urinary retention
• CNS changes: dizziness, drowsiness, hallucinations, euphoria, LOC, pupil reaction
• Allergic reactions: rash, urticaria
• Respiratory dysfunction: respiratory depression, character, rate, rhythm of respirations; notify prescriber if <10/min, shallow
• Need for pain medication, physical dependence

Administer:
• Undiluted 5 mg or less over 2-3 min
• With antiemetic if nausea, vomiting occur
• When pain is beginning to return; determine dosage interval by patient response

Perform/provide:
• Storage in light-resistant area at room temp
• Assistance with ambulation
• Safety measures: top side rails, night-light, call bell in easy reach

Evaluate:
• Therapeutic response: decrease in pain

Teach patient/family:
• To report any symptoms of CNS changes, allergic reactions
• That physical dependency may result after extended use
• That withdrawal symptoms may occur: nausea, vomiting, cramps, fever, faintness, anorexia

Treatment of overdose: Naloxone 0.2-0.8 mg IV, O_2, IV fluids, vasopressors

---

diazepam (℞)
(dye-az'-e-pam)
Apo-Diazepam*, Diazemuls*, diazepam, Diazepam Intensol, Novo-Diapam*, PMS-Diazepam*, Valium, Valrelease, Vivol*, Zetran
Func. class.: Antianxiety
Chem. class.: Benzodiazepine

Controlled Substance Schedule IV
Action: Potentiates the actions of GABA, especially in limbic system, reticular formation; enhances pre-

sympathetic inhibition, inhibits spinal polysynaptic afferent paths

Uses: Anxiety, acute alcohol withdrawal, adjunct in seizure disorders; preoperatively as a relaxant, skeletal muscle relaxation; rectally for acute repetitive seizures

Investigational uses: Panic attacks

Dosage and routes:

Anxiety/convulsive disorders

• *Adult:* **PO** 2-10 mg bid-qid; **EXT REL** 15-30 mg qd

• *Geriatric:* **PO** 1-2 mg qd-bid, increase slowly as needed

• *Child >6 mo:* **PO** 1-2.5 mg tid-qid

Muscle relaxation

• *Geriatric:* **PO** 2-5 mg bid-qid

Tetanic muscle spasms

• *Child <5 yr:* **IM/IV** 5-10 mg q3-4h prn

• *Infant >30 days:* **IM/IV** 1-2 mg q3-4h prn

Status epilepticus

• *Adult:* **IV BOL** 5-20 mg, 2 mg/min, may repeat q5-10min, not to exceed 60 mg; may repeat in 30 min if seizures reappear

• *Child:* **IV BOL** 0.1-0.3 mg/kg (1 mg/min over 3 min); may repeat q15min × 2 doses

• *Adult:* **RECT** 0.2 mg/kg, may repeat 4-12 hr later

• *Child 6-11 yr:* **RECT** 0.3 mg/kg, may repeat 4-12 hr later

• *Child 2-5 yr:* **RECT** 0.5 mg/kg, may repeat 4-12 hr later

Available forms: Tabs 2, 5, 10 mg; caps ext rel 15 mg; inj emulsified 5 mg/ml; oral sol 5 mg/5 ml, 5 mg/ml; gel, rectal delivery system 10, 15, 20 mg, twin packs

Side effects/adverse reactions:

HEMA: **Neutropenia**

RESP: **Respiratory depression**

CNS: Dizziness, drowsiness, confusion, headache, anxiety, tremors, stimulation, fatigue, depression, insomnia, hallucinations

CV: Orthostatic hypotension, **ECG**

*changes, **tachycardia,*** hypotension

EENT: Blurred vision, tinnitus, mydriasis

GI: Constipation, dry mouth, nausea, vomiting, anorexia, diarrhea

INTEG: Rash, dermatitis, itching

Contraindications: Hypersensitivity to benzodiazepines, narrow-angle glaucoma, psychosis, pregnancy (D), lactation

Precautions: Elderly, debilitated, hepatic disease, renal disease

Pharmacokinetics:

PO: Rapidly absorbed; onset ½ hr, duration 2-3 hr

IM: Onset 15-30 min, duration 1-1½ hr; absorption slow and erratic

IV: Onset 1-5 min, duration 15 min Metabolized by liver, excreted by kidneys, crosses placenta, excreted in breast milk, crosses the blood-brain barrier; half-life 20-50 hr, more effective by mouth

Interactions:

• Increased effects of both drugs: barbiturates

• Increased digoxin level, toxicity: digoxin

• Increased diazepam adverse reactions: cimetidine

• Decreased effects of diazepam: oral contraceptives, rifampin, valproic acid, disulfiram, isoniazid, propranolol

• Increased CNS depression: CNS depressants, alcohol

• Drug/smoking: decreased diazepam effect

🍃 Increased action of diazepam: kava

Lab test interferences:

Increase: AST/ALT, serum bilirubin

False increase: 17-OHCS

Decrease: RAIU

NURSING CONSIDERATIONS

Assess:

• B/P (lying, standing), pulse; respiratory rate; if systolic B/P drops

---

◆ = Nursing alert   🍃 = Herb-drug interaction   🚫 = Do not crush

20 mm Hg, hold drug, notify prescriber; respirations q5-15min if given IV

• Blood studies: CBC during long-term therapy; blood dyscrasias (rare)

• Degree of anxiety; what precipitates anxiety and whether drug controls symptoms

• For alcohol withdrawal symptoms, including hallucinations (visual, auditory), delirium, irritability, agitation, fine to coarse tremors

• For seizure control and type, duration, intensity of convulsions

• Hepatic studies: AST, ALT, bilirubin, creatinine, LDH, alk phosphatase

• IV site for thrombosis or phlebitis, which may occur rapidly

• Mental status: mood, sensorium, affect, sleeping pattern, drowsiness, dizziness

• Physical dependency, withdrawal symptoms: headache, nausea, vomiting, muscle pain, weakness after long-term use

• Suicidal tendencies

Administer:

• With food or milk for GI symptoms; crushed if patient is unable to swallow medication whole; do not crush ext rel capsules

• Sugarless gum, hard candy, frequent sips of water for dry mouth

• Reduced opioid dose by ⅓ if given concomitantly with diazepam

IV

• Into large vein; give IV 5 mg or less/1 min or total dose over 3 min or more (children, infants); continuous infusion is not recommended

Additive compatibilities: Netilmicin, verapamil

Syringe compatibilities: Cimetidine

Y-site compatibilities: Cefmetazole, dobutamine, nafcillin, quinidine, sufentanil

Perform/provide:

• Assistance with ambulation during beginning therapy, for drowsiness, dizziness, safety measures

• Check to see PO medication has been swallowed

Evaluate:

• Therapeutic response: decreased anxiety, restlessness, insomnia

Teach patient/family:

• That drug may be taken with food

• That drug is not to be used for everyday stress or used longer than 4 mo unless directed by prescriber; no more than prescribed amount; may be habit forming

• To avoid OTC preparations unless approved by prescriber

• To avoid driving, activities that require alertness; drowsiness may occur

• To avoid alcohol, other psychotropic medications unless directed by prescriber; that smoking may decrease diazepam effect

• Not to discontinue medication abruptly after long-term use

• To rise slowly or fainting may occur, especially in elderly

• That drowsiness may worsen at beginning of treatment

• To avoid use during pregnancy

🚫 Not to break, crush, or chew ext rel caps

Treatment of overdose: Lavage, VS, supportive care, flumazenil

---

diazoxide (℞)

(dye-az-ox′ide)
diazoxide parenteral, Hyperstat IV
Func. class.: Antihypertensive
Chem. class.: Vasodilator

Action: Vasodilates arteriolar smooth muscle by direct relaxation; a reduction in blood pressure with concomitant increases in heart rate, cardiac output; inhibits release of insulin from the pancreas

Uses: Hypertensive crisis when urgent decrease of diastolic pressure required; increase blood glucose levels in hyperinsulinism

Dosage and routes:

Hypoglycemia

• *Adult and child:* **PO** 3-8 mg/kg/day in 2-3 divided doses q8-12h

• *Infants and neonates:* **PO** 8-15 mg/kg/day in 2-3 divided doses 8-12h

Hypertension

• *Adult:* **IV BOL** 1-3 mg/kg rapidly up to a max of 150 mg in a single injection; dose may be repeated at 5-15 min intervals until desired response is achieved; give IV in 30 sec or less

• *Child:* **IV BOL** 1-2 mg/kg rapidly; administration same as adult, not to exceed 150 mg

Available forms: Caps 50 mg; oral susp 50 mg/ml; inj 15 mg/ml, 300 mg/20 ml

Side effects/adverse reactions:

CV: **Hypotension,** T-wave changes, angina pectoris, palpitations, **supraventricular tachycardia, edema,** rebound hypertension, **shock, MI**

CNS: Headache, sleepiness, euphoria, anxiety, EPS, confusion, tinnitus, blurred vision, dizziness, weakness, **seizures, cerebral ischemia, paralysis**

GI: Nausea, vomiting, dry mouth

INTEG: Rash

HEMA: Decreased hemoglobin, hematocrit, **thrombocytopenia**

GU: Breast tenderness; increased BUN, fluid, electrolyte imbalances; Na, water retention

ENDO: Hyperglycemia in diabetics, transient hyperglycemia in nondiabetics

Contraindications: Hypersensitivity to thiazides, sulfonamides, hypertension of aortic coarctation or AV shunt, pheochromocytoma, dissecting aortic aneurysm

Precautions: Tachycardia, fluid, electrolyte imbalances, pregnancy (C), lactation, impaired cerebral or cardiac circulation, children

Pharmacokinetics:

IV: Onset 1-2 min, peak 5 min, duration 3-12 hr; *PO:* onset 1 hr, peak 8-12 hr, duration 8 hr, half-life 20-36 hr, excreted slowly in urine, crosses blood-brain barrier, placenta

Interactions:

• Severe hypotension: antihypertensives

• Increased hyperuricemic, antihypertensive effects of diazoxide: thiazide diuretics

• Hyperglycemia: sulfonylureas

• Decreased anticonvulsant effect: hydantoins

NURSING CONSIDERATIONS

Assess:

• B/P q5min until stabilized, then q1h × 2 hr, then q4h

• Pulse, jugular venous distention q4h

• Electrolytes, blood studies: K, Na, Cl, CO_2, CBC, serum glucose

• Weight daily, I&O

• Edema in feet, legs daily

• Skin turgor, dryness of mucous membranes for hydration status

• Rales, dyspnea, orthopnea

• IV site for extravasation, rate

• Signs of CHF: dyspnea, edema, wet rales

• Postural hypotension, take B/P sitting, standing

Administer:

• Undiluted; give over ½ min or less

• To patient in recumbent position; keep in that position for 1 hr after administration

Syringe compatibilities: Heparin

Perform/provide:

• Storage protected from light

Evaluate:
• Therapeutic response: decreased B/P, primarily diastolic pressure
Treatment of overdose: Dopamine, or norepinephrine for hypotension, Trendelenburg maneuver

---

diclofenac (℞)

(dye-kloe'fen-ak)
Cataflam, diclofenac, Voltaren, Voltaren Rapide*, Voltaren SR, Voltaren XR
Func. class.: Nonsteroidal antiinflammatory
Chem. class.: Phenylacetic acid

Action: Inhibits prostaglandin synthesis by decreasing enzyme needed for biosynthesis; analgesic, antiinflammatory, antipyretic

Uses: Acute, chronic rheumatoid arthritis, osteoarthritis; ankylosing spondylitis, analgesia, primary dysmenorrhea; ophth: postoperative inflammation after cataract extraction

Dosage and routes:
Osteoarthritis
• *Adult:* PO 100-150 mg/day in 2-3 divided doses
Rheumatoid arthritis
• *Adult:* PO 150-200 mg/day in 2-4 divided doses
Ankylosing spondylitis
• *Adult:* PO 100-125 mg/day in 4-5 divided doses, give 25 mg qid and 25 mg hs if needed
Postcataract surgery
• *Adult:* OPHTH 1 gtt of 0.1% sol qid × 2 wk 24 hr post surgery
Analgesia/primary dysmenorrhea
• *Adult:* PO 50 mg tid, max 150 mg/day (Cataflam)
Available forms: Tabs enteric coated 25, 50, 75, 100 mg tabs, ext rel 100 mg; tabs 50 mg (potassium); ophth sol 1%; suppositories: 50*, 100 mg*

Side effects/adverse reactions:
GI: Nausea, anorexia, vomiting, diarrhea, ***jaundice, cholestatic hepatitis,*** constipation, flatulence, cramps, dry mouth, peptic ulcer, GI bleeding, ***hepatotoxicity***
CNS: Dizziness, headache, drowsiness, fatigue, tremors, confusion, insomnia, anxiety, depression, nervousness, paresthesia, muscle weakness
CV: ***CHF,*** tachycardia, peripheral edema, palpitations, ***dysrhythmias,*** hypotension, hypertension, fluid retention
INTEG: Purpura, rash, pruritus, sweating, erythema, petechiae, photosensitivity, alopecia
*GU: **Nephrotoxicity: dysuria, hematuria, oliguria, azotemia, cystitis, UTI***
*HEMA: **Blood dyscrasias,*** epistaxis, bruising
EENT: Tinnitus, hearing loss, blurred vision, ***laryngeal edema***
RESP: Dyspnea, hemoptysis, pharyngitis, ***bronchospasm,*** rhinitis, shortness of breath
Contraindications: Hypersensitivity to aspirin, iodides, other nonsteroidal antiinflammatory agents, asthma
Precautions: Pregnancy (B); lactation, children, bleeding disorders, GI disorders, cardiac disorders, hypersensitivity to other antiinflammatory agents, CrCl <30 ml/min
Pharmacokinetics:
PO: Peak 2-3 hr, elimination half-life 1-2 hr, 90% bound to plasma proteins, metabolized in liver to metabolite, excreted in urine
Interactions:
• Decreased antihypertensive effect: β-blockers, diuretics
• Increased anticoagulant effect: anticoagulants
• Increased toxicity: phenytoin, lithium, cyclosporine, methotrexate

---

• Increased GI side effects: aspirin, other NSAIDs
• GI toxicity: aspirin
• Hyperkalemia: potassium-sparing diuretics
• Need for dosage adjustment: antidiabetics

NURSING CONSIDERATIONS
Assess:
• Blood counts during therapy; watch for decreasing platelets; if low, therapy may need to be discontinued, restarted after hematologic recovery
• LFTs and uric acid periodically
◆ Blood dyscrasias (thrombocytopenia): bruising, fatigue, bleeding, poor healing
Evaluate:
• Therapeutic response: decreased inflammation in joints, decreased inflammation after cataract surgery
Teach patient/family:
• That drug must be continued for prescribed time to be effective
• To report bleeding, bruising, fatigue, malaise; blood dyscrasias do occur
🚫 Not to break, crush, or chew enteric products
• To avoid aspirin, alcoholic beverages
• To take with food, milk, or antacids to avoid GI upset, to swallow whole
• To use caution when driving; drowsiness, dizziness may occur
• To take with a full glass of water to enhance absorption
• To report hepatotoxicity: flu symptoms, nausea, vomiting, jaundice, pruritus, lethargy
• To use sunscreen to prevent photosensitivity
• To avoid use in 3rd trimester of pregnancy

---

dicloxacillin (℞)
(dye-klox-a-sill′-in)
dicloxacillin sodium, Dycill, Dynapen, Pathocil
Func. class.: Antiinfective
Chem. class.: Penicillinase-resistant penicillin

Action: Interferes with cell wall replication of susceptible organisms; osmotically unstable cell wall swells, bursts from osmotic pressure
Uses: Effective for gram-positive cocci *(Staphylococcus aureus, Streptococcus pyogenes, S. viridans, S. faecalis, S. bovis, S. pneumoniae),* infections caused by penicillinase-producing *Staphylococcus*
Dosage and routes:
• *Adult:* **PO** 0.5-4 g/day in divided doses q6h
• *Child:* **PO** 12.5-50 mg/kg in divided doses q6h, max 4 g/day
Available forms: Caps 125, 250, 500 mg; powder for oral susp 62.5 mg/ 5 ml
Side effects/adverse reactions:
HEMA: Anemia, increased bleeding time, *bone marrow depression, granulocytopenia*
GI: Nausea, vomiting, diarrhea, increased AST, ALT, abdominal pain, glossitis, *pseudomembranous colitis*
GU: **Oliguria, proteinuria, hematuria,** *vaginitis, moniliasis, **glomerulonephritis***
CNS: Lethargy, hallucinations, anxiety, depression, twitching, *coma, convulsions*
SYST: **Anaphylaxis**
Contraindications: Hypersensitivity to penicillins; neonates
Precautions: Hypersensitivity to cephalosporins, pregnancy (B), lactation, severe renal or hepatic disease

---

◆ = Nursing alert   🌿 = Herb-drug interaction   🚫 = Do not crush

Pharmacokinetics:
PO: Peak 1 hr, duration 4-6 hr, half-life 30-60 min; metabolized in liver; excreted in urine, bile, breast milk; crosses placenta

Interactions:
• Increased dicloxacillin concentrations: aspirin, probenecid
• Increased effect of anticoagulants
• Decreased action of oral contraceptives

🌿 Delayed/reduced absorption: khat, separate by ≥2 hr

Lab test interferences:
False positive: Urine glucose, urine protein

NURSING CONSIDERATIONS
Assess:
• I&O ratio; report hematuria, oliguria, since penicillin in high doses is nephrotoxic

◆ Any patient with compromised renal system, since drug is excreted slowly in poor renal system function; toxicity may occur rapidly
• Blood studies: WBC, RBC, Hgb, Hct, bleeding time
• Renal studies: urinalysis, protein, blood
• C&S before drug therapy; drug may be given as soon as culture is taken
• WBC and differential, ALT, AST, BUN, creatinine for patients on long-term therapy
• Bowel pattern before, during treatment
• Skin eruptions after administration of penicillin to 1 wk after discontinuing drug
• Respiratory status: rate, character, wheezing, tightness in chest
• Allergies before initiation of treatment, reaction of each medication; highlight allergies on chart in red

Administer:
• Drug after C&S
• On an empty stomach with a full glass of water

• Susp after shaking well before each dose

Perform/provide:
• Adrenalin, suction, tracheostomy set, endotracheal intubation equipment
• Adequate fluid intake (2 L) during diarrhea episodes
• Scratch test to assess allergy after securing order from prescriber; usually done when penicillin is only drug of choice
• Storage in tight container; after reconstituting, store in refrigerator up to 2 wk

Evaluate:
• Therapeutic response: absence of fever, draining wounds

Teach patient/family:
• All aspects of drug therapy, including need to complete course of medication to ensure organism death (10-14 days); culture may be taken after completed course
• To report sore throat, fever, fatigue; may indicate superinfection

🚫 Not to break, crush, or chew caps
• To wear or carry Medic Alert ID if allergic to penicillins
• To notify prescriber of diarrhea

Treatment of anaphylaxis: Withdraw drug; maintain airway; administer epinephrine, aminophylline, O$_2$, IV corticosteroids

dicyclomine (R)

(dye-sye'kloe-meen)

Antispas, Bentyl, Bentylol*, Byclomine, Dibent, dicyclomine HCL, Dilomine, Di-Spaz, Formulex*, Lomine*, Neoquess, Or-Tyl, Spasmoject

Func. class.: Gastrointestinal anticholinergic

Chem. class.: Synthetic tertiary amine

Action: Inhibits muscarinic actions of acetylcholine at postganglionic parasympathetic neuroeffector sites

Uses: Treatment of peptic ulcer disease in combination with other drugs; infant colic, urinary incontinence

Dosage and routes:
• *Adult:* **PO** 10-20 mg tid-qid; **IM** 20 mg q4-6h
• *Child >2 yr:* **PO** 10 mg tid-qid
• *Child 6 mo-2 yr:* **PO** 5 mg tid-qid
Available forms: Caps 10, 20 mg; tabs 20 mg; syr 10 mg/5 ml; inj 10 mg/ml

Side effects/adverse reactions:
CNS: Confusion, stimulation in elderly, headache, insomnia, dizziness, drowsiness, anxiety, weakness, hallucination; *seizures, coma* (child <3 mo)
GI: Dry mouth, constipation, paralytic ileus, heartburn, nausea, vomiting, dysphagia, absence of taste
GU: Hesitancy, retention, impotence
CV: Palpitations, tachycardia
EENT: Blurred vision, photophobia, mydriasis, cycloplegia, increased ocular tension
INTEG: Urticaria, rash, pruritus, anhidrosis, fever, allergic reactions

Contraindications: Hypersensitivity to anticholinergics, narrow-angle glaucoma, GI obstruction, myasthenia gravis, paralytic ileus, GI atony, toxic megacolon

Precautions: Hyperthyroidism, coronary artery disease, dysrhythmias, CHF, ulcerative colitis, hypertension, hiatal hernia, hepatic disease, renal disease, pregnancy (B), lactation, urinary retention, prostatic hypertrophy

Pharmacokinetics:
PO: Onset 1-2 hr, duration 3-4 hr; metabolized by liver; excreted in urine

Interactions:
• Increased adverse reactions: amantadine, tricylic antidepressants, MAOIs, H_1-antihistamines, antiparkinsonian agents, meperidine, phenothiazines, procainamide, quinidine
• Decreased effect of levodopa, ketoconazole

NURSING CONSIDERATIONS
Assess:
• VS, cardiac status: checking for dysrhythmias, increased rate, palpitations
• For urinary retention or hesitancy
• GI complaints: pain, bleeding (frank or occult), nausea, vomiting, anorexia
• Anticholinergic effects in the elderly: urinary retention, constipation, delirium
Administer:
• ½-1 hr ac for better absorption
• Decreased dose to elderly patients; metabolism may be slowed
• Gum, hard candy, frequent rinsing of mouth for dry oral cavity
Perform/provide:
• Storage in tight container protected from light
• Increased fluids, bulk, exercise to decrease constipation
Evaluate:
• Therapeutic response: absence of epigastric pain, bleeding, nausea, vomiting

◆ = Nursing alert   🖊 = Herb-drug interaction   Ⓢ = Do not crush

Teach patient/family:

🚫 Not to break, crush, or chew caps

• To avoid driving, other hazardous activities until stabilized on medication; may cause blurred vision

• To avoid alcohol, other CNS depressants; will enhance sedating properties of this drug

• To avoid hot environments; stroke may occur; drug suppresses perspiration

• To use sunglasses when outside to prevent photophobia

• To drink plenty of fluids

• To report dysphagia

---

didanosine (℞)

(dye-dan′oh-seen)

ddI, dideoxyinosine, Videx

Func. class.: Antiviral

Chem. class.: Synthetic purine nucleoside of deoxyadenosine

Action: Nucleoside analog incorporating into cellular DNA by viral reverse transcriptase, thereby terminating the cellular DNA chain

Uses: Advanced HIV, AIDS infections in adults and children who have been unable to use zidovudine or who have not responded to treatment

Dosage and routes:

• Reduce dosage CrCl <60 ml/min

• *Adult:* PO **>75 kg,** 300 mg bid tabs, or 375 mg bid buffered pwd; 50-74 kg, 200 mg bid tabs, or 250 mg bid buffered pwd

• *Adult:* **PO 35-49 kg,** 125 mg bid tabs, or 167 mg bid buffered pwd

• *Child:* PO tabs 90-120 mg/m^2 q12h; buffered pwd packets 112.5-150 mg/m^2 q12h; **PO (child BSA 1.1-1.4 m^2)** tab 100 mg q8-12h; recon pedi pwd 125 mg q8-12h; **PO (child BSA 0.8-1 m^2)** tabs 75 mg q8-12h; recon pedi pwd 94 mg q8-12h; **PO (child BSA 0.5-0.7 m^2)** tabs 50 mg q8-12h; recon pedi pwd 62 mg q8-12h; **PO (child BSA <0.4 m^2)** tabs 25 mg q8-12h; recon pedi pwd 31 mg q8-12h

Available forms: Tabs, buffered, chewable/dispersible 25, 50, 100, 150 mg; pwd for oral sol, buffered 100, 167, 250, 375 mg/packet; pwd for oral sol, pedi 2, 4 g

Side effects/adverse reactions:

GI: ***Pancreatitis,*** *diarrhea, nausea,* vomiting, *abdominal pain,* constipation, stomatitis, dyspepsia, liver abnormalities, flatulence, taste perversion, dry mouth, oral thrush, melena, increased ALT, AST, alk phosphatase, amylase, ***hepatic failure***

GU: Increased bilirubin, uric acid

CNS: **Peripheral neuropathy, seizures,** confusion, *anxiety,* hypertonia, abnormal thinking, asthenia, *insomnia,* ***CNS depression,*** pain, dizziness, chills, fever

RESP: Cough, pneumonia, dyspnea, asthma, epistaxis, hypoventilation, sinusitis

INTEG: *Rash, pruritus,* alopecia, ecchymosis, hemorrhage, petechiae, sweating

MS: Myalgia, arthritis, myopathy, muscular atrophy

CV: Hypertension, vasodilation, dysrhythmia, syncope, ***CHF,*** palpitation

EENT: Ear pain, otitis, photophobia, visual impairment, retinal depigmentation

HEMA: ***Leukopenia, granulocytopenia, thrombocytopenia, anemia***

Contraindications: Hypersensitivity

Precautions: Renal, hepatic disease, pregnancy (B), lactation, children, sodium-restricted diets, elevated amylase, preexistant peripheral neuropathy, phenylketonuria, hyperuricemia

Pharmacokinetics:

PO: Elimination half-life 1.62 hr, extensive metabolism is thought to occur; administration within 5 min of food will decrease absorption

Interactions:

• Decreased absorption: ketoconazole, dapsone

• Increased side effects from: magnesium, aluminum antacids

• Decreased concentrations of fluoroquinolone, itraconazole, tetracyclines

• Drug/food: any food decreases rate of absorption

NURSING CONSIDERATIONS
Assess:

• Peripheral neuropathy: tingling or pain in hands and feet, distal numbness

• Pancreatitis: abdominal pain, nausea, vomiting, elevated liver enzymes; drug should be discontinued, since condition can be fatal

• Children by dilated retinal examination q6mo to rule out retinal depigmentation

• CBC, differential, platelet count qmo; withhold drug if WBC is <4000 or platelet count is <75,000; notify prescriber of results; alk phosphatase, monitor amylase

• Renal function studies: BUN, serum uric acid, urine CrCl before, during therapy

• Temp q4h, may indicate beginning infection

• Liver function tests before, during therapy (bilirubin, AST, ALT) as needed or qmo

Administer:

• Pediatric powder for oral sol after preparation by pharmacist; dilution is required using purified USP water, then antacid (10 mg/ml), refrigerate, shake before use

Perform/provide:

• Cleanup of powdered products; use wet mop or damp sponge

Evaluate:

• Therapeutic response: absence of infection; symptoms of HIV

Teach patient/family:

• To take on an empty stomach; not to take dapsone at same time as ddI; do not mix powder with fruit juice; chew tab or crush and dissolve in water; drink powder immediately after mixing

• To report signs of infection: increased temp, sore throat, flu symptoms

• To report signs of anemia: fatigue, headache, faintness, shortness of breath, irritability

• To report bleeding; avoid use of razors, commercial mouthwash

• That hair may be lost during therapy (rare); a wig or hairpiece may make patient feel better

---

diethylstilbestrol (℞)
(dye-eth-il-stil-bess′trol)
(stilboestrol)
DES
diethylstilbestrol diphosphate (℞)
DES, Honvol*, Stiphostrol
Func. class.: Estrogen
Chem. class.: Nonsteroidal synthetic estrogen

Action: Needed for adequate functioning of female reproductive system, it affects release of pituitary gonadotropins, inhibits ovulation, adequate calcium use in bone structures

Uses: Breast cancer, prostatic cancer, vasomotor symptoms of menopause

---

◆ = Nursing alert   🖊 = Herb-drug interaction   ⊘ = Do not crush

Dosage and routes:
Prostatic cancer
• *Adult:* **PO** 1-3 mg qd, then 1 mg qd; **PO** 50-200 mg tid (diphosphate); **IM** 5 mg 2×/wk, then 4 mg 2×/wk; **IV** 500 mg-1 g qd × 5 days, then 250-500 mg 1-2×/wk

Breast cancer (postmenopausal)
• *Adult:* **PO** 15 mg qd

Available forms: Diethylstilbestrol: Tabs 1, 5 mg; diethylstilbestrol diphosphate tab 50 mg; inj 0.25 g

Side effects/adverse reactions:

CNS: Dizziness, headache, migraines, depression

CV: Hypotension, thrombophlebitis, edema, *thromboembolism, stroke, pulmonary embolism, myocardial infarction*

GI: Nausea, vomiting, diarrhea, anorexia, pancreatitis, cramps, constipation, increased appetite, increased weight, *cholestatic jaundice, hepatic adenoma*

EENT: Contact lens intolerance, increased myopia, astigmatism

GU: Amenorrhea, cervical erosion, breakthrough bleeding, dysmenorrhea, vaginal candidiasis, breast changes, *gynecomastia, testicular atrophy, impotence, increased risk of breast cancer/endometrial cancer*

INTEG: Rash, urticaria, acne, hirsutism, alopecia, oily skin, seborrhea, purpura, melasma

META: Folic acid deficiency, hypercalcemia, hyperglycemia

Contraindications: Premenopausal breast cancer, thromboembolic disorders, reproductive cancer, genital bleeding (abnormal, undiagnosed), pregnancy (X), lactation

Precautions: Hypertension, asthma, blood dyscrasias, gallbladder disease, CHF, diabetes mellitus, bone disease blocking agents, MI

Interactions:
• Decreased action of anticoagulants, oral hypoglycemics, tamoxifen
• Toxicity: tricyclics, cyclosporine, dantrolene, hepatotoxics
• Decreased action of diethylstilbestrol: anticonvulsants, barbiturates, rifampin
• Increased action of: corticosteroids
• Drug/food: increased caffeine level
• Drug/smoking: increased CV reactions

🌿 Possible additive hormonal effect: alfalfa

Lab test interferences:

Increase: T_4, serum Na, platelet aggregability, thyroxine-binding globulin (TBG), prothrombin; factors VII, VIII, IX, X; triglycerides

Decrease: Serum folate, serum triglyceride, T_3 resin uptake test, glucose tolerance test, antithrombin III, metyrapone test

False positive: LE prep, antinuclear antibodies

NURSING CONSIDERATIONS
Assess:
• Blood glucose in patient with diabetes; blood glucose may rise
• If female patient has an intact uterus
• Weight daily, notify prescriber of weekly weight gain >5 lb; if increase, diuretic may be ordered
• B/P, watch for increase caused by H_2O and Na retention
• Liver function studies, including AST, ALT, bilirubin, alk phosphatase
• Edema, hypertension, cardiac symptoms, jaundice
• Mental status: affect, mood, behavioral changes, aggression
Administer:
• IV after diluting in 300 ml dextrose or NS sol; give at 1-2 ml/min

---

× 15 min; may increase rate to complete infusion 1 hr after starting
• Titrated dose; use lowest effective dose
• In one dose in AM for prostatic cancer
• With food, milk for GI symptoms
• With a progesterone for 10-13 day/mo for female patients with an intact uterus
Evaluate:
• Therapeutic response: absence of breast engorgement, reversal of menopause or decrease in tumor size in prostatic cancer
Teach patient/family:
• To weigh weekly, report gain >5 lb
• To report immediately breast lumps, vaginal bleeding, edema, jaundice, dark urine, clay-colored stools, dyspnea, headache, blurred vision, abdominal pain, numbness or stiffness in legs, chest pain; male to report impotence or gynecomastia
• To check with prescriber before taking any OTC drugs
• To use nonhormonal contraception during treatment
• That antidiabetic medication may need to be adjusted in diabetic patients

---

diflunisal (Ŗ)
(dye-floo'ni-sal)
diflunisal, Dolobid
Func. class.: Nonsteroidal antiinflammatory/analgesic (nonopioid)
Chem. class.: Salicylate derivative

Action: May block pain impulses in CNS that occur in response to inhibition of prostaglandin synthesis; antipyretic action results from inhibition of hypothalamic heat-regulating center to produce vasodilation to allow heat dissipation
Uses: Mild to moderate pain or fever including arthritis; 3-4 times more potent than aspirin
Dosage and routes:
• *Adult:* PO loading dose 1 g; then 500-1000 mg/day in 2 divided doses, q12h, not to exceed 1500 mg/day
• *Geriatric:* ½ adult dose
Available forms: Tabs 250, 500 mg
Side effects/adverse reactions:
CNS: Stimulation, drowsiness, dizziness, confusion, *headache,* flushing, hallucinations, ***coma***
GI: Nausea, vomiting, GI bleeding, diarrhea, heartburn, anorexia
INTEG: Rash, urticaria, bruising, ***Stevens-Johnson syndrome***
EENT: Blurred vision, decreased acuity, corneal deposits
GU: Hematuria, ***interstitial nephritis***
Contraindications: Hypersensitivity to salicylates, GI bleeding, bleeding disorders, children <12 yr, vit K deficiency
Precautions: Anemia, hepatic disease, renal disease, Hodgkin's disease, pregnancy (C), lactation
Pharmacokinetics:
PO: Onset 15-30 min, peak 2-3 hr, half-life 10-12 hr; metabolized by liver; excreted by kidneys; crosses placenta; 99% protein bound; excreted in breast milk
Interactions:
• Decreased effects of diflunisal: antacids, steroids, salicylates; urinary alkalizers
• Increased blood loss: alcohol, heparin
• Increased effects of: anticoagulants, insulin, methotrexate, hydrochlorothiazide, acetaminophen, thrombolytics, indomethacin
• Decreased effects of: probenecid, sulindac

◆ = Nursing alert   ∅ = Herb-drug interaction   ⊘ = Do not crush

Lab test interferences:

Increase: Coagulation, liver function studies, serum uric acid, amylase, CO_2, urinary protein

NURSING CONSIDERATIONS
Assess:

• Pain: frequency, intensity, characteristics, relief after med

• For asthma, aspirin hypersensitivity, nasal polyps that may develop hypersensitivity reactions

• Hepatotoxicity: dark urine; clay-colored stools; jaundice of skin, sclera; itching; abdominal pain; fever; diarrhea (long-term therapy)

• Allergic reactions: rash, urticaria; drug may have to be discontinued

• Renal dysfunction: decreased urine output

• Ototoxicity: tinnitus, ringing, roaring in ears; audiometric testing is needed before, after long-term therapy

• Visual changes: blurring, halos, corneal, retinal damage

• Edema in feet, ankles, legs

Administer:

• To patient whole

• With food, milk for gastric symptoms

Evaluate:

• Therapeutic response: decreased pain, stiffness of joints

Teach patient/family:

◆ To report any symptoms of hepatotoxicity, renal toxicity, visual changes, ototoxicity, allergic reactions (long-term therapy)

• Not to exceed recommended dosage; acute poisoning may result

• To read label on other OTC drugs; many contain aspirin

• That therapeutic response takes 2 wk (arthritis)

Treatment of overdose: Lavage, activated charcoal, monitor electrolytes, VS

---

digitoxin (R)
(di-ji-tox′in)
Crystodigin, digitoxin
Func. class.: Antidysrhythmic, cardiac glycoside, cardiotonic
Chem. class.: Digitalis preparation

D

Action: Inhibits sodium-potassium ATPase, which makes more calcium available for contractile proteins, resulting in increased cardiac output

Uses: CHF, atrial fibrillation, atrial flutter, atrial tachycardia

Dosage and routes:

• *Adult and child >12 yr:* **PO** 1.2-1.6 mg initially (loading); give in divided doses over 24 hr; 150 µg qd; maintenance dose: 0.05-0.3 mg qd, usual 0.15 mg qd; rapid loading dose 0.6 mg, then 0.4 mg, then 0.2 mg q4-6h; slow loading dose 0.2 mg/bid × 4 days, then maintenance

• *Child <1 yr:* 0.045 mg/kg

• *Child 1-2 yr:* 0.04 mg/kg

• *Child >2 yr:* 0.03 mg/kg (0.75 mg/m^2); maintenance: 10% of digitalizing dose

Available forms: Tabs 100 (0.1 mg), 200 µg (0.2 mg)

Side effects/adverse reactions:

CNS: Headache, drowsiness, apathy, confusion, disorientation, fatigue, depression, hallucinations

*CV: **Dysrhythmias,** hypotension, bradycardia, **AV block***

GI: Nausea, vomiting, anorexia, abdominal pain, diarrhea

EENT: Blurred vision, yellow-green halos, photophobia, diplopia

MS: Muscular weakness

Contraindications: Hypersensitivity to digitalis, ventricular fibrillation, ventricular tachycardia, ca-

---

rotid sinus syndrome, 2nd- or 3rd-degree heart block

Precautions: Hepatic disease, acute MI, AV block, hypokalemia, hypomagnesemia, sinus node disease, lactation, severe respiratory disease, hypothyroidism, elderly, pregnancy (C), lactation

Pharmacokinetics:

PO: Onset 1-4 hr, peak 4-12 hr; duration 2-3 wk, half-life 4-20 days; metabolized in liver; excreted in urine

Interactions:

• Hypokalemia: thiazides
• Increased blood levels: spironolactone
• Decreased effects: hydantoins, aminoglutethimide, rifampin, phenylbutazone, barbiturates, cholestyramine, colestipol
• Toxicity: adrenergics, diuretics, succinylcholine, quinidine, thioamines
• Decreased level of digitoxin: thyroid agents

🟋 Increased action: aloe, buckthorn bark/berry, cascara sagrada bark, senna pod/leaf, Siberian ginseng, quinine
🟋 Dysrhythmias: ephedra
🟋 Bradycardia: Indian snakeroot
🟋 Cardiac toxicity: hawthorn
🟋 Digitoxin toxicity: licorice
🟋 Decreased digitoxin absorption: psyllium

Lab test interferences:

Increase: CPK

NURSING CONSIDERATIONS

Assess:

• Apical pulse for 1 min before giving drug; if pulse <60, take again in 1 hr; if <60, call prescriber
• Electrolytes: K, Na, Cl, Ca; renal function studies: BUN, creatinine; blood studies: ALT, AST, bilirubin
• Monitor drug levels (therapeutic level 9-25 ng/ml)

• Cardiac status: apical pulse, character, rate, rhythm

Administer:

• K supplements if ordered for K levels <3.0 mg/dl

Evaluate:

• Therapeutic response: decreased weight, edema, pulse, respiration and increased urine output

Teach patient/family:

• Not to stop drug abruptly; teach all aspects of drug, digitalis toxicity; to keep tabs in container protected from light
• To avoid OTC medications; many adverse interactions
• To notify prescriber of loss of appetite, lower stomach pain, diarrhea, weakness, drowsiness, headache, blurred or yellow vision, rash, depression

Treatment of overdose: Discontinue drug, administer K, digoxin immune FAB, monitor ECG

---

digoxin (℞)

(di-jox'in)

digoxin, Lanoxicaps, Lanoxin, Novo-Digoxin*

Func. class.: Inotropic, antidysrhythmic, cardiac glycoside

Chem. class.: Digitalis preparation

Action: Inhibits the sodium-potassium ATPase, which makes more calcium available for contractile proteins, resulting in increased cardiac output

Uses: CHF, atrial fibrillation, atrial flutter, atrial tachycardia, cardiogenic shock, paroxysmal atrial tachycardia, rapid digitalization in these disorders

Dosage and routes:

• *Adult:* **IV** *digitalizing dose* 0.6-1.0 mg given as 50% of the dose

---

◆ = Nursing alert   🟋 = Herb-drug interaction   🚫 = Do not crush initially, additional fractions given at 4-8 hr intervals; **PO digitalizing dose** 0.75-1.25 mg given as 50% of the dose initially, additional fractions given at 4-8 hr intervals; **maintenance** 0.063-0.5 mg/day (tabs), or 0.350-0.5 mg/day (gelatin cap)

• *Child >10 yr:* **IV digitalizing dose** 8-12 µg/kg given as 50% of the dose initially, additional fractions given at 4-8 hr intervals; **PO digitalizing dose** 0.01-0.015 mg/kg given as 50% of the dose initially, additional fractions given at 6-8 hr intervals; **maintenance** 25%-35% of the loading dose qd as a single dose

• *Child 5-10 yr:* **IV digitalizing dose** 0.015-0.03 mg/kg given as 50% of the dose initially, additional fractions given at 4-8 hr intervals; **PO digitalizing dose** 0.02-0.035 mg/kg given as 50% of the dose initially, additional fractions given at 6-8 hr intervals; **maintenance** 25%-35% of the loading dose qd in 2 divided doses

• *Child 2-5 yr:* **IV digitalizing dose** 0.025-0.035 mg/kg given as 50% of the dose initially, additional fractions given at 4-8 hr intervals; **PO digitalizing dose** 0.03-0.04 mg/kg given as 50% of the dose initially, additional fractions given at 6-8 hr intervals; **maintenance** 25%-35% of the loading dose qd in 2 divided doses

• *Child 1-2 yr:* **IV digitalizing dose** 0.03-0.05 mg/kg given as 50% of the dose initially, additional fractions given at 4-8 hr intervals; **PO digitalizing dose** 0.035-0.06 mg/kg given as 50% of the dose initially, additional fractions given at 4-8 hr intervals; **maintenance** 25%-35% of the loading dose qd in 2 divided doses

• *Infants:* **IV digitalizing dose** 0.02-0.03 mg/kg given as 50% of the dose initially, additional fractions given at 4-8 hr intervals; **PO digitalizing dose** 0.025-0.035 mg/kg given as 50% of the dose initially, additional fractions given at 6-8 hr intervals; **maintenance** 25%-35% of the loading dose qd in 2 divided doses

• *Infants, premature:* **IV digitalizing dose** 0.015-0.025 mg/kg given as 50% of the dose initially, additional fractions given at 4-8 hr intervals; **PO digitalizing dose** 0.02-0.03 mg/kg given as 50% of the dose initially, additional fractions given at 6-8 hr intervals; **maintenance** 20%-30% of the loading dose qd in 2 divided doses

Available forms: Caps 0.05, 0.1, 0.2 mg; elix 0.05 mg/ml; tabs 0.125, 0.25, 0.5 mg; inj 0.5*, 0.25 mg/ml: pediatric inj 0.01 mg/ml

Side effects/adverse reactions:
CNS: Headache, drowsiness, apathy, confusion, disorientation, fatigue, depression, hallucinations
*CV: **Dysrhythmias,** hypotension,* bradycardia, **AV block**
EENT: Blurred vision, yellow-green halos, photophobia, diplopia
GI: Nausea, vomiting, anorexia, abdominal pain, diarrhea

Contraindications: Hypersensitivity to digitalis, ventricular fibrillation, ventricular tachycardia, carotid sinus syndrome, 2nd or 3rd degree heart block

Precautions: Renal disease, acute MI, AV block, severe respiratory disease, hypothyroidism, elderly, pregnancy (C), sinus nodal disease, lactation, hypokalemia

Pharmacokinetics:
PO: Onset ½-2 hr, peak 6-8 hr, duration 3-4 days
IV: Onset 5-30 min, peak 1-5 hr, duration variable
Half-life 1.5 days, excreted in urine

Interactions:
• Decreased digoxin absorption: antacids kaolin/pectin
• Hypercalcemia, hypomagnesemia, digitalis toxicity: thiazides, parenteral Ca
• Hypokalemia, digitalis toxicity: diuretics, amphotericin B, carbenicillin, ticarcillin, corticosteroids
• Decreased digoxin level: thyroid agents, cholestyramine, colestipol, metoclopramide
• Increased digoxin blood levels: propantheline, quinidine, verapamil, amiodarone, anticholinergics, diltiazem, nifedipine
• Increased bradycardia: β-adrenergic blockers, antidysrythmics
🌿 Increased action: aloe, buckthorn bark/berry, cascara sagrada bark, senna pod/leaf, Siberian ginseng, quinine
🌿 Dysrhythmias: ephedra
🌿 Bradycardia: Indian snakeroot
🌿 Cardiac toxicity: hawthorn
🌿 Digoxin toxicity: licorice
🌿 Decreased digoxin absorption: psyllium

Lab test interferences:
Increase: CPK

NURSING CONSIDERATIONS
Assess:
• Apical pulse for 1 min before giving drug; if pulse <60 in adult or <90 in an infant, take again in 1 hr; if <60 in adult, call prescriber; note rate, rhythm, character; monitor ECG continuously during parenteral loading dose
• Electrolytes: K, Na, Cl, Mg, Ca; renal function studies: BUN, creatinine; blood studies: ALT, AST, bilirubin, Hct, Hgb before initiating treatment and periodically thereafter
• I&O ratio, daily weights; monitor turgor, lung sounds, edema
• Monitor drug levels (therapeutic level 0.5-2 ng/ml)

• Cardiac status: apical pulse, character, rate, rhythm
Administer:
PO
• PO with or without food; may crush tabs, mix with food/fluids
• K supplements if ordered for K levels <3, or foods high in K: bananas, orange juice
IV
• Undiluted or 1 ml of drug/4 ml sterile H_2O, D_5, or NS; give >5 min through Y-tube or 3-way stopcock; during digitalization close monitoring is necessary
Additive compatibilities: Bretylium, cimetidine, floxacillin, furosemide, lidocaine, ranitidine, verapamil
Syringe compatibilities: Heparin, milrinone
Y-site compatibilities: Amrinone, cefmetazole, ciprofloxacin, cisatracurium, diltiazem, famotidine, meperidine, meropenem, midazolam, milrinone, morphine, potassium chloride, propofol, remifentanil, tacrolimus, vit B/C
Perform/provide:
• Storage protected from light
Evaluate:
• Therapeutic response: decreased weight, edema, pulse, respiration, rales; increased urine output; serum digoxin level (0.5-2 ng/ml)
Teach patient/family:
• Not to stop drug abruptly; teach all aspects of drug, to take exactly as ordered
• To avoid OTC medications, since many adverse drug interactions may occur; do not take antacid at same time
• To notify prescriber of loss of appetite, lower stomach pain, diarrhea, weakness, drowsiness, headache, blurred or yellow vision, rash, depression, toxicity

---

◆ = Nursing alert   🌿 = Herb-drug interaction   ⊘ = Do not crush

• The toxic symptoms of this drug and when to notify prescriber

• To maintain a sodium-restricted diet as ordered

🚫 Not to break, crush, or chew caps

• To report shortness of breath, difficulty breathing, weight gain, edema, persistent cough

Treatment of overdose: Discontinue drug; give K; monitor ECG; give adrenergic-blocking agent, digoxin immune FAB

digoxin immune FAB (ovine) (Ŗ)

(di-jox'in im-myoon' FAB)
Digibind
Func. class.: Antidote—digoxin specific

Action: Antibody fragments bind to free digoxin or digitoxin to reverse toxicity by not allowing digoxin or digitoxin to bind to sites of action
Uses: Life-threatening digoxin or digitoxin toxicity
Dosage and routes:
Digoxin toxicity
• *Adult:* **IV** dose (mg) = dose ingested (mg) × serum digoxin conc × 5.6 × wt in kg ÷ 1000; if ingested amount is unknown, give 800 mg **IV**; if digoxin liquid caps, **IV,** do not multiply ingested dose by 0.8
Digitoxin
• Body load in mg = serum digitoxin conc × 0.56 × wt in kg ÷ 1000
Available forms: Inj 38 mg/vial (binds 0.5 mg digoxin or digitoxin)
Side effects/adverse reactions:
CV: ***CHF,*** ventricular rate increase, ***atrial fibrillation,*** low cardiac output
RESP: ***Impaired respiratory function,*** rapid respiratory rate
META: ***Hypokalemia***

MISC: ***Anaphylaxis***
INTEG: *Hypersensitivity,* allergic reactions, facial swelling, redness
Contraindications: Mild digoxin toxicity, hypersensitivity
Precautions: Children, lactation, cardiac disease, renal disease, pregnancy (C), allergy to ovine proteins
Pharmacokinetics:
IV: Peaks after completion of infusion, onset 30 min (variable); not known if crosses placenta, breast milk; half-life biphasic—14-20 hr; prolonged in renal disease; excreted by kidneys
Interactions:
• Considered incompatible with all drugs in syringe or sol
Lab test interferences:
Interference: Immunoassay digoxin
NURSING CONSIDERATIONS
Assess:
• Hypokalemia: ST depression, flat T waves, presence of U wave, ventricular dysrhythmia; K levels may decrease rapidly
Administer:
• After diluting 38 mg/4 ml of sterile H_2O for inj 10 mg/ml mix; may be further diluted with normal saline, sol should be clear, colorless
• By bolus if cardiac arrest is imminent or IV over 30 min using a 0.22 μm filter
Perform/provide:
• Storage of reconstituted sol for up to 4 hr in refrigerator
Evaluate:
• Therapeutic response: correction of digoxin toxicity; check digoxin levels 0.5-2 ng/ml; digitoxin level 9-25 ng/ml
Teach patient/family:
• The purpose of medication; to report fever, chills, itching, swelling, dyspnea
• To tell patient to notify anyone in dental or medical care that this drug is being taken

---

dihydroergotamine (Ŗ)
(dye-hye-droe-er-got′a-meen)
D.H.E. 45,
Dihydroergotamine-Sandoz*
Func. class.: α-Adrenergic blocker
Chem. class.: Ergot alkaloid (dihydrogenated)

Action: Constricts smooth muscle in periphery, cranial blood vessels; inhibits norepinephrine uptake

Uses: Vascular headache (migraine or histamine)

Dosage and routes:
• *Adult:* **IM/IV** 1 mg; may repeat q1-2h if needed, not to exceed 3 mg/day or 6 mg/wk

Available forms: Inj 1 mg/ml

Side effects/adverse reactions:
CNS: Numbness in fingers, toes, weakness
CV: Transient tachycardia, chest pain, bradycardia, increase or decrease in B/P, *gangrene*
GI: Nausea, vomiting
MS: Muscle pain

Contraindications: Hypersensitivity to ergot preparations, occlusion (peripheral, vascular), CAD, hepatic disease, pregnancy (X), renal disease, peptic ulcer, hypertension, lactation, children, uremia

Pharmacokinetics:
IM: Onset 15-30 min, peak 2 hr, duration 3-4 hr
IV: Onset 5 min, peak 45 min, duration 3-4 hr; half-life 1.3-4 hr

Interactions:
• Ergot toxicity symptoms: macrolide antibiotics
• Increased vasoconstriction: β-blockers
• Incompatible with any drug in syringe or sol

NURSING CONSIDERATIONS
Assess:
• Weight daily, check for peripheral edema in feet, legs
• For stress level, activity, recreation, coping mechanisms
• Neurologic status: LOC, blurring vision, nausea, vomiting, tingling in extremities that precedes headache
• Ingestion of tyramine (pickled products, beer, wine, aged cheese), food additives, preservatives, colorings, artificial sweeteners, chocolate, caffeine; may precipitate these headaches

Administer:
• IV undiluted; give over 3 min
• At beginning of headache; dose must be titrated to patient response
• Only to women who are not pregnant; harm to fetus may occur

Perform/provide:
• Storage in dark area; do not use discolored solutions
• Quiet, calm environment with decreased stimulation for noise, bright light, excessive talking

Evaluate:
• Therapeutic response: decrease in frequency, severity of headache

Teach patient/family:
• Not to use OTC medications; serious drug interactions may occur
• To report side effects: increased vasoconstriction starting with cold extremities, then paresthesia, weakness
• That an increase in headaches may occur when this drug is discontinued after long-term use
◆ To keep drug out of reach of children; death may occur
• Not to use during pregnancy

◆ = Nursing alert   ▰ = Herb-drug interaction   ⊘ = Do not crush

dihydrotachysterol (R)

(dye-hye-droh-tak-iss'ter-ole)
DHT Intensol*, Hytakerol
Func. class.: Parathyroid agent
(calcium regulator)
Chem. class.: Vitamin D analog

Action: Increases intestinal absorption of calcium for bones, increases renal tubular absorption of phosphate; regulates calcium levels by regulating calcitonin, parathyroid hormone

Uses: Renal osteodystrophy, hypoparathyroidism, pseudohypoparathyroidism, familial hypophosphatemia, postoperative tetany

Dosage and routes:
Hypophosphatemia
• *Adult and child:* **PO** 0.5-2 mg qd, maintenance 0.3-1.5 mg qd
Hypoparathyroidism/pseudohypoparathyroidism
• *Adult:* **PO** 0.8-2.4 mg qd × 4 days, maintenance 0.2-2 mg qd regulated by serum calcium levels
• *Child:* **PO** 1-5 mg qd × 1 wk, maintenance 0.2-1 mg qd regulated by serum Ca levels
Renal osteodystrophy
• *Adult:* **PO** 0.1-0.25 mg qd, then 0.2-1 mg/day

Available forms: Tabs 0.125, 0.2, 0.4 mg; caps 0.125 mg; oral sol 0.2, 0.25 mg/5 ml, 0.2 mg/ml* (Intensol)

Side effects/adverse reactions:
EENT: Tinnitus
CNS: Drowsiness, headache, vertigo, fever, lethargy
GI: Nausea, diarrhea, vomiting, jaundice, anorexia, dry mouth, constipation, cramps, metallic taste
MS: Myalgia, arthralgia, decreased bone development
GU: Polyuria, hypercalciuria, hyperphosphatemia, hematuria
CV: **Dysrhythmias,** hypertension

Contraindications: Hypersensitivity, renal disease, hyperphosphatemia, hypercalcemia
Precautions: Pregnancy (C), renal calculi, lactation, CV disease
Pharmacokinetics:
PO: Onset 2 wk; metabolized by liver, excreted in feces (active/inactive)
Interactions:
• Decreased absorption of dihydrotachysterol: cholestyramine, colestipol mineral oil
• Hypercalcemia: thiazide diuretics, calcium supplements
• Cardiac dysrhythmias: cardiac glycosides, verapamil
• Decreased effect of dihydrotachysterol: corticosteroids, phenytoin, barbiturates
Lab test interferences:
False increase: Cholesterol
NURSING CONSIDERATIONS
Assess:
• BUN, urinary Ca, AST, ALT, cholesterol, creatinine, alk phosphatase, uric acid, chlorine, magnesium, electrolytes, urine pH, phosphate; may increase calcium, should be kept at 9-10 mg/dl, vit D 50-135 IU/dl, phosphate 70 mg/dl
• Alk phosphatase; may be decreased
• For increased blood level, since toxic reactions may occur rapidly
• For dry mouth, metallic taste, polyuria, bone pain, muscle weakness, headache, fatigue, tinnitus, change in LOC, irregular pulse, dysrhythmias, increased respirations, anorexia, nausea, vomiting, cramps, diarrhea, constipation; may indicate hypercalcemia
• Renal status: decreased urinary output (oliguria, anuria), edema in extremities, weight gain >5 lb, periorbital edema
• Nutritional status, diet for sources of vit D (milk, some seafood), Ca

(dairy products, dark green vegetables), phosphates (dairy products) must be avoided

Administer:
• PO, may be increased q4wk depending on blood level

Perform/provide:
• Storage in tight, light-resistant containers at room temp
• Restriction of Na, K if required
• Restriction of fluids if required for chronic renal failure

Evaluate:
• Therapeutic response: prevention of bone deficiencies

Teach patient/family:
• The symptoms of hypercalcemia
• About foods rich in calcium, vit D
🚫 Not to break, crush, or chew caps

---

diltiazem (℞)

(dil-tye′a-zem)
Apo-Diltiaz*, Cardizem, Cardizem CD, Cardizem SR, Dilacor-XR, diltiazem, Tiazac

Func. class.: Calcium channel blocker

Chem. class.: Benzothiazepine

Action: Inhibits calcium ion influx across cell membrane during cardiac depolarization; produces relaxation of coronary vascular smooth muscle, dilates coronary arteries, slows SA/AV node conduction times, dilates peripheral arteries

Uses: Angina pectoris due to coronary insufficiency, hypertension, vasospasm; parenteral: atrial fibrillation, flutter, paroxysmal supraventricular tachycardia

Dosage and routes:
• *Adult:* **PO** 30 mg qid, increasing dose gradually to 180-360 mg/day in divided doses or 60-120 mg bid; may increase to 240-360 mg/day

• *Adult:* **IV BOL** 0.25 mg/kg over 2 min initially, then 0.35 mg/kg may be given after 15 min; if no response, may give **CONT INF** 5-15 mg/hr for up to 24 hr
• *Adult:* **PO** (Cardizem CD) qd

Available forms: Tabs 30, 60, 90, 120 mg; caps ext rel 120, 180, 240, 300, 360 mg; cap, sus rel 60, 90, 120, 180, 240 mg; inj 5 mg/ml (5, 10 ml)

Side effects/adverse reactions:
CV: **Dysrhythmia,** *edema,* **CHF,** bradycardia, hypotension, palpitations, **heart block**
GI: *Nausea,* vomiting, diarrhea, gastric upset, *constipation,* increased liver function studies
GU: Nocturia, polyuria, **acute renal failure**
INTEG: *Rash,* pruritus, flushing, photosensitivity
CNS: Headache, fatigue, *drowsiness,* dizziness, depression, weakness, insomnia, tremor, paresthesia

Contraindications: Sick sinus syndrome, 2nd- or 3rd-degree heart block, hypotension less than 90 mm Hg systolic, acute MI, pulmonary congestion

Precautions: CHF, hypotension, hepatic injury, pregnancy (C), lactation, children, renal disease

Pharmacokinetics: Onset 30-60 min; peak 2-3 hr, immediate rel, 6-11 sus rel; half-life 3½-9 hr; metabolized by liver; excreted in urine (96% as metabolites)

Interactions:
• Increased effects of: β-blockers, digoxin, lithium, carbamazepine, cyclosporine, anesthetics
• Increased effects of diltiazem: cimetidine
🌿 Increased hypotensive effects: grapefruit

NURSING CONSIDERATIONS
Assess:

• Cardiac status: B/P, pulse, respiration, ECG and intervals PR, QRS, QT; if systolic B/P <90 mm Hg or HR <60 bpm, hold dose, notify prescriber

Administer:

• Before meals, hs (PO)

IV

• IV undiluted over 2 min or diluted 125 mg/100 ml, 250 mg/250 ml of D_5W, 0.9% NaCl, D_5/0.45% NaCl, give 10 mg/hr, may increase by 5 mg/hr to 15 mg/hr, continue infusion up to 24 hr

Y-site compatibilities: Albumin, amikacin, amphotericin B, aztreonam, bretylium, bumetanide, cefazolin, cefotaxime, cefotetan, cefoxitin, ceftazidime, ceftriaxone, cefuroxime, cimetidine, ciprofloxacin, clindamycin, digoxin, dobutamine, dopamine, doxycycline, epinephrine, erythromycin, esmolol, fentanyl, fluconazole, gentamicin, hetastarch, hydromorphone, imipenem-cilastatin, labetalol, lidocaine, lorazepam, meperidine, metoclopramide, metronidazole, midazolam, milrinone, morphine, multivitamins, nicardipine, nitroglycerin, norepinephrine, oxacillin, penicillin G potassium, pentamidine, piperacillin, potassium chloride, potassium phosphates, ranitidine, sodium nitroprusside, theophylline, ticarcillin, ticarcillin/clavulanate, tobramycin, trimethoprim-sulfamethoxazole, vancomycin, vecuronium

Perform/provide:

• Storage in tight container at room temp

Evaluate:

• Therapeutic response: decreased anginal pain, decreased B/P

Teach patient/family:

• How to take pulse before taking drug; record or graph should be kept

• To avoid hazardous activities until stabilized on drug, dizziness is no longer a problem

• To limit caffeine consumption

• To avoid OTC drugs unless directed by prescriber

• The importance of complying with all areas of medical regimen: diet, exercise, stress reduction, drug therapy

🚫 Not to break, crush, or chew sus rel caps or tabs

• To report dizziness, shortness of breath, palpitations

• Not to discontinue abruptly

• To take with a full glass of water

Treatment of overdose: Defibrillation, atropine for AV block, vasopressor for hypotension

---

dimenhydrinate
(OTC, ℞)

(dye-men-hye′dri-nate)
Apo-Dimenhydrinate*, Calm-X, Children's Dramamine, dimenhydrinate, Dimetabs, Dinate, Dramamine, Dramanate, Dymenate, Gravol*, Gravol L/A*, Hydrate, Nauseatol*, Novo-Dimenate*, PMS-Dimenhydrinate*, Travamine*, Triptone Caplets

Func. class.: Antiemetic, antihistamine, anticholinergic

Chem. class.: H_1-receptor antagonist, ethanolamine derivative

---

Action: Vestibular stimulation is decreased

Uses: Motion sickness, nausea, vomiting

Dosage and routes:

• *Adult:* **PO** 50-100 mg q4h; **IM/IV** 50 mg q4h as needed

• *Child:* **IM/PO** 5 mg/kg divided in 4 equal doses

Available forms: Tabs 50 mg; inj 50 mg/ml; elixir 15 mg/5 ml*; chew tabs 50 mg

Side effects/adverse reactions:

CNS: Drowsiness, restlessness, headache, dizziness, insomnia, confusion, nervousness, tingling, vertigo

GI: Nausea, anorexia, vomiting, *constipation*

CV: Hypertension, *hypotension*, palpitation

INTEG: Rash, urticaria, fever, chills, flushing

EENT: Dry mouth, blurred vision, diplopia, nasal congestion, photosensitivity

*MISC: **Anaphylaxis***

Contraindications: Hypersensitivity to narcotics, shock

Precautions: Children, cardiac dysrhythmias, elderly, asthma, pregnancy (B), lactation, prostatic hypertrophy, bladder-neck obstruction, narrow-angle glaucoma, stenosing peptic ulcer, pyloroduodenal obstruction

Pharmacokinetics:

IM/PO: Duration 4-6 hr

Interactions:

• Increased effect: alcohol, other CNS depressants

⚠ Increased anticholinergic effect: henbane leaf

Lab test interferences:

False negative: Allergy skin testing

NURSING CONSIDERATIONS

Assess:

• VS, B/P; check patients with cardiac disease more often

• Signs of toxicity of other drugs or masking of symptoms of disease: brain tumor, intestinal obstruction

• Observe for drowsiness, dizziness

Administer:

• IM injection in large muscle mass; aspirate to avoid IV administration

• Tablets may be swallowed whole, chewed, or allowed to dissolve

IV

• After diluting 50 mg/10 ml of NaCl inj; give 50 mg or less over 2 min

Additive compatibilities: Amikacin, calcium gluconate, chloramphenicol, corticotropin, erythromycin, heparin, hydroxyzine, methicillin, norepinephrine, penicillin G potassium, pentobarbital, phenobarbital, potassium chloride, prochlorperazine, vancomycin, vit B/C

Syringe compatibilities: Atropine, diphenhydramine, droperidol, fentanyl, heparin, hydromorphone, meperidine, metoclopramide, morphine, pentazocine, perphenazine, ranitidine, scopolamine

Y-site compatibilities: Acyclovir

• Therapeutic response: absence of nausea, vomiting

Teach patient/family:

• That a false-negative result may occur with skin testing; these procedures should not be scheduled for 4 days after discontinuing use

• To avoid hazardous activities, activities requiring alertness; dizziness may occur; instruct patient to request assistance with ambulation

• To avoid alcohol, other depressants

---

dinoprostone (℞)

(dye-noe-prost'one)

Prepidil, Prostin E₂

Func. class.: Oxytocic, abortifacient

Chem. class.: Prostaglandin E₂

Action: Stimulates uterine contractions, causing abortion; acts within 30 hr for complete abortion

Uses: Abortion during 2nd trimester, benign hydatidiform mole, expulsion of uterine contents in fetal deaths to 28 wk, missed abortion, to efface and dilate the cervix in pregnancy at term

---

⬦ = Nursing alert   ⚠ = Herb-drug interaction   ⊘ = Do not crush

Dosage and routes:
• *Adult:* **VAG SUPP** 20 mg, repeat q3-5h until abortion occurs, max dose is 240 mg
• *Adult:* **GEL** warm to room temp, choose correct length shielded catheter (10 or 20 mm), fill catheter by pushing plunger; patient should remain recumbent for 15-30 min
Available forms: Vag supp 20 mg; gel 0.5 mg/3 g (prefilled syringe)
Side effects/adverse reactions:
CNS: Headache, dizziness, chills, fever
CV: Hypotension, ***dysrhythmias***
GI: Nausea, vomiting, diarrhea
GU: Vaginitis, vaginal pain, vulvitis, vaginismus
INTEG: Rash, skin color changes
MS: Leg cramps, joint swelling, weakness
EENT: Blurred vision
INSERT: Uterine hyperstimulation, fever, nausea, vomiting, diarrhea, abdominal pain
GEL: Uterine contractile abnormality, GI side effects, back pain, fever
FETAL: Bradycardia (i.e., deceleration)
Contraindications: Hypersensitivity, uterine fibrosis, cervical stenosis, pelvic surgery, pelvic inflammatory disease, respiratory disease
Precautions: Hepatic disease, renal disease, cardiac disease, asthma, anemia, jaundice, diabetes mellitus, convulsive disorders, hypertension, hypotension, pregnancy (C)
Interactions
• Increased effect: other oxytocics
• Decreased oxytocic effect: alcohol
⚫ Hypertension: ephedra
Pharmacokinetics:
SUPP: Onset 10 min, duration 2-3 hr; metabolized in spleen, kidney, lungs; excreted in urine
NURSING CONSIDERATIONS
Assess:
• Dilation, effacement of cervix and uterine contraction, fetal heart tones, check for contractions over 1 min
• For fever that occurs ½ hr after suppository insertion (abortion)
• Respiratory rate, rhythm, depth; notify prescriber of abnormalities, pulse, B/P, temp
• Vaginal discharge: check for itching, irritation; indicates vaginal infection
• For fever, chills: increase fluids or give tepid sponge bath or blanket
Administer:
• By gel: after warming to room temp, remove seal from end of syringe, and remove the protective end cap and insert into plunger stopper assembly; make sure patient is in dorsal position
• Antiemetic/antidiarrheal before administration of this drug
Evaluate:
• Therapeutic response: expulsion of fetus
Teach patient/family:
• To remain supine for 10-15 min after insertion
• To report excessive cramping, bleeding, chills, fever
• Some methods of pain, comfort control

diphenhydramine
(OTC, ℞)

(dye-fen-hye′dra-meen)
Allerdryl*, AllerMax*, Aller-
med, Banophen, Beldin, Belix,
Bena-D 10, Bena-D 50, Bena-
dryl, Benadryl 25, Benadryl
Kapseals, Benahist 10, Bena-
hist 50, Ben-Allergin-50,
Benoject-10, Benoject-50,
Benylin Cough, Bydramine,
Compōz, Diphenacen-
50, Diphenadryl, Diphen
Cough, Diphenhist, diphen-
hydramine HCl, Dormarex 2,
Dormin, Fynex, Genahist,
Gen-D-Phen, Hydramine, Hy-
dramyn, Hydril, Hyrexin-50,
Insomnal*, Nidryl, Nighttime
Sleep Aid, Nordryl, Nordryl
Cough, Nytol, Phendry, Sleep-
Eze 3, Sominex 2, Tusstat, Twi-
lite, Uni-Bent Cough, Wehdryl
Func. class.: Antihistamine
Chem. class.: Ethanolamine de-
rivative, H_1-receptor antagonist

Action: Acts on blood vessels, GI,
respiratory system by competing
with histamine for H_1-receptor site;
decreases allergic response by blocking histamine

Uses: Allergy symptoms, rhinitis,
motion sickness, antiparkinsonism,
nighttime sedation, infant colic, nonproductive cough

Dosage and routes:

Renal disease
• CrCl 10-50 ml/min dose q6-12h;
CrCl <10 ml/min dose q12-18h
• *Adult:* **PO** 25-50 mg q4-6h, not to
exceed 400 mg/day; **IM/IV** 10-50
mg, not to exceed 400 mg/day
• *Child >12 kg:* **PO/IM/IV** 5 mg/
kg/day in 4 divided doses, not to
exceed 300 mg/day

Available forms: Caps 25, 50 mg;

tabs 25, 50 mg; liquid 6.25 mg/5 ml;
elix 12.5 mg/5 ml; syr 12.5 mg/5
ml; inj 10, 50 mg/ml

Side effects/adverse reactions:

CNS: Dizziness, drowsiness, poor coordination, fatigue, anxiety, euphoria, confusion, paresthesia, neuritis,
seizures
RESP: Increased thick secretions,
wheezing, chest tightness
HEMA: ***Thrombocytopenia, agranulocytosis, hemolytic anemia***
GI: Dry mouth, nausea, anorexia,
diarrhea
INTEG: Photosensitivity
GU: Retention, dysuria, frequency
EENT: Blurred vision, dilated pupils, tinnitus, nasal stuffiness, dry
nose, throat, mouth
MISC: ***Anaphylaxis***

Contraindications: Hypersensitivity to H_1-receptor antagonist, acute
asthma attack, lower respiratory tract
disease

Precautions: Increased intraocular pressure, renal disease, cardiac
disease, hypertension, bronchial
asthma, seizure disorder, stenosed
peptic ulcers, hyperthyroidism, prostatic hypertrophy, bladder neck obstruction, pregnancy (B), lactation

Pharmacokinetics:

PO: Peak 1-3 hr, duration 4-7 hr;
IM: Onset ½ hr, peak 1-4 hr, duration 4-7 hr; *IV:* Onset immediate,
duration 4-7 hr; metabolized in liver,
excreted by kidneys; crosses placenta, excreted in breast milk; half-
life 2-7 hr

Interactions:

• Increased CNS depression: barbiturates, opiates, hypnotics, tricyclic
antidepressants, alcohol
• Increased effect of diphenhydramine: MAOIs
🌿 Increased anticholinergic effect:
henbane leaf

Lab test interferences:

False negatives: Skin allergy tests

◆ = Nursing alert   🌿 = Herb-drug interaction   ⊘ = Do not crush

NURSING CONSIDERATIONS
Assess:
• Be alert for urinary retention, frequency, dysuria; drug should be discontinued
• CBC during long-term therapy; blood dyscrasias may occur
• Respiratory status: rate, rhythm, increase in bronchial secretions, wheezing, chest tightness

Administer:
• With meals for GI symptoms; absorption may slightly decrease
• Deep IM in large muscle; rotate site
• HS only if using for sleep aid

IV
• Undiluted; give 25 mg/1 min

Additive compatibilities: Amikacin, aminophylline, ascorbic acid, bleomycin, cephapirin, erythromycin, hydrocortisone, lidocaine, methicillin, methyldopa, nafcillin, netilmicin, penicillin G potassium, penicillin G sodium, polymyxin B, vit B/C

Syringe compatibilities: Atropine, butorphanol, chlorpromazine, cimetidine, dimenhydrinate, droperidol, fentanyl, fluphenazine, glycopyrrolate, hydromorphone, hydroxyzine, meperidine, metoclopramide, midazolam, morphine, nalbuphine, pentazocine, perphenazine, prochlorperazine, promazine, promethazine, ranitidine, scopolamine, sufentanil, thiothixene

Y-site compatibilities: Acyclovir, aldesleukin, amifostine, amsacrine, aztreonam, ciprofloxacin, cisatracurium, cisplatin, cladribine, cyclophosphamide, cytarabine, doxorubicin, doxorubicin liposome, famotidine, filgrastim, fluconazole, fludarabine, gallium, granisetron, heparin, hydrocortisone, idarubicin, melphalan, meperidine, meropenem, methotrexate, ondansetron, paclitaxel, piperacillin/tazobactam, potassium chloride, propofol, remifentanil, sargramostim, sufentanil, tacrolimus teniposide, thiotepa, vinorelbine, vit B/C

Perform/provide:
• Hard candy, gum, frequent rinsing of mouth for dryness
• Storage in tight container at room temp

Evaluate:
• Therapeutic response: absence of running or congested nose or rashes, improved sleep

Teach patient/family:
• All aspects of drug use; to notify prescriber of confusion, sedation, hypotension
• To avoid driving, other hazardous activity if drowsiness occurs
• That photosensitivity may occur
• To avoid concurrent use of alcohol, other CNS depressants

Treatment of overdose: Administer ipecac syrup or lavage, diazepam, vasopressors, barbiturates (short-acting)

---

diphenoxylate/atropine (℞)
(dye-fen-ox′ee-late a′troe-peen)
Logene, Lomanate, Lomotil, Lonox
Func. class.: Antidiarrheal
Chem. class.: Phenylpiperidine derivative opiate agonist

Controlled Substance Schedule IV (US)

Action: Inhibits gastric motility by acting on mucosal receptors responsible for peristalsis

Uses: Acute nonspecific and acute exacerbations of chronic functional diarrhea

Dosage and routes:
• *Adult:* **PO** 5 mg qid titrated to

patient response needed, not to exceed 8 tabs/24 hr

• *Child 2-12 yr:* **PO** 0.3-0.4 mg/kg/day in divided dose

Available forms: Tabs 2.5 mg with atropine 0.025 mg; liquid 2.5 mg with atropine 0.025 mg/5 ml

Side effects/adverse reactions:

RESP: **Respiratory depression**

MISC: **Anaphylaxis, angioedema**

CNS: Dizziness, drowsiness, lightheadedness, headache, fatigue, nervousness, insomnia, confusion

GI: Nausea, vomiting, dry mouth, epigastric distress, constipation, **paralytic ileus**

EENT: Burning eyes, blurred vision

Contraindications: Hypersensitivity, pseudomembranous enterocolitis, jaundice, glaucoma, child <2 yr, severe electrolyte imbalances, diarrhea associated with organisms that penetrate intestinal mucosa

Precautions: Hepatic disease, renal disease, ulcerative colitis, pregnancy (C), lactation, severe liver disease

Pharmacokinetics:

PO: Onset 40-60 min, peak 2 hr, duration 3-4 hr, terminal half-life 12-14 hr; metabolized in liver to inactive metabolite; excreted in urine, feces

Interactions:

• Do not use with MAOIs; hypertensive crisis may occur

• Increased action of: alcohol, narcotics, barbiturates, other CNS depressants, anticholinergics

NURSING CONSIDERATIONS

Assess:

• Electrolytes (K, Na, Cl) if on long-term therapy

• Bowel pattern before; for rebound constipation after termination of medication; bowel sounds

• Response after 48 hr; if none, drug should be discontinued

• Abdominal distention, toxic megacolon, which may occur in ulcerative colitis

Administer:

• For 48 hr only; if no response, drug should be discontinued

Evaluate:

• Therapeutic response: decreased diarrhea

Teach patient/family:

• To avoid OTC products unless directed by prescriber; may contain alcohol

• Not to exceed recommended dose

• That drug may be habit forming

• Not to engage in hazardous activities; drowsiness may occur, not to use for longer than 48 hr for acute diarrhea

---

diphtheria and tetanus toxoids and whole-cell pertussis vaccine (DPT, DTP) (℞)

DTwP, Tri-Immunol

diphtheria and tetanus toxoids and acellular pertussis vaccine (℞)

Acel-Imune, DTaP, Tripedin

Func. class.: Vaccine, toxoid

Action: Provide immunity to diphtheria, tetanus, pertussis by stimulating antibody/antitoxin production

Uses: Prevention of diphtheria, tetanus, pertussis

Dosage and routes:

• *Adult:* booster dose q10yr

• *Child >6 wk-6 yr:* **IM** 0.5 ml at 2, 4, 6 mo, 1½ yr; booster needed 0.5 ml at age 6

Available forms: Inj diphtheria 12.5 LfU, tetanus 5 LfU, pertussis 4 U/0.5 ml

---

Side effects/adverse reactions:

GI: Nausea, vomiting, anorexia

INTEG: Skin abscess, urticaria, itching, swelling, erythema, edema at site

CV: Tachycardia, hypotension

MISC: Lymphadenitis, **anaphylaxis,** fever, chills, malaise

CNS: Crying, fretfulness, fever, drowsiness, **seizures, encephalopathy**

MS: Osteomyelitis

Contraindications: Hypersensitivity, active infection, poliomyelitis outbreak, immunosuppression, febrile illness

Precautions: Pregnancy (C)

Interactions:

• Decreased response to toxoid: immunosuppressive agents, antineoplastics, corticosteroids, radiation therapy, alkylating agents

NURSING CONSIDERATIONS

Assess:

• For skin reactions: swelling, rash, urticaria

• For anaphylaxis: inability to breathe, bronchospasm

Administer:

• At least 4 wk apart × 3 doses

• Only with epinephrine 1:1000 on unit to treat laryngospasm

• IM only; not to be given SC (vastus lateralis in infants)

Perform/provide:

• Storage in refrigerator, do not freeze

• Written record of immunization

Evaluate:

• For history of allergies, skin conditions (eczema, psoriasis, dermatitis), reactions to vaccinations

Teach patient/family:

• That does are given at least 4 wk apart × 3 doses; booster need at 10 yr intervals, diphtheria/tetanus

---

dipyridamole (Ŗ)

(dye-peer-id′a-mole)

Apo-Dipyridamole*, dipyridamole*, Novo-Dipiradol*, Persantine, Persantine IV

Func. class.: Coronary vasodilator, antiplatelet

Chem. class.: Nonnitrate

D

Action: Inhibits adenosine uptake, which produces coronary vasodilation; increases oxygen saturation in coronary tissues, coronary blood flow; acts on small resistance vessels with little effect on vascular resistance; may increase development of collateral circulation; decreases platelet aggregation by the inhibition of phosphodiesterase (an enzyme)

Uses: Prevention of transient ischemic attacks, inhibition of platelet adhesion to prevent myocardial reinfarction, thromboembolism, with warfarin in prosthetic heart valves, prevention of coronary bypass graft occlusion with aspirin; possibly effective for long-term therapy of chronic angina pectoris

Dosage and routes:

TIA

• *Adult:* **PO** 50 mg tid, 1 hr ac, not to exceed 400 mg qd

Inhibition of platelet adhesion

• *Adult:* **PO** 50-75 mg qid in combination with aspirin or warfarin; **IV** 570 μg/kg

Available forms: Tabs 25, 50, 75 mg; inj 10 mg/2 ml

Side effects/adverse reactions:

CV: Postural hypotension

CNS: Headache, dizziness, weakness, fainting, syncope

GI: Nausea, vomiting, anorexia, diarrhea

INTEG: Rash, flushing

Contraindications: Hypersensitivity, hypotension
Precautions: Pregnancy (B), lactation
Pharmacokinetics:
PO: Peak 2-2½ hr, duration 6 hr; therapeutic response may take several months; metabolized in liver; excreted in bile; undergoes enterohepatic recirculation
Interactions:
• Prevention of coronary vasodilation: theophylline
• Incompatibility not known
• Additive antiplatelet effects: ASA, NSAID
• Increased bleeding warfarin, heparin

NURSING CONSIDERATIONS
Assess:
• B/P, pulse during treatment until stable; take B/P lying, standing; orthostatic hypotension is common
• Cardiac status: chest pain, what aggravates or ameliorates condition
Administer:
• IV after diluting each 5 mg/2 ml or more D$_5$W, 0.45% NaCl, or 0.9% NaCl to a total vol of 20-50 ml; give over 4 min; do not give undiluted
• On an empty stomach: 1 hr before meals or 2 hr after; give with 8 oz water for better absorption
Perform/provide:
• Storage at room temp
Evaluate:
• Therapeutic response: decreased chest pain (angina), decreased platelet adhesion
Teach patient/family:
• That medication is not cure; may have to be taken continuously in evenly spaced doses only as directed
• That it is necessary to quit smoking to prevent excessive vasoconstriction
• To avoid hazardous activities until stabilized on medication; dizziness may occur
• To rise slowly from sitting or lying to prevent orthostatic hypotension
• Not to use alcohol or OTC medications unless approved by prescriber
Treatment of overdose: Administer IV phenylephrine

---

dirithromycin (℞)
(dye-rith-roe-mye′sin)
Dynabac
Func. class.: Antiinfective
Chem. class.: Macrolide

Action: Binds to 50S ribosomal subunits of susceptible bacteria, suppresses protein synthesis
Uses: Infections of the respiratory tract caused by *Moraxella catarrhalis, Streptococcus* sp., *(S. pneumoniae, S. agalactiae, S. viridans), Legionella pneumophilia, Mycoplasma pneumoniae, Streptococcus pyogenes, Staphylococcus aureus, Bordetella pertussis, Propionibacterium acnes*
Dosage and routes:
• *Adult:* PO 500 mg qd, given for 7-14 days depending on infections
Available forms: Tabs, enteric coated 250 mg
Side effects/adverse reactions:
GI: Abdominal pain, nausea, diarrhea, vomiting, dyspepsia, GI disorders, flatulence, abnormal stools, anorexia, constipation, ***pseudomembranous colitis***
CNS: Headache, dizziness, insomnia
HEMA: Increased platelet count, increased eosinophils
RESP: Cough, dyspnea
INTEG: Pruritus, urticaria
Contraindications: Hypersensitivity to this drug or any other macrolide, or erythromycin, bacteremias

---

◆ = Nursing alert   🥄 = Herb-drug interaction   ⊘ = Do not crush

Precautions: Pregnancy (C), lactation, children, hepatic, renal disease

Pharmacokinetics: Rapidly absorbed, widely distributed, no hepatic metabolism, excreted in bile, feces (up to 97%), plasma half-life 8 hr, terminal 44 hr

Interactions:

• Absorption of dirithromycin slightly enhanced: antacids, H_2-antagonists

• May alter effect of: theophylline

• Drug/food: increased absorption with food

NURSING CONSIDERATIONS

Assess:

• Report hematuria, oliguria in renal disease

• Liver studies: AST, ALT if on long-term therapy

• Renal studies: Urinalysis, protein, blood if on long-term therapy

• C&S before drug therapy; drug may be given as soon as culture is taken; C&S may be repeated after treatment

• Bowel pattern before, during treatment; pseudomembranous colitis may occur

• Skin eruptions, itching

• Respiratory status: rate, character, wheezing, tightness in chest; discontinue drug

• Allergies before treatment, reaction of each medication; place allergies on chart, notify all people giving drugs

Administer:

• Adequate intake of fluids (2 L) during diarrhea episodes

🚫 Whole; do not break, crush, or chew tablets

• With food or within 1 hr of food at same time each day

Perform/provide:

• Storage at room temp, in tight container

Evaluate:

• Therapeutic response: C&S negative for infection

Teach patient/family:

• To take with full glass of water; to give with food

• To report sore throat, fever, fatigue; may indicate superinfection

• To notify prescriber of diarrhea stools, dark urine, pale stools, jaundiced eyes or skin, severe abdominal pain

• To take at evenly spaced intervals; complete dosage regimen

Treatment of hypersensitivity:

Withdraw drug, maintain airway, administer epinephrine, aminophylline, O_2, IV corticosteroids

---

disopyramide (℞)

(dye-soe-peer'a-mide)
disopyramide, Norpace, Norpace CR, Rhythmodan
Func. class.: Antidysrhythmic (Class IA)
Chem. class.: Nonnitrate

Action: Prolongs duration of action potential and effective refractory period; reduces disparity in refractory between normal and infarcted myocardium; prevents increased myocardial excitability and conduction contractility

Uses: PVCs, ventricular tachycardia, supraventricular tachycardia, atrial flutter, fibrillation

Investigational uses: Supraventricular tachycardia (prevention, treatment)

Dosage and routes:

Renal disease:

• CrCl 30-40 ml/min dose q8h; CrCl 15-30 ml/min dose q12h; CrCl <15 ml/min dose q24h

• *Adult:* **PO** 100-200 mg q6h, in renal dysfunction 100 mg q6h; **SUS REL CAPS** 200 mg q12h

- *Child 12-18 yr:* **PO** 6-15 mg/kg/day, in divided doses q6h
- *Child 4-12 yr:* **PO** 10-15 mg/kg/day in divided doses q6h
- *Child 1-4 yr:* **PO** 10-20 mg/kg/day in divided doses q6h
- *Child <1 yr:* **PO** 10-30 mg/kg/day, in divided doses q6h

Available forms: Caps 100, 150 mg (as phosphate); cont rel caps 100, 150 mg; tabs, sus rel 250 mg*

Side effects/adverse reactions:

GU: Urinary retention, hesitancy, impotence

CNS: Headache, dizziness, psychosis, fatigue, depression, paresthesias, anxiety, insomnia

GI: Dry mouth, constipation, nausea, anorexia, flatulence, diarrhea, vomiting

CV: Hypotension, bradycardia, angina, PVCs, tachycardia, increased QRS, QT segments, *cardiac arrest,* edema, weight gain, AV block, *CHF,* syncope, chest pain

META: Hypoglycemia

INTEG: Rash, pruritus, urticaria

MS: Weakness, pain in extremities

EENT: Blurred vision; dry nose, throat, eyes; narrow-angle glaucoma

HEMA: Thrombocytopenia, agranulocytosis, anemia (rare), decreased Hgb, Hct

Contraindications: Hypersensitivity, 2nd- or 3rd-degree block, cardiogenic shock, CHF (uncompensated), sick sinus syndrome, QT prolongation

Precautions: Pregnancy (C), lactation, diabetes mellitus, renal disease, children, hepatic disease, myasthenia gravis, narrow-angle glaucoma, cardiomyopathy, conduction abnormalities

Pharmacokinetics:

PO: Peak 30 min-3 hr, duration 6-12 hr; half-life 4-10 hr; metabolized in liver; excreted in feces, urine, breast milk; crosses placenta

Interactions:

- Increased effects of disopyramide: quinidine, procainamide, propranolol, lidocaine, atenolol, other antidysrhythmics, erythromycin
- Increased side effects of disopyramide: anticholinergics
- Decreased effects of disopyramide: phenytoin, rifampin, phenobarbital

🌿 Increased action: aloe, buckthorn bark/berry, cascara sagrada bark, senna pod/leaf

Lab test interferences:

Increase: Liver enzymes, lipids, BUN, creatinine

Decrease: Hgb/Hct, blood glucose

NURSING CONSIDERATIONS

Assess:

- Apical pulse for 1 min; if less than 60, check again in 1 hr; if still less than 60, notify prescriber
- ECG; check for increased QT, widening QRS; drug should be discontinued
- Weight daily; a rapid weight gain should be reported
- For dehydration or hypovolemia, I&O ratio, electrolytes (Na, K, Cl)
- Liver, kidney function studies (AST, ALT, bilirubin, BUN, creatinine) during treatment
- Diabetics for signs of hypoglycemia (rare)
- B/P continuously for hypotension, hypertension
- For rebound hypertension after 1-2 hr
- Constipation: increased bulk in diet, water, stool softeners, or laxatives needed
- Cardiac rate, respiration: rate, rhythm, character
- Urinary hesitancy, frequency, or a change in I&O ratio; check for edema daily; check for toxicity

Administer:

🚫 Do not break, crush, or chew sus rel cap; give 1 hr before or 2 hr after meals

---

◆ = Nursing alert   🌿 = Herb-drug interaction   🚫 = Do not crush

- Sugar-free gum, frequent sips of water for dry mouth
- Reduced dosage slowly with ECG monitoring

Evaluate:
- Therapeutic response: decreased dysrhythmias

Teach patient/family:
- To take drug exactly as prescribed; if dose is missed, take within 3-4 hr of next dose; do not double dose
- To avoid alcohol, or severe hypotension may occur; to avoid OTC drugs, or serious drug interactions may occur
- To make position change slowly during early therapy to prevent orthostatic hypotension
- To avoid hazardous activities if dizziness or blurred vision occurs
- The importance of complying with drug regimen; tell patient that this drug does not cure condition

Treatment of overdose: O_2, artificial ventilation, ECG, dopamine for circulatory depression, diazepam or thiopental for convulsions, gastric lavage

---

dobutamine (℞)

(doe-byoo'ta-meen)
dobutamine, Dobutrex
Func. class.: Adrenergic direct-acting β_1-agonist
Chem. class.: Catecholamine

Action: Causes increased contractility, increased coronary blood flow and heart rate by acting on β_1-receptors in heart; minor α and β_2 effects

Uses: Cardiac surgery, refractory heart failure, cardiac decompensation

Investigational uses: Cardiogenic shock in children

Unlabeled uses: Congenital heart disease in children undergoing cardiac cath

Dosage and routes:
- *Adult:* **IV INF** 2.5-10 µg/kg/min; may increase to 40 µg/kg/min if needed
- *Child:* **IV INF** 5-20 µg/kg/min over 10 min for cardiac cath
Available forms: Inj 12.5 mg/ml

Side effects/adverse reactions:
CNS: Anxiety, headache, dizziness
CV: Palpitations, tachycardia, hypertension, PVCs, angina
GI: Heartburn, nausea, vomiting
MS: Muscle cramps (leg)

Contraindications: Hypersensitivity, idiopathic hypertrophic subaortic stenosis

Precautions: Pregnancy (B), lactation, children, hypertension

Pharmacokinetics:
IV: Onset 1-2 min, peak 10 min, half-life 2 min; metabolized in liver (inactive metabolites); excreted in urine

Interactions:
- Severe hypertension: guanethidine
- Dysrhythmias: general anesthetics, bretylium
- Decreased action of dobutamine: other β-blockers
- Dysrhythmias: bretylium, general anesthetics
- Increased pressor effect and dysrhythmias: tricyclic antidepressants, MAOIs, oxytocics

NURSING CONSIDERATIONS
Assess:
- Hypovolemia; if present, correct first; administer cardiac glycoside before dobutamine
- Oxygenation/perfusion deficit (check B/P, chest pain, dizziness, loss of consciousness)
- Heart failure: S_3 gallop, dyspnea, neck vein distention, bibasilar crackles in patients with CHF, cardiomyopathy
- ECG during administration con-

tinuously; if B/P increases, drug is decreased; CVP or PWP, cardiac output during infusion
• Serum electrolytes, urine output
◆ Sulfite sensitivity, which may be life-threatening

Administer:
IV
• Diluting each 250 mg/10 ml of sterile H_2O or D_5W for inj; may be further diluted in 50 ml or more given at prescribed rate; should be gradually increased to desired rate; use a CVP catheter or large peripheral vein, use infusion pump, titrate to patient response
• Change IV site q48h
• Plasma expanders for hypovolemia

Additive compatibilities: Amiodarone, atracurium, atropine, dopamine, enalaprilat, epinephrine, flumazenil, hydralazine, isoproterenol, lidocaine, meperidine, meropenem, metaraminol, morphine, nitroglycerin, norepinephrine, phentolamine, phenylephrine, procainamide, propranolol, ranitidine

Syringe compatibilities: Heparin, ranitidine

Y-site compatibilities: Amifostine, amiodarone, amrinone, atracurium, aztreonam, bretylium, calcium chloride, calcium gluconate, ciprofloxacin, cisatracurium, cladribine, diazepam, diltiazem, dopamine, doxorubicin liposome, enalaprilat, epinephrine, famotidine, fentanyl, fluconazole, granisetron, haloperidol, hydromorphone, insulin (regular), labetalol, lidocaine, lorazepam, magnesium sulfate, meperidine, milrinone, morphine, nicardipine, nitroglycerin, norepinephrine, pancuronium, potassium chloride, propofol, ranitidine, remifentanil, sodium nitroprusside, streptokinase, tacrolimus, theophylline, thiotepa,

tolazoline, vecuronium, verapamil, zidovudine

Perform/provide:
• Storage of reconstituted solution for 24 hr if refrigerated

Evaluate:
• Therapeutic response: increased B/P with stabilization, increased urine output

Teach patient/family:
• The reason for drug administration; to report dyspnea, headache, IV site discomfort

Treatment of overdose: Administer a β_1-adrenergic blocker; reduce IV or discontinue, ensure oxygenation/ventilation; for severe tachydysrhythmias (ventricular) give lidocaine or propranolol

---

docusate calcium (℞)
(dok'yoo-sate cal'see-um)
DC Softgels, Pro-Cal-Sof, Sulfalax Calcium, Surfak
docusate sodium (℞)
Colace, Correctol Extra Gentle, Dialose, Diocto, Dioeze, Disonate, Di-Sosul, DOK, DOS, D-S-S, ex-lax, Modane, Regulax SS, Regulex*, Silace
Func. class.: Laxative, emollient
Chem. class.: Anionic surfactant

Action: Increases water, fat penetration in intestine; allows for easier passage of stool
Uses: To soften stools
Dosage and routes:
• *Adult:* **PO** 50-300 mg qd (sodium) or 240 mg (calcium or potassium) prn; **ENEMA** 5 ml (sodium)
• *Child >12 yr:* **ENEMA** 2 ml (sodium)
• *Child 6-12 yr:* **PO** 40-120 mg qd (sodium)

◆ = Nursing alert   *∅* = Herb-drug interaction   ⊘ = Do not crush

• *Child 3-6 yr:* **PO** 20-60 mg qd (sodium)
• *Child <3 yr:* **PO** 10-40 mg qd (sodium)
Available forms: Calcium: caps 50, 240 mg; *sodium:* caps 50, 100, 240, 250 mg; tabs 50, 100 mg; syr 20 mg/5 ml 50, 60/15 ml; liquid 150 mg/15 ml; oral sol 10, 50 mg/ml; enema 283 mg/3.9 cap
Side effects/adverse reactions:
GI: Nausea, anorexia, cramps, diarrhea
INTEG: Rash
EENT: Bitter taste, throat irritation
Contraindications: Hypersensitivity, obstruction, fecal impaction, nausea/vomiting
Precautions: Pregnancy (C), lactation
Pharmacokinetics: Onset 24-72 hr
Interactions:
• Toxicity: mineral oil
NURSING CONSIDERATIONS
Assess:
• Cause of constipation; identify whether fluids, bulk, or exercise are missing from lifestyle
• Cramping, rectal bleeding, nausea, vomiting; if these symptoms occur, drug should be discontinued
Administer:
• In milk, fruit juice to decrease bitter taste
• In morning or evening (oral dose)
Perform/provide:
• Storage in cool environment; do not freeze
Evaluate:
• Therapeutic response: decrease in constipation
Teach patient/family:
🚫 To swallow tabs whole; do not break, crush, or chew
• That normal bowel movements do not always occur daily
• Not to use in presence of abdominal pain, nausea, vomiting

• To notify prescriber if constipation unrelieved or if symptoms of electrolyte imbalance occur: muscle cramps, pain, weakness, dizziness, excessive thirst
• Inform patient that drug may take up to 3 days to soften stools

dofetilide
See appendix a—selected new drugs

dolasetron (℞)
(do-la′se-tron)
Anzemet
Func. class.: Antiemetic
Chem. class.: 5-HT3 receptor antagonist

Action: Prevents nausea, vomiting by blocking serotonin peripherally, centrally, and in the small intestine
Uses: Prevention of nausea, vomiting associated with cancer chemotherapy, radiotherapy, and prevention of postoperative nausea, vomiting
Investigational uses: Radiotherapy-induced nausea/vomiting
Dosage and routes:
Prevention of nausea/vomiting of cancer chemotherapy
• *Adult and child 2-16 yr:* **IV** 1.8 mg/kg as a single dose, ½ hr prior to chemotherapy
• *Adult:* **PO** 100 mg/hr prior to chemotherapy
• *Child 2-16 yr:* **PO** 1.8 mg/kg/hr prior to chemotherapy
Prevention of postoperative nausea/vomiting
• *Adult:* **IV** 12.5 mg as a single dose, 15 min before cessation of anesthesia; **PO** 100 mg 2 hr before surgery (prevention only)
• *Child 2-16 yr:* **IV** 0.35 mg/kg as a single dose, 15 min before cessa-

tion of anesthesia; **PO** 1.2 mg/kg 2 hr before surgery (prevention only)
Available forms: Tabs 50, 100 mg; inj 20 mg/ml (12.5 mg/0.625 ml)
Side effects/adverse reactions:
GI: Diarrhea, constipation, increased AST, ALT, abdominal pain, anorexia
CNS: Headache, dizziness, fatigue, drowsiness
MISC: Rash, **bronchospasm**
GU: Urinary retention, oliguria
CV: **Dysrhythmias,** ECG changes, hypotension, tachycardia, hypertension
Contraindications: Hypersensitivity
Precautions: Pregnancy (B), lactation, children, elderly
Pharmacokinetics: Unknown
Interactions:
• Dysrhythmias: antidysrhythmics
• Increased dolasetron levels: cimetidine
• Decreased dolasetron levels: rifampin
NURSING CONSIDERATIONS
Assess:
• For absence of nausea, vomiting during chemotherapy
• For hypersensitivity reaction: rash, bronchospasm
• For cardiac conduction conditions, electrolyte imbalances, or dysrhythmias
Administer:
• By inj 100 mg/½ min or less or diluted in 50 ml compatible sol; give over 15 min
Perform/provide:
• Storage at room temp 48 hr after dilution
Evaluate:
• Therapeutic response: absence of nausea, vomiting during cancer chemotherapy
Teach patient/family:
• To report diarrhea, constipation, nausea, vomiting, rash, or changes in respirations

• Not to mix product for oral administration in juice until immediately before administration

---

donepezil (℞)
(don-ep-ee′zill)
Aricept
Func. class.: Reversible cholinesterase

Action: Elevates acetylcholine concentrations (cerebral cortex) by slowing degradation of acetylcholine released in cholinergic neurons; does not alter underlying dementia
Uses: Treatment of mild to moderate dementia in Alzheimer's disease
Dosage and routes:
• *Adult:* **PO** 5-10 mg qd hs; may increase to 10 mg qd after 4-6wk
Available forms: Tabs 5, 10 mg
Side effects/adverse reactions:
CNS: Dizziness, *insomnia,* somnolence, *headache,* fatigue, abnormal dreams, syncope, **seizures**
CV: Hypotension or hypertension
GI: Nausea, vomiting, anorexia; *diarrhea*
GU: Urinary frequency, UTI, incontinence
INTEG: Rash, flushing
RESP: Rhinitis, URI, cough, pharyngitis
CV: **Atrial fibrillation**
MS: Cramps, arthritis
Contraindications: Hypersensitivity to this drug or piperidine derivatives
Precautions: Sick sinus syndrome, history of ulcers, GI bleeding, hepatic disease, bladder obstruction, asthma, pregnancy (C), lactation, children, seizures, asthma, COPD
Pharmacokinetics: Well absorbed PO, metabolized to metabolites, elimination half-life 10 hr single dose, 70 hr multiple dosing

Interactions:
- Decreased activity of anticholinergics
- Synergistic effects: succinylcholine, cholinesterase inhibitors, cholinergic agonists
- Increased gastric acid secretions: NSAIDs
- Decreased donepezil effect: carbamazepine, dexamethasone, phenytoin, phenobarbital, rifampin

NURSING CONSIDERATIONS

Assess:
- B/P: hypotension, hypertension
- Mental status: affect, mood, behavioral changes, depression, complete suicide assessment
- GI status: nausea, vomiting, anorexia, diarrhea
- GU status: urinary frequency, incontinence

Administer:
- Between meals; may be given with meals for GI symptoms
- Dosage adjusted to response no more than q6wk

Perform/provide:
- Assistance with ambulation during beginning therapy; dizziness, ataxia may occur

Evaluate:
- Therapeutic response: decrease in confusion, improved mood

Teach patient/family:
- To report side effects: twitching, nausea, vomiting, sweating; indicates overdose
- To use drug exactly as prescribed; at regular intervals, preferably between meals; may be taken with meals for GI upset
- To notify prescriber of nausea, vomiting, diarrhea (dose increase or beginning treatment), or rash
- Not to increase or abruptly decrease dose; serious consequences may result
- That drug is not a cure, relieves symptoms

Treatment of overdose: Withdraw drug, administer tertiary anticholinergics, provide supportive care

---

dopamine (℞)

(doe′pa-meen)
dopamine HCl, Intropin, Revimine*

Func. class.: Adrenergic
Chem. class.: Catecholamine

Action: Causes increased cardiac output; acts on β_1- and α-receptors, causing vasoconstriction in blood vessels; low dose causes renal and mesenteric vasodilation; β_1 stimulation produces inotropic effects with increased cardiac output

Uses: Shock; increased perfusion; hypotension

Unlabeled uses: COPD, RDS in infants

Dosage and routes:
- *Adult:* **IV INF** 2-5 µg/kg/min, not to exceed 50 µg/kg/min, titrate to patient's response
- *Child:* **IV** 5-20 µg/kg/min adjust depending on response

COPD
- *Adult:* **IV** 4 µg/kg/min

CHF
- *Adult:* **IV** 2-5 µg/kg/min

RDS
- *Infant:* **IV** 5 µg/kg/min

Available forms: Inj 40 mg, 160 mg/ml conc for IV inf; 0.8, 1.6, 3.2 mg/ml in D_5W

Side effects/adverse reactions:
CNS: Headache
CV: Palpitations, tachycardia, hypertension, ectopic beats, angina, wide QRS complex, peripheral vasoconstriction
GI: Nausea, vomiting, diarrhea
INTEG: Necrosis, tissue sloughing with extravasation, **gangrene**
RESP: Dyspnea

Contraindications: Hypersensitivity, ventricular fibrillation, tachydysrhythmias, pheochromocytoma
Precautions: Pregnancy (C), lactation, arterial embolism, peripheral vascular disease
Pharmacokinetics:
IV: Onset 5 min, duration <10 min; metabolized in liver, kidney, plasma, excreted in urine (metabolites), half-life 2 min
Interactions:
• Do not use within 2 wk of MAOIs, phenytoin; hypertensive crisis may result
• Dysrhythmias: general anesthetics
• Severe hypertension: ergots
• Decreased action of dopamine: β-blockers, alpha-blockers
• Increased B/P: oxytocics
• Increased pressor effect: tricyclic antidepressants, MAOIs
Lab test interferences:
Increased: Urinary catecholamine, serum glucose

NURSING CONSIDERATIONS
Assess:
• Hypovolemia; if present, correct first
• Oxygenation/perfusion deficit (check B/P, chest pain, dizziness, loss of consciousness)
• Heart failure: S_3 gallop, dyspnea, neck vein distention, bibasilar crackles in patients with CHF, cardiomyopathy
• I&O ratio: if urine output decreases, without decrease in B/P, drug may need to be reduced
• ECG during administration continuously; if B/P increases, drug should be decreased
• B/P and pulse q5min after parenteral route
• CVP or PWP during infusion if possible
• Paresthesias and coldness of extremities; peripheral blood flow may decrease
• Injection site: tissue sloughing; if this occurs, administer phentolamine mixed with NS
Administer:
IV
• Plasma expanders or whole blood for hypovolemia
• IV after diluting 200-400 mg/250-500 ml of D_5W, D_5 0.45% NaCl, D_5 0.9% NaCl, D_5LR, LR
• Parenteral IV dose slowly; after reconstituting, use infusion pump; flush line before infusing; infuse as secondary IV line
Additive compatibilities: Aminophylline, atracurium, bretylium, calcium chloride, cephalothin, chloramphenicol, dobutamine, enalaprilat, flumazenil, heparin, hydrocortisone, kanamycin, lidocaine, meropenem, methylprednisolone, nitroglycerin, oxacillin, potassium chloride, ranitidine, verapamil
Syringe compatibilities: Doxapram, heparin, ranitidine
Y-site compatibilities: Aldesleukin, amifostine, amiodarone, amrinone, atracurium, aztreonam, cefmetazole, cefpirome, ciprofloxacin, cisatracurium, cladribine, diltiazem, dobutamine, doxorubicin liposome, enalaprilat, epinephrine, esmolol, famotidine, fentanyl, fluconazole, foscarnet, granisetron, haloperidol, heparin, hydrocortisone, hydromorphone, labetalol, lidocaine, lorazepam, meperidine, methylprednisolone, metronidazole, midazolam, milrinone, morphine, nicardipine, nitroglycerin, norepinephrine, ondansetron, pancuronium, piperacillin/tazobactam, potassium chloride, propofol, ranitidine, remifentanil, sargramostim, sodium nitroprusside, streptokinase, tacrolimus, theophylline, thiotepa, tolazo-

line, vecuronium, verapamil, vit B/C, warfarin, zidovudine

Perform/provide:
• Storage of reconstituted sol for up to 24 hr if refrigerated
• Do not use discolored sol; protect from light

Evaluate:
• Therapeutic response: increased B/P with stabilization; increased urine output

Teach patient/family:
• The reason for drug administration

Treatment of overdose: Discontinue IV, may give a short-acting α-adrenergic blocker

dornase alfa (℞)
Pulmozyme
Func. class.: Cystic fibrosis agent (orphan drug)

Action: May break down molecules in large amounts of infected sputum; improves air flow, lessens chance of bacterial infection
Uses: Management of cystic fibrosis

Dosage and routes:
• *Adult/child >5 yr:* **INH** 2.5 mg qd
Available forms: Neb 2.5 mg (1 mg/ml)

Side effects/adverse reactions:
RESP: Possibly laryngitis, hoarseness, hemoptysis, transient decrease in pulmonary function
INTEG: Urticaria, rash
MISC: Chest pain

Contraindications: Hypersensitivity
Precautions: Pregnancy (B)
NURSING CONSIDERATIONS
Assess:
• Resp function: B/P, pulse, lung sounds
Administer:
• By nebulization only

Evaluate:
• Therapeutic response: decreased thick tenacious secretions, ease of respirations

Teach patient/family:
• To rinse mouth after use
• About all aspects of drug; avoid smoking, smoke-filled rooms, persons with respiratory infections

doxacurium (℞)
(dox-a-cure′ee-um)
Nuromax
Func. class.: Neuromuscular blocker (nondepolarizing)

Action: Inhibits transmission of nerve impulses by binding with cholinergic receptor sites, antagonizing action of acetylcholine
Uses: Facilitation of endotracheal intubation, skeletal muscle relaxation during mechanical ventilation, surgery, or general anesthesia

Dosage and routes:
• *Adult:* **IV** 0.05 mg/kg; 0.08 mg/kg is used for prolonged neuromuscular blockade; maintenance 0.025 mg/kg
• *Child 2-12 yr:* **IV** 0.03-0.05 mg/kg; may decrease for maintenance dose
Available forms: Inj 1 mg/ml

Side effects/adverse reactions:
*CV: **Decreased B/P, ventricular fibrillation, myocardial infarction, cardiovascular accident***
*RESP: **Prolonged apnea, bronchospasm, wheezing, respiratory depression***
EENT: Diplopia
MS: Weakness, prolonged skeletal muscle relaxation, ***paralysis***
INTEG: Rash, urticaria

Contraindications: Hypersensitivity

Precautions: Pregnancy (C), renal, hepatic disease, lactation, children <3 mo, fluid and electrolyte imbalances, neuromuscular disease, respiratory disease, obesity, elderly, severe burns

Pharmacokinetics: Not metabolized; excretion of unchanged drug in urine and bile

Interactions:

• Increased neuromuscular blockade: aminoglycosides, quinidine, local anesthetics, polymyxin antibiotics, enflurane, isoflurane, tetracyclines, inhalation anesthetics, magnesium, colistin, procainamide, bacitracin, lincomycin, clindamycin, lithium

• Longer onset and shorter duration of doxacurium: phenytoin, carbamazepine

NURSING CONSIDERATIONS

Assess:

• For electrolyte imblances (K, Mg); may lead to increased action of this drug

• Vital signs (B/P, pulse, respirations, airway) until fully recovered; rate, depth, pattern of respirations, strength of hand grip

• I&O ratio; check for urinary retention, frequency, hesitancy

• Recovery: decreased paralysis of face, diaphragm, leg, arm, rest of body

• Allergic reactions: rash, fever, respiratory distress, pruritus; drug should be discontinued

Administer:

IV

• Using nerve stimulator by anesthesiologist to determine neuromuscular blockade

• After succinylcholine effects subside

• Anticholinesterase to reverse neuromuscular blockade

• By slow IV over 1-2 min (only by qualified persons, usually an anesthesiologist)

• Only fresh sol

Solution compatibilities: LR, D$_5$/LR, D$_5$/0.9% NaCl

Y-site compatibilities: Etomidate, thiopental

Perform/provide:

• Storage at room temp; do not freeze

• Reassurance if communication is difficult during recovery from neuromuscular blockade

• Use reconstituted sol within 24 hr

• Frequent (q2h) instillation of artificial tears and covering eyes to prevent drying of cornea

Evaluate:

• Therapeutic response: paralysis of jaw, eyelid, head, neck, rest of body

Treatment of overdose: Neostigmine; monitor VS; may require mechanical ventilation

---

doxapram (℞)

(dox′a-pram)
Dopram
Func. class.: Analeptic

Action: Respiratory stimulation through activation of peripheral carotid chemoreceptor; with higher doses, medullary respiratory centers are stimulated; general CNS stimulation

Uses: Chronic obstructive pulmonary disease (COPD), postanesthesia respiratory stimulation, prevention of acute hypercapnia, drug-induced CNS depression

Dosage and routes:

Postanesthesia

• *Adult:* IV inj 0.5-1 mg/kg, not to exceed 1.5 mg/kg total as a single injection; **IV INF** 250 mg in 250 ml sol, not to exceed 4 mg/kg; run at 1-3 mg/min

Drug-induced CNS depression

• *Adult:* IV priming dose of 2 mg/

◆ = Nursing alert   ⬆ = Herb-drug interaction   ⊘ = Do not crush kg, repeated in 5 min; repeat q1-2h till patient awakes; **IV INF** priming dose 2 mg/kg at 1-3 mg/min, not to exceed 3 g/day

COPD (Hypercapnia)

• *Adult:* **IV INF** 1-2 mg/min, not to exceed 3 mg/min for no longer than 2 hr

Apnea of premature infant

• *Infant:* 2.5-3 mg/kg loading dose followed by infusion of 1 mg/kg/hr
Available forms: Inj 20 mg/ml

Side effects/adverse reactions:

CNS: **Convulsions,** (clonus/generalized), *headache,* restlessness, dizziness, confusion, paresthesias, flushing, sweating, bilateral Babinski's sign, rigidity, depression

GI: Nausea, vomiting, diarrhea, hiccups

GU: Retention, incontinence

CV: Chest pain, hypertension, change in heart rate, lowered T waves, tachycardia, **dysrhythmias**

INTEG: Pruritus, irritation at injection site

EENT: Pupil dilation, sneezing

RESP: **Laryngospasm, bronchospasm,** rebound hypoventilation, dyspnea, cough, tachypnea, hiccups

Contraindications: Hypersensitivity, seizure disorders, severe hypertension, severe bronchial asthma, severe dyspnea, severe cardiac disorders, pneumothorax, pulmonary embolism, severe respiratory disease

Precautions: Bronchial asthma, pheochromocytoma, severe tachycardia, dysrhythmias, pregnancy (B), hypertension, lactation, children

Pharmacokinetics:

IV: Onset 20-40 sec, peak 1-2 min, duration 5-10 min; metabolized by liver; excreted by kidneys (metabolites); half-life 2.5-4 hr

Interactions:

• Synergistic pressor effect: MAOIs, sympathomimetics

• Cardiac dysrhythmias: halothane, cyclopropane, enflurane

NURSING CONSIDERATIONS
Assess:

• BP, heart rate, deep tendon reflexes, ABGs, LOC before administration, q30min

• Po_2, Pco_2, O_2 saturation during treatment

• Hypertension, dysrhythmias, tachycardia, dyspnea, skeletal muscle hyperactivity; may indicate overdosage; discontinue drug

• Respiratory stimulation: increased rate, abnormal rhythm

• Extravasation; change IV site q48h

Administer:
IV

• Undiluted or diluted with equal parts of sterile H_2O for inj; may be diluted 250 mg/250 ml of D_5W, $D_{10}W$ and run as infusion

• IV undiluted over 5 min; IV inf at 1-3 mg/min; adjust for desired respiratory response, using infusion pump IV; if an inf is used after initial dose, start at 1-3 mg/min depending on patient response; D/C after 2 hr; wait 1-2 hr and repeat

• Only after adequate airway is established

• After O_2, IV barbiturates, resuscitative equipment available

Syringe compatibilities: Amikacin, bumetadine, chlorpromazine, cimetidine, cisplatin, cyclophosphamide, dopamine, doxycycline, epinephrine, hydroxyzine, imipramine, isoniazid, lincomycin, methotrexate, netilmicin, phytonadione, pyridoxine, terbutaline, thiamine, tobramycin, vincristine

Perform/provide:

• Placing patient in Sims' position to prevent aspiration of vomitus

• Discontinue infusion if side effects occur; narrow margin of safety

Side effects: *italics* = common; **bold italics** = life-threatening

Evaluate:
• Therapeutic response: increased breathing capacity

Teach patient/family:
• Purpose of medication

Treatment of overdose: Vital signs, lavage, activated charcoal; monitor electrolytes

---

doxazosin (℞)
(dox-ay′zoe-sin)
Cardura
Func. class.: Peripheral α₁-adrenergic blocker
Chem. class.: Quinazoline

Action: Peripheral blood vessels are dilated, peripheral resistance lowered; reduction in blood pressure results from α₁-adrenergic receptors being blocked

Uses: Hypertension, urinary outflow obstruction, symptoms of benign prostatic hyperplasia

Investigational uses: CHF with digoxin and diuretics

Dosage and routes:
BPH
• *Adult:* **PO** 1 mg qd, increase in stepwise manner to 2, 4, 8 mg qd as needed, max 8 mg
• *Adult:* **PO** 1 mg qd, increasing up to 16 mg qd if required; usual range 4-16 mg/day
HTN
• *Geriatric:* **PO** 0.5 mg qhs, gradually increase
Available forms: Tabs 1, 2, 4, 8 mg

Side effects/adverse reactions:
CV: Palpitations, *orthostatic hypotension*, tachycardia, edema, ***dysrhythmias,*** chest pain
CNS: Dizziness, headache, drowsiness, anxiety, depression, vertigo, weakness, fatigue, asthenia
GI: Nausea, vomiting, diarrhea, constipation, abdominal pain

GU: Incontinence, polyuria
EENT: Epistaxis, tinnitus, dry mouth, red sclera, pharyngitis, rhinitis

Contraindications: Hypersensitivity to quinazolines

Precautions: Pregnancy (C), children, lactation, hepatic disease

Pharmacokinetics:
PO: Onset 2 hr, peak 2-6 hr, duration 6-12 hr; half-life 22 hr; metabolized in liver; excreted via bile/feces (<63%) and in urine (9%); extensively protein bound (98%)

Interactions:
• Increased hypotensive effects: β-blockers, verapamil
• Decreased hypotensive effects: indomethacin, NSAIDs
• Decreased effects of clonidine
🍃 Increased doxazosin effect: angelica

NURSING CONSIDERATIONS
Assess:
• B/P (lying, standing) and pulse 2-6 hr after each dose and with each increase; postural effects may occur, rales, dyspnea, orthopnea with B/P; pulse, jugular venous distention q4h
• BUN, uric acid if on long-term therapy
• I&O, weight daily
• Edema in feet, legs daily
• Skin turgor, dryness of mucous membranes for hydration status

Administer:
• Tablets broken, crushed or chewed; if chewed, will be bitter

Perform/provide:
• Storage in tight container in cool environment

Evaluate:
• Therapeutic response: decreased B/P; decreased symptoms of BPH

Teach patient/family:
• That fainting occasionally occurs after first dose; do not drive or op-

---

◆ = Nursing alert   🍃 = Herb-drug interaction   🚫 = Do not crush

erate machinery for 4 hr after first dose or after dosage increase or take first dose hs

• To take 1st dose at hs to decrease orthostatic B/P changes

Treatment of overdose: Administer volume expanders or vasopressors; discontinue drug; place in supine position

---

doxepin (℞)

(dox'e-pin)
Adepin, doxepin HCl, Novo-Doxepin*, Sinequan, Sinequan Concentrate, Triadapin*, Zonolon Topical Cream

Func. class.: Antidepressant, tricyclic

Chem. class.: Dibenzoxepin, tertiary amine

Action: Blocks reuptake of norepinephrine, serotonin into nerve endings, increasing action of norepinephrine, serotonin in nerve cells

Uses: Major depression, anxiety; topical pruritus

Investigational uses: Chronic pain management

Dosage and routes:
• *Adult:* PO 25-75 mg/day, may increase to 300 mg/day for severely ill; **TOP** apply qid × up to 8 days
• *Geriatric:* **PO** 10-25 mg hs, increase qwk by 10-25 mg to desired dose

Available forms: Caps 10, 25, 50, 75, 100, 150 mg; oral conc 10 mg/ml; cream 5%

Side effects/adverse reactions:
HEMA: Agranulocytosis, thrombocytopenia, eosinophilia, leukopenia

CNS: Dizziness, drowsiness, confusion, headache, anxiety, tremors, stimulation, weakness, insomnia, nightmares, EPS (elderly), increased psychiatric symptoms, paresthesia

GI: Diarrhea, dry mouth, nausea, vomiting, *paralytic ileus,* increased appetite, cramps, epigastric distress, jaundice, *hepatitis,* stomatitis, constipation

GU: Urinary retention, acute renal failure

INTEG: Rash, urticaria, sweating, pruritus, photosensitivity

CV: Orthostatic hypotension, ECG changes, tachycardia, hypertension, palpitations

EENT: Blurred vision, tinnitus, mydriasis, ophthalmoplegia, glossitis

Contraindications: Hypersensitivity to tricyclic antidepressants, urinary retention, narrow-angle glaucoma, prostatic hypertrophy

Precautions: Suicidal patients, elderly, pregnancy (C-TOP), UK-PO lactation

Pharmacokinetics:
PO: Steady state 2-8 days; metabolized by liver; excreted by kidneys; crosses placenta; excreted in breast milk; half-life 8-24 hr

Interactions:
• Increased hypertensive action: clonidine, epinephrine, norepinephrine
• Increased doxepin effect: cimetidine, fluoxetine, sertraline
• Increased CNS depression: other CNS depressants
• Hyperpyretic crisis, convulsions, hypertensive episode: MAOI
⬮ Increased anticholinergic effect: belladonna leaf/root, henbane leaf
⬮ Increased action of doxepin: scopolia root, kava

Lab test interferences:
Increase: Serum bilirubin, blood glucose, alk phosphatase

NURSING CONSIDERATIONS
Assess:
• B/P (lying, standing), pulse q4h; if systolic B/P drops 20 mm Hg, hold

---

drug, notify prescriber; take vital signs q4h in patients with cardiovascular disease

• Blood studies: CBC, leukocytes, differential, cardiac enzymes if patient is receiving long-term therapy

• Hepatic studies: AST, ALT, bilirubin

• Weight qwk; appetite may increase with drug

• ECG for flattening of T wave, bundle branch block, AV block, dysrhythmias in cardiac patients; drug should be discontinued gradually several days before surgery

• EPS primarily in elderly: rigidity, dystonia, akathisia

• Mental status: mood, sensorium, affect, suicidal tendencies, increase in psychiatric symptoms: depression, panic

• Urinary retention, constipation; constipation most likely in children, elderly

• Withdrawal symptoms: headache, nausea, vomiting, muscle pain, weakness; not usual unless drug is discontinued abruptly

• Alcohol consumption; if alcohol is consumed, hold dose until morning

Administer:

• Oral conc should be diluted with 120 ml of water, milk, orange, grapefruit, tomato, prune, pineapple juice. Do not mix with grape juice

• Increased fluids, bulk in diet for constipation

• With food, milk for GI symptoms, do not give with carbonated beverages

• Dosage hs for oversedation during day; may take entire dose hs; elderly may not tolerate qd dosing

• Gum, hard candy, or frequent sips of water for dry mouth

• Topically by applying to affected area, rub slightly

Perform/provide:

• Storage in tight container protected from direct sunlight

• Assistance with ambulation during beginning therapy, since drowsiness/dizziness occurs

• Safety measures primarily for elderly

• Checking to see PO medication swallowed

Evaluate:

• Therapeutic response: decreased anxiety, depression

Teach patient/family:

• That therapeutic effects may take 2-3 wk

• To use caution in driving, other activities requiring alertness, because of drowsiness, dizziness, blurred vision

• To avoid alcohol ingestion, other CNS depressants

• Not to discontinue medication quickly after long-term use; may cause nausea, headache, malaise

• To wear sunscreen or large hat, since photosensitivity occurs

Treatment of overdose: ECG monitoring; induce emesis; lavage, activated charcoal; administer anticonvulsant

---

doxercalciferol
See appendix a—selected new drugs

---

doxorubicin (R)
(dox-oh-roo'bi-sin)
Adriamycin PFS, Adriamycin
RDF, Rubex
doxorubicin
liposome (R)
Doxil
Func. class.: Antineoplastic,
antibiotic
Chem. class.: Anthracycline
glycoside

Action: Inhibits DNA synthesis primarily; derived from *Streptomyces peucetius;* replication is decreased by binding to DNA, which causes strand splitting; active throughout entire cell cycle; a vesicant

Uses: Wilms' tumor; bladder, breast, cervical, head, neck, liver, lung, ovarian, prostatic, stomach, testicular, thyroid cancer; Hodgkin's disease; acute lymphoblastic leukemia; myeloblastic leukemia; neuroblastomas; lymphomas; sarcomas

Dosage and routes:

Doxorubicin

• *Adult:* IV 60-75 mg/m^2 q3wk, or 30 mg/m^2 on days 1-3 of 4-wk cycle, not to exceed 550 mg/m^2 cumulative dose; Doxil: Adult IV 20 mg/m^2 q3wk

• *Child:* IV 30 mg/m^2/day × 3 days, may repeat q4wk

Doxorubicin liposome

• *Adult:* IV 20 mg/m^2 q3wk

Available forms: Inj 10, 20, 50, 100, 150 mg; Doxil: liposomal dispersion for inj: 20 mg/ml

Side effects/adverse reactions:

HEMA: **Thrombocytopenia, leukopenia, anemia**

GI: Nausea, vomiting, anorexia, mucositis, **hepatotoxicity**

GU: Impotence, sterility, amenorrhea, gynecomastia, hyperuricemia

INTEG: Rash, necrosis at injection site, dermatitis, reversible alopecia, cellulitis, thrombophlebitis at injection site

CV: Increased B/P, **sinus tachycardia, PVCs,** chest pain, **bradycardia, extrasystoles**

Contraindications: Hypersensitivity, pregnancy (1st trimester) (D), lactation, systemic infections

Precautions: Renal, hepatic, cardiac disease; gout, bone marrow depression (severe)

Pharmacokinetics: Triphasic pattern of elimination; half-life 12 min, 3⅓ hr, 29⅔ hr; metabolized by liver; crosses placenta; excreted in urine, bile, breast milk

Interactions:

• Increased toxicity: other antineoplastics or radiation, mercaptopurine

• Increased risk of hemorrhagic cystitis

• Cardiac toxicity: cyclophosphamide

• Decreased antibody response: live virus vaccine

Lab test interferences:

Increase: Uric acid

NURSING CONSIDERATIONS

Assess:

• CBC, differential, platelet count weekly; withhold drug if WBC is <4000/mm^3 or platelet count is <75,000/mm^3; notify prescriber of these results

• Blood, urine uric acid levels

• Renal function studies: BUN, serum uric acid, urine CrCl, electrolytes before, during therapy

• I&O ratio; report fall in urine output to <30 ml/hr

• Monitor temp q4h; fever may indicate beginning infection

• Liver function tests before, during therapy: bilirubin, AST, ALT, alk phosphatase as needed or monthly; check for jaundice of skin and sclera, dark urine, clay-colored stools, itchy skin, abdominal pain, fever, diarrhea

• ECG; watch for ST-T wave changes, low QRS and T, possible dysrhythmias (sinus tachycardia, heart block, PVCs)

• Bleeding: hematuria, guaiac, bruising, or petechiae, mucosa or orifices q8h

• Effects of alopecia on body image; discuss feelings about body changes

• Inflammation of mucosa, breaks in skin

• Buccal cavity q8h for dryness, sores, ulceration, white patches, oral pain, bleeding, dysphagia

• Alkalosis if severe vomiting is present

• Local irritation, pain, burning at injection site

• GI symptoms: frequency of stools, cramping

• Acidosis, signs of dehydration: rapid respirations, poor skin turgor, decreased urine output, dry skin, restlessness, weakness

• Cardiac status: B/P, pulse, character, rhythm, rate, ABGs, ECG

Administer:

• Antiemetic 30-60 min before giving drug to prevent vomiting

• Allopurinol or sodium bicarbonate to maintain uric acid levels, alkalinization of urine

• Topical or systemic analgesics for pain

• Transfusion for anemia

• Antispasmodic for GI symptoms

IV

◆ Do not interchange doxorubicin with doxorubicin liposome

• Hydrocortisone, dexamethasone, or sodium bicarbonate (1 mEq/1 ml) for extravasation; apply ice compresses

• IV after diluting 10 mg/5 ml of NaCl for inj; another 5 ml of diluent/10 mg is recommended; shake; give over 3-5 min; give through Y-tube of free-flowing 5% dextrose INF or NS

Additive compatibilities: Ondansetron

Syringe compatibilities: Bleomycin, cisplatin, cyclophosphamide, droperidol, leucovorin, methotrexate, metoclopramide, mitomycin, vincristine

Y-site compatibilities: Amifostine, aztreonam, bleomycin, chlorpromazine, cimetidine, cisplatin, cladribine, cyclophosphamide, dexamethasone, diphenhydramine, droperidol, famotidine, filgrastim, fludarabine, fluorouracil, granisetron, hydromorphone, leucovorin, lorazepam, melphalan, methotrexate, methylprednisolone, metoclopramide, mitomycin, morphine, ondansetron, paclitaxel, prochlorperazine, promethazine, propofol, ranitidine, sargramostim, sodium bicarbonate, teniposide, thiotepa, vinblastine, vincristine, vinorelbine

• IV liposome inj (Doxil): dilute dose up to 90 mg/250 ml D_5W, give over ½ hr; do not admix with other sol or meds

Perform/provide:

• Liquid diet: carbonated beverages, geletin may be added if patient is not nauseated or vomiting

• Increased fluid intake to 2-3 L/day to prevent urate, calculi formation

• Rinsing of mouth tid-qid with water, club soda; brushing of teeth bid-tid with soft brush or cotton-tipped applicators for stomatitis; use unwaxed dental floss

• Storage at room temp for 24 hr after reconstituting or 48 hr refrigerated

Evaluate:

• Therapeutic response: decreased tumor size, spread of malignancy

---

◆ = Nursing alert   ✦ = Herb-drug interaction   ⊘ = Do not crush

Teach patient/family:

• To report any complaints, side effects to nurse or prescriber

• That hair may be lost during treatment and wig or hairpiece may make patient feel better; tell patient that new hair may be different in color, texture

• To avoid foods with citric acid, hot or rough texture

• To report any bleeding, white spots, ulcerations in mouth to prescriber; tell patient to examine mouth qd

• That urine and other body fluids may be red-orange for 48 hr

• To avoid crowds and persons with infections when granulocyte count is low

• That contraceptive measures are recommended during therapy

• To avoid vaccinations; reactions may occur

---

doxycycline (℞)

(dox-i-sye'kleen)
Apo-Doxy*, Doryx, Doxy, Doxy-Caps, Doxycin*, doxycycline, Monodox, Novodoxy-clin*, Vibramycin, Vibramycin IV, Vibra-Tabs

Func. class.: Antiinfective
Chem. class.: Tetracycline

Action: Inhibits protein synthesis, prosphorylation in microorganisms by binding to 30S ribosomal subunits, reversibly binding to 50S ribosomal subunits; bacteriostatic

Uses: Syphilis, *Chlamydia trachomatis,* gonorrhea, *Rickettsia,* lymphogranuloma venereum, uncommon gram-negative/positive organisms, malaria prophylaxis, chronic periodontitis, acne

Investigational uses: Traveler's diarrhea, Lyme disease, prevention of chronic bronchitis

Dosage and routes:
• *Adult:* **PO/IV** 100 mg q12h on day 1, then 100 mg/day; **IV** 200 mg in 1-2 inf on day 1, then 100-200 mg/day; delivery syst: 10% for cont rel

• *Child >8 yr:* **PO/IV** 2.2-4.4 mg/kg/day in divided doses q12h

Gonorrhea (uncomplicated) in patients allergic to penicillin
• *Adult:* **PO** 200 mg, then 100 mg hs and 100 mg bid × 3 days or 300 mg, then 300 mg in 1 hr; disseminated; 100 mg **PO** bid × at least 7 days

Malaria prophylaxis
• *Adult:* 100 mg qd 1-2 days prior to travel and daily during travel

C. trachomatis
• *Adult:* **PO** 100 mg bid × 7 days

Syphilis
• *Adult:* **PO** 300 mg/day in divided doses × 10 days

Available forms: Tabs 50, 100 mg; caps 50, 100 mg; syr 50 mg/ml; pwd for inj 100, 200 mg; pwd for oral susp 25 mg/5 ml; Atrigel del syst 10%

Side effects/adverse reactions:
CNS: Fever
HEMA: Eosinophilia, neutropenia, thrombocytopenia, hemolytic anemia
EENT: Dysphagia, glossitis, decreased calcification of deciduous teeth, oral candidiasis
GI: Nausea, abdominal pain, vomiting, diarrhea, anorexia, enterocolitis, *hepatotoxicity,* flatulence, abdominal cramps, gastric burning, stomatitis
CV: Pericarditis
GU: Increased BUN
INTEG: Rash, urticaria, photosensitivity, increased pigmentation, exfoliative dermatitis, pruritus, *angioedema*

Contraindications: Hypersensitivity to tetracyclines, children <8 yr, pregnancy (D)

Precautions: Hepatic disease, lactation

Pharmacokinetics:
PO: Peak 1½-4 hr, half-life 15-22 hr; excreted in bile, 90% protein bound

Interactions:
• Decreased effects of doxycycline: antacids, $NaHCO_3$, dairy products, alkali products, iron, kaolin/pectin, barbiturates, carbamazepine, phenytoin, cimetidine sucralfate, cholestyramine, colestipol
• Increased effect: warfarin
• Decreased effects: penicillins, oral contraceptives
⫸ Increased action: bromelain

Lab test interferences:
False increase: Urinary catecholamines; ALT, AST

NURSING CONSIDERATIONS
Assess:
• I&O ratio
• Blood studies: PT, CBC, AST, ALT, BUN, creatinine
• Signs of infection
• Allergic reactions: rash, itching, pruritus, angioedema
• Nausea, vomiting, diarrhea; administer antiemetic, antacids as ordered
• Overgrowth of infection: fever, malaise, redness, pain, swelling, drainage, perineal itching, diarrhea, changes in cough or sputum
• IV site for phlebitis/thrombosis; drug is highly irritating

Administer:
• After C&S
• 2 hr before or after laxative or iron products; 3 hr after antacid or kaolin-pectin products

IV
• After diluting 100 mg or less/10 ml of sterile H_2O or NS for inj; further dilute with 100-1000 ml of NaCl, D_5, Ringer's LR D_5LR, Normosol-M, Normosol-R in D_5W; run 100 mg or less over 1-4 hr; do not give IM/SC; inf must be completed in 6 hr, when diluted in LR sol, or 12 hr in other sol

Additive compatibilities: Ranitidine

Syringe compatibilities: Doxapram
Y-site compatibilities: Acyclovir, amifostine, amiodarone, aztreonam, cisatracurium, cyclophosphamide, diltiazem, filgrastim, fludarabine, granisetron, hydromorphone, magnesium sulfate, melphalan, meperidine, morphine, ondansetron, perphenazine, propofol, remifentanil, sargramostim, tacrolimus, teniposide, theophylline, thiotepa, vinorelbine

Perform/provide:
• Storage in tight, light-resistant container at room temp

Evaluate:
• Therapeutic response: decreased temp, absence of lesions, negative C&S

Teach patient/family:
• To avoid sun, since burns may occur; sunscreen does not seem to decrease photosensitivity
• That all prescribed medication must be taken to prevent superinfection
🚫 Not to break, crush, or chew caps
• To take with a full glass of water; may take with food

---

droperidol (R)

(droe-per'i-dole)

droperidol, Inapsine

Func. class.: Neuroleptic

Chem. class.: Butyrophenone derivative

Action: Acts on CNS at subcortical levels, produces tranquilization, sleep; antiemetic

Uses: Premedication for surgery; induction, maintenance in general anesthesia; postoperatively for nausea, vomiting

Dosage and routes:

Induction

• *Adult:* **IV/IM** 0.22-0.275 mg/kg given with analgesic or general anesthetic; may give 1.25-2.5 mg additionally

• *Child 2-12 yr:* **IV** 88-165 µg/kg, titrated to response needed

Premedication

• *Adult:* **IM** 2.5-10 mg ½-1 hr before surgery

• *Child 2-12 yr:* **IM** 1-1.5 mg/20-25 lb

Maintaining general anesthesia

• *Adult:* **IV** 1.25-2.5 mg

Regional anesthesia adjunct

• *Adult:* **IV/IM** 2.5-5 mg

Diagnostic procedures without general anesthesia

• *Adult:* **IM** 2.5-10 mg ½-1 hr prior to procedure; 1.25-2.5 mg may be needed

Available forms: Inj 2.5 mg/ml

Side effects/adverse reactions:

RESP: **Laryngospasm, bronchospasm**

CNS: Dystonia, akathisia, flexion of arms, fine tremors, dizziness, anxiety, drowsiness, restlessness, hallucination, depression

CV: *Tachycardia, hypotension*

EENT: Upward rotation of eyes, oculogyric crisis

INTEG: Chills, facial sweating, shivering

Contraindications: Hypersensitivity, child <2 yr, pregnancy (C), lactation

Precautions: Elderly, cardiovascular disease (hypotension, bradydysrhythmias), renal disease, liver disease, Parkinson's disease

Pharmacokinetics:

IM/IV: Onset 3-10 min, peak ½ hr, duration 3-6 hr; metabolized in liver; excreted in urine as metabolites; crosses placenta, half-life 2-3 hr

Interactions:

• Increased CNS depression: alcohol, opiates, barbiturates, antipsychotics, or other CNS depressants

• Increased hypotension: nitrates, antihypertensives

• Increased side effects of lithium

🍇 Increased action: kava

NURSING CONSIDERATIONS

Assess:

• VS q10min during IV administration, q30min after IM dose

• EPS: dystonia, akathisia

◆ For increasing heart rate or decreasing B/P, notify prescriber at once; do not place patient in Trendelenburg position, or sympathetic blockade may occur, causing respiratory arrest

Administer:

• Anticholinergics (benztropine, diphenhydramine) for EPS

• Only with crash cart, resuscitative equipment nearby

• IM deep in large muscle mass

IV

• Undiluted; give through Y-tube at 10 mg or less/min; titrate to patient response; may be given as an infusion by adding dose to 250 ml LR, D₅W, 0.9% NaCl

Syringe compatibilities: Atropine, bleomycin, butorphanol, chlorpromazine, cimetidine, cisplatin, cyclophosphamide, dimenhydrinate, diphenhydramine, doxorubicin, fentanyl, glycopyrrolate, hydroxyzine, meperidine, metoclopramide, midazolam, mitomycin, morphine, nalbuphine, pentazocine, perphenazine, prochlorperazine, promazine, promethazine, scopolamine, vinblastine, vincristine

Y-site compatibilities: Amifostine, aztreonam, bleomycin, cisatracurium, cisplatin, cladribine, cyclophosphamide, cytarabine, doxorubicin, doxorubicin liposome, famotidine, filgrastim, fluconazole, fludarabine, granisetron, hydrocortisone, idarubicin, melphalan, meperidine, metoclopramide, mitomycin, ondansetron, paclitaxel, potassium chloride, propofol, remifentanil, sargramostim, teniposide, thiotepa, vinblastine, vincristine, vinorelbine, vit B/C

Evaluate:

• Therapeutic response: decreased anxiety, absence of vomiting during and after surgery

Teach patient/family:

• To rise slowly from sitting or standing to minimize orthostatic hypotension

---

dyphylline (℞)

(dye'fi-lin)
Dilor, Dyflex-200, Dylline, dyphylline, Lufyllin, Neothylline
Func. class.: Bronchodilator
Chem. class.: Xanthine, ethylenediamide

Action: Relaxes smooth muscle of respiratory system by blocking phosphodiesterase, which increases cyclic AMP; cyclic AMP results in positive inotropic, chronotropic effects, bronchodilation, stimulation of CNS

Uses: Bronchial asthma, bronchospasm in chronic bronchitis, COPD
Dosage and routes:
• *Adult:* **PO** 200-800 mg q6h; **IM** 250-500 mg q6h injected slowly
• *Child >6 yr:* **PO** 4-7 mg/kg/day in 4 divided doses
Available forms: Tabs 200, 400 mg; elix 33.3, 53.3 mg/5 ml; inj 250 mg/ml
Side effects/adverse reactions:
CNS: Anxiety, restlessness, insomnia, dizziness, **convulsions,** headache, light-headedness, muscle twitching
CV: Palpitations, sinus tachycardia, hypotension, flushing, dysrhythmias
GI: Nausea, vomiting, anorexia, dyspepsia, epigastric pain
INTEG: Flushing, urticaria
RESP: Tachypnea
OTHER: Fever, dehydration, **albuminuria,** hyperglycemia
Contraindications: Hypersensitivity to xanthines, tachydysrhythmias
Precautions: Elderly, CHF, cor pulmonale, hepatic disease, active peptic ulcer disease, diabetes mellitus, hyperthyroidism, hypertension, children, renal disease, pregnancy (B), lactation, glaucoma
Pharmacokinetics: Peak 1 hr, halflife 2 hr, excreted in urine unchanged
Interactions:
• Do not mix in syringe with other drugs
• Increased action of dyphylline: cimetidine, propranolol, erythromycin, troleandomycin
• May increase effects of anticoagulants
• Cardiotoxicity: β-blockers
• Increased metabolism: barbiturates, phenytoin
• Decreased elimination of dyphylline: uricosurics
NURSING CONSIDERATIONS
Assess:
• Dyphylline blood levels; toxicity

◆ = Nursing alert   ▧ = Herb-drug interaction   ⊘ = Do not crush

may occur with small increase above 20 μg/ml
• Monitor I&O; diuresis occurs; dehydration may be the result in elderly or children
• Whether theophylline was given recently
• Auscultate lung fields bilaterally; notify prescriber of abnormalities
• Allergic reactions: rash, urticaria; drug should be discontinued

Administer:
• PO after meals to decrease GI symptoms; absorption may be affected
• Avoid IM injection; pain occurs

Perform/provide:
• Storage protected from light, at room temp

Evaluate:
• Therapeutic response: decreased dyspnea, respiratory rate, rhythm

Teach patient/family:
• To check OTC medications, current prescription medications for ephedrine; will increase stimulation; not to drink alcohol or caffeine
• To avoid hazardous activities; dizziness, drowsiness, blurred vision may occur
• For GI upset, to take drug with 8 oz water; avoid taking with food, since absorption may be decreased

---

edrophonium (℞)

(ed-roh-fone′ee-um)
Enlon, Reversol, Tensilon
Func. class.: Cholinergics, anticholinesterase
Chem. class.: Quaternary ammonium compound

Action: Inhibits destruction of acetylcholine, which increases concentration at sites where acetylcholine is released; this facilitates transmission of impulses across myoneural junction

Uses: To diagnose myasthenia gravis; curare antagonist; differentiation of myasthenic crisis from cholinergic crisis

Dosage and routes:
Tensilon test (myasthenia gravis diagnosis)
• *Adult:* IV 1-2 mg over 15-30 sec, then 8 mg if no response; IM 10 mg; if cholinergic reaction occurs, retest after ½ hr with 2 mg IM
• *Child >34 kg:* IV 2 mg; if no response in 45 sec, then 1 mg q45sec, not to exceed 10 mg; IM 5 mg
• *Child <34 kg:* IV 1 mg; if no response in 45 sec, then 1 mg q45sec, not to exceed 5 mg; IM 2 mg
• *Infant:* IV 0.5 mg
Reversal of nondepolarizing neuromuscular blockers
• *Adult:* IV 10 mg over 30-45 sec, may repeat, not to exceed 40 mg
Differentiation of myasthenic crisis from cholinergic crisis
• *Adult:* IV 1 mg, if no response in 1 min, may repeat
Available forms: Inj 10 mg/ml

Side effects/adverse reactions:
INTEG: Rash, urticaria
CNS: Dizziness, headache, sweating, weakness, ***convulsions,*** incoordination, ***paralysis,*** drowsiness, ***loss of consciousness***
GI: Nausea, diarrhea, vomiting, cramps, increased salivary and gastric secretions, dysphagia, increased peristalsis
CV: Dysrhythmias, bradycardia, hypotension, *AV block,* ECG changes, ***cardiac arrest,*** syncope
GU: Urinary frequency, incontinence, urgency
*RESP: **Respiratory depression, bronchospasm, constriction, laryngospasm, respiratory arrest,** dyspnea, increased bronchial secretions*
EENT: Miosis, blurred vision, lacrimation, visual changes

E

Contraindications: Obstruction of intestine, renal system, hypersensitivity

Precautions: Seizure disorders, bronchial asthma, coronary occlusion, hyperthyroidism, dysrhythmias, peptic ulcer, megacolon, poor GI motility, pregnancy (C), bradycardia, hypotension

Pharmacokinetics:
IV: Onset 30-60 sec, duration 6-15 min
IM: Onset 2-10 min, duration 12-45 min

Interactions:
• Decreased action of edrophonium: procainamide, quinidine, atropine, anesthetics, phenothiazines, antihistamines, haloperidol, magnesium, corticosteroids, antidysrhythmics
• Bradycardia: digitalis
• Prolonged action of: depolarizing muscle relaxants

NURSING CONSIDERATIONS
Assess:
• VS, respiration during test; muscle strength
• Diabetic patient carefully, since this drug lowers blood glucose

Administer:
◆ Only with atropine sulfate available for cholinergic crisis
• Only after all other cholinergics have been discontinued

IV, direct
• 2 mg or less over 15-30 sec; as a curare antagonist, over 30-45 sec; or given as continuous infusion in myasthenic crisis

Y-site compatibilities: Heparin, hydrocortisone, potassium chloride, vit B/C

Perform/provide:
• Storage at room temp

Evaluate:
• Therapeutic response: increased muscle strength, hand grasp; improved gait; absence of labored breathing (if severe)

Teach patient/family:
• To wear Medic Alert ID specifying myasthenia gravis, drugs taken

Treatment of overdose: Respiratory support, atropine 1-4 mg (IV)

---

efavirenz (℞)
(ef-ah-veer'enz)
Sustiva
Func. class.: Antiviral
Chem. class.: Nonnucleoside reverse transcriptase inhibitor (NNRTI)

Action: Binds directly to reverse transcriptase and blocks RNA, DNA causing a disruption of the enzyme's site

Uses: HIV-1 in combination with other antivirals

Dosage and routes:
Given in combination with protease inhibitor or nucleoside analog reverse transcriptase inhibitors (NARTIs)
• *Adult:* **PO** 600 mg qd hs
• *Child: 10-<15 kg:* **PO** 200 mg qd hs
• *Child: 15-<20 kg:* **PO** 250 mg qd hs
• *Child: 20-<25 kg:* **PO** 300 mg qd hs
• *Child: 25-<32.5 kg:* **PO** 350 mg qd hs
• *Child: 32.5-<40 kg:* **PO** 400 mg qd hs
• *Child: ≥40 kg:* Adult dose

Available forms: Caps 50, 100, 200 mg

Side effects/adverse reactions:
GU: Hematuria, kidney stones
CNS: Fatigue, impaired concentration, insomnia, abnormal dreams, depression, headache
GI: Diarrhea, abdominal pain, *nausea*
INTEG: Rash, dizziness, ***erythema***

---

multiforme, Stevens-Johnson syndrome, toxic epidermal necrolysis
Contraindication: Hypersensitivity

Precautions: Liver disease, pregnancy (C), lactation, children <3yr, renal disease, myelosuppression

Pharmacokinetics: Well absorbed, metabolized by liver, terminal half-life 52-76 hr

Interactions:
• Decreased efavirenz levels: rifamycins
• Do not give together with benzodiazepines, ergots, midazolam, triazolam
• Decreased levels of: indinavir, saquinavir
• Increased levels of both drugs: ritonavir, estrogens
• Increased levels of: warfarin
• Drug/food: increased absorption: high-fat foods

NURSING CONSIDERATIONS
Assess:
• Signs of infection, anemia
• Liver studies: ALT, AST: renal studies
• C&S before drug therapy; drug may be taken as soon as culture is taken; repeat C&S after treatment; determine the presence of other sexually transmitted disease
• Bowel pattern before, during treatment; if severe abdominal pain with bleeding occurs, drug should be discontinued; monitor hydration
• Skin eruptions; rash, urticaria, itching
• Allergies before treatment, reaction to each medication; place allergies on chart
• CBC, blood chemistry, plasma HIV RNA, absolute CD4+/CD8+ cell counts/%, serum beta-2 microglobulin, serum ICD+24 antigen levels, cholesterol, hepatic enzymes
• Signs of toxicity: severe nausea/vomiting, maculopapular rash

Administer:
• HS to decrease CNS side effects
Teach patient/family:
• To take as prescribed; if dose is missed, take as soon as remembered; do not double dose; take with water, juice; may be taken with or without food
• To make sure health-care provider knows all the medications being taken
• That if severe rash occurs, to notify health-care provider
• Not to breastfeed or become pregnant if taking this drug
• That adverse reactions (rash, dizziness, abnormal dreams, insomnia) lessen after a month
• To avoid hazardous activities if dizziness/drowsiness occur

---

enalapril/ enalaprilat (Ŗ)
(e-nal'a-pril)/(e-nal'a-pril-at)
Vasotec, Vasotec IV
Func. class.: Antihypertensive
Chem. class.: Angiotensin-converting enzyme inhibitor

Action: Selectively suppresses renin-angiotensin-aldosterone system; inhibits ACE; prevents conversion of angiotensin I to angiotensin II, dilation of arterial, venous vessels

Uses: Hypertension, systolic CHF, diabetic neuropathy, post MI, left ventricular dysfunction

Dosage and routes:
Hypertension
• *Adult:* **PO** 5 mg/day, may increase or decrease to desired response range 10-40 mg/day; **IV** 1.25 mg q6h over 5 min
• *Child:* **PO** 0.1 mg/kg/day in 1-2 divided doses, max 0.5 mg/kg/day
• *Child:* **IV** 5-10 µg/kg/dose q8-24h

Patients on diuretics

• *Adult:* **IV** 0.625 mg over 5 min, may give additional doses of 1.25 mg q6h

Renal impairment

• *Adult:* **PO** 2.5 mg qd (CrCl <30 ml/min) increase gradually; **IV** CrCl >30 ml/min 1.25 mg q6h; CrCl <30 ml/min 0.625 mg as one time dose, increase as per B/P

CHF

• *Adult:* **PO** 5-20 mg/day in 2 divided doses

Available forms: Tabs 2.5, 5, 10, 20 mg; inj 1.25 mg/ml

Side effects/adverse reactions:

CV: Hypotension, chest pain, tachycardia, **dysrhythmias,** syncope

CNS: Insomnia, dizziness, paresthesias, headache, fatigue, anxiety

GI: Nausea, vomiting, colitis, cramps, diarrhea, constipation, flatulence, dry mouth, loss of taste

INTEG: Rash, purpura, alopecia, hyperhidrosis

HEMA: Agranulocytosis, neutropenia

EENT: Tinnitus, visual changes, sore throat, double vision, dry burning eyes

GU: Proteinuria, renal failure, increased frequency of polyuria or oliguria

RESP: Dyspnea, dry cough, rales, angioedema

META: Hyperkalemia

Contraindications: Hypersensitivity, history of angioedema, pregnancy (D) 2nd and 3rd trimester

Precautions: Renal disease, hyperkalemia, pregnancy (C) 1st trimester, lactation, hepatic failure, dehydration, bilateral renal artery stenosis

Pharmacokinetics:

PO: Peak 4-6 hr; half-life 1½ hr; metabolized by liver to active metabolite, excreted in urine

IV: Onset 5-15 min, peak up to 4 hr

Interactions:

• Hypersensitivity: allopurinol

• Severe hypotension: diuretics, other antihypertensives

• Decreased effects of enalapril: aspirin, antacids

• Increased K levels: salt substitutes, K-sparing diuretics, K supplements

• May increase effects of ergots, neuromuscular blocking agents, antihypertensives, hypoglycemics, barbiturates, reserpine, levodopa, lithium

• Effects may be increased by phenothiazines, diuretics, phenytoin, quinidine, nifedipine

Lab test interferences:

Interference: Glucose/insulin tolerance tests

NURSING CONSIDERATIONS

Assess:

• B/P, pulse q4h; note rate, rhythm, quality

• Electrolytes: K, Na, Cl during 1st 2 wk of therapy

• Baselines in renal, liver function tests before therapy begins and 1 wk into therapy

• Edema in feet, legs daily

• Skin turgor, dryness of mucous membranes for hydration status

• Symptoms of CHF: edema, dyspnea, wet rales

Administer:

IV, direct/int inf

• Undiluted over 5 min, use diluent provided or 50 ml D$_5$W, 0.9% NaCl, 0.9% NaCl in D$_5$W or LR, Isolyte E, give through Y-tube of free-flowing inf of 0.9% NaCl, D$_5$W, LR, Isolyte E

Additive compatibilities: Dobutamine, dopamine, heparin, meropenem, nitroglycerin, nitroprusside, potassium chloride

Y-site compatibilities: Allopurinol, amifostine, amikacin, aminophylline, ampicillin, ampicillin/sul-

---

◆ = Nursing alert   ∥ = Herb-drug interaction   Ⓢ = Do not crush bactam, aztreonam, butorphanol, calcium gluconate, cefazolin, cefoperazone, ceftazidime, ceftizoxime, chloramphenicol, cimetidine, cisatracurium, cladribine, clindamycin, dextran 40, dobutamine, dopamine, doxorubicin liposome, erythromycin, esmolol, famotidine, fentanyl, filgrastim, ganciclovir, gentamicin, granisetron, heparin, hetastarch, hydrocortisone, labetalol, lidocaine, magnesium sulfate, melphalan, meropenem, methylprednisolone, metronidazole, morphine, nafcillin, nicardipine, nitroprusside, penicillin G potassium, phenobarbital, piperacillin, piperacillin/tazobactam, potassium chloride, potassium phosphate, propofol, ranitidine, remifentanil, teniposide, thiotepa, tobramycin, trimethoprim/sulfamethoxazole, vancomycin, vinorelbine

Evaluate:

• Therapeutic response: decreased B/P

Teach patient/family:

• Not to use OTC (cough, cold, or allergy) products unless directed by prescriber; to avoid salt substitutes
• To avoid sunlight or wear sunscreen for photosensitivity
• To comply with dosage schedule, even if feeling better
• To notify prescriber of mouth sores, sore throat, fever, swelling of hands or feet, irregular heartbeat, chest pain, signs of angioedema
• That excessive perspiration, dehydration, vomiting, diarrhea may lead to fall in blood pressure; consult prescriber if these occur
• That drug may cause dizziness, fainting; light-headedness may occur during 1st few days of therapy
• That drug may cause skin rash or impaired perspiration; angioedema may occur and to D/C if it occurs
• Not to discontinue drug abruptly
• That CV adverse reactions may reoccur
• To rise slowly to sitting or standing position to minimize orthostatic hypotension

Treatment of overdose: Lavage, IV atropine for bradycardia, IV theophylline for bronchospasm, digitalis, O_2, diuretic for cardiac failure

enoxacin (Ŗ)
(e-nox′a-sin)
Penetrex
Func. class.: Antiinfective
Chem. class.: Fluoroquinolone

Action: Inhibits the enzyme that repairs bacterial DNA, thereby preventing bacterial replication; DNA-gyrase inhibitor

Uses: Uncomplicated urethral or cervical gonorrhea, uncomplicated and complicated UTI; effective against staphylococci, *Aeromonas* sp., *Citrobacter* sp., *Enterobacter* sp., *Escherichia coli, Haemophilus ducreyi, Klebsiella* sp., *Morganella morganii, Neisseria gonorrheae, Proteus vulgaris, Proteus mirabilis, Providencia* sp., *Pseudomonas aeruginosa, Serratia*

Dosage and routes:

Gonorrhea
• *Adult:* **PO** 400 mg as a single dose
Uncomplicated UTI
• *Adult:* **PO** 200 mg q12h × 7 days
Complicated UTI
• *Adult:* **PO** 400 mg q12h × 14 days
Renal disease
• CrCl <30 ml/min give initial dose, then give 50% of dose q12h
Available forms: Tabs 200, 400 mg

Side effects/adverse reactions:

CNS: Dizziness, headache, fatigue, somnolence, depression, insomnia, anxiety, *seizures*

GI: Diarrhea, nausea, vomiting, anorexia, flatulence, heartburn, abdominal pain, dry mouth, increased AST, ALT

INTEG: Rash, pruritus, photosensitivity

EENT: Visual disturbances, dizziness

Contraindications: Hypersensitivity to quinolones

Precautions: Pregnancy (C), lactation, children, elderly, renal disease, seizure disorders

Pharmacokinetics:

PO: Peak 1 hr, half-life 3-6 hr, steady state 2 days; excreted in urine as unchanged drug, metabolites

Interactions:

• Increased levels of: aminophylline, cyclosporine, theophylline, use cautiously

• Decreased absorption of enoxacin: antacids with magnesium, aluminum; iron salts, sucralfate, bismuth subsalicylate

• Increased digoxin levels: digoxin, monitor for toxicity

• Drug/food: decreased absorption with food

NURSING CONSIDERATIONS

Assess:

• Kidney, liver function studies: BUN, creatinine, AST, ALT

• I&O ratio, urine pH; <5.5 is ideal

• CNS symptoms: insomnia, vertigo, headache, agitation, confusion

• Allergic reactions: rash, flushing, urticaria, pruritus

Administer:

• After clean-catch urine for C&S

• 2 hr before or 2 hr after antacids, zinc, iron, calcium

Perform/provide:

• Limited intake of alkaline foods, drugs; milk, dairy products, peanuts, vegetables, alkaline actacids, sodium bicarbonate

Evaluate:

• Therapeutic response: negative C&S, absence of symptoms of infection

Teach patient/family:

• That fluids must be increased to 3 L/day to avoid crystallization in kidneys

• If dizziness occurs, to ambulate, perform activities with assistance

• Not to take within 2 hr of antacids, calcium, iron, milk, sucralfate

• To use sunscreen, protective clothing for photosensitivity

• To complete full course of drug therapy, take 1 hr ac or 2 hr pc

• To contact prescriber if adverse reactions occur or if inflammation or pain of tendon occurs

---

enoxaparin (℞)

(ee-nox′a-par-in)
Lovenox
Func. class.: Anticoagulant
Chem. class.: Unfractionated porcine heparin

Action: Prevents conversion of fibrinogen to fibrin and prothrombin to thrombin by enhancing inhibitory effects of antithrombin III; produces higher ratio of antifactor Xa to antifactor IIa

Uses: Prevention of deep-vein thrombosis, pulmonary emboli in hip and knee replacement

Dosage and routes:

Hip/knee replacement

• *Adult:* SC 30 mg bid given 12-24 hr post-op for 7-10 days, provided that hemostasis has been established

Abdominal surgery

• *Adult:* SC 40 mg qd × 7-10 days to prevent thromboembolic complications

• Prevention of ischemic complica-

 = Nursing alert   = Herb-drug interaction   ⊘ = Do not crush

tions in unstable angina/non-Q-wave MI with aspirin

• *Adult:* SC 1 mg/kg q12h until stable with aspirin 100-325 mg qd

Available forms: Inj 30 mg/0.3 ml, 40 mg/0.4 ml, 60 mg/0.6 ml, 80 mg/0.8 ml, 100 mg/1 ml

Side effects/adverse reactions:

CNS: Fever, confusion

GI: Nausea

SYST: Edema, peripheral edema

HEMA: **Hypochromic anemia, thrombocytopenia,** bleeding

CV: **Cardiac toxicity**

INTEG: Ecchymosis

Contraindications: Hypersensitivity to this drug, heparin, or pork; hemophilia, leukemia with bleeding, peptic ulcer disease, thrombocytopenic purpura, heparin-induced thrombocytopenia

Precautions: Alcoholism, elderly, pregnancy (B), hepatic disease (severe), renal disease (severe), blood dyscrasias, severe hypertension, subacute bacterial endocarditis, acute nephritis, lactation, children

Pharmacokinetics:

SC: Maximum antithrombin activity (3-5 hr), elimination half-life 4½ hr

Interactions:

• Increased action of enoxaparin: anticoagulants, salicylates, NSAIDs, antiplatelets

• Increased hypoprothrombinemia: plicamycin, valproic acid

• Do not mix with other drugs or infusion fluids

⚡ Increased risk of bleeding: bromelain, cinchona bark

Lab test interferences:

Decrease: Platelet count

Increase: AST, ALT

NURSING CONSIDERATIONS

Assess:

• Blood studies (Hct, platelets, occult blood in stools), anti-Xa; thrombocytopenia may occur

• Bleeding gums, petechiae, ecchymosis, black tarry stools, hematuria

• For neuro symptoms in patients who have received spinal anesthesia

Administer:

• Only after screening patient for bleeding disorders

• SC only; do not give IM

• To recumbent patient; give SC; rotate inj sites (left/right anterolateral, left/right posterolateral abdominal wall)

• Insert whole length of needle into skin fold held with thumb and forefinger

◆ Only this drug when ordered; not interchangeable with heparin

• At same time each day to maintain steady blood levels

• Do not massage area or aspirate when giving SC injection

• Avoiding all IM injections that may cause bleeding

Perform/provide:

• Storage at 77° F (25° C); do not freeze

Evaluate:

• Therapeutic response: prevention of deep vein thrombosis

Teach patient/family:

• To use soft-bristle toothbrush to avoid bleeding gums, to use electric razor

• To report any signs of bleeding: gums, under skin, urine, stools

• To avoid OTC drugs containing aspirin

Treatment of overdose: Protamine SO₄ 1% sol; dose should equal dose of enoxaparin

entacapone
See appendix a—selected new drugs

ephedrine (℞)

(e-fed'rin)

ephedrine sulfate

Func. class.: Bronchodilator, adrenergic, mixed direct and indirect effects

Chem. class.: Phenylisopropylamine

Action: Causes increased contractility and heart rate by acting on β-receptors in the heart; also acts on α-receptors, causing vasoconstriction in blood vessels

Uses: Shock; increased perfusion; hypotension, bronchodilation

Dosage and routes:

Vasopressor

• *Adult:* **IM/SC** 25-50 mg, not to exceed 150 mg/24 hr; **IV** 10-25 mg, not to exceed 150 mg/24 hr

• *Child:* **SC/IV** 3 mg/kg/day or 25-100 mg/m²/day in divided doses q4-6h

Bronchodilator

• *Adult:* **PO** 25-50 mg bid-qid, not to exceed 400 mg/day; **IM/SC** 12.5-25 mg

• *Child 6-12yr:* 6.25-12.5 mg q4h, max 75 mg/24 hr

• *Child >2 yr:* **PO** 2-3 mg/kg/day or 100 mg/m²/day in 4-6 divided doses

Orthostatic hypotension

• *Adult:* **PO** 25 mg qd-qid

• *Child:* **PO** 3 mg/kg/day in 4-6 divided doses

Stimulation

• *Adult:* **PO** 25-50 mg q3-4h prn

• *Child:* **PO** 3 mg/kg/day or 100 mg/m²/day in divided doses

Labor

• *Adult:* Administer **IV** dose to maintain B/P at or <1³⁰⁄₈₀ mm Hg

Available forms: Inj 25, 30, 50 mg/ml; caps 25, 50 mg

Side effects/adverse reactions:

CNS: Tremors, anxiety, insomnia, headache, dizziness, confusion, hallucinations, ***convulsions, CNS depression, cerebral hemorrhage***

GU: Dysuria, urinary retention

CV: Palpitations, tachycardia, hypertension, chest pain, ***dysrhythmias***

GI: Anorexia, nausea, vomiting

*RESP: **Dyspnea***

Contraindications: Hypersensitivity to sympathomimetics, narrow-angle glaucoma, nonanaphylactic shock during general anesthesia

Precautions: Pregnancy (C), lactation, cardiac disorders, hyperthyroidism, diabetes mellitus, prostatic hypertrophy

Pharmacokinetics:

PO: Onset 15-60 min, duration 2-4 hr

IV: Onset 5 min, duration 2 hr

Metabolized in liver; excreted in urine (unchanged), breast milk; crosses blood-brain barrier, placenta

Interactions:

• Severe hypertension: oxytocics

• Do not use with MAOIs or tricyclic antidepressants; hypertensive crisis may occur

• Decreased effect of ephedrine: methyldopa, urinary acidifiers, rauwolfia alkaloids, alpha-adrenergic blockers, diuretics

• Increased effect of ephedrine: urinary alkalizers

• Dysrhythmia: halothane anesthetics, cardiac glycosides, levodopa

• Decreased effect of guanethidine

 Increased action of ephedrine: ephedra

NURSING CONSIDERATIONS

Assess:

• I&O ratio

• ECG continuously during administration; if B/P increases, drug is decreased; B/P and pulse q5min after parenteral route; CVP or PWP during infusion if possible

---

 = Nursing alert   = Herb-drug interaction   ⊘ = Do not crush

• For paresthesias and coldness of extremities; peripheral blood flow may decrease; long-term use may produce a pseudoanxiety state requiring sedative; increased lactic acid with severe metabolic acidosis can occur

• Injection site: tissue sloughing; if this occurs, administer phentolamine mixed with 0.9% NaCl

Administer:

IV, direct

• Through Y-tube or 3-way stopcock; give 10-25 mg slowly; may repeat in 5-10 min

• Plasma expanders for hypovolemia

Additive compatibilities: Chloramphenicol, lidocaine, metaraminol, nafcillin, penicillin G potassium

Solution compatibilities: D_5W, $D_{10}W$, LR, 0.9% NaCl, 0.45% NaCl, Ringer's

Syringe compatibilities: Pentobarbital

Y-site compatibilities: Etomidate, propofol

Perform/provide:

• Storage of reconstituted sol refrigerated no longer than 24 hr

• Do not use discolored sol

Evaluate:

• Therapeutic response: increased B/P with stabilization

Teach patient/family:

• The reason for drug administration

---

epinephrine (℞)

(ep-i-nef′rin)

Adrenalin Chloride, Adrenalin Ana-Guard, AsthmaHaler Mist, AsthmaNefrin, Bronitin Mist, Bronkaid Mist, Epinal, epinephrine, Epinephrine HCI, Epinephrine Pediatric, Epipen Jr., Epitrate, Eppy/N, Glaucon, Medihaler-Epi, microNefrin, Nephron, Primatene Mist, S-2, Sus-Phrine, Vaponefrin

Func. class.: Bronchodilator-adrenergic

Chem. class.: Catecholamine

Action: β_1- and β_2-agonist causing increased levels of cyclic AMP producing bronchodilation, cardiac, and CNS stimulation; large doses cause vasoconstriction; small doses can cause vasodilation via β_2-vascular receptors

Uses: Acute asthmatic attacks, hemostasis, bronchospasm, anaphylaxis, allergic reactions, cardiac arrest, adjunct in anesthesia

Dosage and routes:

Asthma

• *Adult and child:* **INH** 1-2 puffs of 1:100 or 2.25% racemic q15min

Bronchodilator

• *Adult:* **SC** 0.2-0.5 mg q20min-4h, max 1 mg/dose

Anaphylactic shock/vasopressor

• *Adult:* **SC/IM** 0.5 mg, repeat q5min if needed, then **IV; IV** 0.1-0.25 mg, repeat q5-15min or inf 1 µg/min, increase to 4 µg/min if needed

• *Child:* **SC/IM/IV** 10 µg/kg, repeat q5-15min up to 0.3 mg

Anaphylactic reaction/asthma

• *Adult:* **SC/IM** 0.1-0.5 mg, repeat q10-15min, do not exceed 1 mg/dose; epinephrine susp 0.5 mg **SC**, may repeat 0.5-1.5 mg q6h

---

• *Child:* **SC** 0.01 mg/kg, repeat q15min, × 2 doses, then q4h, max 0.5 mg/dose; epinephrine susp 0.025 mg/kg **SC,** may repeat q6h, max 0.75 mg in child ≤30 kg

Cardiac arrest

• *Adult:* **IC, IV,** endotracheal 0.1-1 mg, repeat q5min prn

• *Child:* **IC, IV,** endotracheal 5-10 µg q5min, may use 0.1 µg/kg/min **IV INF** after initial dose

Available forms: Aerosol 0.16 mg/ spray, 0.2 mg/spray, 0.25 mg/spray; inj 1:1000 (1 mg/ml), 1:200 (5 mg/ ml), 0.01 mg/ml (1:100,000), 0.1 mg/ml (1:10,000), 0.5 mg/ml (1: 2000); sol for nebulization 1:100, 1.25%, 2.25% (base)

Side effects/adverse reactions:

CNS: Tremors, anxiety, insomnia, headache, *dizziness,* confusion, hallucinations, *cerebral hemorrhage,* weakness, drowsiness, headache

CV: Palpitations, tachycardia, hypertension, *dysrhythmias,* increased T wave

GI: Anorexia, nausea, vomiting

RESP: Dyspnea

Contraindications: Hypersensitivity to sympathomimetics, narrow-angle glaucoma, nonanaphylactic shock during general anesthesia, OBS, local anesthesia of certain areas, labor, cardiac dilatation, coronary insufficiency, cerebral arteriosclerosis, organic heart disease

Precautions: Pregnancy (C), lactation, cardiac disorders, hyperthyroidism, diabetes mellitus, prostatic hypertrophy

Pharmacokinetics:

SC: Onset 3-5 min, duration 20 min

PO, INH: Onset 1 min

Crosses placenta; metabolized in liver

Interactions:

• Do not use with MAOIs or tricyclic antidepressants; hypertensive crisis may occur

• Toxicity: other sympathomimetics

• Decreased hypertensive effects: α-adrenergic blockers

• Dysrhythmias: bretylium, cardiac glycosides, halothane anesthetics

• Decreased vascular response: diuretics, ergot alkaloids, phenothiazines

• Increased pressor response: guanethidine, antihistamines, levothyroxine

• Severe hypertension: oxytocics

🍃 Increased action of epinephrine: ephedra

NURSING CONSIDERATIONS

Assess:

• ECG during administration continuously; if B/P increases, drug is decreased; B/P and pulse q5min after parenteral route; CVP, ISVR, PCWP during infusion if possible; inadvertent high arterial B/P can result in angina, aortic rupture, cerebral hemorrhage

• Injection site: tissue sloughing; administer phentolamine with NS

• Sulfite sensitivity, which may be life-threatening

Administer:

• Increased dose of insulin in diabetic patients

IV

• Parenteral dose slowly, after reconstituting 1 mg (1:1000 sol)/10 ml or more NS; to prepare a 1:10,000 sol for maintenance, may be further diluted in 500 ml D_5W; give 1 mg or less over 1 min or more through Y-tube or 3-way stopcock; 1 mg = 1 ml of 1:1000 or 10 ml of 1:10,000

Additive compatibilities: Amikacin, cimetidine, dobutamine, floxacillin, furosemide, metaraminol, ranitidine, verapamil

Syringe compatibilities: Doxapram, heparin, milrinone

Y-site compatibilities: Amrinone, atracurium, calcium chloride, cal-

---

◆ = Nursing alert   🍃 = Herb-drug interaction   🚫 = Do not crush

cium gluconate, cisatracurium, diltiazem, dobutamine, dopamine, famotidine, fentanyl, furosemide, heparin, hydrocortisone sodium succinate, hydromorphone, labetalol, lorazepam, midazolam, milrinone, morphine, nicardipine, nitroglycerin, norepinephrine, pancuronium, phytonadione, potassium chloride, propofol, ranitidine, remifentanil, vecuronium, vit B/C, warfarin

Perform/provide:
• Storage of reconstituted sol refrigerated no longer than 24 hr
• Do not use discolored sol

Evaluate:
• Therapeutic response: increased B/P with stabilization or ease of breathing

Teach patient/family:
• The reason for drug administration
• To rinse mouth after use to prevent dryness after inhalation
• Not to take OTC preparations

Treatment of overdose: Administer an α-blocker and a β-blocker

---

epirubicin
See appendix a—selected new drugs

---

epoetin (℞)
(ee-poe′e-tin)
EPO, Epogen, erythropoietin, Procrit
Func. class.: Biologic modifier, hormone
Chem. class.: Amino acid polypeptide

Action: Erythropoietin is one factor controlling rate of red cell production; drug is developed by recombinant DNA technology

Uses: Anemia caused by reduced endogenous erythropoietin production, primarily end-stage renal disease; to correct hemostatic defect in uremia; anemia due to AZT treatment in HIV patients; anemia due to chemotherapy; reduction of allogeneic blood transfusion in surgery patients

Dosage and routes:
Anemia secondary to chemotherapy
• *Adult:* **SC** 150 U/kg 3 ×/wk, may increase after 2 mo up to 300 U/kg 3 ×/wk

Anemia in chronic renal failure
• *Adult:* **SC/IV** 50-100 U/kg 3 ×/wk, then adjust dose by 25 U/kg/dose to maintain Hct; maintenance: 12.5-25 U/kg, titrate to target Hct

Anemia secondary to zidovudine treatment
• *Adult:* **SC/IV** 100 U/kg 3 ×/wk × 2 mo, may increase by 50-100 U/kg q1-2mo, up to 300 U/kg 3 ×/wk

Available forms: Inj 2000, 3000, 4000, 10,000, 20,000 U/ml

Side effects/adverse reactions:
CV: Hypertension, ***hypertensive encephalopathy,*** *headache*
CNS: Seizures, coldness, sweating
MS: Bone pain

Contraindications: Hypersensitivity to mammalian cell–derived products, or human albumin

Precautions: Seizure disorder, uncontrolled hypertension, porphyria, pregnancy (C)

Pharmacokinetics:
IV: Metabolized in body; extent of metabolism unknown; onset of increased reticulocyte count 1-6 wk; peak, immediate

NURSING CONSIDERATIONS
Assess:
• Renal studies: urinalysis, protein, blood, BUN, creatinine
• Blood studies: ferritin, transferrin monthly; transferrin sat ≥20%, fer-

E

ritin ≥100 ng/ml; Hct 2×/wk until stabilized in target range (30%-33%) then at regular intervals; those with endogenous erythropoietin levels of <500 U/L respond to this agent

• B/P; check for rising B/P as Hct rises

• CV status: hypertension may occur rapidly leading to hypertensive encephalopathy

• I&O; report drop in output to <50 ml/hr

• CNS symptoms: coldness, sweating, pain in long bones

Administer:

IV

• Do not shake

• Additional heparin to lower chance of clots

• By direct inj or bolus into IV tubing or venous line at end of dialysis

• Dialysis patients: thrill, bruit of shunts, monitor for circulation impairment

• Decrease dose by 25 U/kg, if Hct increases by 4% in 2 wk

Solution compatibilities: NaCl 0.9%, $D_{10}W$, $D_{10}W$/albumin, sterile water for inj, TPN

Evaluate:

• Therapeutic response: increase in reticulocyte count in 1-6 wk, Hgb/Hct; increased appetite, enhanced sense of well-being

Teach patient/family:

• To avoid driving or hazardous activity during beginning of treatment To monitor B/P

• To take iron supplements, vitamin B_{12}, folic acid as directed

---

eptifibatide (℞)
(ep-tih-fib′ah-tide)
Integrilin
Func. class.: Antiplatelet agent
Chem. class.: Glycoprotein IIb/IIIa inhibitor

Action: Platelet glycoprotein antagonist. this agent reversibly prevents fibrinogen, von Willebrand's factor from binding to the glycoprotein IIb/IIIa receptor, inhibitin platelet aggregation

Uses: Acute coronary syndrome including those with PCI (percutaneous coronary intervention)

Dosage and routes:

Acute coronary syndrome

• *Adult:* **IV BOL** 180 µg/kg as soon as diagnosed, then **IV CONT** 2 µg/kg/min until discharge or CABG up to 72 hr; may decrease inf rate to 0.5 µg/kg/min if undergoing PCI; continue inf for 20-24 hr postprocedure, allowing up to 96 hr of treatment

PCI in patients without acute coronary syndrome

• *Adult:* **IV BOL** 135 µg/kg given immediately before PCI; then 0.5 µg/kg/min × 20-24 hr

Available forms: 2 mg/ml (10 ml), 0.75 mg/ml (100 ml)

Side effects/adverse reactions:

CV: **Stroke,** hypotension

SYST: **Bleeding**

GU: Hematuria

HEMA: **Thrombocytopenia**

Contraindications: Hypersensitivity, active internal bleeding; history of bleeding, stroke within 1 mo; major surgery with severe trauma, severe hypotension, history of intracranial bleeding, intracranial neoplasm, arteriovenous malformation/aneurysm, aortic dissection, dependence on renal dialysis

---

 = Nursing alert   = Herb-drug interaction   ⊘ = Do not crush

Precautions: Bleeding, pregnancy (B), lactation, children, elderly, renal function impairment

Interactions:
• Increased bleeding: aspirin, heparin, NSAIDs, anticoagulants, ticlopidine, clopidogrel, dipyridamole, thrombolytics
• Do not give with platelet receptor inhibitors IIb, IIIa

Pharmacokinetics: half-life 2.5 hr, steady state 4-6 hr, metabolism limited, excretion via kidneys

NURSING CONSIDERATIONS
Assess:
• Platelets, Hgb, Hct, creatinine, PT/APTT baseline INR within 6 hr of loading dose and qd therafter, patients undergoing PCI should have ACT monitored; maintain APTT 50-70 sec unless PCI is to be performed; during PCI, ACT should be 300-350 sec; if platelets drop <100,000/mm^3, obtain additional platelet counts; if thrombocytopenia is confirmed, discontinue drug; also, draw Hct, Hgb, serum creatinine
• ECG continuously
• For bleeding gums, bruising, ecchymosis, petechiae

Administer:
IV
• After withdrawing bolus dose from 10 ml vial, give IV push over 1-2 min; follow bolus dose with continuous inf using pump, give drug undiluted directly from 100 ml vial, spike 100 ml vial with vented infusion set, use caution when centering spike on circle of stopper top

Solution compatibilities: 0.9% NaCl, D$_5$

Perform/provide:
• Discontinuing drug prior to CABG
• All medications PO if possible, avoid IM inj and all catheters

Teach patient/family:
• To report bruising, bleeding, chest pain

---

ergoloid (℞)
(er′goe-loid)
Ergoloid Mesylates, Gerimal, Hydergine, Hydergine LC
Func. class.: Migraine agent
Chem. class.: Ergot alkaloid—amino acid

Action: May increase cerebral metabolism and blood flow

Uses: Dementias: senile, Alzheimer's, multiinfarct, primary progressive

Dosage and routes:
• *Adult:* **PO/SL** 1 mg tid, may increase to 4.5-12 mg/day

Available forms: Tabs SL 0.5, 1 mg; tabs 1 mg; caps 1 mg; liquid 1 mg/ml

Side effects/adverse reactions:
GI: Nausea, vomiting, sublingual irritation

Contraindications: Hypersensitivity to ergot preparations; psychosis

Precautions: Acute intermittent porphyria, pregnancy (C), lactation

Pharmacokinetics:
PO: Peak 1 hr; metabolized in liver; excreted as metabolites in feces; crosses blood-brain barrier; half-life 3½ hr

NURSING CONSIDERATIONS
Assess:
• Weight daily; check for peripheral edema in feet, legs
• B/P and pulse, check regularly
• Neurologic status: LOC, blurring vision, nausea, vomiting, tingling in extremities; underlying and reversible causes of dementia
• Toxicity: dyspnea; hypotension or hypertension; rapid, weak pulse; delirium; nausea; vomiting; bradycardia

Side effects: *italics* = common; ***bold italics*** = life-threatening

Administer:

• With or after meals to avoid GI symptoms

 SL tabs whole; do not break, crush, or chew

• For 6 mo, if no improvement at max dose, D/C drug should be considered

Perform/provide:

• Storage in well-closed container at room temp

Evaluate:

• Therapeutic response: decreased forgetfulness, increased mental alertness and ability for self-care

Teach patient/family:

• To change positions slowly and to move extremities before walking

• To maintain dosage at approved level; not to increase drug

• To report side effects, including increased vasoconstriction starting with cold extremities, then paresthesia, weakness

• That 6 mo treatment may be required; some improvement occurs in 1 mo

◆ To keep drug out of reach of children; death may occur

• Treatment of overdose: Induce emesis if orally ingested, or gastric lavage; administer saline cathartic, keep warm

---

ergonovine (℞)

(er-goe-noe'veen)
ergonovine maleate,
Ergotrate Maleate
Func. class.: Oxytocic
Chem. class.: Ergot alkaloid

Action: Stimulates uterine contractions and vascular smooth muscle, decreases bleeding

Uses: Postpartum or postabortion hemorrhage

Investigational uses: To induce a coronary artery spasm

Dosage and routes:

Oxytocic

• *Adult:* **PO** 0.2-0.4 mg q6-12h; **IM** 0.2 mg q2-4h, not to exceed 5 doses; **IV** 0.2 mg given over 1 min

Induced coronary artery spasm

• *Adult:* **IV** 50 µg q5min up to 400 µg or when chest pain occurs

Available forms: Inj 0.2 mg/ml; tab 0.2 mg

Side effects/adverse reactions:

CNS: Headache, dizziness, fainting

CV: Hypertension, chest pain

GI: Nausea, vomiting

INTEG: Sweating

RESP: Dyspnea

EENT: Tinnitus

GU: Cramping

Contraindications: Hypersensitivity to ergot medication, augmentation of labor, before delivery of placenta, spontaneous abortion (threatened), pelvic inflammatory disease

Precautions: Hepatic disease, renal disease, cardiac disease, asthma, anemia, convulsive disorders, hypertension, glaucoma, obliterative vascular disease

Pharmacokinetics:

IM: Onset 2-5 min, duration 3 hr

IV: Onset immediate, duration 45 min

Metabolized in liver, excreted in urine

Interactions:

• Hypertension: sympathomimetics, ergots

 Hypertension: ephedra

NURSING CONSIDERATIONS

Assess:

• Ergotism: nausea, vomiting, weakness, muscular pain, insensitivity to cold, paresthesias of extremities; drug should be discontinued

• B/P, pulse; watch for change that may indicate hemorrhage

◆ = Nursing alert   = Herb-drug interaction   ⊘ = Do not crush

• Respiratory rate, rhythm, depth; notify prescriber of abnormalities

• Fundal tone, nonphasic contractions; check for relaxation

Administer:

• IM inj deep in large muscle mass; rotate injection sites if additional doses are given

• With emergency equipment available

IV, direct

• Through Y-tube or 3-way stopcock

Additive compatibilities: Amikacin, cephapirin, sodium bicarbonate

Evaluate:

• Therapeutic response: decreased blood loss, severe cramping

Teach patient/family:

• To report increased blood loss, increased temp, or foul-smelling lochia; that cramping is normal

Treatment of overdose: Stop drug, give vasodilators, heparin, dextran

---

ergotamine (℞)

(er-got'a-meen)

Ergomar*

Func. class.: α-Adrenergic blocker

Chem. class.: Ergot alkaloid—amino acid

Action: Constricts smooth muscle in peripheral, cranial blood vessels, relaxes uterine muscle; blocks serotonin release

Uses: Vascular headache (migraine, cluster histamine)

Dosage and routes:

• *Adult:* **SL** 1 tab, may use q30min, max 3 tabs/24 hr

Available forms: SL tabs 2 mg

Side effects/adverse reactions:

CNS: Numbness in fingers, toes, headache, weakness

CV: Transient tachycardia, chest pain,

bradycardia, edema, claudication, increase or decrease in B/P

GI: Nausea, vomiting, diarrhea, abdominal cramps

MS: Muscle pain

Contraindications: Hypersensitivity to ergot preparations, occlusion (peripheral, vascular), CAD, hepatic disease, renal disease, peptic ulcer, hypertension, pregnancy (X), Raynaud's disease, peripheral vascular disease, intermittent claudication

Precautions: Lactation, children, anemia, elderly

Pharmacokinetics:

PO: Peak 30 min-3 hr; metabolized in liver; excreted as metabolites in feces; crosses blood-brain barrier; excreted in breast milk

Interactions:

• Increased risk of ergot toxicity: macrolides

• Increased vasoconstriction: β-blockers

NURSING CONSIDERATIONS

Assess:

• Ergotism: nausea, vomiting, weakness, muscular pain, insensitivity to cold, paresthesia of extremities; drug should be discontinued

• Weight daily, check for peripheral edema in feet, legs

• For stress level, activity, recreation, coping mechanisms

• Neurologic status: LOC, blurring vision, nausea, vomiting, tingling in extremities that occurs preceding the headache

• Ingestion of tyramine foods (pickled products, beer, wine, aged cheese), food additives, preservatives, colorings, artificial sweeteners, chocolate, caffeine; may precipitate headaches

• Toxicity: dyspnea, hypotension or hypertension, rapid, weak pulse, delirium, nausea, vomiting

Administer:

• At beginning of headache; dose must be titrated to patient response
• Not to pregnant women; harm to fetus may occur

Perform/provide:

• Quiet, calm environment with decreased stimulation for noise, bright light, or excessive talking

Evaluate:

• Therapeutic response: decrease in frequency, severity of headache

Teach patient/family:

• Not to use OTC medications; serious drug interactions may occur
• To maintain dose at approved level; not to increase even if drug does not relieve headache
• To report side effects including increased vasoconstriction starting with cold extremities, then paresthesia, weakness
• That an increase in headaches may occur when this drug is discontinued after long-term use
◆ To keep drug out of reach of children; death may occur
• **Treatment of overdose:** Induce emesis or gastric lavage if orally ingested; administer saline cathartic; keep warm

erythromycin base (℞)

(eh-rith-roh-my′sin)

Apo-Erythro*, E-Mycin, Eramycin, Erybid*, Eryc, Ery-Tab, E-Base, Erythromid*, Erythromycin Base Filmtab, Erythromycin Delayed-Release, Novo-Rythro Encap*, PCE Dispertab

erythromycin estolate (℞)

Ilosone, Novo-Rythro*

erythromycin ethylsuccinate (℞)

Apo-Erythro-Es*, E.E.S., Ery Ped, Novo-Rythro*

erythromycin lactobionate (℞)

Erythrocin

erythromycin stearate (℞)

Apo-Erythro-S*
Novo-Rythro*

Func. class.: Antiinfective
Chem. class.: Macrolide

Action: Binds to 50S ribosomal subunits of susceptible bacteria and suppresses protein synthesis

Uses: Infections caused by *Neisseria gonorrhoeae;* mild to moderate respiratory tract, skin, soft tissue infections caused by *Streptococcus pneumoniae, Mycoplasma pneumoniae, Corynebacterium diphtheriae, Bordetella pertussis, Treponema pallidum, Borrelia burgdorferi, Listeria monocytogenes;* syphilis; Legionnaire's disease, *Legionella pneumophila, Chlamydia trachomatis; Haemophilus influenzae* (when used with sulfonamides)

Dosage and routes:

Soft tissue infections

• *Adult:* **PO** 250-500 mg q6h (base, estolate, stearate); **PO** 400-800 mg q6h (ethylsuccinate); **IV INF** 15-20 mg/kg/day (lactobionate) divided q6h

• *Child:* **PO** 30-50 mg/kg/day in divided doses q6h (salts); **IV** 20-40 mg/kg/day in divided doses q6h (lactobionate)

N. gonorrhoeae/PID

• *Adult:* **IV** 500 mg q6h × 3 days (gluceptate, lactobionate), then **PO** 250 mg (base, estolate, stearate) or 400 mg (ethylsuccinate) q6h × 1 wk

Syphilis

• *Adult:* **PO** 30 g in divided doses over 15 days (base, estolate, stearate)

Chlamydia

• *Adult:* **PO** 500 mg q6h × 1 wk or 250 mg qid × 2 wk

• *Infant:* **PO** 50 mg/kg/day in 4 divided doses × 3 wk or more

• *Newborn:* **PO** 50 mg/kg/day in 4 divided doses × 2 wk or more

Intestinal amebiasis

• *Adult:* **PO** 250 mg q6h × 10-14 days (base, estolate, stearate)

• *Child:* **PO** 30-50 mg/kg/day in divided doses q6h × 10-14 days (base, estolate, stearate)

Available forms: Base: tabs, enteric-coated 250, 333, 500 mg; tabs, film-coated 250, 500 mg; caps, enteric-coated 125, 250 mg; estolate: tabs, chewable 125, 250 mg; tabs 500 mg; caps 125, 250 mg; drops 100 mg/ml; susp 125, 250 mg/5 ml; stearate: tabs, film-coated 250, 500 mg; ethylsuccinate: tabs, chewable 200, 400 mg; 100 mg/2.5 ml, 200, 400 mg/5 ml; susp 200, 400 mg; powder for suspension: 100 mg/2.5 ml, 200 and 400 mg/5 ml; powder for inj: 500 mg and 1 g (lactobionate), 250 mg, 500 mg, 1 g (as gluceptate)

Side effects/adverse reactions:
*CV: **Dysrhythmias***
INTEG: Rash, urticaria, pruritus, thrombophlebitis (IV site)

*GI: Nausea, vomiting, diarrhea, **hepatotoxicity,** abdominal pain, stomatitis, heartburn, anorexia, pruritus ani*
GU: Vaginitis, moniliasis
EENT: Hearing loss, tinnitus
*SYST: **Anaphylaxis***

Contraindications: Hypersensitivity, preexisting liver disease (estolate), hepatic disease

Precautions: Pregnancy (B), hepatic disease, lactation

Pharmacokinetics: Peak 4 hr, duration 6 hr, half-life 1-2 hr; metabolized in liver; excreted in bile, feces, protein binding 75%-90%

Interactions:

• Increased action of oral anticoagulants, digoxin, theophylline, methylprednisolone, cyclosporine, bromocriptine, disopyramide, ergots, triazolam, dihydropyridine, calcium antagonists, lovastatin, simvastatin, midazolam, clindamycin

Lab test interferences:

False increase: 17-OHCS/17-KS, AST/ALT

Decrease: Folate assay

NURSING CONSIDERATIONS
Assess:

• I&O ratio; report hematuria, oliguria in renal disease

• Liver studies: AST, ALT

• Renal studies: urinalysis, protein, blood

• C&S before drug therapy; drug may be given as soon as culture is taken; C&S may be repeated after treatment

• Bowel pattern before, during treatment

• Skin eruptions, itching

• Respiratory status: rate, character, wheezing, tightness in chest; discontinue drug if these occur

• Allergies before treatment, reaction of each medication; place allergies on chart in bright red; notify all people giving drugs

Administer:

• Do not give by IM or IV push

• Enteric-coated tablets may be given with food

🚫 Do not break, crush, or chew

• Chewable tabs should be chewed only

IV

• After diluting 500 mg or less/10 ml sterile H_2O without preservatives; dilute further in 80-250 ml of 0.9% NaCl, LR, Normosol-R; may be further diluted to 1 mg/ml and given as continuous infusion; run 1 g or less/100 ml over ½-1 hr; continuous infusion over 6 hr, may require buffers to neutralize pH if dilution is <250 ml, use infusion pump

Additive compatibilities: *Gluceptate:* Calcium gluconate, corticotropin, dimenhydrinate, heparin, hydrocortisone, methicillin, penicillin G potassium, potassium chloride, sodium bicarbonate

Lactobionate: Aminophylline, ampicillin, cimetidine, diphenhydramine, hydrocortisone, lidocaine, methicillin, penicillin G potassium or sodium, pentobarbital, polymyxin B, potassium chloride, prednisolone, prochlorperazine, promazine, ranitidine, sodium bicarbonate, verapamil

Syringe compatibilities: *Lactobionate:* Methicillin

Y-site compatibilities: Acyclovir, amiodarone, cyclophosphamide, diltiazem, enalaprilat, esmolol, famotidine, foscarnet, heparin, hydromorphone, idarubicin, labetalol, lorazepam, magnesium sulfate, meperidine, midazolam, morphine, multivitamins, perphenazine, tacrolimus, theophylline, vit B/C, zidovudine

Perform/provide:

• Storage at room temp; store susp in refrigerator

• Adequate intake of fluids (2 L) during diarrhea episodes

Evaluate:

• Therapeutic response: decreased symptoms of infection

Teach patient/family:

• To take oral drug with full glass of water; with food for GI symptoms

• Not to take with fruit juice

• To report sore throat, fever, fatigue (could indicate superinfection)

• To notify nurse of diarrhea stools, dark urine, pale stools, jaundice of eyes or skin, and severe abdominal pain

• To take at evenly spaced intervals; complete dosage regimen

Treatment of hypersensitivity: Withdraw drug; maintain airway; administer epinephrine, aminophylline, O_2, IV corticosteroids

---

esmolol (℞)

(ez'moe-lole)

Brevibloc

Func. class.: β-Adrenergic blocker (antidysrhythmic II)

Action: Competitively blocks stimulation of β_1-adrenergic receptors in the myocardium; produces negative chronotropic, inotropic activity (decreases rate of SA node discharge, increases recovery time), slows conduction of AV node, decreases heart rate, decreases O_2 consumption in myocardium; also decreases renin-aldosterone-angiotensin system at high doses; inhibits β_2-receptors in bronchial system slightly

Uses: Supraventricular tachycardia, noncompensatory tachycardia, hypertensive crisis

---

Dosage and routes:

• *Adult:* IV loading dose 500 µg/kg/min over 1 min; maintenance 50 µg/kg/min for 4 min; if no response in 5 min, give 2nd loading dose; then increase inf to 100 µg/kg/min for 4 min; if no response, repeat loading dose, then increase maintenance inf by 50 µg/kg/min (max of 200 µg/kg/min), titrate to patient response

• *Child:* IV 50 µg/kg/min, may increase q10min (max 300 µg/kg/min)

Available forms: Inj 10 mg, 250 mg/ml

Side effects/adverse reactions:

INTEG: Induration, inflammation at site, discoloration, edema, erythema, burning pallor, flushing, rash, pruritus, dry skin, alopecia

CNS: Confusion, light-headedness, paresthesia, somnolence, fever, dizziness, fatigue, headache, depression, anxiety, *seizures*

GI: Nausea, vomiting, anorexia, gastric pain, flatulence, constipation, heartburn, bloating

CV: Hypotension, bradycardia, chest pain, peripheral ischemia, shortness of breath, *CHF,* conduction disturbances

GU: Urinary retention, impotence, dysuria

RESP: *Bronchospasm,* dyspnea, cough, wheeziness, nasal stuffiness

Contraindications: 2nd- or 3rd-degree heart block, cardiogenic shock, CHF, cardiac failure, hypersensitivity

Precautions: Hypotension, pregnancy (C), peripheral vascular disease, diabetes, hypoglycemia, thyrotoxicosis, renal disease, lactation

Pharmacokinetics:

Onset very rapid, duration short, half-life 9 min; metabolized by hydrolysis of the ester linkage; excreted via kidneys

Interactions:

• Increased digoxin levels: digoxin
• Increased esmolol levels: morphine
• Reversal of esmolol effects: isoproterenol, norepinephrine, dopamine, dobutamine
• Increased effects of both drugs: disopyramide
• Increased effects of lidocaine

🖉 Potassium deficiency: aloe, buckthorn bark/berry, cascara sagrada bark, senna pod/leaf

Lab test interferences:

Interference: Glucose/insulin tolerance test

NURSING CONSIDERATIONS

Assess:

• I&O ratio, weight daily
• B/P, pulse q4h; note rate, rhythm, quality; rapid changes can cause shock; if systolic <100 or diastolic <60, notify prescriber before giving drug
• ECG continuously during inf, hypotension is common
• Baselines in renal, liver function tests before therapy begins
• Breath sounds and respiratory pattern: wheezing from bronchospasm
• Edema in feet, legs daily
• Skin turgor, dryness of mucous membranes for hydration status

Administer:

• Reduced dosage in cool environment

IV

• IV diluted 5 g/20 ml of D_5W, D_5R, D_5 0.9% NaCl, 0.45% NaCl, LR, D_5 0.45% NaCl, 0.9% NaCl further dilute in the remaining 480 ml (10 mg/ml) and give as infusion; give loading dose over 1 min, then maintenance over 4 min; may repeat loading dose q5min with increased maintenance dose; maintenance dose should not be >200 µg/kg/min and be given up to 48 hr; dose should be

Side effects: *italics* = common; ***bold italics*** = life-threatening

E

tapered at 25 μg/kg/min; use infusion pump

Additive compatibilities: Aminophylline, atracurium, bretylium, heparin

Y-site compatibilities: Amikacin, aminophylline, amiodarone, ampicillin, atracurium, butorphanol, calcium chloride, cefazolin, cefmetazole, cefoperazone, ceftazidime, ceftizoxime, chloramphenicol, cimetidine, cisatracurium, clindamycin, diltiazem, dopamine, enalaprilat, erythromycin, famotidine, fentanyl, gentamicin, heparin, hydrocortisone, insulin (regular), labetalol, magnesium sulfate, methyldopate, metronidazole, midazolam, morphine, nafcillin, nitroglycerin, nitroprusside, norepinephrine, pancuronium, penicillin G potassium, phenytoin, piperacillin, polymyxin B, potassium chloride, potassium phosphate, propofol, ranitidine, remifentanil, streptomycin, tacrolimus, tobramycin, trimethoprim-sulfamethoxazole, vancomycin, vecuronium

Perform/provide:
• Storage protected from light, moisture; in cool environment

Evaluate:
• Therapeutic response: lower B/P immediately, lower heart rate

Teach patient/family:
• To notify prescriber if pain, swelling occurs at IV site

Treatment of overdose: Discontinue drug

estazolam (R)
(ess-taz'oh-lam)
ProSom
Func. class.: Sedative, hypnotic
Chem. class.: Benzodiazepine derivative

Controlled Substance Schedule IV (US)

Action: Produces CNS depression at the limbic, thalamic, hypothalamic levels of the CNS; may be mediated by neurotransmitter γ-aminobutyric acid (GABA); results are sedation, hypnosis, skeletal muscle relaxation, anxiolytic action

Uses: Insomnia

Dosage and routes:
• *Adult:* **PO** 1-2 mg hs
• *Elderly:* **PO** 0.5-1 mg hs

Available forms: Tabs 1, 2 mg

Side effects/adverse reactions:
INTEG: Dermatitis, allergy, sweating, flushing, pruritus
HEMA: **Leukopenia, granulocytopenia (rare)**
CNS: Lethargy, drowsiness, daytime sedation, dizziness, confusion, lightheadedness, headache, anxiety, irritability, weakness, tremors, depression, lack of coordination
GI: Nausea, vomiting, diarrhea, heartburn, abdominal pain, constipation, anorexia, taste alteration
CV: Chest pain, pulse changes, palpitations, tachycardia
MISC: Joint pain, congestion

Contraindications: Hypersensitivity to benzodiazepines, pregnancy (X), sleep apnea

Precautions: Hepatic disease, renal disease, suicidal individuals, drug abuse, elderly, psychosis, child <18 yr, lactation, depression, pulmonary insufficiency

Pharmacokinetics: Onset 15-45 min, peak 1½-2 hr, duration 7-8 hr,

---

◆ = Nursing alert   🍃 = Herb-drug interaction   🚫 = Do not crush

half-life 10-24 hr; metabolized by liver; excreted by kidneys (inactive/active metabolites); crosses placenta; excreted in breast milk

Interactions:
• Increased effects of estazolam: cimetidine, disulfiram, isoniazid, probenecid, oral contraceptives
• Increased CNS depression: alcohol, CNS depressants
• Decreased effect of estazolam: theophylline, rifampin, smoking
• Increased effects of: phenytoin, digoxin

🌿 Increased CNS depression: kava

NURSING CONSIDERATIONS
Assess:
• Blood studies: Hct, Hgb, RBCs (if on long-term therapy)
• For REM rebound if abruptly discontinued after 3 wk of use
• Hepatic studies: AST, ALT, bilirubin before, during long-term therapy
• Mental status: mood, sensorium, affect, memory (long, short)
• Blood dyscrasias: fever, sore throat, bruising, rash, jaundice, epistaxis (rare)
• Type of sleep problem: falling asleep, staying asleep

Administer:
• After removal of cigarettes to prevent fire
• After trying conservative measures for insomnia
• ½-1 hr before hs for sleeplessness
• On empty stomach for fast onset; with food for GI symptoms
• Checking to see PO medication has been swallowed

Perform/provide:
• Assistance with ambulation after receiving dose
• Safety measures: night-light, call bell within easy reach
• Storage in tight container in cool environment

Evaluate:
• Therapeutic response: ability to sleep at night, fewer early AM awakenings

Teach patient/family:
• To avoid driving, other activities requiring alertness until drug is stabilized
• To report palpitations, chest pain
• To notify prescriber if pregnancy is suspected
• To taper drug over 1-2 wk if taken for extended period of time

E

---

esterified estrogens (℞)
Estratab, Menest, Neo-Estrone*
Func. class.: Estrogen
Chem. class.: Nonsteroidal synthetic estrogen

Action: Needed for adequate functioning of female reproductive system; affects release of pituitary gonadotropins, inhibits ovulation, adequate calcium use in bone

Uses: Menopause, prostatic cancer, hypogonadism, female castration, primary ovarian failure, atrophic vaginitis, kraurosis vulvae, osteoporosis, advanced inoperable breast cancer

Dosage and routes:
Menopause
• *Adult:* **PO** 0.3-3.75 mg qd 3 wk on, 1 wk off
Hypogonadism/castration/ovarian failure
• *Adult:* **PO** 2.5 mg qd-tid 3 wk on, 1 wk off
Prostatic cancer
• *Adult:* **PO** 1.25-2.5 mg tid
Breast cancer
• *Adult:* **PO** 10 mg tid × 3 mo or longer
Available forms: Tabs 0.3, 0.625, 1.25, 2.5 mg, film coated tabs 0.3, 0.625, 1.25, 2.5 mg

---

Side effects/adverse reactions:
CNS: Dizziness, headache, migraines, depression
CV: Hypotension, thrombophlebitis, edema, ***thromboembolism, stroke, pulmonary embolism, myocardial infarction***
GI: *Nausea,* vomiting, diarrhea, anorexia, pancreatitis, cramps, constipation, increased appetite, increased weight, ***cholestatic jaundice, hepatic adenoma***
EENT: Contact lens intolerance, increased myopia, astigmatism
GU: Amenorrhea, cervical erosion, breakthrough bleeding, dysmenorrhea, vaginal candidiasis, breast changes, *gynecomastia, testicular atrophy, impotence,* ***increased risk of breast cancer, endometrial cancer***
INTEG: Rash, urticaria, acne, hirsutism, alopecia, oily skin, seborrhea, purpura, melasma
META: Folic acid deficiency, hypercalcemia, hyperglycemia
Contraindications: Breast cancer, thromboembolic disorders, reproductive cancer, genital bleeding (abnormal, undiagnosed), pregnancy (X)
Precautions: Hypertension, asthma, blood dyscrasias, gallbladder disease, CHF, diabetes mellitus, bone disease, depression, migraine headache, convulsive disorders, hepatic disease, renal disease, family history of cancer of breast or reproductive tract
Pharmacokinetics:
PO: Degraded in liver; excreted in urine; crosses placenta; excreted in breast milk
Interactions:
• Decreased action of anticoagulants, oral hypoglycemics, tamoxifen
• Increased toxicity: cyclosporine, dantrolene

• Decreased action of estrogens: anticonvulsants, barbiturates, phenylbutazone, rifampin
• Increased action of corticosteroids
🌿 Increased estrogen level: grapefruit

NURSING CONSIDERATIONS
Assess:
• Blood glucose in patient with diabetes
• Weight daily; notify prescriber of weekly weight gain >5 lb; if increase, diuretic may be ordered
• B/P q4h; watch for increase caused by H_2O and Na retention
• I&O ratio; be alert for decreasing urinary output and increasing edema
• Liver function studies, including AST, ALT, bilirubin, alk phosphatase
• Edema, hypertension, cardiac symptoms, jaundice
• Mental status: affect, mood, behavioral changes, aggression
• Hypercalcemia
• Female patient for intact uterus, if so, progesterone should be added to estrogen therapy to decrease the risk of endometrial cancer
Administer:
• Titrated dose; use lowest effective dose
• With food or milk to decrease GI symptoms
Evaluate:
• Therapeutic response: reversal of menopause symptoms or decrease in tumor size in prostatic cancer
Teach patient/family:
• To weigh weekly, report gain >5 lb
• To check with prescriber before using OTC drugs
◆ To report breast lumps, vaginal bleeding, edema, jaundice, dark urine, clay-colored stools, dyspnea, headache, blurred vision, abdominal pain, numbness or stiffness in

---

◆ = Nursing alert   🌿 = Herb-drug interaction   🚫 = Do not crush

legs, chest pain; male to report impotence or gynecomastia
• To notify prescriber if pregnancy is suspected

---

estradiol/estradiol cypionate/estradiol valerate/estradiol transdermal system/ estradiol hemihydrate (℞)

(ess-tra-dye'ole)
Alora, Cypionate, Delestrogen, dep-Gynogen, Depo Estradiol, Depogen, Dioval 40, Dioval XX, Dura-Estrin, Duragen-10, Duragen-20, Duragen-40, Esclim, Estra-D, Estraderm/Deladiol-40, Estraderm TTS, Estradiol Cypionate, Estradiol Valerate, Estra-L 20, Estra-L 40, Estro-Cyp, Estroject-LA, Estronol-LA/Estrace, FemPatch, Gynogen L.A. "10," Gynogen L.A. "20," Gynogen L.A. "40," L.A.E. 20, Valergen 10, Valergen 20, Valergen 40/ Estrace/Vagifem

Func. class.: Estrogen
Chem. class.: Nonsteroidal synthetic estrogen

Action: Needed for adequate functioning of female reproductive system; affects release of pituitary gonadotropins, inhibits ovulation, adequate calcium use in bone
Uses: Menopause, inoperable breast cancer, prostatic cancer, atrophic vaginitis, kraurosis vulvae, hypogonadism, primary ovarian failure, prevention of osteoporosis
Dosage and routes:
Hormone replacement
• *Adult:* **TD** 0.05-0.1 mg/24 hr, apply 2 ×/wk

Menopause/hypogonadism/castration/ovarian failure
• *Adult:* **PO** 1-2 mg qd 3 wk on, 1 wk off or 5 days on, 2 days off **IM** 1-5 mg q3-4wk (cypionate); 10-20 mg q4wk (valerate)
• *Adult:* **TOP** Estraderm 0.05 mg/24 hr applied 2 ×/wk Climera 0.05 mg/hr applied 1 ×/wk in a cyclic regimen; women with hysterectomy may use continuously
Prostatic cancer
• *Adult:* **IM** 30 mg q1-2wk (valerate); **PO** 1-2 mg tid (oral estradiol)
Breast cancer
• *Adult:* **PO** 10 mg tid × 3 mo or longer
Atropic vaginitis/kraurosis vulvae
• *Adult:* **VAG CREAM** 2-4 g qd × 1-2 wk, then 1 g 1-3 ×/wk cycled; vag tab 1 qd × 2 wk, maintenance 1 tab 2 ×/wk
Available forms: Estradiol tabs 0.5, 1, 2 mg; cypionate inj 5 mg/ml; valerate inj 10, 20, 40 mg/ml; transderm 0.025, 0.0375, 0.05, 0.075, 0.1 mg/24 hr release rate; vag cream 100 µg/g; hemihydrate vag tab 25 µg
Side effects/adverse reactions:
CNS: Dizziness, headache, migraines, depression, *seizures*
CV: Hypotension, thrombophlebitis, edema, *thromboembolism, stroke, pulmonary embolism, myocardial infarction*
GI: Nausea, vomiting, diarrhea, anorexia, pancreatitis, cramps, constipation, increased appetite, increased weight, *cholestatic jaundice, hepatic adenoma*
EENT: Contact lens intolerance, increased myopia, astigmatism
GU: Amenorrhea, cervical erosion, breakthrough bleeding, dysmenorrhea, vaginal candidiasis, breast changes, *gynecomastia, testicular atrophy, impotence, increased risk*

Side effects: *italics* = common; ***bold italics*** = life-threatening

of breast cancer, endometrial cancer

INTEG: Rash, urticaria, acne, hirsutism, alopecia, oily skin, seborrhea, purpura, melasma

META: Folic acid deficiency, hypercalcemia, hyperglycemia

Contraindications: Breast cancer, thromboembolic disorders, reproductive cancer, genital bleeding (abnormal, undiagnosed), pregnancy (X)

Precautions: Hypertension, asthma, blood dyscrasias, gallbladder disease, CHF, diabetes mellitus, bone disease, depression, migraine headache, convulsive disorders, hepatic disease, renal disease, family history of cancer of breast or reproductive tract

Pharmacokinetics:

PO/INJ/TD: Degraded in liver; excreted in urine; crosses placenta; excreted in breast milk

Interactions:

• Decreased action of anticoagulants, oral hypoglycemics, tamoxifen

• Decreased action of estradiol: anticonvulsants, barbiturates, phenylbutazone, rifampin, calcium

• Increased action of: corticosteroids

• Increased toxicity: cyclosporine, dantrolene

🍏 Increased estrogen level: grapefruit

Lab test interferences:

Increase: BSP retention test, PBI, T_4, serum sodium, platelet aggregation, thyroxine-binding globulin (TBG), prothrombin, factors VII, VIII, IX, X, triglycerides

Decrease: Serum folate, serum triglyceride, T_3 resin uptake test, glucose tolerance test, antithrombin III, pregnanediol, metyrapone test

False positive: LE prep, antinuclear antibodies

NURSING CONSIDERATIONS

Assess:

• Blood glucose of diabetic patient

• Weight daily, notify prescriber of weekly weight gain >5 lb; if increase, diuretic may be ordered

• B/P q4h, watch for increase caused by H_2O and Na retention

• I&O ratio; decreasing urinary output, increasing edema

• Liver function studies, including AST, ALT, bilirubin, alk phosphatase

• Hypertension, cardiac symptoms, jaundice, hypercalcemia

• Mental status: affect, mood, behavioral changes, aggression

• Female patient for intact uterus, if so, progesterone should be added to estrogen therapy to decrease risk of endometrial cancer

Administer:

• Titrated dose; use lowest effective dose

• IM inj deeply in large muscle mass

• With food or milk to decrease GI symptoms (oral)

• Apply to trunk of body 2 ×/wk (transdermal)

• On intermittent cycle schedule: 3 wk on, then 1 wk off; if patch falls off, reapply (transdermal)

Evaluate:

• Therapeutic response: reversal of menopause symptoms or decrease in tumor size in prostatic cancer

Teach patient/family:

• To weigh weekly, report gain >5 lb

◆ To report breast lumps, vaginal bleeding, edema, jaundice, dark urine, clay-colored stools, dyspnea, headache, blurred vision, abdominal pain, numbness or stiffness in legs, chest pain; male to report impotence or gynecomastia

---

◆ = Nursing alert   🍏 = Herb-drug interaction   🚫 = Do not crush

estrogenic substances, conjugated/ estrogens, conjugated synthetic A (℞)

C.E.S*, conjugated estrogens*, Premarin, Premarin Intravenous/Cenestin

Func. class.: Estrogen
Chem. class.: Nonsteroidal synthetic estrogen

Action: Needed for adequate functioning of female reproductive system; it affects release of pituitary gonadotropins, inhibits ovulation, adequate calcium use in bone

Uses: Menopause, inoperable breast cancer, prostatic cancer, abnormal uterine bleeding, hypogonadism, primary ovarian failure, osteoporosis

Dosage and routes:
Menopause
• *Adult:* PO 0.3-1.25 mg qd 3 wk on, 1 wk off
Osteoporosis
• *Adult:* PO 0.625 mg qd or in cycle
Atrophic vaginitis
• *Adult:* VAG CREAM 2-4 g ml qd × 21 days, off 7 days, repeat
Prostatic cancer
• *Adult:* PO 1.25-2.5 mg tid
Breast cancer
• *Adult:* PO 10 mg tid × 3 mo or longer
Abnormal uterine bleeding
• *Adult:* IV/IM 25 mg, repeat in 6-12 hr
Castration/primary ovarian failure
• *Adult:* PO 1.25 mg qd 3 wk on, 1 wk off
Hypogonadism
• *Adult:* PO 2.5 mg bid-tid × 20 days/mo
Available forms: Tabs 0.3, 0.625, 0.9, 1.25, 2.5 mg; inj 25 mg/vial; vag cream 0.625 mg/g; synthetic A tabs 0.625, 0.9 mg

Side effects/adverse reactions:
CNS: Dizziness, headache, migraine, depression, *seizures*
CV: Hypotension, thrombophlebitis, edema, *thromboembolism, stroke, pulmonary embolism, myocardial infarction*
GI: Nausea, vomiting, diarrhea, anorexia, pancreatitis, cramps, constipation, increased appetite, increased weight, *cholestatic jaundice, hepatic adenoma*
EENT: Contact lens intolerance, increased myopia, astigmatism
GU: Amenorrhea, cervical erosion, breakthrough bleeding, dysmenorrhea, vaginal candidiasis, breast changes, *gynecomastia, testicular atrophy, impotence, increased risk of breast cancer, endometrial cancer*
INTEG: Rash, urticaria, acne, hirsutism, alopecia, oily skin, seborrhea, purpura, melasma
META: Folic acid deficiency, hypercalcemia, hyperglycemia

Contraindications: Breast cancer, thromboembolic disorders, reproductive cancer, genital bleeding (abnormal, undiagnosed), pregnancy (X), lactation

Precautions: Hypertension, asthma, blood dyscrasias, gallbladder disease, CHF, diabetes mellitus, bone disease, depression, migraine headache, convulsive disorders, hepatic disease, renal disease, family history of cancer of breast or reproductive tract

Pharmacokinetics:
PO/IV/IM: Degraded in liver, excreted in urine, crosses placenta, excreted in breast milk

Interactions:
• Increased toxicity: cyclosporine, dantrolene

• Decreased action of anticoagulants, oral hypoglycemics, tamoxifen

• Decreased action of estrogens: anticonvulsants, barbiturates, phenylbutazone, rifampin

• Increased action of corticosteroids

🌿 Increased estrogen level: grapefruit

NURSING CONSIDERATIONS
Assess:

• Blood glucose if diabetic patient

• Weight daily; notify prescriber of weekly weight gain >5 lb; if increase, diuretic may be ordered

• B/P q4h; watch for increase caused by H_2O and Na retention

• I&O ratio; be alert for decreasing urinary output, increasing edema

• Liver function studies: AST, ALT, bilirubin, alk phosphatase

• Hypertension, cardiac symptoms, jaundice, hypercalcemia

• Mental status: affect, mood, behavioral changes, aggression

• Female patient for intact uterus, if so, progesterone should be added to estrogen therapy to decrease risk of endometrial cancer

Administer:

• Titrated dose, use lowest effective dose

• IM reconstitute after withdrawing >5 ml of air from container and inject sterile diluent on vial side, rotate to dissolve; give injection deep in large muscle mass

• With food or milk to decrease GI symptoms (PO)

IV, direct

• IV, after reconstituting as for IM, inject into distal port of running IV line of D_5W, 0.9% NaCl, LR at 5 mg/min or less

Y-site compatibilities: Heparin/hydrocortisone, potassium chloride, vit B/C

Evaluate:

• Therapeutic response: absence of breast engorgement, reversal of menopause symptoms, or decrease in tumor size in prostatic cancer

Teach patient/family:

• To avoid breastfeeding, since drug is excreted in breast milk

• To weigh weekly, report gain >5 lb

◆ To report breast lumps, vaginal bleeding, edema, jaundice, dark urine, clay-colored stools, dyspnea, headache, blurred vision, abdominal pain, numbness or stiffness in legs, chest pain; male to report impotence or gynecomastia

• To avoid sunlight or wear sunscreen; burns may occur

• To notify prescriber if pregnancy is suspected

---

estrone (R)

(ess'trone)

Aquest, Estrone Aqueous, Estrone-5, Estronol, Femogen Forte*, Kestrone-5, Theelin Aqueous

Func. class.: Estrogen

Chem. class.: Nonsteroidal synthetic estrogen

Action: Needed for adequate functioning of female reproductive system; affects release of pituitary gonadotropins, inhibits ovulation, promotes adequate calcium use in bone structures

Uses: Menopause, prostatic cancer, atrophic vaginitis, hypogonadism, primary ovarian failure, kraurosis vulvae, female castration, osteoporosis

Dosage and routes:

Menopause/atrophic vaginitis

• *Adult:* **IM** 0.1-0.5 mg 2-3 ×/wk

Prostatic cancer

• *Adult:* **IM** 2-4 mg 2-3 ×/wk

◆ = Nursing alert   🌿 = Herb-drug interaction   🚫 = Do not crush

Female hypogonadism/primary ovarian failure
• *Adult:* IM 0.1-1 mg qwk in one dose or divided doses
Available forms: Inj 2, 5 mg/ml
Side effects/adverse reactions:
CNS: Dizziness, headache, migraine, depression
CV: Hypotension, thrombophlebitis, edema, ***thromboembolism, stroke, pulmonary embolism, myocardial infarction***
GI: Nausea, vomiting, diarrhea, anorexia, pancreatitis, cramps, constipation, increased appetite, increased weight, ***cholestatic jaundice,*** hepatic adenoma
EENT: Contact lens intolerance, increased myopia, astigmatism
GU: Amenorrhea, cervical erosion, breakthrough bleeding, dysmenorrhea, vaginal candidiasis, breast changes, *gynecomastia, testicular atrophy, impotence,* **increased risk of breast cancer, endometrial cancer**
INTEG: Rash, urticaria, acne, hirsutism, alopecia, oily skin, seborrhea, purpura, melasma
META: Folic acid deficiency, hypercalcemia, hyperglycemia
Contraindications: Breast cancer, thromboembolic disorders, reproductive cancer, genital bleeding (abnormal, undiagnosed), pregnancy (X)
Precautions: Hypertension, asthma, blood dyscrasias, gallbladder disease, CHF, diabetes mellitus, bone disease, depression, migraine headache, convulsive disorders, hepatic disease, renal disease, family history of cancer of the breast or reproductive tract
Pharmacokinetics:
IM: Degraded in liver; excreted in urine, breast milk; crosses placenta
Interactions:
• Decreased action of anticoagulants, oral hypoglycemics

• Decreased action of estrone: anticonvulsants, barbiturates, phenylbutazone, rifampin
• Increased action of corticosteroids

🖊 Increased estrogen level: grapefruit

NURSING CONSIDERATIONS
Assess:
• Blood glucose in diabetic patient
• Weight daily, notify prescriber of weekly weight gain >5 lb; if increase, diuretic may be ordered
• B/P q4h, watch for increase caused by H_2O, Na retention
• I&O ratio; be alert for decreasing urinary output, increasing edema
• Liver function studies, including AST, ALT, bilirubin, alk phosphatase
• Hypertension, cardiac symptoms, jaundice, hypercalcemia
• Mental status: affect, mood, behavioral changes, aggression
• Female patient for intact uterus, if so, progesterone should be added to estrogen therapy to decrease risk of endometrial cancer
Administer:
• Titrated dose; use lowest effective dose
• IM injection deep in large muscle mass
Evaluate:
• Therapeutic response: absence of breast engorgement, reversal of menopause symptoms, or decrease in tumor size in prostatic cancer
Teach patient/family:
• To weigh weekly, report gain >5 lb
◆ To report breast lumps, vaginal bleeding, edema, jaundice, dark urine, clay-colored stools, dyspnea, headache, blurred vision, abdominal pain, numbness or stiffness in legs, chest pain; male to report impotence or gynecomastia

• To avoid sunlight or wear sunscreen, burns may occur
• To notify prescriber if pregnancy is suspected

---

etanercept (Ŗ)
(eh-tan'er-sept)
Enbrel
Func. class.: Biological

Action: Binds tumor necrosis factor (TNF), which is involved in immune and inflammatory reactions

Uses: Acute, chronic rheumatoid arthritis that has not responded to other treatment

Dosage and routes:
• *Adult:* **SC** 25 mg 2×/wk, may be given with other drugs for rheumatoid arthritis
• *Child 4-17 yr:* **SC** 0.4 mg/kg, max 25 mg, 2×/wk

Available forms: Powder for inj: 25 mg

Side effects/adverse reactions:
GI: Abdominal pain, dyspepsia
CNS: Headache, asthenia, dizziness
INTEG: Rash, *inj site reaction*
RESP: Pharyngitis, cough, URI, non-URI, sinusitis, *rhinitis*

Contraindications: Hypersensitivity, sepsis

Precautions: Pregnancy (B), lactation, children <4 yr

Pharmacokinetics: Elimination half-life 115 hr

Interactions:
• Do not give concurrently with vaccines, immunizations should be brought up to date before treatment

NURSING CONSIDERATIONS
Assess:
• Pain, stiffness, swelling of joints during treatment

Administer:
• After reconstituting 1 ml of supplied diluent, slowly inject diluent into vial, swirl contents, do not

shake, sol should be clear/colorless, do not use if cloudy or discolored
• Do not admix with other sol or medications, do not use filter

Evaluate:
• Therapeutic response: decreased inflammation, pain in joints

Teach patient/family:
• That drug must be continued for prescribed time to be effective
• To use caution when driving; dizziness may occur
• About self-administration if appropriate: inj should be made in thigh, abdomen, upper arm; rotate sites at least 1 in from old site

---

ethacrynate/etha-crynic (Ŗ)
(eth-a-kri'nate)/(eth-a-kri'nik)
Edecrin, Edecrin Sodium
Func. class.: Loop diuretic
Chem. class.: Ketone derivative

Action: Acts on loop of Henle by inhibiting reabsorption of chloride, sodium

Uses: Pulmonary edema, edema in CHF, liver disease, nephrotic syndrome, ascites

Investigational uses: Glaucoma

Dosage and routes:
• *Adult:* **PO** 50-200 mg/day; may give up to 200 mg bid
• *Child:* **PO** 25 mg, increased by 25 mg/day until desired effect occurs

Pulmonary edema
• *Adult:* **IV** 50-100 mg given over several min or 0.5-1 mg/kg

Available forms: Tabs 25, 50 mg; powder for inj 50 mg

Side effects/adverse reactions:
GU: Polyuria, **renal failure,** glycosuria
ELECT: Hypokalemia, hypochloremic alkalosis, hypomagnesemia, hyperuricemia, hypocalcemia, hy-

---

ponatremia, decreased glucose tolerance

CNS: Headache, fatigue, weakness, vertigo

GI: Nausea, ***severe diarrhea,*** dry mouth, vomiting, anorexia, cramps, upset stomach, abdominal pain, ***acute pancreatitis,*** jaundice, ***GI bleeding;*** abdominal distention

EENT: Loss of hearing, ear pain, tinnitus, blurred vision

INTEG: Photosensitivity, *rash*

ENDO: Hyperglycemia

HEMA: ***Thrombocytopenia, agranulocytosis, leukopenia, neutropenia***

Contraindications: Hypersensitivity to sulfonamides, anuria, hypovolemia, lactation, electrolyte depletion, infants

Precautions: Dehydration, ascites, severe renal disease, pregnancy (B), hypoproteinemia

Pharmacokinetics:

PO: Onset ½ hr, peak 2 hr, duration 6-8 hr

IV: Onset 5 min, peak 15-30 min, duration 2 hr

Excreted by kidneys; crosses placenta; half-life 30-70 min

Interactions:

• Increased hypotension: antihypertensives

• Decreased diuretic effect: indomethacin, NSAIDs

• Increased ototoxicity: cisplatin, aminoglycosides, vancomycin

• Increased toxicity: lithium, nondepolarizing skeletal muscle relaxants, cardiac glycosides

• Increased anticoagulant activity: warfarin

NURSING CONSIDERATIONS

Assess:

• Weight, I&O daily to determine fluid loss; effect of drug may be decreased if used qd

• Rate, depth, rhythm of respiration, effect of exertion

• B/P lying, standing; postural hypotension may occur

• Electrolytes: K, Na, Cl; include BUN, blood glucose, CBC, serum creatinine, blood pH, ABGs, uric acid, Ca, Mg, ototoxicity if receiving high IV doses

• Improvement in CVP q8h

• Signs of metabolic alkalosis: drowsiness, restlessness

• Signs of hypokalemia: postural hypotension, malaise, fatigue, tachycardia, leg cramps, weakness

• Rashes, fever qd

• Confusion, especially in elderly; take safety precautions if needed

Administer:

• In AM to avoid interference with sleep if using drug as a diuretic

• K replacement if K less than 3 mg/dl

• With food if nausea occurs; absorption may be decreased slightly

• PO, IV only; do not give IM/SC

IV

• After diluting with 50 ml NaCl inj; give through Y-tube or 3-way stopcock or heplock; give 10 mg or less over 1 min or run infusion over ½ hr; do not add to IV sol

Additive compatibilities: Chlorpromazine, cimetidine, prochlorperazine, promazine

Y-site compatibilities: Heparin/hydrocortisone, potassium chloride, vit B/C

Evaluate:

• Therapeutic response: improvement in edema of feet, legs, sacral area daily if being used in CHF

Teach patient/family:

• To increase fluid intake to 2-3 L/day unless contraindicated; to rise slowly from lying or sitting position

• About adverse reactions: muscle cramps, weakness, nausea, dizziness, diarrhea; if diarrhea occurs drug should be discontinued

• To take with food or milk for GI symptoms
• To take early in day to prevent nocturia
Treatment of overdose: Lavage if taken orally; monitor electrolytes; give dextrose in saline; monitor hydration, CV, renal status

---

ethambutol (R_x)

(e-tham'byoo-tole)
Etibi*, Myambutol*
Func. class.: Antitubercular
Chem. class.: Diisopropylethyl-ene diamide derivative

Action: Inhibits RNA synthesis, decreases tubercle bacilli replication
Uses: Pulmonary tuberculosis, as an adjunct, other mycobacterial infections
Dosage and routes:
• *Adult and child >13 yr:* **PO** 15-25 mg/kg/day as a single dose
Renal disease
• CrCl 10-50 ml/min dose q24-36h; CrCl <10 ml/min dose q48h
Retreatment
• *Adult:* **PO** 25 mg/kg/day as single dose × 2 mo with at least 1 other drug, then decrease to 15 mg/kg/day as single dose, max 2.5 g/day
• *Child:* 15 mg/kg/day
Available forms: Tabs 100, 400 mg
Side effects/adverse reactions:
GI: Abdominal distress, anorexia, nausea, vomiting
INTEG: Dermatitis, pruritus, *toxic epidermal necrolysis*
CNS: Headache, confusion, fever, malaise, dizziness, *disorientation,* hallucinations
EENT: Blurred vision, optic neuritis, photophobia, decreased visual acuity
META: Elevated uric acid, acute gout, liver function impairment

MISC: **Thrombocytopenia,** joint pain, bloody sputum, **anaphylaxis**
Contraindications: Hypersensitivity, optic neuritis, child <13 yr
Precautions: Pregnancy (C), lactation, renal disease, diabetic retinopathy, cataracts, ocular defects, hepatic and hematopoietic disorders
Pharmacokinetics:
PO: Peak 2-4 hr, half-life 3 hr; metabolized in liver; excreted in urine (unchanged drug/inactive metabolites, unchanged drug in feces)
Interactions:
• Delayed absorption of ethambutol: aluminum salts
NURSING CONSIDERATIONS
Assess:
• Liver studies qwk: ALT, AST, bilirubin
• Signs of anemia: Hct, Hgb, fatigue
• Mental status often: affect, mood, behavioral changes; psychosis may occur
• Hepatic status: decreased appetite, jaundice, dark urine, fatigue
• C&S, including sputum, before treatment
Administer:
PO
• With meals to decrease GI symptoms
• Antiemetic if vomiting occurs
• After C&S is completed; qmo to detect resistance
• 2 hr before antacids
Evaluate:
• Therapeutic response: decreased symptoms of TB
Teach patient/family:
• To avoid alcohol products
• That compliance with dosage schedule, duration is necessary
• That scheduled appointments must be kept or relapse may occur

---

• To report any visual changes or rash to physician

---

ethinyl estradiol (℞)
(eth'in-il ess-tra-dye'ole)
Estinyl
Func. class.: Estrogen
Chem. class.: Nonsteroidal synthetic estrogen

Action: Needed for adequate functioning of female reproductive system; affects release of pituitary gonadotropins, inhibits ovulation, promotes adequate calcium use in bone structures

Uses: Menopause, prostatic cancer, atrophic vaginitis, kraurosis vulvae, osteoporosis, breast cancer (5 yr or more after menopause), breast engorgement, hypogonadism

Dosage and routes:

Menopause

• *Adult:* **PO** 0.02-0.5 mg qd 3 wk on, 1 wk off

Prostatic cancer

• *Adult:* **PO** 0.15-2 mg qd

Hypogonadism

• *Adult:* **PO** 0.05 mg qd-tid × 2 wk/mo, then 2 wk progesterone, then 3-6 mo cycles, then 2 mo off

Breast cancer

• *Adult:* **PO** 1 mg tid

Breast engorgement

• *Adult:* **PO** 0.5-1 mg qd × 3 days, then tapered off over 7 days

Available forms: Tabs 0.02, 0.05, 0.5 mg

Side effects/adverse reactions:

CNS: Dizziness, headache, migraine, depression, *seizures*

CV: Hypotension, thrombophlebitis, edema, ***thromboembolism, stroke, pulmonary embolism, myocardial infarction***

GI: Nausea, vomiting, diarrhea, anorexia, pancreatitis, cramps, constipation, increased appetite, increased weight, ***cholestatic jaundice, hepatic adenoma***

EENT: Contact lens intolerance, increased myopia, astigmatism

GU: Amenorrhea, cervical erosion, breakthrough bleeding, dysmenorrhea, vaginal candidiasis, breast changes, *gynecomastia, testicular atrophy, impotence,* ***increased risk of breast cancer, endometrial cancer***

INTEG: Rash, urticaria, acne, hirsutism, alopecia, oily skin, seborrhea, purpura, melasma

META: Folic acid deficiency, hypercalcemia, hyperglycemia

Contraindications: Thromboembolic disorders, reproductive cancer, genital bleeding (abnormal, undiagnosed), pregnancy (X)

Precautions: Hypertension, asthma, blood dyscrasias, gallbladder disease, CHF, diabetes mellitus, bone disease, depression, migraine headache, convulsive disorders, hepatic disease, renal disease, family history of cancer of breast or reproductive tract

Pharmacokinetics:

PO: Degraded in liver; excreted in urine, breast milk; crosses placenta

Interactions:

• Decreased action of anticoagulants, oral hypoglycemics, tamoxifen

• Increased toxicity: cyclosporines, dantrolene

• Decreased action of ethinyl estradiol: anticonvulsants, barbiturates, phenylbutazone, rifampin

• Increased action of corticosteroids

Increased estrogen level: grapefruit

NURSING CONSIDERATIONS

Assess:

• Blood glucose of diabetic patient

• Weight daily, notify prescriber of

weekly weight gain >5 lb; if increase, diuretic may be ordered

• B/P q4h; watch for increase caused by H_2O, Na retention

• I&O ratio; be alert for decreasing urinary output, increasing edema

• Liver function studies: AST, ALT, bilirubin, alk phosphatase

• Hypertension, cardiac symptoms, jaundice, hypercalcemia

• Mental status: affect, mood, behavioral changes, aggression

• Female patients for intact uterus, if so, progesterone should be added to decrease risk of endometrial cancer

Administer:

• Titrated dose; use lowest effective dose

• With food or milk to decrease GI symptoms

Evaluate:

• Therapeutic response: absence of breast engorgement, reversal of menopause symptoms, or decrease in tumor size in prostatic cancer

Teach patient/family:

• To weigh weekly, report gain >5 lb

◆ To report breast lumps, vaginal bleeding, edema, jaundice, dark urine, clay-colored stools, dyspnea, headache, blurred vision, abdominal pain, numbness or stiffness in legs, chest pain; male to report impotence or gynecomastia

• To notify prescriber if pregnancy is suspected

---

ethosuximide (R)

(eth-oh-sux′i-mide)
Zarontin
Func. class.: Anticonvulsant
Chem. class.: Succinimide

Action: Inhibits spike, wave formation in absence seizures (petit mal), decreases amplitude, frequency, duration, spread of discharge in minor motor seizures

Uses: Absence seizures, partial seizures, tonic-clonic seizures

Dosage and routes:

• *Adult and child >6 yr:* **PO** 250 mg bid initially; may increase by 250 mg q4-7d, not to exceed 1.5 g/day

• *Child 3-6 yr:* **PO** 250 mg/day or 125 mg bid; may increase by 250 mg q4-7d, not to exceed 1.5 g/day

Available forms: Caps 250 mg, syr 250 mg/5 ml

Side effects/adverse reactions:

HEMA: **Agranulocytosis, aplastic anemia, thrombocytopenia, leukocytosis, eosinophilia, pancytopenia**

CNS: Drowsiness, dizziness, fatigue, euphoria, lethargy, anxiety, aggressiveness, irritability, depression, insomnia, headache

GI: Nausea, vomiting, heartburn, anorexia, diarrhea, abdominal pain, cramps, dry mouth, constipation, hiccups, weight loss, gum hypertrophy, tongue swelling

GU: Vaginal bleeding; pink, brown urine

INTEG: Urticaria, pruritic erythema, hirsutism, **Stevens-Johnson syndrome**

EENT: Myopia, blurred vision

Contraindications: Hypersensitivity to succinimide derivatives

Precautions: Lactation, pregnancy (C), hepatic disease, renal disease

Pharmacokinetics:

PO: Peak 1-7 hr, steady state 4-7 days; metabolized by liver; excreted in urine, bile, feces; half-life 24-60 hr

Interactions:

• Increased CNS depression: alcohol

• Increased hydantoin levels

• Decreased valproic acid levels

Lab test interferences:

False positive: Direct Coombs' test

Increase: LFTs

◆ = Nursing alert   ∥ = Herb-drug interaction   ⊘ = Do not crush

NURSING CONSIDERATIONS
Assess:
- Renal studies: urinalysis, BUN, urine creatinine
- Blood studies: CBC, Hct, Hgb, reticulocyte counts qwk for 4 wk, then qmo
- Hepatic studies: AST, ALT, bilirubin
- Drug levels during treatment; therapeutic range (40-100 μg/ml)
- Mental status: mood, sensorium, affect, behavioral changes; if mental status changes, notify prescriber
- Eye problems: need for ophthalmic examinations before, during, after treatment (slit lamp, fundoscopy, tonometry)
- Allergic reaction: red, raised rash; exfoliative dermatitis; if these occur, drug should be discontinued
- Blood dyscrasias: fever, sore throat, bruising, rash, jaundice
- ◆ Toxicity: bone marrow depression, nausea, vomiting, ataxia, diplopia, cardiovascular collapse, Stevens-Johnson syndrome

Administer:
- With food, milk to decrease GI symptoms

Perform/provide:
- Hard candy, frequent rinsing, gum for dry mouth
- Assistance with ambulation early in treatment; dizziness occurs
- Seizure precautions: padded side rails, move objects that could harm patient

Evaluate:
- Therapeutic response: decreased seizure activity; document on patient's chart

Teach patient/family:
- To carry ID card or Medic Alert bracelet stating patient's name, drugs taken, condition, prescriber's name, phone number
- To avoid driving, other activities that require alertness
- To avoid alcohol ingestion, CNS depressants; increased sedation may occur
- 🚫 Not to break, crush, or chew caps
- Not to discontinue medication quickly after long-term use; absence seizures may occur
- To continue regular dental checkups to identify gingival hyperplasia
- Symptoms of thrombocytopenia, leukopenia; notify prescriber if these occur

Treatment of overdose: Lavage, activated charcoal; monitor electrolytes, VS

---

etidocaine (R)
(eh-tie′doh-kane)
Duranest HCl
Func. class.: Local anesthetic
Chem. class.: Amide

Action: Competes with calcium for sites in nerve membrane that control sodium transport across cell membrane; decreases rise of depolarization phase of action potential
Uses: Peripheral nerve block, caudal anesthesia, central neural block, vaginal block
Dosage and routes:
- Varies with route of anesthesia
Available forms: Inj 1%, 1.5%
Side effects/adverse reactions:
CNS: Anxiety, restlessness, ***convulsions, loss of consciousness,*** drowsiness, disorientation, tremors, shivering
CV: ***Myocardial depression, cardiac arrest, dysrhythmias,*** bradycardia, hypotension, hypertension, ***fetal bradycardia***
GI: Nausea, vomiting
EENT: Blurred vision, tinnitus, pupil constriction
INTEG: Rash, urticaria, allergic re-

actions, edema, burning, skin discoloration at injection site, tissue necrosis

*RESP: **Status asthmaticus, respiratory arrest, anaphylaxis***

Contraindications: Hypersensitivity, child <12 yr, elderly, severe liver disease

Precautions: Severe drug allergies, pregnancy (B)

Pharmacokinetics: Onset 2-8 min, duration 3-6 hr; metabolized by liver, excreted in urine (metabolites)

Interactions:

• Dysrhythmias: epinephrine, halothane, enflurane
• Hypertension: MAOIs, tricyclic antidepressants, phenothiazines
• Decreased action of etidocaine: chloroprocaine

NURSING CONSIDERATIONS
Assess:

• B/P, pulse, respiration during treatment
• Fetal heart tones during labor
• Allergic reactions: rash, urticaria, itching
• Cardiac status: ECG for dysrhythmias, pulse, B/P during anesthesia

Administer:

• Only with crash cart, resuscitative equipment nearby
• Only drugs without preservatives for epidural or caudal anesthesia

Perform/provide:

• Use of new sol; discard unused portions

Evaluate:

• Therapeutic response: anesthesia necessary for procedure

Treatment of overdose: Airway, O_2, vasopressor, IV fluids, anticonvulsants for seizures

---

etidronate (℞)
(eh-tih-droe'nate)
Didronel, Didronel IV
Func. class.: Parathyroid agent (calcium regulator)
Chem. class.: Diphosphate

Action: Decreases bone resorption and new bone development (accretion)

Uses: Paget's disease, heterotopic ossification, hypercalcemia of malignancy

Dosage and routes:
Paget's disease

• *Adult:* **PO** 5-10 mg/kg/day 2 hr ac with H_2O, not to exceed 20 mg/kg/day, max 6 mo or 11-20 mg/kg/day for max of 3 mo

Heterotopic ossification

• *Adult:* **PO** 20 mg/kg qd × 2 wk, then 10 mg/kg/day for 10 wk, total 12 wk

Hypercalcemia

• *Adult:* **IV** 7.5 mg/kg/day × 3 days, then **PO** 20 mg/kg/day

Heterotopic ossification/hip replacement

• *Adult:* **PO** 20 mg/kg/day × 4 wk before and 3 mo after surgery

Available forms: Tabs 200, 400 mg; inj 50 mg/ml

Side effects/adverse reactions:
GI: Nausea, diarrhea
MS: Bone pain, hypocalcemia, decreased mineralization of nonaffected bones
*GU: **Nephrotoxicity***
*CNS: **Seizures***

Contraindications: Pathologic fractures, children, colitis, severe renal disease with creatinine >5 mg/dl

Precautions: Pregnancy (C), renal disease, lactation, restricted vit D/calcium

Pharmacokinetics: Not metabo-

---

lized; excreted in urine/feces; therapeutic response: 1-3 mo

Interactions:

• Decreased absorption: calcium, aluminum, magnesium antacids/supplements, iron products

• Drug/food: dairy products: decreased absorption

NURSING CONSIDERATIONS

Assess:

• I&O ratio; check for decreased output in renal patients

• BUN, creatinine, uric acid, phosphate chloride, albumin, pH, urine Ca, Mg, alk phosphatase, urinalysis; Ca should be kept at 9-10 mg/dl, vit D 50-135 IU/dl

• Muscle spasm, laryngospasm, paresthesias, facial twitching, colic; may indicate hypocalcemia

• Nutritional status, diet for sources of vit D (milk, some seafood), Ca (dairy products, dark green vegetables), phosphates—adequate intake is necessary

• Persistent nausea or diarrhea

Administer:

• On empty stomach with H_2O 2 hr ac

• Drug therapy should not last longer than 6 mo

• IV after diluting in 250 ml or more NS; give over 2 hr or longer

• Food, especially high in Ca; vitamins with mineral supplements or antacids high in metals should not be given within 2 hr of dose

Evaluate:

• Therapeutic response: management of bone deficiencies, Paget's disease

Teach patient/family:

• To avoid OTC products

• That therapeutic response may take 1-3 mo; effects persist for months after drug is discontinued

• That adequate intake of Ca+, vit D is necessary

etodolac (℞)

(ee-toe'doe-lak)

Lodine, Lodine XL

Func. class.: Nonsteroidal antiinflammatory/nonopioid analgesic

Action: Inhibits prostaglandin synthesis by decreasing an enzyme needed for biosynthesis; analgesic, antiinflammatory, antipyretic

Uses: Mild to moderate pain, osteoarthritis

Dosage and routes:

Osteoarthritis

• *Adult:* **PO** 800-1200 mg/day in divided doses q6-8h initially, then adjust dose to 600-1200 mg/day in divided doses; do not exceed 1200 mg/day; patients <60 kg not to exceed 20 mg/kg

Analgesia

• *Adult:* **PO** 200-400 mg q6-8h prn for acute pain; do not exceed 1200 mg/day; patients <60 kg, not to exceed 20 mg/kg

Available forms: Caps 200, 300 mg; tabs 400, 500 mg; ext rel 400, 600 mg

Side effects/adverse reactions:

CV: Tachycardia, peripheral edema, fluid retention, palpitations, dysrhythmias, CHF

*GU: **Nephrotoxicity:** dysuria, hematuria, oliguria, azotemia, cystitis, urinary tract infection*

*HEMA: **Blood dyscrasias***

INTEG: Erythema, urticaria, purpura, rash, pruritus, sweating, ***Stevens-Johnson syndrome***

*GI: Nausea, anorexia, vomiting, diarrhea, jaundice, **cholestatic hepatitis,** constipation, flatulence, cramps, dry mouth, peptic ulcer, dyspepsia, **GI bleeding***

CNS: Dizziness, headache, drowsiness, fatigue, tremors, confusion, in-

somnia, anxiety, depression, light-headedness, vertigo

EENT: Tinnitus, hearing loss, blurred vision, photophobia

Contraindications: Hypersensitivity; patients in whom aspirin, iodides, or other nonsteroidal antiinflammatories have produced asthma; rhinitis, urticaria, nasal polyps, angioedema, bronchospasm

Precautions: Pregnancy (C); lactation; children; bleeding; GI, cardiac disorders; elderly; renal, hepatic disorders

Pharmacokinetics:
PO: Peak 1-2 hr, serum protein binding >90%, half-life 7 hr; metabolized by liver (metabolites excreted in urine)

Interactions:
• Increased toxicity: cyclosporine, digoxin, lithium, methotrexate, phenytoin
• May increase GI toxicity: aspirin
• Decreased effect of etodolac: antacids
• Decreased effect of: beta-blockers, diuretics

NURSING CONSIDERATIONS
Assess:
• Pain: location, frequency, characteristics; relief after med
• Blood, renal, liver studies: BUN, creatinine, AST, ALT, Hgb, before treatment, periodically thereafter
• For GI bleeding: black stools, hematemesis
• Audiometric, ophthalmic examination before, during, after treatment
• For eye, ear problems: blurred vision, tinnitus; may indicate toxicity
• For asthma, aspirin hypersensitivity, nasal polyps that may be hypersensitive to etodolac

Administer:
PO
• With food to decrease GI symp-

toms, since extent of absorption is not affected by food

Perform/provide:
• Storage at room temp

Evaluate:
• Therapeutic response: decreased pain, stiffness, swelling in joints, ability to move more easily

Teach patient/family:
• To report blurred vision or ringing, roaring in ears; may indicate toxicity

🚫 Not to break, crush, or chew ext rel tabs
• To avoid driving, other hazardous activities if dizziness or drowsiness occurs

◆ To report change in urine pattern, weight increase, edema, pain increase in joints, fever, blood in urine; indicates nephrotoxicity
• That therapeutic effects may take up to 1 mo
• To avoid aspirin, alcoholic beverages while taking this medication

---

etoposide (Rx)
(e-toe-poe′side)
Etopophos, VePesid
Func. class.: Antineoplastic-misc.
Chem. class.: Semisynthetic podophyllotoxin

Action: Inhibits mitotic activity through metaphase to mitosis; also inhibits cells from entering mitosis, depresses DNA, RNA synthesis

Uses: Leukemias, lung, testicular cancer, lymphomas, neuroblastoma, melanoma, ovarian cancer

Dosage and routes:
• *Adult:* **IV** 45-75 mg/m^2/day × 3-5 days given q3-5wk or 200-250 mg/m^2/wk, or 125-140 mg/m^2/day 3 × wk, q5wk

---

◆ = Nursing alert   🍃 = Herb-drug interaction   🚫 = Do not crush

Available forms: Inj 20 mg/ml; caps 50 mg; 113.6 etoposide phosphate = 100 etoposide

Side effects/adverse reactions:

*HEMA: **Thrombocytopenia, leukopenia, myelosuppression, anemia***

*GI: Nausea, vomiting, anorexia, **hepatotoxicity***

INTEG: Rash, alopecia, phlebitis at IV site

*RESP: **Bronchospasm***

CV: Hypotension

CNS: Headache, *fever*

*GU: **Nephrotoxicity***

*SYST: **Anaphylaxis***

Contraindications: Hypersensitivity, bone marrow depression, severe hepatic disease, severe renal disease, bacterial infection, pregnancy (D)

Precautions: Renal disease, hepatic disease, lactation, children, gout

Pharmacokinetics: Half-life 3 hr, terminal 15 hr; metabolized in liver; excreted in urine; crosses placental barrier

Interactions:

• Increased pro-time: warfarin

NURSING CONSIDERATIONS

Assess:

• CBC, differential, platelet count weekly; withhold drug if WBC is <4000 or platelet count is <75,000; notify prescriber

• Renal function studies: BUN, serum uric acid, urine CrCl, electrolytes before, during therapy

• I&O ratio; report fall in urine output to <30 ml/hr; check blood pressure bid and report any significant decrease

• Monitor temp q4h; may indicate beginning infection

• Liver function tests before, during therapy (bilirubin, AST, ALT, LDH) as needed or monthly

• RBC, Hct, Hgb; may be decreased

• Bleeding: hematuria, guaiac stools, bruising or petechiae, mucosa or orifices q8h

• Effects of alopecia on body image; discuss feelings about body changes

• Jaundice of skin and sclera, dark urine, clay-colored stools, itchy skin, abdominal pain, fever, diarrhea

• B/P q15 min during inf, if systolic reading <90 mm Hg, discontinue inf and notify prescriber

• Buccal cavity q8h for dryness, sores or ulceration, white patches, oral pain, bleeding, dysphagia

• Local irritation, pain, burning, discoloration at injection site

• Symptoms indicating severe allergic reaction: rash, pruritus, urticaria, purpuric skin lesions, itching, flushing

◆ Symptoms of anaphylaxis: flushing, restlessness, coughing, difficulty breathing

• Frequency of stools, characteristics: cramping, acidosis; signs of dehydration: rapid respirations, poor skin turgor, decreased urine output, dry skin, restlessness, weakness

Administer:

• Antiemetic 30-60 min before giving drug and prn to prevent vomiting

• Allopurinol or sodium bicarbonate to maintain uric acid levels, alkalinization of urine

• Hyaluronidase 150 U/ml to 1 ml NaCl to infiltration area, ice compress for vesicant activity

• Transfusion for anemia

• Antispasmodic, epinephrine, corticosteroids, antihistamines for reactions

IV (VePesid)

• After diluting 100 mg/250 ml or more D_5W or NaCl to 0.2-0.4 mg/ml, infuse over 30-60 min; phosphate may be given over 5 min-3½ hr; may dilute further to 0.1 mg/ml in 0.9% NaCl, D₅W

Additive compatibilities: Carboplatin, cisplatin, cytarabine, floxuridine, fluorouracil, hydroxyzine, ifosfamide, ondansetron

Y-site compatibilities: Allopurinol, amifostine, aztreonam, cladribine, doxorubicin liposome, fludarabine, granisetron, melphalan, ondansetron, paclitaxel, piperacillin/tazobactam, sargramostim, sodium bicarbonate, teniposide, thiotepa, vinorelbine

Perform/provide:

• Liquid diet: carbonated beverages, Jell-O; dry toast or crackers may be added if patient is not nauseated or vomiting

• Increase fluid intake to 2-3 L/day to prevent urate deposits, calculi formation

• Diet low in purines: organ meats (kidney, liver), dried beans, peas to maintain alkaline urine

• Nutritious diet with iron, vitamin supplements

Evaluate:

• Therapeutic response: decreased tumor size, spread of malignancy

Teach patient/family:

• To report any complaints or side effects to nurse or prescriber

• To report any changes in breathing or coughing

• That hair may be lost during treatment; a wig or hairpiece may make patient feel better; tell patient that new hair may be different in color, texture

---

exemestane
See appendix a—selected new drugs

---

factor IX complex (human)/factor IV (℞)

Alpha-Nine SD, Benefix, Konyne 80, Mononine, Profilnine/Alpha Nine, Proplex SX-T, Proplex T

Func. class.: Hemostatic
Chem. class.: Factors II, VII, IX, X

Action: Causes an increase in blood levels of clotting factors II, VII, IX, X; factor IX (human) has IX activity

Uses: Hemophilia B (Christmas disease), factor IX deficiency, anticoagulant reversal, control of bleeding in patients with factor VIII inhibitors, reversal of overdose of anticoagulants in emergencies

Dosage and routes:
Factor IX complex (human) bleeding in hemophilia B

• *Adult and child:* **IV** establish 25% of normal factor IX or 60-75 U/kg, then 10-20 U/kg/day 1-2 ×/wk

Prophylaxis for bleeding in hemophilia B

• *Adult and child:* **IV** 10-20 U/kg 1-2 ×/wk

Bleeding in hemophilia A/inhibitors of factor VIII (Proplex T, Konyne 80)

• *Adult and child:* **IV** 75 U/kg, repeat in 12 hr

Oral anticoagulant reversal

• *Adult and child:* **IV** 15 U/kg

Factor VII deficiency (use Proplex T only)

• *Adult and child:* **IV** 0.5 U/kg × weight (kg) × desired factor IX increase (% of normal); repeat q4-6h if needed

---

Factor IX (human) minor-moderate hemorrhage

Use only Alpha Nine, Alpha-Nine SD

• *Adult and child:* **IV** dose to increase factor IX level to 20%-30% in one dose

Serious hemorrhage

• *Adult and child:* **IV** dose to increase factor IX to 30%-50% as daily inf

Minor hemorrhage (mononine only)

• *Adult and child:* **IV** dose to increase factor IX to 15%-25% (20-30 U/kg), repeat in 24 hr if needed

Major hemorrhage

• *Adult and child:* **IV** dose to increase factor IX to 25%-50% (75 U/kg) q18-30h × 10 days or less

Available forms: Inj (number of units noted on label)

Side effects/adverse reactions:

GI: Nausea, vomiting, abdominal cramps, jaundice, *viral hepatitis*

INTEG: Rash, flushing, *urticaria*

CNS: Headache, dizziness, malaise, paresthesia, *lethargy, chills, fever, flushing*

HEMA: **Thrombosis, hemolysis, AIDS, DIC**

CV: Hypotension, tachycardia, *MI, venous thrombosis, pulmonary embolism*

RESP: **Bronchospasm**

Contraindications: Hypersensitivity, hepatic disease, DIC, elective surgery, mild factor IX deficiency

Precautions: Neonates/infants, pregnancy (C)

Pharmacokinetics:

IV: Half-life factor VII–3-6 hr, factor IX–24-36 hr; rapidly cleared from plasma

Interactions:

• Incompatible with protein products

◆Increased risk of thrombosis: aminocaproic acid; do not administer

NURSING CONSIDERATIONS
Assess:

• Blood studies (coagulation factors assays by % normal: 5% prevents spontaneous hemorrhage, 30%-50% for surgery, 80%-100% for severe hemorrhage)

• Increased B/P, pulse

• For bleeding q15-30min, immobilize and apply ice to affected joints

• I&O; if urine becomes orange or red, notify prescriber

• Allergic or pyrogenic reaction: fever, chills, rash, itching, slow infusion rate if not severe

◆ DIC: bleeding, ecchymosis, hypersensitivity, changes in coagulation tests

Administer:

• Hepatitis B vaccine before administration

• IV after warming to room temp 3 ml/min or less, with plastic syringe only; do not admix

• After dilution with provided diluent, 50 U/ml or 25 U/ml; do not exceed 10 ml/min; decrease rate if fever, headache, flushing, tingling occur

• After crossmatch if patient has blood type A, B, AB, to determine incompatibility with factor

Perform/provide:

• Storage of reconstituted sol for 3 hr at room temp or up to 2 yr refrigeration (powder); check expiration date

Evaluate:

• Therapeutic response: prevention of hemorrhage

Teach patient/family:

• To report any signs of bleeding: gums, under skin, urine, stools, emesis

• The risk of viral hepatitis, AIDS; to be tested q2-3mo for HIV, even though risk is low

• That immunization for hepatitis B may be given first

• To carry ID identifying disease; avoid salicylates, inform other health professionals of condition

---

famciclovir (℞)
(fam-cy'clo-veer)
Famvir
Func. class.: Antiviral
Chem. class.: Guanosine nucleoside

Action: Inhibits DNA polymerase and viral DNA synthesis by conversion of this guanosine nucleoside to penciclovir

Uses: Treatment of acute herpes zoster, genital herpes; recurrent herpes in HIV patients

Dosage and routes:
• *Adult:* **PO** 500 mg q8h
Renal dose: CrCl ≥60 ml/min, 500 mg q8h; 40-59 ml/min, 500 mg q12h; 20-39 ml/min, 500 mg q24h
Recurrent mucocutaneous herpes simplex
• *Adult:* **PO** 500 bid × 1 wk
Available forms: Tabs 125, 250, 500 mg

Side effects/adverse reactions:
MS: Back pain, arthralgia
GU: Decreased sperm count
CNS: Headache, fatigue, dizziness, paresthesia, somnolence, fever
RESP: Pharyngitis, sinusitis
GI: Nausea, vomiting, diarrhea, constipation, *abdominal pain, anorexia*
INTEG: Pruritus

Contraindications: Hypersensitivity to this drug, penciclovir
Precautions: Renal disease, pregnancy (B), hypersensitivity to acyclovir, ganciclovir, lactation
Pharmacokinetics: Unknown
Interactions:
• Decreased renal excretion: theophylline, probenecid, digoxin
• Decreased metabolism: cimetidine

NURSING CONSIDERATIONS
Assess:
• For number, distribution of lesions; burning, itching, pain, which are early symptoms of herpes infection
• Renal function studies: urine CrCl, BUN before and during treatment if decreased renal function; dose may have to be lowered
• Bowel pattern before, during treatment; diarrhea may occur
Administer:
• With or without meals; absorption does not appear to be lowered when taken with food
• Within 72 hr of the appearance of rash in herpes zoster
Evaluate:
• Therapeutic response: decreased size, spread of lesions
Teach patient/family:
• How to recognize beginning infection
• How to prevent spread of infection
• The reason for medication, expected results

---

famotidine (OTC, ℞)
(fa-moe'ti-deen)
Mylanta AR, Pepcid, Pepcid AC, Pepcid IV
Func. class.: H₂-histamine receptor antagonist

Action: Competitively inhibits histamine at histamine H_2-receptor site, decreasing gastric secretion while pepsin remains at a stable level

Uses: Short-term treatment of active duodenal ulcer, maintenance therapy for duodenal ulcer, Zollinger-Ellison syndrome, multiple endocrine adenomas, gastric ulcers; gastroesophageal reflux disease, heartburn

---

◆ = Nursing alert   🌿 = Herb-drug interaction   ⊘ = Do not crush

Dosage and routes:
Renal disease
• CrCl <10 ml/min 20 mg hs or dose q36-48h
Duodenal ulcer
• *Adult:* **PO** 40 mg qd hs × 4-8 wk, then 20 mg qd hs if needed (maintenance); **IV** 20 mg q12h if unable to take **PO**
Hypersecretory conditions
• *Adult:* **PO** 20 mg q6h; may give 160 mg q6h if needed; **IV** 20 mg q12h if unable to take **PO**
Heartburn relief/prevention
• *Adult:* **PO** 10 mg with water or 1 hr before eating
Available forms: Tabs 10, 20, 40 mg; powder for oral susp 40 mg/5 ml; inj 10 mg/ml, 20 mg/50 ml 0.9% NaCl
Side effects/adverse reactions:
*HEMA: **Thrombocytopenia***
CNS: Headache, dizziness, paresthesia, *seizure,* depression, anxiety, somnolence, insomnia, fever
EENT: Taste change, tinnitus, orbital edema
GI: Constipation, nausea, vomiting, anorexia, cramps, abnormal liver enzymes
INTEG: Rash
MS: Myalgia, arthralgia
*RESP: **Bronchospasm***
Contraindications: Hypersensitivity
Precautions: Pregnancy (B), lactation, children <12 yr, severe renal disease, severe hepatic function, elderly
Pharmacokinetics: Absorption 50% (PO)
PO: Onset 30-60 min, duration 6-12 hr, peak 1-3 hr
IV: Onset immediate, peak 30-60 min, duration 6-12 hr, plasma protein-binding 15%-20%; metabolized in liver 30% (active metabolites), 70% excreted by kidneys, half-life 2½-3½ hr

Interactions:
• Decreased absorption: ketoconazole
• Decreased absorption of famotidine: antacids
NURSING CONSIDERATIONS
Assess:
• Blood counts during therapy; watch for decreasing platelets; if low, therapy may have to be discontinued and restarted after hematologic recovery
• For bleeding, hematuria, hematuresis, occult blood in stools; abdominal pain
• Blood dyscrasias (thrombocytopenia): bruising, fatigue, bleeding, poor healing
Administer:
• Antacids 1 hr before or 2 hr after famotidine; may be given with foods or liquids
• After shaking oral suspension
IV, direct
• After diluting 2 ml of drug (10 mg/ml) in 0.9% NaCl to total volume of 5-10 ml; inject over 2 min to prevent hypotension
IV, int inf
• After diluting 20 mg (2 ml) of drug in 100 ml of LR, 0.9% NaCl, D_5W, $D_{10}W$; run over 15-30 min
Additive compatibilities: Cefazolin, cefmetazole, flumazenil, vancomycin
Y-site compatibilities: Acyclovir, allopurinol, amifostine, aminophylline, amphotericin, ampicillin, ampicillin/sulbactam, amrinone, amsacrine, atropine, aztreonam, bretylium, calcium gluconate, cefazolin, cefoperazone, cefotaxime, cefotetan, cefoxitin, ceftazidime, ceftizoxime, ceftriaxone, cefuroxime, cephalothin, cephapirin, chlorpromazine, cisatracurium, cisplatin, cladribine, cyclophosphamide, cytarabine, dexamethasone, dextran 40, digoxin, diphenhydramine, dob-

utamine, dopamine, doxorubicin, doxorubicin liposome, droperidol, enalaprilat, epinephrine, erythromycin, esmolol, filgrastim, fluconazole, fludarabine, folic acid, gentamicin, granisetron, haloperidol, heparin, hydrocortisone, hydromorphone, hydroxyzine, imipenem/cilastatin, insulin (regular), isoproterenol, labetalol, lidocaine, lorazepam, magnesium sulfate, melphalan, meperidine, methotrexate, methylprednisolone, metoclopramide, mezlocillin, midazolam, morphine, nafcillin, nitroglycerin, nitroprusside, norepinephrine, ondansetron, oxacillin, paclitaxel, perphenazine, phenylephrine, phenytoin, phytonadione, piperacillin, potassium chloride/phosphate, procainamide, propofol, remifentanil, sargramostim, sodium bicarbonate, teniposide, theophylline, thiamine, thiotepa, ticarcillin, ticarcillin/clavulanate, verapamil, vinorelbine

Perform/provide:
• Storage in cool environment (oral); IV sol is stable for 48 hr at room temp; do not use discolored sol; discard unused oral sol after 1 mo

Evaluate:
• Therapeutic response: decreased abdominal pain

Teach patient/family:
• That drug must be continued for prescribed time in prescribed method to be effective; do not double dose
• To report bleeding, bruising, fatigue, malaise, since blood dyscrasias occur
• About possibility of decreased libido, reversible after discontinuing therapy
• To avoid irritating foods, alcohol, aspirin, and extreme temp of foods that may irritate GI system
• That smoking should be avoided; diminishes effectiveness of drug

• To avoid tasks requiring alertness; dizziness, drowsiness may occur
• To increase bulk and fluids in the diet to prevent constipation

---

fat emulsions (℞)

Intralipid 10%, Intralipid 20%, Liposyn II 10%, Liposyn II 20%, Liposyn III 10%, Liposyn III 20%, Soyacal 20%

Func. class.: Caloric
Chem. class.: Fatty acid, long chain

Action: Needed for energy, heat production; consist of neutral triglycerides, primarily unsaturated fatty acids

Uses: Increase calorie intake, fatty acid deficiency, prevention

Dosage and routes:
Deficiency
• *Adult and child:* **IV** 8%-10% of required calorie intake (intralipid)
Adjunct to TPN
• *Adult:* **IV** 1 ml/min over 15-30 min (10%) or 0.5 ml/min over 15-30 min (20%); may increase to 500 ml over 4-8 hr if no adverse reactions occur; not to exceed 2.5 g/kg
• *Child:* **IV** 0.1 ml/min over 10-15 min (10%) or 0.05 ml/min over 10-15 min (20%); may increase to 1 g/kg over 4 hr if no adverse reactions occur; not to exceed 4 g/kg
Prevention of deficiency
• *Adult:* **IV** 500 ml 2 ×/wk (10%), given 1 ml/min for 30 min, not to exceed 500 ml over 6 hr
• *Child:* **IV** 5-10 ml/kg/day (10%), given 0.1 ml/min for 30 min, not to exceed 100 ml/hr

Available forms: Inj 10% (50, 100, 200, 250, 500 ml), 20% (50, 100, 200, 250, 500 ml)

Side effects/adverse reactions:
CNS: Dizziness, headache, drowsiness, *focal seizures*

---

*CV: **Shock***

GI: Nausea, vomiting, ***hepatomegaly***

RESP: Dyspnea, ***fat in lung tissue***

HEMA: ***Hyperlipemia, hypercoagulation, thrombocytopenia, leukopenia, leukocytosis***

Contraindications: Hypersensitivity, hyperlipemia, lipid necrosis, acute pancreatitis accompanied by hyperlipemia, hyperbilirubinemia of the newborn

Precautions: Severe liver disease, diabetes mellitus, thrombocytopenia, gastric ulcers, premature and term newborns, pregnancy (C), sepsis

NURSING CONSIDERATIONS
Assess:

• Triglycerides, free fatty acid levels, platelet counts daily to prevent fat overload, thrombocytopenia

• Liver function studies: AST, ALT Hct, Hgb; notify prescriber if abnormal

• Nutritional status: calorie count by dietitian; monitor weight daily

Administer:
IV, int inf

• At 10% (1 ml/min); 20% (0.5 ml/min) initially × 15-30 min, may increase 10% (120 ml/hr); 20% (62.5 ml/hr) if no adverse reaction; do not give more than 500 ml on first day

• After changing IV tubing at each infusion: infection may occur with old tubing

• With infusion pump at prescribed rate; do not use in-line filter sized for lipid emulsion; clogging will occur

Additive compatibilities: Cefamandole, chloramphenicol, cimetidine, cyclosporine, diphenhydramine, famotidine, heparin, hydrocortisone, multivitamins, nizatidine, penicillin G potassium

Y-site compatibilities: Ampicillin, cefamandole, cefazolin, cefoxitin, cephapirin, clindamycin, digoxin, dopamine, erythromycin, furosemide, gentamicin, IL-2, isoproterenol, kanamycin, lidocaine, norepinephrine, oxacillin, penicillin G potassium, ticarcillin, tobramycin

Perform/provide:

• Do not use mixed sol if separated or oily looking

Evaluate:

• Therapeutic response: increased weight

Teach patient/family:

• The reason for use of lipids

F

---

felodipine (℞)

(fell-oh′di-peen)
Plendil, Renedil*

Func. class.: Antihypertensive, calcium channel blocker
Chem. class.: Dihydropyridine

Action: Inhibits calcium ion influx across cell membrane, resulting in dilation of peripheral arteries

Uses: Essential hypertension, alone or with other antihypertensives

Dosage and routes:

• *Adult:* **PO** 5 mg qd initially, usual range 5-10 mg qd; do not exceed 20 mg qd; do not adjust dosage at intervals of <2 wk

• *Geriatric:* **PO** 2.5 mg qd

Hepatic disease

• **PO** 2.5-5 mg, max 10 mg/day

Available forms: Ext rel tabs 2.5, 5, 10 mg

Side effects/adverse reactions:

*CV: **Dysrhythmia**,* edema, ***CHF,*** hypotension, palpitations, ***MI, pulmonary edema,*** tachycardia, syncope, AV block, angina

GI: Nausea, vomiting, diarrhea, gastric upset, constipation, increased liver function studies, dry mouth

GU: Nocturia, polyuria

INTEG: Rash, pruritus

MISC: Flushing, sexual difficulties, cough, nasal congestion, shortness of breath, wheezing, epistaxis, respiratory infection, chest pain

CNS: Headache, fatigue, drowsiness, dizziness, anxiety, depression, nervousness, insomnia, lightheadedness, paresthesia, tinnitus, psychosis, somnolence

HEMA: Anemia

Contraindications: Hypersensitivity, sick sinus syndrome, 2nd- or 3rd-degree heart block

Precautions: CHF, hypotension <90 mm Hg systolic, hepatic injury, pregnancy (C), lactation, children, renal disease, elderly

Pharmacokinetics: Peak plasma levels 2.5-5 hr; highly protein bound, >99% metabolized in liver, 0.5% excreted unchanged in urine; elimination half-life 11-16 hr

Interactions:
• Decreased felodipine levels: anticonvulsants
• Decreased theophylline level: theophylline
• Increased felodipine level: cimetidine, ranitidine
🍷 Increased felodipine level: grapefruit juice

NURSING CONSIDERATIONS
Assess:
• Cardiac status: B/P, pulse, respiration, ECG

Administer:
• Once daily as whole tab

Evaluate:
• Therapeutic response: decreased B/P

Teach patient/family:
🚫 To swallow whole; do not break, crush, or chew
• To avoid hazardous activities until stabilized on drug, dizziness is no longer a problem
• To avoid OTC drugs unless directed by a prescriber, to limit caffeine consumption

• The importance of complying with all areas of medical regimen: diet, exercise, stress reduction, drug therapy

Treatment of overdose: Defibrillation, atropine for AV block, vasopressor for hypotension

---

fenofibrate (micronized) (℞)
(fen-oh-fee′brate)
Tricor
Func. class.: Antilipemic
Chem. class.: Aryloxisobutyric acid derivative

Action: Inhibits biosynthesis of low-density and very low-density lipoproteins, which are responsible for triglyceride development; mobilizes triglycerides from tissue; increases excretion of neutral sterols

Uses: Types IV, V hyperlipidemia that do not respond to other treatment

Dosage and routes:
• *Adult:* PO 67 mg/day

Available forms: Caps 67 mg

Side effects/adverse reactions:
CNS: Fatigue, weakness, drowsiness, dizziness
CV: Angina, *dysrhythmias*
GI: Nausea, vomiting, dyspepsia, increased liver enzymes, flatulence, hepatomegaly, gastritis
GU: Dysuria, proteinuria, oliguria
INTEG: Rash, urticaria, pruritus
MISC: Polyphagia, weight gain
MS: Myalgias, arthralgias

Contraindications: Severe hepatic disease, severe renal disease, primary biliary cirrhosis

Precautions: Peptic ulcer, pregnancy (C), lactation, pancreatitis

Pharmacokinetics: Peak 6-8h

◆ = Nursing alert   🌿 = Herb-drug interaction   🚫 = Do not crush

Interactions:

• Decreased fenofibrate elimination: immunosuppressants, nephrotoxics
• Decreased absorption of fenofibrate: bile acid sequestrants
• Do not use with HMG-CoA reductase inhibitors, no data available
• Increased anticoagulant effects: oral anticoagulants
• Drug/food: decreased absorption

NURSING CONSIDERATIONS
Assess:

• Lipid levels, LFTs baseline and periodically during treatment
• Pancreatitis, renal failure, rhabdomyolyis, myositis, drug should be discontinued

Administer:

• Drug with meals if GI symptoms occur

Evaluate:

• Therapeutic response: decreased triglycerides, diarrhea, pruritus (excess bile acids)
• Bowel pattern daily; increase bulk, water in diet if constipation develops

Teach patient/family:

• That compliance is needed, since toxicity may result if doses are missed
• That risk factors should be decreased: high-fat diet, smoking, alcohol consumption, absence of exercise
• That birth control should be practiced while on this drug
• To report GU symptoms: decreased libido, impotence, dysuria, proteinuria, oliguria, hematuria
🚫 Not to break, crush, or chew caps

---

fenoldopam (Ŗ)
(feh-nahl'doh-pam)
Corlopam
Func. class.: Antihypertensive
Chem. class.: Vasodilator

Action: Antagonizes D_1-like dopamine receptors; binds to α_2-adrenoceptors; increases renal blood flow
Uses: Hypertensive crisis when urgent decrease of pressure required; including malignant hypertension
Dosage and routes:

• *Adult:* **CONT IV** titrate initial dose upward or downward no more frequently than q15min; increments should range between 0.05-0.1 μg/kg/min; initial doses of 0.03-0.1 μg/kg/min titrated slowly result in less reflex tachycardia
Available forms: Inj conc 10 mg/ml
Side effects/adverse reactions:
CNS: Headache, anxiety, dizziness
CV: **Hypotension,** ST-T-wave changes, angina pectoris, palpitations, **MI, ischemic heart disease**
GI: Nausea, vomiting, constipation, diarrhea
HEMA: **Leukocytosis,** bleeding
META: Increased BUN, glucose, LDH, creatinine, hypokalemia
Contraindications: Hypersensitivity, sulfite sensitivity
Precautions: Tachycardia, pregnancy (B), lactation, children, intraocular pressure, hypokalemia
Pharmacokinetics: Elimination half-life 5 min, steady state 20 min
Interactions:

• Increased hypotension: avoid use with β-blockers

NURSING CONSIDERATIONS
Assess:

• B/P q5min until stabilized, then q1h × 2 hr, then q4h
• Pulse, jugular venous distension q4h

- Electrolytes, blood studies: K, Na, Cl, CO_2, CBC, serum glucose
- Weight daily, I&O
- Edema in feet, legs daily
- Skin turgor, dryness of mucous membranes for hydration status
- Rales, dyspnea, orthopnea
- IV site for extravasation, rate
- Postural hypotension, take B/P sitting, standing

Administer:

IV

- After diluting contents of ampules in 0.9% NaCl, or 5% dextrose inj (40 μg/ml); then add 4 ml of conc (40 mg of drug/1000 ml); 2 ml of conc (20 mg of drug/500 ml); 1 ml of conc (10 mg of drug/250 ml)
- To patient in recumbent position; keep in that position for 1 hr after administration

Perform/provide;

- Diluted sol is stable in normal light/temp for 24 hr

Evaluate:

- Therapeutic response: decreased B/P

Teach patient/family:

- To change positions slowly to prevent orthostatic hypotension
- To report dyspnea, chest pain, bleeding

---

fenoprofen (Ŗ)

(fen-oh-proe′fen)

fenoprofen, Nalfon

Func. class.: Nonsteroidal antiinflammatory/nonopioid analgesic

Chem. class.: Propionic acid derivative

Action: Inhibits prostaglandin synthesis by decreasing enzyme needed for biosynthesis; analgesic, antiinflammatory, antipyretic

Uses: Mild to moderate pain, osteoarthritis, rheumatoid arthritis, acute gout, arthritis, ankylosing spondylitis, inflammation, dysmenorrhea

Dosage and routes:

Pain

- *Adult:* **PO** 200 mg q4-6h prn

Arthritis

- *Adult:* **PO** 300-600 mg qid, not to exceed 3.2 g/day

Available forms: Caps 200, 300 mg; tabs 600 mg

Side effects/adverse reactions:

GI: Nausea, anorexia, vomiting, diarrhea, jaundice, ***cholestatic hepatitis***, constipation, flatulence, cramps, dry mouth, peptic ulcer

CNS: Dizziness, headache, drowsiness, fatigue, tremors, confusion, insomnia, anxiety, depression

CV: ***Tachycardia***, peripheral edema, palpitations, ***dysrhythmias***

INTEG: Purpura, rash, pruritus, sweating

GU: ***Nephrotoxicity: dysuria, hematuria, oliguria, azotemia***

HEMA: ***Blood dyscrasias***

EENT: Tinnitus, hearing loss, blurred vision

Contraindications: Hypersensitivity, asthma, severe renal disease, severe hepatic disease

Precautions: Pregnancy (B) 1st and 2nd trimester, lactation, children, bleeding disorders, GI disorders, cardiac disorders, hypersensitivity to other antiinflammatory agents, elderly, CrCl <30 ml/min, hypertension

Pharmacokinetics:

PO: Peak 2 hr, half-life 2-4 hr; metabolized in liver; excreted in urine (metabolites), breast milk; 99% plasma protein binding

Interactions:

- Decreased fenoprofen effect: phenobarbital
- Increased effects of: oral anticoagulants, sulfonylureas

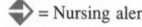 = Nursing alert   ▒ = Herb-drug interaction   ⊘ = Do not crush

• Increased GI toxicity: aspirin
• Decreased effect of: diuretics
• Increased GI reactions: corticosteroids, alcohol

NURSING CONSIDERATIONS
Assess:
• Renal, liver, blood studies: BUN, creatinine, AST, ALT, Hgb, before treatment, periodically thereafter
• Audiometric, ophthalmic examination before, during, after treatment
• For eye, ear problems: blurred vision, tinnitus; may indicate toxicity
Administer:
• With food for GI symptoms; however, best to take on empty stomach to facilitate absorption
Perform/provide:
• Storage at room temp
Evaluate:
• Therapeutic response: decreased pain, stiffness in joints, decreased swelling in joints, ability to move more easily
Teach patient/family:
• To report blurred vision, ringing, roaring in ears; may indicate toxicity
• To avoid driving, other hazardous activities if dizziness, drowsiness occurs
• To report change in urine pattern, increased weight, edema, increased pain in joints, fever, blood in urine; indicates nephrotoxicity
• To report GI bleeding symptoms; GI toxicity can occur
• That therapeutic effects may take up to 1 mo, to take as prescribed
• To take with a full glass of water to enhance absorption, avoid taking with food
• To avoid concurrent use of alcohol, aspirin, acetaminophen, other OTC meds without consulting prescriber
Ⓢ Not to break, crush, or chew caps

fentanyl (℞)
(fen'ta-nill)
Actiq, Fentanyl, Fentanyl Oralet, Sublimaze
Func. class.: Narcotic analgesic
Chem. class.: Opiate, synthetic phenylpiperidine derivative

Controlled Substance Schedule II

Action: Inhibits ascending pain pathways in CNS, increases pain threshold, alters pain perception by binding to opiate receptors
Uses: Preoperatively, postoperatively; adjunct to general anesthetic, when combined with droperidol; Fentanyl Oralet—anesthesia as premedication, conscious sedation; Actiq—breakthrough cancer pain
Dosage and routes:
Anesthetic
• *Adult:* **IV** 0.05-0.1 mg q2-3 min prn
Preoperatively
• *Adult:* **IM** 0.05-0.1 mg q30-60 min before surgery
Postoperatively
• *Adult:* **IM** 0.05-0.1 mg q1-2h prn
Fentanyl Oralet
• *Adult:* Transmucosal 5 μg/kg = fentanyl IM 0.75-1.25 μg/kg, do not exceed 5 μg/kg
• *Child:* Transmucosal may need doses of 5-15 μg/kg; must be watched continuously for hypoventilation
Actiq
• *Adult:* Transmucosal 200 μg, redose if needed 15 min after completion of 1st dose, do not give more than 2 doses during titration period; when a successful dose is found, have patient consume ≤4 U/day
Available forms: Inj 0.05 mg/ml; lozenges 100, 200, 300, 400 μg; lozenges on a stick 200, 400, 600, 800, 1200, 1600 μg

Side effects/adverse reactions:
CNS: Dizziness, delirium, euphoria
GI: Nausea, vomiting
MS: Muscle rigidity
EENT: Blurred vision, miosis
CV: **Bradycardia, arrest,** hypotension or hypertension
RESP: **Respiratory depression, arrest, laryngospasm**
Contraindications: Hypersensitivity to opiates, myasthenia gravis
Precautions: Elderly, respiratory depression, increased intracranial pressure, seizure disorders, severe respiratory disorders, cardiac dysrhythmias, pregnancy (C), lactation
Pharmacokinetics:
IM: Onset 7-8 min, peak 30 min, duration 1-2 hr
IV: Onset immediate, peak 3-5 min, duration ½-1 hr; metabolized by liver; excreted by kidneys; crosses placenta; excreted in breast milk; half-life 1½-6 hr; 80% bound to plasma proteins
Interactions:

• Effects may be increased with other CNS depressants: alcohol, narcotics, sedative/hypnotics, antipsychotics, skeletal muscle relaxants

⟋ Increased action: kava
NURSING CONSIDERATIONS
Assess:

• VS after parenteral route; note muscle rigidity, drug history, liver, kidney function test
• CNS changes: dizziness, drowsiness, hallucinations, euphoria, LOC, pupil reaction
• Allergic reactions: rash, urticaria
• Respiratory dysfunction: respiratory depression, character, rate, rhythm; notify prescriber if respirations are <10/min
Administer:

• By injection (IM, IV); give slowly to prevent rigidity

• Only with resuscitative equipment available
IV

• IV undiluted by anesthesiologist or diluted with 5 ml or more sterile H_2O or 0.9% NaCl given through Y-tube or 3-way stopcock at 0.1 mg or less/1-2 min
Additive compatibilities: Bupivacaine
Solution compatibilities: D_5W, 0.9% NaCl
Syringe compatibilities: Atracurium, atropine, bupivacaine/ketamine, butorphanol, chlorpromazine, cimetidine, clonidine/lidocaine, dimenhydrinate, diphenhydramine, droperidol, heparin, hydromorphone, hydroxyzine, meperidine, metoclopramide, midazolam, morphine, pentazocine, perphenazine, prochlorperazine, promazine, promethazine, ranitidine, scopolamine
Y-site compatibilities: Amphotericin B cholesteryl, atracurium, cisatracurium, diltiazem, dobutamine, dopamine, enalaprilat, epinephrine, esmolol, etomidate, furosemide, heparin, hydrocortisone, hydromorphone, labetalol, lorazepam, midazolam, milrinone, morphine, nafcillin, nicardipine, nitroglycerin, norepinephrine, pancuronium, potassium chloride, propofol, ranitidine, remifentanil, sargramostim, thiopental, vecuronium, vit B/C
Transmucosal

• Remove foil just before administration, instruct patient to place under tongue and suck, not chew (Oralet); place between cheek and lower gum, moving it back and forth and suck, not chew (Actiq); all products not used or partially used should be flushed down the toilet
Perform/provide:

• Storage in light-resistant area at room temp

⬥ = Nursing alert　　　⟋ = Herb-drug interaction　　　⊘ = Do not crush

• Coughing, turning, deep breathing for postoperative patients
• Safety measures: side rails, nightlight, call bell within reach
Evaluate:
• Therapeutic response: induction of anesthesia, breakthrough cancer pain

---

fentanyl/droperidol combination (℞)
(fen'ta-nil)/(droe-per'i-dole)
Innovar
Func. class.: General anesthetic, narcotic analgesic
Chem. class.: Phenylpiperone derivative

Controlled Substance Schedule II
Action: Action at subcortical levels to reduce motor activity, produces analgesia
Uses: Premedication, adjunct to general anesthesia, maintenance of anesthesia
Dosage and routes:
Induction
• *Adult:* IV 1 ml/20-25 lb
• *Child:* IV 0.5 ml/20 lb
Premedication
• *Adult:* IM 0.5-2 ml 45-60 min before surgery or procedure
• *Child:* IM 0.25 ml/20 lb 45-60 min before surgery or procedure
Available forms: Inj 0.05 mg fentanyl, 2.5 mg droperidol/ml
Side effects/adverse reactions:
RESP: **Laryngospasm, bronchospasm, respiratory arrest**
CNS: Dystonia, akathisia, *flexion of arms, fine tremors, dizziness, anxiety, drowsiness, restlessness, hallucination, depression, muscular rigidity,* EPS
CV: Tachycardia, hypotension, circulatory depression
EENT: Upward rotation of eyes, oculogyric crisis, blurred vision

INTEG: Chills, facial sweating, shivering, diaphoresis
GI: Nausea, vomiting
Contraindications: Hypersensitivity, child <2 yr, myasthenia gravis
Precautions: Elderly, increased intracranial pressure, cardiovascular disease (bradydysrhythmias), renal disease, liver disease, Parkinson's disease, COPD, pregnancy (C)
Pharmacokinetics:
IV: Onset 20 sec, peak 2-10 min, duration ½-2 hr; tranquilizing effect may last up to 12 hr
IM: Onset 7 min, duration 1-2 hr; metabolized in liver; excreted in urine metabolites (90%)
Interactions:
• Increased CNS depression: alcohol, narcotics, barbiturates, antipsychotics, other CNS depressants
• Decreased effects of amphetamines, anticonvulsants, anticoagulants
• Increased intraocular pressure: anticholinergics, antiparkinson drugs
• Increased side effects of lithium
🍃 Increased action: kava
NURSING CONSIDERATIONS
Assess:
• VS q10min during IV administration, q30min after IM dose
• Liver functions test and BUN, creatinine, Paco$_2$
• Rigidity of skeletal muscles
• EPS: dystonia, akathisia
• Increasing heart rate or decreasing B/P by >10% from baseline; notify prescriber at once; do not place patient in Trendelenburg position or sympathetic blockade may occur, causing respiratory arrest
Administer:
• Anticholinergics (benztropine, diphenhydramine) for EPS
• Only with crash cart, resuscitative equipment nearby; narcotic antagonist for severe respiratory depression, cardiac monitor

---

IV

• IV direct undiluted through Y-tube or 3-way stopcock; give each 1 ml undiluted drug/1min or more; 0.1 ml/kg may be diluted in 250 ml D$_5$W and given as IV INF over 5-10 min; titrate to response

Additive compatibilities: Sodium bicarbonate

Syringe compatibilities: Benzquinamide, glycopyrrolate

Y-site compatibilities: Hydrocortisone, potassium chloride, vit B/C

Perform/provide:

• Slow movement of patient to avoid orthostatic hypotension

Evaluate:

• Therapeutic response: decreased anxiety, absence of vomiting, maintenance of anesthesia

Teach patient/family:

• To use deep breathing, turning, coughing after surgery to prevent increased secretions in lungs

---

fentanyl transdermal (℞)

Duragesic-25, Duragesic-50, Duragesic-75, Duragesic-100

Func. class.: Narcotic analgesic

Chem. class.: Opiate, synthetic phenylpiperidine

Controlled Substance Schedule II

Action: Inhibits ascending pain pathways in CNS, increases pain threshold, alters pain perception by binding to opiate receptors

Uses: Management of chronic pain for those requiring opioid analgesia

Dosage and routes:

• *Adult:* 25 µg/hr; may increase until pain relief occurs; apply patch to flat surface on upper torso and wear for 72 hr; apply new patch on different site for continued relief

Available forms: Patch 2.5, 5, 7.5, 10 mg/hr

Side effects/adverse reactions:

CNS: Dizziness, delirium, euphoria, light-headedness, sedation, dysphoria, agitation, anxiety

GI: Nausea, vomiting, diarrhea, cramps

EENT: Blurred vision, miosis

CV: Bradycardia, *cardiac arrest,* hypotension or hypertension, facial flushing, chills

*RESP: **Respiratory depression, laryngospasm, bronchospasm;*** depresses cough; hypoventilation

Contraindications: Hypersensitivity to opiates, myasthenia gravis, children <12 yr, patient <18 yr with weight <110 lb

Precautions: Elderly, respiratory depression, increased intracranial pressure, seizure disorders, severe respiratory disorders, cardiac dysrhythmias, pregnancy (C), fever

Interactions:

• Effects may be increased with other CNS depressants: alcohol, narcotics, sedative/hypnotics, antipsychotics, skeletal muscle relaxants

 Increased action: kava

NURSING CONSIDERATIONS

Assess:

• Pain control; check for duration, site, character of pain, fever; use pain and sedation scoring

• CNS changes: dizziness, drowsiness, hallucinations, euphoria, LOC, pupil reaction

• Allergic reactions: rash, urticaria

• Respiratory dysfunction: respiratory depression, character, rate, rhythm; notify prescriber if respirations are <10/min

Administer:

• q72h for continuous pain relief; dosage is adjusted after at least two applications

• Give short-acting analgesics until patch takes effect (24 hr)

◆ = Nursing alert   = Herb-drug interaction   🚫 = Do not crush

Perform/provide:

• Safety measures: side rails, nightlight, call bell within reach

Evaluate:

• Therapeutic response: decreased pain

Teach patient/family:

• To avoid activities that require alertness

---

ferrous fumarate (℞)
Femiron, Feostat, Feostat Drops, Hemocyte, Ircon, Nephro-Fer, Novofumar*, Palafer*, Span-FF
ferrous gluconate (℞)
Fergon, Fertinic*, Novoferrogluc*
ferrous sulfate (℞)
Apo-Ferrous Sulfate*, ED-IN-SOL, Feosol, Fer-gen-sol, Fer-Iron Drops, Fero-Grad, Mol-Iron
ferrous sulfate, dried (℞)
Fe⁵⁰, Feosol, Feratab, Novoferrosulfa*, PMS-Ferrous Sulfate, Slow Fe
ferric gluconate complex (℞)
Ferrlecit
Func. class.: Hematinic
Chem. class.: Iron preparation

Action: Replaces iron stores needed for red blood cell development, energy and O_2 transport, utilization; fumarate contains 33% elemental iron; gluconate, 12%; sulfate, 20%; iron, 30%; ferrous sulfate exsiccated

Uses: Iron deficiency anemia, prophylaxis for iron deficiency in pregnancy

Dosage and routes:

Fumarate

• *Adult:* **PO** 200 mg tid-qid

• *Child 2-12 yr:* **PO** 3 mg/kg/day (elemental iron) tid-qid

• *Child 6 mo-2 yr:* **PO** up to 6 mg/kg/day (elemental iron) tid-qid; **PO** 6 mg/kg/day in 3-4 divided doses

• *Infant:* **PO** 10-25 mg/day (elemental iron) in 3-4 divided doses

Gluconate

• *Adult:* **PO** 200-600 mg tid

• *Child 6-12 yr:* **PO** 300-900 mg qd

• *Child <6 yr:* **PO** 100-300 mg qd

Sulfate

• *Adult:* **PO** 0.75-1.5 g/day in divided doses tid

• *Child 6-12 yr:* **PO** 600 mg/day in divided doses

Pregnancy

• *Adult:* **PO** 300-600 mg/day in divided doses

Complex

Adult IV Inf (125 mg) 10 ml/100 ml of NaCl for Inj given over 1 hr

Available forms:

Fumarate

Tabs 63, 195, 200, 324, 325 mg; tabs chewable 100 mg; tabs cont rel 300 mg; oral susp 100 mg/5 ml, 45 mg/0.6 ml

Gluconate

Tabs 300, 320, 325 mg; caps 86, 325, 435 mg; tabs film-coated 300 mg; elix 300 mg/5 ml

Sulfate

Tabs, 195, 300, 325 mg; tabs enteric-coated 325 mg; tabs ext rel, time-rel caps, 525 mg

Dried

Tabs, 200 mg; tabs ext rel 160 mg; caplets ext rel 160 mg

Complex

Inj. 62.5 mg/5 ml (12.5 mg/ml)

Side effects/adverse reactions:

GI: Nausea, constipation, epigastric pain, black and red tarry stools, vomiting, diarrhea

INTEG: Temporarily discolored tooth enamel and eyes

Contraindications: Hypersensitivity, ulcerative colitis/regional enteritis, hemosiderosis/hemochromatosis, peptic ulcer disease, hemolytic anemia, cirrhosis

Precautions: Anemia (long-term), pregnancy (A)

Pharmacokinetics:

PO: Excreted in feces, urine, skin, breast milk; enters bloodstream; bound to transferrin; crosses placenta

Interactions:

• Decreased absorption of: penicillamine, levodopa, methyldopa, fluoroquinolones, L-thyroxine, tetracycline

• Decreased absorption of iron preparations: antacids, cimetidine, cholestyramine, vit E

• Increased action of iron preparation: ascorbic acid, chloramphenicol

• Drug/food: decreased absorption: dairy products, caffeine, eggs

Lab test interferences:

False positive: Occult blood

NURSING CONSIDERATIONS
Assess:

• Blood studies: Hct, Hgb, reticulocytes, bilirubin before treatment, at least monthly

◆ Toxicity: nausea, vomiting, diarrhea (green, then tarry stools), hematemesis, pallor, cyanosis, shock, coma

• Elimination; if constipation occurs, increase water, bulk, activity

• Nutrition: amount of iron in diet (meat, dark green leafy vegetables, dried beans, dried fruits, eggs)

• Cause of iron loss or anemia, including salicylates, sulfonamides, antimalarials, quinidine

Administer:

• Between meals for best absorption; may give with juice; do not give with antacids or milk, delay at least 1 hr; if GI symptoms occur, give pc even if absorption is decreased; eggs, milk products, chocolate, caffeine interfere with absorption

• Liquid through plastic straw to avoid discoloration of tooth enamel; dilute thoroughly

• At least 1 hr before hs, since corrosion may occur in stomach

• For <6 mo for anemia

Perform/provide:

• Storage in tight, light-resistant container

Evaluate:

• Therapeutic response: improvement in Hct, Hgb, reticulocytes; decreased fatigue, weakness

Teach patient/family:

• That iron will change stools black or dark green

• That iron poisoning may occur if increased beyond recommended level

🚫 To swallow tab whole; not to break, crush, or chew unless labeled as chewable

• To keep out of reach of children

• Not to substitute one iron salt for another; elemental iron content differs (e.g., 300 mg ferrous fumarate contains about 100 mg elemental iron; 300 mg ferrous gluconate contains only about 30 mg elemental iron)

• To avoid reclining position for 15-30 min after taking drug to avoid esophageal corrosion

• To follow diet high in iron

Treatment of overdose: Induce vomiting; give eggs, milk until lavage can be done

---

◆ = Nursing alert   ▮ = Herb-drug interaction   🚫 = Do not crush

fexofenadine (℞)

(fex-oh-fi′na-deen)
Allegra
Func. class.: Antihistamine
Chem. class.: Piperidine, peripherally selective

Action: Acts on blood vessels, GI, respiratory system by competing with histamine for H_1-receptor site; decreases allergic response by blocking pharmacologic effects of histamine

Uses: Rhinitis, allergy symptoms

Dosage and routes:
• *Adult and child >12 yr:* 60 mg bid

Renal dose:
• CrCl <80 ml/min 60 mg qd

Available forms: Caps 60 mg

Side effects/adverse reactions:

GU: Frequency, dysuria, urinary retention, impotence

HEMA: **Hemolytic anemia, thrombocytopenia, leukopenia, agranulocytosis, pancytopenia**

RESP: Thickening of bronchial secretions, dry nose, throat

GI: Nausea, diarrhea, abdominal pain, vomiting, constipation

CNS: Headache, stimulation, drowsiness, sedation, fatigue, confusion, blurred vision, tinnitus, restlessness, tremors, paradoxical excitation in children or elderly

INTEG: Rash, eczema, photosensitivity, urticaria

CV: Hypotension, palpitations, bradycardia, tachycardia, *dysrhythmias* (rare)

Contraindications: Hypersensitivity, newborn or premature infants, lactation, severe hepatic disease

Precautions: Pregnancy (C), elderly, children, respiratory disease, narrow-angle glaucoma, prostatic hypertrophy, bladder neck obstruction, asthma

Pharmacokinetics: Well absorbed; onset 3-5 min, peak 1-2 hr, duration 8-12 hr

Interactions:
• Increased CNS depression: alcohol, other CNS depressants
🖉 Increased anticholinergic effect: henbane leaf

Lab test interferences:
False negative: Skin allergy tests

NURSING CONSIDERATIONS

Assess:
• I&O ratio: be alert for urinary retention, frequency, dysuria, especially elderly; drug should be discontinued if these occur
• Respiratory status: rate, rhythm, increase in bronchial secretions, wheezing, chest tightness

Administer:
• On empty stomach 1 hr before or 2 hr after meals

Perform/provide:
• Hard candy, gum, frequent rinsing of mouth for dryness
• Storage in tight, light-resistant container

Evaluate:
• Therapeutic response: absence of running or congested nose or rashes

Teach patient/family:
• All aspects of drug use; to notify prescriber if confusion, sedation, hypotension occur
• To avoid driving, other hazardous activity if drowsiness occurs
• To avoid alcohol, other CNS depressants
• Not to exceed recommended dose; dysrhythmias may occur
🚫 Not to break, crush, or chew caps

Treatment of overdose: Administer ipecac syrup or lavage, diazepam, vasopressors, barbiturates (short-acting)

fibrinolysin/
desoxy-
ribonuclease (R)

(fye-brin-oh-lye'sin)/(dez-ox-ee-rye-boo-nuke'lee-ase)
Elase
Func. class.: Enzyme
Chem. class.: Proteolytic, bovine

Action: Dissolves fibrin in clots and fibrinous exudates; attacks DNA in areas of disintegrating cells
Uses: Debridement of wounds, vaginitis, cervicitis, ulcerative colitis; 2nd-, 3rd-degree burns; irrigating wounds, topically
Dosage and routes:
Debridement/intravaginally
• *Adult:* **OINT** 5 g × 5 applications
Irrigating
• *Adult:* **IRIG** dilution depends on type of wound
Available forms: Fibrinolysin with desoxyribonuclease 666.6 U/g; powder for reconstitution fibrinolysin 25 U/desoxyribonuclease 15,000 U
Side effects/adverse reactions:
INTEG: Hyperemia
Contraindications: Hypersensitivity to bovine or mercury products, hematoma
Precautions: Pregnancy (C)
NURSING CONSIDERATIONS
Assess:
• For signs of irritation and inflammation; drug should be discontinued
• Wound: drainage, color, odor, size, depth
Administer:
• After reconstituting with 10 ml sterile NaCl sol; use only fresh sol
• After removing necrotic debris, dry eschar
• Wet dressing by mixing 1 vial Elase/10-50 ml NS; saturate gauze with sol; pack area; remove in 6-8 hr; repeat tid-qid
Perform/provide:
• Cleansing of wound using aseptic technique; cover with drug, then dressing; change at least qid
Evaluate:
• Therapeutic response: decrease in wound scarring, tissue necrosis

filgrastim (R)

(fill-grass'stim)
G-CSF, granulocyte colony stimulator, Neupogen
Func. class.: Biologic modifier
Chem. class.: Granulocyte colony-stimulating factor

Action: Stimulates proliferation and differentiation of neutrophils
Uses: To decrease infection in patients receiving antineoplastics that are myelosuppressive; to increase WBC in patients with drug-induced neutropenia; bone marrow transplantation
Dosage and routes:
• *Adult and child:* **IV/SC** 5 µg/kg/day in a single dose; may increase by 5 µg/kg in each chemotherapy cycle; give qd for up to 2 wk until the absolute neutrophil count (ANC) is 10,000/mm^3; response to G-CSF is much greater with **SC** than **IV** therapy
Available forms: Inj 300 µg/ml
Side effects/adverse reactions:
RESP: Respiratory distress syndrome
CNS: Fever
*HEMA: **Thrombocytopenia***
INTEG: Alopecia, exacerbation of skin conditions
MS: Osteoporosis, skeletal pain
GI: Nausea, vomiting, diarrhea, mucositis, anorexia
Contraindications: Hypersensitivity to proteins of *E. coli*

◆ = Nursing alert   🖋 = Herb-drug interaction   🚫 = Do not crush

Precautions: Pregnancy (C), lactation, cardiac conditions, children, myeloid malignancies

Pharmacokinetics:

IV: Onset 5-60 min, peak 24 hr, duration up to a week

SC: Onset 5-60 min, peak 2-8 hr, duration up to a week

Interactions:

• Do not use this drug concomitantly with antineoplastics

Lab test interferences:

Increase: Uric acid, lactate dehydrogenase, alk phosphatase

NURSING CONSIDERATIONS

Assess:

• Blood studies: CBC, platelet count before treatment and twice weekly; neutrophil counts may be increased for 2 days after therapy

Administer:

• Using single-use vials; after dose is withdrawn, do not reenter vial

• For 2 wk or until ANC is 10,000/mm³ after the expected chemotherapy neutrophil nadir

Cont IV inf

• Dilute in D_5W to a conc of >15 μg/ml, vial is for one-time use; give over 15-30 min (chemotherapy); over 4-24 hr (bone marrow transplantation); do not use 0.9% NaCl to dilute drug

Y-site compatibilities: Acyclovir, allopurinol, amikacin, aminophylline, ampicillin, ampicillin/sulbactam, aztreonam, bleomycin, bumetanide, buprenorphine, butorphanol, calcium gluconate, carboplatin, carmustine, cefazolin, cefotetan, ceftazidime, chlorpromazine, cimetidine, cisplatin, cyclophosphamide, cytarabine, dacarbazine, daunorubicin, dexamethasone, diphenhydramine, doxorubicin, doxycycline, droperidol, enalaprilat, famotidine, floxuridine, fluconazole, fludarabine, gallium, ganciclovir, granisetron, haloperidol, hydrocortisone, hydromorphone, hydroxyzine, idarubicin, ifosfamide, leucovorin, lorazepam, mechlorethamine, melphalan, meperidine, mesna, methotrexate, metoclopramide, miconazole, minocycline, mitoxantrone, morphine, nalbuphine, netilmicin, ondansetron, plicamycin, potassium chloride, promethazine, ranitidine, sodium bicarbonate, streptozocin, ticarcillin, ticarcillin/clavulanate, tobramycin, trimethoprim-sulfamethoxazole, vancomycin, vinblastine, vincristine, vinorelbine, zidovudine

Perform/provide:

• Storage in refrigerator; do not freeze; may store at room temp up to 6 hr

• Avoid shaking

Evaluate:

• Therapeutic response: absence of infection

Teach patient/family:

• The technique for self-administration: dose, side effects, disposal of containers and needles; provide instruction sheet

---

finasteride (�)

(fin-ass′te-ride)

Proscar, Propecia

Func. class.: Hormone, androgen inhibitor

Chem. class.: 5-α-reductase inhibitor

Action: Inhibits 5-α-reductase and reduction in DHT; DHT induces androgenic effects by binding to androgen receptors in the cell nuclei of the prostate gland, liver, skin; prevents development of BHP

Uses: Symptomatic benign prostatic hyperplasia (Proscar); male-pattern baldness (Propecia)

Side effects: *italics* = common; ***bold italics*** = life-threatening

Dosage and routes:
Proscar
• *Adult:* **PO** 5 mg qd × 6-12 mo
Propecia
• *Adult:* **PO** 1 mg qd
Available forms: Tabs 1, 5 mg
Side effects/adverse reactions:
GU: Impotence, decreased libido, decreased volume of ejaculate
Contraindications: Hypersensitivity, children, women who are pregnant or may become pregnant should not handle tabs, pregnancy (X)
Precautions: Large residual urinary volume, severely diminished urinary flow, liver function abnormalities
Pharmacokinetics: Bioavailability 63%, plasma protein binding 90%; metabolized in the liver; excreted in urine (metabolites) 39%, feces (57%); crosses blood-brain barrier; peak 1-2 hr, duration 24 hr
Interactions:

• Increases theophylline clearance
NURSING CONSIDERATIONS
Assess:

• Urinary patterns, residual urinary volume, severely diminished urinary flow

• PSA levels and digital rectal exam prior to initiating therapy and periodically thereafter

• Liver function studies prior to treatment; extensively metabolized in liver
Administer:

• Without regard to meals

• For a minimum of 6 mo; not all patients will respond
Perform/provide:

• Storage <86° F (30° C); protect from light; keep container tightly closed
Evaluate:

• Therapeutic response: increased urinary flow, decreased postvoiding dribbling, frequency, nocturia

Teach patient/family:

• Pregnant women or women who may become pregnant should not touch crushed tabs or come into contact with semen of a patient taking this drug; may adversely affect developing male fetus

• That volume of ejaculate may be decreased during treatment; impotence and decreased libido may also occur

• Propecia results may not occur for 3 mo

• Proscar results may not occur for 6-12 mo

---

flavoxate (℞)
(fla-vox′ate)
Urispas
Func. class.: Spasmolytic
Chem. class.: Flavone derivative

Action: Relaxes smooth muscles in urinary tract
Uses: Relief of nocturia, incontinence, suprapubic pain, dysuria, frequency associated with urologic conditions (symptomatic only)
Dosage and routes:
• *Adult and child >12 yr:* **PO** 100-200 mg tid-qid
Available forms: Tabs 100 mg
Side effects/adverse reactions:
HEMA: **Leukopenia, eosinophilia**
CNS: Anxiety, restlessness, dizziness, **convulsions,** headache, drowsiness, confusion, decreased concentration
CV: Palpitations, sinus tachycardia, hypotension
GI: Nausea, vomiting, anorexia, abdominal pain, constipation
GU: Dysuria
INTEG: Urticaria, dermatitis
EENT: Blurred vision, increased intraocular tension, dry mouth, throat

---

Contraindications: Hypersensitivity, GI obstruction, GI hemorrhage, GU obstruction

Precautions: Pregnancy (B), lactation, suspected glaucoma, children <12 yr, elderly

Pharmacokinetics: Excreted in urine, peak 2 hr

NURSING CONSIDERATIONS
Assess:

• Urinary status: dysuria, frequency, nocturia, incontinence

• Allergic reactions: rash, urticaria; drug should be discontinued

Evaluate:

• Therapeutic response: decreased dysuria

Teach patient/family:

• To avoid hazardous activities; dizziness may occur; to avoid exercise and hot weather, which may precipitate heat stroke

---

flecainide (℞)
(flek-ay′nide)
Tambocor
Func. class.: Antidysrhythmic (Class IC)

Action: Decreases conduction in all parts of the heart, with greatest effect on His-Purkinje system, which stabilizes cardiac membrane

Uses: Life-threatening ventricular dysrhythmias, sustained ventricular tachycardia, supraventricular tachydysrhythmias

Dosage and routes:

• *Adult:* PO 50-100 mg q12h; may increase q4d by 50 mg q12h to desired response, not to exceed 400 mg/day

Renal disease

• CrCl <35 ml/min dose 50%-75%

Available forms: Tabs 50, 100, 150 mg

Side effects/adverse reactions:

CNS: Headache, dizziness, involuntary movement, confusion, psychosis, restlessness, irritability, paresthesias, ataxia, flushing, somnolence, depression, anxiety, malaise

EENT: Tinnitus, *blurred vision,* hearing loss

GI: Nausea, vomiting, anorexia, constipation, abdominal pain, flatulence, change in taste

CV: Hypotension, bradycardia, angina, PVCs, **heart block, cardiovascular collapse, arrest,** dysrhythmias, **CHF, fatal ventricular tachycardia**

RESP: Dyspnea, **respiratory depression**

INTEG: Rash, urticaria, edema, swelling

HEMA: Leukopenia, thrombocytopenia

GU: Impotence, decreased libido, polyuria, urinary retention

Contraindications: Hypersensitivity, severe heart block, cardiogenic shock, nonsustained ventricular dysrhythmias, frequent PVCs, non-life-threatening dysrhythmias

Precautions: Pregnancy (C), lactation, children, renal disease, liver disease, CHF, respiratory depression, myasthenia gravis

Pharmacokinetics:

PO: Peak 3 hr; half-life 12-27 hr; metabolized by liver; excreted unchanged by kidneys (10%); excreted in breast milk

Interactions:

• Increased levels of both drugs: beta-blockers

• Increased level of flecainide: amiodarone, cimetidine

• Increased negative inotropic effects: disopyramide, verapamil

• Increased digoxin level: digoxin

• Increased or decreased effect: alkalinizing agents, acidifying agents

�ов Potassium deficiency: aloe, buckthorn bark/berry, cascara sagrada bark, senna pod/leaf

---

Lab test interferences:
Increase: CPK

NURSING CONSIDERATIONS
Assess:
• For hypokalemia, hyperkalemia before administration; correct electrolytes
• Blood levels: trough (0.2-1 µg/ml)
• B/P, ECG continuously for fluctuations
⬥ Malignant hyperthermia: tachypnea, tachycardia, changes in B/P, increased temp
• Cardiac rate, respiration: monitor rate, rhythm, character, continuously
• Respiratory status: rate, rhythm, lung fields for rales
• CNS effects: dizziness, confusion, psychosis, paresthesias, convulsions; drug should be discontinued
• Increased respiration, increased pulse; drug should be discontinued
Administer:
• Reduced dosage as soon as dysrhythmia is controlled
Evaluate:
• Therapeutic response: decreased dysrhythmias
Teach patient/family:
• To change position slowly from lying or sitting to standing to minimize orthostatic hypotension
• To take as prescribed, not to skip or double dose
• To avoid hazardous activities that require alertness until response is known
Treatment of overdose: O_2, artificial ventilation, ECG, dopamine for circulatory depression, diazepam or thiopental for convulsions, treat ventricular dysrhythmias

---

fluconazole (R)
(floo-kon'a-zole)
Diflucan
Func. class.: Antifungal

Action: Inhibits ergosterol biosynthesis, causes direct damage to membrane phospholipids
Uses: Oropharyngeal candidiasis in AIDS patients, chronic mucocutaneous candidiasis, urinary candidiasis, cryptococcal meningitis
Dosage and routes:
Renal disease
• CrCl 11-50 ml/min dose 50%
Vaginal candidiasis
• *Adult:* PO 150 mg as a single dose
Serious fungal infections
• *Adult:* PO/IV 50-400 mg initially, then 200 mg qd for 4 wk
• *Child:* 6-12 mg/kg/day
Oropharyngeal candidiasis
• *Adult:* PO/IV 200 mg initially, then 100 mg qd for at least 2 wk
• *Child:* 3 mg/kg/day
Available forms: Tabs 50, 100, 150, 200 mg; inj 200, 400 mg/200 ml; powder for oral susp 10 mg, 40 mg/ml
Side effects/adverse reactions:
GI: Nausea, vomiting, diarrhea, cramping, flatus, increased AST, ALT, *hepatotoxicity*
CNS: Headache
INTEG: Stevens-Johnson syndrome
Contraindications: Hypersensitivity
Precautions: Renal disease, pregnancy (C), lactation
Pharmacokinetics: Peak 2-4 hr, bioavailability (PO) 90%, excreted unchanged in urine 80%
Interactions:
• Potentiation of anticoagulation: warfarin
• Increased plasma concentrations: cyclosporine, phenytoin, theophylline

---

⬥ = Nursing alert   🖊 = Herb-drug interaction   🚫 = Do not crush

• Increased LFTs: sulfonylureas, isoniazid, phenytoin, rifampin, valproic acid
• Hypoglycemia: oral antidiabetics
• Increased metabolism of fluconazole: rifampin
• Increased effect of zidovudine

NURSING CONSIDERATIONS
Assess:
• VS q15-30min during first infusion; note changes in pulse, B/P
• I&O ratio; watch for decreasing urinary output, change in specific gravity; discontinue drug to prevent renal damage
• Weight weekly; if weight gain >2 lb/wk and edema is present, renal damage should be considered
◆ Renal toxicity: increasing BUN, serum creatinine; if BUN is >40 mg/dl or if serum creatinine is >3 mg/dl, drug may be discontinued or dosage reduced
• For hepatotoxicity: increasing AST, ALT, periodically alk phosphatase, bilirubin

Administer:
• Drug only after C&S confirms organism, drug needed to treat condition

IV
• After diluting according to package directions; run at 200 mg/hr or less; do not use plastic containers in connections; check for bag leaks
• Using an infusion pump check for extravasation and necrosis q2h

Additive compatibilities: Acyclovir, amikacin, amphotericin B, cefazolin, ceftazidime, clindamycin, gentamicin, heparin, meropenem, metronidazole, morphine, piperacillin, potassium chloride, theophylline

Y-site compatibilities: Acyclovir, aldesleukin, allopurinol, amifostine, amikacin, aminophylline, ampicillin/sulbactam, aztreonam, benztropine, cefazolin, cefepime, cefotetan, cefoxitin, chlorpromazine, cimetidine, cisatracurium, dexamethasone, diphenhydramine, dobutamine, dopamine, doxorubicin liposome, droperidol, famotidine, filgrastim, fludarabine, foscarnet, gallium, ganciclovir, gentamicin, granisetron, heparin, hydrocortisone, immune globulin, leucovorin, lorazepam, melphalan, meperidine, meropenem, metoclopramide, metronidazole, midazolam, morphine, nafcillin, nitroglycerin, ondansetron, oxacillin, paclitaxel, pancuronium, penicillin G potassium, phenytoin, piperacillin/tazobactam, prochlorperazine, promethazine, propofol, ranitidine, remifentanil, sargramostim, tacrolimus, teniposide, theophylline, thiotepa, ticarcillin/clavulanate, tobramycin, vancomycin, vecuronium, vinorelbine, zidovudine

Perform/provide:
• Storage protected from moisture and light, diluted sol is stable 24 hr

Evaluate:
• Therapeutic response: decreasing oral candidiasis, fever, malaise, rash; negative C&S for infection organism

Teach patient/family:
• That long-term therapy may be needed to clear infection
• That medication may be taken with food to reduce GI effects
• To consider using alternative contraception if using oral contraceptives

F

flucytosine (℞)

(floo-sye'toe-seen)
Ancobon, Ancotil*, 5-FC
Func. class.: Antifungal
Chem. class.: Pyrimidine (fluorinated)

Action: Converted to fluorouracil after entering fungi; inhibits RNA, DNA synthesis; synergistic action when used with amphotericin B in some fungal infections

Uses: *Candida* infections (septicemia, endocarditis, pulmonary, UTI), *Cryptococcus* (meningitis, pulmonary, urinary tract infections)

Dosage and routes:
Renal disease
• CrCl 10-50 ml/min give q16h; CrCl <10 ml/min give q24h
• *Adult and child >50 kg:* **PO** 50-150 mg/kg/day q6h
• *Adult and child <50 kg:* **PO** 1.5-4.5 g/m²/day or 50-100 mg/kg/day in 4 divided doses

Available forms: Caps 250, 500 mg
Side effects/adverse reactions:
INTEG: Rash
CNS: Headache, confusion, dizziness, sedation, vertigo
GI: Nausea, vomiting, anorexia, diarrhea, abdominal distention, cramps, enterocolitis; increased AST, ALT, alk phosphatase; ***bowel perforation*** (rare)
*HEMA: **Thrombocytopenia, agranulocytosis, anemia, leukopenia, pancytopenia***
GU: Increased BUN, creatinine
Contraindications: Hypersensitivity

Precautions: Renal disease, impaired hepatic function, bone marrow depression, blood dyscrasias, radiation/chemotherapy, pregnancy (C), lactation

Pharmacokinetics:
PO: Peak 2½-6 hr, half-life 3-6 hr, excreted in urine (unchanged), well distributed to CSF, aqueous humor, joints
Interactions:
• Synergism: amphotericin B
Lab test interferences:
False increase: Creatinine

NURSING CONSIDERATIONS
Assess:
• VS q15-30min during first infusion; note changes in pulse, B/P
• Blood studies: CBC, including platelets
• Drug level during treatment (therapeutic level 25-100 μg/ml); if renal impairment is present, level usually kept <100 μg/ml
 For renal toxicity: increasing BUN, serum creatinine; if serum creatinine >1.7 mg/100 dl, dosage may be reduced
• For hepatotoxicity: increasing AST, ALT, alk phosphatase
• For allergic reaction: dermatitis, rash; drug should be discontinued, antihistamines (mild reaction) or epinephrine (severe reaction) administered
• For blood dyscrasias, fatigue, bruising, malaise, dark urine
Administer:
• Drug only after C&S confirms organism, drug needed to treat condition
• Few caps at a time with food to decrease nausea, vomiting over 15 min
Perform/provide:
• Symptomatic treatment as ordered for adverse reactions: aspirin, antihistamines, antiemetics, antispasmodics
• Storage in tight, light-resistant container at room temp
Evaluate:
• Therapeutic response: decreased

 = Nursing alert   = Herb-drug interaction   🚫 = Do not crush

fever, malaise, rash, negative C&S for infecting organism
Teach patient/family:
• That long-term therapy may be needed to clear infection (1-2 mo depending on type of infection)
• To report symptoms of blood dyscrasias: fatigue, bruising, malaise, dark urine
🚫 Not to break, crush, or chew caps

---

fludrocortisone (℞)
(floo-droe-kor'ti-sone)
Florinef
Func. class.: Corticosteroid
Chem. class.: Mineralocorticoid

Action: Promotes increased reabsorption of sodium and loss of potassium, water, hydrogen from distal renal tubules
Uses: Adrenal insufficiency, salt-losing adrenogenital syndrome
Dosage and routes:
• *Adult:* **PO** 0.1-0.2 mg qd
• *Child:* **PO** 0.05-0.1 mg/day
Available forms: Tabs 0.1 mg
Side effects/adverse reactions:
CNS: Flushing, sweating, headache
*CV: Hypertension, **circulatory collapse, thrombophlebitis, embolism,*** tachycardia
MS: Fractures, osteoporosis, weakness
Contraindications: Hypersensitivity, acute glomerulonephritis, amebiasis
Precautions: Pregnancy (C), osteoporosis, CHF, lactation
Pharmacokinetics:
PO: Half-life 3.5 hr, metabolized by liver, excreted in urine
Interactions:
• Decreased action of fludrocortisone: cholestyramine, colestipol, barbiturates, rifampin, ephedrine, phenytoin, theophylline
• Decreased potassium levels: thiazides, potassium-wasting drugs
• Increased B/P: sodium-containing food or medication
🌿 Potassium deficiency: aloe, buckthorn, cascara sagrada, senna
Lab test interferences:
Increase: Potassium, sodium
Decrease: Hct
NURSING CONSIDERATIONS
Assess:
• Weight daily; notify prescriber of weekly gain >5 lb
• B/P q4h, pulse; notify prescriber if chest pain occurs
• I&O ratio; be alert for decreasing urinary output, increasing edema
• K depletion: paresthesias, fatigue, nausea, vomiting, depression, polyuria, dysrhythmias, weakness
• Edema, hypertension, cardiac symptoms
Administer:
• Titrated dose; use lowest effective dose
• With food or milk to decrease GI symptoms
Perform/provide:
• Assistance with ambulation in patient with bone tissue disease to prevent fractures
Evaluate:
• Therapeutic response: correction of adrenal insufficiency
Teach patient/family:
• That ID as steroid user should be carried
• Not to discontinue this medication abruptly
• To notify health-care provider of muscle cramps, weight gain, edema, nausea

F

flumazenil (℞)

(flu-maz′e-nill)
Anexate*, Romazicon

Func. class.: Antidote: Benzodiazepine receptor antagonist
Chem. class.: Imidazobenzodiazepine derivative

Action: Antagonizes actions of benzodiazepines on CNS, competitively inhibits activity at benzodiazepine recognition site on GABA/benzodiazepine receptor complex

Uses: Reversal of sedative effects of benzodiazepines

Dosage and routes:
Reversal of conscious sedation or in general anesthesia
• *Adult:* **IV** 0.2 mg given over 15 sec; wait 45 sec, then give 0.2 mg if consciousness does not occur; may be repeated at 60-sec intervals prn (max 3 mg/hr)
• *Child:* **IV** 10 μg (0.01 mg)/kg; cumulative dose of 1 mg or less
Management of suspected benzodiazepine overdose
• *Adult:* **IV** 0.2 mg given over 30 sec; wait 30 sec, then give 0.3 mg over 30 sec if consciousness does not occur; further doses of 0.5 mg can be given over 30 sec at intervals of 1 min up to cumulative dose of 3 mg
• *Child:* **IV** 100 μg (0.1 mg)/kg; cumulative dose of 1 mg or less
Available forms: Inj 0.1 mg/ml
Side effects/adverse reactions:
EENT: Abnormal vision, blurred vision, tinnitus
CV: Hypertension, palpitations, cutaneous vasodilation, *dysrhythmias,* bradycardia, tachycardia, chest pain
GI: Nausea, vomiting, hiccups
CNS: Dizziness, agitation, emotional lability, confusion, *convulsions,* somnolence

SYST: Headache, injection site pain, increased sweating, fatigue, rigors
Contraindications: Hypersensitivity to this drug or benzodiazepines, serious cyclic antidepressant overdose, patients given benzodiazepine for control of life-threatening condition
Precautions: Pregnancy (C), lactation, children, elderly, renal disease, seizure disorders, head injury, labor/delivery, hepatic disease, hypoventilation, panic disorder, drug & alcohol dependency, ambulatory patients
Pharmacokinetics: Terminal half-life 41-79 min; metabolized in liver
Interactions:
• Toxicity: mixed drug overdosage
NURSING CONSIDERATIONS
Assess:
• Cardiac status using continuous monitoring
• For seizures; protect patient from injury
• GI symptoms: nausea, vomiting; place in side-lying position to prevent aspiration
• Allergic reactions: flushing, rash, urticaria, pruritus
Administer:
• Check airway and IV access before administration
IV, direct
• Give undiluted or diluted with 0.9% NaCl, D_5W, LR, give over 15 sec
Additive compatibilities: Aminophylline, cimetidine, dobutamine, dopamine, famotidine, heparin, lidocaine, procainamide, ranitidine
Solution compatibilities: D_5W
Evaluate:
• Therapeutic response: decreased sedation, respiratory depression, toxicity
Teach patient/family:
• That amnesia may continue
• Not to engage in hazardous activities for 18-24 hr after discharge

◆ = Nursing alert　　🖋 = Herb-drug interaction　　🚫 = Do not crush

• Not to take any alcohol or non-prescription drugs for 18-24 hr

flunisolide (R)
(floo-nis'oh-lide)
AeroBid, Nasalide, Rhinalar*
Func. class.: Misc. respiratory drug
Chem. class.: Glucocorticoid

Action: Decreases inflammation by suppression of migration of polymorphonuclear leukocytes, fibroblasts, reversal of increased capillary permeability and lysosomal stabilization; does not depress hypothalamus

Uses: Rhinitis, allergies, nasal polyps

Dosage and routes:
• *Adult and child >6 yr:* **SPRAY** 2 puffs bid, not to exceed 4 puffs bid
Available forms: Nasal sol 25 µg/metered dose (Nasalide), 250 µg/metered dose (AeroBid)

Side effects/adverse reactions:
CNS: Headache, nervousness, restlessness
EENT: Hoarseness, *Candida* infection of oral cavity, sore throat
GI: Nausea, vomiting, dry mouth

Contraindications: Hypersensitivity, child <6 yr

Precautions: Nonasthmatic bronchial disease; bacterial, fungal, viral infections of mouth, throat, lungs; respiratory TB; untreated fungal, bacterial, or viral infections; pregnancy (C), glaucoma

Pharmacokinetics:
INH: Duration 1 hr

NURSING CONSIDERATIONS
Assess:
• Infection: increased temp, WBC, even after withdrawal of medication; drug masks infection

Administer:
• Titrated dose; use lowest effective dose

Evaluate:
• Therapeutic response: ease of respirations, decreased inflammation

Teach patient/family:
• To use gum: rinse mouth after each dose
• That ID as steroid user should be carried
• To notify prescriber if therapeutic response decreases; dosage adjustment may be needed
• The proper administration technique; shake well before use
• The importance of compliance to therapy
• Teach patient about cushingoid symptoms
• The symptoms of adrenal insufficiency: nausea, anorexia, fatigue, dizziness, dyspnea, weakness, joint pain

fluoride (PO) (R)
(floor'ide)
Fluor-A-Day*, Fluoride Loz, Fluoritab, Flura-Loz, Karidium, Luride, Pediaflor, Pharmaflur, Phos-Flur, Solu-Flur*

fluoride (top) (R)
ACT, Fluorigard, Fluorinse, Gel Kam, Gel-Tin, Karigel, MouthKote, Stop, Thera-Flur
Func. class.: Trace elements
Chem. class.: Fluoride ion

Action: Needed for hard tooth enamel and for resistance to periodontal disease; reduces acid production by dental bacteria

Uses: Prevention of dental caries, osteoporosis

Dosage and routes:
• *Adult and child >12 yr:* **Top** 10

ml 0.2% sol qd after brushing teeth, rinse mouth for >1 min with sol
• *Child 6-12 yr:* **Top** 5 ml 0.2% sol
• *Child >3 yr:* **PO** 1 mg qd
• *Child <3 yr:* **PO** 0.5 mg qd

Available forms: Tabs chewable 0.5, 1 mg; tabs 1 mg, tabs effervescent 10 mg; drops 0.125, 0.25, 0.5 mg/drop; rinse supplements 0.2 mg/ml, rinse 0.01%, 0.02%, 0.04%, 0.09%; gel 0.1%, 0.5%; lozenges 1 mg; sol 0.2 mg/ml

Side effects/adverse reactions:
*ACUTE OVERDOSE: **Black tarry stools, bloody vomit, diarrhea, decreased respiration, increased salivation, watery eyes***
*CHRONIC OVERDOSE: **Hypocalcemia and tetany, respiratory arrest, sores in mouth, constipation, loss of appetite, nausea, vomiting, weight loss, discoloration of teeth*** (white, black, brown)

Contraindications: Hypersensitivity, pregnancy (NR)
Precautions: Child <6 yr
Pharmacokinetics:
PO: Excreted in urine and feces; crosses placenta, breast milk
Interactions:
• Drug/food: avoid use with dairy products

NURSING CONSIDERATIONS
Assess:
• For mottling of teeth, during treatment
Administer:
• Drops after meals with fluids or undiluted tabs; may be chewed; do not swallow whole; may be given with water or juice; avoid milk
Evaluate:
• Therapeutic response: absence of dental caries
Teach patient/family:
• To monitor children using gel or rinse; not to be swallowed
• Not to drink, eat, or rinse mouth for at least ½ hr

• Not to use during pregnancy
• To apply after brushing and flossing hs
• To store out of children's reach

---

fluorouracil (5-fluorouracil) (℞)
(flure-oh-yoor′a-sil)
Adrucil, Efudex, Fluoroplex, 5-FU
Func. class.: Antineoplastic, antimetabolite
Chem. class.: Pyrimidine antagonist

Action: Inhibits DNA synthesis; interferes with cell replication by competitively inhibiting thymidylate synthesis, S phase of cell cycle–specific vesicant

Uses: Cancer of breast, colon, rectum, stomach, pancreas, multiple actinic keratoses, superficial basal cell carcinomas

Dosage and routes:
• *Adult:* **IV** 12 mg/kg/day × 4 days, not to exceed 800 mg/day; may repeat with 6 mg/kg on day 6, 8, 10, 12; maintenance is 10-15 mg/kg/wk as a single dose, not to exceed 1 g/wk
Actinic/solar keratoses
• *Adult:* **Top** 1% cream/sol 1-2 ×/day
Superficial basal cell carcinoma
• *Adult:* **Top** 5% sol 2 ×/day × 3-12 wk

Available forms: Inj 50 mg/ml; cream 1%, 5%; sol 1%, 2%, 5%

Side effects/adverse reactions:
CV: Myocardial ischemia, angina
*HEMA: **Thrombocytopenia, leukopenia, myelosuppression, anemia, agranulocytosis***
GI: Anorexia, stomatitis, diarrhea, nausea, vomiting, ***hemorrhage,*** enteritis glossitis
*GU: **Renal failure***
EENT: Epistaxis

INTEG: Rash, fever
CNS: Lethargy, malaise, weakness
Contraindications: Hypersensitivity, myelosuppression, pregnancy (D), poor nutritional status, serious infections
Precautions: Renal disease, hepatic disease, bone marrow depression, angina, lactation, children
Pharmacokinetics: Half-life 10-20 min, 20 hr terminal; metabolized in the liver; excreted in the urine; crosses blood-brain barrier
Interactions:
• Increased toxicity: radiation or other antineoplastics
Lab test interferences:
Increase: Liver function studies, 6-HIAA
Decrease: Albumin
NURSING CONSIDERATIONS
Assess:
• CBC, differential, platelet count weekly; withhold drug if WBC is <3500/mm^3 or platelet count is <100,000/mm^3; notify prescriber of these results; drug should be discontinued
• Renal function studies: BUN, serum uric acid, urine CrCl, electrolytes before, during therapy
• I&O ratio; report fall in urine output to <30 ml/hr
• Temp q4h; fever may indicate beginning infection
• Liver function tests before, during therapy: bilirubin, alk phosphatase, AST, ALT, LDH; prn or qmo
• Bleeding: hematuria, guaiac, bruising or petechiae, mucosa or orifices q8h
• Inflammation of mucosa, breaks in skin
• Buccal cavity q8h for dryness, sores or ulceration, white patches, oral pain, bleeding, dysphagia
• Symptoms indicating severe allergic reaction: rash, urticaria, itching, flushing

• GI symptoms: frequency of stools, cramping
• Acidosis, signs of dehydration: rapid respirations, poor skin turgor, decreased urine output, dry skin, restlessness, weakness
Administer:
• Antiemetic 30-60 min before giving drug to prevent vomiting and for several days thereafter
IV
• Undiluted; may inject through Y-tube or 3-way stopcock; give over 1-3 min; may be diluted in NS, D$_5$W, given over 2-8 hr as IV INF
Additive compatibilities: Bleomycin, cephalothin, cyclophosphamide, etoposide, floxuridine, hydromorphone, ifosfamide, methotrexate, mitoxantrone, prednisolone, vincristine
Solution compatibilities: Amino acids 4.25%/D$_{25}$, D$_5$/LR, D$_{3.3}$/0.3 NaCl, D$_5$W, 0.9% NaCl, TPN #23
Syringe compatibilities: Bleomycin, cisplatin, cyclophosphamide, furosemide, heparin, leucovorin, methotrexate, metoclopramide, mitomycin, vinblastine, vincristine
Y-site compatibilities: Allopurinol, amifostine, aztreonam, bleomycin, cefepime, cisplatin, cyclophosphamide, doxorubicin, doxorubicin liposome, fludarabine, furosemide, granisetron, heparin, hydrocortisone, leucovorin, mannitol, melphalan, methotrexate, metoclopramide, mitomycin, paclitaxel, piperacillin/tazobactam, potassium chloride, propofol, sargramostim, teniposide, thiotepa, vinblastine, vincristine, vit B/C
Topical
• Wear gloves when applying; may use with a loose dressing
Perform/provide:
• Protection from light
• Strict asepsis, protective isolation if WBC levels are low

• Increase fluid intake to 2-3 L/day to prevent dehydration, unless contraindicated

• Changing of IV site q48h

• Rinsing of mouth tid-qid with water, club soda; brushing of teeth bid-tid with soft brush or cotton-tipped applicator for stomatitis; use unwaxed dental floss

• Nutritious diet with iron, vitamin supplements, low fiber, few dairy products, especially when combined with radiotherapy as ordered

Evaluate:

• Therapeutic response: decreased tumor size, spread of malignancy

Teach patient/family:

• To avoid foods with citric acid, hot or rough texture if stomatitis is present; to drink adequate fluids

• To report stomatitis: any bleeding, white spots, ulcerations in mouth; tell patient to examine mouth qd, report symptoms

• To report signs of infection: fever, sore throat, flulike symptoms

• To report signs of anemia: fatigue, headache, faintness, shortness of breath, irritability

• To report bleeding: avoid use of razors, commercial mouthwash

• To avoid use of aspirin products or ibuprofen

• To use contraception during therapy (men and women)

---

fluoxetine (R)

(floo-ox'eh-teen)

Prozac

Func. class.: Antidepressant, SSRI

Action: Inhibits CNS neuron uptake of serotonin but not of norepinephrine

Uses: Major depressive disorder, obsessive-compulsive disorder (OCD), bulimia nervosa

Investigational uses: Alcoholism, anorexia nervosa, ADHD, bipolar II affective disorder, borderline personality disorder, cataplexy, narcolepsy, kleptomania, migraine, obesity, posttraumatic stress disorder, schizophrenia, Tourette syndrome, trichotillomania, levodopa-induced dyskinesia, social phobia

Dosage and routes:

Depression/obsessive-compulsive disorder

• *Adult:* **PO** 20 mg qd in AM; after 4 wk if no clinical improvement is noted, dose may be increased to 20 mg bid in AM, PM, not to exceed 80 mg/day

• *Geriatric:* **PO** 10 mg/day, increase as needed

• *Child 5-18 yr:* **PO** 5-10 mg/kg/day, max 20 mg/day

Bulimia nervosa

• *Adult:* **PO** 60 mg/day in AM

Available forms: Pulvules 10, 20 mg; liquid 20 mg/5 ml

Side effects/adverse reactions:

CNS: Headache, nervousness, insomnia, drowsiness, anxiety, tremor, dizziness, fatigue, sedation, poor concentration, abnormal dreams, agitation, **convulsions,** *apathy, euphoria, hallucinations, delusions, psychosis*

GI: Nausea, diarrhea, dry mouth, anorexia, dyspepsia, constipation, cramps, vomiting, taste changes, flatulence, decreased appetite

INTEG: Sweating, rash, pruritus, acne, alopecia, urticaria

RESP: Infection, pharyngitis, nasal congestion, sinus headache, sinusitis, cough, dyspnea, bronchitis, asthma, hyperventilation, pneumonia

CV: Hot flashes, palpitations, angina pectoris, **hemorrhage,** *hypertension,* **tachycardia,** *first-degree AV*

◆ = Nursing alert　　🖋 = Herb-drug interaction　　🚫 = Do not crush

block, ***bradycardia, MI, thrombophlebitis***

MS: Pain, arthritis, twitching

GU: Dysmenorrhea, decreased libido, urinary frequency, UTI, amenorrhea, cystitis, impotence, urine retention

EENT: Visual changes, ear/eye pain, photophobia, tinnitus

SYST: Asthenia, viral infection, fever, allergy, chills

Contraindications: Hypersensitivity

Precautions: Pregnancy (B), lactation, children, elderly, diabetes mellitus

Pharmacokinetics:

PO: Peak 6-8 hr; metabolized in liver; excreted in urine; half-life 1-384 hr; steady state 28-35 days, protein binding 94%

Interactions:

• Do not use MAOIs with or 14 days prior to fluoxetine

• Increased side effects: highly protein-bound drugs

• Increased effect: haloperidol

• Decreased fluoxetine effect: cyproheptadine

• Increased half-life of: diazepam

• Increased levels or toxicity of: carbamazepine, lithium, digoxin, warfarin, phenytoin

• Increased levels of: tricyclic antidepressants, phenothiazines

• Paradoxical worsening of OCD: buspirone

• Increased CNS depression: alcohol, antidepressants, opioids, sedatives

⊘ Increased action: kava

⊘ St. John's wort: Do not use together

Lab test interferences:

Increase: Serum bilirubin, blood glucose, alk phosphatase

Decrease: VMA, 5-HIAA

False increase: Urinary catecholamines

NURSING CONSIDERATIONS

Assess:

• Mental status: mood, sensorium, affect, suicidal tendencies, increase in psychiatric symptoms, depression, panic

• B/P (lying/standing), pulse q4h; if systolic B/P drops 20 mm Hg, hold drug, notify prescriber; take vital signs q4h in patients with cardiovascular disease

• Blood studies: CBC, leukocytes, differential, cardiac enzymes if patient is receiving long-term therapy; check platelets; bleeding can occur

• Hepatic studies: AST, ALT, bilirubin, creatinine

• Weight qwk; appetite may decrease with drug

• ECG for flattening of T wave, bundle branch, AV block, dysrhythmias in cardiac patients

• Alcohol consumption; if alcohol is consumed, hold dose until AM

Administer:

• With food or milk for GI symptoms

• Crushed if patient is unable to swallow medication whole

• Dosage hs if oversedation occurs during the day; may take entire dose hs; elderly may not tolerate once/day dosing

• Gum, hard candy, frequent sips of water for dry mouth

Perform/provide:

• Storage at room temp; do not freeze

• Assistance with ambulation during therapy, since drowsiness, dizziness occur

• Safety measures primarily in elderly

• Checking to see if PO medication swallowed

Evaluate:

• Therapeutic response: decreased depression, symptoms of OCD

Teach patient/family:
• That therapeutic effect may take 1-4 wk
• To use caution in driving, other activities requiring alertness because of drowsiness, dizziness, blurred vision
• To use sunscreen to prevent photosensitivity
• To avoid alcohol ingestion, other CNS depressants
• To notify prescriber if pregnant or plan to become pregnant or breastfeed

---

fluoxymesterone (R)

(floo-ox-ee-mess′te-rone)
Fluoxymesterone, Halotestin
Func. class.: Androgenic anabolic steroid
Chem. class.: Halogenated testosterone derivative

Action: Increases weight by building body tissue, increases potassium, phosphorus, chloride, nitrogen levels, bone development
Uses: Impotence from testicular deficiency, hypogonadism; breast engorgement; palliative treatment of female breast cancer
Dosage and routes:
Hypogonadism/impotence
• *Adult:* **PO** 2-10 mg qd
Breast engorgement
• *Adult:* **PO** 2.5 mg qd, then 5-10 mg qd × 5 days
Breast cancer
• *Adult:* **PO** 15-30 mg qd in divided doses until therapeutic effect occurs, then dosage should be reduced
Available forms: Tabs 2, 5, 10 mg
Side effects/adverse reactions:
INTEG: Rash, acneiform lesions; oily hair, skin; flushing, sweating, acne vulgaris, alopecia, hirsutism
CNS: Dizziness, headache, fatigue, tremors, paresthesias, flushing, sweating, anxiety, lability, insomnia
MS: Cramps, spasms, carpal tunnel syndrome
CV: Increased B/P
GU: Hematuria, amenorrhea, vaginitis, decreased libido, decreased breast size, clitoral hypertrophy, testicular atrophy
GI: Nausea, vomiting, constipation, weight gain, ***cholestatic jaundice***
EENT: Conjunctional edema, nasal congestion
ENDO: Abnormal GTT
Contraindications: Severe renal, severe cardiac, severe hepatic disease, hypersensitivity, pregnancy (X), lactation, genital bleeding (abnormal), children
Precautions: Diabetes mellitus, CV disease, MI
Pharmacokinetics:
PO: Metabolized in liver; excreted in urine; crosses placenta; excreted in breast milk
Interactions:
• Hepatotoxicity: other hepatotoxic agents
• Increased PT: anticoagulants
• Altered dosage requirements: oral antidiabetics, insulin
Lab test interferences:
Increase: Serum cholesterol, blood glucose, urine glucose
Decrease: Serum Ca; serum K, T_4, T_3; thyroid ^{131}I uptake test, urine 17-OHCS, 17-KS, PBI, BSP

NURSING CONSIDERATIONS
Assess:
• Weight daily; notify prescriber if weekly weight gain is >5 lb
• B/P q4h
• I&O ratio; be alert for decreasing urinary output, increasing edema
• Growth rate in children; growth rate may be uneven (linear/bone growth) if used for extended periods

---

◆ = Nursing alert   ✷ = Herb-drug interaction   ⊘ = Do not crush

- Electrolytes: K, Na, Cl, cholesterol
- Liver function studies: ALT, AST, bilirubin
- Edema, hypertension, cardiac symptoms, jaundice
- Mental status: affect, mood, behavioral changes, aggression
- Signs of masculinization in female: increased libido, deepening of voice, breast tissue, enlarged clitoris, menstrual irregularities; male: gynecomastia, impotence, testicular atrophy
- Hypercalcemia: lethargy, polyuria, polydipsia, nausea, vomiting, constipation; drug may have to be decreased
- Altered glucose level in diabetics, dosage may need to be changed

Administer:
- Titrated dose, use lowest effective dose
- With food or milk to decrease GI symptoms

Perform/provide:
- Diet with increased calories, protein; decrease Na if edema occurs

Evaluate:
- Therapeutic response: increased appetite, stamina

Teach patient/family:
- That drug must be combined with complete health plan: diet, rest, exercise
- To notify prescriber if therapeutic response decreases
- Not to discontinue abruptly
- About change in gender characteristics
- That females need to report menstrual irregularities, if pregnancy is suspected
- That 1-3 mo course is necessary for response in breast cancer
- That steroids should not be used for bodybuilding

fluphenazine decanoate (℞)
(floo-fen'a-zeen)
Modecate Concentrate*, Prolixin Decanoate
fluphenazine enanthate (℞)
Moditen Enanthate*, Prolixin Enanthate
fluphenazine hydrochloride (℞)
Apo-Fluphenazine*, Moditen HCL*, Moditen HCl-H.P.*, Permitil*, Prolixin
Func. class.: Antipsychotic, neuroleptic
Chem. class.: Phenothiazine, piperazine

Action: Depresses cerebral cortex, hypothalamus, limbic system, which control activity and aggression; blocks neurotransmission produced by dopamine at synapse; exhibits strong α-adrenergic and anticholinergic blocking action; mechanism for antipsychotic effects is unclear
Uses: Psychotic disorders, schizophrenia
Dosage and routes:
Enanthate, decanoate
- *Adult and child >12 yr:* **SC** 12.5-25 mg q1-3wk
HCl
- *Adult:* **PO** 2.5-10 mg, in divided doses q6-8h, not to exceed 20 mg qd; **IM** initially 1.25 mg then 2.5-10 mg in divided doses q6-8h
- *Child:* **PO** 0.25-3.5 mg qd in divided doses q4-6h, max 10 mg/qd
Available forms: HCl tabs 1, 2.5, 5, 10 mg; elix 2.5 mg/5 ml; conc 5 mg/ml; inj 2.5 mg/ml; enanthate, decanoate, depot inj 25 mg/ml
Side effects/adverse reactions:
RESP: Laryngospasm, dyspnea, ***respiratory depression***

CNS: EPS: pseudoparkinsonism, akathisia, dystonia, tardive dyskinesia, drowsiness, headache, seizures, neuroleptic malignant syndrome

HEMA: Anemia, *leukopenia, leukocytosis, agranulocytosis, aplastic anemia, thrombocytopenia*

INTEG: Rash, photosensitivity, dermatitis

EENT: Blurred vision, glaucoma, dry eyes

GI: Dry mouth, nausea, vomiting, anorexia, constipation, diarrhea, jaundice, weight gain, *paralytic ileus, hepatitis*

GU: Urinary retention, urinary frequency, enuresis, impotence, amenorrhea, gynecomastia

CV: Orthostatic hypotension, hypertension, *cardiac arrest,* ECG changes, *tachycardia*

Contraindications: Hypersensitivity, circulatory collapse, liver damage, cerebral arteriosclerosis, coronary disease, severe hypertension/hypotension, blood dyscrasias, coma, child <12 yr, brain damage, bone marrow depression, alcohol and barbiturate withdrawal

Precautions: Pregnancy (C), lactation, seizure disorders, hypertension, hepatic disease, cardiac disease, elderly

Pharmacokinetics:

PO/IM (HCl): Onset 1 hr, peak 2-4 hr, duration 6-8 hr

SC (enanthate): Onset 1-2 days, peak 2-3 days, duration 1-3 wk, half-life 3.5-4 days; decanoate: onset 1-3 days, peak 1-2 days, duration over 4 wk, single-dose half-life 6.8-9.6 days; multiple dose, 14.3 days; metabolized by liver; excreted in urine (metabolites); crosses placenta; enters breast milk

Interactions:

• Oversedation: other CNS depressants, alcohol, barbiturate anesthetics

• Toxicity: epinephrine

• Decreased effects of levodopa, lithium

• Decreased effects of fluphenazine: smoking, barbiturates

• Increased anticholinergic effects: anticholinergics

🌿 Increased anticholinergic effect: henbane leaf

🌿 Possible increased action: kava

Lab test interferences:

Increase: Liver function tests, cardiac enzymes, cholesterol, blood glucose, prolactin, bilirubin, PBI, cholinesterase

Decrease: Hormones (blood and urine)

False positive: Pregnancy tests, PKU urinary steroids, 17-OHCS, pregnancy tests

NURSING CONSIDERATIONS

Assess:

• Swallowing of PO medication; check for hoarding, giving of medication to other patients

• I&O ratio; palpate bladder if low urinary output occurs

• Bilirubin, CBC, liver function studies monthly

• Urinalysis is recommended before and during prolonged therapy

• Affect, orientation, LOC, reflexes, gait, coordination, sleep pattern disturbances

• B/P standing and lying; take pulse and respirations q4h during initial treatment; establish baseline before starting treatment; report drops of 30 mm Hg

• Dizziness, faintness, palpitations, tachycardia on rising

• EPS including akathisia (inability to sit still, no pattern to movements), tardive dyskinesia (bizarre movements of jaw, mouth, tongue, extremities), pseudoparkinsonism (rigidity, tremors, pill rolling, shuffling gait)

• Skin turgor qd

• Constipation, urinary retention qd; if these occur, increase bulk, H_2O in diet

Administer:

• Concentrate with juice, milk, or uncaffeinated drinks

• Antiparkinsonian agent if EPS occur

• IM inj into large muscle mass; to minimize postural hypotension, give injection and have patient remain seated or recumbent for ½ hr

• Use dry needle, or solution will become cloudy; use 21 G or larger due to viscosity

Syringe compatibilities: Benztropine, diphenhydramine, hydroxyzine

Perform/provide:

• Decreased sensory input by dimming lights, avoiding loud noises

• Supervised ambulation until stabilized on medication; do not involve in strenuous exercise; fainting is possible; patient should not stand still for long periods

• Increased fluids to prevent constipation

• Sips of water, candy, gum for dry mouth

• Storage in tight, light-resistant container in cool environment

Evaluate:

• Therapeutic response: decrease in emotional excitement, hallucinations, delusions, paranoia, reorganization of patterns of thought, speech

Teach patient/family:

• That orthostatic hypotension occurs often; to rise from sitting or lying position gradually; avoid hazardous activities until stabilized on medication

• To avoid hot tubs, hot showers, tub baths, since hypotension may occur; that in hot weather, heat stroke may occur; take extra precautions to stay cool

⬥ To avoid abrupt withdrawal of this drug, or EPS may result; drug should be withdrawn slowly

• To avoid OTC preparations (cough, hay fever, cold) unless approved by prescriber; serious drug interactions may occur; avoid use with alcohol, CNS depressants; increased drowsiness may occur

• To use a sunscreen to prevent burns

• About importance of compliance with drug regimen

• About EPS and necessity for meticulous oral hygiene, since oral candidiasis may occur

• To report sore throat, malaise, fever, bleeding, mouth sores; if these occur, CBC should be drawn and drug discontinued

• That urine may turn pink to reddish-brown

Treatment of overdose: Lavage; if orally ingested, provide an airway; *do not induce vomiting*

---

flurazepam (R)

(flure-az′e-pam)
Apo-Flurazepam*, Dalmane, flurazepam, Novo-Flupam*
Func. class.: Sedative/hypnotic
Chem. class.: Benzodiazepine derivative

Controlled Substance Schedule IV (USA), Schedule F (Canada)

Action: Produces CNS depression at the limbic, thalamic, hypothalamic levels of CNS; may be mediated by neurotransmitter γ-aminobutyric acid (GABA); results are sedation, hypnosis, skeletal muscle relaxation, anticonvulsant activity, anxiolytic action

Uses: Insomnia

Dosage and routes:
• *Adult:* **PO** 15-30 mg hs; may repeat dose once if needed
• *Elderly:* **PO** 15 mg hs; may increase if needed
Available forms: Caps 15, 30 mg
Side effects/adverse reactions:
HEMA: **Leukopenia, granulocytopenia** (rare)
CNS: Lethargy, drowsiness, daytime sedation, dizziness, confusion, lightheadedness, headache, anxiety, irritability
GI: Nausea, vomiting, diarrhea, heartburn, abdominal pain, constipation
CV: Chest pain, pulse changes
Contraindications: Hypersensitivity to benzodiazepines, pregnancy, lactation, intermittent porphyria, uncontrolled pain, pregnancy (X)
Precautions: Anemia, hepatic disease, renal disease, suicidal individuals, drug abuse, elderly, psychosis, child <15 yr
Pharmacokinetics:
PO: Onset 15-45 min, duration 7-8 hr; metabolized by liver; excreted by kidneys (inactive/active metabolites); crosses placenta; excreted in breast milk; half-life 47-100 hr, additional 100 hr for active metabolites
Interactions:
• Increased effects of flurazepam: cimetidine, disulfiram, probenicid, isoniazid
• Increased action of both drugs: alcohol, CNS depressants
• Decreased effect of flurazepam: antacids, theophylline, rifampin, smoking
🌿 Increased action: kava
Lab test interferences:
Increase: AST, ALT, serum bilirubin
False increase: Urinary 17-OHCS
Decrease: RAI uptake

NURSING CONSIDERATIONS
Assess:
• Blood studies: Hct, Hgb, RBC (if on long-term therapy)
• Hepatic studies: AST, ALT, bilirubin
• Mental status: mood, sensorium, affect, memory (long, short)
◆ Blood dyscrasias: fever, sore throat, bruising, rash, jaundice, epistaxis (rare)
• Type of sleep problem: falling asleep, staying asleep
Administer:
• After removal of cigarettes to prevent fires
• After trying conservative measures for insomnia
• ½-1 hr before hs for sleeplessness
• On empty stomach for fast onset, but may be taken with food if GI symptoms occur
Perform/provide:
• Assistance with ambulation after receiving dose
• Safety measures: night-light, call bell within easy reach
• Checking to see if PO medication has been swallowed
• Storage in tight container in cool environment
Evaluate:
• Therapeutic response: ability to sleep at night, decreased amount of early morning awakening if taking drug for insomnia
Teach patient/family:
• To avoid driving or other activities requiring alertness until drug is stabilized
• To avoid alcohol ingestion or CNS depressants; serious CNS depression may result
• That effects may take 2 nights for benefits to be noticed
• Alternative measures to improve sleep: reading, exercise several hr before hs, warm bath, warm milk, TV, self-hypnosis, deep breathing

---

◆ = Nursing alert   🌿 = Herb-drug interaction   🚫 = Do not crush

• That hangover is common in elderly

🚫 Not to break, crush, or chew caps

Treatment of overdose: Lavage, activated charcoal; monitor electrolytes, vital signs

---

flutamide (℞)

(floo'-ta-mide)
Euflex*, Eulexin
Func. class.: Antineoplastic, hormone
Chem. class.: Antiandrogen

Action: Interferes with testosterone uptake in the nucleus or testosterone activity in target tissues; arrests tumor growth in androgen-sensitive tissue, i.e., prostate gland

Uses: Metastatic prostatic carcinoma, stage D2 in combination with LHRH agonistic analogs (leuprolide)

Dosage and routes:
• *Adult:* **PO** 250 mg q8h tid, for a daily dosage of 750 mg

Available forms: Caps 125, 250* mg

Side effects/adverse reactions:
CNS: Hot flashes, drowsiness, confusion, depression, anxiety, paresthesia
GU: Decreased libido, impotence, gynecomastia
GI: Diarrhea, nausea, vomiting, increased liver function studies, **hepatitis,** anorexia
*HEMA: **Leukopenia, thrombocytopenia, hemolytic anemia***
INTEG: Irritation at site, rash, photosensitivity
MISC: Edema, neuromuscular and pulmonary symptoms, hypertension
Contraindications: Hypersensitivity, pregnancy (D)
Pharmacokinetics: Rapidly and

completely absorbed; excreted in urine and feces as metabolites; half-life 6 hr, geriatric half-life 8 hr; 94% bound to plasma proteins

NURSING CONSIDERATIONS
Assess:
• Liver function studies: AST, ALT, alk phosphatase, which may be elevated; monitor CBC
• For CNS symptoms including: drowsiness, confusion, depression, anxiety
Evaluate:
• Therapeutic response: decrease in prostatic tumor size, decrease in spread of cancer
Teach patient/family:
🚫 Not to break, crush, or chew caps
• To report side effects: decreased libido, impotence, breast enlargement, hot flashes, diarrhea
• That this drug is taken with leuprolide for medical castration

---

fluvastatin (℞)

(flu'vah-stay-tin)
Lescol
Func. class.: Antilipidemic
Chem. class.: Synthetically derived fermentation product

Action: Inhibits HMG-CoA reductase enzyme, which reduces cholesterol synthesis

Uses: As an adjunct in primary hypercholesterolemia (types Ia, Ib), coronary atherosclerosis in CAD

Dosage and routes:
• *Adult:* **PO** 20-40 mg qd in PM initially, usual range 20-80 mg, not to exceed 80 mg; should be given in 2 doses (40 mg AM, 40 mg PM); dosage adjustments may be made in 4 wk intervals or more

Available forms: Caps 20, 40 mg
Side effects/adverse reactions:
INTEG: Rash, pruritus

GI: Nausea, constipation, diarrhea, dyspepsia, flatus, *liver dysfunction,* pancreatitis

EENT: Lens opacities

MS: Myalgia, *myositis, rhabdomyolysis*

CNS: Headache, dizziness, insomnia

MISC: Fatigue, influenza

HEMA: Thrombocytopenia, hemolytic anemia, leukopenia

RESP: Upper respiratory infection, rhinitis, cough, pharyngitis, sinusitis

Contraindications: Hypersensitivity, pregnancy (X), lactation, active liver disease

Precautions: Past liver disease, alcoholism, severe acute infections, trauma, hypotension, uncontrolled seizure disorders, severe metabolic disorders, electrolyte imbalance

Pharmacokinetics: Metabolized in liver, highly protein bound, excreted primarily in feces, half-life <1 hr

Interactions:

• Increased effects of warfarin

• Increased myalgia, myositis: cyclosporine, gemfibrozil, niacin, erythromycin

• Increased serum level of digoxin

• Decreased effects of fluvastatin: bile acid sequestrants, propranolol, nicotinic acid, digoxin, rifampin, alcohol, after a meal within 1 hr of taking drug

NURSING CONSIDERATIONS
Assess:

• Fasting lipid profile (cholesterol, LDL, HDL, TG) q8wk, then q3-6 mo when stable

• Liver function studies q1-2mo during the first 1½ yr of treatment; AST, ALT, liver function tests may be increased

• Renal studies in patients with compromised renal system: BUN, I&O ratio, creatinine

• Eyes with slit lamp before, 1 mo after treatment begins, annually; lens opacities may occur

Perform/provide:

• Storage in cool environment in tight container protected from light

Evaluate:

• Therapeutic response: decrease in cholesterol to desired level after 8 wk

Teach patient/family:

• That blood work will be necessary during treatment

• To report severe GI symptoms, headache

• That previously prescribed regimen will continue: low-cholesterol diet, exercise program

🚫 Not to break, crush, or chew caps

• To report suspected pregnancy, not to use during pregnancy

---

fluvoxamine (℞)
(flu-vox′a-meen)
Luvox
Func. class.: Antidepressant-SSRI

Action: Inhibits CNS neuron uptake of serotonin but not of norepinephrine

Uses: Obsessive-compulsive disorder

Investigational uses: Depression

Dosage and routes:

• *Adult:* **PO** 50 mg hs, increase by 50 mg at 4-7 day intervals, max 300 mg

Available forms: Tabs 50, 100 mg

Side effects/adverse reactions:

CNS: Headache, drowsiness, dizziness, convulsions, sleep disorders

*GI: Nausea, anorexia, constipation, **hepatotoxicity,** vomiting, diarrhea*

INTEG: Rash, sweating

GU: Decreased libido

Contraindications: Hypersensitivity

Precautions: Pregnancy (C), lactation, children, elderly

Pharmacokinetics: Crosses blood-brain barrier, 77% protein binding, metabolism by the liver, terminal half-life 16.9 hr, peak 2-8 hr

Interactions:

• Increased CNS depression: alcohol, barbiturates, benzodiazepines

• Increased toxicity: tricyclic antidepressants, theophylline, lithium

◆ Fatal reaction: MAO inhibitors

• Drug/smoking: Increased metabolism, decreased effects

/ **Increased effect, possible fatal reaction: St. John's wort**

/ Increased effect: kava

NURSING CONSIDERATIONS

Assess:

• Hepatic studies: AST, ALT, bilirubin

• Mental status: mood, sensorium, affect, suicidal tendencies; increase in psychiatric symptoms: depression, panic

• Constipation; most likely in elderly

◆ For withdrawal symptoms: headache, nausea, vomiting, muscle pain, weakness; not usual unless discontinued abruptly

Administer:

• With food, milk for GI symptoms

Perform/provide:

• Storage at room temp; do not freeze

Evaluate:

• Therapeutic response: decrease in depression

Teach patient/family:

• That therapeutic effects may take 2-3 wk

• To use caution in driving, other activities requiring alertness because of drowsiness, dizziness that may occur

• Not to discontinue medication quickly after long-term use: may cause nausea, headache, malaise

• To increase bulk in diet if constipation occurs, especially elderly

• To take gum; hard, sugarless candy; or frequent sips of water for dry mouth

---

folic acid (vit B$_9$) (OTC)

(foe′lik a′sid)
Apo-Folic*, Folate, Folvite, Novofolacid*, Vitamin B$_9$
Func. class.: Vit B complex group

Action: Needed for erythropoiesis; increases RBC, WBC, platelet formation in megaloblastic anemias

Uses: Megaloblastic or macrocytic anemia caused by folic acid deficiency; liver disease, alcoholism, hemolysis, intestinal obstruction, pregnancy

Dosage and routes:

Therapeutic dose

• *Adult and child:* **PO/IM/SC/IV** up to 1 mg qd

Maintenance dose

• *Adult and child >4 yr:* **PO/IM/IV/SC** 0.4 mg/day

• *Pregnant and lactating:* **PO/IM/IV/SC** 0.8 mg/day

• *Child <4 yr:* **PO/IM/IV/SC** 0.3 mg/day

Available forms: Tabs 0.4, 0.8, 1 mg; inj 5 mg/ml

Side effects/adverse reactions:

RESP: **Bronchospasm**

INTEG: Flushing

Contraindications: Hypersensitivity, anemias other than megaloblastic/macrocytic anemia, vit B$_{12}$ deficiency anemia, uncorrected pernicious anemia

Precautions: Pregnancy (A)

Pharmacokinetics:

PO: Peak ½-1 hr; bound to plasma proteins; excreted in breast milk;

---

metabolized by liver; excreted in urine (small amounts)

Interactions:
• Decreased folate levels: chloramphenicol, aspirin, methotrexate, oral contraceptives, sulfasalazine
• Increased metabolism of phenobarbital, hydantoins

NURSING CONSIDERATIONS
Assess:
• For fatigue, dyspnea, weakness, SOB that are signs of megaloblastic anemia
• Hgb, Hct, and reticulocyte count
• Folate levels: 6-15 µg/ml
• Nutritional status: bran, yeast, dried beans, nuts, fruits, fresh vegetables, asparagus
• Drugs currently taken: alcohol, oral contraceptives, hydantoins, trimethoprim; these drugs may cause increased folic acid use by body and contribute to a deficiency

Administer:
IV
• Direct undiluted 5 mg or less/1 min or may be added to most IV sol or TPN

Solution compatibilities: $D_{20}W$
Y-site compatibilities: Famotidine

Perform/provide:
• Storage in light-resistant container

Evaluate:
• Therapeutic response: increased weight, oriented well-being; absence of fatigue

Teach patient/family:
• To take drug exactly as prescribed
• To notify prescriber of side effects

follitropin alfa/ follitropin beta (℞)
(fol'ee-tro-pin)
Gonal-F/Follistim
Func. class.: Ovulation stimulant
Chem. class.: Gonadotropin

Action: Stimulates ovarian follicular growth in primary ovarian failure

Uses: Induction of ovulation, assisted reproductive technologies (in vitro fertilization)

Dosage and routes:
Ovulation induction
• **SC** 75 IU, may increase by 37.5 IU after 2 wk, may increase again after 1 wk by 37.5 IU; treatment should not exceed 35 days unless a serum estradiol rise indicates imminent follicular development

Follicle stimulation
• *Adult:* **SC** 150 IU/day on day 2 or 3 of the follicular phase, should not exceed 10 days

Available forms: Gonal-F: 75 IU, 150 IU; Follistim: powder for inj 75 IU

Side effects/adverse reactions:
CNS: Malaise
GI: Nausea, vomiting, constipation, increased appetite, abdominal pain
INTEG: Rash, dermatitis, urticaria, alopecia
GU: Polyuria, urinary frequency, **birth defects, spontaneous abortion,** multiple ovulation, breast pain

Contraindications: Hypersensitivity, pregnancy (X), undiagnosed vaginal bleeding, intracranial lesion, ovarian cyst not caused by polycystic ovarian disease

Precautions: Lactation, arterial thromboembolism

Pharmacokinetics: Metabolized in liver, excreted in feces, stored in fat

---

◆ = Nursing alert   ⁄ = Herb-drug interaction   ⊘ = Do not crush

NURSING CONSIDERATIONS
Administer:
- At same time qd to maintain drug level
- After dissolving contents of ampule in 1-2 ml of sterile saline, give immediately, discard unused portion

Evaluate:
- Therapeutic response: ovulation, pregnancy

Teach patient/family:
- That multiple births are common after taking this drug
- To notify prescriber of low abdominal pain; may indicate ovarian cyst, cyst rupture
- The proper method of taking, recording basal body temp to determine whether ovulation has occurred
- That if ovulation can be determined (there is a slight decrease in temp, then a sharp increase for ovulation), to attempt coitus 3 days before and qod until after ovulation
- That if pregnancy is suspected, to notify prescriber immediately

---

foscarnet (℞)
(foss-kar'net)
Foscavir
Func. class.: Antiviral
Chem. class.: Inorganic pyrophosphate organic analog

Action: Antiviral activity is produced by selective inhibition at the pyrophosphate binding site on virus-specific DNA polymerases and reverse transcriptases at concentrations that do not affect cellular DNA polymerases

Uses: Treatment of CMV retinitis, HSV infections, used with ganciclovir for relapsing patients

Dosage and routes:
- *Adult:* **IV INF** 60 mg/kg given over at least 1 hr, q8h × 2-3 wk initially, then 90-120 mg/kg/day over 2 hr, usually give with at least 750-1000 ml **NS** qd

In renal abnormalities:
- *Adult:* **IV**
Male:

$$\frac{140 - age}{serum\ creatinine \times 72} = CrCl$$

Female: $0.85 \times$ above value
Dose based on table provided in package insert

Available forms: Inj 24 mg/ml

Side effects/adverse reactions:
CNS: Fever, dizziness, *headache*, *seizures, fatigue,* neuropathy, tremor, ataxia, vertigo, dementia, stupor, EEG abnormalities, vertigo, *coma,* abnormal gait, hypertonia, EPS, hemiparesis, *paralysis,* hyperreflexia, paraplegia, *tetany,* hyporeflexia, neuralgia, neuritis, *cerebral edema, paresthesia,* depression, *confusion, anxiety,* insomnia, somnolence, amnesia, hallucinations, agitation
GI: Nausea, *vomiting, diarrhea, anorexia,* abdominal pain, constipation, dysphagia, rectal hemorrhage, dry mouth, melena, flatulence, ulcerative stomatitis, pancreatitis, enteritis, enterocolitis, glossitis, proctitis, stomatitis, increased amylases, gastroenteritis, *pseudomembranous colitis,* duodenal ulcer, *paralytic ileus, esophageal ulceration,* abnormal A-G ratio, increased AST, ALT, cholecystitis, *hepatitis,* dyspepsia, tenesmus, hepatosplenomegaly, jaundice
INTEG: Rash, sweating, pruritus, skin ulceration, seborrhea, skin discoloration, alopecia, acne, dermatitis, pain/inflammation at injection site, facial edema, dry skin, urticaria
HEMA: Anemia, *granulocytopenia, leukopenia, thrombocytopenia,* platelet abnormalities, *thrombosis, pulmonary embolism, coagulation disorders, decreased prothrombin,*

Side effects: *italics* = common; ***bold italics*** = life-threatening

hypochromic anemia, pancytopenia, hemolysis, leukocytosis, lymphadenopathy, epistaxis, lymphopenia
SYST: Hypokalemia, hypocalcemia, hypomagnesemia; increased alk phosphatase, LDH, BUN; acidosis, hypophosphatemia, hyperphosphatemia, dehydration, glycosuria, increased CPK, hypervolemia, infection, *sepsis, death, ascites,* hyponatremia, hypochloremia, hypercalcemia
GU: Acute renal failure, decreased CrCl and increased serum creatinine, *glomerulonephritis, toxic nephropathy, nephrosis, renal tubular disorders, pyelonephritis, uremia, hematuria, albuminuria,* dysuria, polyuria
RESP: Coughing, dyspnea, pneumonia, sinusitis, pharyngitis, *pulmonary infiltration,* stridor, *pneumothorax, hemoptysis, bronchospasm,* bronchitis, *respiratory depression, pleural effusion, pulmonary hemorrhage,* rhinitis
EENT: Visual field defects, vocal cord paralysis, speech disorders, taste perversion, eye pain, conjunctivitis, tinnitus, otitis
CV: Hypertension, palpitations, ECG abnormalities, 1st degree AV block, nonspecific ST-T segment changes, hypotension, cerebrovascular disorder, cardiomyopathy, *cardiac arrest,* bradycardia, dysrhythmias
MS: Arthralgia, myalgia
Contraindications: Hypersensitivity, CrCl <0.4 ml/min/kg
Precautions: Pregnancy (C), lactation, children, elderly, renal disease, seizure disorders, electrolyte/mineral imbalances, severe anemia
Pharmacokinetics: 14%-17% plasma protein bound, half-life 2-8 hr in normal renal function
Interactions:
• Nephrotoxicity: aminoglycosides, amphotericin B, IV pentamidine

• Hypocalcemia: pentamidine
• Seizures: ciprofloxacin
• Increased anemia: zidovudine
NURSING CONSIDERATIONS
Assess:
• Culture should be done prior to treatment (blood, urine, throat)
• Ophthalmic exam should confirm diagnosis
• Kidney, liver function studies: BUN, creatinine, AST, ALT
• I&O ratio, urine pH
• Blood counts q2wk; watch for decreasing granulocytes, Hgb; if low, therapy may have to be discontinued and restarted after hematologic recovery; blood transfusions may be required
• GI symptoms: nausea, vomiting, diarrhea; severe symptoms may necessitate discontinuing drug
• Electrolytes and minerals: Ca, P, Mg, Na, K; watch closely for tetany during first administration
◆ Blood dyscrasias (anemia, granulocytopenia); bruising, fatigue, bleeding, poor healing
• Allergic reactions: flushing, rash, urticaria, pruritus
Administer:
• Increased fluids before and during drug administration to induce diuresis and minimize renal toxicity
IV, int inf
• Using infusion device, at no more than 1 mg/kg/min; do not give by rapid or bolus IV; give by CVP or peripheral vein; standard 24 mg/ml sol may be used without dilution if using by CVP; dilute the 24 mg/ml sol to 12 mg/ml with D_5W or NS if using peripheral vein
Y-site compatibilities: Aldesleukin, amikacin, aminophylline, ampicillin, aztreonam, benzquinamide, cefazolin, cefoperazone, cefoxitin, ceftazidime, ceftizoxime, ceftriaxone, cefuroxime, chloramphenicol, cimetidine, clindamycin, dexameth-

◆ = Nursing alert   ⧫ = Herb-drug interaction   ⊘ = Do not crush asone, dopamine, erythromycin, fluconazole, flucytosine, furosemide, gentamicin, heparin, hydrocortisone, hydromorphone, hydroxyzine, imipenem-cilastatin, metoclopramide, metronidazole, miconazole, morphine, nafcillin, oxacillin, penicillin G potassium, phenytoin, piperacillin, ranitidine, ticarcillin/clavulanate, tobramycin

Perform/provide:
• Regular ophthalmologic exams
• Close monitoring during therapy for tingling, numbness, paresthesias; if these occur, stop infusion, obtain lab sample for electrolytes

Evaluate:
• Therapeutic response: improvement in CMV retinitis

Teach patient/family:
• To call prescriber if sore throat, swollen lymph nodes, malaise, fever occur, since other infections may occur
• To report perioral tingling, numbness in extremities, and paresthesias
• That serious drug interactions may occur if OTC products are ingested; check first with prescriber
• That drug is not a cure but will control symptoms

---

fosfomycin (℞)

(foss-foe-mye'sin)
Monurol
Func. class.: Urinary antiinfective

Action: Interferes with protein synthesis in bacterial cell by binding to ribosomal subunit, causing misreading of the genetic code; inaccurate peptide sequence forms in protein chain, causing bacterial death
Uses: Infections of the urinary tract caused by *E. faecalis, E. coli*

Dosage and routes:
• *Adult >18 yr:* 1 sachet with or without food, always mix with water before ingesting
Available forms: Single-dose sachet (3 g fosfomycin), orange flavored

Side effects/adverse reactions:
GU: Vaginitis, dysuria, hematuria, menstrual disorder
CNS: Headache, dizziness, fever, insomnia, somnolence, migraine, asthenia, nervousness
GI: Nausea, vomiting, anorexia, constipation, dry mouth, flatulence, increased SGPT; *diarrhea,* dyspepsia
INTEG: Rash, pruritus

Contraindications: Hypersensitivity

Precautions: Pregnancy (B), children <12 yr, lactation, renal disease
Pharmacokinetics: Rapidly absorbed, not bound to plasma proteins, excreted unchanged in urine/feces, half-life 4-8 hr

Interactions:
• Increased urinary excretion of fosfomycin: metoclopramide

NURSING CONSIDERATIONS

Assess:
• Urine pH, urine should be kept alkaline
• Overgrowth of infections: fever, pain
• C&S before starting treatment to identify infecting organism

Administer:
• PO, pour contents of sachet into 3-4 oz (½ cup) of water, stir to dissolve, use cold water, take immediately
• Only a single dose is necessary
• 1 hr ac or 2 hr pc antacids or calcium

Perform/provide:
• Adequate fluids of 2-3 L/day, unless contraindicated
• Storage at 59°-86° F (15°-30° C)

Evaluate:

• Therapeutic response: absence of fever, negative C&S after treatment

Teach patient/family:

• Give patient directions to dissolve sachet, caution patient not to take in dry form

---

fosinopril (℞)

(foss'in-oh-pril)
Monopril

Func. class.: Antihypertensive
Chem. class.: Angiotensin-converting enzyme (ACE) inhibitor

Action: Selectively suppresses renin-angiotensin-aldosterone system; inhibits ACE; prevents conversion of angiotensin I to angiotensin II; results in dilation of arterial, venous vessels

Uses: Hypertension, alone or in combination with thiazide diuretics, systolic CHF

Dosage and routes:

• *Adult:* **PO** 10 mg qd initially, then 20-40 mg/day divided bid or qd

Renal dose

5 mg qd

Available forms: Tabs 10, 20 mg

Side effects/adverse reactions:

CV: Hypotension, chest pain, palpitations, angina, orthostatic hypotension

GU: Proteinuria, increased BUN, creatinine, decreased libido

HEMA: Decreased Hct, Hgb; *eosinophilia, leukopenia, neutropenia*

INTEG: Angioedema, rash, flushing, sweating, photosensitivity, pruritus

RESP: Cough, sinusitis, dyspnea, *bronchospasm*

META: Hyperkalemia

GI: Nausea, constipation, vomiting, diarrhea

CNS: Insomnia, paresthesia, head-*ache, dizziness,* fatigue, memory disturbance, tremor, mood change

MS: Arthralgia, myalgia

Contraindications: Hypersensitivity to ACE inhibitors, pregnancy (D) 2nd/3rd trimester, lactation, children

Precautions: Impaired liver function, hypovolemia, blood dyscrasias, CHF, COPD, asthma, elderly

Pharmacokinetics:

PO: Peak 3 hr; serum protein binding 97%; half-life 12 hr; metabolized by liver (metabolites excreted in urine, feces)

Interactions:

• Increased hypotension: diuretics, other antihypertensives, ganglionic blockers, adrenergic blockers

• Increased toxicity: vasodilators, hydralazine, prazosin, K-sparing diuretics, sympathomimetics

• Decreased absorption: antacids

• Decreased antihypertensive effect: indomethacin

• Increased serum levels of digoxin, lithium

Lab test interferences:

False positive: Urine acetone

NURSING CONSIDERATIONS

Assess:

• Blood studies: neutrophils, decreased platelets

• B/P, orthostatic hypotension, syncope

• Renal studies: protein, BUN, creatinine; increased levels may indicate nephrotic syndrome

• Baselines in renal, liver function tests before therapy begins

• K levels, although hyperkalemia rarely occurs

• Edema in feet, legs daily

• Allergic reactions: rash, fever, pruritus, urticaria; drug should be discontinued if antihistamines fail to help

---

⬇ = Nursing alert   🌿 = Herb-drug interaction   🚫 = Do not crush

Administer:
• IV infusion of 0.9% NaCl (as ordered) to expand fluid volume if severe hypotension occurs

Perform/provide:
• Storage in tight container at 86° F (30° C) or less
• Supine position for severe hypotension

Evaluate:
• Therapeutic response: decrease in B/P

Teach patient/family:
• Not to discontinue drug abruptly
• Not to use OTC products (cough, cold, allergy) unless directed by prescriber; not to use salt substitutes containing potassium without consulting prescriber
• The importance of complying with dosage schedule, even if feeling better
• To rise slowly to sitting or standing position to minimize orthostatic hypotension
• To notify prescriber of mouth sores, sore throat, fever, swelling of hands or feet, irregular heartbeat, chest pain
• To report excessive perspiration, dehydration, vomiting, diarrhea; may lead to fall in B/P
• That drug may cause dizziness, fainting, light-headedness during first few days of therapy
• That drug may cause skin rash or impaired perspiration
• How to take B/P; normal readings for age group

Treatment of overdose: 0.9% NaCl IV INF, hemodialysis

fosphenytoin (R)
(foss-fen'i-toy-in)
Cerebyx
Func. class.: Anticonvulsant
Chem. class.: Hydantoin

Action: Inhibits spread of seizure activity in motor cortex by altering ion transport; increases AV conduction

Uses: Generalized tonic-clonic seizures; status epilepticus

Dosage and routes:

Status epilepticus
• *Adult and child:* **IV** loading dose 15-20 mg PE/kg given at 100-150 mg PE/min

Nonemergent/maintenance dosing
• *Adult and child:* **IV** loading dose 10-20 mg PE/kg; maintenance dosing 4-6 mg PE/kg/day given at a rate of <150 mg PE/min

Available forms: Inj 150 mg (100 mg phenytoin equiv), 750 mg (500 mg phenytoin equiv)

Side effects/adverse reactions:

CNS: Drowsiness, dizziness, insomnia, paresthesias, depression, suicidal tendencies, aggression, headache, confusion

CV: Hypotension, ***ventricular fibrillation***

EENT: Nystagmus, diplopia, blurred vision

GI: Nausea, vomiting, constipation, anorexia, weight loss, hepatitis, jaundice, gingival hyperplasia

GU: Nephritis, urine discoloration

*HEMA: **Agranulocytosis, leukopenia, aplastic anemia, thrombocytopenia, megaloblastic anemia***

INTEG: Rash, lupus erythematosus, ***Stevens-Johnson syndrome,*** hirsutism

SYST: Hypocalcemia

Contraindications: Hypersensitiv-

F

Side effects: *italics* = common; ***bold italics*** = life-threatening

ity, psychiatric conditions, pregnancy (D), bradycardia, SA and AV block, Stokes-Adams syndrome

Precautions: Allergies, hepatic disease, renal disease

Pharmacokinetics: Metabolized by liver, excreted by kidneys

Interactions:

• Decreased effects of fosphenytoin: alcohol (chronic use), antihistamines, antacids, antineoplastics, CNS depressants, rifampin, folic acid, carbamazepine, reserpine, tricyclics

• Increased fosphenytoin level: cimetidine, amiodarone, chloramphenicol, estrogens, H_2 antagonists, phenothiazines, salicylates, sulfonamides

Lab test interferences:

Decrease: Dexamethasone, metyrapone test serum, PBI, urinary steroids

Increase: Glucose, alk phosphatase

NURSING CONSIDERATIONS

Assess:

• Drug level: toxic level 30-50 μg/ml

• Blood studies: CBC, platelets q2 wk until stabilized, then qmo × 12 mo, then q3mo; discontinue drug if neutrophils <1600/mm^3

• Mental status: mood, sensorium, affect, memory (long, short)

• Seizure activity including type, location, duration, and character; provide seizure precaution

• Renal studies; urinalysis, BUN, urine creatine

• Hepatic studies: ALT, AST, bilirubin, creatinine

• Allergic reaction: red raised rash; if this occurs, drug should be discontinued

• For toxicity: bone marrow depression, nausea, vomiting, ataxia, diplopia, cardiovascular collapse, slurred speech, confusion

• Respiratory depression; rate, depth, character of respirations

◆ Blood dyscrasias: fever, sore throat, bruising, rash, jaundice

• Continuous monitoring of ECG, B/P, respiratory function

• Rash, discontinue as soon as rash develops, serious adverse reactions such as Stevens-Johnson syndrome can occur

Administer:

IV

• Dilute in D_5 or 0.9% NaCl 1.5-25 mg PE/ml, give <150 mg PE/min

Y-site compatibilities: Esmolol, famotidine, foscarnet

Additive compatibilities: Potassium chloride

Solution compatibilities: D_5W, $D_{10}W$, amino acid inj 10%, D_5LR, D_5/0.9% NaCl, Plasmalyte A, LR, sterile water for inj

Evaluate:

• Therapeutic response: decrease in severity of seizures

Teach patient/family:

• The reason for and expected outcome of treatment

• Not to use machinery or engage in hazardous activity, as drowsiness, dizziness may occur

• To carry medical ID denoting drug use

• To notify prescriber of rash, bleeding, bruising, slurred speech, jaundice of skin or eyes, joint pain, nausea, vomiting, severe headaches

• To keep all medical appointments, including lab work, physical assessment

---

◆ = Nursing alert   ⫻ = Herb-drug interaction   ⊘ = Do not crush

furosemide (℞)

(fur-oh'se-mide)
Fumide, Furomide M.D., furosemide, Lasix, Luramide, Novosemide*, Uritol*
Func. class.: Loop diuretic
Chem. class.: Sulfonamide derivative

Action: Inhibits reabsorption of sodium and chloride at proximal and distal tubule and in the loop of Henle

Uses: Pulmonary edema; edema in CHF, liver disease, nephrotic syndrome, ascites, hypertension

Investigational uses: Hypercalcemia in malignancy

Dosage and routes:

• *Adult:* **PO** 20-80 mg/day in AM; may give another dose in 6 hr up to 600 mg/day; **IM/IV** 20-40 mg, increased by 20 mg q2h until desired response

• *Child:* **PO/IM/IV** 2 mg/kg; may increase by 1-2 mg/kg/q6-8h up to 6 mg/kg

Pulmonary edema

• *Adult:* **IV** 40 mg given over several min, repeated in 1 hr; increase to 80 mg if needed

Hypertensive crisis/acute renal failure

• *Adult:* **IV** 100-200 mg over 1-2 min

Available forms: Tabs 20, 40, 80 mg; oral sol 10 mg/ml, 40 mg/5 ml; inj 10 mg/ml

Side effects/adverse reactions:

CNS: Headache, fatigue, weakness, vertigo, paresthesias

CV: Orthostatic hypotension, chest pain, ECG changes, *circulatory collapse*

EENT: Loss of hearing, ear pain, tinnitus, blurred vision

ELECT: Hypokalemia, hypochloremic alkalosis, hypomagnesemia, hyperuricemia, hypocalcemia, hyponatremia, metabolic alkalosis

ENDO: Hyperglycemia

GI: Nausea, diarrhea, dry mouth, vomiting, anorexia, cramps, oral, gastric irritations, pancreatitis

*GU: Polyuria, **renal failure,*** glycosuria

*HEMA: **Thrombocytopenia, agranulocytosis, leukopenia, neutropenia, anemia***

INTEG: Rash, pruritus, purpura, ***Stevens-Johnson syndrome,*** sweating, photosensitivity, urticaria

MS: Cramps, stiffness

Contraindications: Hypersensitivity to sulfonamides, anuria, hypovolemia, infants, lactation, electrolyte depletion

Precautions: Diabetes mellitus, dehydration, severe renal disease, pregnancy (C), cirrhosis, ascites

Pharmacokinetics:

PO: Onset 1 hr, peak 1-2 hr, duration 6-8 hr; absorbed 70%

IV: Onset 5 min, peak ½ hr, duration 2 hr (metabolized by the liver 30%) Excreted in urine, some as unchanged drug, feces; crosses placenta; excreted in breast milk; half-life ½-1 hr

Interactions:

• Increased toxicity: lithium, nondepolarizing skeletal muscle relaxants, digitalis

• Increased K action of antihypertensives, oral anticoagulants, nitrates

• Increased ototoxicity: aminoglycosides, cisplatin, vancomycin

• Decreased antihypertensive effect of furosemide: indomethacin, metolazone

Lab test interferences:

Interference: GTT

NURSING CONSIDERATIONS

Assess:

• Signs of metabolic alkalosis: drowsiness, restlessness

- Signs of hypokalemia: postural hypotension, malaise, fatigue, tachycardia, leg cramps, weakness
- Rashes, temp elevation qd
- Confusion, especially in elderly; take safety precautions if needed
- Hearing, including tinnitus and hearing loss, when giving high doses for extended periods
- Weight, I&O qd to determine fluid loss; effect of drug may be decreased if used qd
- Rate, depth, rhythm of respiration, effect of exertion, lung sounds
- B/P lying, standing; postural hypotension may occur
- Electrolytes: K, Na, Cl; include BUN, blood sugar, CBC, serum creatinine, blood pH, ABGs, uric acid, Ca, Mg
- Skin turgor, edema, condition of mucous membranes in mouth and nose
- Glucose in urine if patient is diabetic
- Allergies to sulfonamides, thiazides

Administer:
- In AM to avoid interference with sleep if using drug as a diuretic
- K replacement if K <3 mg/dL
- PO with food if nausea occurs; absorption may be decreased slightly; tabs may be crushed

IV
- Undiluted; may be given through Y-tube or 3-way stopcock; give 20 mg or less/min; may be added to NS or D_5W if large doses are required and given as IV INF, not to exceed 4 mg/min; use infusion pump

Additive compatibilities: Amikacin, aminophylline, ampicillin, atropine, bumetanide, calcium gluconate, cefamandole, cefoperazone, cefuroxime, cimetidine, cloxacillin, dexamethasone, diamorphine, digoxin, epinephrine, heparin, isosorbide, kanamycin, lidocaine, meropenem, morphine, nitroglycerin, penicillin G, potassium chloride, ranitidine, scopolamine, sodium bicarbonate, theophylline, tobramycin, verapamil

Syringe compatibilities: Bleomycin, cisplatin, cyclophosphamide, fluorouracil, heparin, leucovorin, methotrexate, mitomycin

Y-site compatibilities: Allopurinol, amifostine, amikacin, amphotericin B cholesteryl, aztreonam, bleomycin, cefepime, cefmetazole, cisplatin, cladribine, cyclophosphamide, cytarabine, doxorubicin liposome, epinephrine, fentanyl, fludarabine, fluorouracil, foscarnet, gallium, granisetron, heparin, hydrocortisone, hydromorphone, indomethacin, kanamycin, leucovorin, lorazepam, melphalan, meropenem, methotrexate, mitomycin, nitroglycerin, norepinephrine, paclitaxel, piperacillin/tazobactam, potassium chloride, propofol, ranitidine, remifentanil, sargramostim, tacrolimus, teniposide, thiotepa, tobramycin, tolazoline, vit B/C

Evaluate:
- Therapeutic response: improvement in edema of feet, legs, sacral area daily if medication is being used for CHF

Teach patient/family:
- To discuss the need for a high-K diet or K replacement with prescriber
- To increase fluid intake 2-3 L/day unless contraindicated
- To rise slowly from lying or sitting position; orthostatic hypotension may occur
- To recognize adverse reactions that may occur: muscle cramps, weakness, nausea, dizziness
- Regarding entire regimen, including exercise, diet, stress relief for hypertension

• To take with food or milk for GI symptoms
• To use sunscreen or protective clothing to prevent photosensitivity
• To take early in day to prevent sleeplessness
• To avoid OTC medication unless directed by prescriber

Treatment of overdose: Lavage if taken orally; monitor electrolytes; administer dextrose in saline; monitor hydration, CV, renal status

---

gabapentin (R)

(gab'a-pen-tin)
Neurontin
Func. class.: Anticonvulsant

Action: Mechanism unknown; may increase seizure threshold; structurally similar to GABA; gabapentin binding sites in neocortex, hippocampus

Uses: Adjunct treatment of partial seizures, with or without generalization in adults

Investigational uses: Chronic pain

Dosage and routes:
• *Adult:* **PO** 900-1800 mg/day in 3 divided doses; may titrate by giving 300 mg on the first day, 300 mg bid on second day, 300 mg tid on third day; may increase to 1800 mg/day by adding 300 mg on subsequent days

Available forms: Caps 100, 300, 400 mg

Side effects/adverse reactions:

CNS: Dizziness, fatigue, anxiety, somnolence, ataxia, amnesia, abnormal thinking, unsteady gait, depression

CV: Vasodilation

EENT: Dry mouth, blurred vision, diplopia

GI: Constipation, increased appetite, dental abnormalities

GU: Impotence, bleeding, *UTI*

HEMA: **Leukopenia,** decreased WBC

INTEG: Pruritus, abrasion

MS: Myalgia

RESP: Rhinitis, pharyngitis, coughing

Contraindications: Hypersensitivity to this drug

Precautions: Hepatic disease, renal disease, pregnancy (C), lactation, children <12 yr, elderly

Pharmacokinetics: Largely unbound to plasma proteins; not metabolized; excreted in urine (unchanged); elimination half-life 5-7 hr

Interactions:
• Decreased levels of gabapentin: antacids

Lab test interferences:

False-positive: Urinary protein using Ames N-multistix SG

NURSING CONSIDERATIONS

Assess:
• Renal studies: urinalysis, BUN, urine creatinine q3mo
• Hepatic studies: ALT, AST, bilirubin
• Description of seizures; location, duration, characteristics
• Mental status: mood, sensorium, affect, behavioral changes; if mental status changes, notify prescriber
• Eye problems, need for ophthalmic examinations before, during, after treatment (slit lamp, fundoscopy, tonometry)
• Allergic reaction: purpura, red raised rash; if these occur, drug should be discontinued
• Pain: location, duration, characteristics if using for chronic pain

Administer:
• At least 2 hr pc with antacids
• Caps may be opened and contents put in applesauce or dissolved in juice

Perform/provide:
• Storage at room temp away from heat and light

Side effects: *italics* = common; ***bold italics*** = life-threatening

• Hard candy, frequent rinsing of mouth, gum for dry mouth

• Assistance with ambulation during early part of treatment; dizziness occurs

• Seizure precautions: padded side rails; move objects that may harm patient

• Increased fluids, bulk in diet for constipation

Evaluate:

• Therapeutic response: decreased seizure activity; decrease in chronic pain

Teach patient/family:

• To carry Medic Alert ID stating patient's name, drugs taken, condition, prescriber's name and phone number

• To avoid driving, other activities that require alertness: dizziness, drowsiness may occur

• Not to discontinue medication quickly after long-term use, taper over ≥1 wk

🚫 Not to crush or chew caps

Treatment of overdose: Lavage, VS

---

gallamine (℞)

(gal'a-meen)
Flaxedil

Func. class.: Neuromuscular blocker (nondepolarizing)

Action: Inhibits transmission of nerve impulses by binding with cholinergic receptor sites, antagonizing action of acetylcholine

Uses: Facilitation of endotracheal intubation, skeletal muscle relaxation during mechanical ventilation, surgery, general anesthesia

Dosage and routes:

• *Adult and child >1 mo:* **IV** 1 mg/kg, not to exceed 100 mg, then 0.5-1 mg/kg q30-40min

• *Child <1 mo, >5 kg:* **IV** 0.25-0.75 mg/kg, then 0.01-0.05 mg/kg q30-40min

Available forms: Inj 20 mg/ml

Side effects/adverse reactions:

CV: Bradycardia, tachycardia, increased, decreased B/P

*RESP: **Prolonged apnea, bronchospasm, cyanosis, respiratory depression***

EENT: Increased secretions

INTEG: Rash, flushing, pruritus, urticaria

*CNS: **Malignant hyperthermia***

GI: Decreased motility

Contraindications: Hypersensitivity to iodides

Precautions: Pregnancy (C), thyroid disease, collagen disease, cardiac disease, lactation, children <2 yr, electrolyte imbalances, dehydration, neuromuscular disease (myasthenia gravis), respiratory disease, renal disease

Pharmacokinetics:

IV: Onset 2 min, duration 20-30 min; half-life 2 min, 29 min (terminal); excreted in urine, feces (metabolites); crosses placenta

Interactions:

• Increased neuromuscular blockade: aminoglycosides, clindamycin, lincomycin, quinidine, local anesthetics, polymyxin antibiotics, lithium, narcotic analgesics, thiazides, enflurane, isoflurane; used with cyclopropane, may provoke ventricular dysrhythmias

• Dysrhythmias: theophylline

• Incompatible with anesthetics, barbiturates in sol; incompatible with any other drug in syringe

NURSING CONSIDERATIONS

Assess:

• For electrolyte imbalances (K, Mg); may lead to increased action of this drug

• Vital signs (B/P, pulse, respirations, airway) q15min until fully re-

---

◆ = Nursing alert   🍃 = Herb-drug interaction   🚫 = Do not crush

covered; rate, depth, pattern of respirations, strength of hand grip
• I&O ratio; check for urinary retention, frequency, hesitancy
• Recovery: decreased paralysis of face, diaphragm, leg, arm, rest of body
• Allergic reactions: rash, fever, respiratory distress, pruritus; drug should be discontinued

Administer:
• Using nerve stimulator by anesthesiologist to determine neuromuscular blockade
• Anticholinesterase to reverse neuromuscular blockade
• IV undiluted over 1-2 min (only by qualified person, usually an anesthesiologist)
• Only slightly discolored sol

Perform/provide:
• Storage in light-resistant, cool area
• Reassurance if communication is difficult during recovery from neuromuscular blockade

Evaluate:
• Therapeutic response: paralysis of jaw, eyelid, head, neck, rest of body

Treatment of overdose: Edrophonium or neostigmine, atropine; monitor VS; may require mechanical ventilation

gallium (R̶)
(gal'ee-um)
Ganite
Func. class.: Electrolyte modifier
Chem. class.: Hypocalcemic drug

Action: Lowers serum calcium levels by inhibiting calcium resorption from bone
Uses: Cancer-related hypercalcemia

Dosage and routes:
• *Adult:* **IV** 100-200 mg/m^2 qd × 5 days; infuse over 24 hr
Available forms: 25 mg/ml inj
Side effects/adverse reactions:
HEMA: **Anemia, leukopenia**
CV: Tachycardia
EENT: Blurred vision, optic neuritis, hearing loss
GU: **Nephrotoxicity,** increased BUN, creatinine
META: *Hypophosphatemia,* hypocalcemia, decreased serum bicarbonate
Contraindications: Hypersensitivity, severe renal disease
Precautions: Pregnancy (C), lactation, children, mild renal disease
Pharmacokinetics:
IV: Onset 12-24 hr, peak 5 days, duration 8 days
Interactions:
• Increased nephrotoxicity: aminoglycosides, amphotericin B

NURSING CONSIDERATIONS
Assess:
• Renal status: BUN, creatinine, urine output; if creatinine level is 2.5 mg/dl or more, drug should be discontinued
• Monitor Ca, phosphate, bicarbonate, since all levels may be decreased and supplements of phosphate may be needed
• For hypercalcemia: nausea, vomiting, fatigue, weakness, thirst, dehydration, dysrhythmias, change in mental status
• For hypocalcemia: dysrhythmias; paresthesia; twitching; colic; laryngospasm; Trousseau's, Chvostek's sign; tremors
• For hypophosphatemia: confusion, decreased reflexes, joint stiffness and pain, portal hypotension

Administer:
IV
• Adequate hydration with IV saline, 2 L/day during treatment

• After dilution of dose/1 L 0.9% NaCl or D_5W, run over 24 hr, use infusion pump

Y-site compatibilities: Acyclovir, allopurinol, amifostine, aminophylline, ampicillin/sulbactam, aztreonam, cefazolin, ceftazidime, ceftriaxone, cimetidine, ciprofloxacin, cladribine, cyclophosphamide, dexamethasone, diphenhydramine, filgrastim, fluconazole, furosemide, granisetron, heparin, hydrocortisone, ifosfamide, magnesium sulfate, mannitol, melphalan, meperidine, mesna, methotrexate, metoclopramide, ondansetron, piperacillin, piperacillin/tazobactam, potassium chloride, ranitidine, sodium bicarbonate, teniposide, thiotepa, ticarcillin/clavulanate, trimethoprim-sulfamethoxazole, vancomycin, vinorelbine

Perform/provide:

• Storage of solution 48 hr at room temp, 1 wk in refrigerator

Evaluate:

• Therapeutic response: decreased serum Ca levels

Teach patient/family:

• To follow dietary guidelines given by prescriber, including adequate Ca (dairy products, broccoli) and vit D (fortified milk, grain products, fish oil)

---

ganciclovir (DHPG) (Ŗ)
(gan-sye′kloe-vir)
Cytovene, Vitrasert
Func. class.: Antiviral
Chem. class.: Synthetic nucleoside analog

Action: Inhibits replication of herpesviruses in vitro, in vivo by selective inhibition of the human CMV DNA polymerase and by direct incorporation into viral DNA

Uses: Cytomegalovirus (CMV) retinitis in immunocompromised persons, including those with AIDS, after indirect ophthalmoscopy confirms diagnosis

Dosage and routes:

• Reduce dose in renal disease CrCl <70 ml/min

Prevention of CMV

• *Adult:* **IV** 5 mg/kg q12h × 1-2 wk, then 5 mg/kg/day or 6 mg/kg × 5 days/wk

Induction treatment

• *Adult:* **IV** 5 mg/kg given over 1 hr, q12h × 2-3 wk

Maintenance treatment

• *Adult:* **IV INF** 5 mg/kg given over 1 hr, qd × 7 days/wk; or 6 mg/kg qd × 5 days/wk; **INTRAVITERAL** 200 μg qwk; **PO** 1000 mg tid with food or 500 mg q3h while awake

• Dosage must be reduced in renal impairment

Available forms: Powder 500 mg/vial; caps 250, 500 mg; implant, intraviteral 4.5 mg

Side effects/adverse reactions:

*HEMA: **Granulocytopenia, thrombocytopenia, irreversible neutropenia, anemia, eosinophilia***

*GI: Abnormal LFTs, nausea, vomiting, anorexia, diarrhea, abdominal pain, **hemorrhage***

INTEG: Rash, alopecia, pruritus, urticaria, pain at site, phlebitis

*CNS: Fever, chills, **coma**, confusion, abnormal thoughts, dizziness, bizarre dreams, headache, psychosis, tremors, somnolence, paresthesia, weakness, **seizures***

CV: Dysrhythmia, hypertension/hypotension

RESP: Dyspnea

EENT: Retinal detachment in CMV retinitis

*GU: **Hematuria**, increased creatinine, BUN*

Contraindications: Hypersensitivity to acyclovir or ganciclovir, absolute neutrophil count <500, platelet count <25,000

Precautions: Preexisting cytopenias, renal function impairment, pregnancy (C), lactation, children <6 mo, elderly

Pharmacokinetics: Half-life 3-4½ hr; excreted by kidneys (unchanged); crosses blood-brain barrier, CSF

Interactions:

• Decreased renal clearance of ganciclovir: probenecid

• Increased toxicity: dapsone, pentamidine, flucytosine, vincristine, vinblastine, adriamycin, doxorubicin, amphotericin B, trimethoprim-sulfa combinations, or other nucleoside analogs, cyclosporine

• Severe granulocytopenia: zidovudine; do not give together

• Increased seizures: imipenem/cilastatin

NURSING CONSIDERATIONS

Assess:

• For leukopenia/neutropenia/thrombocytopenia: WBCs, platelets q2d during 2 ×/d dosing and then q1wk

• For leukopenia with qd WBC count in patients with prior leukopenia with other nucleoside analogs or for whom leukopenia counts are <1000 cells/mm³ at start of treatment

• Serum creatinine or CrCl ≥ q2wk

Administer:

PO

• With food

IV

• Mixed in biologic cabinet, using gown, gloves, mask

• IV after diluting 500 mg/10 ml sterile H₂O for injection (50 mg/ml); shake; further dilute in 100 ml D₅W, 0.9% NaCl, LR and run over 1 hr; use infusion pump

• Slowly; do not give by bolus IV, IM, SC injection

• Using diluted sol within 12 hr; do not refrigerate or freeze

Y-site compatibilities: Allopurinol, amphotericin B cholesteryl, cisplatin, cyclophosphamide, doxorubicin liposome, enalaprilat, filgrastim, fluconazole, granisetron, melphalan, methotrexate, paclitaxel, propofol, remifentanil, tacrolimus, teniposide, thiotepa

Evaluate:

• Therapeutic response: decreased symptoms of CMV

Teach patient/family:

• That drug does not cure condition, that regular ophthalmologic examinations are necessary

• That major toxicities may necessitate discontinuing drug

• To use contraception during treatment and that infertility may occur; men should use barrier contraception for 90 days after treatment

• To take PO with food

• To report infection: fever, chills, sore throat; blood dyscrasias: bruising, bleeding, petechiae

• To avoid crowds, persons with respiratory infections

• To use sunscreen to prevent burns

---

ganirelix
See appendix a—selected new drugs

---

gatifloxacin
See appendix a—selected new drugs

---

gemcitabine (R)
(jem-sit′a-been)
Gemzar
Func class: Misc. antineoplastic
Chem class: Nucleoside analog

Action: Exhibits antitumor activity by killing cells undergoing DNA

Side effects: *italics* = common; ***bold italics*** = life-threatening

synthesis (S-phase) and blocking G1/ S-phase boundary

Uses: Adenocarcinoma of the pancreas (nonresectable Stage II, III, or metastatic Stage IV); non–small cell lung cancer (Stage IIIA or B, IV); in combination with cisplatin for inoperable, advanced, or metastatic non–small cell lung cancer

Dosage and routes:

• *Adult:* IV 1000 mg/m^2 given over ½ hr qwk × 7 wk, then 1 wk rest period; subsequent cycles should be infused once qwk × 3 wk out of every 4 wk

Non–small cell lung cancer
4-wk schedule:

• *Adult:* IV 1000 mg/m^2 given over ½ hr on days 1, 8, 15, of each 28-day cycle. Give cisplatin **IV** 100 mg/m^2 on day 1 after gemcitabine
3-wk schedule:

• *Adult:* IV 1250 mg/m^2 given over ½ hr on days 1, 8 of each 21-day cycle. Give cisplatin 100 mg/m^2 after the inf of gemcitabine on day 1

Available forms: Lyophilized powder 20 mg/ml

Side effects/adverse reactions:
GI: Diarrhea, nausea, vomiting, anorexia, constipation, stomatitis
INTEG: Irritation at site, rash, alopecia
HEMA: **Leukopenia, anemia, neutropenia, thrombocytopenia**
OTHER: Dyspnea, fever, **hemorrhage**, infection

Contraindications: Hypersensitivity, pregnancy (D)

Precautions: Lactation, children, elderly, myelosuppression, irradiation

Pharmacokinetics: Half-life 42-79 min

Interactions:

• Increased bleeding: NSAIDs, alcohol, salicylates

• Increased myelosuppression, di-

arrhea: other antineoplastics, radiation

NURSING CONSIDERATIONS
Assess:

• CBC, differential, platelet count weekly; withhold drug if WBC is <3500/mm^3, or platelet count <100,000/mm^3; notify prescriber of these results; drug should be discontinued

• Blood dyscrasias: bruising, bleeding, petechiae

• I&O nutritional intake

• Hepatic/renal studies

• Food preferences: list likes, dislikes

• Buccal cavity q8h for dryness, sores, or ulceration, white patches, oral pain, bleeding, dysphagia

• GI symptoms: frequency of stools; cramping

• Signs of dehydration: rapid respirations, poor skin turgor, decreased urine output, dry skin, restlessness, weakness

Administer:
IV

• After reconstituting with 0.9% NaCl 5 ml/200 mg vial of drug or 25 ml/1 g of drug, shake = 40 mg/ml may be further diluted with 0.9% NaCl to conc as low as 0.1 mg/ml

Perform/provide:

• Increased fluid intake to 2-3 L/day to prevent dehydration, unless contraindicated

• Changing of IV site q48h

• Rinsing of mouth tid-qid with water, club soda; brushing of teeth bid-tid with soft brush or cotton-tipped applicator for stomatitis; use unwaxed dental floss

• Nutritious diet with iron, vitamin supplement, low fiber, few dairy products

Evaluate:

• Therapeutic response: decrease in tumor size, decrease in spread of cancer

---

Teach patient/family:

• To avoid foods with citric acid or hot or rough texture if stomatitis is present; to drink adequate fluids

• To avoid use with NSAIDs, alcohol, salicylates

• To report stomatitis; any bleeding, white spots, ulcerations in mouth; tell patient to examine mouth qd, report symptoms

• To report signs of anemia: fatigue, headache, faintness, shortness of breath, irritability

• To use contraception during therapy

Treatment of overdose: Induce vomiting, provide supportive care

---

gemfibrozil (℞)

(jem-fi′broe-zil)
Lopid
Func. class.: Antilipemic
Chem. class.: Aryloxisobutyric acid derivative

Action: Inhibits biosynthesis of VLDL, decreases triglycerides, increases HDL

Uses: Type II, III/IV, V hyperlipidemia as adjunct with diet therapy

Dosage and routes:

• *Adult:* **PO** 1200 mg in divided doses bid 30 min before meals

Available forms: Tabs 600 mg; caps 300 mg*

Side effects/adverse reactions:

GI: Nausea, vomiting, dyspepsia, diarrhea, abdominal pain

INTEG: Rash, urticaria, pruritus

HEMA: **Leukopenia, anemia, eosinophilia, thrombocytopenia**

CNS: Dizziness, blurred vision

MISC: Taste perversion

Contraindications: Severe hepatic disease, preexisting gallbladder disease, severe renal disease, primary biliary cirrhosis, hypersensitivity

Precautions: Monitor hematologic and hepatic function, pregnancy (C), lactation

Pharmacokinetics:

PO: Peak 1-2 hr; plasma protein binding >90%; half-life 1½ hr; excreted in urine; metabolized in liver

Interactions:

• May increase anticoagulant properties: oral anticoagulants

• Increased risk of myositis, myalgia: lovastatin

Lab test interferences:

Increase: Liver function studies, CPK, BSP, thymol turbidity, glucose

Decrease: Hgb, Hct, WBC

NURSING CONSIDERATIONS

Assess:

• Triglycerides, cholesterol; if cholesterol increases, drug should be discontinued

• Renal studies, LFTs, CBC if patient is on long-term therapy; if LFTs increase, therapy should be discontinued

• Bowel pattern daily; increase bulk, water in diet if constipation develops, especially in elderly

Administer:

PO

• 30 min before morning and evening meals

Evaluate:

• Therapeutic response: decreased cholesterol, triglyceride levels

Teach patient/family:

• That compliance is needed for positive results; do not double or skip dose

• That risk factors should be decreased: high-fat diet, smoking, alcohol consumption, absence of exercise

• To notify prescriber of diarrhea, nausea, vomiting, chills, fever, sore throat

🚫 Not to break, crush, or chew caps

---

gentamicin (R)

(jen-ta-mye'sin)
Alcomicin*, Apogen*, Cidomycin*, Garamycin, Garamycin Intrathecal, Garamycin IV Piggyback, Garamycin Pediatric, gentamicin sulfate, Gentamicin Sulfate IV Piggyback, Jenamicin, Pediatric Gentamicin Sulfate

Func. class.: Antiinfective
Chem. class.: Aminoglycoside

Action: Interferes with protein synthesis in bacterial cell by binding to ribosomal subunit, causing misreading of genetic code; inaccurate peptide sequence forms in protein chain, causing bacterial death

Uses: Severe systemic infections of CNS, respiratory, GI, urinary tract, bone, skin, soft tissues caused by susceptible strains of *Proteus aeruginosa, Proteus, Klebsiella, Serratia, Escherichia coli, Enterobacter, Citrobacter, Staphylococcus, Shigella, Salmonella, Acinetobacter,* acute PID

Dosage and routes:
Severe systemic infections
• *Adult:* **IV INF** 3-5 mg/kg/day in 3 divided doses q8h; dilute in 50-200 ml **NS** or D₅W given over 30 min-1 hr; **IM** 3 mg/kg/day in divided doses q8h
• *Adult:* **INTRATHECAL** 4-8 mg qd
• *Child:* **IV/IM** 2-2.5 mg/kg q8h
• *Neonate and infant:* **IV/IM** 2.5 mg/kg q8-12h
• *Neonate <1 wk:* 2.5 mg/kg q12-24h
• *Infant and child >3 mo:* **INTRATHECAL** 1-2 mg qd
Once daily dosing/extended interval dosing
• *Adult:* **IV** 5-7 mg/kg/dose, adjust according to levels

Dental/respiratory procedures, GI/GU surgery (prophylaxis endocarditis)
• *Adult:* **IM** 1.5 mg/kg ½-1 hr before procedure with ampicillin
• *Child:* **IM** 2.5 mg/kg ½-1 hr before procedure with ampicillin
Available forms: Inj 10, 40, 60, 80, 100 mg; intrathecal 2 mg/ml
Side effects/adverse reactions:
GU: **Oliguria, hematuria, renal damage, azotemia, renal failure, nephrotoxicity**
CNS: Confusion, depression, numbness, tremors, **convulsions,** muscle twitching, **neurotoxicity,** dizziness, vertigo
EENT: **Ototoxicity,** deafness, visual disturbances, tinnitus
HEMA: **Agranulocytosis, thrombocytopenia, leukopenia, eosinophilia,** anemia
GI: Nausea, vomiting, anorexia; increased ALT, AST, bilirubin; hepatomegaly, **hepatic necrosis,** splenomegaly
CV: Hypotension, hypertension, palpitations
INTEG: Rash, burning, urticaria, dermatitis, alopecia
Contraindications: Severe renal disease, hypersensitivity
Precautions: Neonates, mild renal disease, pregnancy (C), hearing deficits, myasthenia gravis, lactation, elderly, Parkinson's disease
Pharmacokinetics:
IM: Onset rapid, peak 1-2 hr
IV: Onset immediate, peak 1-2 hr; plasma half-life 1-2 hr, infants 6-7 hr; duration 6-8 hr; not metabolized; excreted unchanged in urine; crosses placental barrier; poor penetration into CSF
Interactions:
• Increased ototoxicity, neurotoxicity, nephrotoxicity: other aminogly-

---

◆ = Nursing alert   ∥ = Herb-drug interaction   ⊘ = Do not crush

cosides, amphotericin B, polymyxin, vancomycin, ethacrynic acid, furosemide, mannitol, methoxyflurane, cisplatin, cephalosporins, penicillins

• Increased effects: nondepolarizing neuromuscular blockers

NURSING CONSIDERATIONS
Assess:

• Weight before treatment; calculation of dosage is usually based on ideal body weight, but may be calculated on actual body weight

• I&O ratio, urinalysis daily for proteinuria, cells, casts; report sudden change in urine output; toxicity is increased in patients with decreased renal function if high doses are given

• VS during infusion; watch for hypotension, change in pulse

• IV site for thrombophlebitis, including pain, redness, swelling, q30min, change site if needed; discontinue, apply warm compresses to site

• Serum peak, drawn at 30-60 min after IV INF or 60 min after IM inj, and trough level drawn just before next dose; blood level should be 2-4 times bacteriostatic level; peak = 4-12 µg/ml, trough = 1-2 µg/ml

• Urine pH if drug is used for UTI; urine should be kept alkaline

• Renal impairment by securing urine for CrCl testing, BUN, serum creatinine; lower dosage should be given in renal impairment (CrCl <80 ml/min)

• Deafness by audiometric testing, ringing, roaring in ears, vertigo; assess hearing before, during, after treatment

• Dehydration: high specific gravity, decrease in skin turgor, dry mucous membranes, dark urine

• Overgrowth of infection including fever, malaise, redness, pain, swelling, perineal itching, diarrhea, stomatitis, change in cough or sputum

• C&S before starting treatment to identify infecting organism

• Vestibular dysfunction: nausea, vomiting, dizziness, headache; drug should be discontinued if severe

• Injection sites for redness, swelling, abscesses; use warm compresses at site

Administer:

• IM inj in large muscle mass; rotate injection sites

• Drug in evenly spaced doses to maintain blood level

• Bicarbonate to alkalinize urine if ordered for UTI, as drug is most active in alkaline environment

IV

• After diluting in 50-200 ml NS or D_5W; sol concentration should be 1 mg/ml or less; decrease vol of diluent in child; maintain 0.1% sol run over ½-1 hr (adults) or up to 2 hr (children); flush IV line with NS or D_5W after administration

Additive compatibilities: Atracurium, aztreonam, bleomycin, cefoxitin, cimetidine, ciprofloxacin, fluconazole, meropenem, methicillin, metronidazole, ofloxacin, penicillin G sodium, ranitidine, verapamil

Syringe compatibilities: Clindamycin, methicillin, penicillin G sodium

Y-site compatibilities: Acyclovir, amifostine, amiodarone, amsacrine, atracurium, aztreonam, cefpirome, ciprofloxacin, cyclophosphamide, cytarabine, diltiazem, enalaprilat, esmolol, famotidine, filgrastim, fluconazole, fludarabine, foscarnet, granisetron, hydromorphone, IL-2, insulin, labetalol, lorazepam, magnesium sulfate, melphalan, meperidine, meropenem, midazolam, morphine, multivitamins, ondansetron, paclitaxel, pancuronium, perphenazine, sargramostim, tacrolimus, teniposide, theophylline, thiotepa, tolazine, vecuronium, vinorelbine, vit B/C, zidovudine

Perform/provide:

• Adequate fluids of 2-3 L/day, unless contraindicated, to prevent irritation of tubules

• Supervised ambulation, other safety measures with vestibular dysfunction

Evaluate:

• Therapeutic response: absence of fever, draining wounds, negative C&S after treatment

Teach patient/family:

• To report headache, dizziness, symptoms of overgrowth of infection, renal impairment

• To report loss of hearing, ringing, roaring in ears, or feeling of fullness in head

---

glatiramer (℞)
(glah-tear′a-meer)
Copaxone
Func. class.: MS agent

Action: Unknown, may modify the immune responses responsible for multiple sclerosis

Uses: Reduction of the frequency of relapses in patients with relapsing-remitting multiple sclerosis

Dosage and routes:

• *Adult:* **SC** 20 mg/day

Available forms: Inj 20 mg/ml

Side effects/adverse reactions:

CV: Migraine, palpitations, syncope, tachycardia, vasodilation

GI: Nausea, vomiting, diarrhea, anorexia, gastroenteritis

HEMA: Ecchymosis, lymphadenopathy

META: Edema, weight gain

MS: Arthralgia

CNS: Anxiety, hypertonia, tremor, vertigo, speech disorder, agitation, confusion

RESP: Bronchitis, dyspnea

INTEG: Pruritus, rash, sweating, urticaria, erythema

EENT: Ear pain

GU: Urinary urgency, dysmenorrhea, vaginal moniliasis

Contraindications: Hypersensitivity to this drug or mannitol

Precautions: Immune disorders, renal disease, pregnancy (B), lactation

Pharmacokinetics: Unknown

NURSING CONSIDERATIONS

Assess:

• Blood, renal, hepatic studies: prior to treatment

• For CNS symptoms: anxiety, confusion, vertigo

• GI status: diarrhea, vomiting, abdominal pain, gastroenteritis

• Cardiac status: tachycardia, palpitations, vasodilation, chest pain

Administer:

• SC route

• Using a sterile syringe/needle to transfer the supplied diluent into the vial, rotate vial gently, do not shake; withdraw medication using a syringe with 27 G needle; administer SC into hip, thigh, arm; discard unused portion

• Use SC route only; do not give IM or IV

• Do not use sol that contains precipitate or is discolored

• Use immediately

Evaluate:

• Therapeutic response: decreased symptoms of multiple sclerosis

Teach patient/family:

• Give written, detailed instructions about the drug; provide initial and return demonstrations on inj procedure; give information on use and disposal of drug

• That blurred vision, sweating may occur

◆ = Nursing alert   ∥ = Herb-drug interaction   ⊘ = Do not crush

- That irregular menses, dysmenorrhea, or metrorrhagia as well as breast pain may occur; use contraception during treatment
- That if pregnancy is suspected, or if nursing, notify prescriber
- Not to change dosing or to stop taking drug without advice of prescriber

glipizide (℞)
(glip-i'zide)
Glucotrol, Glucotrol XL
glimepiride
(glye-me'pi-ride)
Amaryl
Func. class: Antidiabetic
Chem. class.: Sulfonylurea
(2nd generation)

Action: Causes functioning β-cells in pancreas to release insulin, leading to drop in blood glucose levels; may improve insulin binding to insulin receptors or increase the number of insulin receptors with prolonged administration; may also reduce basal hepatic glucose secretion; not effective if patient lacks functioning β-cells

Uses: Stable adult-onset diabetes mellitus (type II) NIDDM
Dosage and routes:
Glipizide
- *Adult:* PO 5 mg initially, then increase to desired response; max 40 mg/day in divided doses or 15 mg/dose
- *Elderly/hepatic disease:* PO 2.5 mg initially, then increase to desired response; max 40 mg/day in divided doses or 15 mg/dose
Glimepiride
- *Adult:* PO 1-2 mg qd, then increase q1-2wk up to 8 mg/day
Renal dose:
Adult: PO 1 mg qd with breakfast, may titrate upward as needed

Available forms: glipizide: tabs 5, 10 mg scored; ext rel tab 10 mg; glimepiride: tabs 1, 2, 4 mg
Side effects/adverse reactions:
CNS: Headache, weakness, dizziness, drowsiness, tinnitus, fatigue, vertigo
*GI: **Hepatotoxicity, cholestatic jaundice,** nausea, vomiting, diarrhea,* heartburn
*HEMA: **Leukopenia, thrombocytopenia, agranulocytosis, aplastic anemia;** increased AST, ALT, alk phosphatase; **pancytopenia, hemolytic anemia***
INTEG: Rash, allergic reactions, pruritus, urticaria, eczema, photosensitivity, erythema
*ENDO: **Hypoglycemia***
Contraindications: Hypersensitivity to sulfonylureas, juvenile or brittle diabetes
Precautions: Pregnancy (C), elderly, cardiac disease, severe renal disease, severe hepatic disease, thyroid disease
Pharmacokinetics:
PO: Completely absorbed by GI route, onset 1-1½ hr, peak 1-3 hr, duration 10-24 hr, half-life 2-4 hr; metabolized in liver; excreted in urine; 90%-95% is plasma protein bound
Interactions:
- Increased action of: digitalis, glycosides
- Increased hypoglycemic effects: insulin, MAOIs, cimetidine, chloramphenicol, guanethidine, methyldopa, nonsteroidal antiinflammatories, salicylates, probenecid, androgens, anticoagulants, clofibrate, fenfluramine, fluconazole, gemfibrozil, histamine H_2 antagonists, magnesium salts, phenylbutazone, sulfinpyrazone, sulfonamides, tricyclic antidepressants, urinary acidifiers

• Effectiveness may be decreased: thiazide diuretics, rifampin, isoniazid, beta-blockers, cholestyramine, diazoxide, hydantoins, urinary alkalinizers, charcoal

◢ Decreased hypoglycemic effect: broom, buchu, dandelion, juniper

◢ Increased or decreased hypoglycemic effect: chromium, fenugreek, ginseng

◢ Increased glucose tolerance: karela

NURSING CONSIDERATIONS
Assess:
• Blood, urine glucose levels during treatment to determine diabetes control
• Hypo/hyperglycemic reaction that can occur soon after meals

Administer:
• Drug 30 min before meals

Perform/provide:
• Storage in tight, light-resistant container at room temp

Evaluate:
• Therapeutic response: decrease in polyuria, polydipsia, polyphagia, clear sensorium, absence of dizziness, stable gait

Teach patient/family:
• Not to drink alcohol; explain disulfiram reaction
• To check for symptoms of cholestatic jaundice: dark urine, pruritus, yellow sclera; prescriber should be notified
• To use a capillary blood glucose test while on this drug
• To test blood glucose levels tid
• The symptoms of hypo/hyperglycemia, what to do about each; to have glucagon emergency kit available
• That drug must be continued on daily basis; explain consequence of discontinuing drug abruptly
• To take drug in morning to prevent hypoglycemic reactions at night

• To avoid OTC medications unless ordered by prescriber
• That diabetes is a lifelong illness; drug will not cure disease
• That all food in diet plan must be eaten to prevent hypoglycemia
• To carry Medic Alert ID for emergency purposes
• To test urine for glucose/ketones tid if this drug is replacing insulin
• To continue weight control, dietary restrictions, exercise, hygiene

Treatment of overdose: Glucose 25 g IV via dextrose 50% solution 50 ml or 1 mg glucagon

---

glyburide (℞)
(glye′byoor-ide)
DiaBeta*, Euglucon*, Glynase PresTab, Micronase
Func. class.: Antidiabetic
Chem. class.: Sulfonylurea (2nd generation)

Action: Causes functioning β-cells in pancreas to release insulin, leading to drop in blood glucose levels; may improve insulin binding to insulin receptors and increase number of insulin receptors with prolonged administration; may also reduce basal hepatic glucose secretion; not effective if patient lacks functioning β-cells

Uses: Stable adult-onset diabetes mellitus (type II) NIDDM

Dosage and routes:
DiaBeta/Micronase
• *Adult:* **PO** 2.5-5 mg initially, then increased to desired response
• *Elderly:* **PO** 1.25 mg initially, then increased to desired response; max 20 mg/day, maintenance 1.25-20 mg/qd; tabs, micronized
Glynase PresTab
• *Adult:* **PO** 1.5-3 mg/day initially, may increase by 1.5 mg/wk

---

◆ = Nursing alert   *◢* = Herb-drug interaction   ◐ = Do not crush

• *Elderly:* **PO** 0.75-3 mg/day, may increase by 1.5 mg/wk

Available forms: Tabs 1.25, 2.5, 3, 5 mg; (Glynase PresTab) 1.5, 3, 6 mg

Side effects/adverse reactions:

CNS: Headache, weakness, paresthesia, tinnitus, fatigue, vertigo

GI: Nausea, fullness, heartburn, *hepatotoxicity, cholestatic jaundice,* vomiting, diarrhea

*HEMA: **Leukopenia, thrombocytopenia, agranulocytosis, aplastic anemia,*** increased AST, ALT, alk phosphatase

INTEG: Rash, allergic reactions, pruritus, urticaria, eczema, photosensitivity, erythema

*ENDO: **Hypoglycemia***

MS: Joint pain

Contraindications: Hypersensitivity to sulfonylureas, juvenile or brittle diabetes

Precautions: Pregnancy (B), elderly, cardiac disease, severe renal disease, severe hepatic disease, thyroid disease, severe hypoglycemic reactions

Pharmacokinetics:

PO: Completely absorbed by GI route; onset 2-4 hr, peak 4 hr, duration 24 hr; half-life 10 hr; metabolized in liver; excreted in urine, feces (metabolites); crosses placenta; 90%-95% is plasma protein bound

Interactions:

• Both drugs' effects may be decreased: diazoxide

• Increased level: digoxin

• Increased hypoglycemic effects: insulin, MAOIs, oral anticoagulants, chloramphenicol, guanethidine, methyldopa, NSAIDs, salicylates, probenecid, androgens, fenfluramine, fluconazole, gemfibrozil, histamine H_2 antagonists, magnesium salts, phenylbutazone, sulfinpyrazone, sulfonamides, tricyclic antidepressants, urinary acidifiers

• Decreased action of glyburide: thiazide diuretics, rifampin, isoniazid, beta-blockers, cholestyramine, diazoxide, hydantoins, urinary alkalinizers, charcoal

⚕ Decreased hypoglycemic effect: broom, buchu, dandelion, juniper

⚕ Increased or decreased hypoglycemic effect: chromium, fenugreek, ginseng

⚕ Increased glucose tolerance: karela

NURSING CONSIDERATIONS

Assess:

• Hypo/hyperglycemic reaction that can occur soon after meals

Administer:

• With breakfast

Perform/provide:

• Storage in tight container in cool environment

Evaluate:

• Therapeutic response: decrease in polyuria, polydipsia, polyphagia, clear sensorium, absence of dizziness, stable gait

Teach patient/family:

• To check for symptoms of cholestatic jaundice: dark urine, pruritus, jaundiced sclera; if these occur, notify prescriber

• To use a capillary blood glucose test while on this drug

• The symptoms of hypo/hyperglycemia, what to do about each

• That drug must be continued on daily basis; explain consequence of discontinuing drug abruptly

• To take drug in morning to prevent hypoglycemic reactions at night

• To avoid OTC medications unless ordered by prescriber

• That diabetes is a lifelong illness; drug will not cure disease

• That all food included in diet plan must be eaten to prevent hypoglycemia; to have glucagon emergency kit available

G

• To carry a Medic Alert ID for emergency purposes

Treatment of overdose: Glucose 25 g IV via dextrose 50% sol, 50 ml or 1 mg glucagon

---

glycerin (OTC)

(gli′ser-in)
Fleet Babylax, Glycerin USP, Glycerol, Osmoglyn, Sani-Supp
Func. class.: Laxative, hyperosmotic
Chem. class.: Trihydric alcohol

Action: Increases osmotic pressure, draws fluid into colon, lumen from extravascular spaces to intravascular

Uses: Constipation, intraocular pressure reduction

Dosage and routes:
Laxative
• *Adult and child >6 yr:* **RECT SUPP** 3 g; **ENEMA** 5-15 ml
• *Child <6 yr:* **RECT SUPP** 1-1.5 g; **ENEMA** 2-5 ml
Intraocular pressure reduction
• *Adult:* **PO** 1-1.5 g/kg once, then may be given 500 mg/kg q6h
• *Child:* **PO** 1-1.5 g/kg once, then 500 mg/kg 4-8 hr after first dose
Available forms: Rect sol 4 ml/applicator; supp; oral sol 0.6 g/ml
Side effects/adverse reactions:
CNS: Headache, confusion, ***convulsions***
GI: Nausea, vomiting, diarrhea
META: Dehydration
Contraindications: Hypersensitivity
Precautions: Pregnancy (C)
NURSING CONSIDERATIONS
Assess:
• Cause of constipation; identify whether fluids, bulk, or exercise is missing from lifestyle
• Cramping, rectal bleeding, nausea, vomiting; if these symptoms occur, drug should be discontinued

Administer:
• Insert supp; may cause evacuation in ½ hr
• Enema: use 4 ml applicator; patient should be in side-lying position
• Pour oral sol over cracked ice and sip through a straw
• To prevent cerebral dehydration, headache, patient should be recumbent during and after administration
Perform/provide:
• Storage in cool environment; do not freeze
Evaluate:
• Therapeutic response: decrease in constipation
Teach patient/family:
• Not to use laxatives for long-term therapy; bowel tone will be lost
• That normal bowel movements do not always occur daily
• Not to use in presence of abdominal pain, nausea, vomiting
• To notify prescriber if constipation unrelieved or if symptoms of electrolyte imbalance occur: muscle cramps, pain, weakness, dizziness, excessive thirst

---

glycopyrrolate (R)

(glye-koe-pye′roe-late)
glycopyrrolate, Robinul, Robinul Forte
Func. class.: Cholinergic blocker
Chem. class.: Quaternary ammonium compound

Action: Inhibits the action of acetylcholine at receptor sites in autonomic nervous system, which controls secretions, free acids in stomach

Uses: Decreased secretions before surgery, reversal of neuromuscular

---

blockade, peptic ulcer disease, irritable bowel syndrome

Dosage and routes:

Preoperatively

• *Adult:* **IM** 0.002 mg/kg ½-1 hr before surgery

• *Child 2-12 yr:* **IM** 0.002-0.004 mg/kg

• *Child <2 yr:* **IM** 0.004 mg/kg

Control of secretions

• *Child:* **PO** 40-100 µg/kg/dose q3-4×/day

Reversal of neuromuscular blockade

• *Adult and child:* **IV** 0.2 mg for each 1 mg of neostigmine or 5 mg **IV** of pyridostigmine simultaneously

GI disorders

• *Adult:* **PO** 1-2 mg bid-tid; **IM/IV** 0.1-0.2 mg tid-qid, titrated to patient response

Available forms: Tabs 1, 2 mg; inj 0.2 mg/ml

Side effects/adverse reactions:

INTEG: Urticaria, allergic reactions

MISC: Suppression of lactation, nasal congestion, decreased sweating

CNS: Confusion, anxiety, restlessness, irritability, delusions, hallucinations, headache, sedation, depression, incoherence, dizziness, lethargy, flushing, weakness

EENT: Blurred vision, photophobia, dilated pupils, difficulty swallowing, increased intraocular pressure, mydriasis, cycloplegia

CV: Palpitations, tachycardia, postural hypotension, paradoxical bradycardia

GI: Dryness of mouth, constipation, nausea, vomiting, abdominal distress, paralytic ileus, altered taste perception

SYST: **Anaphylaxis**

GU: Urinary hesitancy, retention, impotence

Contraindications: Hypersensitivity, narrow-angle glaucoma, myasthenia gravis, GI/GU obstruction, child <3 yr, tachycardia, myocardial ischemia, hepatic disease, ulcerative colitis, toxic megacolon

Precautions: Pregnancy (B), elderly, lactation, prostatic hypertrophy, renal disease, CHF, pulmonary disease, hyperthyroidism

Pharmacokinetics:

PO: Peak 1 hr, duration 8-12 hr

IM: Peak 30-45 min, duration 2-7 hr

IV: Peak 10-15 min, duration 2-7 hr; excreted in urine (50%), (unchanged); half-life 1-2 hr

Interactions:

• Increased anticholinergic effect: alcohol, antihistamines, phenothiazines, amantadine, tricyclics

• Decreased absorption of glycopyrrolate: antacids, antidiarrheals

NURSING CONSIDERATIONS

Assess:

• I&O ratio; retention commonly causes decreased urinary output

• Urinary hesitancy, retention: palpate bladder if retention occurs

• Constipation; increase fluids, bulk, exercise if this occurs

• For tolerance over long-term therapy; dose may have to be increased or changed

• Mental status: affect, mood, CNS depression, worsening of mental symptoms during early therapy

Administer:

• Parenteral dose with patient recumbent to prevent postural hypotension

• Parenteral dose slowly; keep in bed for at least 1 hr after dose; monitor vital signs

• After checking dose carefully; even slight overdose may lead to toxicity

• With or after meals to prevent GI upset; may give with fluids other than water

IV

• Undiluted, give through a Y-tube or 3-way stopcock; give 0.2 mg or less over 1-2 min

Syringe compatibilities: Atropine, benzquinamide, chlorpromazine, cimetidine, codeine, diphenhydramine, droperidol, droperidol/fentanyl, hydromorphone, hydroxyzine, levorphanol, lidocaine, meperidine, meperidine/promethazine, midazolam, morphine, nalbuphine, neostigmine, oxymorphone, procaine, prochlorperazine, promazine, promethazine, pyridostigmine, ranitidine, scopolamine, triflupromazine, trimethobenzamide

Y-site compatibilities: Propofol

Perform/provide:
• Storage at room temp
• Hard candy, frequent drinks, sugarless gum to relieve dry mouth

Evaluate:
• Therapeutic response: decreased secretions

Teach patient/family:
• Not to discontinue this drug abruptly; to taper off over 1 wk; to take PO ½-1 hr ac
• To avoid driving, other hazardous activities; drowsiness may occur
• To avoid OTC medication: cough, cold preparations with alcohol, antihistamines unless directed by prescriber

---

goserelin (R)
(goe'se-rel-lin)
Zoladex

Func. class.: Gonadotropin-releasing hormone

Chem. class.: Synthetic decapeptide analog of LHRH

Action: Inhibitor of pituitary gonadotropin secretion; initially increases LH and FSH, with increases in testosterone, reduction in sex steroid levels

Uses: Advanced prostate cancer (10.8 mg), endometriosis, advanced breast cancer, endometrial thinning (3.6 mg)

Dosage and routes:
• *Adult:* SC 3.6 mg q28d

Available forms: Depot inj 3.6, 10.8 mg

Side effects/adverse reactions:
CNS: Headaches, **spinal cord compression,** anxiety, depression
CV: **Dysrhythmia, cerebrovascular accident,** hypertension, **MI,** chest pain
ENDO: Gynecomastia, breast tenderness, hot flashes
GI: Nausea, vomiting, constipation, diarrhea, ulcer
GU: Spotting, breakthrough bleeding, decreased libido, renal insufficiency, urinary obstruction, urinary tract infection
INTEG: Rash, pain on injection
MS: Osteoneuralgia

Contraindications: Hypersensitivity to LHRH, LHRH-agonist analogs, pregnancy (D)—breast cancer, (X)—endometriosis, lactation, nondiagnosed vaginal bleeding

Pharmacokinetics: Peak serum concentrations in 14-28 days; half-life 4½ hr

Lab test interferences:
Increase: Alk phosphatase, estradiol, FSH, LH, testosterone levels
Decrease: Testosterone levels, progesterone

NURSING CONSIDERATIONS
Assess:
• I&O ratios; palpate bladder for distention in urinary obstruction
• For relief of bone pain (back pain)

Administer:
• SC using implant, inserted by qualified person into upper subcutaneous tissue in abdominal wall q28d or q12wk (10.8 mg)

Evaluate:
• Therapeutic response: more normal levels of prostate-specific antigen, acid phosphatase, alk phos-

---

◆ = Nursing alert　　　⫶ = Herb-drug interaction　　　⊘ = Do not crush phatase; testosterone level of <25 ng/dl

Teach patient/family:
• That gynecomastia and postmenopausal symptoms may occur but will decrease after treatment is discontinued

---

granisetron (Rx)
(grane-iss'e-tron)
Kytril
Func. class.: Antiemetic
Chem. class.: 5-HT₃ receptor antagonist

Action: Prevents nausea, vomiting by blocking serotonin peripherally, centrally, and in the small intestine

Uses: Prevention of nausea, vomiting associated with cancer chemotherapy including high-dose cisplatin

Dosage and routes:
• *Adult and child:* **IV** 10 μg/kg over 5 min, 30 min before the start of cancer chemotherapy; *adult* **PO** 1 mg bid, give first dose 1 hr before chemotherapy and next dose 12 hr after first

Available forms: Inj 1 mg/ml; tab 1 mg

Side effects/adverse reactions:
CNS: Headache, asthenia, anxiety, dizziness
CV: Hypertension
GI: Diarrhea, *constipation,* increased AST, ALT, *nausea*
HEMA: **Leukopenia,** anemia, ***thrombocytopenia***
MISC: Rash, ***bronchospasm***

Contraindications: Hypersensitivity

Precautions: Pregnancy (B), lactation, children, elderly

Pharmacokinetics: Metabolized in liver to an active metabolite, half-life 10-12 hr

NURSING CONSIDERATIONS
Assess:
• For absence of nausea, vomiting during chemotherapy
• Hypersensitive reaction: rash, bronchospasm

Administer:
IV, direct
• Dilute in 0.9% NaCl for inj or D₅W (20-50 ml); give over 5 min; ½ hr before chemotherapy

Additive compatibilities: Dexamethasone, methylprednisolone

Solution compatibilities: D₅W, 0.9% NaCl

Y-site compatibilities: Acyclovir, allopurinol, amifostine, amikacin, aminophylline, amphotericin B cholesteryl, ampicillin, ampicillin/sulbactam, amsacrine, aztreonam, bleomycin, bumetanide, buprenorphine, butorphanol, calcium gluconate, carboplatin, carmustine, cefazolin, cefepime, cefonicid, cefoperazone, cefotaxime, cefotetan, cefoxitin, ceftazidime, ceftizoxime, ceftriaxone, cefuroxime, chlorpromazine, cimetidine, ciprofloxacin, cisplatin, cladribine, clindamycin, cyclophosphamide, cytarabine, dacarbazine, dactinomycin, daunorubicin, dexamethasone, diphenhydramine, dobutamine, dopamine, doxorubicin, doxorubicin liposome, doxycycline, droperidol, enalaprilat, etoposide, famotidine, filgrastim, fluconazole, fluorouracil, floxuridine, fludarabine, furosemide, gallium, ganciclovir, gentamicin, haloperidol, heparin hydrocortisone, hydromorphone, hydroxyzine, idarubicin, ifosfamide, imipenem-cilastatin, leucovorin, lorazepam, magnesium sulfate, melphalan, meperidine, mesna, methotrexate, methylprednisolone, metoclopramide, metronidazole, mezlocillin, miconazole, minocycline, mitomycin, mitoxantrone, morphine, nalbuphine, netilmicin, ofloxacin, paclitaxel, piperacillin, piperacillin/tazobactam, plicamycin, potassium chloride, prochlorperazine, promethazine, propofol, ranitidine, sargramostim, sodium bicarbonate, streptozocin, teniposide, thiotepa, ticarcillin, ticarcillin/clavulanate, tobramycin, trimethoprim - sulfamethoxazole, vancomycin, vinblastine, vincristine, vinorelbine, zidovudine

Perform/provide:

• Storage at room temp for 24 hr after dilution

Evaluate:

• Therapeutic response: absence of nausea, vomiting during cancer chemotherapy

Teach patient/family:

• To report diarrhea, constipation, rash, changes in respirations

---

griseofulvin microsize (℞)
(gris-ee-oh-ful'vin)
Fulvicin-U/F, Grifulvin V, Grisactin, Grisovin-FP*
griseofulvin ultramicrosize (℞)
Fulvicin P/G, Grisactin Ultra, Gris-PEG
Func. class.: Antifungal
Chem. class.: Penicillium griseofulvum derivative

Action: Arrests fungal cell division at metaphase; binds to human keratin, making it resistant to disease

Uses: Mycotic infections: tinea corporis, tinea pedis, tinea cruris, tinea barbae, tinea capitis, tinea unguium if caused by *Epidermophyton, Microsporum, Trichophyton*

Dosage and routes:

• *Adult:* **PO** 500-1000 mg qd in single or divided doses (microsize), 125-165 mg bid (ultramicrosize) or 250-330 mg qd; may need 500-660 mg in divided doses for severe infections

• *Child:* **PO** 10 mg/kg/day or 30 mg/m^2/day (microsize) or 5 mg/kg/day (ultramicrosize)

Available forms: Microcaps 125, 250 mg; tabs 250, 500 mg; oral susp 125 mg/ml; ultratabs 125, 165, 250, 330 mg

Side effects/adverse reactions:

INTEG: Rash, urticaria, photosensitivity, lichen planus

CNS: Headache, peripheral neuritis, paresthesias, confusion, dizziness, fatigue

EENT: Transient hearing loss

GU: Proteinuria, cylinduria, precipitate porphyria, increased thirst

GI: Nausea, vomiting, anorexia, diarrhea, cramps, dry mouth, flatulence, ***bleeding***

*HEMA: **Leukopenia, granulocytopenia, neutropenia, monocytosis***

Contraindications: Hypersensitivity, porphyria, hepatic disease, lupus erythematosus

Precautions: Penicillin sensitivity, pregnancy (C)

Pharmacokinetics:

PO: Peak 4 hr, half-life 9-24 hr, metabolized in liver; excreted in urine (inactive metabolites), feces, perspiration

Interactions:

• Tachycardia: alcohol

• Decreased action of griseofulvin: barbiturates

• Decreased action of warfarin, cyclosporine, salicylates, oral contraceptives

• Drug/food: increased absorption: High-fat foods

NURSING CONSIDERATIONS

Assess:

• I&O ratio

• Liver studies qwk (ALT, AST, bilirubin, alk phosphatase)

⬥ = Nursing alert   ⫻ = Herb-drug interaction   ⊘ = Do not crush

• Renal studies: BUN, serum creatinine
• Blood studies: CBC, platelets, q2wk
• For history of penicillin allergy; may be cross-sensitive to this drug

◆ For renal toxicity: increasing BUN, serum creatinine, proteinuria, cylindruria
• For blood dyscrasias: fatigue, malaise, dark urine, bruising
• Use only when topical treatment is ineffective

Administer:
• Drug carefully, making sure there is no confusion with dosage form (microsize vs ultramicrosize)
• With meals to decrease GI symptoms; fatty meals for better absorption
• Until three separate cultures are negative for infective organism

Perform/provide:
• Storage in tight, light-resistant container at room temp

Evaluate:
• Therapeutic response: decreased rash, negative C&S for infecting organism

Teach patient/family:
• That long-term therapy may be needed to clear infection (2 wk-6 mo depending on organism)
• Proper hygiene: hand-washing technique, nail care, use of concomitant topical agents if prescribed
• The importance of compliance even after feeling better
• To avoid alcohol, since nausea, vomiting, hypertension may occur
• To use sunscreen or avoid direct sunlight to prevent photosensitivity
• To notify prescriber of sore throat, fever, skin rash, which may indicate overgrowth of organisms
• To use nonhormonal contraception

guaifenesin (OTC, ℞)
(gwye-fen′e-sin)
Amonidrin, Anti-tuss, Balminil*, Breonesin, Fenesin, Gee-Gee, Genatuss, GG-Cen, Glyate, Glycotuss, Glytuss, guaifenesin, Guiatuss, Halotussin, Humibid, Humibid L.A., Hytuss, Hytuss ZX, Malotuss, Monafed, Mytussin, Naldecon Senior EX, Resyl*, Robitussin, Scot-Tussin Expectorant, Sinumist-SR, UniTussin
Func. class.: Expectorant

Action: Acts as an expectorant by stimulating a gastric mucosal reflex to increase the production of lung mucus

Uses: Dry, nonproductive cough

Dosage and routes:
• *Adult:* **PO** 100-400 mg q4-6h, not to exceed 1.2 g/day; **EXT REL** 600-1200 mg q12h, not to exceed 2.4 g/day
• *Child 6-12 yr:* **PO** 100-200 mg q4h; 600 mg q12h (**EXT REL**) not to exceed 1.2 g/day
• *Child 2-6 yr:* **PO** 50-100 mg q4h; not to exceed 600 mg/day

Available forms: Tabs 100, 200 mg; tabs, ext rel 600 mg; caps 200 mg; caps, ext rel: 300 mg; syr 100, 200 mg/5 ml

Side effects/adverse reactions:
CNS: Drowsiness
GI: Nausea, anorexia, vomiting

Contraindications: Hypersensitivity, persistent cough

Precautions: Pregnancy (C)

NURSING CONSIDERATIONS

Assess:
• Cough: type, frequency, character, including sputum; fluids should be increased to 2 L/day

Perform/provide:
• Storage at room temp

• Increased fluids, room humidification to liquefy secretions
Evaluate:
• Therapeutic response: absence of cough
Teach patient/family:
• To avoid driving, other hazardous activities if drowsiness occurs (rare)
• To avoid smoking, smoke-filled room, perfumes, dust, environmental pollutants, cleansers

---

guanabenz (℞)
(gwan'a-benz)
Wytensin
Func. class.: Antihypertensive
Chem. class.: Central α_2-adrenergic agonist

Action: Stimulates central α_2-adrenergic receptors in the CNS resulting in decreased sympathetic outflow from brain with decreased peripheral resistance
Uses: Hypertension
Dosage and routes:
• *Adult:* **PO** 4 mg bid, increasing in increments of 4-8 mg/day q1-2wk, not to exceed 32 mg bid
Available forms: Tabs 4, 8 mg
Side effects/adverse reactions:
RESP: Dyspnea
CV: Severe rebound hypertension, chest pain, *dysrhythmias,* palpitations, hypotension
CNS: Drowsiness, dizziness, sedation, headache, depression, weakness
EENT: Nasal congestion, blurred vision
GI: Nausea, diarrhea, constipation, dry mouth, anorexia, abnormal taste
GU: Impotence, urinary frequency, gynecomastia
MS: Backache, extremities pain
Contraindications: Hypersensitivity to guanabenz

Precautions: Pregnancy (C), lactation, children <12 yr, severe coronary insufficiency, recent myocardial infarction, cerebrovascular disease, severe hepatic or renal failure, elderly
Pharmacokinetics:
PO: Onset 1 hr, peak 2-4 hr; half-life 4-14 hr; excreted in urine
Interactions:
• Increased hypotension: diuretics, other antihypertensives
• Do not use with MAOIs
• Increased orthostatic hypotension: alcohol, opioids
• Decreased hypotensive effect: tricyclic antidepressants, phenothiazines, ephedrine
NURSING CONSIDERATIONS
Assess:
• Renal studies: protein, BUN, creatinine; watch for increased levels
• Baselines in renal, liver function tests before therapy begins
• B/P during beginning treatment, periodically thereafter
• Edema in feet and legs daily
• Allergic reaction: rash, fever, pruritus, urticaria; drug should be discontinued if antihistamines fail to help
• Renal symptoms: polyuria, oliguria, frequency
Administer:
• In AM, at hs
Evaluate:
• Therapeutic response: decrease in B/P
Teach patient/family:
• To avoid hazardous activities; sedation may occur
• Not to discontinue drug abruptly, or withdrawal symptoms may occur: anxiety, increased B/P, headache, insomnia, increased pulse, tremors, nausea, sweating
• Not to use OTC (cough, cold, or allergy) products unless directed by prescriber

◆ = Nursing alert   ⫘ = Herb-drug interaction   ⊘ = Do not crush

• The importance of complying with dosage schedule even if feeling better

• To notify prescriber of swelling of hands or feet, irregular heartbeat, chest pain

• About excessive perspiration, dehydration, vomiting, diarrhea; may lead to fall in blood pressure; consult prescriber if these occur

• That drug may cause dizziness, fainting; light-headedness may occur during first few days of therapy

• That compliance is necessary; not to skip or stop drug unless directed by prescriber

• That drug may cause skin rash or impaired perspiration

Treatment of overdose: Administer vasopressor, discontinue drug; supine position

---

guanadrel (℞)

(gwahn'a-drel)

Hylorel

Func. class.: Antihypertensive

Chem. class.: Adrenergic blocker, peripheral guanethidine derivative

Action: Inhibits sympathetic vasoconstriction by inhibiting release of norepinephrine, depletes norepinephrine stores in adrenergic nerve endings, adrenal medulla

Uses: Hypertension (moderate to severe as an adjunct)

Dosage and routes:

• *Adult:* **PO** 5 mg bid, adjusted to desired response weekly or monthly; may need 20-75 mg/day in divided doses; higher doses are given tid or qid

• *Geriatric:* **PO** 5 mg/day, titrate as needed

Renal dose

• CrCl 10-50 ml/min dose q12-24h; CrCl <10 ml/min dose q24-48h

Available forms: Tabs 10, 25 mg

Side effects/adverse reactions:

CV: Orthostatic hypotension, **bradycardia, CHF,** palpitations, chest pain, **tachycardia, dysrhythmias**

CNS: Drowsiness, fatigue, weakness, feeling of faintness, insomnia, dizziness, mental changes, memory loss, hallucinations, *depression,* anxiety, *confusion, paresthesias, headache*

GI: Nausea, cramps, diarrhea, constipation, dry mouth, anorexia, indigestion

INTEG: Rash, purpura, alopecia

EENT: Nasal stuffiness, tinnitus, visual changes, sore throat, double vision, dry, burning eyes

GU: Ejaculation failure, impotence, dysuria, nocturia, urinary frequency

RESP: **Bronchospasm,** dyspnea, cough, rales, SOB

MS: Leg cramps, aching, pain, inflammation

Contraindications: Hypersensitivity, pheochromocytoma, lactation, CHF, child <18 yr

Precautions: Elderly, pregnancy (B), bronchial asthma, peptic ulcer, electrolyte imbalances, vascular disease

Pharmacokinetics:

PO: Onset 0.5-2 hr, peak 4-6 hr, duration 8 hr; half-life 10-12 hr; metabolized in liver 50%; excreted in urine (50% unchanged)

Interactions:

• Increased hypotension: diuretics, other antihypertensives

• Do not use with MAOIs

• Increased orthostatic hypotension: alcohol, opioids

• Decreased hypotensive effect: tricyclic antidepressants, phenothiazines, ephedrine

NURSING CONSIDERATIONS

Assess:

• Renal function studies in renal impairment (BUN, creatinine)

- Bleeding time; check for ecchymosis, thrombocytopenia, purpura
- I&O in renal disease patient
- Cardiac status: B/P lying and standing, pulse; watch for hypotension
- Edema in feet, legs daily; take weight daily
- Skin turgor, dryness of mucous membranes for hydration status
- Symptoms of CHF: edema, dyspnea, wet rales

Perform/provide:
- Storage in airtight container

Evaluate:
- Therapeutic response: decreased B/P

Teach patient/family:
- To avoid driving and performing hazardous activities if drowsiness occurs
- Not to discontinue drug abruptly
- Not to use OTC cough, cold preparations unless directed by prescriber
- To report bradycardia, dizziness, confusion, depression, fever, or sore throat
- That impotence, gynecomastia may occur but are reversible
- To rise slowly to sitting or standing position to minimize orthostatic hypotension
- That therapeutic effect may take 2-4 wk

---

guanethidine (℞)
(gwahn-eth'i-deen)
Apo-Guanethidine*, guanethidine sulfate*, Ismelin
Func. class.: Antihypertensive
Chem. class.: Antiadrenergic agent, peripheral

Action: Inhibits norepinephrine release, depleting norepinephrine stores in adrenergic nerve endings

Uses: Moderate to severe hypertension

Dosage and routes:
- *Adult:* **PO** 10-12.5 mg qd, increase by 10 mg qwk; may require 25-50 mg qd
- *Adult:* (hospitalized) 25-50 mg; may increase by 25-50 mg/day or every other day
- *Child:* **PO** 0.2 mg/kg/day; (6 mg/m^2/day) increase q7-10d, 0.2 mg/kg or 6 mg/m^2/day not to exceed 3000 µg/kg/24 hr

Available forms: Tabs 10, 25 mg
Side effects/adverse reactions:
CV: Orthostatic hypotension, dizziness, weakness, bradycardia, **CHF,** fatigue, angina, heart block, chest paresthesia
CNS: Depression
GI: Nausea, vomiting, *diarrhea,* constipation, dry mouth, weight gain, anorexia, abdominal pain
INTEG: Dermatitis, loss of scalp hair
EENT: Nasal congestion, ptosis, blurred vision
GU: Ejaculation failure, impotence, nocturia, edema, *urinary retention,* increased BUN, *urinary frequency*
RESP: Dyspnea, cough, shortness of breath
Contraindications: Hypersensitivity, pheochromocytoma, recent MI, CHF, cardiac failure, sinus bradycardia
Precautions: Pregnancy (C), lactation, peptic ulcer, asthma
Pharmacokinetics:
PO: Therapeutic level 1-3 wk; half-life 5 days; metabolized by liver; excreted in urine (metabolites), breast milk
Interactions:
- Increased hypotension: diuretics, other antihypertensives
- Do not use with MAOIs
- Increased orthostatic hypotension: alcohol

◆ = Nursing alert   ▥ = Herb-drug interaction   ⃠ = Do not crush

• Decreased hypotensive effect: tricyclic antidepressants, phenothiazines, ephedrine, oral contraceptives, doxepin, haloperidol, amphetamines

Lab test interferences:

Increase: BUN

Decrease: Blood glucose, VMA excretion, urinary norepinephrine

NURSING CONSIDERATIONS

Assess:

• Renal function studies in renal impairment (BUN, creatinine)

• Bleeding time; check for ecchymosis, thrombocytopenia, purpura

• I&O in renal disease patient

• Cardiac status: B/P, pulse; watch for hypotension

• Edema in feet, legs daily; take weight daily

• Skin turgor, dryness of mucous membranes for hydration status

• Symptoms of CHF: edema, dyspnea, wet rales

Evaluate:

• Therapeutic response: decreased B/P

Teach patient/family:

• To avoid driving, hazardous activities if drowsiness occurs

• Not to discontinue drug abruptly

• Not to use OTC cough, cold preparations unless directed by prescriber

• To report bradycardia, dizziness, confusion, depression, fever, sore throat

• That impotence, gynecomastia may occur but are reversible

• To rise slowly to sitting or standing position to minimize orthostatic hypotension; more common in AM, hot weather, during exercise, or when using alcohol

• That therapeutic effect may take 2-4 wk

• To notify prescriber of severe diarrhea

Treatment of overdose: Lavage, vasopressors given cautiously

---

guanfacine (R)

(gwahn'fa-seen)

Tenex

Func. class.: Antihypertensive

Chem. class.: α₂-adrenergic receptor agonist

Action: Stimulates central α-adrenergic receptors, resulting in decreased sympathetic outflow from brain

Uses: Hypertension in individual using a thiazide diuretic

Dosage and routes:

• *Adult:* **PO** 1 mg/day hs; may increase dose in 2-3 wk to 2-3 mg/day

Available forms: Tabs 1 mg

Side effects/adverse reactions:

GI: Dry mouth, constipation, cramps, nausea, diarrhea

CNS: Somnolence, dizziness, headache, fatigue

GU: Impotence, urinary incontinence

EENT: Taste change, tinnitus, vision change, rhinitis, nasal congestion

MS: Leg cramps

RESP: Dyspnea

INTEG: Dermatitis, pruritus, purpura

CV: Bradycardia, chest pain

Contraindications: Hypersensitivity

Precautions: Pregnancy (B), lactation, children <12 yr, severe coronary insufficiency, recent MI, renal or hepatic disease, CVA, elderly

Pharmacokinetics: Peak 1-4 hr; 70% bound to plasma proteins; half-life 17 hr; eliminated via kidneys unchanged and as metabolites

Interactions:

• Increased sedation: CNS depressants, other antihypertensives

---

• Decreased hypotensive effect: tricyclic antidepressants

NURSING CONSIDERATIONS
Assess:
• Blood studies: neutrophils, decrease in platelets
• Baselines in renal, liver function tests before therapy begins
• B/P before, during, after treatment; notify prescriber of significant changes
• Edema in feet, legs daily
• Allergic reaction: rash, fever, pruritus, urticaria; drug should be discontinued if antihistamines fail to help
• Symptoms of CHF: edema, dyspnea, wet rales, B/P
• Renal symptoms: polyuria, oliguria, urinary frequency

Perform/provide:
• Storage of tablets in airtight container

Evaluate:
• Therapeutic response: decreased B/P in hypertension

Teach patient/family:
• To avoid hazardous activities
• Not to discontinue drug abruptly or withdrawal symptoms may occur: anxiety, increased B/P, headache, insomnia, increased pulse, tremors, nausea, sweating
• Not to use OTC (cough, cold, or allergy) products unless directed by prescriber
• To avoid sunlight or to wear sunscreen; photosensitivity may occur
• The importance of complying with dosage schedule even if feeling better

haemophilus b conjugate vaccine, diphtheria CRM$_{197}$ protein conjugate (HbOC) (℞)
(hee-moef'ih-lus)
HibTITER
haemophilus b conjugate vaccine, diphtheria toxoid conjugate (PRP-D)
ProHIBIT
haemophilus b conjugate vaccine, meningococcal protein conjugate (PRP-OMP) (℞)
Pedvax HIB
Func. class.: Vaccine
Chem. class.: H. influenzae capsular polysaccharide

Action: Stimulates antibody production to *H. influenzae b*
Uses: Polysaccharide immunization of children 2-6 yr against *H. influenzae b,* conjugate immunization of child 2, 4, 6 mo; 6 mo dose not needed in Pedvax HIB; booster at 12-18 mo against invasive disease of *H. influenzae b*

Dosage and routes:
• *Child:* **SC** 0.5 ml (polysaccharide), **IM** 0.5 mg (conjugate)
Available forms: Polysaccharide powder for injection 25 µg/0.5 ml after reconstituting; conjugate powder for inj 25 µg polysaccharide and 18 µg conjugated diphtheria toxoid/0.5 ml

Side effects/adverse reactions:
INTEG: Redness, soreness at injection site, rash
SYST: Low-grade fever, acute febrile reactions

Contraindications: Hypersensitivity, febrile illness, active infection
Precautions: Pregnancy (C)
Lab test interferences:
Interference: Latex agglutination, countercurrent immunoelectrophoresis
Interactions:
• Decreased antibody response: other vaccines, immunosuppressants
NURSING CONSIDERATIONS
Assess:
• For skin reactions: swelling, rash, urticaria
• For anaphylaxis: inability to breathe, bronchospasm
• For history of allergies, skin conditions (eczema, psoriasis, dermatitis), reactions to vaccinations
Administer:
• After diluting with 0.6 ml diluent, which will yield 10 doses of 0.5 ml
• Only with epinephrine 1:1000 on unit to treat laryngospasm
• Only by SC or IM route
Perform/provide:
• Storage in refrigerator
• Written record of immunization
Teach patient/family:
• That discomfort may occur at site, acetaminophen can be given

---

halofantrine (℞)
(hay-loh-fan'trin)
Halfan
Func. class.: Antimalarial
Chem. class.: Phenanthrenemethanol

Action: Inhibits parasite replications, transcription of DNA to RNA by forming complexes with DNA of parasite
Uses: Mild to moderate malaria
Dosage and routes:
• *Adult:* **PO** 500 mg q6h × 3 doses; may need to repeat after 1 wk
Available forms: Tabs 250 mg

Side effects/adverse reactions:
*CV: **Dysrhythmias***
GI: Nausea, vomiting, anorexia, diarrhea
Contraindications: Hypersensitivity
Precautions: Severe GI disease, severe hepatic disease, cardiac dysrhythmias
Pharmacokinetics: Metabolized in liver; excreted by kidneys
Interactions:
Unknown
NURSING CONSIDERATIONS
Assess:
• Monitor B/P, pulse, watch for tachycardia
• Monitor liver studies qwk: ALT, AST, bilirubin
Administer:
PO
• 1 hr before or 2 hr after meals at same time each day to maintain level
Perform/provide:
• Storage in tight, light-resistant container
Evaluate:
• Therapeutic response: C&S—negative; decreased symptoms of malaria
Teach patient/family:
• Advise patient to take exactly as prescribed, to take full course that is prescribed

haloperidol (℞)

(hal-oh-pehr′ih-dol)
Apo-Haloperidol*, Haldol,
Novo-Peridol*, Peridol*

haloperidol decanoate (℞)

Haldol Decanoate, Haldol
LA*

haloperidol lactate (℞)

Haldol, Haloperidol Injection,
Haloperidol Intensol

Func. class.: Antipsychotic,
neuroleptic

Chem. class.: Butyrophenone

Action: Depresses cerebral cortex, hypothalamus, limbic system, which control activity and aggression; blocks neurotransmission produced by dopamine at synapse; exhibits strong α-adrenergic, anticholinergic blocking action; mechanism for antipsychotic effects unclear

Uses: Psychotic disorders, control of tics, vocal utterances in Gilles de la Tourette's syndrome, short-term treatment of hyperactive children showing excessive motor activity, prolonged parenteral therapy in chronic schizophrenia, control of severe nausea and vomiting in chemotherapy, organic mental syndrome with psychotic features, hiccups (short-term)

Dosage and routes:

Psychosis

• *Adult:* **PO** 0.5-5 mg bid or tid initially depending on severity of condition; dose is increased to desired dose, max 100 mg/day; **IM** 2-5 mg q1-8h

• *Geriatric:* 0.25-0.5 mg qd-bid, titrate q3-4 days by 0.25-0.5 mg/dose

• *Child 3-12 yr:* **PO/IM** 0.05-0.15 mg/kg/day

• *Decanoate:* Initial dose **IM** is 10-15 mg × daily oral dose at 4 wk interval; do not administer **IV**; not to exceed 100 mg

Chronic schizophrenia

• *Adult:* **IM** 10-15 times **PO** dose q4wk (decanoate)

• *Child 3-12 yr:* **PO/IM** 0.05-0.15 mg/kg/day

Tics/vocal utterances

• *Adult:* **PO** 0.5-5 mg bid or tid, increased until desired response occurs

• *Child 3-12 yr:* **PO** 0.05-0.075 mg/kg/day

Hyperactive children

• *Child 3-12 yr:* **PO** 0.05-0.075 mg/kg/day

Available forms: Tabs 0.5, 1, 2, 5, 10, 20 mg; lactate conc 2 mg/ml; inj 5 mg/ml, decanoate 50 mg base/ml, 100 mg base/ml

Side effects/adverse reactions:

RESP: **Laryngospasm,** dyspnea, *respiratory depression*

CNS: EPS: pseudoparkinsonism, akathisia, dystonia, tardive dyskinesia, drowsiness, headache, seizures, neuroleptic malignant syndrome, confusion

INTEG: Rash, photosensitivity, dermatitis

EENT: Blurred vision, glaucoma, dry eyes

GI: Dry mouth, nausea, vomiting, anorexia, constipation, diarrhea, jaundice, weight gain, *ileus, hepatitis*

GU: Urinary retention, urinary frequency, enuresis, impotence, amenorrhea, gynecomastia

CV: Orthostatic hypotension, hypertension, *cardiac arrest,* ECG changes, *tachycardia*

Contraindications: Hypersensitivity, blood dyscrasias, coma, child <3 yr, brain damage, bone marrow depression, alcohol and barbiturate withdrawal states, Parkinson's disease, angina, epilepsy, urinary retention, narrow-angle glaucoma

Precautions: Pregnancy (C), lactation, seizure disorders, hypertension, hepatic disease, cardiac disease, elderly

Pharmacokinetics:

PO: Onset erratic, peak 2-6 hr, half-life 24 hr

IM: Onset 15-30 min, peak 15-20 min, half-life 21 hr

IM (Decanoate): Peak 4-11 days, half-life 3 wk

Metabolized by liver; excreted in urine, bile; crosses placenta; enters breast milk

Interactions:

• Oversedation: other CNS depressants, alcohol, barbiturate anesthetics

• Toxicity: epinephrine

• Toxicity: lithium

• Decreased effects of lithium, levodopa

• Increased effects of both drugs: β-adrenergic blockers, alcohol

• Increased anticholinergic effects: anticholinergics

• Decreased effects of haloperidol: phenobarbital

🖉 Increased action: kava

Lab test interferences:

Increase: Liver function tests, cardiac enzymes, cholesterol, blood glucose, prolactin, bilirubin, PBI, cholinesterase

Decrease: Hormones (blood, urine)

False positive: Pregnancy tests, PKU

False negative: Urinary steroids

NURSING CONSIDERATIONS

Assess:

• Swallowing of PO medication; check for hoarding or giving of medication to other patients

• I&O ratio; palpate bladder if low urinary output occurs

• Bilirubin, CBC, liver function studies monthly

• Urinalysis is recommended before and during prolonged therapy

• For depression in bipolar patients; rapid mood swings may occur with this drug

• Affect, orientation, LOC, reflexes, gait, coordination, sleep pattern disturbances

• B/P standing and lying; take pulse and respirations q4h during initial treatment; establish baseline before starting treatment; report drops of 30 mm Hg

• Dizziness, faintness, palpitations, tachycardia on rising

• EPS including akathisia (inability to sit still, no pattern to movements), tardive dyskinesia (bizarre movements of jaw, mouth, tongue, extremities), pseudoparkinsonism (rigidity, tremors, pill rolling, shuffling gait)

• Skin turgor daily

◆ For neuroleptic malignant syndrome: hyperthermia, muscle rigidity, altered mental status, increased CPK

• Constipation, urinary retention daily; if these occur, increase bulk, water in diet

Administer:

• Reduced dose to elderly

• Antiparkinsonian agent, to be used if EPS occur

• IM inj into large muscle mass, use 21G, 2″ needle; give no more than 3 ml/inj site; patient should remain recumbent for ½ hr

• Oral liquid: use calibrated dropper; do not mix in coffee or tea

• PO with food or milk

Solution compatibilities: D₅W

Syringe compatibilities: Hydromorphone, sufentanil

Y-site compatibilities: Amifostine, amsacrine, aztreonam, cimetidine, cisatracurium, cladribine, dobutamine, dopamine, doxorubicin liposome, famotidine, filgrastim, fludarabine, granisetron, lidocaine, lorazepam, melphalan, midazolam, nitroglycerin, norepinephrine, ondansetron, paclitaxel, phenylephrine, propofol, remifentanil, sufentanil, tacrolimus, teniposide, theophylline, thiotepa, vinorelbine

Perform/provide:

• Decreased sensory input by dimming lights, avoiding loud noises

• Supervised ambulation until stabilized on medication; do not involve in strenuous exercise program because fainting is possible; patient should not stand still for long periods

• Increased fluids to prevent constipation

• Sips of water, candy, gum for dry mouth

• Storage in tight, light-resistant container

Evaluate:

• Therapeutic response: decrease in emotional excitement, hallucinations, delusions, paranoia, reorganization of patterns of thought, speech, improvement in specific behaviors

Teach patient/family:

• That orthostatic hypotension occurs often and to rise from sitting or lying position gradually

• To avoid hazardous activities until stabilized on medication

• To remain lying down after IM inj for at least 30 min

• To avoid hot tubs, hot showers, tub baths, since hypotension may occur

• To avoid abrupt withdrawal of this drug, or EPS may result; drug should be withdrawn slowly

• To avoid OTC preparations (cough, hay fever, cold) unless approved by prescriber, since serious drug interactions may occur; avoid use with alcohol, CNS depressants; increased drowsiness may occur

• To use a sunscreen to prevent burns

• Regarding compliance with drug regimen

• About EPS and necessity for meticulous oral hygiene, since oral candidiasis may occur

• To report impaired vision, jaundice, tremors, muscle twitching

• That in hot weather, heat stroke may occur; take extra precautions to stay cool

Treatment of overdose: Activated charcoal, lavage if orally ingested; provide an airway; do not induce vomiting

---

heparin (℞)

(hep′a-rin)

Calcilean*, Calciparine*, Hepalean*, Heparin Leo*, Heparin Lock Flush, heparin sodium, Heparin Sodium and 0.45% Sodium Chloride, Heparin Sodium and 0.9% Sodium Chloride, Hep-Lock, Hep-Lock U/P, Liquaemin Sodium

Func. class.: Anticoagulant

Action: Prevents conversion of fibrinogen to fibrin and prothrombin to thrombin by enhancing inhibitory effects of antithrombin III

Uses: Deep-vein thrombosis, pulmonary emboli, myocardial infarction, open heart surgery, disseminated intravascular clotting syndrome, atrial fibrillation with embolization, as an anticoagulant in transfusion and dialysis procedures, prevention of DVT/PE

Dosage and routes:

Deep-vein thrombosis/MI

• *Adult:* **IV PUSH** 5000-7000 U q4h then titrated to PTT or ACT level; **IV BOL** 5000-7500 U, then **IV INF; IV INF** after bolus dose, then 1000 U/hr titrated to PTT or ACT level

• *Child:* **IV INF** 50 U/kg, mainte-

◆ = Nursing alert   ∥ = Herb-drug interaction   ⊘ = Do not crush

nance 100 U/kg q4h or 20,000 U/m² qd

Pulmonary embolism
• *Adult:* **IV PUSH** 7500-10,000 U q4h then titrated to PTT or ACT level; **IV BOL** 7500-10,000, then **IV INF; IV INF** after bolus dose, then 1000 U/hr titrated to PTT or ACT level
• *Child:* **IV INF** 50 U/kg, maintenance 100 U/kg q4h or 20,000 U/m² qd

Open heart surgery
• *Adult:* **IV INF** 150-300 U/kg

Prophylaxis for DVT/PE
• *Adult:* **SC** 5,000 U q8-12h

Heparin flush
• *Adult and child:* **IV** 10-100 U

Available forms:
Sodium carpaject: 5000 U/ml; disposable inj: 1000, 2500, 5000, 7500, 10,000, 15,000, 20,000, 40,000 U/ml; unit dose: 1000, 5000, 10,000, 20,000, 40,000 U/ml; vials: 1000, 2000, 2500, 5000, 7500, 10,000, 20,000, 40,000 U/ml; disposable syringes flush: 10 U/ml; vials: 100 U/ml; calcium inj: 5000 U/0.2 ml; ampules: 12,500 U/0.5 ml; 20,000 U/0.8 ml

Side effects/adverse reactions:
CNS: Fever, chills
GI: Diarrhea, nausea, vomiting, anorexia, stomatitis, abdominal cramps, *hepatitis*
GU: Hematuria
HEMA: Hemorrhage, thrombocytopenia
SYST: Anaphylaxis
INTEG: Rash, dermatitis, urticaria, alopecia, pruritus

Contraindications: Hypersensitivity, hemophilia, leukemia with bleeding, peptic ulcer disease, thrombocytopenic purpura, hepatic disease (severe), renal disease (severe), blood dyscrasias, severe hypertension, subacute bacterial endocarditis, acute nephritis

Precautions: Alcoholism, elderly, pregnancy (C)

Pharmacokinetics: Well absorbed (SC)
IV: Peak 5 min, duration 2-6 hr
SC: Onset 20-60 min, duration 8-12 hr
Half-life 1½ hr, excreted in urine, 95% bound to plasma proteins, does not cross placenta or alter breast milk; removed from the system via the lymph and spleen

Interactions:
• Decreased action of corticosteroids
• Increased action of diazepam
• Decreased action of heparin: digitalis, tetracyclines, antihistamines
• Increased action of heparin: oral anticoagulants, salicylates, dextran, steroids, nonsteroidal antiinflammatories
✒ Increased risk of bleeding: bromelain, cinchona bark

Lab test interferences:
False increase: T_3 uptake, serum thyroxine, BSP
Decrease: Uric acid
False negative: ^{125}I fibrinogen uptake

NURSING CONSIDERATIONS
Assess:
• Blood studies (Hct, occult blood in stools) q3mo
• Partial prothrombin time, which should be 1.5-2 × control, PTT often done qd, also APTT, ACT
• Platelet count q2-3d; thrombocytopenia may occur on 4th day of treatment
◆ Bleeding gums, petechiae, ecchymosis, black tarry stools, hematuria, epistaxis, decrease in Hct, B/P; indicate bleeding and possible hemorrhage
• Fever, skin rash, urticaria
• Needed dosage change q1-2wk

Administer:

• At same time each day to maintain steady blood levels

• SC deep with 25G ⅜″ needle; do not massage area or aspirate when giving SC injection; give in abdomen between pelvic bones, rotate sites; do not pull back on plunger, leave in for 10 sec; apply gentle pressure for 1 min

• Changing needles is not recommended

• Avoiding all IM injections that may cause bleeding

IV

• Diluted in 0.9% NaCl, dextrose, Ringer's sol and given by direct, intermittent, or continuous infusion; give 1000 U or less over 1 min; then 5000 U or less over 1 min; infusion may run from 4-24 hr; use infusion pump

• Blood after adding 7500 U/100 ml NaCl inj, add 6-8 ml of this sol/100 ml of whole blood

Additive compatibilities: Aminophylline, amphotericin, ascorbic acid, bleomycin, calcium gluconate, cefepime, cephapirin, chloramphenicol, clindamycin, cloxacillin, colistimethate, dimenhydrinate, dopamine, enalaprilat, erythromycin gluceptate, esmolol, floxacillin, fluconazole, flumazenil, furosemide, hydrocortisone, isoproterenol, lidocaine, lincomycin, magnesium sulfate, meropenem, methyldopate, methylprednisolone, metronidazole/sodium bicarbonate, nafcillin, norepinephrine, octreotide, penicillin G, potassium chloride, prednisolone, promazine, ranitidine, sodium bicarbonate, verapamil, vit B, vit B/C

Syringe compatibilities: Aminophylline, amphotericin B, ampicillin, atropine, azlocillin, bleomycin, cefamandole, cefazolin, cefoperazone, cefotaxime, cefoxitin, chloramphenicol, cimetidine, cisplatin, clindamycin, cyclophosphamide, diazoxide, digoxin, dimenhydrinate, dobutamine, dopamine, epinephrine, fentanyl, fluorouracil, furosemide, leucovorin, lidocaine, lincomycin, methotrexate, metoclopramide, mezlocillin, mitomycin, moxalactam, nafcillin, naloxone, neostigmine, nitroglycerin, norepinephrine, pancuronium, penicillin G, phenobarbital, piperacillin, sodium nitroprusside, succinylcholine, trimethoprim-sulfamethoxazole, verapamil, vincristine

Y-site compatibilities: Acyclovir, aldesleukin, allopurinol, amifostine, aminophylline, ampicillin, ampicillin/sulbactam, atracurium, atropine, aztreonam, betamethasone, bleomycin, calcium gluconate, cefazolin, cefotetan, cefotiam, ceftazidime, ceftriaxone, cephalothin, cephapirin, chlordiazepoxide, chlorpromazine, cimetidine, cisplatin, cladribine, clindamycin, conjugated estrogens, cyanocobalamin, cyclophosphamide, cytarabine, dexamethasone, digoxin, diphenhydramine, dopamine, doxorubicin liposome, edrophonium, enalaprilat, epinephrine, erythromycin, esmolol, ethacrynate, famotidine, fentanyl, fluconazole, fludarabine, fluorouracil, foscarnet, furosemide, gallium, granisetron, hydralazine, hydrocortisone, hydromorphone, insulin (regular), isoproterenol, kanamycin, leucovorin, lidocaine, lorazepam, magnesium sulfate, melphalan, menadiol, meperidine, meropenem, methicillin, methotrexate, methoxamine, methyldopate, methylergonovine, metoclopramide, metronidazole, midazolam, milrinone, minocycline, mitomycin, morphine, nafcillin, neostigmine, nitroglycerin, nitroprusside, norepinephrine, ondansetron, oxacillin, oxytocin, paclitaxel, pancuronium, penicillin G potassium, pentazocine, phytonadione, piperacillin, piperacillin/tazobactam, potassium chloride, prednisolone, procainamide, prochlorperazine, propofol, propranolol, pyridostigmine, ranitidine, remifentanil, sargramostim, scopolamine, sodium bicarbonate, streptokinase, succinylcholine, tacrolimus, teniposide, theophylline, thiopental, thiotepa, ticarcillin, ticarcillin/clavulanate, trimethobenzamide, vecuronium, vinblastine, vincristine, vinorelbine, warfarin, zidovudine

Perform/provide:
• Storage in tight container
Evaluate:
• Therapeutic response: decrease of deep-vein thrombosis, PTT 1.5-2.5 × control, free flowing IV
Teach patient/family:
• To avoid OTC preparations that may cause serious drug interactions unless directed by prescriber
• That drug may be held during active bleeding (menstruation), depending on condition
• To use soft-bristle toothbrush to avoid bleeding gums, avoid contact sports, use electric razor, avoid IM injection
• To carry a Medic Alert ID identifying drug taken
• To report any signs of bleeding: gums, under skin, urine, stools
Treatment of overdose: Withdraw drug, protamine SO₄ 1:1 solution

---

hepatitis B immune globulin (℞)
Gammagee, Hep-B, H-BIG, HyperHep
Func. class.: Immune globulin

Action: Provides passive immunity to hepatitis B
Uses: Prevention of hepatitis B virus in exposed patients, including passive immunity in neonates born to HB$_s$Ag+ mother

Dosage and routes:
• *Adult and child:* **IM** 0.06 ml/kg within 1 wk of exposure, repeat after 4 wk, if patient refuses hepatitis B vaccine
• *Neonates:* **IM** 0.5 ml within 12 hr of birth
Available forms: 1, 4, 5 ml vials; 0.5 ml single dose syringe

Side effects/adverse reactions:
INTEG: Soreness at injection site, urticaria, erythema, swelling
SYST: Induration
CNS: Headache, dizziness, fever
GI: Nausea, vomiting
*SYST: **Anaphylaxis, angioedema***
Contraindications: Hypersensitivity to immune globulins, coagulation disorders
Precautions: Pregnancy (C), elderly, lactation, children; active infection, IgA deficiency

NURSING CONSIDERATIONS
Assess:
• For history of allergies, skin conditions (eczema, psoriasis, dermatitis), reactions to vaccinations
• For skin reactions: rash, induration, urticaria
◆ For anaphylaxis: inability to breathe, bronchospasm, hypotension, wheezing, diaphoresis, fever, flushing
Administer:
• After rotating vial; do not shake
• Only with epinephrine 1:1000 on unit to treat laryngospasm
• In deltoid for better absorption (adult)
Perform/provide:
• Written record of immunization
• Comfort measures
Evaluate:
• Prevention of hepatitis B

H

Teach patient/family:
• That discomfort may occur at site
• To report any rash, wheezing, inability to breathe immediately

---

hetastarch (R)
(het´a-starch)
Hespan
Func. class.: Plasma expander
Chem. class.: Synthetic polymer

Action: Similar to human albumin, which expands plasma volume by colloidal osmotic pressure

Uses: Plasma volume expander, leukapheresis

Dosage and routes:
• *Adult:* **IV INF** 500-1000 ml (30-60 g), total dose not to exceed 1500 ml/day, not to exceed 20 ml/kg/hr (hemorrhagic shock)

Leukapheresis
• *Adult:* **IV INF** 250-700 ml infused at 1:8 ratio with whole blood, may be repeated 2/wk up to 10 treatments

Available forms: 6% hetastarch/0.9% NaCl inj

Side effects/adverse reactions:
HEMA: Decreased hematocrit, platelet function, increased bleeding/coagulation times, increased sed rate
INTEG: Rash, urticaria, pruritus, angioedema, chills, fever, flushing, peripheral edema
RESP: Wheezing, dyspnea, ***bronchospasm, pulmonary edema***
GI: Nausea, vomiting
EENT: Periorbital edema
SYST: ***Anaphylaxis***
CNS: Headache

Contraindications: Hypersensitivity, severe bleeding disorders, renal failure, CHF (severe)

Precautions: Pregnancy (C), liver disease, pulmonary edema

Pharmacokinetics:
IV: Expands blood volume 1-2 × amount infused, excreted in urine

Lab test interferences:
False increase: Bilirubin

NURSING CONSIDERATIONS
Assess:
• VS q5min × 30 min; CVP during infusion (5-10 cm H_2O normal range), PCWP
• Monitor CBC with differential, Hgb, Hct, pro-time, PTT, platelet count, clotting time during treatment; Hct may drop; do not allow to drop >30% by vol
• Urine output q1h, watch for increase in urinary output, which is common; if output does not increase, infusion should be decreased or discontinued
• I&O ratio and specific gravity, urine osmolarity; if specific gravity is very low, renal clearance is low; drug should be discontinued
• Allergy: rash, urticaria, pruritus, wheezing, dyspnea, bronchospasm; drug should be discontinued immediately
◆ For circulatory overload: increased pulse, respirations, SOB, wheezing, chest tightness, chest pain
• For dehydration after infusion: decreased output, fever, poor skin turgor, increased specific gravity, dry skin

Administer:
IV
• INF undiluted, run at 20 ml/kg/hr (1.2 g/kg); reduced rate in septic shock, burns

Additive compatibilities: Cloxacillin, fosphenytoin

Y-site compatibilities: Cimetidine, diltiazem, enalaprilat
• Storage at room temp; discard unused portion, do not freeze, do not use if turbid or deep brown or if precipitate forms

---

◆ = Nursing alert   🖋 = Herb-drug interaction   Ⓢ = Do not crush

Evaluate:
• Therapeutic response: increased plasma volume
Teach patient/family:
• When to notify prescriber

---

hyaluronidase (℞)

(hye-al-yoor-on'i-dase)
Wydase
Func. class.: Enzyme

Action: Hydrolyzes hyaluronic acid within areas filled with exudates
Uses: Hypodermoclysis, subcutaneous urography; adjunct to dispersion of other drugs
Dosage and routes:
Adjunct
• *Adult and child:* **INJ** 150 U with other drug
Urography
• *Adult and child:* **SC** 75 U over scapula, then contrast medium injected at same site
Hypodermoclysis
• *Adult and child >3 yr:* **SC** 150 U/L of lysis sol
Available forms: Inj 150 U/ml
Side effects/adverse reactions:
INTEG: Rash, urticaria, itching
OTHER: Overhydration (hyperdermoclysis)
Contraindications: Hypersensitivity to bovine products, CHF, hypoproteinemia, around infected/inflamed or cancerous area
Precautions: Pregnancy (C)
Interactions:
• Systemic reactions: local anesthetics
NURSING CONSIDERATIONS
Assess:
• Site before administration (hypodermoclysis)
• For overhydration in child <3 yr
Administer:
• After test dose: 0.02 ml of 150 U/ml sol is injected; if wheal develops or itching occurs, test is positive
• Right after mixing; sol is unstable
• To child <3 yr, not exceeding 200 ml; in neonates, not exceeding 2 ml/min
Additive compatibilities: Amikacin, sodium bicarbonate
Syringe compatibilities: Pentobarbital, thiopental
Perform/provide:
• Protection from heat
Evaluate:
• Therapeutic response: absence of swelling, pain after hypodermoclysis
Teach patient/family:
• Reason for drug and expected results

---

hydralazine (℞)

(hye-dral'a-zeen)
Alazine, Apresoline,
hydralazine HCl, Novo-
Hylazin*, Pralzine, Rolzine,
Supres*
Func. class.: Antihypertensive, direct-acting peripheral vasodilator
Chem. class.: Phthalazine

Action: Vasodilates arteriolar smooth muscle by direct relaxation; reduction in blood pressure with reflex increases in cardiac function
Uses: Essential hypertension; *parenteral:* severe essential hypertension, CHF
Dosage and routes:
• *Adult:* **PO** 10 mg qid 2-4 days, then 25 mg for rest of first wk, then 50 mg qid individualized to desired response, not to exceed 300 mg qd; **IV/IM BOL** 20-40 mg q4-6h, administer **PO** as soon as possible; **IM** 20-40 mg q4-6h
• *Child:* **PO** 0.75-3 mg/kg/day in 4 divided doses, max 7.5 mg/kg/24

hr; **IV BOL** 0.1-0.2 mg/kg q4-6h;
IM 0.1-0.2 mg/kg q4-6h
Available forms: Inj 20 mg/ml; tabs
10, 25, 50, 100 mg
Side effects/adverse reactions:
MISC: Nasal congestion, muscle
cramps, *lupuslike symptoms*
CV: Palpitations, reflex tachycardia, angina, **shock,** edema, rebound
hypertension
*CNS: Headache, tremors, dizziness,
anxiety,* peripheral neuritis, depression
GI: Nausea, vomiting, anorexia, diarrhea, constipation
INTEG: Rash, pruritus
HEMA: **Leukopenia, agranulocytosis,** anemia, **thrombocytopenia**
GU: Impotence, urinary retention,
Na, H_2O retention
Contraindications: Hypersensitivity to hydralazines, coronary artery
disease, mitral valvular rheumatic
heart disease, rheumatic heart disease
Precautions: Pregnancy (C), CVA,
advanced renal disease, elderly
Pharmacokinetics:
PO: Onset 20-30 min, peak 1 hr,
duration 2-4 hr
IM: Onset 5-10 min, peak 1 hr, duration 2-4 hr
IV: Onset 5-20 min, peak 10-80 min,
duration 2-6 hr; half-life 2-8 hr; metabolized by liver; less than 10%
present in urine
Interactions:
• Increased tachycardia, angina:
sympathomimetics (epinephrine,
norepinephrine)
• Increased effects of β-blockers
• Severe hypotension: MAOIs
NURSING CONSIDERATIONS
Assess:
• B/P q5min × 2 hr, then q1h × 2 hr,
then q4h
• Pulse, jugular venous distention
q4h

• Electrolytes, blood studies: K, Na,
Cl, CO_2, CBC, serum glucose
• Weight daily, I&O
• LE prep, ANA titer before starting
therapy and during treatment; assess for fever, joint pain, rash, sore
throat (lupus-like symptoms); notify prescriber
• Edema in feet, legs daily
• Skin turgor, dryness of mucous
membranes for hydration status
• Rales, dyspnea, orthopnea
• IV site for extravasation, rate
• Fever, joint pain, tachycardia, palpitations, headache, nausea
• Mental status: affect, mood, behavior, anxiety; check for personality changes
Administer:
• Give with meals (PO) to enhance
absorption
• To recumbent patient, keep for 1
hr after administration
IV
• IV undiluted; give through Y-tube
or 3-way stopcock each 10 mg ≤min
Additive compatibilities: Dobutamine
Y-site compatibilities: Heparin, hydrocortisone, potassium chloride, verapamil, vit B/C
Evaluate:
• Therapeutic response: decreased
B/P
Teach patient/family:
• To take with food to increase bioavailability (PO)
• To avoid OTC preparations unless
directed by prescriber
• To notify prescriber if chest pain,
severe fatigue, fever, muscle or joint
pain occurs
• To rise slowly to prevent orthostatic hypotension
• To notify prescriber if pregnancy
is suspected
Treatment of overdose: Administer vasopressors, volume expanders

◆ = Nursing alert   ⫰ = Herb-drug interaction   ⊘ = Do not crush for shock; if PO, lavage or give activated charcoal, digitalization

hydrochlorothiazide (℞)

(hye-droe-klor-oh-thye'a-zide)
Diaqua, Diuchlor H*, Esidrix,
Ezide, Hydro-Chlor,
hydrochlorothiazide,
HydroDiuril, Hydromal,
Hydro-Par, Hydro-T,
Hydrozide*, Microzide, Neo-
Codema*, Novohydrazide*,
Oretic, Thiuretic, Urozide*

Func. class.: Thiazide diuretic,
antihypertensive
Chem. class.: Sulfonamide derivative

Action: Acts on distal tubule and
cortical thick ascending limb of loop
of Henle by increasing excretion of
water, sodium, chloride, potassium
Uses: Edema, hypertension, diuresis, CHF; edema in corticosteroid,
estrogen therapy
Dosage and routes:
• *Adult:* **PO** 25-100 mg/day
• *Geriatric:* **PO** 12.5 mg/day, initially
• *Child >6 mo:* **PO** 2 mg/kg/day in
divided doses
• *Child <6 mo:* **PO** up to 4 mg/kg/
day in divided doses
Available forms: Tabs 25, 50, 100
mg; sol 50 mg/5 ml, 100 mg/ml
Side effects/adverse reactions:
GU: Urinary frequency, polyuria,
uremia, glucosuria, hyperurecemia
CNS: Drowsiness, paresthesia, depression, headache, *dizziness, fatigue, weakness,* fever
GI: Nausea, vomiting, anorexia, constipation, diarrhea, cramps, pancreatitis, GI irritation, ***hepatitis***
EENT: Blurred vision
INTEG: Rash, urticaria, purpura, photosensitivity, alopecia, erythema
multiforme
META: Hyperglycemia, hyperuricemia, increased creatinine, BUN
*HEMA: **Aplastic anemia, hemolytic
anemia, leukopenia, agranulocytosis, thrombocytopenia, neutropenia***
CV: Irregular pulse, orthostatic hypotension, palpitations, volume depletion, allergic myocarditis
ELECT: Hypokalemia, hypercalcemia, hyponatremia, hypochloremia,
hypomagnesemia
Contraindications: Hypersensitivity to thiazides or sulfonamides, anuria, renal decompensation, hypomagnesemia
Precautions: Hypokalemia, renal
disease, pregnancy (B), lactation,
hepatic disease, gout, COPD, lupus erythematosus, diabetes mellitus, hyperlipidemia, CrCl <25 ml/
min
Pharmacokinetics:
PO: Onset 2 hr, peak 4 hr, duration
6-12 hr, half-life 6-15 hr; excreted
unchanged by kidneys; crosses placenta; enters breast milk
Interactions:
• Increased toxicity of lithium, nondepolarizing skeletal muscle relaxants, cardiac glycosides
• Decreased effects of antidiabetics
• Decreased absorption of thiazides: cholestyramine, colestipol
• Increased risk of renal failure:
NSAIDs
• Hyperglycemia, hyperuricemia,
increased antihypertensives: diazoxide
• Hypokalemia: glucocorticoids,
amphotericin B
• Increased effects: loop diuretics
⍟ Potassium deficiency: aloe, buckthorn bark/berry, cascara sagrada
bark, licorice root, senna pod/leaf

H

Lab test interferences:
Increase: BSP retention, amylase, parathyroid test
Decrease: PBI, PSP

NURSING CONSIDERATIONS
Assess:
• Weight, I&O daily to determine fluid loss; effect of drug may be decreased if used qd
• Rate, depth, rhythm of respiration, effect of exertion
• B/P lying, standing; postural hypotension may occur
• Electrolytes: K, Mg, Na, Cl; include BUN, blood sugar, CBC, serum creatinine, blood pH, ABGs, uric acid, Ca; renal function
• Glucose in urine if patient is diabetic
• Signs of metabolic alkalosis: drowsiness, restlessness
• Signs of hypokalemia: postural hypotension, malaise, fatigue, tachycardia, leg cramps, weakness, dehydration
• Rashes, temp qd
• Confusion, especially in elderly; take safety precautions if needed
Administer:
• In AM to avoid interference with sleep if using drug as a diuretic
• K replacement if K <3 mg/dl
• With food; if nausea occurs, absorption may be decreased slightly
Evaluate:
• Therapeutic response: improvement in edema of feet, legs, sacral area qd, decreased B/P
Teach patient/family:
• To increase fluid intake to 2-3 L/day unless contraindicated; to rise slowly from lying or sitting position
• To notify prescriber of muscle weakness, cramps, nausea, dizziness
• That drug may be taken with food or milk
• To use sunscreen for photosensitivity

• That blood sugar may be increased in diabetics
• To take early in day to avoid nocturia
Treatment of overdose: Lavage if taken orally; monitor electrolytes; administer dextrose in saline; monitor hydration, CV, renal status

---

hydrocodone (R)
(hye-droe-koe′done)
Hycodan, Robidone*,
Tussigon
Func. class.: Antitussive opioid analgesic
Chem. class.: Opiate

Controlled Substance Schedule III
Action: Acts directly on cough center in medulla to suppress cough; binds to opiate receptors in CNS to reduce pain
Uses: Hyperactive and nonproductive cough, mild pain
Dosage and routes:
• *Adult:* **PO** 5 mg q4h prn
• *Child:* **PO** 1.25-5 mg q4h prn or 0.2 mg/kg q3-4h
Available forms: Syrup 5 mg/5 ml; tabs 5 mg (long-acting)
Side effects/adverse reactions:
CNS: **Drowsiness**, dizziness, lightheadedness, confusion, headache, sedation, euphoria, dysphoria, weakness, hallucinations, disorientation, mood changes, dependence, ***convulsions***
GI: Nausea, vomiting, anorexia, constipation, cramps, dry mouth
GU: Increased urinary output, dysuria, urinary retention
INTEG: Rash, urticaria, flushing, pruritus
EENT: Tinnitus, blurred vision, miosis, diplopia
CV: Palpitations, tachycardia, bradycardia, change in B/P, ***circulatory depression,*** syncope

---

⬦ = Nursing alert   🌿 = Herb-drug interaction   🚫 = Do not crush

*RESP: **Respiratory depression***
Contraindications: Hypersensitivity, addiction (narcotic)
Precautions: Addictive personality, pregnancy (C), lactation, increased intracranial pressure, MI (acute), severe heart disease, respiratory depression, hepatic disease, renal disease, child <18 yr
Pharmacokinetics: Onset 10-20 min, duration 4-6 hr, half-life 3½-4½ hr; metabolized in liver; excreted in urine; crosses placenta
Interactions:
• Increased CNS depression: alcohol, narcotics, sedative/hypnotics, phenothiazines, skeletal muscle relaxants, general anesthetics, tricyclic antidepressants
Lab test interferences:
Increase: Amylase, lipase
NURSING CONSIDERATIONS
Assess:
• Pain: intensity, type, location, and other characteristics
• CNS changes: dizziness, drowsiness, hallucinations, euphoria, LOC, pupil reaction
• Allergic reactions: rash, urticaria
• Cough and respiratory dysfunction: respiratory depression, character, rate, rhythm; notify prescriber if respirations are <10/min
• Need for pain medication, physical dependence
Administer:
• With antiemetic after meals if nausea or vomiting occurs
Perform/provide:
• Storage in light-resistant area at room temp
• Assistance with ambulation
• Safety measures: night-light, call bell within easy reach
Evaluate:
• Therapeutic response: decrease in pain or cough

Teach patient/family:
• To report any symptoms of CNS changes, allergic reactions
• That physical dependency may result when used for extended periods
• That withdrawal symptoms may occur: nausea, vomiting, cramps, fever, faintness, anorexia
🚫 Not to break, crush, or chew tabs
Treatment of overdose: Naloxone HCl (Narcan) 0.2-0.8 mg IV, O₂, IV fluids, vasopressors

H

---

hydrocortisone (℞)
(hy-dro-kor′tih-sone)
Cortef, Cortenema, Hydrocortone
hydrocortisone acetate (℞)
Cortifoam, Hydrocortone Acetate
hydrocortisone cypionate (℞)
Cortef
hydrocortisone sodium phosphate (℞)
Hydrocortone Phosphate
hydrocortisone sodium succinate (℞)
A-hydroCort, Solu-Cortef
Func. class.: Corticosteroid
Chem. class.: Short-acting glucocorticoid

Action: Decreases inflammation by suppression of migration of polymorphonuclear leukocytes, fibroblasts, reversal of increased capillary permeability and lysosomal stabilization
Uses: Severe inflammation, septic shock, adrenal insufficiency, ulcerative colitis, collagen disorders
Dosage and routes:
Adrenal insufficiency/inflammation
• *Adult:* **PO** 5-30 mg bid-qid; **IM/IV**

100-250 mg (succinate), then 50-100 mg **IM** as needed; **IM/IV** 15-240 mg q12h (phosphate)

Shock

• *Adult:* 500 mg-2 g q2-6h (succinate)

• *Child:* **IM/IV** 0.186-1 mg/kg bid-tid (succinate)

Colitis

• *Adult:* **ENEMA** 100 mg nightly for 21 days

Available forms: Tabs 5, 10, 20 mg; inj 25, 50 mg/ml; enema 100 mg/60 ml; acetate-inj 25*, 50 mg/ml*, enema 10% aerosol foam; supp 25 mg; cypionate-oral susp 10 mg/5 ml; phosphate-inj 50 mg/ml; succinate inj 100 mg*, 250 mg*, 500 mg*, 1000 mg/vial*

Side effects/adverse reactions:

CNS: Depression, flushing, sweating, headache, mood changes

CV: Hypertension, circulatory collapse, thrombophlebitis, embolism, tachycardia, edema

EENT: Fungal infections, increased intraocular pressure, blurred vision

GI: Diarrhea, nausea, abdominal distention, *GI hemorrhage,* increased appetite, *pancreatitis*

HEMA: Thrombocytopenia

INTEG: Acne, poor wound healing, ecchymosis, petechiae

MS: Fractures, osteoporosis, weakness

Contraindications: Psychosis, hypersensitivity, idiopathic thrombocytopenia, acute glomerulonephritis, amebiasis, fungal infections, nonasthmatic bronchial disease, child <2 yr, AIDS, TB

Precautions: Pregnancy (C), lactation, diabetes mellitus, glaucoma, osteoporosis, seizure disorders, ulcerative colitis, CHF, myasthenia gravis, renal disease, esophagitis, peptic ulcer

Pharmacokinetics:

PO: Onset 1-2 hr, peak 1 hr, duration 1-1½ days

IM/IV: Onset 20 min, peak 4-8 hr, duration 1-1½ days

RECT: Onset 3-5 days

Metabolized by liver, excreted in urine (17-OHCS, 17-KS), crosses placenta

Interactions:

• Decreased action of hydrocortisone: cholestyramine, colestipol, barbiturates, rifampin, ephedrine, phenytoin, theophylline

• Decreased effects of anticoagulants, anticonvulsants, antidiabetics, toxoids, vaccines

• Increased side effects: alcohol, amphotericin B, digitalis, cyclosporine, diuretics

• Risk of GI bleeding: salicylates, NSAIDs

🍵 Potassium deficiency: aloe, buckthorn, cascara sagrada, senna

Lab test interferences:

Increase: Cholesterol, Na, blood glucose, uric acid, Ca, urine glucose

Decrease: Ca, K, T$_4$, T$_3$, thyroid ^{131}I uptake test, urine 17-OHCS, 17-KS, PBI

False negative: Skin allergy tests

NURSING CONSIDERATIONS

Assess:

• K, blood sugar, urine glucose while on long-term therapy; hypokalemia and hyperglycemia

• Weight daily, notify prescriber of weekly gain >5 lb

• B/P q4h, pulse; notify prescriber of chest pain

• I&O ratio; be alert for decreasing urinary output, increasing edema

• Plasma cortisol levels during long-term therapy (normal level: 138-635 nmol/L SI units when drawn at 8 AM)

• Infection: increased temp, WBC, even after withdrawal of medication; drug masks infection

---

◆ = Nursing alert   🍵 = Herb-drug interaction   🚫 = Do not crush

• K depletion: paresthesias, fatigue, nausea, vomiting, depression, polyuria, dysrhythmias, weakness
• Edema, hypertension, cardiac symptoms
• Mental status: affect, mood, behavioral changes, aggression
Administer:
• Daily dose in AM for better results
• IM inj deep in large muscle mass; rotate sites; avoid deltoid; use 21G needle
• In one dose in AM to prevent adrenal suppression; avoid SC administration; may damage tissue
• With food or milk for GI symptoms (PO)
• Rectal: telling patient to retain for 20 min if possible
IV
• Phosphate: IV undiluted or added to dextrose or saline inj and given by infusion; give 25 mg or less/min
• Succinate: IV in mix-o-vial, or reconstitute 250 mg or less/2 ml bacteriostatic H_2O for inj; mix gently; give direct IV over 1 min or more; may be further diluted in 100, 250, 500, or 1000 ml of D_5W, D_5 0.9%, NaCl 0.9% given over ordered rate
Sodium phosphate preparations
Additive compatibilities: Amikacin, amphotericin B, bleomycin, cephapirin, metaraminol, sodium bicarbonate, verapamil
Syringe compatibilities: Metoclopramide
Y-site compatibilities: Allopurinol, amifostine, aztreonam, cefepime, cladribine, famotidine, filgrastim, fluconazole, fludarabine, granisetron, melphalan, ondansetron, paclitaxel, piperacillin/tazobactam, teniposide, thiotepa, vinorelbine
Sodium succinate preparations
Additive compatibilities: Amikacin, aminophylline, amphotericin B, calcium chloride, calcium gluconate, cephalothin, cephapirin, chlor-amphenicol, clindamycin, cloxacillin, corticotropin, daunorubicin, diphenhydramine, dopamine, erythromycin, floxacillin, lidocaine, magnesium sulfate, mephentermine, metronidazole/sodium bicarbonate, mitomycin, mitoxantrone, netilmicin, netilmicin/potassium chloride, norepinephrine, penicillin G potassium/sodium, piperacillin, polymyxin B, potassium chloride, sodium bicarbonate, theophylline, thiopental, vancomycin, verapamil, vit B/C
Syringe compatibilities: Metoclopramide, thiopental
Y-site compatibilities: Acyclovir, allopurinol, amifostine, aminophylline, amphotericin B cholesteryl, ampicillin, amrinone, amsacrine, atracurium, atropine, aztreonam, betamethasone, calcium gluconate, cefepime, cefmetazole, cephalothin, cephapirin, chlordiazepoxide, chlorpromazine, cisatracurium, cladribine, cyanocobalamin, cytarabine, dexamethasone, digoxin, diphenhydramine, dopamine, doxorubicin liposome, droperidol, edrophonium, enalaprilat, epinephrine, esmolol, estrogens conjugated, ethacrynate, famotidine, fentanyl, fentanyl/droperidol, filgrastim, fludarabine, fluorouracil, foscarnet, furosemide, gallium, granisetron, heparin, hydralazine, insulin (regular), isoproterenol, kanamycin, lidocaine, lorazepam, magnesium sulfate, melphalan, menadiol, meperidine, methicillin, methoxamine, methylergonovine, minocycline, morphine, neostigmine, norepinephrine, ondansetron, oxacillin, oxytocin, paclitaxel, pancuronium, penicillin G potassium, pentazocine, phytonadione, piperacillin/tazobactam, prednisolone, procainamide, prochlorperazine, propofol, propranolol, pyridostigmine, remifentanil, sco-

H

polamine, sodium bicarbonate, succinylcholine, tacrolimus, teniposide, theophylline, thiotepa, trimethaphan, trimethobenzamide, vecuronium, vinorelbine

Perform/provide:

• Assistance with ambulation in patient with bone tissue disease to prevent fractures

Evaluate:

• Therapeutic response: ease of respirations, decreased inflammation

Teach patient/family:

• That ID as steroid user should be carried

• To notify prescriber if therapeutic response decreases; dosage adjustment may be needed; of signs of infection

• Not to discontinue abruptly, or adrenal crisis can result; drug should be tapered off

• To avoid OTC products: salicylates, alcohol in cough products, cold preparations unless directed by prescriber

• About cushingoid symptoms of adrenal insufficiency: nausea, anorexia, fatigue, dizziness, dyspnea, weakness, joint pain

---

hydromorphone (℞)

(hye-droe-mor'fone)
Dilaudid, Dilaudid HP,
hydromorphone HCl
Func. class.: Narcotic analgesic
Chem. class.: Opiate, semisynthetic phenanthrene

Controlled Substance Schedule II
Action: Inhibits ascending pain pathways in CNS, increases pain threshold, alters pain perception
Uses: Moderate to severe pain
Dosage and routes:

• *Adult:* **PO** 1-6 mg q4-6h prn; **IM/SC/IV** 2-4 mg q4-6h; **RECT** 3 mg hs prn

• *Geriatric:* **PO** 1-2 mg q4-6h
• *Child:* 0.5 mg q3-4h prn
Available forms: Inj 1, 2, 3, 4, 10 mg/ml; tabs 1, 2, 3, 4, 8 mg; supp 3 mg; oral sol 5 mg/5 ml; syrup 1 mg/5 ml
Side effects/adverse reactions:
CNS: Drowsiness, dizziness, confusion, headache, sedation, euphoria
GI: Nausea, vomiting, anorexia, constipation, cramps
GU: Increased urinary output, dysuria, urinary retention
INTEG: Rash, urticaria, bruising, flushing, diaphoresis, pruritus
EENT: Tinnitus, blurred vision, miosis, diplopia
CV: Palpitations, bradycardia, change in B/P
*RESP: **Respiratory depression***
Contraindications: Hypersensitivity, addiction (narcotic)
Precautions: Addictive personality, pregnancy (C), lactation, increased intracranial pressure, MI (acute), severe heart disease, respiratory depression, hepatic disease, renal disease, child <18 yr
Pharmacokinetics: Onset 15-30 min, peak ½-1 hr, duration 4-5 hr; metabolized by liver; excreted by kidneys; crosses placenta; excreted in breast milk, half-life 2-3 hr
Interactions:
• Effects may be increased with other CNS depressants: alcohol, opiates, sedative/hypnotics, antipsychotics, skeletal muscle relaxants
🍵 Increased action: kava
Lab test interferences:
Increase: Amylase
NURSING CONSIDERATIONS
Assess:
• I&O ratio; check for decreasing output; may indicate urinary retention
• CNS changes: dizziness, drowsiness, hallucinations, euphoria, LOC, pupil reaction

---

◆ = Nursing alert   🍵 = Herb-drug interaction   🚫 = Do not crush

• Allergic reactions: rash, urticaria
• Respiratory dysfunction: respiratory depression, character, rate, rhythm; notify prescriber if respirations are <10/min
• Need for pain medication, physical dependence
• Pain control, sedation by scoring
Administer:
• With antiemetic if nausea, vomiting occur
• When pain is beginning to return; determine interval by response
• Rotate inj sites when giving SC
IV
• Direct diluted with 5 ml sterile H_2O or NS; give through Y-tube or 3-way stopcock; give 2 mg or less/5 min
• IV INF: Dilute each 0.1-1 mg/ml NS (0.1-1 mg/ml), deliver by narcotic syringe infusor; may be diluted in D_5W, D_5/NaCl, 0.45% NaCl, or NS for larger amounts and delivery through an infusion pump
Additive compatibilities: Bupivacaine, fluorouracil, midazolam, ondansetron, promethazine, verapamil
Solution compatibilities: D_5W, D_5/0.45% NaCl, D_5/0.9% NaCl, D_5/LR, D_5/Ringer's sol, 0.45% NaCl, 0.9% NaCl, Ringer's and lactated Ringer's sol
Syringe compatibilities: Atropine, bupivacaine, ceftazidime, chlorpromazine, cimetidine, dimenhydrinate, diphenhydramine, fentanyl, glycopyrrolate, haloperidol, hydroxyzine, lorazepam, midazolam, pentazocine, pentobarbital, prochlorperazine, promethazine, ranitidine, scopolamine, tetracaine, thiethylperazine, trimethobenzamide
Y-site compatibilities: Acyclovir, allopurinol, amifostine, amikacin, amsacrine, aztreonam, cefamandole, cefazolin, cefepime, cefmetazole, cefoperazone, cefotaxime, cefoxitin, ceftazidime, ceftizoxime, cefuroxime, cephalothin, cephapirin, chloramphenicol, cisatracurium, cisplatin, cladribine, clindamycin, cyclophosphamide, cytarabine, diltiazem, dobutamine, dopamine, doxorubicin, doxorubicin liposome, doxycycline, epinephrine, erythromycin lactobionate, famotidine, fentanyl, filgrastim, fludarabine, foscarnet, furosemide, gentamicin, granisetron, heparin, kanamycin, labetalol, lorazepam, magnesium sulfate, melphalan, methotrexate, metronidazole, mezlocillin, midazolam, milrinone, morphine, moxalactam, nafcillin, nicardipine, nitroglycerin, norepinephrine, ondansetron, oxacillin, paclitaxel, penicillin G potassium, piperacillin, piperacillin/tazobactam, propofol, ranitidine, remifentanil, teniposide, thiotepa, ticarcillin, tobramycin, trimethoprim-sulfamethoxazole, vancomycin, vecuronium, vinorelbine
Perform/provide:
• Storage in light-resistant area at room temp
• Assistance with ambulation
• Safety measures: side rails, nightlight, call bell within easy reach
Evaluate:
• Therapeutic response: decrease in pain
Teach patient/family:
• To report any symptoms of CNS changes, allergic reactions
• That physical dependency may result when used for extended periods
• That withdrawal symptoms may occur: nausea, vomiting, cramps, fever, faintness, anorexia
Treatment of overdose: Naloxone HCl (Narcan) 0.2-0.8 mg IV, O_2, IV fluids, vasopressors

H

**hydromorphone/
guaifenesin/
alcohol (℞)**
(hye-droe-mor′fone)
Dilaudid Cough Syrup
Func. class.: Antitussive, narcotic
Chem. class.: Phenanthrene derivative, guaifenesin

Controlled Substance Schedule II
Action: Increases respiratory tract fluid by decreasing surface tension, adhesiveness, which increases removal of mucus; analgesic, antitussive
Uses: Cough
Dosage and routes:
• *Adult:* PO 1 mg q3-4h prn
Available forms: Syr 1 mg/5 ml
Side effects/adverse reactions:
CNS: Dizziness, drowsiness
GI: Nausea, constipation, vomiting, anorexia
CV: Hypotension
INTEG: Urticaria, rash
*RESP: **Respiratory depression***
Contraindications: Hypersensitivity, increased intracranial pressure, status asthmaticus
Precautions: Hypothyroidism, Addison's disease, CNS depression, brain tumor, asthma, hepatic disease, renal disease, COPD, psychosis, alcoholism, convulsive disorders, pregnancy (C), lactation
Pharmacokinetics: Metabolized by liver; half-life 2-4 hr
• Enhanced CNS depression: barbiturates, narcotics, antipsychotics, antidepressants
⍦ Increased action: kava
NURSING CONSIDERATIONS
Assess:
• VS, cardiac status, including hypotension
• Respiratory rate, depth
• Cough: type, frequency, character, including sputum
Administer:
• Decreased dose to elderly patients; metabolism may be slowed
Perform/provide:
• Storage at room temp
• Increased fluids, bulk, exercise to decrease constipation
Evaluate:
• Therapeutic response: absence of cough
Teach patient/family:
• To avoid driving, other hazardous activities until patient stabilized on medication if drowsiness occurs
• To avoid alcohol, other CNS depressants; will enhance sedating properties of this drug

**hydroxocobalamin
(vit B₁₂) (℞)**
(hye-drox′-o-ko-bal′a-min)
Acti-B$_{12}$*, Alphamin, Hydrobexan, Hydro-Crysti 12, Hydroxo-12, hydroxycobalamin, LA-12
Func. class.: Vitamin
Chem. class.: B$_{12}$—water-soluble vitamin

Action: Needed for adequate nerve functioning, protein and carbohydrate metabolism, normal growth, RBC development
Uses: Vit B$_{12}$ deficiency, pernicious anemia, vit B$_{12}$ malabsorption syndrome, Schilling test
Dosage and routes:
RDA levels
• *Adult and child ≥12 yr:* 2 µg
• *Pregnancy:* 2.2 µg
• *Lactation:* 2.6 µg
• *Child 7-11 yr:* 1.4 µg
• *Child 4-6 yr:* 1 µg
• *Child 6 mo-1 yr:* 0.5 µg
• *Neonate to 6 mo:* 0.3 µg

⬥ = Nursing alert   ⍦ = Herb-drug interaction   ⊘ = Do not crush

Vitamin B₁₂ deficiency

Adult: **IM** 30-100 µg qd × 5-10 days, maintenance 100-200 mg **IM** qmo

Child: **IM** 1-30 µg qd × 5-10 days, maintenance 60 µg **IM** qmo or more often

Pernicious anemia/malabsorption syndrome

• *Adult:* **IM** 100-1000 µg qd × 2 wk, then 100-1000 µg **IM** qmo

• *Child:* **IM** 1000-5000 µg × 2 wk or more given in 100-500 µg doses, then 60 µg **IM/SC** qmo

Schilling test

• *Adult and child:* **IM** 1000 µg in one dose

Available forms: Inj 1000 µg/ml

Side effects/adverse reactions:

CNS: Flushing, optic nerve atrophy

GI: Diarrhea

*CV: **CHF**, peripheral vascular thrombosis, **pulmonary edema***

INTEG: Itching, rash

Contraindications: Hypersensitivity, optic nerve atrophy, cardiac disease

Precautions: Pregnancy (A), (C) if used above RDA level, lactation, children

Pharmacokinetics: Stored in liver, kidneys, stomach; 50%-90% excreted in urine; crosses placenta, breast milk

Interactions:

• Decreased absorption of hydroxocobalamin: aminoglycosides, anticonvulsants, colchicine, chloramphenicol, antineoplastics, cimetidine, alcohol, vit C, K preparations

Lab test interferences:

False positive: Intrinsic factor

NURSING CONSIDERATIONS

Assess:

• K levels during beginning treatment

• CBC for increased reticulocyte count during first week of therapy, followed by increase in RBC and hemoglobin

• For pulmonary edema or worsening of CHF in cardiac patients

Administer:

• By IM inj for pernicious anemia unless contraindicated

Evaluate:

• Therapeutic response: decreased anorexia, dyspnea on excretion, palpitations, paresthesias, psychosis, visual disturbances

Teach patient/family:

• That treatment must continue for life in pernicious anemia

• The importance of a well-balanced diet

H

---

hydroxychloroquine (℞)

(hye-drox-ee-klor′oh-kwin)

Plaquenil

Func. class.: Antimalarial

Chem. class.: 4-Aminoquinoline derivative

Action: Inhibits parasite replications, transcription of DNA to RNA by forming complexes with DNA in parasite

Uses: Malaria caused by *P. vivax, P. malariae, P. ovale, P. falciparum* (some strains): lupus erythematosus, rheumatoid arthritis

Dosage and routes:

Malaria

• *Adult and child:* **PO** 5 (base) mg/kg/wk on same day of week, not to exceed 400 mg (310 mg base); treatment should begin 2 wk before entering endemic area, continue 8 wk after leaving; if treatment begins after exposure, 800 mg (620 mg base) for adult, 10 mg/kg for children in 2 divided doses 6 hr apart

Lupus erythematosus

• *Adult:* **PO** 400 mg (310 mg base) qd-bid; length depends on patient

response; maintenance 200-400 mg (155-310 mg base) qd
• *Child:* PO 3-5 mg (base)/kg/day max 400 mg/day

Rheumatoid arthritis

• *Adult:* PO 400-600 mg (310-465 mg base) qd, then 200-300 mg (155-310 mg base) qd after good response

Available forms: Tabs 200 mg (base 155 mg)

Side effects/adverse reactions:

CV: Hypotension, heart block, *asystole with syncope*

INTEG: Pruritus, pigmentation changes, skin eruptions, lichen planus-like eruptions, eczema, *exfoliative dermatitis,* alopecia

CNS: Headache, stimulation, fatigue, irritability, *convulsions,* bad dreams, dizziness, confusion, psychosis, decreased reflexes

EENT: Blurred vision, corneal changes, retinal changes, difficulty focusing, tinnitus, vertigo, deafness, photophobia, corneal edema

GI: Nausea, vomiting, anorexia, diarrhea, cramps

HEMA: Thrombocytopenia, agranulocytosis, hemolytic anemia, leukopenia

Contraindications: Hypersensitivity, retinal field changes, porphyria, children (long-term)

Precautions: Blood dyscrasias, severe GI disease, neurologic disease, alcoholism, hepatic disease, G6PD deficiency, psoriasis, eczema, pregnancy (C), lactation

Pharmacokinetics:

PO: Peak 1-2 hr, half-life 3-5 days; metabolized in liver; excreted in urine, feces, breast milk; crosses placenta

Interactions:

• Decreased action of hydroxychloroquine: Mg or Al compounds
• Increased levels of digoxin

• Increased antibody titer: rabies vaccine

NURSING CONSIDERATIONS
Assess:

• Ophthalmic test if long-term treatment or drug dosage >150 mg/day
• Liver studies qwk: AST, ALT, bilirubin
• Blood studies: CBC, platelets; WBC, RBC, platelets may be decreased
• For decreased reflexes: knee, ankle
• ECG during therapy
• Watch for depression of T waves, widening of QRS complex
• Allergic reactions: pruritus, rash, urticaria
• Blood dyscrasias: malaise, fever, bruising, bleeding (rare)
• For ototoxicity (tinnitus, vertigo, change in hearing); audiometric testing should be done before, after treatment

◆ For toxicity: blurring vision, difficulty focusing, headache, dizziness, knee, ankle reflexes; drug should be discontinued immediately

Administer:

PO

• Before or after meals or with milk; at same time each day to maintain drug level

Perform/provide:

• Storage in tight, light-resistant container at room temp; keep injection in cool environment

Evaluate:

• Therapeutic response: decreased symptoms of malaria, lupus erythematosus, rheumatoid arthritis

Teach patient/family:

• To use sunglasses in bright sunlight to decrease photophobia
• That urine may turn rust or brown
• To report hearing, visual problems, fever, fatigue, bruising, bleeding, which may indicate blood dyscrasias

Treatment of overdose: Induce vomiting; gastric lavage; administer barbiturate (ultrashort-acting), vasopressor, ammonium chloride; tracheostomy may be necessary

---

hydroxyurea (R)
(hye-drox'ee-yoo-ree-ah)
Droxia, Hydrea
Func. class.: Antineoplastic, antimetabolite
Chem. class.: Synthetic urea analog

Action: Acts by inhibiting DNA synthesis without interfering with RNA or protein synthesis; incorporates thymidine into DNA, causing direct damage to DNA strands; S phase specific of cell cycle

Uses: Melanoma, chronic myelocytic leukemia, recurrent or metastatic ovarian cancer, squamous cell carcinoma of the head and neck, sickle cell anemia, psoriasis

Dosage and routes:
Renal disease
• CrCl 10-50 ml/min dose 50%; CrCl <10 ml/min dose 20%
Solid tumors
• *Adult:* **PO** 80 mg/kg as a single dose q3d or 20-30 mg/kg as a single dose qd
In combination with radiation
• *Adult:* **PO** 80 mg/kg as a single dose q3d; should be started 7 days before irradiation
Resistant chronic myelocytic leukemia
• *Adult:* **PO** 20-30 mg/kg/day as a single daily dose
Available forms: Caps 200, 300, 400, 500 mg

Side effects/adverse reactions:
*HEMA: **Leukopenia, anemia, thrombocytopenia***
GI: Nausea, vomiting, anorexia, diarrhea, stomatitis, constipation

GU: Increased BUN, uric acid, creatinine, temporary renal function impairment
INTEG: Rash, urticaria, pruritus, dry skin
CV: Angina, ischemia
CNS: Headache, confusion, hallucinations, dizziness, ***convulsions***

Contraindications: Hypersensitivity, leukopenia (<2500/mm^3), thrombocytopenia (<100,000/mm^3), anemia (severe), pregnancy (D), lactation

Precautions: Renal disease (severe)
Pharmacokinetics: Readily absorbed when taken orally, peak level in 2 hr; degraded in liver; excreted in urine, almost totally eliminated in 24 hr; readily crosses blood-brain barrier

Interactions:
• Increased toxicity: radiation or other antineoplastics

Lab test interferences:
Increase: Renal function studies

NURSING CONSIDERATIONS
Assess:
• CBC, differential, platelet count qwk; withhold drug if WBC is <3500/mm^3 or platelet count is <100,000/mm^3; notify prescriber; drug should be discontinued
• Renal function studies: BUN, serum uric acid, urine CrCl, electrolytes before, during therapy
• I&O ratio; report fall in urine output to <30 ml/hr
• Monitor temp q4h; fever may indicate beginning infection
• Liver function tests before, during therapy: bilirubin, alk phosphatase, AST, ALT, LDH; prn or qmo
• B/P q3-4h; check for chest pain; angina, ischemia may occur
• Bleeding: hematuria, guaiac, bruising or petechiae, mucosa or orifices q8h
• Food preferences; list likes, dislikes

• Inflammation of mucosa, breaks in skin
• Buccal cavity q8h for dryness, sores or ulceration, white patches, oral pain, bleeding, dysphagia
• Symptoms indicating severe allergic reaction: rash, urticaria, itching, flushing
• Neurotoxicity: headaches, hallucinations, convulsions, dizziness

Administer:
• Allopurinol or $NaHCO_3$ concurrently to prevent high uric acid levels; extra fluids
• Antiemetic 30-60 min before giving drug and prn
• Antibiotics for prophylaxis of infection
• Transfusion for anemia

Perform/provide:
• Rinsing of mouth tid-qid with water, club soda; brushing of teeth bid-tid with soft brush or cotton-tipped applicators for stomatitis; use unwaxed dental floss
• Nutritious diet with iron, vitamin supplements as ordered

Evaluate:
• Therapeutic response: decreased tumor size, spread of malignancy

Teach patient/family:
🚫 Not to break, crush, or chew caps
• To report signs of infection: elevated temp, sore throat, flulike symptoms
• To report signs of anemia: fatigue, headache, faintness, shortness of breath, irritability
• To report bleeding: avoid use of razors, commercial mouthwash
• To avoid use of aspirin products, ibuprofen
• To avoid foods with citric acid, hot or rough texture if stomatitis is present
• To report stomatitis: any bleeding, white spots, ulcerations in the mouth; tell patient to examine mouth qd, report symptoms
• That contraceptive measures are recommended during therapy
• To notify prescriber of fever, chills, sore throat, nausea, vomiting, anorexia, diarrhea, bleeding, bruising; may indicate blood dyscrasias

---

hydroxyzine (℞)

(hye-drox'i-zeen)
Apo-Hydroxyzine*, Atarax, Atarax 100, hydroxyzine HCl, hydroxyzine pamoate, Multipax*, Novohydroxyzine*, Vistaril, Vistazine 50
Func. class.: Antianxiety/antihistamine/sedative-hypnotic
Chem. class.: Piperazine derivative

Action: Depresses subcortical levels of CNS, including limbic system, reticular formation
Uses: Anxiety preoperatively, postoperatively to prevent nausea, vomiting, to potentiate narcotic analgesics; sedation; pruritus

Dosage and routes:
• *Adult:* **PO** 25-100 mg tid-qid
• *Geriatric:* **PO** 10 mg tid-qid (pruritus)
• *Child >6 yr:* 50-100 mg/day in divided doses
• *Child <6 yr:* 50 mg/day in divided doses

Preoperatively/postoperatively
• *Adult:* **IM** 25-100 mg q4-6h
• *Child:* **IM** 0.5-1.1 mg/kg q4-6h
Available forms: Tabs 10, 25, 50, 100 mg; caps 25, 50, 100 mg; syr 10 mg/5 ml; oral susp 25 mg/5 ml; inj 25, 50 mg/ml

Side effects/adverse reactions:
CV: Hypotension
CNS: Dizziness, drowsiness, confu-

◆ = Nursing alert   🖊 = Herb-drug interaction   🚫 = Do not crush

sion, headache, tremors, fatigue, depression, *convulsions*
GI: Dry mouth
Contraindications: Hypersensitivity to this drug or cetirizine, early pregnancy, lactation, acute asthma
Precautions: Elderly, debilitated, hepatic disease, renal disease, narrow-angle glaucoma, COPD, prostatic hypertrophy, pregnancy (C)
Pharmacokinetics:
PO: Onset 15-30 min, duration 4-6 hr, half-life 3 hr, metabolized by liver, excreted by kidneys
Interactions:
• Increased CNS depressant effect: barbiturates, opioids, analgesics, alcohol
�herb Increased anticholinergic effect: henbane leaf
🌿 Increased action: kava

NURSING CONSIDERATIONS
Assess:
• B/P (lying, standing), pulse; if systolic B/P drops 20 mm Hg, hold drug, notify prescriber
• Mental status: mood, sensorium, affect
• Increased sedation
Administer:
• By Z-track injection in large muscle for IM to decrease pain, chance of necrosis, never give IV/SC
• With food or milk for GI symptoms (PO)
• Crushed if patient is unable to swallow medication whole
• Gum, hard candy, frequent sips of water for dry mouth
Additive compatibilities: Cisplatin, cyclophosphamide, cytarabine, dimenhydrinate, etoposide, lidocaine, mesna, methotrexate, nafcillin
Syringe compatibilities: Atropine, atropine/meperidine, benzquinamide, bupivacaine, butorphanol, chlorpromazine, cimetidine, codeine, diphenhydramine, doxapram, droperidol, fentanyl, fluphenazine,

glycopyrrolate, hydromorphone, lidocaine, meperidine, meperidine/atropine, methotrimeprazine, metoclopramide, midazolam, morphine, nalbuphine, oxymorphone, pentazocine, perphenazine, procaine, prochlorperazine, promazine, promethazine, scopolamine, sufentanil, thiothixene
Y-site compatibilities: Aztreonam, ciprofloxacin, cisatracurium, cladribine, famotidine, filgrastim, foscarnet, granisetron, melphalan, ondansetron, propofol, remifentanil, sufentanil, teniposide, thiotepa, vinorelbine
Perform/provide:
• Assistance with ambulation during beginning therapy, since drowsiness/dizziness occurs
• Safety measures, including side rails
• Checking to see if PO medication has been swallowed
Evaluate:
• Therapeutic response: decreased anxiety
Teach patient/family:
• That medication is not to be used for everyday stress or used longer than 4 mo
• To avoid OTC preparations (cold, cough, hay fever) unless approved by prescriber
• To avoid driving, activities that require alertness
• To avoid alcohol ingestion, other psychotropic medications
• Not to discontinue medication quickly after long-term use
• To rise slowly or fainting may occur
Treatment of overdose: Lavage if orally ingested; VS, supportive care; IV norepinephrine for hypotension

H

---

hyoscyamine (℞)

(hye-oh-sye′a-meen)
Anaspaz, Cystospaz, Cystospaz-M, Gastrosed, Levsin, Levsin Drops, Levsinex Timecaps, Neoquess

Func. class.: Anticholinergic
Chem. class.: Belladonna alkaloid

Action: Inhibits muscarinic actions of acetylcholine at postganglionic parasympathetic neuroeffector sites

Uses: Treatment of peptic ulcer disease in combination with other drugs; other GI disorders, other spastic disorders, urinary incontinence

Dosage and routes:
• *Adult:* **PO/SL** 0.125-0.25 mg tid-qid ac, hs; **TIME REL** 0.375 q12h; **IM/SC/IV** 0.25-0.5 mg q6h
• *Child 2-10 yr:* ½ adult dose
• *Child <2 yr:* ¼ adult dose

Available forms: Tabs 0.125, 0.13, 0.15 mg; caps time rel 0.375 mg; sol 0.125 mg/ml; elix 0.125 mg/5 ml; inj 0.5 mg/ml

Side effects/adverse reactions:
CNS: Confusion, stimulation in elderly, headache, insomnia, dizziness, drowsiness, anxiety, weakness, hallucination
GI: Dry mouth, constipation, paralytic ileus, heartburn, nausea, vomiting, dysphagia, absence of taste
GU: Urinary hesitancy, retention, impotence
CV: Palpitations, tachycardia
EENT: Blurred vision, photophobia, mydriasis, cycloplegia, increased ocular tension
INTEG: Urticaria, rash, pruritus, anhidrosis, fever, allergic reactions

Contraindications: Hypersensitivity to anticholinergics, narrow-angle glaucoma, GI obstruction, myasthenia gravis, paralytic ileus, GI atony, toxic megacolon, prostatic hypertrophy

Precautions: Hyperthyroidism, coronary artery disease, dysrhythmias, CHF, ulcerative colitis, hypertension, hiatal hernia, hepatic disease, renal disease, pregnancy (C), urinary retention, elderly

Pharmacokinetics:
PO: Duration 4-6 hr; metabolized by liver; excreted in urine; half-life 3.5 hr

Interactions:
• Decreased effect of hyoscyamine: antacids
• Increased anticholinergic effect: amantadine, tricyclic antidepressants, MAOIs, H_1-antihistamines
• Decreased effect of phenothiazines, levodopa, ketoconazole

NURSING CONSIDERATIONS

Assess:
• VS, cardiac status: checking for dysrhythmias, increased rate, palpitations
• I&O ratio; check for urinary retention or hesitancy
• GI complaints: pain, bleeding (frank or occult), nausea, vomiting, anorexia

Administer:
• ½ hr ac for better absorption
• Decreased dose to elderly patients; metabolism may be slowed
• Gum, hard candy, frequent rinsing of mouth for dryness of oral cavity

Perform/provide:
• Storage in tight container protected from light
• Increased fluids, bulk, exercise to decrease constipation

Evaluate:
• Therapeutic response: absence of epigastric pain, bleeding, nausea, vomiting

Teach patient/family:
• To avoid driving, other hazardous activities until stabilized on medication

 = Nursing alert   🖋 = Herb-drug interaction   ⊘ = Do not crush

• To avoid alcohol or other CNS depressants; will enhance sedating properties of this drug

• To avoid hot environments; heat stroke may occur; drug suppresses perspiration

• To use sunglasses when outside to prevent photophobia; may cause blurred vision

🚫 Not to break, crush, or chew time rel caps

---

ibuprofen (OTC, ℞)

(eye-byoo-proe′fen)

Aches-N-Pain, Actiprofen*, Advil, Amersol*, Apo-Ibuprofen*, Children's Advil, Excedrin IS, Genpril, Haltran, Ibuprin, ibuprofen, Ibuprohm, IBU-Tab, Medipren, Menadol, Midol-200, Motrin, Motrin IB, Motrin Junior Strength, Novoprofen*, Nuprin, Pamprin-IB, Rufen, Saleto-200, Saleto-400, Saleto-600, Saleto-800, Trendar

Func. class.: Nonsteroidal antiinflammatory

Chem. class.: Propionic acid derivative

Action: Inhibits prostaglandin synthesis by decreasing enzyme needed for biosynthesis; analgesic, antiinflammatory, antipyretic

Uses: Rheumatoid arthritis, osteoarthritis, primary dysmenorrhea, gout, dental pain, musculoskeletal disorders, fever

Dosage and routes:

Analgesic

• *Adult:* **PO** 200-400 mg q4-6h, not to exceed 3.2 g/day

• *Child:* **PO** 4-10 mg/kg/dose q6-8h

Antipyretic

• *Child 6 mo-12 yr:* **PO** 5 mg/kg (temp <102.5° F or 39.2° C), 10 mg/kg, (temp >102.5° F), may repeat q4-6h, max 40 mg/kg/day

Antiinflammatory

• *Adult:* **PO** 300-800 mg tid-qid, max 3.2 g/day

• *Child:* **PO** 30-40 mg/kg/day in 3-4 divided doses, max 50 mg/kg/day

Available forms: Tabs 100, 200, 300, 400, 600, 800 mg; oral susp 40 mg/ml, 100 mg/5 ml; tabs, chew 50, 100 mg; drops 40 mg/ml

Side effects/adverse reactions:

CV: Tachycardia, peripheral edema, palpitations, dysrhythmias

CNS: Headache, dizziness, drowsiness, fatigue, tremors, confusion, insomnia, anxiety, depression

EENT: Tinnitus, hearing loss, blurred vision

GI: Nausea, anorexia, vomiting, diarrhea, jaundice, ***cholestatic hepatitis,*** constipation, flatulence, cramps, dry mouth, peptic ulcer

*GU: **Nephrotoxicity:*** dysuria, hematuria, oliguria, azotemia

*HEMA: **Blood dyscrasias,*** increased bleeding time

INTEG: Purpura, rash, pruritus, sweating

Contraindications: Hypersensitivity, asthma, severe renal disease, severe hepatic disease

Precautions: Pregnancy (B) 1st and 2nd trimester, lactation, children, bleeding disorders, GI disorders, cardiac disorders, hypersensitivity to other antiinflammatory agents, elderly, CHF, CrCl <25 ml/min

Pharmacokinetics: Well absorbed (PO)

PO: Onset ½ hr; peak 1-2 hr, half-life 2-4 hr, metabolized in liver (inactive metabolites), excreted in urine (inactive metabolites), 90%-99% plasma protein binding, does not enter breast milk

Interactions:

• Decreased effect of: antihypertensives, thiazides, furosemide

• Decreased ibuprofen: aspirin

• Increased toxicity: digoxin, lithium, oral anticoagulants, cyclosporine

• Increased GI reactions: aspirin, corticosteroids

NURSING CONSIDERATIONS
Assess:

• Renal, liver, blood studies: BUN, creatinine, AST, ALT, Hgb, before treatment, periodically thereafter

• Pain: note type, duration, location and intensity with ROM 1 hr after administration

• Audiometric, ophthalmic examination before, during, after treatment; for eye, ear problems: blurred vision, tinnitus; may indicate toxicity

• Fever: temp before and 1 hr after administration

• Cardiac status: edema (peripheral), tachycardia, palpitations; monitor B/P, pulse for character, quality, rhythm especially in patients with cardiac disease/elderly

• For history of peptic ulcer disorder; asthma, aspirin, hypersensitivity, check closely for hypersensitivity reactions

Administer:

• With food, milk, or antacid to decrease GI symptoms; however, best to take on empty stomach to facilitate absorption; if nausea and vomiting occur/persist, notify prescriber

Perform/provide:

• Storage at room temp

Evaluate:

• Therapeutic response: decreased pain, stiffness in joints; decreased swelling in joints; ability to move more easily; reduction in fever or menstrual cramping

Teach patient/family:

• To report blurred vision, ringing, roaring in ears; may indicate toxicity; eye and hearing tests should be done during long-term therapy

• To avoid driving, other hazardous activities if dizziness or drowsiness occurs

⬥To report change in urine pattern, increased weight, edema, increased pain in joints, fever, blood in urine; indicate nephrotoxicity

• That therapeutic inflammatory effects may take up to 1 mo

• To avoid alcohol, salicylates; bleeding may occur in arthritis

• To use sunscreen to prevent photosensitivity

---

ibutilide (℞)
(eye-byoo'tih-lide)
Corvert
Func. class.: Antidysrhythmic
(Class III)

Action: Prolongs duration of action potential and effective refractory period, noncompetitive α- and β-adrenergic inhibition

Uses: Atrial fibrillation/flutter

Dosage and routes:

• *Adult:* **IV INF** (≥60 kg) 1 vial (1 mg) given over 10 min; **IV INF** (<60 kg) 0.01 mg/kg given over 10 min

Available forms: Inj 0.1 mg/ml

Side effects/adverse reactions:

CNS: Headache

GI: Nausea

CV: Hypotension, bradycardia, sinus arrest, CHF, dysrhythmias, hypertension, extrasystoles, ventricular tachycardia, bundle branch block, AV block

Contraindications: Hypersensitivity

Precautions: Sinus node dysfunction, 2nd- or 3rd-degree AV block, electrolyte imbalances, pregnancy (C), bradycardia, lactation, children <18 yr, renal/hepatic disease, elderly

Pharmacokinetics:

PO: Onset 1-3 wk, peak 2-10 hr;

⬥ = Nursing alert   ⫽ = Herb-drug interaction   ⊘ = Do not crush

half-life 15-100 days; metabolized by liver, excreted by kidneys
Interactions:

• Prodysrhythmia: phenothiazines, tricyclics, tetracycline, antidepressants, H₁-receptor antagonists

• Increased levels of digitalis, quinidine, procainamide, flecainide, disopyramide, phenytoin

🖊 Increased action: aloe, buckthorn, cascara sagrada, senna

NURSING CONSIDERATIONS
Assess:

• I&O ratio; electrolytes: (K, Na, Cl)

• Liver function studies: AST, ALT, bilirubin, alk phosphatase

• ECG continuously to determine drug effectiveness, measure PR, QRS, QT intervals, check for PVCs, other dysrhythmias, discontinue if atrial fibrillation/flutter ceases

• For dehydration or hypovolemia

• For rebound hypertension after 1-2 hr

• Cardiac rate, respiration: rate, rhythm, character, chest pain

Administer:
IV

• Undiluted or diluted in 50 ml 0.9% NaCl, or D₅W (0.017 mg/ml) give over 10 min

• Solution is stable for 48 hr refrigerated or 24 hr, room temp

• Do not admix with other solution, drugs

• Reduced dosage slowly with ECG monitoring

Evaluate:

• Therapeutic response: decrease in atrial fibrillation/flutter

Teach patient/family:

• To report side effects immediately

• Reason for medication

---

idarubicin (℞)
(eye-dah-roob′ih-sin)
Idamycin
Func. class.: Antineoplastic, antibiotic
Chem. class.: Anthracycline glycoside

Action: Inhibits DNS synthesis by binding to DNA, a vesicant derived from daunorubicin by binding to DNA, which causes strand splitting; cell cycle specific (S phase)

Uses: Used in combination with other antineoplastics for acute myelocytic leukemia in adults

Dosage and routes:

• *Adult:* **IV** 12 mg/m²/day × 3 days in combination with cytosine

Available forms: Inj 5, 10 mg vials

Side effects/adverse reactions:

*HEMA: **Thrombocytopenia, leukopenia, anemia***

GI: Nausea, vomiting, abdominal pain, mucositis, diarrhea, ***hepatotoxicity***

INTEG: Rash, extravasation, dermatitis, reversible alopecia, urticaria, thrombophlebitis at injection site

*CV: **Dysrhythmias, CHF, pericarditis, myocarditis,** peripheral edema*

CNS: Fever, chills, headache

Contraindications: Hypersensitivity, pregnancy (D), lactation

Precautions: Renal and hepatic disease, gout, bone marrow depression, children

Pharmacokinetics: Half-life 22 hr; metabolized by liver; crosses placenta; excreted in bile, urine (primarily as metabolites)

Interactions:

• Increased toxicity: other antineoplastics or radiation

• Decreased antibody response: live virus vaccines

Lab test interferences:

Increase: Uric acid

NURSING CONSIDERATIONS
Assess:

• CBC, differential, platelet count weekly; withhold drug if WBC is <4000/mm³ or platelet count is <75,000/mm³; notify prescriber of these results

• Blood, urine, uric acid levels

• Renal function studies: BUN, serum uric acid, urine CrCl, electrolytes before, during therapy

• I&O ratio; report fall in urine output to <30 ml/hr

• Monitor temp q4h; fever may indicate beginning infection

• Liver function tests before, during therapy: bilirubin, AST, ALT, alk phosphatase prn or qmo; check for jaundice of skin, sclera, dark urine, clay-colored stools, itchy skin, abdominal pain, fever, diarrhea

• Cardiac toxicity: CHF, dysrhythmias, cardiomyopathy; cardiac studies should be done before and periodically during treatment: ECG, chest x-ray

• ECG: watch for ST-T wave changes, low QRS and T, possible dysrhythmias (sinus tachycardia, heart block, PVCs)

• Bleeding: hematuria, guaiac stools, bruising or petechiae, mucosa or orifices q8h

• Effects of alopecia on body image; discuss feelings about body changes

• Inflammation of mucosa, breaks in skin

• Buccal cavity q8h for dryness, sores, ulceration, white patches, oral pain, bleeding, dysphagia

• Local irritation, pain, burning at injection site

• GI symptoms: frequency of stools, cramping

• Acidosis, signs of dehydration: rapid respirations, poor skin turgor, decreased urine output, dry skin, restlessness, weakness

Administer:

• Allopurinol or sodium bicarbonate to reduce uric acid levels, alkalinization of urine

• Transfusion for anemia

• Hydrocortisone for extravasation; apply ice compress after stopping infusion

IV, direct

• After preparing in biologic cabinet wearing gown, gloves, mask

• Antiemetic 30-60 min before giving drug and 6-10 hr after treatment to prevent vomiting

• After reconstituting 5 mg vial with 5 ml 0.9% NaCl (1 mg/1 ml); give over 10-15 min through Y-tube or 3-way stopcock of inf of D₅ or NS; discard unused portion

Solution compatibilities: D₃.₃/0.3% NaCl, D₅/0.9% NaCl, D₅W, LR, 0.9% NaCl

Y-site compatibilities: Amifostine, amikacin, aztreonam, cimetidine, cladribine, cyclophosphamide, cytarabine, diphenhydramine, droperidol, erythromycin, filgrastim, granisetron, imipenem/cisplatin, magnesium sulfate, mannitol, melphalan, metoclopramide, potassium chloride, ranitidine, sargramostim, thiotepa, vinorelbine

Perform/provide:

• Strict hand-washing technique, gloves, protective clothing

• Liquid diet: carbonated beverages, gelatin may be added if patient is not nauseated or vomiting

• Increase fluid intake to 2-3 L/day to prevent urate and calculi formation

• Diet low in purines: absence of organ meats (kidney, liver), dried beans, peas to reduce uric acid level

• Rinsing of mouth tid-qid with water, club soda; brushing of teeth tid-

---

⬥ = Nursing alert   = Herb-drug interaction   🚫 = Do not crush qid with soft brush or cotton-tipped applicators for stomatitis; use unwaxed dental floss

• Storage at room temp for 3 days after reconstituting or 7 days refrigerated

Evaluate:

• Therapeutic response: decreased tumor size, spread of malignancy

Teach patient/family:

• To report any complaints, side effects to nurse or prescriber

• That hair may be lost during treatment and wig or hairpiece may make patient feel better; tell patient that new hair may be different in color, texture

• To avoid foods with citric acid, hot or rough texture

• To report any bleeding, white spots, ulcerations in mouth; tell patient to examine mouth qd

• That urine may be red-orange for 48 hr

• To use contraception during treatment with this drug and for ≥4 mo after treatment

---

ifosfamide (℞)

(i-foss'fa-mide)

Ifex

Func. class.: Antineoplastic alkylating agent

Chem. class.: Nitrogen mustard

Action: Alkylates DNA, RNA, inhibits enzymes that allow synthesis of amino acids in proteins; also responsible for cross-linking DNA strands; activity is not cell cycle stage specific

Uses: Testicular cancer

Dosage and routes:

• *Adult:* **IV** 1.2 g/m²/day × 5 days, repeat course q3wk, given with mesna

Available forms: Inj 1, 3 g

Side effects/adverse reactions:

CNS: Facial paresthesia, fever, malaise, somnolence, confusion, depression, hallucinations, dizziness, disorientation, ***seizures, coma***

GI: Nausea, vomiting, anorexia, ***hepatotoxicity,*** stomatitis, constipation

INTEG: Dermatitis, alopecia, pain at injection site

GU: ***Hematuria, nephrotoxicity, hemorrhagic cystitis,*** dysuria, urinary frequency

HEMA: ***Thrombocytopenia, leukopenia, anemia***

Contraindications: Hypersensitivity, bone marrow suppression, pregnancy (D)

Precautions: Renal disease, lactation, children

Pharmacokinetics: Metabolized by liver; saturation occurs at high doses; excreted in urine; half-life 7-15 hr

Interactions:

• Increased myelosuppression: other antineoplastics, radiation

• Decreased antibody response: live virus vaccines

• Increased toxicity: barbiturates, allopurinol

NURSING CONSIDERATIONS

Assess:

• Liver function studies before, during therapy (bilirubin, AST, ALT, LDH) as needed or monthly

• CBC, differential, platelet count weekly; withhold drug if WBC <2000 or platelet count <50,000; notify prescriber

• Monitor temp q4h (may indicate beginning infection)

• Blood dyscrasias (anemia, granulocytopenia); bruising, fatigue, bleeding, poor healing

• Allergic reactions: dermatitis, exfoliative dermatitis, pruritus, urticaria

---

• I&O ratio; monitor for hematuria; hemorrhagic cystitis can occur; increase fluids to 3L/day

• Neuro symptoms: hallucinations, confusion, disorientation, drug should be discontinued

• Bleeding: hematuria, guaiac, bruising or petechiae, mucosa or orifices q8h

• Jaundice of skin, sclera, dark urine, clay-colored stools, itchy skin, abdominal pain, fever, diarrhea

Administer:

• Antiemetic 30-60 min before giving drug to prevent vomiting

• Antibiotics for prophylaxis of infection

• Always give with mesna to prevent ifosfamide-induced hemorrhagic cystitis

IV

• After diluting 1 g/20 ml sterile or bacteriostatic H_2O for inj with parabens or benzyl only; shake; may be diluted further with D_5W, LR, NS, sterile H_2O for inj; 1 g/20 ml = 50 mg/ml; 1 g/50ml = 20 mg/ml; 1 g/200 ml = 5 mg/ml; give over ≥ 30 min; may also give as cont inf over 72 hr

Additive compatibilities: Carboplatin, cisplatin, etoposide, fluorouracil, mesna

Syringe compatibilities: Mesna

Y-site compatibilities: Allopurinol, amifostine, amphotericin B cholesteryl, aztreonam, doxorubicin liposome, filgrastim, fludarabine, gallium, granisetron, melphalan, ondansetron, paclitaxel, piperacillin/ tazobactam, propofol, sargramostim, sodium bicarbonate, teniposide, thiotepa, vinorelbine

Perform/provide:

• Storage of powder at room temp

• Increase fluid intake to 3 L/day to prevent hemorrhagic cystitis

• Warm compresses at injection site for inflammation

Evaluate:

• Therapeutic response: decrease in size and spread of tumor

Teach patient/family:

• To notify prescriber of sore throat, swollen lymph nodes, malaise, fever; other infections may occur

• Not to have vaccinations during treatment

• That hair may be lost during treatment; a wig or hairpiece may make the patient feel better; new hair may be different in color, texture

• To report signs of anemia: fatigue, headache, faintness, shortness of breath, irritability

• To report bleeding; avoid use of razors, commercial mouthwash

• To avoid use of aspirin products, NSAIDs, ibuprofen, hemorrhage can occur

• To use contraceptive measures during therapy

• To avoid crowds, those with infections

---

imipenem/cilastatin (℞)
(i-me-pen′em sye-la-stat′in)
Primaxin IM, Primaxin IV
Func. class.: Antiinfective-misc. penicillin

Action: Interferes with cell wall replication of susceptible organisms; osmotically unstable cell wall swells, bursts from osmotic pressure; addition of cilastatin prevents renal inactivation that occurs with high urinary concentrations of imipenem

Uses: Serious infections caused by gram-positive: *Streptococcus pneumoniae*, group A β-hemolytic streptococci, *Staphylococcus aureus*, enterococcus; gram-negative: *Klebsiella, Proteus, Escherichia coli, Acinetobacter, Serratia, Pseudomonas aeruginosa, Salmonella, Shigella*

◆ = Nursing alert   ∥ = Herb-drug interaction   ⊘ = Do not crush

Dosage and routes:
• Renal adjustment is needed at CrCl <70 ml/min
• *Adult:* **IV** 250-500 mg q6h; severe infections may require 1 g q6h; may give **IM** q12h (total daily **IM** dosage >1500 mg not recommended); mild to moderate infections
• *Child:* **IV** 600-100 mg/kg/day, max 4 g/day
Available forms: Inj 250, 500 mg (IV); inj 500, 750 mg (IM)
Side effects/adverse reactions:
CNS: Fever, somnolence, *seizures,* confusion, dizziness, weakness, myoclonia
*GI: Diarrhea, nausea, vomiting, **pseudomembranous colitis, hepatitis,*** glossitis
CV: Hypotension, palpitations
*HEMA: **Eosinophilia, neutropenia,*** decreased Hgb, Hct
INTEG: Rash, urticaria, pruritus, pain at injection site, phlebitis, erythema at injection site
*SYST: **Anaphylaxis***
RESP: Chest discomfort, dyspnea, hyperventilation
Contraindications: Hypersensitivity, IM hypersensitivity to local anesthetics of the amide type
Precautions: Pregnancy (C), lactation, elderly, hypersensitivity to penicillins, seizure disorders, renal disease, children
Pharmacokinetics:
IV: Onset immediate, peak ½-1 hr, half-life 1 hr; 70%-80% excreted unchanged in urine
Interactions:
• Increased imipenem plasma levels: probenecid
• Increased toxicity: beta-lactam antibiotics
• Increased risk of seizures: ganciclovir
Lab test interferences:
Increase: AST, ALT, LDH, BUN, alk phosphatase, bilirubin, creatinine
False positive: Direct Coombs' test
NURSING CONSIDERATIONS
Assess:
• For infection: increased temp, WBC, characteristics of wounds, sputum, urine culture or stool culture
• Sensitivity to penicillin, other cephalosporins
• Renal disease: lower dose may be required
• Bowel pattern qd; if severe diarrhea occurs, drug should be discontinued; may indicate pseudomembranous colitis
• Allergic reactions: rash, urticaria, pruritus, wheezing, laryngeal edema; may occur few days after therapy begins; have epinephrine, antihistamine, emergency equipment available
• Overgrowth of infection: perineal itching, fever, malaise, redness, pain, swelling, drainage, rash, diarrhea, change in cough, sputum
Administer:
• After C&S is taken
IV
• After reconstitution of 250 or 500 mg with 10 ml of diluent and shake; add to at least 100 ml of same inf sol
• 250-500 mg over 20-30 min; 1 g over 40-60 min; give through Y-tube or 3-way stopcock; do not give by IV bolus or if cloudy
Y-site compatibilities: Acyclovir, amifostine, aztreonam, cefepime, cisatracurium, diltiazem, famotidine, fludarabine, foscarnet, granisetron, idarubicin, insulin (regular), melphalan, methotrexate, ondansetron, propofol, remifentanil, tacrolimus, teniposide, thiotepa, vinorelbine, zidovudine
Evaluate:
• Therapeutic response: negative

C&S; absence of signs and symptoms of infection

Teach patient/family:

• To report severe diarrhea; may indicate pseudomembranous colitis

• To report sore throat, bruising, bleeding, joint pain; may indicate blood dyscrasias (rare)

Treatment of anaphylaxis: Epinephrine, antihistamines; resuscitate if needed

---

imipramine (℞)

(im-ip′ra-meen)

Apo-Imipramine*, imipramine HCl*, Impril*, Janimine, Novo-Pramine*, SK-Pramine, Tofranil, Tofranil PM, Tipramine

Func. class.: Antidepressant—tricyclic

Chem. class.: Dibenzazepine—tertiary amine

Action: Blocks reuptake of norepinephrine, serotonin into nerve endings, increasing action of norepinephrine, serotonin in nerve cells

Uses: Depression, enuresis in children

Investigational uses: Chronic pain, migraine headaches, cluster headaches as adjunct, incontinence

Dosage and routes:

• *Adult:* **PO/IM** 75-100 mg/day in divided doses, may increase by 25-50 mg to 200 mg, not to exceed 300 mg/day; may give daily dose hs

• *Geriatric:* **PO** 25 mg hs, may increase to 100 mg/day in divided doses

• *Child:* **PO** 25-75 mg/day

Enuresis

• *Child:* **PO** 10 mg at hs, max 50 mg

Available forms: Tabs 10, 25, 50 mg; inj 25 mg/2 ml; caps 75, 100, 125, 150 mg

Side effects/adverse reactions:

HEMA: **Agranulocytosis, thrombocytopenia, eosinophilia, leukopenia**

CNS: Dizziness, drowsiness, confusion, headache, anxiety, tremors, stimulation, weakness, insomnia, nightmares, EPS (elderly), increased psychiatric symptoms, paresthesia

GI: Diarrhea, dry mouth, nausea, vomiting, *paralytic ileus;* increased appetite; cramps, epigastric distress, jaundice, *hepatitis,* stomatitis

GU: Retention, **acute renal failure**

INTEG: Rash, urticaria, sweating, pruritus, photosensitivity

CV: Orthostatic hypotension, ECG changes, tachycardia, hypertension, palpitations

EENT: Blurred vision, tinnitus, mydriasis

Contraindications: Hypersensitivity to tricyclic antidepressants, recovery phase of MI, convulsive disorders, prostatic hypertrophy

Precautions: Suicidal patients, severe depression, increased intraocular pressure, narrow-angle glaucoma, urinary retention, cardiac disease, hepatic disease, hyperthyroidism, electroshock therapy, elective surgery, elderly, pregnancy (C), lactation

Pharmacokinetics:

PO: Steady state 2-5 days; metabolized by liver; excreted in urine, breast milk, feces; crosses placenta; half-life 6-20 hr

Interactions:

• Decreased effects of guanethidine, clonidine, indirect-acting sympathomimetics (ephedrine)

• Increased effects of direct-acting sympathomimetics (epinephrine), alcohol, barbiturates, benzodiazepines, CNS depressants

• Hyperpyretic crisis, convulsions, hypertensive episode: MAOI (pargyline [Eutonyl])

⚠ Increased anticholinergic effect: belladonna, henbane

⚠ Increased action of imipramine: scopolia, kava

Lab test interferences:

Increase: Serum bilirubin, alk phosphatase, blood glucose

Decrease: 5-HIAA, VMA, urinary catecholamines

NURSING CONSIDERATIONS

Assess:

• B/P (lying, standing), pulse q4h; if systolic B/P drops 20 mm Hg, hold drug, notify prescriber; take vital signs q4h in patients with cardiovascular disease

• Blood studies: CBC, leukocytes, differential, cardiac enzymes if patient is receiving long-term therapy

• Hepatic studies: AST, ALT, bilirubin

• Weight qwk; appetite may increase with drug

• ECG for flattening of T wave, bundle branch block, AV block, dysrhythmias in cardiac patients

• EPS primarily in elderly: rigidity, dystonia, akathisia

• Mental status: mood, sensorium, affect, suicidal tendencies, increase in psychiatric symptoms: depression, panic

• Urinary retention, constipation; constipation is more likely to occur in children, elderly

◆Withdrawal symptoms: headache, nausea, vomiting, muscle pain, weakness; not usual unless drug discontinued abruptly

• Alcohol consumption; if alcohol is consumed, hold dose until morning

Administer:

• Increased fluids, bulk in diet for constipation, urinary retention

• With food or milk for GI symptoms

• Dosage hs if oversedation occurs during day; may take entire dose hs; elderly may not tolerate once/day dosing

• Gum, hard candy, or frequent sips of water for dry mouth

• In IM route after running warm water over ampule to dissolve crystals

Syringe compatibilities: Doxapram

Y-site compatibilities: Cladribine

Perform/provide:

• Storage in tight container at room temp; do not freeze

• Assistance with ambulation during beginning therapy, since drowsiness/dizziness occurs

• Safety measures, primarily in elderly

• Checking to see if PO medication swallowed

Evaluate:

• Therapeutic response: decreased depression, enuresis, pain

Teach patient/family:

• That therapeutic effects may take 2-3 wk

• That drug is dispensed in small amounts because of suicide potential, especially in beginning of therapy

• To use caution in driving, other activities requiring alertness because of drowsiness, dizziness, blurred vision

• To avoid alcohol ingestion, other CNS depressants

• Not to discontinue medication quickly after long-term use; may cause nausea, headache, malaise

• To wear sunscreen or large hat, since photosensitivity occurs

🚫 Not to break, crush, or chew caps

Treatment of overdose: ECG monitoring; induce emesis; lavage, activated charcoal; administer anticonvulsant

---

Side effects: *italics* = common; ***bold italics*** = life-threatening

immune globulin (R)
Gamimune N, Gammagard
S/D, gamma globulin,
Gammar–P IV, Iveegam,
Polygam, Polygam S/D,
Sandoglobulin,
Venoglobulin-I,
Venoglobulin-S
Func. class.: Immune serum
Chem. class.: IgG

Action: Provides passive immunity to hepatitis A, measles, varicella, rubella, immune globulin deficiency; contains gamma globulin antibodies (IgG)

Uses: Immunodeficiency syndrome, B-cell chronic lymphocytic leukemia, Kawasaki syndrome, bone marrow transplantation, pediatric HIV infection, agammaglobulinemia, hepatitis A, B exposure, measles exposure, measles vaccine complications, purpura, rubella exposure, chickenpox exposure

Dosage and routes:
• *Adult:* IM 30-50 ml qmo; IV 100 mg/kg qmo, 0.01-0.02 ml/kg/min × ½ hr (Gamimune N); IV 200 mg/kg qmo, 0.05-1 ml/min × 15-30 min, then increase to 1.5-2.5 ml/min (Sandoglobulin)
• *Child:* IM 20-40 ml qmo
Hepatitis A exposure
• *Adult and child:* IM 0.02-0.04 ml/kg or 0.1 mg/kg if treatment is delayed
Hepatitis B exposure
• *Adult and child:* IM 0.06 ml/kg within 1 wk, qmo
Measles (postexposure)
• *Child:* IM 0.25 ml/kg within 6 days
Immunoglobulin deficiency
• *Adult and child:* IM 1.3 ml/kg, then 0.66 ml/kg after 2-4 wk and q2-4wk thereafter

Idiopathic thrombocytopenia, purpura
• *Adult and child:* IV 0.4 g/kg × 5 days or 1 g/kg/day × 1-2 days
Kawasaki syndrome
• *Child:* PO 2 g/kg as a single dose
Available forms: Inj 2, 10 ml/vial; 5% sol 0.5, 1, 2.5, 3, 6, 10 g vials
Side effects/adverse reactions:
INTEG: Pain at injection site, rash, pruritus, chills, chest pain
MS: Arthralgia
SYST: Lymphadenopathy, *anaphylaxis*
CNS: Headache, fatigue, malaise
GI: Abdominal pain
Contraindications: Hypersensitivity
Precautions: Pregnancy (C)
Interactions:
• Do not administer live virus vaccines within 3 mo of this drug
NURSING CONSIDERATIONS
Assess:
• For exposure date: this drug should be given within 6 days of measles, 7 days of hepatitis B, 14 days of hepatitis A
• For anaphylaxis: diaphoresis, wheezing, chest tightness, hypotension
Administer:
• IM ≤3 ml in one site, use large muscle mass
• Only with epinephrine 1:1000, resuscitative equipment available
• Only within 2 wk of exposure to hepatitis A
IV
• Gamimune N: IV undiluted or dilute with D₅; give 0.01 ml/kg/min; may increase to 0.02-0.04 ml/kg/min
• Sandoglobulin: IV diluted with provided diluent; give 0.5-1 ml/min × 15-30 min; may increase to 1.5-2.5 ml/min
• Venoglobulin-I: (50 mg/ml sol) give 0.01-0.02 ml/kg/min; if no ad-

◆ = Nursing alert   ∅ = Herb-drug interaction   ⊘ = Do not crush

verse reaction in ½ hr, increase to 0.04 ml/kg/min, store at room temp
• Gammagard: reconstitute with sterile H_2O for inj (50 mg protein/ml); give 0.5 ml/kg/hr, may increase to 4 ml/kg/hr, use infusion set provided
• Gammar-IV: give 0.01 ml/kg/min (50 mg/ml sol) × 15-30 min, may increase to 0.02 ml/kg/min, may increase to 0.03-0.06 ml/kg/min
Y-site compatibilities: Fluconazole, sargramostim
Perform/provide:
• Storage at 36°-46° F (2°-8° C)
Evaluate:
• Prevention of infection, increased platelets
Teach patient/family:
• That passive immunity is temporary
• The treatment of anaphylaxis: epinephrine, diphenhydramine, O_2, vasopressors, corticosteroids

---

indapamide (℞)
(in-dap'a-mide)
indapamide, Lozide*, Lozol
Func. class.: Diuretic—thiazide-like, antihypertensive
Chem. class.: Indoline

Action: Acts on proximal section of distal renal tubule and thick ascending loop of Henle by inhibiting reabsorption of sodium; may act by direct vasodilation caused by blocking of calcium channel
Uses: Edema of CHF, hypertension, diuresis
Dosage and routes:
Edema
• *Adult:* **PO** 2.5 mg qd in AM; may be increased to 5 mg qd if needed
Antihypertensive
• *Adult:* 1.25-5 mg qd; may increase to 5 mg/day over 8 wk

Available forms: Tabs 1.25, 2.5 mg
Side effects/adverse reactions:
GU: Polyuria, nocturia, urinary frequency, impotence
ELECT: Hypochloremic alkalosis, hypomagnesemia, hyperuricemia, hypercalcemia, hyponatremia, hypokalemia, hyperglycemia
CNS: Headache, dizziness, fatigue, weakness, nervousness, agitation, extremity numbness, depression
GI: Nausea, diarrhea, dry mouth, vomiting, anorexia, cramps, constipation, abdominal pain
EENT: Blurred vision, nasal congestion, increased intraocular pressure
INTEG: Rash, pruritus
MS: Cramps
CV: Orthostatic hypotension, volume depletion, palpitations, dysrhythmias, PVCs
Contraindications: Hypersensitivity, anuria, hepatic coma
Precautions: Hypokalemia, dehydration, ascites, hepatic disease, severe renal disease, pregnancy (B), lactation, CrCl <25 ml/min (not effective)
Pharmacokinetics:
PO: Onset 1-2 hr, peak 2 hr, duration up to 36 hr; excreted in urine, feces; half-life 14-18 hr
Interactions:
• Hyperglycemia: diazoxide
• Increased toxicity of: muscle relaxants, steroids, lithium, digitalis
• Decreased K: steroids, amphotericin B
• Decreased effects: antidiabetics, antigout agents, anticoagulants
• Decreased absorption: cholestyramine, colestipol
• Decreased hypotensive effect: indomethacin, NSAIDs
🖉 Potassium deficiency: aloe, buckthorn, cascara sagrada, licorice, senna

---

Lab test interferences:

Increase: Ca, parathyroid test glucose, uric acid

NURSING CONSIDERATIONS
Assess:

• Weight daily, I&O daily to determine fluid loss; effect of drug may be decreased if used qd

• Rate, depth, rhythm of respiration, effect of exertion

• B/P lying, standing; postural hypotension may occur

• Electrolytes: K, Mg, Na, Cl: include BUN, CBC, serum creatinine, blood pH, ABGs, uric acid, Ca, glucose

• Signs of metabolic alkalosis, hypokalemia

• Rashes, fever qd

• Confusion, especially in elderly; take safety precautions if needed

• Hydration: skin turgor, thirst, dry mucous membranes

Administer:

• In AM to avoid interference with sleep

• With food; if nausea occurs, absorption may be decreased slightly

Evaluate:

• Therapeutic response: improvement in edema of feet, legs, sacral area daily, decreased B/P

Teach patient/family:

• Diet high in K; to rise slowly from lying or sitting position

• To recognize adverse reactions: muscle cramps, weakness, nausea, dizziness

• To take with food or milk for GI symptoms

• To use sunscreen for photosensitivity

• To take early in day to prevent nocturia

Treatment of overdose: Lavage if taken orally; monitor electrolytes, administer IV fluids; monitor hydration, CV, renal status

---

indinavir (℞)

(en-den'a-veer)

Crixivan

Func. class.: Antiviral

Chem. class.: Synthetic peptide-like substrate analog

Action: Inhibits human immunodeficiency virus (HIV) protease; this prevents maturation of the infectious virus

Uses: HIV alone or in combination

Dosage and routes:

• Reduce dose in mild/moderate hepatic impairment and ketoconazole co-administration

• *Adult:* **PO** 800 mg q8h; if given with ddI, give 1 hr apart on empty stomach

Available forms: Caps 200, 400 mg

Side effects/adverse reactions:

GI: Diarrhea, abdominal pain, nausea, vomiting, anorexia, dry mouth

CNS: Headache, insomnia, dizziness, somnolence

INTEG: Rash

MS: Pain

OTHER: Asthenia

Contraindications: Hypersensitivity

Precautions: Liver disease, pregnancy (C), lactation, children, renal disease

Pharmacokinetics: Unknown

Interactions:

• Increase indinavir levels: ketoconazole

• Decreased indinavir levels: rifamycins

• Increased levels of both drugs: clarithromycin, zidovudine

• Increased levels of isoniazid, oral contraceptives

◆Life-threatening dysrhythmias: ergots, midazolam, rifampin, triazolam

---

◆ = Nursing alert   ⧳ = Herb-drug interaction   ⊘ = Do not crush

• Drug/food: increased absorption: high-fat, grapefruit, high protein

NURSING CONSIDERATIONS
Assess:
• Signs of infection, anemia
• Liver studies: ALT, AST
• The presence of other sexually transmitted diseases
• Bowel pattern before, during treatment; if severe abdominal pain with bleeding occurs, drug should be discontinued; monitor hydration
• Skin eruptions; rash, urticaria, itching
• Allergies before treatment, reaction of each medication; place allergies on chart

Administer:
• With water, 1 hr ac or 2 hr pc

Teach patient/family:
• To take as prescribed; if dose is missed, take as soon as remembered up to 1 hr before next dose; do not double dose
🚫 Not to break, crush, or chew caps
• That drug must be taken in equal intervals around the clock to maintain blood levels for duration of therapy

---

indomethacin (℞)

(in-doe-meth′a-sin)
Apo-Indomethacin*, Indameth*, Indocid*, Indocin, Indocin IV, Indocin PDA*, Indocin SR, indomethacin, Novomethacin*

Func. class.: Nonsteroidal antiinflammatory (NSAID)

Chem. class.: Propionic acid derivative

Action: Inhibits prostaglandin synthesis by decreasing enzyme needed for biosynthesis; analgesic, antiinflammatory, antipyretic

Uses: Rheumatoid arthritis, ankylosing rheumatoid spondylitis, acute gouty arthritis, closure of patent ductus arteriosus in premature infants

Dosage and routes:

Arthritis/antiinflammatory
• *Adult:* **PO/RECT** 25-50 mg bid; may increase by 25 mg/day qwk, not to exceed 200 mg/day; **SUS REL** 75 mg qd, may increase to 75 mg bid

Acute arthritis
• *Adult:* **PO/RECT** 50 mg tid; use only for acute attack, then reduce dose

Patent ductus arteriosus
Longer or repeated treatment courses may be necessary for very premature infants
• *Infant <2 days:* **IV** 0.2 mg/kg, then 0.1 mg/kg q12-24h
• *Infant 2-7 days:* **IV** 0.2 mg/kg, then 0.2 mg × 2 doses after 12, 24 hr
• *Infant >7 days:* **IV** 0.2 mg/kg, then 0.25 mg/kg × 2 doses after 12, 24 hr

Available forms: Caps 25, 50 mg; caps ext rel 75 mg; susp 25 mg/5 ml; rec supp 50 mg; inj 1 mg vial

Side effects/adverse reactions:

GI: Nausea, anorexia, *vomiting,* diarrhea, jaundice, **cholestatic hepatitis,** *constipation,* flatulence, cramps, dry mouth, peptic ulcer, *ulceration, perforation, GI bleeding*

CNS: Dizziness, drowsiness, fatigue, tremors, confusion, insomnia, anxiety, depression, headache

CV: Tachycardia, peripheral edema, palpitations, dysrhythmias, hypertension

INTEG: Purpura, rash, pruritus, sweating

GU: **Nephrotoxicity: dysuria, hematuria, oliguria, azotemia**

HEMA: **Blood dyscrasias,** prolonged bleeding

EENT: Tinnitus, hearing loss, blurred vision

Contraindications: Hypersensitivity, asthma, severe renal disease, severe hepatic disease, ulcer disease

Precautions: Pregnancy, lactation, children, bleeding disorders, GI disorders, cardiac disorders, hypersensitivity to other antiinflammatory agents, pregnancy (B) 1st and 2nd trimesters, lactation, depression

Pharmacokinetics:

PO: Onset 1-2 hr, peak 3 hr, duration 4-6 hr; metabolized in liver, kidneys; excreted in urine, bile, feces; crosses placenta; excreted in breast milk; 99% plasma protein binding

Interactions:

• Increased effect of: digoxin, penicillamine, phenytoin

• Decreased effect of antihypertensives

• Decreased levels of indomethacin: aspirin

• Toxicity: lithium, methotrexate, cyclosporine, aminoglycosides, aspirin, corticosteroids, triamterene, alcohol

• Increased risk of bleeding: anticoagulants

NURSING CONSIDERATIONS

Assess:

• Renal, liver, blood studies: BUN, creatinine, AST, ALT, Hgb, before treatment, periodically thereafter; if renal function has decreased, do not give subsequent doses

• Audiometric, ophthalmic exam before, during, after treatment

• For eye, ear problems: blurred vision, tinnitus; may indicate toxicity

• For confusion, mood changes, hallucinations, especially in elderly

Administer:

PO

• With food to decrease GI symptoms and prevent ulcerations; do not crush, chew, or break sus rel cap

IV

• After diluting 1 mg/ml or more NS or sterile H_2O for inj without preservative; give over 20-30 min to avoid dramatic shift in cerebral blood flow

Y-site compatibilities: Furosemide, insulin (regular), potassium chloride, sodium bicarbonate, sodium nitroprusside

Perform/provide:

• Storage at room temp

Evaluate:

• Therapeutic response: decreased pain, stiffness in joints, decreased swelling in joints, ability to move more easily

Teach patient/family:

• To report blurred vision, ringing, roaring in ears; may indicate toxicity

• To avoid driving, other hazardous activities if dizziness, drowsiness occurs

• To report change in urine pattern, increased weight, edema, increased pain in joints, fever, blood in urine; indicate nephrotoxicity; to report mood changes: anxiety, depression

• That therapeutic antiinflammatory effects may take up to 1 mo

• To avoid alcohol, NSAIDs, salicylates; bleeding may occur

Ⓝ Not to break, crush, or chew sus rel or reg caps

• To use sunscreen to prevent photosensitivity

---

infliximab

(in-fliks′ih-mab)

Remicade

Func. class.: Monoclonal antibody

Action: Monoclonal antibody that neutralizes the activity of tumor necrosis factor alpha (TNF α) found

◆ = Nursing alert   ✐ = Herb-drug interaction   Ⓝ = Do not crush in Crohn's disease; decreased infiltration of inflammatory cells

Uses: Crohn's disease, fistulizing; moderate-severe

Dosage and routes:

Crohn's disease (moderate-severe)
• *Adult:* **IV INF** 5 mg/kg

Crohn's disease (fistulizing)
• *Adult:* **IV INF** 5 mg/kg initially, then repeat dose 2 wk, 6 wk after 1st dose

Available forms: Powder for inj 100 mg

Side effects/adverse reactions:

SYST: ***Anaphylaxis***

GI: Nausea, vomiting, abdominal pain, stomatitis, constipation, dyspepsia, flatulence

CNS: Headache, dizziness, depression, vertigo, fatigue, anxiety, fever

HEMA: ***Anemia***

INTEG: Rash, dermatitis, urticaria, dry skin, sweating, flushing, hematoma, pruritus

RESP: URI, pharyngitis, bronchitis, cough, dyspnea, sinusitis

MS: Myalgia, back pain, arthralgia

GU: Dysuria, urinary frequency

CV: Chest pain, hyper- and hypotension, ***tachycardia***

Contraindications: hypersensitivity to murines

Precautions: Pregnancy (C), lactation, children, elderly

Pharmacokinetics: Distributed to vascular compartment, half-life 9.5 days

NURSING CONSIDERATIONS

Assess:
• GI symptoms: nausea, vomiting, abdominal pain
• Take periodic blood counts (CBC)
• CV status: B/P, pulse, chest pain
• Allergic reaction: rash, dermatitis, urticaria, dyspnea, hypotension, fever, chills; discontinue if severe, administer epinephrine, corticosteroids, antihistamines

Administer:

IV INF
• Immediately after reconstitution; reconstitute with 10 ml of sterile water for inj, further dilute total dose/ 250 ml of 0.9% NaCl inj to a total conc. of between 0.4 and 4 mg/ml; use 21G or smaller needle for reconstitution, direct sterile water at glass wall of vial, gently swirl
• Give over ≥2 hr, use polyethylene-lined infusion with in-line, sterile, low-protein-bind filter

Perform/provide:
• Refrigerated storage, do not freeze

Evaluate:
• Therapeutic response: absence of fever, mucus in stools

Teach patient/family:
• Not to breastfeed while taking this drug
• To notify prescriber of GI symptoms, hypersensitivity reactions

---

influenza virus vaccine, trivalent A & B (whole virus/split virus) (Ŗ)

Fluogen, FluShield, Fluviral*, Fluvirin, Fluzone, influenza virus vaccine, Trivalent

Func. class.: Vaccine

Action: Produces antibodies to influenza virus; split virus vaccine causes less adverse reactions

Uses: Prevention of Russian, Chile, Philippine influenza

Dosage and routes:
• *Adult and child >12 yr:* **IM** 0.5 ml in 1 dose
• *Child 3-12 yr:* **IM** 0.5 ml, repeat in 1 mo (split) unless 1978-1985 vaccine was given
• *Child 6 mo to 3 yr:* **IM** 0.25 ml, repeat in 1 mo (split) unless 1978-1985 vaccine was given

---

Available forms: Inj IM (varies)

Side effects/adverse reactions:

CNS: Fever, Guillain-Barré syndrome

INTEG: Urticaria, induration, erythema

SYST: **Anaphylaxis,** malaise

MS: Myalgia

Contraindications: Hypersensitivity, active infection; chicken, egg allergy, Guillain-Barré syndrome

Precautions: Elderly, immunosuppression, pregnancy (B)

NURSING CONSIDERATIONS

Assess:

• For skin reactions: rash, induration, erythema

• For anaphylaxis: inability to breathe, bronchospasm

Administer:

• Only with epinephrine 1:1000 on unit to treat laryngospasm

• Only IM

Perform/provide:

• Written record of immunization

• At least 2 mo after measles virus vaccine; do not administer at same time as DPT

Evaluate:

• For history of allergies, skin conditions (eczema, psoriasis, dermatitis), reactions to vaccinations

---

insulin, analog injection (lispro) (℞)
Humalog

insulin, isophane suspension (NPH) (℞)
Humulin N, Iletin NPH*, Iletin II NPH*, Novolin ge NPH*, Novolin N, Novolin N PenFill, Novolin N Prefilled, NPH Iletin I, NPH Iletin II, NPH-N

insulin, isophane suspension and regular insulin (℞)
Humulin 70/30, Humalin 30/70*, Novolin 70/30, Novolin 70/30 PenFill, Novolin 70/30 Prefilled, Novolin ge 30/70*

insulin, regular (℞)
Humulin R*, Iletin I*, Iletin II*, Novolin ge Toronto*, Novolin R, Novolin R Velosulin, Novolin R PenFill, Novolin R Prefilled, Regular Ilentin I, II, Regular Purified Pork Insulin, Velosulin Human BR

insulin, zinc suspension (Lente) (℞)
Humulin L, Iletin*, Iletin II*, Lente Ilentin I, Lente Iletin II, Lente L, Novolin ge Lente*, Novolin L

insulin, zinc suspension extended (Ultralente) (℞)
Humulin U Ultralente, Humulin U*, Novolin ge Ultralente*

isophane insulin suspension and insulin injection (℞)
Humalin 50/50, Novolin 50/50*

Func. class.: Pancreatic hormone
Chem. class.: Exogenous unmodified insulin

Action: Decreases blood sugar; by transport of insulin into cells and the conversion of glucose to glycogen, indirectly increases blood pyruvate and lactate, decreases phosphate and potassium; insulin may be beef, pork, human (processed by recombinant DNA technologies)

Uses: Adult-onset diabetes, juvenile diabetes, ketoacidosis types I and II, type II (non–insulin-dependent) diabetes mellitus, type I (insulin-dependent) diabetes mellitus

Dosage and routes:
Insulin, isophane, suspension
• *Adult:* **SC** dosage individualized by blood, urine glucose; usual dose 7-26 U/day; may increase by 2-10 U/day if needed

Regular insulin (ketoacidosis)
• *Adult:* **IV** 5-10 U, then 5-10 U/hr until desired response, then switch to **SC** dose; **IV**/inf 2-12 U (50 U/500 ml of normal saline)
• *Child:* **IV** 0.1 U/kg

Replacement
• *Adult and child:* **SC** 0.5-1 U/kg/day qid given 30 min ac
• *Adolescent:* **SC** 0.8-1.2 mg/kg/day; this dosage is used during rapid growth

Available forms: NPH Inj 100 U/ml; regular inj 100 U/ml; zinc susp 100 U/ml; insulin analog inj 100 U/ml; insulin zinc susp, ext (Ultralente) 100 U/ml; isophane insulin/insulin inj 100 U/ml; insulin lispro 100 U/ml 1.5 ml cartridges

Side effects/adverse reactions:
EENT: Blurred vision, dry mouth
INTEG: Flushing, rash, urticaria, warmth, *lipodystrophy,* lipohypertrophy, swelling, redness
META: Hypoglycemia, rebound hyperglycemia (Somogyi effect 12-72 hr or longer)
SYST: ***Anaphylaxis***

Contraindications: Hypersensitivity to protamine
Precautions: Pregnancy (B)
Pharmacokinetics:
SC (lispro): Onset rapid, peak ½-1 hr, duration 3-4 hr
SC (NPH): Onset 1-2 hr, peak 4-12 hr, duration 18-24 hr
SC (regular susp): Onset ½ hr, peak 4-8 hr, duration 12-24 hr
SC (regular): Onset ½-1 hr, peak 2-4 hr, duration 5-7 hr
IV (regular): Onset 10-30 min, peak 10-30 min, duration ½-1 hr
SC (regular conc): Onset ½-1 hr, peak 2-5 hr, duration 5-7 hr
SC (zinc susp): Onset 1-2 ½ hr, peak 7-15 hr, duration 12-24 hr
SC (zinc susp conc): Onset 4-8 hr, peak 10-30 hr, duration, 7-36 hr
SC (zinc susp prompt): Onset 1-1 ½ hr, peak 5-10 hr, duration 12-16 hr
Metabolized by liver, muscle, kidneys; excreted in urine

Interactions:
• Increased hypoglycemia: salicylate, alcohol, β-blockers, anabolic steroids, fenfluramine, phenylbutazone, sulfinpyrazone, guanethidine, oral hypoglycemics, MAOIs, tetracycline
• Decreased hypoglycemia: thiazides, thyroid hormones, oral contraceptives, corticosteroids, estrogens, dobutamine, epinephrine
🌿 Decreased hypoglycemic effect: broom, buchu, dandelion, juniper
🌿 Decreased or increased hypoglycemic effect: chromium, fenugreek, ginseng
🌿 Increased glucose tolerance: karela

Lab test interferences:
Increase: VMA
Decrease: K, Ca
Interference: Liver function studies, thyroid function studies

---

NURSING CONSIDERATIONS
Assess:

• Fasting blood glucose, 2 hr PP (80-150 mg/dl, normal fasting level; 70-130 mg/dl, normal 2 hr level); also glycosylated Hgb may be drawn to identify treatment effectiveness

• Urine ketones during illness; insulin requirements may increase during stress, illness, surgery

• For hypoglycemic reaction that can occur during peak time (sweating, weakness, dizziness, chills, confusion, headache, nausea, rapid weak pulse, fatigue, tachycardia, memory lapses, slurred speech, staggering gait, anxiety, tremors, hunger)

• For hyperglycemia: acetone breath, polyuria, fatigue, polydipsia, flushed, dry skin, lethargy

Administer:

SC

• After warming to room temp by rotating in palms to prevent injecting cold insulin; use only insulin syringes with markings or syringe matching U/ml; rotate inj sites within one area: abdomen, upper back, thighs, upper arm, buttocks; keep record of sites

• Increased dosages if tolerance occurs; give human insulin to those allergic to beef or pork

• Do not use if cloudy, thick, or discolored

• Lispro: 15 min ac

IV

• IV direct, undiluted via vein, Y-site, 3-way stopcock; give at 50 U/min or less

• By cont inf after diluting with IV sol and run at prescribed rate; use IV inf pump for correct dosing; give reduced dose at serum glucose level of 250 mg/100 ml

Additive compatibilities: Bretylium, cimetidine, lidocaine, meropenem, ranitidine, verapamil

Syringe compatibilities: Metoclopramide

Y-site compatibilities: Amiodarone, ampicillin, ampicillin/sulbactam, aztreonam, cefazolin, cefotetan, dobutamine, esmolol, famotidine, gentamicin, heparin, heparin/hydrocortisone, imipenem/cilastatin, indomethacin, magnesium sulfate, meperidine, meropenem, midazolam, morphine, nitroglycerin, oxytocin, pentobarbital, potassium chloride, propofol, ritodrine, sodium bicarbonate, sodium nitroprusside, tacrolimus, terbutaline, ticarcillin, ticarcillin/clavulanate, tobramycin, vancomycin, vit B/C

Perform/provide:

• Store at room temp for <1 mo; keep away from heat and sunlight; refrigerate all other supply; do not use if discolored; do not freeze—IV route, regular only

Evaluate:

• Therapeutic response: decrease in polyuria, polydipsia, polyphagia, clear sensorium, absence of dizziness, stable gait

Teach patient/family:

• That blurred vision occurs; not to change corrective lens until vision is stabilized 1-2 mo

• To keep insulin, equipment available at all times

• That drug does not cure diabetes but controls symptoms

• To carry Medic Alert ID as diabetic

• To recognize hypoglycemia reaction: headache, tremors, fatigue, weakness

• The dosage, route, mixing instructions, if any diet restrictions, disease process

• To carry candy or lump sugar to treat hypoglycemia

• The symptoms of ketoacidosis: nausea, thirst, polyuria, dry mouth, decreased B/P, dry, flushed skin, acetone breath, drowsiness, Kussmaul respirations

• That a plan is necessary for diet, exercise; all food on diet should be eaten; exercise routine should not vary

• About blood glucose testing; make sure patient is able to determine glucose level

• To avoid OTC drugs unless directed by prescriber

Treatment of overdose: Glucose 25g IV, via dextrose 50% sol, 50 ml or glucagon 1 mg

---

interferon alfa-2a/ interferon alfa-2b (℞)

(in-ter-feer´on)
Roferon-a/Intron-a
Func. class.: Misc. antineoplastic
Chem. class.: Protein product

Action: Antiviral action inhibits viral replication by reprogramming virus; antitumor action suppresses cell proliferation; immunomodulating action phagocytizes target cells; may also inhibit virus replication in virus-infested cells

Uses: Hairy cell leukemia in persons >18 yr, condylomata acuminata, malignant melanoma, AIDS (use phase II with zidovudine), chronic hepatitis B, C

Investigational uses: Bladder tumors, carcinoid tumors, non-Hodgkin's lymphoma, essential thrombocytopenia, cytomegaloviruses, herpes simplex

Dosage and routes:
alfa-2a
• *Adult:* **SC/IM** 3 million IU × 16-24 wk, then 3 million IU 3 ×/wk maintenance
alfa-2b
Chronic hepatitis B
• 30-35 million IU/wk **SC/IM** as 5

million IU/day or 10 million IU/ 3 × /wk × 16 wk
Hairy cell leukemia
• 2 million IU/m² 3 ×/wk; if severe adverse reactions occur, dose should be skipped or reduced by ½
Condylomata acuminata
• 1 million IU/lesion 3 × /wk × 3 wk
Kaposi's sarcoma
• 30 million IU/m² 3 × /wk
Available forms: alfa-2a inj 3, 6, 36 million IU/ml; alfa-2b inj 3, 5, 10, 18, 25 million U/vial, powder for inj 5, 10, 18, 25, 50 million U/vial
Side effects/adverse reactions:
CNS: Dizziness, confusion, numbness, paresthesias, hallucinations, **convulsions, coma,** amnesia, anxiety, mood changes
CV: Edema, hypotension, hypertension, chest pain, palpitations, dysrhythmias, ***CHF, MI, CVA***
INTEG: Rash, dry skin, itching, alopecia, flushing, photosensitivity
GI: Weight loss, taste changes
GU: Impotence
MISC: Flulike syndrome; fever, fatigue, myalgias, headache, chills
Contraindications: Hypersensitivity
Precautions: Severe hypotension, dysrhythmia, tachycardia, pregnancy (C), lactation, children, severe renal or hepatic disease, convulsion disorder
Pharmacokinetics: Half-life (interferon alfa-2a) 3.7-8.5 hr, peak 3-4 hr; half-life (interferon alfa-2b) 2-7 hr, peak 6-8 hr
interferon alpha-2b
Interactions:
• Increased theophylline levels: aminophylline
• Increased neutropenia: zidovudine
Lab test interferences:
Interference: AST, ALT, LDH, alk phosphatase, WBC, platelets, granulocytes, creatinine

---

NURSING CONSIDERATIONS
Assess:

• For symptoms of infection; chills, fever, headache; may be masked by drug fever

• CNS reaction: LOC, mental status, dizziness, confusion, paresthesia, slurred speech

• Cardiac status: Lung sounds; ECG before and during treatment, especially in those with cardiac disease

• Bone marrow depression: bruising, bleeding, blood in stools, urine, sputum, emesis

• Mental status: depression, suicidal thoughts, hallucinations, amnesia

Administer:

alfa-2a

• SC/IM after reconstituting 18 million U/3 ml of diluent provided (6 million U/ml)

• 36 million U/ml is used for Kaposi's sarcoma only

alfa-2b

• IM/SC after reconstituting 3-5 million IU/1 ml, 10 million IU/2 ml, 25 million IU/5 ml, of diluent provided, mix gently

• Intralesional after reconstituting 10 million IU/1 ml bacteriostatic water for inj; no more than 5 lesions can safely be treated at a time

• At hs to minimize side effects

• Acetaminophen as ordered to alleviate fever and headache

Perform/provide:

• Storage of reconstituted sol for 1 mo in refrigerator

• Increased fluid intake to 2-3 L/day

Evaluate:

• Therapeutic response: decrease in size, number of lesions

Teach patient/family:

• To take acetaminophen for fever

• To avoid hazardous tasks, since confusion, dizziness may occur; avoid prolonged sunlight, use sunscreen

• That brands of this drug should not be changed; each form is different, with different doses

• That fatigue is common; activity may have to be altered to take hs to minimize flulike symptoms

• Not to become pregnant while taking drug; possible mutagenic effects

• To report signs of infection: sore throat, fever, diarrhea, vomiting

• That impotence may occur during treatment but is temporary

• That emotional lability is common; notify prescriber if severe or incapacitating

---

interferon alfacon-1
(℞)

(in-ter-feer′on al′fa-kon)

Infergen

Func. class.: Recombinant type I interferon

Action: Induces biologic responses and has antiviral, antiproliferative and immunomodulatory effects

Uses: Chronic hepatitis C infections

Investigational uses: Hairy cell leukemia when used with G-CSF

Dosage and routes:

• *Adult:* **SC** 9 µg as a single inj 3×/wk × 24 wk

Available forms: Inj 9 µg, 15 µg

Side effects/adverse reactions:

CNS: Headache, fatigue, fever, rigors, insomnia, dizziness

GI: Abdominal pain, nausea, diarrhea, anorexia, dyspepsia, vomiting, constipation, flatulence, hemorrhoids, decreased salivation

MS: Back, limb, neck skeletal pain

GU: Dysmenorrhea, vaginitis, menstrual disorders

INTEG: Alopecia, pruritus, rash, erythema, dry skin

EENT: Tinnitus, earache, conjunctivitis, eye pain

◆ = Nursing alert　　🖉 = Herb-drug interaction　　Ⓢ = Do not crush

HEMA: ***Granulocytopenia, thrombocytopenia, leukopenia,*** ecchymosis

CV: Hypertension, palpitation

PSYCH: Nervousness, depression, anxiety, lability, abnormal thinking

RESP: Pharyngitis, upper respiratory infection, cough, sinusitis, rhinitis, respiratory tract congestion, epistaxis, dyspnea, bronchitis

Contraindications: Hypersensitivity to alpha interferons, or products from *E. coli*

Precautions: Thyroid disorders, myelosuppression, hepatic, cardiac disease, lactation, children <18 yr

Pharmacokinetics: Peak 24-36 hr

Interactions:
• None known

NURSING CONSIDERATIONS

Assess:
• Platelet counts, heme concentration, ANC, serum creatinine concentration, albumin, bilirubin, TSH, T4
• For myelosuppression, hold dose if neutrophil count is <500 × 10^6^/L or if platelets are <50 × 10^9^/L
• For hypersensitivity: discontinue immediately if hypersensitivity occurs

Evaluate:
• Therapeutic response: decreased chronic hepatitis C signs/symptoms

Teach patient/family:
• Provide patient or family member with written, detailed information about drug

---

interferon alfa-n 1 lymphoblastoid

See appendix a—selected new drugs

---

interferon alfa-n 3 (℞)

(in-ter-feer′on)
Alferon N

Func. class.: Antineoplastic
Chem. class.: Human interferon α-protein

Action: Binds interferon to membrane receptors on cell surface with high specificity; this produces protein synthesis, inhibition of virus replication, suppression of cell proliferation, increased phagocytosis

Uses: Condylomata acuminata (venereal/genital warts)

Dosage and routes:
• *Adult:* 0.05 ml (250,000 IU) per wart, given 2 × /wk × 8 wk; not to exceed 0.5 ml (2.5 million IU); inject into base of wart

Available forms: Inj 5 m IU/l ml vial with 3.3 mg/ml phenol and 1 mg/ml human albumin

Side effects/adverse reactions:

CNS: Fever, headache, sweating, vasovagal reaction, chills, fatigue, dizziness, insomnia, sleepiness, depression

GI: Nausea, vomiting, heartburn, diarrhea, constipation, anorexia, stomatitis, dry mouth

MS: Myalgias, arthralgia, back pain

INTEG: Pain at injection site, pruritus

CV: Chest pain, hypotension

Contraindications: Hypersensitivity to this product, egg protein, IgG, neomycin

Precautions: Pregnancy (C), lactation, children, CHF, angina (unstable), COPD, diabetes mellitus with ketoacidosis, hemophilia, pulmonary embolism, thrombophlebitis, bone marrow depression, convulsive disorder

Pharmacokinetics: Unable to detect

Lab test interferences:
Interference: AST, ALT, LDH, alk phosphatase, WBC, platelets, granulocytes, creatinine

NURSING CONSIDERATIONS
Assess:
• For symptoms of infection; may be masked by drug fever
• CNS reaction: LOC, mental status, dizziness, confusion
• For body image disturbance
Administer:
• Acetaminophen to alleviate fever and headache
Perform/provide:
• Storage of reconstituted sol for 1 mo in refrigerator
• Increased fluid intake to 2-3 L/day
Evaluate:
• Therapeutic response: decrease in wart size
Teach patient/family:
• To avoid hazardous tasks, since confusion, dizziness may occur
• That brands of this drug should not be changed; each form is different, with different doses
• That fatigue is common; activity may have to be altered
• Not to become pregnant while taking drug; possible mutagenic effects
• To report signs of infection: sore throat, fever, diarrhea, vomiting
• To recognize the signs of hypersensitivity: liver, urticaria, wheezing, dyspnea; notify prescriber immediately

---

interferon beta-1a
(in-ter-feer′on)
Avonex
interferon beta-1b (℞)
Betaseron
Func. class.: Multiple sclerosis agent
Chem. class.: *E. coli* derivative

Action: Antiviral, immunoregulatory; action not clearly understood; biologic response modifying properties mediated through specific receptors on cells, inducing expression of interferon-induced gene products

Uses: Ambulatory patients with relapsing or remitting multiple sclerosis

Investigational uses: May be useful in treatment of AIDS, AIDS-related Kaposi's sarcoma, malignant melanoma, metastatic renal cell carcinoma, cutaneous T cell lymphoma, acute non-A, non-B hepatitis

Dosage and routes:
interferon beta-1a
• *Adult:* **IM** 30 µg qwk
interferon beta-1b
Relapsing/remitting multiple sclerosis
• *Adult:* **SC** 0.25 mg (8 IU) qod
Available forms: beta-1a 33 µg (6.6 million IU/vial); beta-1b powder for inj lyophilized 0.3 mg (9.6 mIU)

Side effects/adverse reactions:
CNS: Headache, fever, pain, chills, mental changes, hypertonia, **suicide attempts**
CV: Migraine, palpitations, hypertension, tachycardia, peripheral vascular disorders
EENT: Conjunctivitis, blurred vision
GI: Diarrhea, constipation, vomiting, abdominal pain
GU: Dysmenorrhea, irregular men-

⬥ = Nursing alert   ▰ = Herb-drug interaction   ⊘ = Do not crush *ses, metrorrhagia,* cystitis, breast pain

HEMA: **Decreased lymphocytes, ANC, WBC;** lymphadenopathy

INTEG: Sweating, inj site reaction

MS: Myalgia, **myasthenia**

RESP: Sinusitis, dyspnea

Contraindications: Hypersensitivity to natural or recombinant interferon-β or human albumin

Precautions: Pregnancy (C), lactation, child <18 yr, chronic progressive MS, depression, mental disorders

NURSING CONSIDERATIONS
Assess:

• Blood, renal, hepatic studies: CBC, differential, platelet counts, BUN, creatinine ALT, urinalysis; if absolute neutrophil count < 750/mm^3, or if AST/ALT is 10 × normal, drug is discontinued

• CNS symptoms: headache, fatigue, depression

• GI status: diarrhea or constipation, vomiting, abdominal pain

• Cardiac status: increased B/P, tachycardia

• Mental status: depression, depersonalization, suicidal thoughts, insomnia

• For multiple sclerosis symptoms

Administer:

• Acetaminophen for fever, headache

• SC only

Interferon beta-1a

• Reconstitute with 1.1 ml diluent, swirl, give within 6 hr

Interferon beta-1b

• Reconstitute by injecting diluent provided (1.2 ml) into vial, swirl (8 mIU/ml), use 27G needle for inj

Perform/provide:

• Storage in refrigerator; do not freeze

Evaluate:

• Therapeutic response: decreased symptoms of multiple sclerosis

Teach patient/family:

• To provide patient or family member with written, detailed information about the drug

• That blurred vision, sweating may occur

• That female patients may experience irregular menses, dysmenorrhea, or metrorrhagia as well as breast pain

• To use sunscreen to prevent photosensitivity

• To notify prescriber if pregnancy is suspected

• Inj technique and care of equipment

• To notify prescriber of increased temp, chills, muscle soreness, fatigue

---

interferon gamma-1b (R̶)
(in-ter-feer′on)
Actimmune
Func. class.: Biologic response modifier
Chem. class.: Lymphokine, interleukin type

Action: Species-specific protein synthesized in response to viruses, potent phagocyte-activating effects; can mediate killing of *S. aureus, T. gondii, L. donovani, L. monocytogenes, M. avium-intracellulare;* enhances oxidative metabolism of macrophages, enhances antibody-dependent cellular cytotoxicity

Uses: Serious infections associated with chronic granulomatous disease

Dosage and routes:

• *Adult:* SC 50 µg/m^2 (1.5 million U/m^2) for patients with surface area >0.5 m^2; 1.5 µg/kg/dose for patient with surface area <0.5 m^2; give Monday, Wednesday, Friday for 3 × /wk dosing

Side effects: *italics* = common; **bold italics** = life-threatening

Available forms: Inj 100 µg (3 million U)/single-dose vial

Side effects/adverse reactions:

GI: Nausea, anorexia, abdominal pain, weight loss, diarrhea, vomiting

CNS: Headache, fatigue, depression, fever, chills

INTEG: Rash, pain at injection site

MS: Myalgia, arthralgia

Contraindications: Hypersensitivity to interferon gamma, *E. coli*-derived products

Precautions: Pregnancy (C), cardiac disease, seizure disorders, CNS disorders, myelosuppression, lactation, children

Pharmacokinetics:

SC: Dose absorbed 89%, elimination half-life 5.9 hr, peak 7 hr

Interactions:

• Increased myelosuppression: other myelosuppressive agents

NURSING CONSIDERATIONS

Assess:

• Blood, renal, hepatic studies: CBC, differential, platelet counts, BUN, creatinine, ALT, urinalysis

• CNS symptoms: headache, fatigue, depression

Administer:

• At hs to minimize adverse reactions; administer acetaminophen for fever, headache

• 50% of dose if severe reactions occur or discontinue treatment until reactions subside

• In right and left deltoid and anterior thigh

• Warm to room temp before use; do not leave at room temp over 12 hr (unopened vial)

Perform/provide:

• Storage in refrigerator upon receipt; do not freeze; do not shake

Evaluate:

• Therapeutic response: decreased serious infections, improvement in existing infections and inflammatory conditions

Teach patient/family:

• The method of administration if family members will be giving medication

• Provide patient or family member with written, detailed information about drug

---

ipecac syrup (R̶, OTC)
(ip′e-kak)

Func. class.: Emetic

Chem. class.: Cephaelis ipecacuanha derivative

Action: Acts on chemoreceptor trigger zone to induce vomiting; irritates gastric mucosa

Uses: In poisoning to induce vomiting

Dosage and routes:

• *Adult:* PO 15-30 ml, then 200-300 ml water; repeat 1×, if vomiting does not occur within 20 min

• *Child >1 yr:* PO 15 ml, then 200-300 ml water

• *Child 6-12 mo:* PO 5-10 ml, then 100-200 ml water; may repeat dose if needed

Available forms: Liq

Side effects/adverse reactions:

CNS: Depression, convulsions, coma

GI: Nausea, vomiting, bloody diarrhea

CV: Circulatory failure, atrial fibrillation, fatal myocarditis, dysrhythmias

Contraindications: Hypersensitivity, unconscious/semiconscious, depressed gag reflex, poisoning with petroleum products or caustic substances, convulsions

Precautions: Lactation, pregnancy (C)

Pharmacokinetics:

PO: Onset 15-30 min

⬥ = Nursing alert   🌿 = Herb-drug interaction   Ⓝ = Do not crush

Interactions:

• Do not administer with activated charcoal, other antiemetics; effect will be decreased

• Drug/food: decreased effect: dairy products

• Increased abdominal distention: carbonated drinks

NURSING CONSIDERATIONS
Assess:

• VS, B/P; check patients with cardiac disease more often

• Type of poisoning; do not administer if petroleum products or caustic substances have been ingested: kerosene, gasoline, lye, Drano

• Respiratory status before, during, after administration; check rate, rhythm, character; respiratory depression can occur rapidly with elderly or debilitated patients

Administer:

◆ Ipecac syrup, not ipecac fluid, which is 14 times stronger; death may occur

• Activated charcoal after vomiting completed; may begin lavage after 10-15 min after 2 doses of ipecac syrup with no result

Evaluate:

• Therapeutic response: vomiting

---

ipratropium (℞)

(i-pra-troe′pee-um)

Atrovent

Func. class.: Anticholinergic, bronchodilator

Chem. class.: Synthetic quaternary ammonium compound

Action: Inhibits interaction of acetylcholine at receptor sites on the bronchial smooth muscle, resulting in decreased cGMP and bronchodilation

Uses: Bronchodilation during bronchospasm in those with COPD; rhinorrhea in children 6-11 yr (nasal spray)

Dosage and routes:

• *Adult:* 2 **INH** 4 × day, not to exceed 12 **INH**/24 hr; sol 500 μg (1 unit dose) given 3-4 ×/day

• *Child 6-11 yr:* Nasal 1 spray in each nostril

Available forms: Aerosol 18 μg/actuation; nasal spray 0.03%, 0.06%; sol for inh 0.02%

Side effects/adverse reactions:

GI: Nausea, vomiting, cramps

EENT: Dry mouth, blurred vision

CNS: Anxiety, dizziness, headache, nervousness

RESP: Cough, worsening of symptoms, **bronchospasms**

INTEG: Rash

CV: Palpitation

Contraindications: Hypersensitivity to this drug, atropine, soya lecithin

Precautions: Pregnancy (B), lactation, children <12 yr, narrow-angle glaucoma, prostatic hypertrophy, bladder neck obstruction

Pharmacokinetics: Half-life 2 hr; does not cross blood-brain barrier

NURSING CONSIDERATIONS
Assess:

• For palpitations; if severe, drug may have to be changed

• For tolerance over long-term therapy; dose may have to be increased or changed

Administer:

Nebulizer

• Use sol in nebulizer with a mouthpiece rather than a face mask

Nasal spray

• Priming pump initially requires 7 actuations of the pump, priming again is not necessary if used regularly

Perform/provide:

• Storage at room temp

• Hard candy, frequent drinks, sugarless gum to relieve dry mouth

---

Evaluate:

• Therapeutic response: ability to breathe adequately

Teach patient/family:

• That compliance is necessary with number of inhalations/24 hr, or overdose may occur; spacer device in the elderly

• To shake before using

• The correct method of inhalation and cleaning of equipment daily

---

irbesartan (℞)

(er-be-sar′tan)

Avapro

Func. class.: Antihypertensive

Chem. class.: Angiotensin II receptor blocker (Type AT_1)

Action: Blocks the vasoconstrictor and aldosterone-secreting effects of angiotensin II; selectively blocks the binding of angiotensin II to the AT_1 receptor found in tissues

Uses: Hypertension, alone or in combination

Investigational uses: Heart failure, hypertensive patients with diabetic nephropathy caused by type II diabetes

Dosages and routes:

• *Adult:* **PO** 150 mg qd; may be increased to 300 mg qd

Available forms: 75, 150, 300 mg

Side effects/adverse reactions:

CNS: Dizziness, anxiety, headache, fatigue

GI: Diarrhea, dyspepsia

RESP: Cough, upper respiratory infection

Contraindications: Hypersensitivity, pregnancy (D) 2nd and 3rd trimester

Precautions: Hypersensitivity to ACE inhibitors; pregnancy (C) 1st trimester, lactation, children, elderly, renal disease

Pharmacokinetics: Extensively metabolized, half-life 11-15 hr, highly bound to plasma proteins, excreted in urine and feces

NURSING CONSIDERATIONS

Assess:

• B/P, pulse q4h; note rate, rhythm, quality

• Electrolytes: K, Na, Cl

• Baselines in renal, liver function tests before therapy begins

• Edema in feet, legs qd

• Skin turgor, dryness of mucous membranes for hydration status

Administer:

• Without regard to meals

• IV 0.9% NaCl and place supine for severe hypotension

Evaluate:

• Therapeutic response: decreased B/P

Teach patient/family:

• To comply with dosage schedule, even if feeling better

• That drug may cause dizziness, fainting; light-headedness may occur

• To rise slowly to sitting or standing position to minimize orthostatic hypotension

• To notify prescriber if pregnancy is suspected

---

irinotecan (℞)

(ear-een-oh-tee′kan)

Camptosar

Func. class.: Antineoplastic hormone

Chem. class.: Topoisomerase inhibitor

Action: Cytotoxic by producing damage to double-strand DNA during DNA synthesis

Uses: Metastatic carcinoma of the colon or rectum

Dosage and routes:

• *Adult:* **IV** 125 mg/m² given over

⬥ = Nursing alert   🌿 = Herb-drug interaction   🚫 = Do not crush

1½ hr qwk × 4 wk, then 2 wk rest period, may be repeated; 4 wk or 2 wk off, dosage adjustments may be made to 150 mg/m² (high) or 50 mg/m² (low); adjustments should be made in increments of 25-50 mg/m² depending on patient's tolerance

Available forms: Inj 20 mg/ml

Side effects/adverse reactions:

CNS: Fever, headache, chills, dizziness

GI: Diarrhea, nausea, vomiting, anorexia, constipation, cramps, flatus, stomatitis, dyspepsia

INTEG: Irritation at site, rash, sweating

HEMA: **Leukopenia, anemia, neutropenia**

RESP: Dyspnea, increased cough, rhinitis

CV: Vasodilation

MISC: Edema, asthenia, weight loss

Contraindications: Hypersensitivity, pregnancy (D)

Precautions: Lactation, children, elderly, myelosuppression, irradiation

Pharmacokinetics: Rapidly and completely absorbed; excreted in urine and bile as metabolites; half-life 10 hr, bound to plasma proteins 30%-68%

Interactions:

• Increased myelosuppression, diarrhea: other antineoplastics, radiation

• Increased lymphocytopenia: dexamethasone

• Increased akathisia: prochlorperazine

• Increased dehydration: diuretics

NURSING CONSIDERATIONS

Assess:

• For CNS symptoms: fever, headache, chills, dizziness

• CBC, differential, platelet count weekly; withhold drug if WBC is <2000/mm³, or platelet count <100,000/mm³, Hgb ≤9 g/dl, neutrophil ≤1000/mm³; notify prescriber of these results; drug should be discontinued, and colony-stimulating factor given

• Buccal cavity q8h for dryness, sores, or ulceration, white patches, oral pain, bleeding, dysphagia

• GI symptoms: frequency of stools; cramping

• Signs of dehydration: rapid respirations, poor skin turgor, decreased urine output, dry skin, restlessness, weakness

• Bone marrow depression: bruising, bleeding, blood in stools, urine, sputum, emesis

Administer:

• Antiemetics and dexamethasone 10 mg at least ½ hr before antineoplastics

• After preparing in biologic cabinet using gloves, mask, gown

IV

• By intermittent inf after diluting with 0.9% NaCl or D₅ (0.12-1.1 mg/ml) give over 1½ hr

• Do not admix with other solutions or medications

Perform/provide:

• Increased fluid intake to 2-3 L/day to prevent dehydration, unless contraindicated

• Changing of IV site q48h

• Rinsing of mouth tid-qid with water, club soda; brushing of teeth bid-tid with soft brush or cotton-tipped applicator for stomatitis; use unwaxed dental floss

• Nutritious diet with iron, vitamin supplement, low fiber, few dairy products

Evaluate:

• Therapeutic response: decrease in tumor size, decrease in spread of cancer

Teach patient/family:

• To avoid foods with citric acid or hot or rough texture if stomatitis is present; to drink adequate fluids

• To report stomatitis; any bleeding, white spots, ulcerations in mouth; tell patient to examine mouth qd, report symptoms

• To report signs of anemia: fatigue, headache, faintness, shortness of breath, irritability

• To use contraception during therapy

• To avoid salicylates, NSAIDs, alcohol, bleeding may occur

• About alopecia, that when hair grows back, it will be different texture, thickness

• To avoid vaccinations while taking this drug

• To report diarrhea that occurs 24 hr after administration, severe dehydration can occur rapidly

Treatment of overdose: Induce vomiting, provide supportive care

---

iron dextran (℞)
DexFerrum, Imferon, In Fed
Func. class.: Hematinic
Chem. class.: Ferric hydroxide complex with dextran

Action: Iron is carried by transferrin to the bone marrow, where it is incorporated into hemoglobin

Uses: Iron deficiency anemia

Dosage and routes:

• *Adult and child:* **IM** 0.5 ml as a test dose by Z-track, then no more than the following per day:

• *Adult <50 kg:* **IM** 100 mg

• *Adult >50 kg:* **IM** 250 mg

• *Infant <5 kg:* **IM** 25 mg

• *Child <5-9 kg:* **IM** 50 mg

• *Adult:* **IV** 0.5 ml (25 mg) test dose, then 100 mg qd after 2-3 days; give 25 mg test dose, wait 5 min, then infuse over 6-12 hr or use equation that follows:

$$\frac{0.3 \times \text{wt (lb)} \times \dfrac{100\text{-Hgb (g/dl)} \times 100}{14.8}}{} = \text{mg iron}$$

<30 lb (66 kg) should be given 80% of above formula dose

Available forms: Inj 50 mg/ml

Side effects/adverse reactions:

CNS: Headache, paresthesia, dizziness, shivering, weakness, *seizures*

GI: Nausea, vomiting, metallic taste, abdominal pain

INTEG: Rash, pruritus, urticaria, fever, sweating, chills, brown skin discoloration, pain at injection site, necrosis, sterile abscesses, phlebitis

CV: Chest pain, *shock,* hypotension, tachycardia

RESP: Dyspnea

HEMA: **Leukocytosis**

OTHER: **Anaphylaxis**

Contraindications: Hypersensitivity, all anemias excluding iron deficiency anemia, hepatic disease

Precautions: Acute renal disease, children, asthma, lactation, rheumatoid arthritis (IV), infants <4 mo, pregnancy (C)

Pharmacokinetics:

IM: Excreted in feces, urine, bile, breast milk; crosses placenta; most absorbed through lymphatics; can be gradually absorbed over weeks/months from fixed locations

Interactions:

• Decreased reticulocyte response: chloramphenicol

• Increased toxicity: oral iron—do not use

• Decreased absorption of fluoroquinolones, penicillamine

Lab test interferences:

False increase: Serum bilirubin

False decrease: Serum Ca

False positive: ^{99m}Tc diphosphate bone scan, iron test (large doses >2 ml)

⬥ = Nursing alert   🌿 = Herb-drug interaction   ⊘ = Do not crush

NURSING CONSIDERATIONS
Assess:

• Blood studies: Hct, Hgb, reticulocytes, transferrin, plasma iron concentrations, ferritin, total iron-binding, bilirubin before treatment, at least monthly

• Allergy: anaphylaxis, rash, pruritus, fever, chills, wheezing; notify prescriber immediately, keep emergency equipment available

• Cardiac status: anginal pain, hypotension, tachycardia

• Nutrition: amount of iron in diet (meat, dark green leafy vegetables, dried beans, dried fruits, eggs)

• Cause of iron loss or anemia, including use of salicylates, sulfonamides

• Toxicity: nausea, vomiting, diarrhea, fever, abdominal pain (early symptoms), cyanotic-looking lips, nailbeds, seizures, CV collapse (late symptoms)

Administer:

• D/C oral iron before parenteral; give only after test dose of 25 mg by preferred route; wait at least 1 hr before giving remaining portion

• IM deeply in large muscle mass; use Z-track method and a 19-20G 2-3"; needle; ensure needle is long enough to place drug deep in muscle, change needles after withdrawing drug and before injecting to prevent skin, tissue staining

◆ Only with epinephrine available in case of anaphylactic reaction during dose

IV

• IV after flushing with 10 ml 0.9% NaCl; give undiluted; may be diluted in 50-250 ml NS for infusion; give 1 ml (50 mg) or less over 1 min or more; flush line after use with 10 ml 0.9% NaCl; patient should remain recumbent for ½-1 hr

• IV injection requires single-dose vial without preservative; verify on label IV use is approved

Additive compatibilities: Netilmicin

Solution compatibility: TPN #211

Perform/provide:

• Storage at room temp in cool environment

• Recumbent position 30 min after IV injection to prevent orthostatic hypotension

• Therapeutic response: increased serum iron levels, Hct, Hgb

Teach patient/family:

• That iron poisoning may occur if increased beyond recommended level; not to take oral iron preparation

• That delayed reaction may occur 1-2 days after administration and last 3-4 days (IV) 3-7 days (IM); report fever, chills, malaise, muscle, joint aches, nausea, vomiting, backache

Treatment of overdose: Discontinue drug, treat allergic reaction, give diphenhydramine or epinephrine as needed, give iron-chelating drug in acute poisoning

---

isoniazid (℞)

(eye-soe-nye'a-zid)
INH, isoniazid, Isotamine*, Laniazid, Laniazid C.T., Nydrazid, PMS-Isoniazid*, Tubizid

Func. class.: Antitubercular
Chem. class.: Isonicotinic acid hydrazide

Action: Bactericidal interference with lipid, nucleic acid biosynthesis
Uses: Treatment, prevention of tuberculosis
Dosage and routes:
Treatment
• *Adult:* **PO/IM** 5 mg/kg qd as

---

single dose for 9 mo to 2 yr, not to exceed 300 mg/day

• *Child and infant:* **PO/IM** 10-20 mg/kg qd as single dose for 18-24 mo, not to exceed 300 mg/day

Prevention

• *Adult:* **PO** 300 mg qd as single dose × 12 mo

• *Child and infant:* **PO/IM** 10 mg/kg qd as single dose for 12 mo, not to exceed 300 mg/day

Available forms: Tabs 50, 100, 300 mg; inj 100 mg/ml; powder, syr 50 mg/5 ml

Side effects/adverse reactions:
Hypersensitivity: fever, skin eruptions, lymphadenopathy, vasculitis
CNS: Peripheral neuropathy, dizziness, memory impairment, *toxic encephalopathy, convulsions,* psychosis
EENT: Blurred vision, optic neuritis
HEMA: Agranulocytosis, hemolytic, aplastic anemia, thrombocytopenia, eosinophilia, methemoglobinemia
MISC: Dyspnea, B_6 deficiency, pellagra, hyperglycemia, metabolic acidosis, gynecomastia, rheumatic syndrome, SLE-like syndrome
GI: Nausea, vomiting, epigastric distress, *jaundice, fatal hepatitis*
Contraindications: Hypersensitivity, acute liver disease
Precautions: Pregnancy (C), renal disease, diabetic retinopathy, cataracts, ocular defects, hepatic disease, child <13 yr
Pharmacokinetics:
PO: Peak 1-2 hr, duration 6-8 hr
IM: Peak 45-60 min
Metabolized in liver; excreted in urine (metabolites); crosses placenta; excreted in breast milk
Interactions:
• Increased toxicity: tyramine foods, alcohol, cycloserine, ethionamide, rifampin, carbamazepine, warfarin, phenytoin, benzodiazepines

• Decreased absorption: aluminum antacids
• Decreased effectiveness of BCG vaccine, ketoconazole
NURSING CONSIDERATIONS
Assess:
• Liver studies qwk: ALT, AST, bilirubin
• Renal status: before, qmo: BUN, creatinine, output, sp gr, urinalysis
• Mental status often: affect, mood, behavioral changes; psychosis may occur
• Hepatic status: decreased appetite, jaundice, dark urine, fatigue
Administer:
• PO with meals to decrease GI symptoms; better to take on empty stomach 1 hr ac or 2 hr pc
• Antiemetic if vomiting occurs
• After C&S is completed; qmo to detect resistance
• IM deep in large muscle mass, massage, rotate inj site
Evaluate:
• Therapeutic response: decreased symptoms of TB
Teach patient/family:
• That compliance with dosage schedule, duration is necessary, not to skip or double dose
• That scheduled appointments must be kept or relapse may occur
• To avoid alcohol while taking drug, may increase risk of hepatic injury
• That if diabetic, use blood glucose monitor to obtain correct result
• To report weakness, fatigue, loss of appetite, nausea, vomiting, jaundice of skin or eyes, tingling/ numbness of hands/feet
Treatment of Overdose:
Pyridoxine

---

isoproterenol (℞)

(eye-soe-proe-ter′e-nole)
Aerolone, Dispos-a-
Medisoproterenol HCl, Isoproterenol HCl, Isuprel, Isuprel
Glossets, Isuprel Mistometer,
Medihaler-Iso, Vapo-Iso

Func. class.: β-adrenergic agonist

Chem. class.: Catecholamine

Action: Has β_1 and β_2 action; relaxes bronchial smooth muscle and dilates the trachea and main bronchi by increasing levels of cAMP, which relaxes smooth muscles; causes increased contractility and heart rate by acting on β-receptors in heart

Uses: Bronchospasm, asthma, heart block, ventricular dysrhythmias, shock

Dosage and routes:

Asthma, bronchospasm

• *Adult:* **SL** 10-20 mg q6-8h; **INH** 1 puff, may repeat in 2-5 min, maintenance 1-2 puffs 4-6 × /day; **IV** 10-20 µg during anesthesia

• *Child:* **SL** 5-10 mg q6-8h; **INH** 1 puff, may repeat in 2-5 min, maintenance 1-2 puffs 4-6 × /day

Heart block/ventricular dysrhythmias

• *Adult:* **IV** 0.02-0.06, then 0.01-0.2 mg or 5 µg/min HCl; 0.2 mg, then 0.02-1 mg as needed HCl

Shock

• *Adult:* **IV INF** 0.5-5 µg/min 1 mg/ 500 ml D_5W, titrate to B/P, CVP, hourly urine output

Available forms: Sol for nebulization 1:400 (0.25%), 1:200 (0.5%), 1:100 (1%); aerosol 0.25%, 0.2%; pwd for inh 0.1 mg/cart; inj 1:5000 (0.2 mg/ml); glossets (SL) 10, 15 mg

Side effects/adverse reactions:

CNS: Tremors, anxiety, insomnia, headache, dizziness, stimulation

CV: Palpitations, tachycardia, hypertension, ***cardiac arrest***

GI: Nausea, vomiting

RESP: Bronchial irritation, edema, dryness of oropharynx, ***bronchospasms*** (overuse)

META: Hyperglycemia

Contraindications: Hypersensitivity to sympathomimetics, narrow-angle glaucoma

Precautions: Pregnancy (C), cardiac disorders, hyperthyroidism, diabetes mellitus, prostatic hypertrophy, elderly

Pharmacokinetics:

IV: Onset rapid, duration 10 min

INH/SL: Onset 1-2 hr

RECT: Onset 2-4 hr

Metabolized in liver, lungs, GI tract

Interactions:

• Increased effects of both drugs: other sympathomimetics

• Decreased action when used with β-blockers

NURSING CONSIDERATIONS

Assess:

• Resp function: B/P, pulse, lung sounds

• Blood studies (CBC, WBC, differential), since blood dyscrasias may occur (rare)

• I&O ratio; check for urinary retention, frequency, hesitancy

• For paresthesias and coldness of extremities; peripheral blood flow may decrease

• Injection site: tissue sloughing; administer phentolamine mixed with 0.9% NaCl

Administer:

• With meals for GI symptoms

• SL ≤ q3-4h or no more than tid

IV

• Direct dilute 0.2 mg/10 ml 0.9% NaCl (1:50,000 sol); give over 1 min; IV INF 2 mg (1:5000 sol)/500 ml of D_5W; run each 1 ml (1:250,000) sol/min; may be increased; use infusion pump, intra-cardiac, 1:5000 sol undiluted

Additive compatibilities: Atracurium, calcium chloride, calcium gluceptate, cephalothin, cimetidine, dobutamine, floxacillin, heparin, magnesium sulfate, multivitamins, netilmicin, potassium chloride, ranitidine, succinylchloride, verapamil, vit B/C

Syringe compatibilities: Ranitidine

Y-site compatibilities: Amiodarone, amrinone, atracurium, bretylium, cisatracurium, famotidine, heparin, hydrocortisone, pancuronium, potassium chloride, propofol, remifentanil, tacrolimus, vecuronium, vit B/C

Perform/provide:
• Storage at room temp; do not use discolored sol

Evaluate:
• Therapeutic response: increased B/P with stabilization, ease of breathing

Teach patient/family:
• To rinse mouth after use
• Use of inhaler; review package insert with patient; to avoid getting aerosol in eyes; to wash inhaler in warm water and dry qd
• Use of spacer device in elderly
• About all aspects of drug; avoid smoking, smoke-filled rooms, persons with respiratory infections

Treatment of overdose: Administer a β-blocker

isosorbide dinitrate (℞)
(eye-soe-sor′bide)
Apo-ISDN*, Cedocard-SR*, Coronex*, Dilatrate-SR, ISDN, Iso-Bid, Isonate, Isorbid, Isordil, Isordil Tembids, Isordil Titradose, Isosorbide Dinitrate, Isotrate Timecelles, Novasorbide, Sorbitrate, Sorbitrate SA

isosorbide mononitrate
(eye-soe-sor′bide)
Imdur, ISMO, Monoket
Func. class.: Antianginal, vasodilator
Chem. class.: Nitrate

Action: Decreases preload, afterload, which is responsible for decreasing left ventricular end-diastolic pressure, systemic vascular resistance and reducing cardiac O_2 demand

Uses: Chronic stable angina pectoris, prophylaxis of angina pain

Dosage and routes:
Dinitrate
• *Adult:* **PO** 5-40 mg qid; **SL** 2.5-10 mg, may repeat q2-3h; **CHEW TAB** 5-10 mg prn or q2-3h as prophylaxis; **SUS REL** 40-80 mg q8-12h
Mononitrate
• *Adult:* **PO** 10-20 mg bid, 7 hr apart; Imdur: initiate at 30-60 mg/day as a single dose, increase q3d as needed

Available forms:
Dinitrate: Caps sus rel 40 mg; tabs 5, 10, 20, 30, 40 mg; chew tabs 5, 10 mg; SL tabs 2.5, 5, 10 mg; ext rel tab 40, 60 mg
Mononitrate: Tabs 20 mg; (ISMO, Monoket) 10, 20 mg; ext rel (Imdur) 30, 60, 120 mg

Side effects/adverse reactions:
MISC: Twitching, hemolytic anemia, *methemoglobinemia*

CV: Postural hypotension, tachycardia, **collapse,** syncope
GI: Nausea, vomiting
INTEG: Pallor, sweating, rash
CNS: Vascular headache, flushing, dizziness, weakness, faintness
Contraindications: Hypersensitivity to this drug or nitrates, severe anemia, increased intracranial pressure, cerebral hemorrhage, acute MI
Precautions: Postural hypotension, pregnancy (C), lactation, children
Pharmacokinetics:
mononitrate
Sus action: Duration 6-8 hr
dinitrate
PO: Onset 15-30 min, duration 4-6 hr
SL: Onset 2-5 min, duration 1-4 hr
CHEW TAB: Onset 3 min, duration ½-3 hr
Metabolized by liver, excreted in urine as metabolites (80%-100%)
Interactions:
• Increased effects: β-blockers, diuretics, antihypertensives, alcohol, calcium channel blockers, phenothiazines
NURSING CONSIDERATIONS
Assess:
• B/P, pulse, respirations during beginning therapy
• Pain: duration, time started, activity being performed, character
• Tolerance if taken over long period
• Headache, light-headedness, decreased B/P; may indicate a need for decreased dosage
Administer:
• After checking expiration date
Ⓝ Do not break, crush, or chew sus rel caps, SL tabs
• PO with 8 oz H_2O on empty stomach; do not crush SR or SL drug
• SL tabs should be placed under the tongue until dissolved

Evaluate:
• Therapeutic response: decrease or prevention of anginal pain
Teach patient/family:
• To leave tabs in original container
• To avoid alcohol products
• That drug may cause headache, but tolerance usually develops; taking with meals may reduce or eliminate headache
• That drug may be taken before stressful activity (exercise, sexual activity)
• That SL may sting when drug comes in contact with mucous membranes
• To avoid hazardous activities if dizziness occurs
• The importance of complying with complete medical regimen
• To make position changes slowly to prevent orthostatic hypotension
Ⓝ Not to crush, chew sus rel caps, SL tabs

isradipine (R)
(is-ra'di-peen)
DynaCirc, DynaCirc CR
Func. class.: Antihypertensive, calcium channel blocker
Chem. class.: Dihydropyridine

Action: Inhibits calcium ion influx across cell membrane during cardiac depolarization; produces relaxation of coronary vascular smooth muscle, peripheral vascular smooth muscle; dilates coronary vascular arteries; increases myocardial oxygen delivery in patients with vasospastic angina
Uses: Essential hypertension, angina pectoris, vasospastic angina
Dosage and routes:
• *Adult:* PO 2.5 mg bid; increase at 3-4 wk intervals up to 10 mg bid or 5 mg qd cont rel may be increased q2-4wk, max 20 mg/day

Available forms: Caps 2.5, 5 mg, cont rel tabs 5, 10 mg

Side effects/adverse reactions:

*HEMA: **Thrombocytopenia, leukopenia, anemia***

CV: Peripheral edema, tachycardia, hypotension, chest pain, ***CHF, dysrhythmias***

GI: Nausea, vomiting, diarrhea, gastric upset, constipation, ***hepatitis***

GU: Nocturia, polyuria, ***acute renal failure***

INTEG: Rash, pruritus, urticaria, photosensitivity, hair loss

CNS: Headache, fatigue, dizziness, fainting, sleep disturbances

MISC: Flushing, ***Stevens-Johnson syndrome***

Contraindications: Sick sinus syndrome, 2nd- or 3rd-degree heart block, hypotension less than 90 mm Hg systolic, hypersensitivity

Precautions: CHF, hypotension, hepatic disease, pregnancy (C), lactation, children, renal disease, elderly

Pharmacokinetics: Metabolized in liver; metabolites excreted in urine, feces; secreted in breast milk, peak plasma levels at 2-3 hr

Interactions:

• Decreased antihypertensive effect: NSAIDs

• Increased effects: digitalis, neuromuscular blocking agents, cyclosporine

• Increased effects of isradipine: cimetidine, carbamazepine

NURSING CONSIDERATIONS

Assess:

• Renal, hepatic, electrolytes prior to and during treatment

• B/P, pulse rate, chest pain; monitor ECG periodically during therapy

• Cardiac status: B/P, pulse, respiration, ECG; assess anginal pain, precipitating, ameliorating factors

Evaluate:

• Therapeutic response: decreased anginal pain, decreased B/P

Teach patient/family:

🚫 Not to break, crush, or chew cont rel tabs

• To avoid hazardous activities until stabilized on drug, dizziness is no longer a problem

• To limit caffeine consumption

• To avoid OTC drugs unless directed by prescriber

• The importance of compliance in all areas of medical regimen: diet, exercise, stress reduction, drug therapy

• To notify prescriber of irregular heartbeat, shortness of breath, swelling of feet and hands, pronounced dizziness, constipation, nausea, hypotension

Treatment of overdose: Defibrillation, β-agonists, IV Ca inotropic agents, diuretics, atropine for AV block, vasopressor for hypotension

---

itraconazole (℞)

(it-ra-con′a-zol)

Sporanox

Func. class.: Antifungal, systemic

Chem. class.: Triazole derivative

Action: Alters cell membranes and inhibits several fungal enzymes

Uses: Systemic candidiasis, chronic mucocandidiasis, oral thrush, candiduria, coccidioidomycosis, histoplasmosis, chromomycosis, paracoccidioidomycosis, blastomycosis (pulmonary and extrapulmonary), onychomycosis

Investigational uses: Dermatophytoses, pityriasis versicolor, sebopsoriasis, vaginal candidiasis, cryptococcus, subcutaneous mycoses, dimorphic infections, leish-

---

◆ = Nursing alert   ⏐ = Herb-drug interaction   🚫 = Do not crush maniasis, fungal keratitis, alternariosis, zygomycosis

Dosage and routes:

• *Adult:* **PO** 200 mg qd with food; may increase to 400 mg qd if needed; life-threatening infections may require a loading dose of 200 mg tid × 3 days; **IV** 200 mg bid × 4 doses, then 200 mg qd, give each dose over 1 hr

• *Child:* **PO** 3-5 mg/kg/day

Available forms: Caps 100 mg; oral sol 10 mg/ml; inj 10 mg/ml

Side effects/adverse reactions:

CV: Hypertension

GU: Gynecomastia, impotence, decreased libido

INTEG: Pruritus, fever, *rash,*

CNS: Headache, dizziness, insomnia, somnolence, depression

GI: Nausea, vomiting, anorexia, diarrhea, cramps, abdominal pain, flatulence, ***GI bleeding, hepatotoxicity***

MISC: Edema, fatigue, malaise, hypokalemia, tinnitus

Contraindications: Hypersensitivity, lactation, fungal meningitis, coadministration with terfenadine

Precautions: Hepatic disease, achlorhydria or hypochlorhydria (drug-induced), children, pregnancy (C)

Pharmacokinetics:

PO: Peak 3-5 hr, half-life 64 hr; metabolized in liver; excreted in bile, feces; requires acid pH for absorption; distributed poorly to CSF; highly protein bound

Interactions:

• Edema: calcium channel blockers

• Increased sedation: triazolam, oral midazolam

• Increased digoxin levels: digoxin

• Tinnitus, hearing loss: quinidine

• Increased levels of: tacrolimus, buspirone

• Hepatotoxicity: other hepatotoxic drugs

• Itraconazole increases levels of cyclosporine

• Decreased action of itraconazole: antacids, H_2-receptor antagonists, rifamycins, didanosine

• Increased anticoagulant effect: warfarin

• Severe hypoglycemia: oral hypoglycemics

• Concomitant administration with phenytoin may result in decreased levels of itraconazole; effects of phenytoin may be increased

NURSING CONSIDERATIONS

Assess:

• I&O ratio

• Liver studies (ALT, AST, bilirubin) if on long-term therapy

• For allergic reaction: rash, photosensitivity, urticaria, dermatitis

◆ For hepatotoxicity: nausea, vomiting, jaundice, clay-colored stools, fatigue

Administer:

• In the presence of acid products only; do not use alkaline products or antacids within 2 hr of drug; may give coffee, tea, acidic fruit juices

• IV: after adding full contents 25 ml to 50 ml NaCl, mix gently, use flow control device, give over 1 hr; use separate line, flush after use

• Oral sol: patient should swish in mouth vigorously

• With hydrochloric acid if achlorhydria is present

• Oral sol and caps are not interchangeable on a mg/mg basis

Perform/provide:

• Storage in tight container at room temp

Evaluate:

• Therapeutic response: decreased fever, malaise, rash, negative C&S for infecting organism

Teach patient/family:

• That long-term therapy may be needed to clear infection (1 wk-6 mo depending on infection)

• To avoid hazardous activities if dizziness occurs

• To take 2 hr ac administration of other drugs that increase gastric pH (antacids, H_2-blockers, omeprazole, sucralfate, anticholinergics) to notify health-care provider of all medications taken; to take after a full meal (caps), on empty stomach (oral sol)

• The importance of compliance with drug regimen

• To notify prescriber of GI symptoms, signs of liver dysfunction (fatigue, nausea, anorexia, vomiting, dark urine, pale stools)

Ⓝ Not to break, crush, or chew caps; not to use oral sol, caps interchangeably

---

kanamycin (℞)

(kan-a-mye'sin)
kanamycin sulfate, Kantrex
Func. class.: Antiinfective
Chem. class.: Aminoglycoside

Action: Interferes with protein synthesis in bacterial cell by binding to the 30s ribosomal subunit, causing inaccurate peptide sequence to form in protein chain, causing bacterial death

Uses: Severe systemic infections of CNS, respiratory, GI, urinary tract, bone, skin, soft tissues caused by *Escherichia coli, Acinetobacter, Proteus, Klebsiella pneumoniae, Pseudomonas aeruginosa;* also used as adjunct in hepatic coma, peritonitis, preoperatively to sterilize bowel; decreases ammonia-producing bacteria in bowel and intraperitoneally after fecal spill during surgery

Dosage and routes:
Severe systemic infections
• *Adult and child:* IV INF 15 mg/kg/d in divided doses q8-12h; diluted 500 mg/200 ml of NS or D_5W given over 30-60 min, not to exceed 1.5 g/d; IM 15 mg/kg/d in divided doses q8-12h, not to exceed 1.5 g/d, irrigation not to exceed 1.5 g/d
Hepatic coma
• *Adult:* PO 8-12 g/d in divided doses
Preoperative bowel sterilization
• *Adult:* PO 1 g qh × 4 doses, then q6h × 36-72 hr
Available forms: Inj 75, 500 mg/2 ml, 1 g/3 ml; cap 500 mg
Side effects/adverse reactions:
*GU: **Oliguria, hematuria, renal damage, azotemia, renal failure, nephrotoxicity***
CNS: Confusion, depression, numbness, tremors, ***convulsions,*** muscle twitching, ***neurotoxicity***
RESP: Respiratory depression
*EENT: **Ototoxicity,** deafness, visual disturbances, dizziness, vertigo, tinnitus
*HEMA: **Agranulocytosis, thrombocytopenia, leukopenia, eosinophilia, anemia***
GI: Nausea, vomiting, anorexia, increased ALT, AST, bilirubin, hepatomegaly, ***hepatic necrosis,*** splenomegaly
CV: Hypotension
INTEG: Rash, burning, urticaria, dermatitis, alopecia
Contraindications: Bowel obstruction, severe renal disease, hypersensitivity, pregnancy (D)
Precautions: Neonates, myasthenia gravis, hearing deficits, mild renal disease, lactation, Parkinson's disease
Pharmacokinetics:
PO: Not absorbed
IM: Onset rapid, peak 1-2 hr
IV: Onset immediate, peak 1-2 hr

Plasma half-life 2-3 hr; not metabolized; excreted unchanged in urine; crosses placenta; poor penetration into CSF

Interactions:

• Increased ototoxicity, neurotoxicity, nephrotoxicity: other aminoglycosides, amphotericin B, polymyxin, vancomycin, ethacrynic acid, furosemide, mannitol, methoxyflurane, cisplatin, cephalosporins, bacitracin, penicillins

• Increased effects: nondepolarizing muscle relaxants, succinylcholine

• Decreased effects of oral anticoagulants

NURSING CONSIDERATIONS
Assess:

• Weight before treatment; dosage is usually calculated on ideal body weight, but may be calculated on actual body weight

• I&O ratio, urinalysis daily for proteinuria, cells, casts; report sudden change in urine output

• VS during infusion; watch for hypotension, change in pulse

• IV site for thrombophlebitis, including pain, redness, swelling q30min; change site if needed; apply warm compresses to discontinued site

• Serum peak, drawn at 30-60 min after IV infusion or 60 min after IM injection; trough level drawn just before next dose; blood level should be 2-4 × bacteriostatic level; trough = 5-10 mEq/ml, peak = <30 mEq/ml

• Urine pH if drug is used for UTI; urine should be kept alkaline

• Renal impairment by CrCl, BUN, serum creatinine testing of urine; lower dosage should be given in renal impairment (CrCl <80 ml/min)

• Deafness by audiometric testing, ringing, roaring in ears, vertigo; assess hearing before, during, after treatment

• Dehydration: high specific gravity, decrease in skin turgor, dry mucous membranes, dark urine

• Superinfection: fever, malaise, redness, pain, swelling, perineal itching, diarrhea, stomatitis, change in cough, sputum

• C&S before starting treatment to identify infecting organism

• Vestibular dysfunction: nausea, vomiting, dizziness, headache; drug should be discontinued if severe

• Injection sites for redness, swelling, abscesses; use warm compresses at site

Administer:

• IM inj in large muscle mass; rotate injection sites

• Penicillins at least 1 hr before or after this drug

• Drug in evenly spaced doses to maintain blood level

• Bicarbonate to alkalinize urine if ordered in treating UTI, as drug is most active in alkaline environment

IV

• After diluting 500 mg or less/100 ml of D_5W, D_5/NaCl, 0.9% NaCl, LR or more; give 3-4 ml/min or less; flush line after use

Additive compatibilities: Ascorbic acid, cefoxitin, chloramphenicol, clindamycin, dopamine, furosemide, penicillin G potassium, penicillin G sodium, polymyxin B, sodium bicarbonate, vit B/C; admixing is not recommended

Syringe compatibilities: Penicillin G sodium

Y-site compatibilities: Cyclophosphamide, furosemide, heparin with hydrocortisone, hydromorphone, magnesium sulfate, meperidine, morphine, perphenazine, potassium chloride, vit B/C

Perform/provide:

• Adequate fluids of 2-3 L/day unless contraindicated to prevent irritation of tubules

• Flush of IV line with NS or D₅W after infusion

• Supervised ambulation, other safety measures with vestibular dysfunction

Evaluate:

• Therapeutic effect: absence of fever, draining wounds, negative C&S after treatment

Teach patient/family:

• To report headache, dizziness, symptoms of overgrowth of infection, renal impairment

• To report loss of hearing, ringing, roaring in ears or feeling of fullness in head

Treatment of overdose: Hemodialysis; monitor serum levels of drug

g/5 ml, pectin 43 mg/5 ml; kaolin 0.98 g/5 ml, pectin 21.7 mg/5 ml

Side effects/adverse reactions:

GI: Constipation (chronic use)

Precautions: Pregnancy (C)

Interactions:

• Decreased action of all other drugs

NURSING CONSIDERATIONS

Assess:

• Bowel pattern before; for rebound constipation, after; bowel sounds

• For dehydration in children

Administer:

• After shaking suspension

• For 48 hr only

Evaluate:

• Therapeutic response: decreased diarrhea

Teach patient/family:

• Not to exceed recommended dose

• To shake well before administration

• To take all other medications ≥2 hr apart

---

kaolin, pectin (OTC)

(kay'oh-lin, pek'tin)

Donnagel-MB*, Kaodene, Kao-Spen, Kapectolin

Func. class.: Antidiarrheal

Chem. class.: Hydrous magnesium aluminum silicate

Action: Decreases gastric motility, H₂O content of stool; adsorbent, demulcent

Uses: Diarrhea (cause undetermined)

Dosage and routes:

• *Adult:* PO 60-120 ml (30 ml conc) after each loose BM

• *Child >12 yr:* PO 60 ml after each loose BM

• *Child 6-12 yr:* PO 30-60 ml (15 ml conc) after each loose BM

• *Child 3-6 yr:* PO 15-30 ml (7.5 ml conc) after each loose BM

Available forms: Susp kaolin 0.87

---

ketoconazole (℞)

(kee-toe-koe'na-zole)

Nizoral

Func. class.: Antifungal

Chem. class.: Imidazole derivative

Action: Alters cell membranes and inhibits several fungal enzymes

Uses: Systemic candidiasis, chronic mucocandidiasis, oral thrush, candiduria, coccidioidomycosis, histoplasmosis, chromomycosis, paracoccidioidomycosis, blastomycosis; tinea cruris, tinea corporis, tinea versicolor, *Pityrosporum ovale*

Investigational uses: Cushing's syndrome, advanced prostatic cancer

Dosage and routes:

• *Adult:* PO 200-400 mg qd for 1-2 wk (candidiasis), 6 wk (other infections)

◆ = Nursing alert   ∥ = Herb-drug interaction   ⊘ = Do not crush

• *Child:* **PO:** >2 yr: 3.3-6.6 mg/kg/day as single daily dose; <2 yr, daily dose not established
• *Adult and child:* **TOP** 2% cream applied qd or bid
• *Adult:* Shampoo massage into scalp 1 min, reapply × 3 min, rinse, continue treatment 2 ×/wk × 1 mo, no more than q3d

Available forms: Tabs 200 mg; oral susp 100 mg/5 ml*, cream 2%, shampoo 2%

Side effects/adverse reactions:
GU: Gynecomastia, impotence
INTEG: Pruritus, fever, chills, photophobia, rash, dermatitis, purpura, urticaria
CNS: Headache, dizziness, somnolence
SYST: **Anaphylaxis**
GI: Nausea, vomiting, anorexia, diarrhea, abdominal pain, **hepatotoxicity**
HEMA: **Thrombocytopenia, leukopenia, hemolytic anemia**

Contraindications: Hypersensitivity, lactation, fungal meningitis; coadministration with terfenadine
Precautions: Renal disease, hepatic disease, achlorhydria (drug-induced), pregnancy (C), children <2 yr, other hepatotoxic agents including terfenadine
Pharmacokinetics:
PO: Peak 1-2 hr, half-life 2 hr, terminal 8 hr; metabolized in liver; excreted in bile, feces; requires acid pH for absorption; distributed poorly to CSF; highly protein bound
Interactions:
• Hepatotoxicity: other hepatotoxic drugs (including terfenadine)
• Ketoconazole increases concentration of cyclosporine
• Decreased action of ketoconazole: antacids, H$_2$-receptor antagonists, anticholinergics, isoniazid, rifampin

• Increased anticoagulant effect: warfarin, anticoagulants
• Ketoconazole may decrease theophylline effect
• Inhibited metabolism: paclitaxel
⧬ Decreased ketoconazole action: Yew

NURSING CONSIDERATIONS
Assess:
• For infection symptoms before and after treatment
• I&O ratio
• Liver studies (ALT, AST, bilirubin) if on long-term therapy
• For allergic reaction: rash, photosensitivity, urticaria, dermatitis
◆ For hepatotoxicity: nausea, vomiting, jaundice, clay-colored stools, fatigue
Administer:
• In the presence of acid products only; do not use alkaline products, proton pump inhibitors, H$_2$-antagonists, antacids within 2 hr of drug; may give coffee, tea, acidic fruit juices, cola
• With food to decrease GI symptoms
• With HCl if achlorhydria is present; dissolve tab/4 ml of aqueous sol 0.2 N HCl, use straw to avoid contact, rinse with water afterward and swallow
Perform/provide:
• Storage in tight container at room temp
Evaluate:
• Therapeutic response: decreased fever, malaise, rash, negative C&S for infecting organism, absence of scaling
Teach patient/family:
• That long-term therapy may be needed to clear infection (1 wk-6 mo depending on infection)
• To avoid hazardous activities if dizziness occurs
• To take 2 hr ac administration of

K

other drugs that increase gastric pH (antacids, H₂-blockers, omeprazole, sucralfate, anticholinergics)
• The importance of compliance with drug regimen
• To notify prescriber of GI symptoms, signs of liver dysfunction (fatigue, nausea, anorexia, vomiting, dark urine, pale stools)
• Use sunglasses to prevent photophobia

---

ketoprofen (otc, ℞)

(ke-toe-proe'fen)
Actron, Apo-Keto*, Apo-Keto-E*, ketoprofen, Orudis, Orudis-E*, Orudis-KT, Orudis-SR*, Oruvail, Rhodis*

Func. class.: Nonsteroidal antiinflammatory (NSAID)
Chem. class.: Propionic acid derivative

Action: Inhibits prostaglandin synthesis by decreasing enzyme needed for biosynthesis; analgesic, antiinflammatory, antipyretic
Uses: Mild to moderate pain, osteoarthritis, rheumatoid arthritis, dysmenorrhea
Dosage and routes:
Antiinflammatory
• *Adult:* PO 150-300 mg in divided doses tid-qid, not to exceed 300 mg/day or ext rel 150-200 mg qd
Analgesic
• *Adult:* PO 25-50 mg q6-8h
Available forms: Caps 12.5, 25, 50, 75 mg; ext rel cap 100, 150, 200 mg
Side effects/adverse reactions:
GI: Nausea, anorexia, vomiting, diarrhea, jaundice, *cholestatic hepatitis,* constipation, flatulence, cramps, dry mouth, peptic ulcer
*CNS: Dizziness, drowsiness, fatigue, tremors, confusion, insomnia, anxiety, depression, headache

CV: Tachycardia, peripheral edema, palpitations, dysrhythmias, hypertension
INTEG: Purpura, rash, pruritus, sweating
GU: Nephrotoxicity: dysuria, hematuria, oliguria, azotemia
HEMA: Blood dyscrasias
EENT: Tinnitus, hearing loss, blurred vision
Contraindications: Hypersensitivity, asthma, severe renal disease, severe hepatic disease, ulcer disease
Precautions: Pregnancy (B) 1st trimester, lactation, children, bleeding disorders, GI disorders, cardiac disorders, hypersensitivity to other antiinflammatory agents, elderly
Pharmacokinetics:
PO: Peak 2 hr, half-life 2-4 hr; metabolized in liver; excreted in urine (metabolites); excreted in breast milk; 99% plasma protein binding
Interactions:
• Increased toxicity: cyclosporine, lithium, methotrexate, phenytoin, alcohol
• Increased risk of bleeding: warfarin
• Increased levels of ketoprofen: aspirin, probenecid
• Decreased effect of: diuretics, antihypertensives
• Increased adverse GI reactions: aspirin, corticosteroids
NURSING CONSIDERATIONS
Assess:
• For pain: type, location, intensity, ROM before and 1-2 hr after treatment
• Renal, liver, blood studies: BUN, creatinine, AST, ALT, Hgb, before treatment, periodically thereafter
• For aspirin sensitivity, asthma; these patients may be more likely to develop hypersensitivity to NSAIDs
• Audiometric, ophthalmic examination before, during, after treatment

---

◆ = Nursing alert   ▮ = Herb-drug interaction   Ⓢ = Do not crush

- For eye, ear problems: blurred vision, tinnitus; may indicate toxicity
- For GI bleeding: blood in sputum, emesis, stools

Administer:

🚫 Whole; do not crush, break, or chew ext rel caps

- With food to decrease GI symptoms; however, best to take on empty stomach to facilitate absorption

Perform/provide:

- Storage at room temp

Evaluate:

- Therapeutic response: decreased pain, stiffness in joints, decreased swelling in joints, ability to move more easily; decreased fever

Teach patient/family:

- To report blurred vision, ringing, roaring in ears; may indicate toxicity
- To avoid driving, other hazardous activities if dizziness, drowsiness occurs, especially elderly
- To report change in urine pattern, increased weight, edema, increased pain in joints, fever, blood in urine; indicate nephrotoxicity; rash, itching, blurred vision, ringing in the ears, flulike symptoms
- That therapeutic effects may take up to 1 mo, to take with 8 oz of water and sit upright for ½ hr after administration to prevent GI irritation
- To avoid aspirin, alcohol, steroids
- To wear sunscreen to prevent photosensitivity

ketorolac (R)

(kee-toe'role-ak)
Acular, Toradol

Func. class.: Nonsteroidal antiinflammatory/nonopioid analgesic

Chem. class.: Pyrrolo-pyrrole

Action: Inhibits prostaglandin synthesis by decreasing an enzyme needed for biosynthesis; analgesic, antiinflammatory, antipyretic effects

Uses: Mild to moderate pain; seasonal allergic conjunctivitis (ophth)

Dosage and routes:

- *Adult (multiple dosing):* **IV BOL/IM** 30 mg q6h max 120 mg/day, with transition of 20 mg **PO** (1st dose), then 10 mg q4-6h; *≥65 yr, renal impairment, or weight <50 kg:* 15 mg q6h, max 60 mg
- *Adult (single dosing):* **IV BOL/IM** 30 mg **IV** or 60 mg **IM,** then 20 mg transition dose, not to exceed 40 mg/day then 10 mg q4-6h; *≥65 yr, renal impairment, or weight <50 kg:* give 30 mg **IM** or 15 mg **IV**
- *Adult:* **OPHTH** 1 gtt qid

Available forms: Inj 15, 30 mg/ml (prefilled syringes); ophth 0.5% sol; tab 10 mg

Side effects/adverse reactions:

CV: Hypertension, flushing, syncope, pallor, edema, vasodilation

CNS: Dizziness, *drowsiness,* tremors

EENT: Tinnitus, hearing loss, blurred vision

GI: Nausea, anorexia, vomiting, diarrhea, constipation, flatulence, cramps, dry mouth, peptic ulcer, ***GI bleeding, perforation***, taste change

GU: ***Nephrotoxicity: dysuria, hematuria, oliguria, azotemia***

HEMA: ***Blood dyscrasias,*** prolonged bleeding

K

INTEG: Purpura, rash, pruritus, sweating

Contraindications: Hypersensitivity, asthma, severe renal disease, severe hepatic disease, peptic ulcer disease, L&D, lactation, CV bleeding

Precautions: Pregnancy (C), children, bleeding disorders, GI disorders, cardiac disorders, hypersensitivity to other antiinflammatory agents, elderly, CrCl <25 ml/min

Pharmacokinetics:

PO: Peak 2-3 hr, duration 4-6 hr

IM: Peak 50 min, half-life 6 hr enters breast milk, <50% metabolized by liver, excreted by kidneys

Interactions:

• Increased toxicity: methotrexate, lithium

• Increased risk of bleeding: anticoagulants, salicylates

• Decreased effects: antihypertensives, diuretics

• Increased renal impairment: ACE inhibitors

• Compatible in 0.9% NaCl, D_5, Ringer's, LR, Plasmalate

NURSING CONSIDERATIONS

Assess:

• Patients with aspirin sensitivity, asthma; may be more likely to develop hypersensitivity to NSAIDs

• For pain: type, location, intensity, ROM before and 1 hr after treatment

• Eyes: redness, swelling, tearing, itching (ophth)

• Renal, liver, blood studies: BUN, creatinine, AST, ALT, Hgb before treatment, periodically thereafter; check for dehydration

• Bleeding times; check for bruising, bleeding; test for occult blood in urine

• For eye, ear problems: blurred vision, tinnitus (may indicate toxicity)

◆ Hepatic dysfunction: jaundice, yellow sclera and skin, clay-colored stools

• Audiometric, ophthalmic exam before, during, after treatment

• GI bleeding: blood in sputum, emesis, stools

Administer:

• IM/IV for 5 days or less; continue therapy with PO

IV

• Give undiluted over ≥15 sec

Solution compatibility: D_5W, 0.9% NaCl, LR

Syringe compatibilities: Sufentanil

Y-site compatibilities: Cisatracurium, remifentanil, sufentanil

Perform/provide:

• Storage at room temp

Evaluate:

• Therapeutic response: decreased pain, stiffness, swelling in joints, ability to move more easily; decreased ocular itching (ophth)

Teach patient/family:

• To report blurred vision or ringing, roaring in ears (may indicate toxicity)

• To avoid driving, other hazardous activities if dizziness or drowsiness occurs

• To report change in urine pattern, weight increase, edema, pain increase in joints, fever, blood in urine (indicates nephrotoxicity)

• To avoid alcohol, salicylates, other NSAIDs, acetaminophen

• This drug may cause redness, burning if soft contact lenses are worn (ophth)

◆ = Nursing alert   🖋 = Herb-drug interaction   🚫 = Do not crush

labetalol (℞)

(la-bet'a-lole)
Normodyne, Trandate
Func. class.: Antihypertensive
Chem. class.: α/β-blocker

Action: Produces decreases in B/P without reflex tachycardia or significant reduction in heart rate through mixture of α-blocking, β-blocking effects; elevated plasma renins are reduced

Uses: Mild to moderate hypertension; treatment of severe hypertension (IV)

Investigational uses: Angina pectoris (PO), hypotension during surgery (IV)

Dosage and routes:
Hypertension
• *Adult:* **PO** 100 mg bid; may be given with a diuretic; may increase to 200 mg bid after 2 days; may continue to increase q1-3 days; max 400 mg bid

Hypertensive crisis
• *Adult:* **IV INF** 200 mg/160 ml D₅W, run at 2 ml/min; stop infusion at desired response, repeat q6-8h as needed; **IV BOL** 20 mg over 2 min, may repeat 40-80 mg q10min, not to exceed 300 mg

Available forms: Tabs 100, 200, 300 mg; inj 5 mg/ml in 20 ml amps

Side effects/adverse reactions:
CV: Orthostatic hypotension, bradycardia, CHF, chest pain, ventricular dysrhythmias, AV block
CNS: Dizziness, mental changes, drowsiness, fatigue, headache, catatonia, depression, anxiety, nightmares, paresthesias, lethargy
GI: Nausea, vomiting, diarrhea
INTEG: Rash, alopecia, urticaria, pruritus, fever
HEMA: Agranulocytosis, thrombocytopenia, purpura (rare)

EENT: Tinnitus, visual changes, sore throat, double vision, dry, burning eyes
GU: Impotence, dysuria, ejaculatory failure
RESP: Bronchospasm, dyspnea, wheezing

Contraindications: Hypersensitivity to β-blockers, cardiogenic shock, heart block (2nd or 3rd degree), sinus bradycardia, CHF, bronchial asthma

Precautions: Major surgery, pregnancy (C), lactation, diabetes mellitus, renal disease, thyroid disease, COPD, well-compensated heart failure, CAD, nonallergic bronchospasm, elderly, hepatic disease

Pharmacokinetics:
PO: Onset ½-2 hr, peak 2-4 hr, duration 8-12 hr
IV: Onset 5 min, peak 15 min, duration 2-4 hr
Half-life 6-8 hr; metabolized by liver (metabolites inactive); excreted in urine; crosses placenta; excreted in breast milk

Interactions:
• Do not use within 2 wk of MAOIs
• Decreased effects of labetalol: thyroid hormones
• Myocardial depression: hydantoins, general anesthetics, verapamil
• Increased hypotension: diuretics, other antihypertensives, cimetidine, nitroglycerin, alcohol
• Decreased effects: sympathomimetics, lidocaine, indomethacin, theophylline, cimetidine, beta-blockers, bronchodilators, xanthines
• Decreased antihypertensive effect: NSAIDs
• Increased bradycardia: cardiac glycosides
• Increased hypoglycemia: insulin, oral antidiabetics

Lab test interferences:
False increase: Urinary catecholamines

NURSING CONSIDERATIONS
Assess:

• I&O, weight daily; fluid overload: weight gain, jugular venous distention, edema, rales in lungs

• B/P during beginning treatment, periodically thereafter, pulse q4h; note rate, rhythm, quality

• Apical/radial pulse before administration; notify prescriber of any significant changes

• Baselines in renal, liver function tests before therapy begins

• Edema in feet, legs daily

• Skin turgor, dryness of mucous membranes for hydration status

Administer:

• PO ac, hs; tab may be crushed or swallowed whole

• Reduced dosage in renal dysfunction

IV

• Undiluted or diluted in LR, D₅W, D₅ in 0.2%, 0.9%, 0.33% NaCl or Ringer's inj; give undiluted 20 mg or less/2 min; infusion is titrated to patient response; 200 mg of drug/160 ml sol = 1 mg/ml; 300 mg of drug/240 ml sol = 1 mg/ml; 200 mg of drug/250 ml sol = 2 mg/3 ml; use infusion pump

• Keeping patient recumbent during and for 3 hr after administration

Solution compatibilities: D₅R, D₅LR, D₂ ₁/₂/0.45% NaCl, D₅/0.2% NaCl, D₅/0.33% NaCl, D₅0.9% NaCl, D₅W, Ringer's, LR

Y-site compatibilities: Amikacin, aminophylline, amiodarone, ampicillin, butorphanol, calcium gluconate, cefazolin, ceftazidime, ceftizoxime, chloramphenicol, cimetidine, clindamycin, diltiazem, dobutamine, dopamine, enalaprilat, epinephrine, erythromycin, esmolol, famotidine, fentanyl, gentamicin, hydromorphone, lidocaine, lorazepam, magnesium sulfate, meperidine, met-

ronidazole, midazolam, milrinone, morphine, nicardipine, nitroglycerin, norepinephrine, nitroprusside, oxacillin, penicillin G potassium, piperacillin, potassium chloride, potassium phosphate, propofol, ranitidine, sodium acetate, tobramycin, trimethoprim-sulfamethoxazole, vancomycin, vecuronium

Perform/provide:

• Storage in dry area at room temp; do not freeze

Evaluate:

• Therapeutic response: decreased B/P after 1-2 wk

Teach patient/family:

• Not to discontinue drug abruptly; taper over 2 wk; may cause precipitate angina

• Not to use OTC products containing α-adrenergic stimulants (nasal decongestants, OTC cold preparations) unless directed by prescriber

• To report bradycardia, dizziness, confusion, depression, fever

• To take pulse at home, advise when to notify prescriber

• To avoid alcohol, smoking, Na intake

• To comply with weight control, dietary adjustments, modified exercise program

• To carry Medic Alert ID to identify drug, allergies

• To avoid hazardous activities if dizziness is present

• To report symptoms of CHF: difficulty breathing, especially on exertion or when lying down, night cough, swelling of extremities

• To take medication at bedtime to prevent effect of orthostatic hypotension

• To wear support hose to minimize effects of orthostatic hypotension

Treatment of overdose: Lavage, IV atropine for bradycardia, IV theophylline for bronchospasm, digi-

---

◆ = Nursing alert   ⧸ = Herb-drug interaction   ⊘ = Do not crush talis, O_2, diuretic for cardiac failure; hemodialysis is useful for removal, hypotension; administer vasopressor (norepinephrine)

---

lactulose (℞)

(lak'tyoo-lose)
Cephulac, Cholac, Chronulac, Constilac, Constulose, Duphalac, Emulose, Enulose Lactulax*

Func. class.: Laxative; ammonia detoxicant (hyperosmotic)
Chem. class.: Lactose synthetic derivative

Action: Prevents absorption of ammonia in colon; increases water in stool

Uses: Chronic constipation, portal-systemic encephalopathy in patients with hepatic disease

Dosages and routes:
Constipation
• *Adult:* **PO** 15-60 ml qd
• *Child:* **PO** 7.5 ml qd
Encephalopathy
• *Adult:* **PO** 20-30 g tid or qid until stools are soft; **RETENTION ENEMA** 30-45 ml in 100 ml of fluid
• *Infant:* 2.5-10 ml/day in divided doses
• *Child:* 40-90 ml/day in divided doses given 2-4 ×/day
Available forms: Syrup 10 g/15 ml

Side effects/adverse reactions:
GI: Nausea, vomiting, anorexia, abdominal cramps, diarrhea, flatulence, distention, belching

Contraindications: Hypersensitivity, low-galactose diet

Precautions: Pregnancy (B), lactation, diabetes mellitus, elderly, debilitated patients

Pharmacokinetics: Metabolized in intestine, excreted by kidneys; onset 1-2 days, peak unknown, duration unknown

Interactions:
• Decreased effects of lactulose: neomycin, other oral antiinfectives

NURSING CONSIDERATIONS
Assess:
• Stool: amount, color, consistency
• Blood ammonia level (30-70 mg/100 ml); may decrease ammonia level by 25%-50%
• Blood, urine electrolytes if drug is used often; may cause diarrhea, hypokalemia, hyponatremia
• I&O ratio to identify fluid loss
• Cause of constipation; determine whether fluids, bulk, or exercise is missing from lifestyle
• Cramping, rectal bleeding, nausea, vomiting; if these symptoms occur, drug should be discontinued
• Clearing of confusion, lethargy, restlessness, irritability if portal-systemic encephalopathy

Administer:
PO
• With 8 oz fruit juice, water, milk to increase palatability of oral form
RECT
• Retention enema by diluting 300 ml lactose/700 ml of water; administer by rectal balloon catheter
• Increased fluids to 2 L/day; do not give with other laxatives; if diarrhea occurs, reduce dosage

Evaluate:
• Therapeutic response: decreased constipation, decreased blood ammonia level, clearing of mental state

Teach patient/family:
• Not to use laxatives long-term
• To dilute with water or fruit juice to counteract sweet taste
• To store in cool environment; do not freeze
• To take on an empty stomach for rapid action
• To report diarrhea; may indicate overdose

L

---

* = Canada only   Side effects: *italics* = common; ***bold italics*** = life-threatening

lamivudine (℞)

(lam-i-voo'deen)
Epivir, Epivir-HBV, 3TC
Func. class.: Antiviral
Chem. class.: Nucleoside reverse transcriptase inhibitor

Action: Inhibits replication of HIV virus by incorporating into cellular DNA by viral reverse transcriptase, thereby terminating cellular DNA chain

Uses: HIV infection in combination with zidovudine (Epivir); chronic hepatitis B (Epivir-HBV)

Dosage and routes:

• Dosage reduction needed in renal disease (CrCl <50 ml/min)

• *Adult and adolescent (12-16 yr):* **PO** 150 mg bid with zidovudine; <50 kg (110 lbs): **PO** 2 mg/kg bid with zidovudine

• *Child 3 mo to 12 yr:* **PO** 4 mg/kg bid, may be given 150 mg bid with zidovudine

Hepatitis B

• *Adult:* **PO** 100 mg qd

Available forms: Tabs 150 mg; oral sol 5, 10 mg/ml; tabs: 100 mg (Epivir-HBV)

Side effects/adverse reactions:

HEMA: **Neutropenia, anemia, thrombocytopenia**

CNS: Fever, headache, malaise, dizziness, insomnia, depression, fatigue, chills

GI: Nausea, vomiting, diarrhea, anorexia, cramps, dyspepsia, ***pancreatitis (pediatrics)***

RESP: Cough

EENT: Taste change, hearing loss, photophobia

INTEG: Rash

MS: Myalgia, arthralgia, pain

Contraindications: Hypersensitivity

Precautions: Granulocyte count <1000/mm^3 or Hgb <9.5 g/dl, pregnancy (C), lactation, children, renal disease, severe hepatic function, pancreatitis

Pharmacokinetics: Rapidly absorbed, distributed to extravascular space, excreted unchanged in urine

Interactions:

• Increased level of zidovudine when given with lamivudine

• Increased level of lamivudine: trimethoprim-sulfamethoxazole

NURSING CONSIDERATIONS

Assess:

• Blood counts q2wk; watch for neutropenia, thrombocytopenia, Hgb, CD4, viral load; if low, therapy may have to be discontinued and restarted after hematologic recovery; blood transfusions may be required

• Liver studies: AST, ALT, bilirubin; amylase, lipase, triglycerides, CD4, viral load periodically during treatment

• Children for pancreatitis

Administer:

• PO bid

Perform/provide:

• With other antiretrovirals only

• Storage in cool environment; protect from light

Evaluate:

• Blood dyscrasias: bruising, fatigue, bleeding, poor healing

Teach patient/family:

• That GI complaints, insomnia resolve after 3-4 wk of treatment

• That drug is not a cure for HIV, but will control symptoms

• To notify prescriber of sore throat, swollen lymph nodes, malaise, fever; other infections may occur

• That patient is still infective, may pass HIV virus on to others

• That follow-up visits must be continued since serious toxicity may occur; blood counts must be done q2wk

◆ = Nursing alert   🖉 = Herb-drug interaction   ⊘ = Do not crush

• That drug must be taken twice a day, even if patient feels better
• That other drugs may be necessary to prevent other infections
• That drug may cause fainting or dizziness

---

lamotrigine (R)

(la-mot'ri-geen)

Lamictal, Lamictal Chewable

Func. class.: Anticonvulsant

Chem. class.: Phenyltriazine

Action: Unknown, may inhibit voltage-sensitive sodium channels

Uses: Adjunct in the treatment of partial seizures; children with Lennox-Gastaut syndrome

Investigational uses: Generalized tonic-clonic, absence, atypical absence and myoclonic seizures; refractory bipolar disorder

Dosage and routes:

Monotherapy

• *Adult:* 50 mg/day for wk 1-2, then increase to 100 mg divided bid for wk 3-4; maintenance, 300-500 mg/day

• *Child:* 2 mg/kg/day in 2 divided doses × 2 wks, then 10 mg/kg/day, max 15 mg/kg/day or 400 mg/day

Multiple therapy

• *Adult:* 25 mg qod wk 1-4, then 150 mg/day in divided doses

• *Child:* 0.1-0.2 mg/kg/day initially, then increase q2wk as needed to 2 mg/kg/day or 150 mg/day

Available forms: Tabs 25, 100, 150, 200 mg; chew dispersible tabs 5, 25 mg

Side effects/adverse reactions:

CNS: Dizziness, ataxia, *headache,* fever, insomnia, tremor, depression, anxiety

EENT: Nystagmus, *diplopia, blurred vision*

GI: Nausea, vomiting, anorexia, abdominal pain, **hepatotoxicity**

GU: Dysmenorrhea

INTEG: **Rash (potentially life-threatening),** alopecia, photosensitivity

SYST: **Stevens-Johnson syndrome**

Contraindications: Hypersensitivity

Precautions: Pregnancy (C), lactation, child <16 yr, renal, hepatic disease

Pharmacokinetics: Half-life varies depending on dose

Interactions:

• Increased metabolic clearance of lamotrigine: carbamazepine, phenobarbital, phenytoin, primidone

• Decreased metabolic clearance of lamotrigine: valproic acid

NURSING CONSIDERATIONS

Assess:

• For seizure activity: duration, type, intensity, halo before seizure

◆ For rash (Stevens-Johnson syndrome or toxic epidermal necrolysis) in pediatric patients, drug should be discontinued at first sign of rash

Administer:

• Chewable dispersible tabs

• Swallow whole, chew, or dispersed in water or diluted fruit juice; if chewed, drink a small amt of water

Evaluate:

• Therapeutic response: decrease in severity of seizures

Teach patient/family:

• To take PO doses divided with or after meals to decrease adverse effects, not to discontinue drug abruptly; seizures may occur

• To avoid hazardous activities until stabilized on drug

• To carry Medic Alert ID, to notify prescriber of skin rash or increased seizure activity, to use sunscreen and protective clothing if photosensitivity occurs

• To notify prescriber if pregnant or intend to become pregnant

---

lansoprazole (℞)
(lan-so-prey′zole)
Prevacid
Func. class.: Antiulcer, proton pump inhibitor
Chem. class.: Benzimidazole

Action: Suppresses gastric secretion by inhibiting hydrogen/potassium ATPase enzyme system in gastric parietal cell; characterized as gastric acid pump inhibitor, since it blocks final step of acid production

Uses: Gastroesophageal reflux disease (GERD), severe erosive esophagitis, poorly responsive systemic GERD, pathologic hypersecretory conditions (Zollinger-Ellison syndrome, systemic mastocytosis, multiple endocrine adenomas); possibly effective for treatment of duodenal, gastric ulcers, maintenance of healed duodenal ulcers

Dosage and routes:
NG tube
• *Adult:* Use intact granules mixed in 40 ml of apple juice and injected through **NG** tube, then flush with apple juice
Duodenal ulcer
• *Adult:* **PO** 15 mg qd before eating for 4 wk, then 15 mg qd to maintain healing of ulcers; associated with *H. pylori*—30 mg lansoprazole, 500 mg clarithromycin, 1 g amoxicillin bid × 14 days or 30 mg lansoprazole, 1 g amoxicillin tid × 14 days
Erosive esophagitis
• *Adult:* **PO** 30 mg qd before eating for up to 8 wk, may use another 8 wk course if needed
Pathologic hypersecretory conditions
• *Adult:* **PO** 60 mg qd, may give up to 90 mg bid

Available forms: Caps, del rel 15, 30 mg
Side effects/adverse reactions:
CNS: Headache, dizziness, confusion, agitation, amnesia, depression
GI: Diarrhea, abdominal pain, vomiting, nausea, constipation, flatulence, acid regurgitation, anorexia, irritable colon
RESP: Upper respiratory infections, cough, epistaxis, asthma, bronchitis, dyspnea
INTEG: Rash, urticaria, pruritus, alopecia
META: Weight gain/loss, gout
EENT: Tinnitus, taste perversion, deafness, eye pain, otitis media
CV: Chest pain, angina, tachycardia, bradycardia, palpitations, **CVA,** hypertension/hypotension, **MI, shock,** vasodilation
GU: **Hematuria,** glycosuria, impotence, kidney calculus, breast enlargement
HEMA: **Hemolysis,** anemia
Contraindications: Hypersensitivity
Precautions: Pregnancy (B), lactation, children
Pharmacokinetics: Absorption after granules leave stomach—rapid; plasma half-life 1½ hr, protein binding 97%, extensively metabolized in liver, excreted in urine, feces; clearance decreased in the elderly, renal and hepatic impairment
Interactions:
• Delayed absorption of lansoprazole: sucralfate
• May be decreased absorption of ketoconazole, ampicillin, iron, digoxin

NURSING CONSIDERATIONS
Assess:
• GI system: bowel sounds q8h, abdomen for pain, swelling, anorexia
• Hepatic enzymes: AST, ALT, alk phosphatase during treatment

---

◆ = Nursing alert　　🌿 = Herb-drug interaction　　🚫 = Do not crush

Administer:

🚫 Before eating; swallow capsule whole; do not break, crush, or chew caps

Evaluate:

• Therapeutic response: absence of epigastric pain, swelling, fullness

Teach patient/family:

• To report severe diarrhea; drug may have to be discontinued

• That diabetic patient should know that hypoglycemia may occur

• To avoid hazardous activities; dizziness may occur

• To avoid alcohol, salicylates, ibuprofen; may cause GI irritation

---

leflunomide (℞)

(leh-floo'noh-mide)

Arava

Chem. class.: Pyrimidine synthesis inhibitor

Action: Inhibits an enzyme involved in pyrimidine synthesis and has antiproliferative effect

Uses: Rheumatoid arthritis

Dosage and routes:

• *Adult:* **PO** loading dose 100 mg/day × 3 days, maintenance 20 mg/day, may be decreased to 10 mg/day if not well tolerated

• *Available forms:* Tabs 10, 20, 100 mg

Side effects/adverse reactions:

GI: Nausea, anorexia, vomiting, constipation, flatulence, diarrhea, elevated LFTs

CNS: Dizziness, insomnia, depression, paresthesia, anxiety, migraine, neuralgia

CV: Palpitations, hypertension, chest pain, angina pectoris, peripheral edema

INTEG: Rash, pruritus, alopecia, acne, hematoma, herpes infections

RESP: Pharyngitis, rhinitis, bronchitis, cough, respiratory infection, pneumonia, sinusitis

EENT: Pharyngitis, oral candidiasis, stomatitis, dry mouth, blurred vision

HEMA: Anemia, ecchymosis, hyperlipidemia

Contraindications: Hypersensitivity, pregnancy (X), lactation

Precautions: Hepatic, renal disorders

Pharmacokinetics:

PO: metabolized in liver to metabolite, excreted in urine

Interactions:

• Increased NSAIDs effect: NSAIDs

• Increased side effects of leflunomide: hepatotoxic agents, methotrexate

• Increased rifampin levels: rifampin

• Decreased effect of leflunomide: charcoal, cholestyramine

NURSING CONSIDERATIONS

Assess:

• Liver function studies: if ALT elevations are > twofold ULN, reduce dose to 10 mg/day

Administer:

PO

• With food for GI upset

Evaluate:

• Therapeutic response: decreased inflammation, pain in joints

Teach patient/family:

• That drug must be continued for prescribed time to be effective

• To take with food, milk, or antacids to avoid GI upset

• To use caution when driving; drowsiness, dizziness may occur

• To take with a full glass of water to enhance absorption

• To avoid pregnancy while taking this drug; not to breastfeed while taking this drug; men should also discontinue drug and begin leflunomide removal protocol if a pregnancy is planned

lepirudin (R)

(lep-ih-roo'din)
Refludan

Func. class.: Anticoagulant
Chem. class.: Hirudin

Action: Direct inhibitor of thrombin that is highly specific

Uses: Heparin-induced thrombocytopenia and other thromboembolic conditions

Dosage and routes:
• *Adult:* **IV** 0.4 mg/kg (≤110 kg) over 15-20 sec; then 0.15 mg/kg (≤110 kg/hr) as a cont inf for 2-10 days or longer

Available forms: Powder for inj 50 mg

Side effects/adverse reactions:
CV: **Heart failure, pericardial effusion, ventricular fibrillation**
SYST: **Multiorgan failure, sepsis**
CNS: Fever
GI: GI bleeding, abnormal LFTs
GU: **Hematuria,** abnormal kidney function
HEMA: **Hemorrhage, thrombocytopenia**
RESP: Pneumonia
INTEG: Allergic skin reactions

Contraindications: Hypersensitivity to hirudins

Precautions: Intracranial bleeding, renal function impairment, lactation, children, hepatic disease, pregnancy (B)

Pharmacokinetics: May be metabolized by the release of amino acids during catabolism; 50% unchanged in urine

Interactions:
• Increased risk of bleeding: warfarin derivatives
• Increased action of lepirudin: thrombolytics

NURSING CONSIDERATIONS
Assess:
• Obtain baseline in APTT before treatment; do not start treatment if APTT ratio ≥ 2.5, then APTT 4 hr after initiation of treatment and at least qd thereafter, if APTT above target, stop inf for 2 hr, then restart at 50%, take APTT in 4 hr; if below target, increase inf rate by 20%, take APTT in 4 hr, do not exceed inf rate of 0.21 mg/kg/hr without checking for coagulation abnormalities
• APTT, which should be 1.5-2.5 × control
 Bleeding gums, petechiae, ecchymosis, black tarry stools, hematuria/epistaxis, B/P, vaginal bleeding and possible hemorrhage
• Fever, skin rash, urticaria

Administer:
• Avoiding all IM injections that may cause bleeding
• After reconstitution and further dilution under sterile conditions; use water for inj or 0.9% NaCl; for further dilution 0.9% NaCl or D₅; for rapid and complete reconstitution, inject 1 ml of diluent into vial and shake gently, use immediately, warm to room temp before use

IV BOL
• Use sol with conc. of 5 mg/ml, reconstitute 5 mg (1 vial)/1 ml of water for inj or 0.9% NaCl, use body wt for correct calculation as to wt

IV INF
• Use sol with a conc. of 0.2 or 0.4 mg/ml; reconstitute 100 mg (2 vials) with 1 ml each (2 ml) water for inj or 0.9% NaCl, transfer to inf bag with either 500 or 250 ml of 0.9% NaCl or D₅

Evaluate:
• Therapeutic response

Teach patient/family:
• To use soft-bristle toothbrush to avoid bleeding gums, avoid contact

---

◆ = Nursing alert   ✿ = Herb-drug interaction   ⊘ = Do not crush

sports, use electric razor, avoid IM injection
• To report any signs of bleeding: gums, under skin, urine, stools

letrozole (℞)

(let'tro-zohl)
Femara
Func. class.: Antineoplastic, nonsteroidal aromatase inhibitor

Action: Binds to the heme group of aromatase. Inhibits conversion of androgens to estrogens to reduce plasma estrogen levels. 30% of breast cancers decrease in size when deprived of estrogen
Uses: Metastatic breast cancer in postmenopausal women
Dosage and routes:
• *Adult:* **PO** 2.5 mg qd
Available forms: Tabs 2.5 mg
Side effects/adverse reactions:
RESP: Dyspnea, cough
*GI: Nausea, vomiting, anorexia, **hepatotoxicity,** constipation, heartburn, diarrhea*
INTEG: Rash, pruritus, alopecia, sweating, hot flashes
CV: Hypertension
CNS: Headache, lethargy, somnolence, dizziness, depression, anxiety
Contraindications: Hypersensitivity, pregnancy (D)
Precautions: Hepatic disease, respiratory disease
Pharmacokinetics: Metabolized in liver, excreted in urine
Interactions: Unknown
NURSING CONSIDERATIONS
Assess:
• Renal function studies: BUN, serum uric acid, urine CrCl, electrolytes before, during therapy
• I&O ratio; report fall in urine output to <30 ml/hr
• Monitor temp q4h; may indicate beginning infection
• Liver function tests before, during therapy (bilirubin, AST, ALT, LDH) as needed or monthly
• RBC, Hct, Hgb, since these may be decreased, lymphocyte count, thyroid function tests
• Jaundiced skin, sclera, dark urine, clay-colored stools, itchy skin, abdominal pain, fever, diarrhea
Perform/provide:
• Liquid diet, including cola, Jell-O; dry toast or crackers as ordered may be added if patient is not nauseated or vomiting
• Nutritious diet with iron and vitamin supplements as ordered
Evaluate:
• Therapeutic response: decrease in size of tumor
Teach patient/family:
• To report any complaints, side effects to nurse or prescriber
• To avoid self-administration of corticosteroids
• That drowsiness may occur and to avoid driving or operating heavy machinery

leucovorin (℞)

(loo-koe-vor'in)
leucovorin calcium,
Wellcovorin
Func. class.: Vitamin, folic acid/methotrexate antagonist antidote
Chem. class.: Tetrahydrofolic acid derivative

Action: Needed for normal growth patterns; prevents toxicity during antineoplastic therapy by protecting normal cells
Uses: Megaloblastic or macrocytic anemia caused by folic acid defi-

ciency, overdose of folic acid antagonist, methotrexate toxicity, toxicity caused by pyrimethamine or trimethoprim, pneumocystosis, toxoplasmosis

Dosage and routes:

Megaloblastic anemia caused by enzyme deficiency
• *Adult and child:* **PO/IV/IM** up to 1 mg/day

Megaloblastic anemia caused by deficiency of folate
• *Adult and child:* **IM** 1 mg or less qd until adequate response

Methotrexate toxicity
• *Adult and child:* **PO/IM/IV** given 6-24 hr after dose of methotrexate 10 mg/m², then 10 mg/m² q6h × 72 hr

Pyrimethamine toxicity
• *Adult and child:* **PO/IM** 5 mg qd

Trimethoprim toxicity
• *Adult and child:* **PO/IM** 400 mg qd

Available forms: Tabs 5, 10, 15, 25 mg; inj 3, 5 mg/ml; powder for inj 10 mg/ml

Side effects/adverse reactions:
RESP: Wheezing
INTEG: Rash, pruritus, erythema, thrombocytosis, urticaria

Contraindications: Hypersensitivity, anemias other than megaloblastic not associated with vit B_{12} deficiency

Precautions: Pregnancy (C)

Interactions:
• Decreased folate levels: chloramphenicol
• Increased metabolism of phenobarbital, hydantoins

NURSING CONSIDERATIONS
Assess:
• CrCl before leucovorin rescue and qd to detect nephrotoxicity
• I&O; watch for nausea and vomiting

• Nutritional status: bran, yeast, dried beans, nuts, fruits, fresh vegetables, asparagus, which have high folic acid levels
• Other drugs taken: alcohol, hydantoins, trimethoprim may cause increased folic acid use by body

Administer:
• Within 1 hr of folic acid antagonist

IM
• No reconstitution needed

IV
• For IV reconstitute 50 mg/5 ml bacteriostatic or sterile H_2O for inj (10 mg/ml) or (100 mg/10 ml); use immediately if sterile H_2O is used
• Give by direct IV over 160 mg/min or less (16 ml of 10 mg/ml sol/min)
• Give by intermittent inf after diluting in 100-500 ml of 0.9% NaCl, D_5W, $D_{10}W$, LR, Ringer's sol

Additive compatibilities: Cisplatin, cisplatin/floxuridine, floxuridine

Syringe compatibilities: Bleomycin, cisplatin, cyclophosphamide, doxorubicin, fluorouracil, furosemide, heparin, methotrexate, metoclopramide, mitomycin, vinblastine, vincristine

Y-site compatibilities: Amifostine, aztreonam, bleomycin, cefepime, cisplatin, cladribine, cyclophosphamide, doxorubicin, doxorubicin liposome, filgrastim, fluconazole, fluorouracil, furosemide, granisetron, heparin, methotrexate, metoclopramide, mitomycin, piperacillin/tazobactam, tacrolimus, teniposide, thiotepa, vinblastine, vincristine

Perform/provide:
• Increase fluid intake if used to treat folic acid inhibitor overdose
• Protection from light and heat

Evaluate:
• Therapeutic response: increased weight; improved orientation, well-being; absence of fatigue

---

 = Nursing alert   ⫽ = Herb-drug interaction   ⊘ = Do not crush

Teach patient/family:
• For leucovorin rescue have patient drink 3 L fluid qd of rescue
• For folic acid deficiency eat folic acid rich foods: bran, yeast, dried beans, nuts, fresh, green leafy vegetables
• To take drug exactly as prescribed
• To notify prescriber of side effects
• To report signs of hyposensitivity reaction immediately

---

leuprolide (℞)

(loo-proe'lide)
Leupron Depo Ped, Lupron, Lupron Depot, Lupron Depot-3 month
Func. class.: Antineoplastic hormone
Chem. class.: Gonadotropin-releasing hormone

Action: Causes initial increase in circulating levels of LH, FSH; continuous administration results in decreased LH, FSH; in men, testosterone is reduced to castrate levels; in premenopausal women, estrogen is reduced to menopausal levels

Uses: Metastatic prostate cancer, management of endometriosis, central precocious puberty

Dosage and routes:
Prostate cancer
• *Adult:* SC 1 mg/day; IM 7.5 mg/dose qmo
Endometriosis/fibroids
• *Adult:* IM 3.75 mg qmo
Central precocious puberty
• *Child:* SC 50 mg/kg/day; may increase by 10 µg/kg/day as needed
• *Child >37.5 kg:* IM 15 mg q4wk
• *Child 25-37.5 kg:* IM 11.25 mg q4wk
• *Child ≤25 kg:* 7.5 mg q4wk

Available forms: Inj (depot) 3.75 mg, 7.5 mg single dose, multiple dose vials (5 mg/ml), single-use kit 11.25 mg vial, pediatric depot 7.5, 11.25, 15 mg; 3 mo depot 22.5 mg single use

Side effects/adverse reactions:
GU: Edema, hot flashes, impotence, decreased libido, amenorrhea, vaginal dryness, gynecomastia
CV: **MI, pulmonary emboli, dysrhythmias**
GI: Anorexia, diarrhea, **GI bleeding**

Contraindications: Hypersensitivity to GnRH or analogs, thromboembolic disorders, pregnancy (X), lactation, undiagnosed vaginal bleeding

Precautions: Edema, hepatic disease, CVA, MI, seizures, hypertension, diabetes mellitus

Pharmacokinetics:
SC: Onset 1-2 wk, peak 2-4 wk; absorbed rapidly (SC), slowly (IM depot); half-life 3 hr

NURSING CONSIDERATIONS
Assess:
• For symptoms of endometriosis (lower abdominal pain)/fibroids before, during, and after treatment
• Liver function tests before, during therapy (bilirubin, AST, ALT, LDH) as needed or monthly, PSA in prostate cancer
• Pituitary gonadotropic and gonadal function during therapy and 4-8 wk after therapy is decreased
• Worsening of signs and symptoms; normal during beginning therapy
• Fatigue, increased pulse, pallor, lethargy
• Edema in feet, joints; stomach pain; shaking
◆ Symptoms indicating severe allergic reaction: rash, pruritus, urticaria, purpuric skin lesions, itching, flushing
• For central precocious puberty (CPP) if treatment is for this condition; secondary S4 characteristics to child <9 yr, estradiol/testosterone

---

Side effects: *italics* = common; **bold italics** = life-threatening

levels, GnRH test, tomography of head, adrenal steroids, chorionic gonadotropin, wrist x-ray, height, weight

Administer:
• IM/SC using syringe and drug packaged together, give deep in large muscle mass, rotate sites
• Use depot IM only
• Reconstitute vial (single dose)/1 ml of diluent, shake, use immediately

Perform/provide:
• Nutritious diet with iron, vitamin supplements as ordered
• Storage in tight container at room temp

Evaluate:
• Therapeutic response: decreased tumor size and spread of malignancy

Teach patient/family:
• To notify prescriber if menstruation continues; menstruation should stop
• To use a nonhormonal method of contraception during therapy
• That bone pain will disappear after 1 wk
• To report any complaints, side effects to nurse or prescriber
• How to prepare, give; to rotate sites for SC injections
• To keep accurate records of dose
• That tumor flare may occur: increase in size of tumor, increased bone pain, will subside rapidly; may take analgesics for pain; premenopausal women must use mechanical birth control; ovulation may be induced

---

levalbuterol

See appendix a—selected new drugs

---

levamisole (R)

(leh-vam′ih-sole)

Ergamisol

Func. class.: Antineoplastic-immunomodulator

Action: May increase the action of macrophages, monocytes, T cells, which will restore immune function; complete action unknown

Uses: Treatment of Dukes' stage C colon cancer given with fluorouracil after surgical resection

Investigational uses: Malignant melanoma (advanced)

Dosage and routes:
• *Adult:* **PO** 50 mg q8h × 3 days; begin treatment at least 1 wk but no more than 4 wk after resection; given with fluorouracil 450 mg/m²/day; **IV** given daily × 5 days beginning 21-34 days after resection; maintenance is 50 mg q8h × 3 days q2wk × 1 yr; given with fluorouracil 45 mg/m²/day by **IV** push qwk starting 28 days after the initial 5-day course × 1 yr

Available forms: Tabs 50 mg

Side effects/adverse reactions:
CNS: Dizziness, headache, paresthesia, somnolence, depression, anxiety, fatigue, fever, mental changes, ataxia, insomnia
GI: Nausea, vomiting, anorexia, diarrhea, stomatitis, constipation, flatulence, dyspepsia, abdominal pain
INTEG: Rash, pruritus, alopecia, dermatitis, urticaria
HEMA: **Granulocytopenia, leukopenia, thrombocytopenia**
CV: Chest pain, edema
META: Hyperbilirubinemia
EENT: Blurred vision, conjunctivitis
OTHER: Rigors, infection, altered sense of smell, arthralgia, myalgia
Contraindications: Hypersensitivity

 = Nursing alert   ⫸ = Herb-drug interaction   ⊘ = Do not crush

Precautions: Pregnancy (C), lactation, children, blood dyscrasias

Pharmacokinetics: Peak 1½-2 hr, elimination half-life 3-4 hr; metabolized by the liver

Interactions:
• Increased plasma level, toxicity: phenytoin
• Disulfiram-like reaction: alcohol
• Increased bone marrow depression: radiation, other antineoplastic
• Increased effects of warfarin

NURSING CONSIDERATIONS
Assess:
• Kidney, liver function studies: BUN, creatinine, AST, ALT, alk phosphatase, bilirubin
• Baseline blood counts with differential, platelets, electrolyte, repeat q3mo for 1 yr; if platelets are <100,000/mm^3, therapy should be discontinued and restarted after recovery; fluorouracil should not be given if WBC is 2500-3500/mm^3; after WBC is >3500/mm^3, dose should be reduced by 20%; if WBC <2500/mm^3 for 10 days, discontinue levamisole
• Stomatitis or GI symptoms: drug may have to be discontinued; then start fluorouracil 28 days after the start of first course
◆ Blood dyscrasias (anemia, granulocytopenia); bruising, fatigue, bleeding, poor healing
• Allergic reactions: dermatitis, exfoliative dermatitis, pruritus, urticaria

Administer:
• 7-20 days after surgery; start fluorouracil with second course of levamisole; begin no sooner than 21 days and no later than 35 days after surgery; if levamisole therapy begins 21-30 days after resection, fluorouracil should be given with first course; apply pressure to venipuncture sites for 10 min, especially if platelets are low

Evaluate:
• Therapeutic response: decrease in size and spread of tumor

Teach patient/family:
• To call prescriber if sore throat, swollen lymph nodes, malaise, fever occur, since other infections may occur
• To use contraception during therapy and 4 mo after
• To avoid alcohol; disulfiram-like reaction can occur; also to avoid tyramine-containing products
• To avoid use of products containing aspirin, ibuprofen; to report bleeding
• To report signs of anemia or CNS reactions
• That hair may be lost during treatment; a wig or hairpiece may be worn

L

levetiracetam
See appendix a—selected new drugs

levobupivacaine
See appendix a—selected new drugs

levodopa (℞)
(lee′voe-doe-pa)
Dopar, Larodopa, L-Dopa
Func. class.: Antiparkinson agent
Chem. class.: Catecholamine

Action: Decarboxylation to dopamine, which increases dopamine levels in brain

Uses: Parkinsonism

Dosage and routes:
• *Adult:* **PO** 0.5-1 g qd divided bid-qid with meals; may increase by up to 0.75 g q3-7d not to exceed 8 g/day unless closely supervised

---

Side effects: *italics* = common; ***bold italics*** = life-threatening

Available forms: Caps 100, 250, 500 mg; tabs 100, 250, 500 mg

Side effects/adverse reactions:

*HEMA: **Hemolytic anemia, leukopenia, agranulocytosis***

CNS: Involuntary choreiform movements, hand tremors, fatigue, headache, anxiety, twitching, numbness, weakness, confusion, agitation, insomnia, nightmares, psychosis, hallucination, hypomania, severe depression, dizziness

GI: Nausea, vomiting, anorexia, abdominal distress, dry mouth, flatulence, dysphagia, bitter taste, diarrhea, constipation

INTEG: Rash, sweating, alopecia

CV: Orthostatic hypotension, tachycardia, hypertension, palpitation

EENT: Blurred vision, diplopia, dilated pupils

MISC: Urinary retention, incontinence, weight change, dark urine

Contraindications: Hypersensitivity, narrow-angle glaucoma, undiagnosed skin lesions

Precautions: Renal disease, cardiac disease, hepatic disease, respiratory disease, MI with dysrhythmias, convulsions, peptic ulcer, pregnancy (C), asthma, endocrine disease, affective disorders, psychosis, lactation, children <12 yr, peptic ulcer

Pharmacokinetics:

PO: Peak 1-3 hr, excreted in urine (metabolites)

Interactions:

• Hypertensive crisis: MAOIs, furazolidone

• Decreased effects of levodopa: anticholinergics, hydantoins, methionine, papaverine, pyridoxine, benzodiazepines

• Increased effects of levodopa: antacids, metoclopramide

• Drug/food: decreased levodopa absorption: high-protein foods

• Increased pyridoxine will decrease levodopa effect

🗲 Decreased action of levodopa, increased EPS: Indian snakeroot

🗲 Increased parkinsonian symptoms: kava

Lab test interferences:

False positive: Urine ketones, urine glucose, Coombs' test

False negative: Urine glucose (glucose oxidase)

False increase: Uric acid, urine protein

Decrease: VMA

NURSING CONSIDERATIONS

Assess:

• Liver function enzymes: AST, ALT, alk phosphatase, LDH, bilirubin, CBC

• Involuntary movements in parkinsonism: akinesia, tremors, staggering gait, muscle rigidity, drooling

◆ Levodopa toxicity: mental, personality changes, increased twitching, grimacing, tongue protrusion

• B/P, respiration during initial treatment; hypo/hypertension should be reported

• Mental status: affect, mood, behavioral changes, depression; complete suicide assessment

Administer:

• Drug until NPO before surgery

• Adjust dosage to patient response

• With meals; limit protein taken with drug

• Only after MAOIs have been discontinued for 2 wk

Perform/provide:

• Assistance with ambulation during beginning therapy

• Testing for diabetes mellitus, acromegaly if on long-term therapy

Evaluate:

• Therapeutic response: decrease in akathisia, increased mood

Teach patient/family:

• That therapeutic effects may take several wk to a few mo

◆ = Nursing alert   🗲 = Herb-drug interaction   🚫 = Do not crush

• To change positions slowly to prevent orthostatic hypotension
• To report side effects: twitching, eye spasms; indicate overdose
• To use drug exactly as prescribed; if drug is discontinued abruptly, parkinsonian crisis may occur
• That urine, sweat may darken
• To avoid vit B_6 preparations, vitamin-fortified foods containing B_6; these foods can reverse effects of levodopa

---

levofloxacin (℞)

(lee-voh-floks′a-sin)
Levaquin
Func. class.: Antiinfective
Chem. class.: Fluoroquinolone

Action: Interferes with conversion of intermediate DNA fragments into high-molecular-weight DNA in bacteria; DNA gyrase inhibitor
Uses: Acute sinusitis, acute chronic bronchitis, community-acquired pneumonia, uncomplicated skin infections, complicated UTI, acute pyelonephritis caused by *Streptococcus pneumoniae, Haemophilus influenzae, H. parainfluenzae, Moraxella catarrhalis*
Dosage and routes:
• *Adult:* **IV INF** 500 mg by slow inf over 1 hr q24h × 7-14 days depending on infection; **PO:** 500 mg q24h × 7-14 days depending on infection
Renal disease
• CrCl 20-49 ml/min initial 500 mg, then 250 mg, q24h; CrCl 10-19 ml/min 250 or 500 mg, depending on condition; then 250 mg q48h
Available forms: Single use vials (500 mg); 25 mg/ml 20 ml vials; premixed flexible containers; tabs 250, 500 mg
Side effects/adverse reactions:
MISC: Hypoglycemia, hypersensitivity, *anaphylaxis, multisystem organ failure*
CNS: Headache, dizziness, *insomnia,* anxiety, *seizures,* encephalopathy, paresthesia
CV: Chest pain, palpitations, vasodilation
HEMA: Eosinophilia, *hemolytic anemia,* lymphopenia
RESP: Pneumonitis
GI: Nausea, flatulence, *vomiting,* diarrhea, abdominal pain, *pseudomembranous colitis*
GU: Vaginitis, crystalluria
INTEG: Rash, pruritus, *photosensitivity, Stevens-Johnson syndrome*
Contraindications: Hypersensitivity to quinolones, photosensitivity
Precautions: Pregnancy (C), lactation, children
Pharmacokinetics: Metabolized in liver, excreted in urine unchanged, half-life 6-8 hr
Interactions:
• Decreased absorption of levofloxacin: antacids containing aluminum, magnesium; sucralfate, zinc, iron
• Altered blood glucose levels: antidiabetic agents
• Increased CNS stimulation, seizures: NSAIDs
• May decrease clearance of: theophylline
• Increased risk of bleeding: warfarin and derivatives
• Do not use with magnesium in the same IV line
Lab test interferences:
Decrease: Glucose, lymphocytes
NURSING CONSIDERATIONS
Assess:
• For previous sensitivity reaction
• For signs and symptoms of infection: characteristics of sputum, WBC >10,000/mm^3, fever; obtain baseline information before and during treatment

---

• C&S before beginning drug therapy to identify if correct treatment has been initiated

◆ For allergic reactions: rash, urticaria, pruritus, chills, fever, joint pain; may occur a few days after therapy begins; epinephrine and resuscitation equipment should be available for anaphylactic reaction

• Bowel pattern qd; if severe diarrhea occurs, drug should be discontinued

• For overgrowth of infection: perineal itching, fever, malaise, redness, pain, swelling, drainage, rash, diarrhea, change in cough, sputum

Administer:

• PO 4 hr before or 2 hr after antacids, iron, calcium, zinc

IV

• Only by slow IV infusion over 1 hr

• Discard any unused sol in the single-dose vial

• Using premix, tear outer wrap at notch and remove sol container, check for leaks, close control clamps; remove cover from port at bottom of container, insert pin into port with a twist; suspend container from hanger, squeeze and release drip chamber to proper fluid level, open flow control to expel air, close clamp; regulate rate with flow control clamps

Solution compatibilities: 0.9% NaCl, D_5W, D_5/0.9% NaCl, D_5LR, D_5/0.45% NaCl, sodium lactate

Evaluate:

• Therapeutic response: absence of signs/symptoms of infection (WBC <10,000/mm³, temp WNL)

Teach patient/family:

• To contact prescriber if vaginal itching, loose, foul-smelling stools, furry tongue occur (may indicate superinfection); report itching, rash, pruritus, urticaria

• To notify prescriber of diarrhea with blood or pus

• To take 4 hr before or 2 hr after antacids, iron, calcium, zinc products

• To complete full course of therapy

---

levomethadyl (℞)

(lev-oh-meth′ah-dil)

ORLAMM

Func. class.: Opiate agonist analgesic

Action: Depresses pain impulse transmission at the spinal cord level by interacting with opioid receptors

Uses: Management of opiate dependency

Dosage and routes:

Opiate withdrawal

• Usually given 3×/wk (Monday, Wednesday, Friday or Tuesday, Thursday, Saturday)

• *Initial dose:* 20-40 mg each dose at 48 or 72 hr; may be adjusted in increments of 5-10 mg until steady state occurs (1-2 wk); patients dependent on methadone may require larger doses

• *Maintenance:* 60-90 mg 3×/wk

• *Transfer to methadone:* Initial treatment given after 48 hr; may give increased or decreased (5-10 mg) in the daily methadone dose (symptoms of withdrawal)

Available forms: Oral sol 10 mg/ml

Side effects/adverse reactions:

CNS: Drowsiness, dizziness, confusion, headache, sedation, euphoria

CV: Palpitations, bradycardia, change in B/P

EENT: Tinnitus, blurred vision, miosis, diplopia

GI: Nausea, vomiting, anorexia, constipation, cramps, biliary tract spasm

GU: Increased urinary output, dysuria, urinary retention

◆ = Nursing alert   ✐ = Herb-drug interaction   ⊘ = Do not crush

INTEG: Rash, urticaria, bruising, flushing, diaphoresis, pruritus
*RESP: **Respiratory depression***
Contraindications: Hypersensitivity
Precautions: Addictive personality, pregnancy (C), lactation, increased intracranial pressure, MI (acute), severe heart disease, respiratory depression, hepatic disease, renal disease, child <18 yr
Pharmacokinetics:
PO: Onset 30-60 min, duration 6-8 hr, cumulative 22-48 hr
Metabolized by liver, excreted by kidneys, crosses placenta, excreted in breast milk
Interactions:
• Increased effects with other CNS depressants: alcohol, narcotics, sedative/hypnotics, antipsychotics, skeletal muscle relaxants, rifampin, phenytoin
NURSING CONSIDERATIONS
Assess:
• I&O ratio; check for decreasing output; may indicate urinary retention
Administer:
• With antiemetic for nausea, vomiting
Perform/provide:
• Storage in light-resistant container at room temp
Evaluate:
• Therapeutic response: decreased dependence on opiate
• CNS changes: dizziness, drowsiness, hallucinations, euphoria, LOC, pupil reaction
• Allergic reactions: rash, urticaria
• Respiratory dysfunction: depression, character, rate, rhythm
Teach patient/family:
• To report any symptoms of CNS changes, allergic reactions
• That physical dependency may result after extended period of use
• That withdrawal symptoms may

occur: nausea, vomiting, cramps, fever, faintness, anorexia
• To avoid pregnancy; if suspected, notify prescriber
• To use contraception during treatment

---

levonorgestrel implant (℞)
(lee-voe-nor-jess′trel)
Norplant System
Func. class.: Contraceptive system
Chem. class.: Synthetic progestin

Action: As a progestin, transforms proliferative endometrium into secretory endometrium; inhibits secretion of pituitary gonadotropins, which prevents follicular maturation and ovulation
Uses: Prevention of pregnancy for 5 yr
Dosage and routes:
• *Adult:* 6 caps subdermally implanted in the upper arm during first 7 days after onset of menses
Available forms: Kit of 6 caps, 36 mg/cap
Side effects/adverse reactions:
CNS: Dizziness, headache, nervousness
GU: Amenorrhea, cervical erosion, breakthrough bleeding, dysmenorrhea, vaginal candidiasis, breast changes, vaginitis
GI: Nausea, abdominal discomfort
INTEG: Alopecia, dermatitis, hirsutism, acne, hypertrichosis, infection at site, pain/itching at site
OTHER: Change in appetite, weight gain
Contraindications: Hypersensitivity, pregnancy (X), thrombophlebitis, undiagnosed genital bleeding,

liver tumors, breast carcinoma, liver disease

Precautions: Depression, psychosis, lactation, fluid retention, contact lens wearers

Pharmacokinetics: Max concentration at 24 hr

Interactions:

• Decreased contraception: phenytoin, carbamazepine

NURSING CONSIDERATIONS
Assess:

• Blood studies: cholesterol, triglycerides; may be increased or decreased; sex hormone—binding globulin, thyroxine, T_3 uptake

• Menstrual irregularities: spotting, prolonged bleeding, amenorrhea; usually diminish

• For jaundice, thrombophlebitis; implants should be removed

• For acne, dermatitis, hirsutism, alopecia

Administer:

• 8 cm (3 in) above the crease of the elbow; implantation should be during first 7 days after onset of menses; implantation should be fanlike, 15 degrees apart

Evaluate:

• Therapeutic response: absence of pregnancy

Teach patient/family:

• That if vision problems occur, an ophthalmologist should be seen

• That physical examinations are necessary

---

levorphanol (℞)

(lee-vor'fa-nole)
Levo-Dromoran, Levorphan
Func. class.: Opioid analgesic (agonist)
Chem. class.: Opiate, synthetic morphine derivative

Controlled Substance Schedule II
Action: Depresses pain impulse transmission at the spinal cord level by interacting with opioid receptors

Uses: Moderate to severe pain

Dosage and routes:

• *Adult:* **PO/SC/IV** 2-3 mg q4-5h prn; **PCA** 0.1 mg/ml

Available forms: Inj 2 mg/ml; tabs 2 mg

Side effects/adverse reactions:

CNS: Drowsiness, dizziness, confusion, headache, sedation, euphoria

GI: Nausea, vomiting, anorexia, constipation, cramps

GU: Urinary retention, dysuria

INTEG: Rash, urticaria, diaphoresis, pruritus

EENT: Tinnitus, blurred vision, miosis, diplopia

CV: Palpitations, bradycardia, change in B/P

*RESP: **Respiratory depression***

Contraindications: Hypersensitivity, addiction (narcotic)

Precautions: Addictive personality, pregnancy (B), lactation, increased intracranial pressure, MI (acute), severe heart disease, respiratory depression, hepatic disease, renal disease, child <18 yr

Pharmacokinetics:

PO: Onset up to ½-1½ hr, peak ½-1 hr, duration 6-8 hr

SC: Peak ½-1 hr, duration 6-8 hr

IV: Peak 20 min, duration 6-8 hr; metabolized by liver; excreted by kidneys; crosses placenta; excreted in breast milk; half-life 12-16 hr

Interactions:

• Do not use with MAOIs, severe reactions have occurred

• Effects may be increased with other CNS depressants: alcohol, narcotics, sedative/hypnotics, antipsychotics, skeletal muscle relaxants

• Decreased analgesia: pentazocine, nalbuphine

🌿 Increased action: kava

◆ = Nursing alert　　🌿 = Herb-drug interaction　　⊘ = Do not crush

Lab test interferences:
Increase: Amylase

NURSING CONSIDERATIONS
Assess:
• I&O ratio; check for decreasing output; may indicate urinary retention
• CNS changes: dizziness, drowsiness, hallucinations, euphoria, LOC, pupil reaction
• Allergic reactions: rash, urticaria
• Respiratory dysfunction: respiratory depression, character, rate, rhythm; notify prescriber if respirations are <10/min
• Need for pain medication, physical dependence

Administer:
• With antiemetic if nausea, vomiting occur
• When pain is beginning to return; determine dosage interval by patient response

IV
• IV directly through Y-tube or 3-way stopcock over 5 min; do not give rapidly; circulatory collapse may occur

Solution compatibility: TPN 212-215

Syringe compatibilities: Glycopyrrolate, propofol

Perform/provide:
• Storage in light-resistant area at room temp
• Assistance with ambulation
• Safety measures: side rails, nightlight, call bell within easy reach

Evaluate:
• Therapeutic response: decrease in pain

Teach patient/family:
• To report any symptoms of CNS changes, allergic reactions
• That physical dependency may result from extended period of use
• That the following withdrawal symptoms may occur: nausea, vomiting, cramps, fever, faintness, anorexia

Treatment of overdose: Naloxone (Narcan) 0.2-0.8 mg IV, O₂, IV fluids, vasopressors

---

levothyroxine (T₄) (℞)
(lee-voe-thye-rox′een)
Eltroxin*, Levo-T, Levoxyl, Levothroid, levothyroxine sodium, Levoxine, PMS-Levothyroxine Sodium*, Synthroid, T₄
Func. class.: Thyroid hormone
Chem. class.: Levoisomer of thyroxine

Action: Increases metabolic rate, controls protein synthesis, increases cardiac output, renal blood flow, O₂ consumption, body temp, blood volume, growth, development at cellular level

Uses: Hypothyroidism, myxedema coma, thyroid hormone replacement, congenital hypothyroidism, thyrotoxicosis, congenital hypothyroidism, some types of thyroid cancer

Dosage and routes:
Severe hypothyroidism
• *Adult:* **PO** 12.5-50 µg qd, increased by 50-100 µg q1-4 wk until desired response, maintenance dose 75-125 µg qd; **IM/IV** 50-100 µg/day as a single dose
• *Child >12 yr:* **PO** 2-3 µg/kg/day as a single dose AM
• *Child 6-12 yr:* **PO** 4-5 µg/kg/day as a single dose AM
• *Child 1-5 yr:* **PO** 5-6 µg/kg/day as a single dose AM
• *Child 6-12 mo:* **PO** 6-8 µg/kg/day as a single dose AM
• *Child to 6 mo:* **PO** 8-10 µg/kg/day as a single dose AM

Myxedema coma
• *Adult:* **IV** 200-500 µg, may increase by 100-300 µg after 24 hr;

place on oral medication as soon as possible

Available forms: Inj 50, 200, 500 μg/vial; tabs 0.025, 0.05, 0.075, 0.088, 0.1, 0.112, 0.125, 0.137, 0.15, 0.175, 0.2, 0.3 mg

Side effects/adverse reactions:

CNS: Anxiety, insomnia, tremors, headache, ***thyroid storm***

CV: Tachycardia, palpitations, angina, dysrhythmias, hypertension, ***cardiac arrest***

GI: Nausea, diarrhea, increased or decreased appetite, cramps

MISC: Menstrual irregularities, weight loss, sweating, heat intolerance, fever

Contraindications: Adrenal insufficiency, myocardial infarction, thyrotoxicosis, hypersensitivity to beef, alcohol intolerance (inj only)

Precautions: Elderly, angina pectoris, hypertension, ischemia, cardiac disease, pregnancy (A), lactation

Pharmacokinetics:

PO: Onset unknown, peak 1-3 wk, duration 1-3 wk

IV: Onset 6-8 hr, peak 24 hr, duration unknown

Half-life 6-7 days; distributed throughout body tissues

Interactions:

• Decreased absorption of levothyroxine: cholestyramine

• Increased effects of anticoagulants, sympathomimetics, tricyclic antidepressants

• Decreased effects of digitalis drugs, insulin, hypoglycemics

• Decreased effects of levothyroxine: estrogens

• Considered to be incompatible in syringe with all other drugs

🌿 Do not give with bugleweed

Lab test interferences:

Increase: CPK, LDH, AST, PBI, blood glucose

Decrease: TSH, ^{131}I uptake test, uric acid, triglycerides

NURSING CONSIDERATIONS

Assess:

• B/P, pulse periodically during treatment

• Weight qd in same clothing, using same scale, at same time of day

• Height, growth rate of a child

• T$_3$, T$_4$, FTIs, which are decreased; radioimmunoassay of TSH, which is increased; radio uptake, which is increased if patient is on too low a dose of medication

• Pro-time may require decreased anticoagulant; check for bleeding, bruising

• Increased nervousness, excitability, irritability, which may indicate too high dose of medication, usually after 1-3 wk of treatment

• Cardiac status: angina, palpitation, chest pain, change in VS

Administer:

• IV after diluting with provided diluent 0.5 mg/5 ml; shake; give through Y-tube or 3-way stopcock; give 0.1 mg or less over 1 min; do not add to IV inf; 0.1 mg = 1 ml

• In AM if possible as a single dose to decrease sleeplessness

• At same time each day to maintain drug level

• Only for hormone imbalances; not to be used for obesity, male infertility, menstrual conditions, lethargy

• Lowest dose that relieves symptoms; lower dose to the elderly and in cardiac diseases

• Crushed and mixed with water, nonsoy formula, or breast milk for infants/children

Perform/provide:

• Storage in tight, light-resistant container; sol should be discarded if not used immediately

• Withdrawal of medication 4 wk before RAIU test

◆ = Nursing alert   🌿 = Herb-drug interaction   🚫 = Do not crush

Evaluate:

• Therapeutic response: absence of depression; increased weight loss, diuresis, pulse, appetite; absence of constipation, peripheral edema, cold intolerance; pale, cool, dry skin; brittle nails, alopecia, coarse hair, menorrhagia, night blindness, paresthesias, syncope, stupor, coma, rosy cheeks

Teach patient/family:

• That hair loss will occur in child, is temporary

• To report excitability, irritability, anxiety, which indicate overdose

• Not to switch brands unless approved by prescriber

• That drug may be discontinued after giving birth, thyroid panel evaluated after 1-2 mo

• That hypothyroid child will show almost immediate behavior/personality change

• That drug is not to be taken to reduce weight

• To avoid OTC preparations with iodine; read labels

• To avoid iodine food, iodized salt, soybeans, tofu, turnips, some seafood, some bread

• That drug is not a cure but controls symptoms and treatment is lifelong

---

lidocaine (℞)

(lye'doe-kane)

Anestacon, Baylocaine, L-Caine, Lidocaine HCl IV for Cardiac Arrhythmias, Lidopen Auto-Injector, Xylocaine HCl IM for Cardiac Arrythmias, Xylocaine HCl IV for Cardiac Arrhythmias

Func. class.: Antidysrhythmic (Class Ib)

Chem. class.: Aminoacyl amide

Action: Increases electrical stimulation threshold of ventricle, His-Purkinje system, which stabilizes cardiac membrane, decreases automaticity

Uses: Ventricular tachycardia, ventricular dysrhythmias during cardiac surgery, myocardial infarction, digitalis toxicity, cardiac catheterization

Dosage and routes:

• *Adult:* **IV BOL** 50-100 mg (1 mg/kg) over 2-3 min, repeat q3-5min, not to exceed 300 mg in 1 hr; begin **IV INF; IV INF** 20-50 μg/kg/min; **IM** 200-300 mg (4.3 mg/kg) in deltoid muscle, may repeat in 1-1½ hr if needed

• *Elderly, CHF, reduced liver function:* **IV BOL** give ½ adult dose

• *Child:* **IV BOL** 1 mg/kg, then **IV INF** 30 μg/kg/min

Available forms: IV INF 0.2% (2 mg/ml), 0.4% (4 mg/ml), 0.8% (8 mg/ml); IV ad 4% (40 mg/ml), 10% (100 mg/ml), 20% (200 mg/ml); IV dir 1% (10 mg/ml), 2% (20 mg/ml); IM 10% 300 mg/ml

Side effects/adverse reactions:

CNS: Headache, dizziness, involuntary movement, confusion, tremor, drowsiness, euphoria, ***convulsions***

EENT: Tinnitus, blurred vision

GI: Nausea, vomiting, anorexia

CV: Hypotension, bradycardia, **heart block, cardiovascular collapse, arrest**

RESP: Dyspnea, *respiratory depression*

INTEG: Rash, urticaria, edema, swelling

MISC: Febrile response, phlebitis at injection site

Contraindications: Hypersensitivity to amides, severe heart block, supraventricular dysrhythmias, Adams-Stokes syndrome, Wolff-Parkinson-White syndrome

Precautions: Pregnancy (B), lactation, children, renal disease, liver disease, CHF, respiratory depression, malignant hyperthermia

Pharmacokinetics:

IV: Onset 2 min, duration 20 min

IM: Onset 5-15 min, duration 1½ hr; half-life 8 min, 1-2 hr (terminal); metabolized in liver; excreted in urine; crosses placenta

Interactions:

• Increased neuromuscular blockade of neuromuscular blockers, tubocurarine

• Increased effects of lidocaine: cimetidine, phenytoin, propranolol, metoprolol

• Decreased effects of lidocaine: barbiturates

⌀ Increased action of lidocaine: aloe, buckthorn, cascara sagrada, senna

Lab test interferences:

Increase: CPK

NURSING CONSIDERATIONS
Assess:

• ECG continuously to determine increased PR or QRS segments; if these develop, discontinue or reduce rate; watch for increased ventricular ectopic beats; may have to rebolus

• IV infusion rate using infusion pump; run at less than 4 mg/min

• Blood levels (therapeutic level: 1.5-6 µg/ml)

• B/P continuously for fluctuations in cardiac rate

• I&O ratio, electrolytes (K, Na, Cl)

◆ Malignant hyperthermia: tachypnea, tachycardia, changes in B/P, increased temp

• Respiratory status: rate, rhythm, lung fields for rales, watch for respiratory depression

• CNS effects: dizziness, confusion, psychosis, paresthesias, convulsions; drug should be discontinued

• Lung fields, bilateral rales may occur in CHF patient

• Increased respiration, increased pulse; drug should be discontinued

Administer:

• IM injection in deltoid; aspirate to avoid intravascular administration; check site daily for infiltration or extravasation

IV

• Bolus undiluted (1%, 2% only) give 50 mg or less over 1 min or dilute 1 g/250-500 ml of D_5W; titrate to patient response; use infusion pump; pediatric inf is 120 mg of lidocaine/100 ml D_5W; 1-2.5 ml/kg/hr = 20-50 µg/kg/min; use only 1%, 2% sol for IV bol

Additive compatibilities: Alteplase, aminophylline, amiodarone, atracurium, bretylium, calcium chloride, calcium gluceptate, calcium gluconate, chloramphenicol, chlorothiazide, cimetidine, dexamethasone, digoxin, diphenhydramine, dobutamine, dopamine, ephedrine, erythromycin lactobionate, floxacillin, flumazenil, furosemide, heparin, hydrocortisone, hydroxyzine, insulin (regular), mephentermine, metaraminol, nafcillin, nitroglycerin, penicillin G potassium, pentobarbital, phenylephrine, potassium chloride, procainamide, prochlorperazine, promazine, ranitidine, sodium bicarbonate, sodium lactate, theophylline, verapamil, vit B/C

Solution compatibilities: D_5W, D_5/0.9% NaCl, D_5/0.45% NaCl, D_5/LR, LR, 0.9% NaCl, 0.45% NaCl

Syringe compatibilities: Cloxacillin, glycopyrrolate, heparin, hydroxyzine, methicillin, metoclopramide, milrinone, moxalactam, nalbuphine

Y-site compatibilities: Alteplase, amiodarone, amrinone, cefazolin, ciprofloxacin, cisatracurium, diltiazem, dobutamine, dopamine, enalaprilat, etomidate, famotidine, haloperidol, heparin, heparin/hydrocortisone, labetalol, meperidine, morphine, nitroglycerin, nitroprusside, potassium chloride, propofol, remifentanil, streptokinase, theophylline, vit B/C, warfarin

Evaluate:
• Therapeutic response: decreased dysrhythmias

Teach patient/family:
• The use of automatic lidocaine injection device if ordered

Treatment of overdose: O_2, artificial ventilation, ECG; administer dopamine for circulatory depression, diazepam or thiopental for convulsions; decrease drug if needed

---

lindane (Rx)

(lin′dane)

GBH*, G-Well*, Kwell, Kwellada*, Kwildane, lindane, Scabene, Thionex

Func. class.: Scabicide, pediculicide

Chem. class.: Chlorinated hydrocarbon (synthetic)

Action: Stimulates nervous system of arthropods, resulting in seizures, death of organism

Uses: Scabies, lice (head/pubic/body), nits

Dosage and routes:
Lice
• *Adult and child:* **CREAM/LOTION** wash area with soap, water; remove visible crusts; apply to skin surfaces; remove with soap, water in 8-12 hr; may reapply in 1 wk if needed; shampoo using 30 ml: work into lather, rub for 5 min, rinse, dry with towel; comb with fine-toothed comb to remove nits

Scabies
• *Adult and child:* **TOP** apply 1% cream/lotion to skin, neck to bottom of feet, toes, repeat in 1 wk prn

Available forms: Lotion, shampoo, cream (1%)

Side effects/adverse reactions:
INTEG: Pruritus, rash, irritation, contact dermatitis
GI: Nausea, vomiting, diarrhea, liver damage (inhalation of vapors)
HEMA: ***Aplastic anemia*** (chronic inhalation of vapors)
CV: ***Ventricular fibrillation*** (chronic inhalation of vapors)
GU: ***Kidney damage*** (chronic inhalation of vapors)
CNS: Tremors, ***convulsions,*** stimulation, dizziness (chronic inhalation of vapors)

Contraindications: Hypersensitivity; premature neonate; patients with known seizure disorders; inflammation of skin, abrasions, or breaks in skin

Precautions: Pregnancy (B); avoid contact with eyes; children <10 yr, infants, lactation

Interactions:
• Oils may enhance absorption; if an oil-based hair dressing is used, shampoo, rinse, dry hair before applying lindane shampoo

NURSING CONSIDERATIONS
Assess:
• Head, hair for lice and nits before

L

and after treatment; if scabies are present check all skin surfaces

• Identify source of infection: school, family, sexual contacts

Administer:

• To body areas, scalp only; do not apply to face, lips, mouth, eyes, any mucous membrane, anus, or meatus

• Topical corticosteroids as ordered to decrease contact dermatitis

• Antihistamines

• Lotions of menthol or phenol to control itching

• Topical antibiotics for infection

Perform/provide:

• Isolation until areas on skin, scalp have cleared and treatment is completed

• Removal of nits by using a fine-toothed comb rinsed in vinegar after treatment; use gloves

Evaluate:

• Therapeutic response: decreased crusts, nits, brownish trails on skin, itching papules in skin folds, decreased itching after several wk

Teach patient/family:

• To wash all inhabitants' clothing, using insecticide; preventive treatment may be required of all persons living in same house, using lotion or shampoo to decrease spread of infection; use rubber gloves when applying drug

• That itching may continue for 4-6 wk

• That drug must be reapplied if accidentally washed off, or treatment will be ineffective

• Not to apply to face; if accidental contact with eyes occurs, flush with water

• To treat sexual contacts simultaneously

Treatment of ingestion: Gastric lavage, saline laxatives, IV diazepam (Valium) for convulsions

---

liothyronine (T$_3$) (℞)
(lye-oh-thye′roe-neen)
Cytomel, liothyronine sodium, Triostat
Func. class.: Thyroid hormone
Chem. class.: Synthetic T$_3$

Action: Increases metabolic rates, cardiac output, O$_2$ consumption, body temp, blood volume, growth, development at cellular level

Uses: Hypothyroidism, myxedema coma, thyroid hormone replacement, congenital hypothyroidism, nontoxic goiter, T$_3$ suppression test

Dosage and routes:

• *Adult:* **PO** 25 µg qd, increased by 12.5-25 µg q1-2wk until desired response, maintenance dose 25-75 µg qd

• *Geriatric:* **PO** 5 µg/day, increase by 5 µg/day q1-2wk

Congenital hypothyroidism

• *Child >3 yr:* **PO** 50-100 µg qd

• *Child <3 yr:* **PO** 5 µg qd, increased by 5 µg q3-4d titrated to response

Myxedema, severe hypothyroidism

• *Adult:* **PO** 5 µg qd; may increase by 5-10 µg q1-2wk; maintenance dose 50-100 µg qd

Nontoxic goiter

• *Adult:* **PO** 5 µg qd, increased by 12.5-25 µg q1-2wk; maintenance dose 75 µg qd

Suppression test

• *Adult:* **PO** 75-100 µg qd × 1 wk; radioactive ^{131}I is given before and after 1 wk dose

Available forms: Tabs 5, 25, 50 µg; inj 10 µg/ml

Side effects/adverse reactions:

CNS: Insomnia, tremors, headache, **thyroid storm**

CV: Tachycardia, palpitations, angina, dysrhythmias, hypertension, **cardiac arrest**

◆ = Nursing alert　　　🌿 = Herb-drug interaction　　　⊘ = Do not crush

GI: Nausea, diarrhea, increased or decreased appetite, cramps

MISC: Menstrual irregularities, weight loss, sweating, heat intolerance, fever

Contraindications: Adrenal insufficiency, myocardial infarction, thyrotoxicosis

Precautions: Elderly, angina pectoris, hypertension, ischemia, cardiac disease, pregnancy (A), lactation

Pharmacokinetics:

PO/IV: Peak 12-48 hr, duration 72 hr, half-life 6-7 days

Interactions:

• Decreased absorption of liothyronine: cholestyramine

• Increased effects of anticoagulants, sympathomimetics, tricyclic antidepressants

• Decreased effects of digitalis drugs, insulin, hypoglycemics

• Decreased effects of liothyronine: estrogens

⊘ Do not use with bugleweed

Lab test interferences:

Increase: CPK, LDH, AST, PBI, blood glucose

Decrease: TSH, ^{131}I uptake test, uric acid, triglycerides

NURSING CONSIDERATIONS

Assess:

• B/P, pulse, periodically during treatment

• Weight qd in same clothing, using same scale, at same time of day

• Height, growth rate of child

• T_3, T_4, which are decreased; radioimmunoassay of TSH, which is increased; radio uptake, which is increased if patient is on too low a dose of medication

• Pro-time may require decreased anticoagulant; check for bleeding, bruising

• Increased nervousness, excitability, irritability, which may indicate too high dose of medication, usually after 1-3 wk of treatment

• Cardiac status: angina, palpitation, chest pain, change in VS

Administer:

• In AM if possible as a single dose to decrease sleeplessness

• At same time each day to maintain drug level

• Only for hormone imbalances; not to be used for obesity, male infertility, menstrual conditions, lethargy

• Lowest dose that relieves symptoms

• Liothyronine after discontinuing other thyroid preparation

Perform/provide:

• Removal of medication 4 wk before RAIU test

Evaluate:

• Therapeutic response: absence of depression; increased weight loss, diuresis, pulse, appetite; absence of constipation, peripheral edema, cold intolerance; pale, cool, dry skin; brittle nails, alopecia, coarse hair, menorrhagia, night blindness, paresthesia, syncope, stupor, coma, rosy cheeks

Teach patient/family:

• That hair loss will occur in child but is temporary

• To report excitability, irritability, anxiety, which indicates overdose

• Not to switch brands unless approved by prescriber

• That hypothyroid child will show almost immediate behavior/personality change

• That drug is not to be taken to reduce weight

• To avoid OTC preparations with iodine; read labels

• To avoid iodine food, iodized salt, soybeans, tofu, turnips, some seafood, some bread

• That drug controls symptoms but does not cure; treatment is lifelong

liotrix (℞)

(lye'oh-trix)
Euthroid, Thyrolar, T₃/T₄
Func. class.: Thyroid hormone
Chem. class.: Levothyroxine/
liothyronine (synthetic T_4, T_3)

Action: Increases metabolic rates, cardiac output, O_2 consumption, body temp, blood volume, growth, development at cellular level

Uses: Hypothyroidism, thyroid hormone replacement

Dosage and routes:

• *Adult and child:* **PO** 15-30 mg qd, increased by 15-30 mg q1-2wk until desired response; may increase by 15-30 mg q2wk in child

• *Elderly:* **PO** 15 mg initially, increase q2-4wk by 15 mg until desired response

Available forms: Euthroid- ½, 1, 2, 3 gr; Thyrolar- ¼, ½, 1, 2, 3 gr; ½ gr = 30 mg

Side effects/adverse reactions:

CNS: Insomnia, tremors, headache, **thyroid storm**

CV: Tachycardia, palpitations, angina, dysrhythmias, hypertension, **cardiac arrest**

GI: Nausea, diarrhea, increased or decreased appetite, cramps

MISC: Menstrual irregularities, weight loss, sweating, heat intolerance, fever

Contraindications: Adrenal insufficiency, myocardial infarction, thyrotoxicosis

Precautions: Elderly, angina pectoris, hypertension, ischemia, cardiac disease, pregnancy (A), lactation

Pharmacokinetics:

PO (T_4): Onset unknown, peak 1-3 wk, duration 1-3 wk

PO (T_3): Onset unknown, peak 24-72 hr, duration 72 hr, half-life 1 wk

Interactions:

• Decreased absorption of liotrix: cholestyramine, colestipol

• Increased effects of anticoagulants, sympathomimetics, tricyclic antidepressants, catecholamines

• Decreased effects of digitalis, insulin, hypoglycemics

• Decreased effects of liotrix: estrogens

⌀ Do not use with bugleweed

Lab test interferences:

Increase: CPK, LDH, AST, PBI, blood glucose

Decrease: TSH, ^{131}I uptake test, uric acid, triglycerides

NURSING CONSIDERATIONS

Assess:

• B/P, pulse periodically during treatment

• Weight qd in same clothing, using same scale, at same time of day

• Height, growth rate of child

• T_3, T_4, FTIs, which are decreased; radioimmunoassay of TSH, which is increased; radio uptake, which is increased if patient is on too low a dose of medication

• Pro-time may require decreased anticoagulant; check for bleeding, bruising

• Increased nervousness, excitability, irritability, which may indicate too high dose of medication, usually after 1-3 wk of treatment

• Cardiac status: angina, palpitation, chest pain, change in VS

Administer:

• In AM if possible as a single dose to decrease sleeplessness

• At same time each day to maintain drug level

• Only for hormone imbalances; not to be used for obesity, male infertility, menstrual conditions, lethargy

• Lowest dose that relieves symptoms

 = Nursing alert   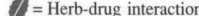 = Herb-drug interaction   ⃠ = Do not crush

Perform/provide:

• Withdrawal of medication 4 wk before RAIU test

• Storage in airtight, light-resistant container

Evaluate:

• Therapeutic response: absence of depression; increased weight loss, diuresis, pulse, appetite; absence of constipation, peripheral edema, cold intolerance; pale, cool, dry skin; brittle nails, coarse hair, menorrhagia, night blindness, paresthesias, syncope, stupor, coma, rosy cheeks

Teach patient/family:

• That hair loss will occur in child, is temporary

• To report excitability, irritability, anxiety, which indicate overdose

• Not to switch brands unless approved by prescriber

• That hypothyroid child will show almost immediate behavior/personality change

• That drug is not to be taken to reduce weight

• To avoid OTC preparations with iodine; read labels

• To avoid iodine food, iodized salt, soybeans, tofu, turnips, some seafood, some bread

• That drug does not cure, but controls symptoms, treatment is lifelong

---

lisinopril (℞)

(lyse-in'oh-pril)

Prinivil, Zestril

Func. class.: Antihypertensive, angiotensin converting enzyme inhibitor (ACE)

Chem. class.: Enalaprilat lysine analog

Action: Selectively suppresses renin-angiotensin-aldosterone system; inhibits ACE, preventing conversion of angiotensin I to angiotensin II

Uses: Mild to moderate hypertension, adjunctive therapy of systolic CHF

Dosage and routes:

Hypertension

• *Adult:* **PO** 10-40 mg qd; may increase to 80 mg qd if required

• *Geriatric:* **PO** 2.5-5 mg/day, increase q7 days

CHF

• *Adult:* **PO** 5 mg initially with diuretics/digitalis

Available forms: Tabs 2.5, 5, 10, 20, 40 mg

Side effects/adverse reactions:

GI: Nausea, vomiting, anorexia, constipation, flatulence, GI irritation

GU: **Proteinuria, renal insufficiency,** sexual dysfunction, impotence

HEMA: **Agranulocytopenia,** neutropenia

INTEG: Rash, pruritus

CNS: *Vertigo,* depression, **stroke,** insomnia, paresthesias, headache, *fatigue,* asthenia

EENT: Blurred vision, nasal congestion

SYST: **Angioedema**

RESP: Dry cough, dyspnea

Contraindications: Hypersensitivity, pregnancy (D) 2nd/3rd trimesters

Precautions: Pregnancy (C) 1st trimester, lactation, renal disease, hyperkalemia, renal artery stenosis

Pharmacokinetics: Onset 1 hr, peak 6-8 hr, duration 24 hr, excreted unchanged in urine

Interactions:

• Increased hypotensive effect: diuretics, other hypertensives, probenecid

• Decreased effects of lisinopril: aspirin, indomethacin

• Increased K levels: K salt substitutes, K-sparing diuretics, K supplements
• Increased effects of antihypertensives, reserpine, diuretics
• Increased hypersensitivity reactions: allopurinol
• Drug/food: high-potassium diet (bananas, orange juice, avocados, nuts, spinach) should be avoided; hyperkalemia may occur
Lab test interferences:
Interference: Glucose/insulin tolerance tests
NURSING CONSIDERATIONS
Assess:
• B/P, pulse q4h; note rate, rhythm, quality
• Electrolytes: K, Na, Cl
• Apical/pedal pulse before administration; notify prescriber of any significant changes
• Baselines in renal, liver function tests before therapy begins
• Edema in feet, legs qd
• Skin turgor, dryness of mucous membranes for hydration status
• Symptoms of CHF: edema, dyspnea, wet rales
Evaluate:
• Therapeutic response: decreased B/P, CHF symptoms
Teach patient/family:
• Not to discontinue drug abruptly
• To rise slowly to sitting or standing position to minimize orthostatic hypotension
• To avoid increasing K in the diet
Treatment of overdose: Lavage, IV atropine for bradycardia, IV theophylline for bronchospasm, digitalis, O_2, diuretic for cardiac failure

lithium (℞)
(li'thee-um)
Carbolith*, Cibalith-S, Duralith*, Eskalith, Eskalith-CR, Lithane, lithium carbonate, Lithizine*, Lithonate, Lithotabs
Func. class.: Antimanic
Chem. class.: Alkali metal ion salt

Action: May alter sodium, potassium ion transport across cell membrane in nerve, muscle cells; may balance biogenic amines of norepinephrine, serotonin in CNS areas involved in emotional responses
Uses: Manic-depressive illness (manic phase), prevention of bipolar manic-depressive psychosis
Dosage and routes:
• *Adult:* PO 300-600 mg tid, maintenance 300 mg tid or qid; slow rel tabs 300 mg bid; dose should be individualized to maintain blood levels at 0.5-1.5 mEq/L
• *Geriatric:* PO 300 mg bid, increase q7 days by 300 mg to desired dose
Renal dose
• **PO** CrCl 10-50 ml/min 50%-75% of dose; CrCl <10 ml/min 25%-50% of dose
• *Child:* **PO** 15-20 mg (0.4-0.5 mEq)/kg/day in 2-3 divided doses, increase as needed, do not exceed adult doses
Available forms: Caps 300, 600 mg; tabs 300 mg; tabs cont rel 450 mg; syr 300 mg/5 ml (8 mEq/5 ml); cap slow rel 300 mg*
Side effects/adverse reactions:
CNS: Headache, drowsiness, dizziness, tremors, twitching, ataxia, *seizure,* slurred speech, restlessness, confusion, stupor, memory loss, clonic movements, fatigue
GI: Dry mouth, anorexia, nausea,

vomiting, diarrhea, incontinence, abdominal pain, metallic taste
*GU: **Polyuria, glycosuria, proteinuria, albuminuria,*** urinary incontinence, polydipsia, edema
CV: Hypotension, ECG changes, ***dysrhythmias, circulatory collapse,*** edema
INTEG: Drying of hair, alopecia, rash, pruritus, hyperkeratosis, acneiform lesions, folliculitis
*HEMA: **Leukocytosis***
EENT: Tinnitus, blurred vision
ENDO: Hyponatremia, hypothyroidism, goiter, hyperglycemia, hyperthyroidism
MS: Muscle weakness
Contraindications: Hepatic disease, renal disease, brain trauma, OBS, pregnancy (D), lactation, children <12 yr, schizophrenia, severe cardiac disease, severe renal disease, severe dehydration
Precautions: Elderly, thyroid disease, seizure disorders, diabetes mellitus, systemic infection, urinary retention
Pharmacokinetics:
PO: Onset rapid, peak ½-4 hr, half-life 18-36 hr depending on age; crosses blood-brain barrier; 80% of filtered lithium is reabsorbed by the renal tubules, excreted in urine; crosses placenta; enters breast milk; well absorbed by oral method
Interactions:
• Increased hypothyroid effects: antithyroid agents, calcium iodide, potassium iodide, iodinated glycerol
• Neurotoxicity: haloperidol, thioridazine
• Increased effects of neuromuscular blocking agents, phenothiazines
• Increased renal clearance: sodium bicarbonate, acetazolamide, mannitol, aminophylline
• Increased toxicity: indomethacin, diuretics, nonsteroidal antiinflammatories, losartan

• Decreased effects of lithium: theophyllines, urea, urinary alkalinizers
• Increased lithium effect/toxicity: carbamazepine, fluoxetine, methyldopa, NSAIDs, thiazide diuretics, probenecid
• Drug/food: significant changes in sodium intake will alter lithium excretion
⚕ Increased effects of lithium, increased toxicity: broom, buchu, dandelion, juniper
Lab test interferences:
Increase: K excretion, urine glucose, blood glucose, protein, BUN
Decrease: VMA, T_3, T_4, PBI, ^{131}I
NURSING CONSIDERATIONS
Assess:
• Weight qd; check for and report edema in legs, ankles, wrists
• Na intake; decreased Na intake with decreased fluid intake may lead to lithium retention; increased Na and fluids may decrease lithium retention
• Skin turgor at least qd
• Urine for albuminuria, glycosuria, uric acid during beginning treatment, q2mo thereafter
• Neuro status: LOC, gait, motor reflexes, hand tremors
• Serum lithium levels qwk initially, then q2mo (therapeutic level: 0.5-1.5 mEq/L)
Administer:
• Reduced dose to elderly
• With meals to avoid GI upset
• Adequate fluids (2-3 L/day) to prevent dehydration during initial treatment, 1-2 L/day during maintenance
Evaluate:
• Therapeutic response: decrease in excitement, manic phase
Teach patient/family:
• The symptoms of minor toxicity: vomiting, diarrhea, poor coordination, fine motor tremors, weakness, lassitude; major toxicity: coarse

tremors, severe thirst, tinnitus, diluted urine

• To monitor urine specific gravity, emphasize need for follow-up care to determine lithium levels

• That contraception is necessary, since lithium may harm fetus

• Not to operate machinery until lithium levels are stable

• That beneficial effects may take 1-3 wk

• About drugs that interact with lithium (provide list) and discuss need for adequate stable intake of salt and fluids

🚫 Not to break, crush, or chew caps

Treatment of overdose: Induce emesis or lavage, maintain airway, respiratory function; dialysis for severe intoxication

---

lomefloxacin (℞)

(lo-meh-flox'a-sin)
Maxaquin
Func. class.: Antiinfective
Chem. class.: Fluoroquinolone

Action: Interferes with conversion of intermediate DNA fragments into high-molecular-weight DNA in bacteria; DNA gyrase inhibitor

Uses: Treatment of lower respiratory tract infections (pneumonia, bronchitis), genitourinary infections (prostatitis, UTIs), preoperatively to reduce UTIs in transurethral surgical procedures; gram-negative bacteria: *Aeromonas, Citrobacter, Enterobacter, Escherichia coli, Haemophilus influenzae, Klebsiella, Legionella, Moraxella catarrhalis, Morganella morganii, Proteus vulgaris, P. mirabilis, Providencia alcalifaciens, P. rettgeri, Pseudomonas aeruginosa, Serratia;* gram-positive bacteria: *Staphylococcus aureus, S. epidermidis, S. saprophyticus*

Dosage and routes:
• *Adult:* **PO** 400 mg/day × 7-14 days depending on type of infection
In renal impairment
• *Adult:* **PO** 200 mg/day
Surgical prophylaxis
• *Adult:* **PO** 400 mg 2-6 hr before surgery
Available forms: Tabs 400 mg
Side effects/adverse reactions:
CNS: Dizziness, headache, somnolence, depression, insomnia, nervousness, confusion, agitation
GI: Diarrhea, *nausea,* vomiting, anorexia, flatulence, heartburn, dry mouth; increased AST, ALT; constipation, abdominal pain, oral thrush, glossitis, stomatitis
INTEG: Rash, pruritus, urticaria, *photosensitivity*
EENT: Visual disturbances
Contraindications: Hypersensitivity to quinolones
Precautions: Pregnancy (C), lactation, children, elderly, renal disease, seizure disorders, excessive exposure to sunlight
Pharmacokinetics:
PO: Peak 1-2 hr, half-life 6-8 hr; excreted in urine as active drug, metabolites
Interactions:
• Decreased absorption: antacids, sucralfate, give 4 hr ac or 2 hr pc
• May increase CNS stimulation, seizures: NSAIDs
• May increase toxicity of lomefloxacin: cimetidine, probenecid
• Increased levels: cyclosporine, warfarin, watch for toxicity
NURSING CONSIDERATIONS
Assess:
• Kidney, liver function studies: BUN, creatinine, AST, ALT
• I&O ratio; urine pH, <5.5 is ideal
• CNS symptoms: insomnia, vertigo, headache, agitation, confusion

---

⬥ = Nursing alert   🖋 = Herb-drug interaction   🚫 = Do not crush

- Allergic reactions: rash, flushing, urticaria, pruritus

Administer:

- After clean-catch urine for C&S
- 2 hr before or 2 hrs after antacids, iron, calcium, zinc products

Evaluate:

- Therapeutic response: negative C&S, absence of signs/symptoms of infection

Teach patient/family:

- That fluids must be increased to 3 L/day to avoid crystallization in kidneys
- That if dizziness or light-headedness occurs, to ambulate, perform activities with assistance
- To complete full course of drug therapy
- To contact prescriber if adverse reactions occur
- To avoid iron- or mineral-containing supplements or antacids within 2 hr before and after dosing
- That photosensitivity may occur and sunscreen should be used

---

lomustine (℞)

(loe-mus′teen)
CCNU, CeeNU
Func. class.: Antineoplastic alkylating agent
Chem. class.: Nitrosourea

Action: Responsible for crosslinking DNA strands, which leads to cell death; activity is not cell cycle phase specific

Uses: Hodgkin's disease, lymphomas, melanomas, multiple myeloma; brain, lung, bladder, kidney, colon cancer

Investigational uses: Brain, breast, renal, GI tract, bronchogenic carcinoma; melanomas

Dosage and routes:

- *Adult:* **PO** 130 mg/m^2 as a single dose q6wk; titrate dose to WBC; do not give repeat dose unless WBC >4000/mm^3, platelet count >100,000/mm^3

Available forms: Caps 10, 40, 100 mg

Side effects/adverse reactions:

HEMA: ***Thrombocytopenia, leukopenia, myelosuppression, anemia***

GI: Nausea, vomiting, anorexia, stomatitis, ***hepatotoxicity***

GU: ***Azotemia, renal failure***

INTEG: Burning at injection site

RESP: ***Fibrosis, pulmonary infiltrate***

Contraindications: Hypersensitivity, leukopenia, thrombocytopenia, pregnancy (D)

Precautions: Radiation therapy

Pharmacokinetics: Metabolized in liver, excreted in urine; half-life 16-48 hr; 50% protein bound; crosses blood-brain barrier; appears in breast milk

Interactions:

- Increased toxicity: barbiturates, phenytoin, chloral hydrate
- Increased metabolism of lomustine: phenobarbital
- Potentiation of lomustine: succinylcholine
- Increased bone marrow depression: allopurinol

NURSING CONSIDERATIONS

Assess:

- CBC, differential, platelet count qwk; withhold drug if WBC <4000/mm^3 or platelet count <100,000/mm^3; notify prescriber
- Pulmonary function tests, chest x-ray films before, during therapy; chest film should be obtained q2wk during treatment
- Renal function studies: BUN, serum uric acid, urine CrCl before, during therapy
- I&O ratio; report fall in urine output of 30 ml/hr

• Monitor temp q4h (may indicate beginning infection); no rectal temps
• Liver function tests before, during therapy (bilirubin, AST, ALT, LDH) as needed or monthly
• Bleeding: hematuria, guaiac, bruising or petechiae, mucosa or orifices q8h
• Dyspnea, rales, unproductive cough, chest pain, tachypnea
• Food preferences; list likes, dislikes
• Jaundiced skin and sclera, dark urine, clay-colored stools, itchy skin, abdominal pain, fever, diarrhea
• Inflammation of mucosa, breaks in skin
• Buccal cavity q8h for dryness, sores or ulceration, white patches, oral pain, bleeding, dysphagia
• Local irritation, pain, burning, discoloration at injection site
◆ Symptoms indicating severe allergic reaction: rash, pruritus, urticaria, purpuric skin lesions, itching, flushing

Administer:
• Antiemetic 30-60 min before giving drug to prevent vomiting
• Antibiotics for prophylaxis of infection

Perform/provide:
• Storage in tight container at room temp
• Strict medical asepsis, protective isolation if WBC levels are low
• Deep-breathing exercises with patient tid-qid; place in semi-Fowler's position
• Increase fluid intake to 2-3 L/day to prevent urate deposits, calculi formation
• Rinsing of mouth tid-qid with water, club soda; brushing of teeth bid-tid with soft brush or cotton-tipped applicators for stomatitis; use unwaxed dental floss

Evaluate:
• Therapeutic response: decreased tumor size, spread of malignancy

Teach patient/family:
• About protective isolation
• To report any changes in breathing or coughing
• To avoid foods with citric acid, hot or rough texture if buccal inflammation is present
• To report any bleeding, white spots, or ulcerations in mouth to prescriber; tell patient to examine mouth qd
• To report signs of infection: fever, sore throat, flulike symptoms
• To report signs of anemia: fatigue, headache, faintness, shortness of breath, irritability
• To avoid use of razors, commercial mouthwash
• To avoid use of aspirin products or ibuprofen

---

loperamide (OTC, R)
(loe-per'a-mide)
A-D Kaopectate II Caplets, loperamide solution, Imodium, Imodium A-D, Imodium A-D Caplet, loperamide, Maalox Antidiarrheal Caplets, Pepto Diarrhea Control
Func. class.: Antidiarrheal
Chem. class.: Piperidine derivative

Action: Direct action on intestinal muscles to decrease GI peristalsis; reduces volume, increases bulk, electrolytes not lost
Uses: Diarrhea (cause undetermined), chronic diarrhea, ileostomy discharge
Dosage and routes:
• *Adult:* **PO** 4 mg, then 2 mg after each loose stool, not to exceed 16 mg/day
• *Child 2-5 yr:* **PO** 1 mg then 0.1 mg/kg after each loose stool

---

◆ = Nursing alert   🖋 = Herb-drug interaction   🚫 = Do not crush

• *Child 5-8 yr:* **PO** 2 mg bid on day 1, then 0.1 mg/kg after each loose stool

• *Child 8-12 yr:* **PO** 2 mg tid on day 1, then 0.1 mg/kg after each loose stool

Available forms: Caps 2 mg; liq 1 mg/5 ml; tabs 2 mg

Side effects/adverse reactions:

CNS: Dizziness, drowsiness, fatigue, fever

GI: Nausea, dry mouth, vomiting, constipation, abdominal pain, anorexia, ***toxic megacolon***

INTEG: Rash

Contraindications: Hypersensitivity, severe ulcerative colitis, pseudomembranous colitis, acute diarrhea associated with *E. coli*

Precautions: Pregnancy (B), lactation, children <2 yr, liver disease, dehydration, bacterial disease

Pharmacokinetics:

PO: Onset ½-1 hr, duration 4-5 hr, half-life 7-14 hr; metabolized in liver; excreted in feces as unchanged drug; small amount in urine

Interactions:

• Do not mix oral sol with other sols

NURSING CONSIDERATIONS

Assess:

• Stools: volume, color, characteristics

• Electrolytes (K, Na, Cl) if on long-term therapy

• Skin turgor q8h if dehydration is suspected

• Bowel pattern before; for rebound constipation

• Response after 48 hr; if no response, drug should be discontinued

• Dehydration in children

• Abdominal distention, toxic megacolon; may occur in ulcerative colitis

Administer:

• For 48 hr only

Perform/provide:

• Storage in tight container

Evaluate:

• Therapeutic response: decreased diarrhea

Teach patient/family:

• To avoid OTC products unless directed by prescriber

• That ostomy patient may take this drug for extended time

• That if drowsiness occurs, not to operate machinery

• To use hard candy, sips of water for dry mouth

🚫 Not to break, crush, or chew caps

---

loracarbef
See cephalosporins—2nd generation

---

loratadine (℞)

(lor-a′ti-deen)

Claritin, Claritin Reditabs

Func. class.: Antihistamine, 2nd generation

Chem. class.: Selective histamine (H₁)-receptor antagonist

Action: Binds to peripheral histamine receptors, providing antihistamine action without sedation

Uses: Seasonal rhinitis

Dosage and routes:

• *Adult and child ≥12 yr:* **PO** 10 mg qd

• *Child 6-12 yr:* **PO** 10 mg (10 ml) qd

Available forms: Tabs 10 mg; tabs rapid-disintegrating 10 mg; syr 5 mg/5 ml

Side effects/adverse reactions:

CNS: Sedation (more common with increased doses), headache

Contraindications: Hypersensitivity, acute asthma attacks, lower respiratory tract disease

---

Precautions: Pregnancy (B), increased intraocular pressure, bronchial asthma

Pharmacokinetics: Peak 1½ hr, elimination half-life 8½-28 hr; metabolized in liver to active metabolites, excreted in urine

Interactions:

• Additive CNS depressant effects: alcohol, other CNS depressants

• Increased CV effects: azole antifungals, macrolide antibiotics

• Increased loratadine levels: cimetidine

• Increased anticholinergic/sedative effects: MAOIs

*Increased anticholinergic effect: henbane leaf

NURSING CONSIDERATIONS
Administer:

• Rapid-disintegrating tabs by placing on tongue, then swallow after disintegrated with or without water

• On empty stomach

Perform/provide:

• Storage in tight container at room temp

Evaluate:

• Therapeutic response: absence of running or congested nose

Teach patient/family:

• To avoid driving, other hazardous activities if drowsiness occurs

---

lorazepam (Ŗ)

(lor-a'ze-pam)
Alzapam, Apo-Lorazepam*,
Ativan, Loraz, lorazepam,
Novolorazem*

Func. class.: Sedative, hypnotic;
antianxiety

Chem. class.: Benzodiazepine

Controlled Substance Schedule IV
Action: Potentiates the actions of GABA, especially in system and reticular formation

Uses: Anxiety, irritability in psychiatric or organic disorders, preoperatively, insomnia, adjunct in endoscopic procedures

Investigational uses: Antiemetic prior to chemotherapy, status epilepticus

Dosage and routes:

Anxiety

• *Adult:* **PO** 2-6 mg/day in divided doses, not to exceed 10 mg/day

• *Geriatric:* **PO** 0.5-1 mg/day in divided doses; or 0.5-1 mg hs

• *Child:* **PO** 0.05 mg/kg/dose, q4-8h

Insomnia

• *Adult:* **PO** 2-4 mg hs; only minimally effective after 2 wk continuous therapy

Preoperatively

• *Adult:* **IM** 50 µg/kg 2 hr prior to surgery; **IV** 44 µg/kg 15-20 min prior to surgery

• *Child:* 0.05 mg/kg

Status epilepticus

• *Neonate:* 0.05 mg/kg

• *Child:* 0.1 mg/kg up to 4 mg/dose

Available forms: Tabs 0.5, 1, 2 mg; inj 2, 4 mg/ml; conc sol 2 mg/ml

Side effects/adverse reactions:

CNS: Dizziness, drowsiness, confusion, headache, anxiety, tremors, stimulation, fatigue, depression, insomnia, hallucinations, weakness, unsteadiness

GI: Constipation, dry mouth, nausea, vomiting, anorexia, diarrhea

INTEG: Rash, dermatitis, itching

CV: Orthostatic hypotension, **ECG changes, tachycardia,** hypotension

EENT: Blurred vision, tinnitus, mydriasis

Contraindications: Hypersensitivity to benzodiazepines, narrow-angle glaucoma, psychosis, pregnancy (D), lactation, child <12 yr, history of drug abuse, COPD

Precautions: Elderly, debilitated, hepatic disease, renal disease

---

◆ = Nursing alert   *= Herb-drug interaction   Ⓝ = Do not crush

Pharmacokinetics:
PO: Onset ½ hr, peak 1-6 hr, duration 24-48 hr
IM: Onset 15-30 min, peak 1-1½ hr, duration 24-48 hr
IV: Onset 5-15 min, peak unknown, duration 24-48 hr
Metabolized by liver; excreted by kidneys; crosses placenta, breast milk; half-life 14 hr

Interactions:
• Decreased effects of lorazepam: oral contraceptives, valproic acid
• Increased effects of lorazepam: CNS depressants, alcohol, disulfiram, oral contraceptives
Increased action: kava

Lab test interferences:
Increase: AST, ALT, serum bilirubin
Decrease: RAIU
False increase: 17-OHCS

NURSING CONSIDERATIONS
Assess:
• B/P (lying, standing), pulse; if systolic B/P drops 20 mm Hg, hold drug, notify prescriber; respirations q5-15min if given IV
• Blood studies: CBC during long-term therapy; blood dyscrasias have occurred rarely
• Hepatic studies: AST, ALT, bilirubin, creatinine, LDH, alk phosphatase
• Mental status: mood, sensorium, affect, sleeping pattern, drowsiness, dizziness
• Physical dependency, withdrawal symptoms: headache, nausea, vomiting, muscle pain, weakness, tremors, convulsions, after long-term, excessive use
◆ Suicidal tendencies

Administer:
• With food or milk for GI symptoms
• Crushed if patient is unable to swallow medication whole

• Sugarless gum, hard candy, frequent sips of water for dry mouth
• Deep into large muscle mass (IM inj)
IV
• IV after diluting in equal vol sterile H_2O, 5% dextrose or 0.9% NaCl for inj; give through Y-tube or 3-way stopcock; give at 2 mg or less over 1 min

Syringe compatibilities: Cimetidine, hydromorphone
Y-site compatibilities: Acyclovir, albumin, allopurinol, amifostine, amikacin, amoxicillin, amoxicillin/clavulanate, amphotericin B cholesteryl, amsacrine, atracurium, bumetanide, cefepime, cefmetazole, cefotaxime, ciprofloxacin, cisatracurium, cisplatin, cladribine, clonidine, cyclophosphamide, cytarabine, dexamethasone, diltiazem, dobutamine, dopamine, doxorubicin, doxorubicin liposome, epinephrine, erythromycin, etomidate, famotidine, fentanyl, filgrastim, fluconazole, fludarabine, furosemide, gentamicin, granisetron, haloperidol, heparin, hydrocortisone, hydromorphone, ketanserin, labetalol, melphalan, methotrexate, metronidazole, midazolam, milrinone, morphine, nicardipine, nitroglycerin, norepinephrine, paclitaxel, pancuronium, piperacillin, piperacillin/tazobactam, potassium chloride, propofol, ranitidine, remifentanil, tacrolimus, teniposide, thiotepa, trimethoprim-sulfamethoxazole, vancomycin, vecuronium, vinorelbine, zidovudine

Perform/provide:
• Assistance with ambulation during beginning therapy, since drowsiness/dizziness occurs
• Check to see if PO medication has been swallowed
• Refrigerate parenteral form

Evaluate:

• Therapeutic response: decreased anxiety, restlessness, insomnia

Teach patient/family:

• That drug may be taken with food

• Not to use drug for everyday stress or used longer than 4 mo unless directed by prescriber

• Not to take more than prescribed amount; may be habit forming

• To avoid OTC preparations (cough, cold, hay fever) unless approved by prescriber

• To avoid driving, activities that require alertness, since drowsiness may occur

• To avoid alcohol ingestion, other psychotropic medications, unless directed by prescriber

• Not to discontinue medication abruptly after long-term use

• To rise slowly or fainting may occur, especially elderly

• That drowsiness may worsen at beginning of treatment

• To use birth control if child-bearing age

Treatment of overdose: Lavage, VS, supportive care, flumazenil

---

losartan (R)

(lo-zar′tan)

Cozaar

Func. class.: Antihypertensive

Chem. class.: Angiotensin II receptor (Type AT_1)

Action: Blocks the vasoconstrictor and aldosterone-secreting effects of angiotensin II; selectively blocks the binding of angiotensin II to the AT_1 receptor found in tissues

Uses: Hypertension, alone or in combination

Dosage and routes:

• *Adult:* **PO** 50 mg qd alone or 25 mg qd when used in combination

Hepatic dose

25 mg qd

Available forms: Tabs 25, 50 mg

Side effects/adverse reactions:

CNS: Dizziness, insomnia, anxiety, confusion, abnormal dreams, migraine, tremor, vertigo, task perversion

CV: Angina pectoris, 2nd-degree AV block, *cerebrovascular accident,* hypotension, *myocardial infarction, dysrhythmias*

EENT: Blurred vision, burning eyes, conjunctivitis

GI: Diarrhea, dyspepsia, anorexia, constipation, dry mouth, flatulence, gastritis, vomiting

GU: Impotence, nocturia, urinary frequency, UTI

HEMA: Anemia

INTEG: Alopecia, dermatitis, dry skin, flushing, photosensitivity, rash, pruritus, sweating

META: Gout

MS: Cramps, myalgia, pain, stiffness

RESP: Cough, upper respiratory infection, congestion, dyspnea, bronchitis

Contraindications: Hypersensitivity, pregnancy (D) 2nd and 3rd trimesters

Precautions: Hypersensitivity to ACE inhibitors; Pregnancy (C) 1st trimester; lactation, children, elderly

Pharmacokinetics: Extensively metabolized, half-life 2 hr, metabolite 6-9 hr, highly bound to plasma proteins, excreted in urine and feces

Interactions:

• Increased lithium toxicity: lithium

NURSING CONSIDERATIONS

Assess:

• B/P, pulse q4h; note rate, rhythm, quality

• Electrolytes: K, Na, Cl

• Baselines in renal, liver function tests before therapy begins

---

- Edema in feet, legs qd
- Skin turgor, dryness of mucous membranes for hydration status

Administer:
- Without regard to meals

Evaluate:
- Therapeutic response: decreased B/P

Teach patient/family:
- To avoid sunlight or wear sunscreen if in sunlight; photosensitivity may occur
- To comply with dosage schedule, even if feeling better
- To notify prescriber of mouth sores, fever, swelling of hands or feet, irregular heartbeat, chest pain
- That excessive perspiration, dehydration, vomiting, diarrhea may lead to fall in blood pressure; consult prescriber if these occur
- That drug may cause dizziness, fainting; light-headedness may occur
- To rise slowly to sitting or standing position to minimize orthostatic hypotension

---

lovastatin (Ŗ)
(loh-vah-stat'in)
Mevacor
Func. class.: Antilipemic
Chem. class.: Aspergillus terreus strain derivative

Action: Inhibits HMG-CoA reductase enzyme, which reduces cholesterol synthesis

Uses: As an adjunct in primary hypercholesterolemia (types IIa, IIb), mixed hyperlipidemia, atherosclerosis

Dosage and routes:
(Patient should first be placed on a cholesterol–lowering diet)
- *Adult:* **PO** 20 mg qd with evening meal; may increase to 20-80 mg/day in single or divided doses, not to exceed 80 mg/day; dosage adjustments should be made qmo, reduce dose in renal disease

Available forms: Tabs 10, 20, 40 mg

Side effects/adverse reactions:
*GI: Flatus, nausea, constipation, diarrhea, dyspepsia, abdominal pain, heartburn, **liver dysfunction***
*MS: Muscle cramps, myalgia, **myositis, rhabdomyolysis***
CNS: Dizziness, headache, tremor
INTEG: Rash, pruritus, photosensitivity
*HEMA: **Thrombocytopenia, hemolytic anemia, leukopenia***
EENT: Blurred vision, dysgeusia, lens opacities

Contraindications: Hypersensitivity, pregnancy (X), lactation, active liver disease

Precautions: Past liver disease, alcoholism, severe acute infections, trauma, hypotension, uncontrolled seizure disorders, severe metabolic disorders, electrolyte imbalances, visual disorder, children

Pharmacokinetics:
PO: Peak 2-4 hr, metabolized in liver (metabolites), highly protein bound; excreted in urine, feces; crosses placenta, excreted in breast milk; half-life 3-4 hr

Interactions:
- Increased effects: bile acid sequestrants, warfarin
- Increased myalgia, myositis: cyclosporine, gemfibrozil, niacin
- Decreased antihyperlipidemic effect: propranolol
- Increased bleeding: warfarin
- Drug/food: increased levels of lovastatin with food

Lab test interferences:
Increase: CPK, liver function tests

NURSING CONSIDERATIONS
Assess:
- Fasting cholesterol, LDL, HDL,

triglycerides periodically during treatment

• Liver function studies q1-2mo during the first 1½ yr of treatment; AST, ALT, liver function tests may increase

• Renal function in patients with compromised renal system: BUN, creatinine, I&O ratio

• Eyes with slit lamp before, 1 mo after treatment begins, annually; lens opacities may occur

Administer:

• In evening with meal; if dose is increased, take with breakfast and evening meal

Perform/provide:

• Storage in cool environment in airtight, light-resistant container

Evaluate:

• Therapeutic response: cholesterol at desired level after 8 wk

Teach patient/family:

• To report suspected pregnancy

• That blood work and eye exam will be necessary during treatment

• To report blurred vision, severe GI symptoms, dizziness, headache, muscle pain, weakness

• That previously prescribed regimen will continue: low-cholesterol diet, exercise program

---

loxapine (℞)

(lox'a-peen)
Loxapac*, loxapine succinate*, Loxitane, Loxitane IM, Loxitane-C

Func. class.: Antipsychotic, neuroleptic

Chem. class.: Dibenzoxazepine

Action: Depresses cerebral cortex, hypothalamus, limbic system, which control activity and aggression; blocks neurotransmission produced by dopamine at synapse; exhibits strong α-adrenergic, anticholinergic blocking action; mechanism for antipsychotic effects is unclear

Uses: Psychotic disorders, nonpsychotic symptoms associated with dementia

Investigational uses: Depression, anxiety

Dosage and routes:

• *Adult:* **PO** 10 mg bid-qid initially, may be rapidly increased depending on severity of condition, maintenance 60-100 mg/day; **IM** 12.5-50 mg q4-6h or more until desired response, then start **PO** form

• *Geriatric:* **PO** 5-10 mg qd-bid, increase q4-7 days by 5-10 mg, max 125 mg

Available forms: Caps 5, 10, 25, 50 mg; conc 25 mg/ml; inj 50 mg/ml

Side effects/adverse reactions:

RESP: **Laryngospasm,** dyspnea, **respiratory depression**

CNS: EPS: pseudoparkinsonism, akathisia, dystonia, tardive dyskinesia, drowsiness, headache, seizures, confusion

HEMA: **Anemia, leukopenia, leukocytosis, agranulocytosis**

INTEG: Rash, photosensitivity, dermatitis

EENT: Blurred vision, glaucoma

GI: Dry mouth, nausea, vomiting, anorexia, constipation, diarrhea, jaundice, weight gain

GU: Urinary retention, urinary frequency, enuresis, impotence, amenorrhea, gynecomastia

CV: Orthostatic hypotension, **cardiac arrest,** ECG changes, tachycardia

Contraindications: Hypersensitivity, blood dyscrasias, coma, brain damage, bone marrow depression, alcohol and barbiturate withdrawal states

Precautions: Pregnancy (C), lactation, seizure disorders, hepatic disease, cardiac disease, prostatic hy-

---

◆ = Nursing alert   🖋 = Herb-drug interaction   🚫 = Do not crush

pertrophy, cardiac conditions, child <16 yr, elderly

Pharmacokinetics:

PO: Onset 20-30 min, peak 2-4 hr, duration 12 hr

IM: Onset 15-30 min, peak 15-20 min, duration 12 hr

Metabolized by liver; excreted in urine; crosses placenta; enters breast milk; initial half-life 5 hr; terminal half-life 19 hr

Interactions:

• Toxicity: epinephrine

• Increased EPS: other antipsychotics

• Decreased effects: guanadrel, guanethidine

• Increased CNS depression: MAOIs, antidepressants

⚕ Increased action: kava

NURSING CONSIDERATIONS

Assess:

• Mental status before initial administration

• Swallowing of PO medication; check for hoarding or giving of medication to other patients

• I&O ratio; palpate bladder if low urinary output occurs

• Bilirubin, CBC, liver function studies qmo

• Urinalysis is recommended before and during prolonged therapy

• Affect, orientation, LOC, reflexes, gait, coordination, sleep pattern disturbances

• B/P standing and lying; take pulse and respirations q4h during initial treatment; establish baseline before starting treatment; report drops of 30 mm Hg

• Dizziness, faintness, palpitations, tachycardia on rising

• EPS including akathisia (inability to sit still, no pattern to movements), tardive dyskinesia (bizarre movements of the jaw, mouth, tongue,

extremities), pseudoparkinsonism (rigidity, tremors, pill rolling, shuffling gait)

◆ For neuroleptic malignant syndrome: muscle rigidity, increased CPK, altered mental status, hyperthermia

• Constipation, urinary retention qd; if these occur, increase bulk, water in diet

Administer:

• Reduced dose to elderly

• Antiparkinsonian agent if EPS symptoms occur

IM

• IM injection into large muscle mass

PO

• Concentrate mixed in orange or grapefruit juice

Perform/provide:

• Decreased sensory input by dimming lights, avoiding loud noises

• Supervised ambulation until stabilized on medication; do not involve in strenuous exercise program because fainting is possible; patient should not stand still for long periods

• Increased fluids to prevent constipation

• Sips of water, candy, gum for dry mouth

• Storage in airtight, light-resistant container

Evaluate:

• Therapeutic response: decrease in emotional excitement, hallucinations, delusions, paranoia; reorganization of patterns of thought, speech

Teach patient/family:

• That orthostatic hypotension may occur and to rise from sitting or lying position gradually

• To remain lying down after IM injection for at least 30 min

• To avoid hot tubs, hot showers, tub baths, as hypotension may oc-

L

Side effects: *italics* = common; ***bold italics*** = life-threatening

cur; that in hot weather heat stroke may occur; take extra precautions to stay cool

• To avoid abrupt withdrawal of this drug, or EPS may result; drug should be withdrawn slowly

• To avoid OTC preparations (cough, hay fever, cold) unless approved by prescriber; serious drug interactions may occur; avoid use with alcohol, CNS depressants; increased drowsiness may occur

• To avoid hazardous activities until stabilized on medication

• To use a sunscreen during sun exposure to prevent burns

• About necessity for meticulous oral hygiene, since oral candidiasis may occur

• To report impaired vision, jaundice, tremors, muscle twitching

Treatment of overdose: Lavage if orally ingested; provide an airway

lymphocyte immune globulin (antithymocyte)

See appendix a—selected new drugs

magaldrate (OTC)

(mag′al-drate)
Losapan*, Lowsium, Riopan, Riopan Extra Strength*
Func. class.: Antacid
Chem. class.: Aluminum/magnesium hydroxide

Action: Neutralizes gastric acidity; drug is dissolved in gastric contents; combination of aluminum, magnesium

Uses: Antacid, peptic ulcer disease (adjunct), duodenal, gastric ulcers, reflux esophagitis, hyperacidity, indigestion, heartburn

Dosage and routes:
• *Adult:* **SUSP** 5-10 ml (400-800 mg) with H_2O between meals, hs, not to exceed 100 ml/day
Available forms: Susp 540 mg/5 ml, liquid 540 mg/5 ml
Side effects/adverse reactions:
GI: Constipation, diarrhea
META: Hypermagnesemia, hypophosphatemia
Contraindications: Hypersensitivity to this drug or aluminum
Precautions: Elderly, fluid restriction, decreased GI motility, GI obstruction, dehydration, renal disease, Na-restricted diets, pregnancy (C)
Pharmacokinetics:
PO: Duration 60 min
Interactions:
• Decreased effectiveness of tetracyclines, ketoconazole
• Decreased absorption of anticholinergics, chlordiazepoxide, cimetidine, corticosteroids, iron salts, phenothiazines, phenytoin, salicylates
NURSING CONSIDERATIONS
Assess:
• GI status: location of pain, intensity, characteristics, heartburn, hematemesis
• Serum Mg^{++} levels with impaired renal function
• Constipation: increase bulk in diet if needed
Administer:
• Laxatives or stool softeners if constipation occurs
• After shaking; give between meals and hs
Evaluate:
• Therapeutic response: absence of pain, decreased acidity
Teach patient/family:
• To separate enteric-coated drugs and antacid by 2 hr
• To notify prescriber immediately of coffee-ground emesis, emesis with frank blood, black tarry stools

---

◆ = Nursing alert   ✏ = Herb-drug interaction   ⊘ = Do not crush

magnesium salicylate (OTC, R)
Doan's pills, Magan, Mobidin
Func. class.: Nonnarcotic analgesic
Chem. class.: Salicylate

Action: Blocks pain impulses in CNS that occur in response to inhibition of prostaglandin synthesis; antipyretic action results from inhibition of hypothalamic heat-regulating center to produce vasodilation to allow heat dissipation

Uses: Mild to moderate pain or fever including arthritis, juvenile rheumatoid arthritis

Dosage and routes:
Arthritis
• *Adult:* PO not to exceed 4.8 g/day in divided doses
Pain/fever
• *Adult:* PO 600 mg tid or qid
Available forms: Tabs 325, 545, 600 mg

Side effects/adverse reactions:
*HEMA: **Thrombocytopenia, agranulocytosis, leukopenia, neutropenia, hemolytic anemia,*** increased pro-time
CNS: Stimulation, drowsiness, dizziness, confusion, ***convulsion,*** headache, flushing, hallucinations, ***coma***
*GI: Nausea, vomiting, **GI bleeding,** diarrhea, heartburn,* anorexia, ***hepatitis***
INTEG: Rash, urticaria, bruising
EENT: Tinnitus, hearing loss
CV: Rapid pulse, ***pulmonary edema***
RESP: Wheezing, hyperpnea
ENDO: Hypoglycemia, hyponatremia, hypokalemia

Contraindications: Hypersensitivity to salicylates, GI bleeding, bleeding disorders, children <12 yr, vit K deficiency

Precautions: Anemia, hepatic disease, renal disease, Hodgkin's disease, pregnancy (C), lactation

Pharmacokinetics:
PO: Onset 15-30 min, peak 1-2 hr, duration 4-6 hr; metabolized by liver; excreted by kidneys; crosses placenta; excreted in breast milk; half-life 1-3½ hr

Interactions:
• Decreased effects of magnesium-salicylate: antacids, steroids, urinary alkalizers
• Increased blood loss: alcohol, heparin
• Increased effects of anticoagulants, insulin, methotrexate
• Decreased effects of probenecid, spironolactone, sulfinpyrazone, sulfonylamides
• Toxic effects: PABA
• Decreased blood sugar levels: salicylates

Lab test interferences:
Increase: Coagulation studies, liver function studies, serum uric acid, amylase, CO_2, urinary protein
Decrease: Serum K, cholesterol, blood glucose
Interference: Urine catecholamines, pregnancy test

NURSING CONSIDERATIONS
Assess:
• Liver function studies: AST, ALT, bilirubin, creatinine (long-term therapy)
• Renal function studies: BUN, urine creatinine (long-term therapy)
• Blood studies: CBC, Hct, Hgb, pro-time (long-term therapy)
• I&O ratio; decreasing output may indicate renal failure (long-term therapy)
◆ Hepatotoxicity: dark urine, clay-colored stools, jaundiced skin and sclera, itching, abdominal pain, fever, diarrhea (long-term therapy)
• Allergic reactions: rash, urticaria;

M

if these occur, drug may have to be discontinued

• Renal dysfunction: decreased urine output

• Ototoxicity: tinnitus, ringing, roaring in ears; audiometric testing is needed before, after long-term therapy

• Visual changes: blurring, halos, corneal and retinal damage

• Edema in feet, ankles, legs

• Prior drug history; there are many drug interactions

Administer:

• To patient crushed or whole; chewable tablets may be chewed

• With food or milk to decrease gastric symptoms; give 30 min before or 2 hr after antacids

• With full glass of water

Evaluate:

• Therapeutic response: decreased pain, fever

Teach patient/family:

• To report any symptoms of hepatotoxicity, renal toxicity, visual changes, ototoxicity, allergic reactions, bleeding (long-term therapy)

• Not to exceed recommended dosage; acute poisoning may result

• To read label on other OTC drugs; many contain aspirin

• That therapeutic response takes 2 wk (arthritis)

• To avoid alcohol ingestion; GI bleeding may occur

• That if anticoagulants are given with this drug, both should be discontinued 2 wk before surgery

Treatment of overdose: Lavage, activated charcoal, monitor electrolytes, VS

---

magnesium salts (OTC)
(mag-nee'zee-um)
magnesium chloride, Chloromag, Slo-Mag
magnesium citrate (OTC)
citrate of magnesia, Citroma, CitroMag*, Evac-Q-Mag
magnesium hydroxide (OTC)
Phillips Magnesium Tablets, Phillips' Milk of Magnesia, MOM
magnesium oxide (OTC)
Mag-Ox 400, Maox, Uro-Mag
magnesium sulfate (OTC)
epsom salts
Func. class.: Electrolyte; anticonvulsant; laxative, saline; antacid

---

Action: Increases osmotic pressure, draws fluid into colon, neutralizes HCl

Uses: Constipation, bowel preparation before surgery or exam

Dosage and routes:

Laxative

• *Adult:* **PO** 30-60 ml hs (Milk of Magnesia), 300 mg

• *Adult and child >6 yr:* **PO** 15 g in 8 oz H_2O (magnesium sulfate); **PO** 10-20 ml (Concentrated Milk of Magnesia); **PO** 5-10 oz hs (magnesium citrate)

• *Child 2-6 yr:* 5-15 ml (Milk of Magnesia)

Prevention of magnesium deficiency

• *Adult and child ≥10 yr:* **PO** male: 270-400 mg/day; female: 280-300 mg/day; lactation: 335-350 mg/day; pregnancy 320 mg/day

• *Child 8-10 yr:* **PO** 170 mg/day

• *Child 4-7 yr:* **PO** 120 mg/day
• *Child infant to 4 yr:* 40-80 mg/day
Deficiency
• *Adult:* **PO** 200-400 mg in divided doses tid-qid; **IM** 1 g q6h × 4 doses; **IV** 5 g (severe)
• *Child 6-12 yr:* 3-6 mg/kg/day in divided doses tid-qid
Pre-eclampsia/eclampsia
magnesium sulfate
• *Adult:* **IM/IV** 4-5 g **IV inf;** with 5 g **IM** in each gluteus, then 5 g q4h or 4 g **IV inf,** then 1-2 g/hr **cont inf**
Available forms:
• Chloride: sus rel tabs 535 mg (64 mg Mg) enteric tabs 833 mg (100 mg Mg); inj 200 mg/ml citrate; 240, 296, 300 ml/bottle (77 mEq Mg/ 100 ml)
• Hydroxide: 400 mg/5 ml; conc liquid 800 mg/5 ml, 600 mg (260 Mg)
• Oxide: Tabs 400 mg; caps 140 mg
• Sulfate: Powder for oral; bulk packages; epsom salts, bulk packages; inj 10%, 12.5%, 25%, 50%
Side effects/adverse reactions:
CNS: Muscle weakness, flushing, sweating, confusion, sedation, depressed reflexes, *flaccidity, paralysis,* hypothermia
GI: Nausea, vomiting, anorexia, cramps
CV: Hypotension, heart block, *circulatory collapse*
META: Electrolyte, fluid imbalances
Contraindications: Hypersensitivity, renal diseases, abdominal pain, nausea/vomiting, obstruction, acute surgical abdomen, rectal bleeding
Precautions: Pregnancy (A)
Pharmacokinetics:
PO: Onset 3-6 hr
IM: Onset 1 hr, duration 4 hr
IV: Duration ½ hr
Interactions:
• Increased effect of neuromuscular blockers

• Decreased absorption of tetracyclines, other antiinfectives, nitrofurantoin

NURSING CONSIDERATIONS
Assess:
• I&O ratio; check for decrease in urinary output
• Cause of constipation; lack of fluids, bulk, exercise
• Cramping, rectal bleeding, nausea, vomiting; drug should be discontinued
⬥ Mg toxicity: thirst, confusion, decrease in reflexes
Administer:
• With 8 oz H_2O
IV
• Only when calcium gluconate available for magnesium toxicity
• IV undiluted 1.5 ml of 10% sol over 1 min; may dilute to 20% sol, infuse over 3 hr
• IV at less than 150 mg/min; circulatory collapse may occur
Additive compatibilities: Calcium gluconate, cephalothin, chloramphenicol, cisplatin, heparin, hydrocortisone, isoproterenol, meropenem, methyldopa, norepinephrine, penicillin G potassium, potassium phosphate, verapamil
Y-site compatibilities: Acyclovir, aldesleukin, amifostine, amikacin, ampicillin, aztreonam, cefamandole, cefazolin, cefmetazole, cefoperazone, cefotaxime, cefoxitin, cephalothin, cephapirin, chloramphenicol, cisatracurium, clindamycin, dobutamine, doxycycline, doxorubicin liposome, enalaprilat, erythromycin, esmolol, famotidine, fludarabine, gallium, gentamicin, granisetron, heparin, hydrocortisone, hydromorphone, idarubicin, insulin, kanamycin, labetalol, meperidine, metronidazole, minocycline, morphine, moxalactam, nafcillin, ondansetron, oxacillin, paclitaxel, pen-

M

icillin G potassium, piperacillin, piperacillin/tazobactam, potassium chloride, propofol, remifentanil, sargramostim, thiotepa, ticarcillin, tobramycin, trimethoprim-sulfamethoxazole, vancomycin, vit B complex/C

Evaluate:
• Therapeutic response: decreased constipation

Teach patient/family:
• Not to use laxatives for long-term therapy; bowel tone will be lost
• That chilling helps the taste of magnesium citrate
• To shake suspension well
• To not give at hs as a laxative; may interfere with sleep
• To give citrus fruit after administering to counteract unpleasant taste

---

mannitol (R)
(man'i-tole)
mannitol, Osmitrol, Resectial
Func. class.: Osmotic diuretic
Chem. class.: Hexahydric alcohol

Action: Acts by increasing osmolarity of glomerular filtrate, which raises osmotic pressure of fluid in renal tubules; decrease in reabsorption of water, electrolytes; increase in urinary output, sodium, chloride excretion

Uses: Edema, promote systemic diuresis in cerebral edema, decrease intraocular pressure, improve renal function in acute renal failure, chemical poisoning

Dosage and routes:
Oliguria, prevention
• *Adult:* IV 50-100 g 5%-25% sol
Oliguria, treatment
• *Adult:* IV 300-400 mg/kg 20%-25% sol up to 100 g 15%-20% sol

• *Child:* IV 0.25-2 g/kg as 15%-20% sol run over 2-6 hr
Intraocular pressure/intracranial pressure
• *Adult:* IV 1½-2 g/kg 15%-25% sol over ½-1 hr
• *Child:* IV 1-2 g/kg (30-60 g/m²) as 15%-20% sol run over ½-1 hr
Renal failure
• *Adult:* IV 50-200 g/24 hr, adjusted to maintain output of 30-50 mg/hr
Diuresis in drug intoxication
• *Adult and child >12 yr:* 5%-10% sol continuously up to 200 g IV, while maintaining 100-500 ml urine output/hr
Available forms: Inj 5%, 10%, 15%, 20%; irrigation: 5%

Side effects/adverse reactions:
GU: Marked diuresis, urinary retention, thirst
CNS: Dizziness, headache, ***convulsions, rebound increased ICP,*** confusion
GI: Nausea, vomiting, dry mouth, diarrhea
CV: Edema, thrombophlebitis, hypotension, hypertension, ***tachycardia,*** angina-like chest pains, fever, chills
RESP: Pulmonary congestion
ELECT: Fluid, electrolyte imbalances, *acidosis,* electrolyte loss, dehydration
EENT: Loss of hearing, blurred vision, nasal congestion, decreased intraocular pressure

Contraindications: Active intracranial bleeding, hypersensitivity, anuria, severe pulmonary congestion, edema, severe dehydration, progressive heart, renal failure

Precautions: Dehydration, pregnancy (C), severe renal disease, CHF, lactation

Pharmacokinetics:
IV: Onset 30-60 min for diuresis, ½-1 hr for intraocular pressure, 25

◆ = Nursing alert   ⫽ = Herb-drug interaction   ⊘ = Do not crush

min for cerebrospinal fluid; duration 4-6 hr for intraocular pressure, 3-8 hr for cerebrospinal fluid; excreted in urine, half-life 100 min

Interactions:
• Decreased effect: lithium
• Increased effects of EDTA
• Drug/food: potassium foods: increased hyperkalemia

Lab test interferences:
Interference: Inorganic phosphorus, ethylene glycol

NURSING CONSIDERATIONS
Assess:
• Weight, I&O qd to determine fluid loss; effect of drug may be decreased if used qd; output qh prn
• Rate, depth, rhythm of respiration, effect of exertion
• B/P lying, standing; postural hypotension may occur
• Electrolytes: K, Na, Cl; include BUN, CBC, serum creatinine, blood pH, ABGs, CVP, PAP
• Signs of metabolic acidosis: drowsiness, restlessness
• Signs of hypokalemia: postural hypotension, malaise, fatigue, tachycardia, leg cramps, weakness
• Rashes, temp qd
• Confusion, especially in elderly; take safety precautions if needed
• Hydration including skin turgor, thirst, dry mucous membranes
• For blurred vision, pain in eyes, before and during treatment (increased intraocular pressure); neuro checks, intracranial pressure during treatment (increased intracranial pressure)

Administer:
IV
• In 15%-25% sol with filter; give over ½-1½ hr; rapid infusion may worsen CHF; warm in hot water and shake to dissolve crystals
• Test dose in severe oliguria, 0.2

g/kg over 3-5 min; if no urine increase, give second test dose; if no response, reassess patient
Irrigation:
• 100 ml of 25%/900 ml of sterile water for inj (2.5% sol)

Additive compatibilities: Amikacin, bretylium, cefamandole, cefoxitin, cimetidine, cisplatin, dopamine, fosphenytoin, furosemide, gentamicin, metoclopramide, netilmicin, nizatidine, ofloxacin, ondansetron, sodium bicarbonate, tobramycin, verapamil

Y-site compatibilities: Allopurinol, amifostine, amphotericin B cholesteryl, aztreonam, cisatracurium, cladribine, fludarabine, fluorouracil, gallium, idarubicin, melphalan, ondansetron, paclitaxel, piperacillin, propofol, remifentanil, sargramostim, teniposide, thiotepa, vinorelbine

Evaluate:
• Therapeutic response: improvement in edema of feet, legs, sacral area daily if medication is being used in CHF; decreased intraocular pressure, prevention of hypokalemia, increased excretion of toxic substances; decreased ICP

Teach patient/family:
• To rise slowly from lying or sitting position
• The reason for and method of treatment

Treatment of overdose: Discontinue infusion; correct fluid, electrolyte imbalances; hemodialysis; monitor hydration, CV, renal function

Side effects: *italics* = common; ***bold italics*** = life-threatening

measles, mumps, and rubella vaccine (R̥)
M-M-R-II
Func. class.: Vaccine

Action: Produces antibodies to measles, mumps, rubella

Uses: Prevention of measles, mumps, rubella

Dosage and routes:
• *Adult:* SC 1 vial; 2 vials separated by 1 mo, in person born after 1957
• *Child >15 mo and adult:* SC 0.5 ml

Available forms: Inj SC measles 1000 $TCID_{50}$, mumps 20,000 $TCID_{50}$, rubella 1000 $TCID_{50}$ (0.5 ml)

Side effects/adverse reactions:
CNS: Fever, *subacute sclerosing panencephalitis and blindness associated with optic neuritis,* paresthesias
INTEG: Urticaria, erythema, burning, stinging at injection site
SYST: Lymphadenitis, *anaphylaxis,* malaise, sore throat, headache
MS: Osteomyelitis, arthralgia, arthritis

Contraindications: Hypersensitivity, blood dyscrasias, anemia, active infection, immunosuppression; egg, chicken allergy; pregnancy, febrile illness, neomycin allergy, neoplasms

Precautions: Elderly, lactation, children with TB

Interactions:
• Decreased response to TB skin test
• Decreased immune response: other live virus vaccines

NURSING CONSIDERATIONS
Assess:
• For skin reactions: rash, induration, erythema
• For anaphylaxis: inability to breathe, bronchospasm

Administer:
• Only with epinephrine 1:1000 on unit to treat laryngospasm
• Only SC

Perform/provide:
• Storage at 39° F (4° C); protect from heat, light; do not give within 1 mo of other live virus vaccines
• Written record of immunization

Evaluate:
• For history of allergies, skin disorders (eczema, psoriasis, dermatitis), reactions to vaccinations

Teach patient/family:
• That fever may occur 5-12 days after vaccine given
• That joint pains, tingling in extremities may occur 5-12 days after vaccine given
• That pain and inflammation may occur
• To take acetaminophen for fever

mebendazole (R̥)
(me-ben′da-zole)
Vermox
Func. class.: Anthelmintic
Chem. class.: Carbamate

Action: Inhibits glucose uptake, degeneration of cytoplasmic microtubules in the cell; interferes with absorption, secretory function

Uses: Pinworms, roundworms, hookworms, whipworms, threadworms, pork tapeworms, dwarf tapeworms, beef tapeworms, hydatid cyst

Dosage and routes:
• *Adult and child >2 yr:* PO 100 mg as a single dose or bid × 3 days, depending on type of infection; course may be repeated in 3 wk if needed

Available forms: Tabs, chew 100 mg

Side effects/adverse reactions:
CNS: Dizziness, fever, headache

GI: Transient diarrhea, abdominal pain, nausea, vomiting

Contraindications: Hypersensitivity

Precautions: Child <2 yr, lactation, pregnancy (C) (1st trimester)

Pharmacokinetics:

PO: Peak ½-7 hr; excreted in feces primarily (metabolites), small amount in urine (unchanged); highly bound to plasma proteins

Interactions:

• Decreased effect of mebendazole: carbamazepine, hydantoins

• Drug/food: increased absorption: high-fat meal

NURSING CONSIDERATIONS

Assess:

• Stools during entire treatment; specimens must be sent to lab while still warm, also 1-3 wk after treatment is completed

• For allergic reaction: rash (rare)

• For diarrhea during expulsion of worms; avoid self-contamination with patient's feces

• For infection in other family members, since infection from person to person is common

• Blood studies: AST, ALT, alk phosphatase, BUN, CBC during treatment

Administer:

• May be crushed, chewed, swallowed whole

• PO after meals to avoid GI symptoms, since absorption is not altered by food

• Second course after 3 wk if needed; usually recommended

Perform/provide:

• Storage in tight container

Evaluate:

• Therapeutic response: expulsion of worms and 3 negative stool cultures after completion of treatment

Teach patient/family:

• Proper hygiene after BM, including hand-washing technique; tell patient to avoid putting fingers in mouth; clean fingernails

• That infected person should sleep alone; do not shake bed linen, change bed linen qd, wash in hot water, change and wash undergarments daily

• To clean toilet qd with disinfectant (green soap solution)

• The need for compliance with dosage schedule, duration of treatment

• To wear shoes, wash all fruits and vegetables well before eating; use commercial fruit/vegetable cleaner

• That all members of the family should be treated (pinworms)

---

mechlorethamine (R)

(me-klor-eth′a-meen)

Mustargen, Nitrogen Mustard

Func. class.: Antineoplastic alkylating agent

Chem. class.: Nitrogen mustard

Action: Responsible for cross-linking DNA strands leading to cell death; rapidly degraded, a vesicant; activity is not cell cycle phase-specific

Uses: Hodgkin's disease, leukemias, lymphomas, lymphosarcoma; ovarian, breast, lung carcinoma; neoplastic effusions

Dosage and routes:

• *Adult:* **IV** 0.4 mg/kg or 10 mg/m^2 as 1 dose or 2-4 divided doses over 2-4 days; second course after 3 wk depending on blood cell count

Neoplastic effusions

• *Adult:* **INTRACAVITARY** 10-20 mg, may be 200-400 µg/kg

Available forms: Inj 10 mg

Side effects/adverse reactions:

EENT: Tinnitus, hearing loss

HEMA: ***Thrombocytopenia, leukopenia, agranulocytosis,*** anemia

GI: Nausea, vomiting, diarrhea, stomatitis, weight loss, colitis, ***hepatotoxicity***

CNS: Headache, dizziness, drowsiness, paresthesia, peripheral neuropathy, ***coma***

INTEG: Alopecia, pruritus, herpes zoster, extravasation

Contraindications: Lactation, pregnancy (D), myelosuppression, acute herpes zoster

Precautions: Radiation therapy, chronic lymphocytic leukopenia

Pharmacokinetics: Metabolized in liver, excreted in urine

Interactions:
• Increased toxicity: antineoplastics, radiation
• Blood dyscrasias: amphotericin B

NURSING CONSIDERATIONS
Assess:
• CBC, differential, platelet count qwk; withhold drug if WBC is <1000/mm^3 or platelet count is <75,000/mm^3; notify prescriber
• Renal function studies: BUN, serum uric acid, urine CrCl before, during therapy
• I&O ratio; report fall in urine output of 30 ml/hr
• Monitor temp q4h (may indicate beginning infection); no rectal temps
• Liver function tests before, during therapy (bilirubin, AST, ALT, LDH) as needed or monthly
• Bleeding: hematuria, guaiac, bruising or petechiae, mucosa or orifices q8h
• Jaundiced skin and sclera, dark urine, clay-colored stools, itchy skin, abdominal pain, fever, diarrhea
• Effects of alopecia on body image; discuss feelings about body changes
• Buccal cavity q8h for dryness, sores, ulceration, white patches, oral pain, bleeding, dysphagia
• Local irritation, pain, burning, discoloration at injection site

◆ Symptoms indicating severe allergic reaction: rash, pruritus, urticaria, purpuric skin lesions, itching, flushing

Administer:
• After using guidelines for preparation of cytotoxic drugs
• Antiemetic 30-60 min before giving drug and prn
• IV after diluting 10 mg/10 ml sterile H$_2$O or NaCl; leave needle in vial, shake, withdraw dose, give through Y-tube or 3-way stopcock or directly over 3-5 min
• Watch for infiltration; infiltrate area with isotonic sodium thiosulfate or 1% lidocaine; apply ice for 6-12 hr
• Topical or systemic analgesics for pain
• Local or systemic drugs for infection

Y-site compatibilities: Amifostine, aztreonam, filgrastim, fludarabine, granisetron, melphalan, ondansetron, sargramostim, teniposide, vinorelbine

Perform/provide:
• Storage at room temp in dry form
• Increase fluid intake to 2-3 L/day to prevent urate deposits, calculi formation
• Diet low in purines: organ meats (kidney, liver), dried beans, peas to maintain alkaline urine
• Preparation under hood using gloves and mask
• Rinsing of mouth tid-qid with water, club soda; brushing of teeth bid-tid with soft brush or cotton-tipped applicators for stomatitis; use unwaxed dental floss
• Warm compresses at injection site for inflammation

Evaluate:
• Therapeutic response: decreased tumor size, spread of malignancy

Teach patient/family:
• The rationale for and techniques of protective isolation

◆ = Nursing alert   ⫽ = Herb-drug interaction   ⊗ = Do not crush

• That sterility, amenorrhea can occur; reversible after discontinuing treatment

• That hair may be lost during treatment; a wig or hairpiece may make patient feel better; new hair may be different in color, texture

• To avoid foods with citric acid, hot or rough texture

• To report any bleeding, white spots, or ulcerations in mouth to prescriber; tell patient to examine mouth qd

• To report signs of infection: fever, sore throat, flulike symptoms

• To report signs of anemia: fatigue, headache, faintness, shortness of breath, irritability

• To avoid use of razors, commercial mouthwash

• To avoid use of aspirin products, NSAIDs

• To notify prescriber if pregnancy is suspected; to use contraception during treatment

---

meclizine (OTC, R)
(mek′li-zeen)
Antivert, Antivert/25, Antivert/25 Chewable, Antivert-50, Antrizine, Bonamine*, Bonine, Dizmiss, Dramamine II, meclizine HCl, Meni-D, Ru-Vert-M
Func. class.: Antiemetic, antihistamine, anticholinergic
Chem. class.: H_1-receptor antagonist, piperazine derivative

Action: Acts centrally by blocking chemoreceptor trigger zone, which in turn acts on vomiting center
Uses: Vertigo, motion sickness
Dosage and routes:
• *Adult:* **PO** 25-100 mg qd in divided doses or 1 hr before traveling
Available forms: Tabs 12.5, 25, 50 mg; chew tabs 25 mg; caps 15, 25, 30 mg

Side effects/adverse reactions:
CNS: Drowsiness, fatigue, restlessness, headache, insomnia
CV: Hypotension
GU: Urinary retention
GI: Nausea, anorexia
EENT: Dry mouth, blurred vision
Contraindications: Hypersensitivity to cyclizines, shock
Precautions: Children, narrowangle glaucoma, glaucoma, urinary retention, lactation, prostatic hypertrophy, elderly, pregnancy (B), CV disease, hypertension, seizure disease
Pharmacokinetics:
PO: Duration 8-24 hr, half-life 6 hr
Interactions:
• Increased effect of alcohol, opioids, other CNS depressants
⊘ Increased anticholinergic effect: henbane leaf
Lab test interferences:
False negative: Allergy skin testing
NURSING CONSIDERATIONS
Assess:
• VS, B/P
◆ Signs of toxicity of other drugs or masking of symptoms of disease: brain tumor, intestinal obstruction
• Observe for drowsiness, dizziness, LOC
Administer:
PO
• Tablets may be swallowed whole, chewed, or allowed to dissolve; give with food to decrease GI upset
• Lowest possible dose in elderly, anticholinergic effects
Evaluate:
• Therapeutic response: absence of dizziness, vomiting
Teach patient/family:
• That a false-negative result may occur with skin testing for allergies; these procedures should not be scheduled for 4 days after discontinuing use

• To avoid hazardous activities, activities requiring alertness; dizziness may occur; instruct patient to request assistance with ambulation
• To avoid alcohol, other depressants

---

medroxyprogeste-rone (R)

(me-drox′ee-proe-jess′te-rone)
Amen, Curretab, Cycrin, Depo-Provera, medroxyprogesterone acetate, Provera
Func. class.: Antineoplastic, hormone
Chem. class.: Progesterone derivative

Action: Inhibits secretion of pituitary gonadotropins, which prevents follicular maturation and ovulation; stimulates growth of mammary tissue; antineoplastic action against endometrial cancer

Uses: Uterine bleeding (abnormal), secondary amenorrhea, endometrial cancer, renal cancer, contraceptive, prevent endometrial changes associated with estrogen replacement therapy (ERT)

Investigational uses: Pickwickian syndrome, sleep apnea, hypersomnolence

Dosage and routes:
Secondary amenorrhea
• *Adult:* PO 5-10 mg qd × 5-10 days
Endometrial/renal cancer
• *Adult:* IM 400-1000 mg/wk
Uterine bleeding
• *Adult:* PO 5-10 mg qd × 5-10 days starting on 16th day of menstrual cycle
Contraceptive
• *Adult:* INJ q3mo
With ERT
• *Adult:* PO monophasic 2.5 mg qd; Biphasic 5 mg days 15-28 of cycle

Available forms: Tabs 2.5, 5, 10, 100* mg; inj susp 50*, 100*, 150, 400 mg/ml

Side effects/adverse reactions:
CNS: Dizziness, headache, migraines, depression, fatigue
CV: Hypotension, thrombophlebitis, edema, *thromboembolism, stroke, pulmonary embolism, MI*
GI: Nausea, vomiting, anorexia, cramps, increased weight, *cholestatic jaundice*
EENT: Diplopia
GU: Amenorrhea, cervical erosion, breakthrough bleeding, dysmenorrhea, vaginal candidiasis, breast changes, *gynecomastia, testicular atrophy, impotence,* endometriosis, *spontaneous abortion*
INTEG: Rash, urticaria, acne, hirsutism, alopecia, oily skin, seborrhea, purpura, melasma, photosensitivity
META: Hyperglycemia

Contraindications: Breast cancer, hypersensitivity, thromboembolic disorders, reproductive cancer, genital bleeding (abnormal, undiagnosed), pregnancy (D)

Precautions: Lactation, hypertension, asthma, blood dyscrasias, gallbladder disease, CHF, diabetes mellitus, bone disease, depression, migraine headache, convulsive disorders, hepatic disease, renal disease, family history of cancer of breast or reproductive tract

Pharmacokinetics:
PO: Duration 24 hr, excreted in urine and feces, metabolized in liver

Lab test interferences:
Increase: Alk phosphatase, N (urine), pregnanediol, amino acids
Decrease: GTT, HDL

NURSING CONSIDERATIONS
Assess:
• Weight qd; notify prescriber of weekly weight gain >5 lb
• B/P at beginning of treatment and periodically

◆ = Nursing alert   ✔ = Herb-drug interaction   🚫 = Do not crush

• I&O ratio; be alert for decreasing urinary output, increasing edema
• Liver function studies: ALT, AST, bilirubin, periodically during long-term therapy
• Edema, hypertension, cardiac symptoms, jaundice
• Mental status: affect, mood, behavioral changes, depression
• Hypercalcemia

Administer:
• Titrated dose; use lowest effective dose
• Oil solution deep in large muscle mass (IM), rotate sites
• With food or milk to decrease GI symptoms (PO)

Perform/provide:
• Storage in dark area

Evaluate:
• Therapeutic response: decreased abnormal uterine bleeding, absence of amenorrhea, decrease in size and growth of tumor

Teach patient/family:
• To avoid sunlight or use sunscreen; photosensitivity can occur
• About cushingoid symptoms
• To report breast lumps, vaginal bleeding, edema, jaundice, dark urine, clay-colored stools, dyspnea, headache, blurred vision, abdominal pain, numbness or stiffness in legs, chest pain; male to report impotence or gynecomastia
• To report suspected pregnancy

---

megestrol (℞)

(me-jess'trole)
Megace, megestrol acetate
Func. class.: Antineoplastic
Chem. class.: Hormone, progestin

Action: Affects endometrium by antiluteinizing effect; this is thought to bring about cell death

Uses: Breast, endometrial cancer, renal cell cancer, cachexia

Dosage and routes:
Endometrial/ovarian carcinoma
• *Adult:* PO 40-320 mg/day in divided doses
Breast carcinoma
• *Adult:* PO 40 mg qid
Anorexia (AIDS)
• *Adult:* PO 800 mg qd (oral susp)
Available forms: Tabs 20, 40 mg; oral susp 200 mg/5 ml

Side effects/adverse reactions:
GI: Nausea, vomiting, diarrhea, abdominal cramps, weight gain
GU: Gynecomastia, fluid retention, **hypercalcemia**, vaginal bleeding, discharge, impotence, decreased libido
CV: **Thrombophlebitis, thromboembolism**
INTEG: Alopecia, rash, pruritus, purpura, itching
CNS: Mood swings

Contraindications: Hypersensitivity, pregnancy D (tabs); X (susp)

Pharmacokinetics:
PO: Duration 1-3 days, half-life 60 min; metabolized in liver; excreted in feces, breast milk

Lab test interferences:
Increase: Alk phosphatase, urinary N, urinary pregnanediol, plasma amino acids
False positive: Urine glucose
Decrease: HDL, glucose tolerance test

NURSING CONSIDERATIONS
Assess:
• I&O ratio; weights
• Effects of alopecia on body image; discuss feelings about body changes
◆ Symptoms indicating severe allergic reaction: rash, pruritus, urticaria, purpuric skin lesions, itching, flushing
• Frequency of stools, characteristics: cramping, acidosis, signs of de-

hydration (rapid respirations, poor skin turgor, decreased urine output, dry skin, restlessness, weakness)
• Anorexia, nausea, vomiting, constipation, weakness, loss of muscle tone
• Thrombophlebitis: Homans' sign, edema, pain in calf, thigh, notify prescriber

Administer:
• Diuretics for increased fluids
• Oral susp for AIDS patients

Perform/provide:
• Increase fluid intake to 2-3 L/day to prevent dehydration and maintain normal Ca
• Nutritious diet with iron, vitamin supplements as ordered
• Storage in tight container at room temp

Evaluate:
• Therapeutic response: decreased tumor size, spread of malignancy; weight gain in AIDS patients

Teach patient/family:
• To report vaginal bleeding
• That nonhormonal contraception should be used during and 4 mo after treatment
• That gynecomastia can occur; reversible after discontinuing treatment
• To recognize and report signs of fluid retention, thromboemboli, hepatotoxicity

---

melphalan (R)

(mel'fa-lan)
Alkeran, Alkeran IV, L-PAM, L-Sarcolysin
Func. class.: Antineoplastic, alkylating agent
Chem. class.: Nitrogen mustard

Action: Responsible for crosslinking DNA strands leading to cell death; activity is not cell cycle phase-specific

Uses: Multiple myeloma, malignant melanoma, advanced ovarian cancer

Investigational uses: Breast, testicular, prostate carcinoma; osteogenic sarcoma, chronic myelogenous leukemia

Dosage and routes:
Multiple myeloma
• *Adult:* **PO** 6 mg qd × 2-3 wk; stop drug for 4 wk or until WBC level begins to rise; do not administer if WBC <3000/mm^3 or platelets <100,000/mm^3; may be given 0.15 mg/kg/day × 7 days; wait until platelets and WBCs rise, then 0.05 mg/kg/day

Ovarian carcinoma
• *Adult:* **IV INF** 16 mg/m^2, reduce in renal insufficiency, give over 15-20 min, give at 2 wk intervals × 4 doses, then at 4 wk intervals

Available forms: Tabs 2 mg, powder for inj 50 mg

Side effects/adverse reactions:
HEMA: **Thrombocytopenia, neutropenia, leukopenia,** anemia
GI: Nausea, vomiting, stomatitis, diarrhea
GU: Amenorrhea, hyperuricemia, gonadal suppression
INTEG: Rash, urticaria, alopecia, pruritus
RESP: **Fibrosis, dysplasia**
SYST: **Anaphylaxis,** allergic reactions

Contraindications: Lactation, pregnancy (D), hypersensitivity to this drug or other nitrogen mustards

Precautions: Radiation therapy, bone marrow depression, infections, renal disease, children

Pharmacokinetics: Metabolized in liver, excreted in urine, half-life 1½ hr

Interactions:
• Increased toxicity: antineoplastics, radiation

 = Nursing alert   = Herb-drug interaction   ⃠ = Do not crush

• Decreased antibody response: live virus vaccines
• Increased pulmonary toxicity: carmustine

NURSING CONSIDERATIONS
Assess:

• CBC, differential, platelet count qwk; withhold drug if WBC is <3000/mm³ or platelet count is <100,000/mm³; notify prescriber
• Renal function studies: BUN, serum uric acid, urine CrCl before, during therapy
• I&O ratio; report fall in urine output to 30 ml/hr
• For infection: fever, cough, temperature, sore throat, notify prescriber
• For bleeding: bruising, blood in urine, stools, emesis
• Liver function tests before, during therapy (bilirubin, AST, ALT, LDH) as needed or monthly
• Bleeding: hematuria, guaiac, bruising or petechiae, mucosa or orifices q8h
• Jaundiced skin and sclera, dark urine, clay-colored stools, itchy skin, abdominal pain, fever, diarrhea
• Buccal cavity q8h for dryness, sores, ulceration, white patches, oral pain, bleeding, dysphagia
• Local irritation, pain, burning, discoloration at injection site
◆ Symptoms indicating severe allergic reaction: rash, pruritus, urticaria, purpuric skin lesions, itching, flushing

Administer:

• Antiemetic 30-60 min before giving drug to prevent vomiting
Y-site compatibilities: Acyclovir, amikacin, aminophylline, ampicillin, aztreonam, bleomycin, bumetanide, buprenorphine, butorphanol, calcium gluconate, carboplatin, carmustine, cefazolin, cefepime, cefoperazone, cefotaxime, cefotetan, ceftazidime, ceftizoxime, ceftriaxone, cefuroxime, cimetidine, cisplatin, clindamycin, cyclophosphamide, cytarabine, dacarbazine, dactinomycin, daunorubicin, dexamethasone, diphenhydramine, doxorubicin, doxycycline, droperidol, enalaprilat, etoposide, famotidine, floxuridine, fluconazole, fludarabine, fluorouracil, furosemide, gallium, ganciclovir, gentamicin, granisetron, haloperidol, heparin, hydrocortisone, hydrocortisone sodium phosphate, hydromorphone, hydroxyzine, idarubicin, ifosfamide, imipenem-cilastatin, lorazepam, mannitol, mechlorethamine, meperidine, mesna, methotrexate, methylprednisolone, metoclopramide, metronidazole, miconazole, minocycline, mitomycin, mitoxantrone, morphine, nalbuphine, netilmicin, ondansetron, pentostatin, piperacillin, plicamycin, potassium chloride, prochlorperazine, promethazine, ranitidine, sodium bicarbonate, streptozocin, teniposide, thiotepa, ticarcillin, ticarcillin/clavulanate, tobramycin, trimethoprim-sulfamethoxazole, vancomycin, vinblastine, vincristine, vinorelbine, zidovudine

Perform/provide:

• Storage in airtight, light-resistant container
• Strict medical asepsis, protective isolation if WBC levels are low
• Increase fluid intake to 2-3 L/day to prevent urate deposits, calculi formation
• Diet low in purines: organ meats (kidney, liver), dried beans, peas to maintain alkaline urine
• Rinsing of mouth tid-qid with water, club soda; brushing of teeth bid-tid with soft brush or cotton-tipped applicators for stomatitis; use unwaxed dental floss
• Warm compresses at injection site for inflammation

Evaluate:
• Therapeutic response: decreased tumor size, spread of malignancy
Teach patient/family:
• That sterility, amenorrhea can occur; reversible after discontinuing treatment
• To avoid foods with citric acid, hot or rough texture
• To report any bleeding, white spots, or ulcerations in mouth to prescriber; tell patient to examine mouth qd
• To report signs of infection: fever, sore throat, flulike symptoms
• To report suspected pregnancy; to use contraception during treatment
• To report signs of anemia: fatigue, headache, faintness, shortness of breath, irritability
• To avoid use of razors, commercial mouthwash
• To avoid use of aspirin products, NSAIDs, alcohol

---

menotropins (℞)

(men-oh-troe′pins)

Humegon, Pergonal, Repronex

Func. class.: Gonadotropin

Chem. class.: Exogenous gonadotropin

Action: In women, increases follicular growth, maturation; in men, when given with HCG, stimulates spermatogenesis
Uses: Infertility, anovulation in women, stimulates spermatogenesis in men
Dosage and routes:
Infertility
• *Men:* **IM** 1 ampule 3 × wk with HCG 2000 U 2 × wk × 4 mo
• *Women:* **IM** 75 IU FSH, LH qd × 9-12 days, then 10,000 U HCG 1 day after these drugs; repeat × 2 menstrual cycles, then increase to 150 IU FSH, LH qd × 9-12 days,

then 10,000 U HCG 1 day after these drugs × 2 menstrual cycles
Anovulation
• *Women:* **IM** 75 IU FSH, LH qd × 9-12 days, then 10,000 U HCG 1 day after last dose of these drugs; repeat × 1-3 menstrual cycles
Available forms: Powder for inj lyophilized 75 IU FSH, LH activity 150 IU FSH, LH activity
Side effects/adverse reactions:
CNS: Fever
CV: **Hypovolemia**
RESP: **ARDS, pulmonary embolism, pulmonary infarction**
SYST: **Anaphylaxis**
GI: *Nausea,* vomiting, diarrhea, anorexia
GU: Ovarian enlargement, abdominal distention/pain, multiple births, ovarian hyperstimulation: sudden ovarian enlargement, ascites with or without pain, pleural effusion; gynecomastia in men
HEMA: **Hemoperitoneum, arterial thromboembolism**
Contraindications: Primary ovarian failure, abnormal bleeding, thyroid/adrenal dysfunction, organic intracranial lesion, ovarian cysts, primary testicular failure, pregnancy (X)
NURSING CONSIDERATIONS
Assess:
• Weight qd; notify prescriber if weight increases rapidly
• Estrogen excretion level; if >100 µg/24 hr, drug is withheld; hyperstimulation syndrome may occur
• I&O ratio; be alert for decreasing urinary output
• Ovarian enlargement, abdominal distention/pain; report symptoms immediately
Administer:
IM
• After reconstituting with 1-2 ml sterile saline inj; use immediately

---

⬦ = Nursing alert   ⫽ = Herb-drug interaction   ⃠ = Do not crush

Evaluate:

• Therapeutic response: ovulation, pregnancy

Teach patient/family:

• That multiple births are possible; if pregnancy occurs, usually 4-6 wk after start of treatment

• To keep appointment during treatment qd × 2 wk

---

meperidine (R)

(me-per'i-deen)
Demerol, meperidine, Pethadol, Pethidine
Func. class.: Opiate analgesic
Chem. class.: Phenylpiperidine derivative

Controlled Substance Schedule II
Action: Depresses pain impulse transmission at the spinal cord level by interacting with opioid receptors
Uses: Moderate to severe pain, preoperatively, postoperatively
Dosage and routes:

Pain

• *Adult:* **PO/SC/IM** 50-150 mg q3-4h prn; dose should be decreased if given **IV**

• *Child:* **PO/SC/IM** 1 mg/kg q4-6h prn, not to exceed 100 mg q4h

Labor analgesia

• *Adult:* **SC/IM** 50-100 mg given when contractions are regularly spaced, repeat q1-3h prn

Preoperatively

• *Adult:* **IM/SC** 50-100 mg q30-90 min before surgery; dose should be reduced if given **IV**

• *Child:* **IM/SC** 1-2.2 mg/kg 30-90 min before surgery

Renal disease

• CrCl 10-50 ml/min 75% of dose; CrCl <10 ml/min 50% of dose

Available forms include: Inj 10, 50, 75, 100 mg/ml; tabs 50, 100 mg; syr 50 mg/5 ml

Side effects/adverse reactions:
*CNS: Drowsiness, dizziness, confusion, headache, sedation, euphoria, **increased intracranial pressure**, **seizures***
CV: Palpitations, bradycardia, change in B/P, tachycardia (IV)
EENT: Tinnitus, blurred vision, miosis, diplopia, depressed corneal reflex
GI: Nausea, vomiting, anorexia, constipation, cramps
GU: Urinary retention, dysuria
INTEG: Rash, urticaria, bruising, flushing, diaphoresis, pruritus
*RESP: **Respiratory depression***
Contraindications: Hypersensitivity, addiction (narcotic)
Precautions: Addictive personality, pregnancy (B), lactation, increased intracranial pressure, MI (acute), severe heart disease, respiratory depression, hepatic disease, renal disease, child <18 yr, elderly
Pharmacokinetics:
Absorption 50% (PO), well absorbed IM, SC
PO: Onset 15 min, peak ½-1 hr, duration 2-4 hr
SC/IM: Onset 10 min, peak ½-1 hr, duration 2-4 hr
IV: Onset 5 min, duration 2 hr
Metabolized by liver (to active/inactive metabolites), excreted by kidneys; crosses placenta, excreted in breast milk; half-life 3-4 hr; toxic by-product can result from regular use
Interactions:

• Increased effects with: other CNS depressants, alcohol, opioids, sedative/hypnotics, antipsychotics, skeletal muscle relaxants

◆May cause fatal reaction: MAOIs, procarbazine

Lab test interferences:
Increase: Amylase, lipase

M

NURSING CONSIDERATIONS
Assess:
• Pain: location, type, character; give before pain becomes extreme
• Renal function prior to initiating therapy; poor renal function can lead to accumulation of toxic metabolite and seizures
• I&O ratio; check for decreasing output; may indicate urinary retention
• Need for drug
• For constipation; increase fluids, bulk in diet
• CNS changes: dizziness, drowsiness, hallucinations, euphoria, LOC, pupil reactions
• Allergic reactions: rash, urticaria
• Respiratory dysfunction: depression, character, rate, rhythm; notify prescriber if respirations are <12/min

Administer:
• Patient should remain recumbent for 1 hr after IM/SC route
• With antiemetic for nausea, vomiting
• When pain is beginning to return; determine dosage interval by patient response
• In gradually decreasing dose after long-term use; withdrawal symptoms may occur

IV
• After diluting with 5 ml or more sterile H_2O or NS; give directly over 4-5 min; may be further diluted in sol to 1 mg/ml during anesthesia in D_5W or NS; if diluted in NS, may be given through patient-controlled inf device

Additive compatibilities: Cefazolin, dobutamine, ondansetron, scopolamine, succinylcholine, triflupromazine, verapamil

Syringe compatibilities: Atropine, benzquinamide, butorphanol, chlorpromazine, cimetidine, dimenhydrinate, diphenhydramine, droperidol, fentanyl, glycopyrrolate, hydroxyzine, ketamine, metoclopramide, midazolam, pentazocine, perphenazine, prochlorperazine, promazine, promethazine, ranitidine, scopolamine

Y-site compatibilities: Amifostine, amikacin, ampicillin, atenolol, aztreonam, bumetanide, cefamandole, cefazolin, cefmetazole, cefotaxime, cefotetan, cefoxitin, ceftazidime, ceftizoxime, ceftriaxone, cefuroxime, cephalothin, cephapirin, chloramphenicol, cisatracurium, cladribine, clindamycin, dexamethasone, diltiazem, diphenhydramine, dobutamine, dopamine, doxorubicin liposome, doxycycline, droperidol, erythromycin, famotidine, filgrastim, fluconazole, fludarabine, gallium, gentamicin, granisetron, heparin, hydrocortisone, insulin (regular), kanamycin, labetalol, lidocaine, methyldopate, magnesium sulfate, melphalan, methylprednisolone, metoclopramide, metoprolol, metronidazole, moxalactum, ondansetron, oxacillin, oxytocin, paclitaxel, penicillin G potassium, piperacillin, potassium chloride, propofol, propranolol, ranitidine, remifentanil, sargramostim, teniposide, thiotepa, ticarcillin, ticarcillin/clavulanate, tobramycin, trimethoprimsulfamethoxazole, vancomycin, verapamil, vinorelbine

Perform/provide:
• Storage in light-resistant container at room temp
• Assistance with ambulation
• Safety measures: night-light, call bell within easy reach

Evaluate:
• Therapeutic response: decrease in pain

Teach patient/family:
• To report any symptoms of CNS changes, allergic reactions

 = Nursing alert   = Herb-drug interaction   ⃠ = Do not crush

Acetaminophen/Codeine

Tylenol with Codeine
300/15mg: McNeil

Tylenol with Codeine
300/30mg: McNeil

Tylenol with Codeine
300/60mg: McNeil

Acetaminophen/Hydrocodone

Lorcet Plus
650/7.5mg: Forest

Lorcet
650/10mg: Forest

Vicodin
500/5mg: Knoll

Vicodin ES
750/7.5mg: Knoll

Anexsia
650/7.5mg: Monarch

Lortab
500/5mg: Whitby

Lortab
500/7.5mg: Whitby

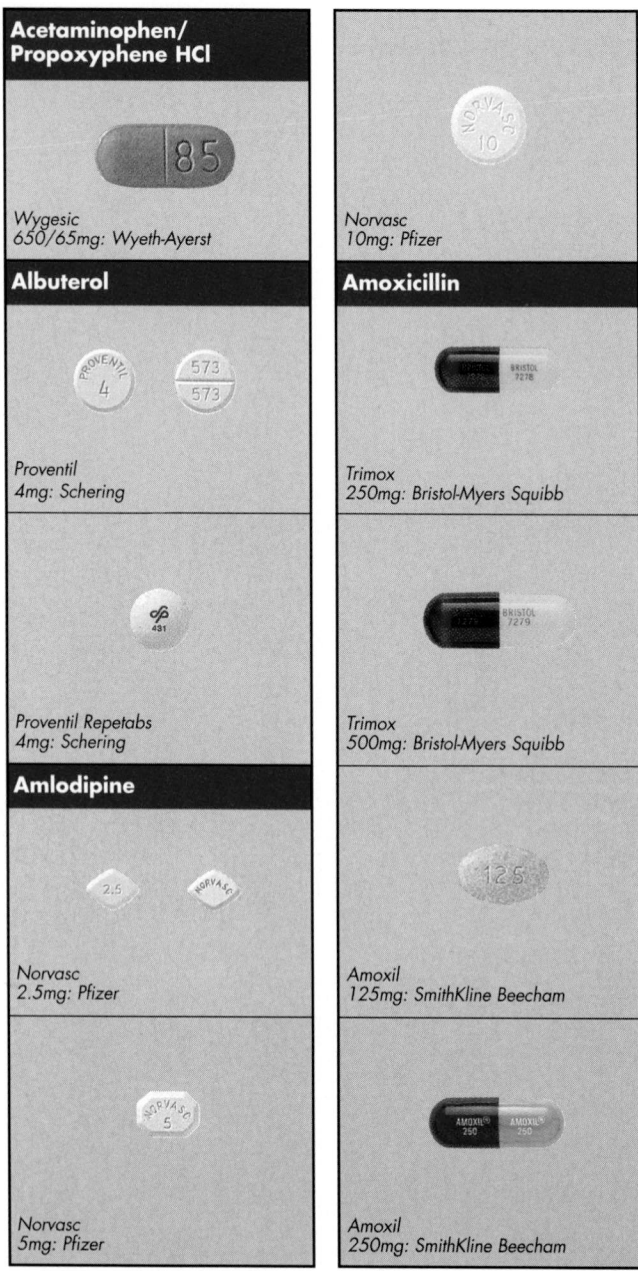

Acetaminophen/ Propoxyphene HCl

*Wygesic
650/65mg: Wyeth-Ayerst*

Albuterol

*Proventil
4mg: Schering*

*Proventil Repetabs
4mg: Schering*

Amlodipine

*Norvasc
2.5mg: Pfizer*

*Norvasc
5mg: Pfizer*

*Norvasc
10mg: Pfizer*

Amoxicillin

*Trimox
250mg: Bristol-Myers Squibb*

*Trimox
500mg: Bristol-Myers Squibb*

*Amoxil
125mg: SmithKline Beecham*

*Amoxil
250mg: SmithKline Beecham*

Amoxil
250mg: SmithKline Beecham

Amoxil
500mg: SmithKline Beecham

Amoxicillin/Clavulanate

Augmentin
125/31.25mg: SmithKline Beecham

Augmentin
250/62.5mg: SmithKline Beecham

Augmentin
250/125mg: SmithKline Beecham

Augmentin
500/125mg: SmithKline Beecham

Augmentin
875/125mg: SmithKline Beecham

Azithromycin

Zithromax
250mg: Pfizer

Zithromax
250mg: Pfizer

Cephalexin

Keflex
250mg: Dista

Keflex
500mg: Dista

Ciprofloxacin HCl

Cipro
250mg: Miles

Cipro
500mg: Miles

Cipro
750mg: Miles

Clarithromycin

Biaxin
250mg: Abbott

Biaxin
500mg: Abbott

Digoxin

Lanoxicaps
0.1mg: Glaxo Wellcome

Diltiazem HCl

Cardizem
30mg: Hoechst Marion Roussel

Cardizem
60mg: Hoechst Marion Roussel

Cardizem
90mg: Hoechst Marion Roussel

Cardizem CD
120mg: Hoechst Marion Roussel

Cardizem CD
180mg: Hoechst Marion Roussel

Cardizem CD
240mg: Hoechst Marion Roussel

Dilacor XR
180mg: Rhone-Poulenc Rorer

Dilacor XR
240mg: Rhone-Poulenc Rorer

Enalapril

Vasotec
2.5mg: Merck

Vasotec
5mg: Merck

Vasotec
10mg: Merck

Vasotec
20mg: Merck

Estrogens, Conjugated

Premarin
0.3mg: Wyeth-Ayerst

Premarin
0.625mg: Wyeth-Ayerst

Premarin
0.9mg: Wyeth-Ayerst

Premarin
1.25mg: Wyeth-Ayerst

Premarin
2.5mg: Wyeth-Ayerst

**Estrogens, Conjugated/
Medroxyprogesterone**

Prempro
0.625/2.5mg: Wyeth-Ayerst

Premphase
0.625/5mg: Wyeth-Ayerst

Fluoxetine HCl

Prozac
10mg: Dista

Prozac
20mg: Dista

Furosemide

Lasix
20mg: Hoechst Marion Roussel

Lasix
40mg: Hoechst Marion Roussel

Lasix
80mg: Hoechst Marion Roussel

Generic
20mg: Rugby

Generic
40mg: Rugby

Generic
80mg: Rugby

Levothyroxine

Levothroid
0.025mg: Forest

Levothroid
0.05mg: Forest

Levothroid
0.075mg: Forest

Levothroid
0.088mg: Forest

Levothroid
0.1mg: Forest

Levothroid
0.112mg: Forest

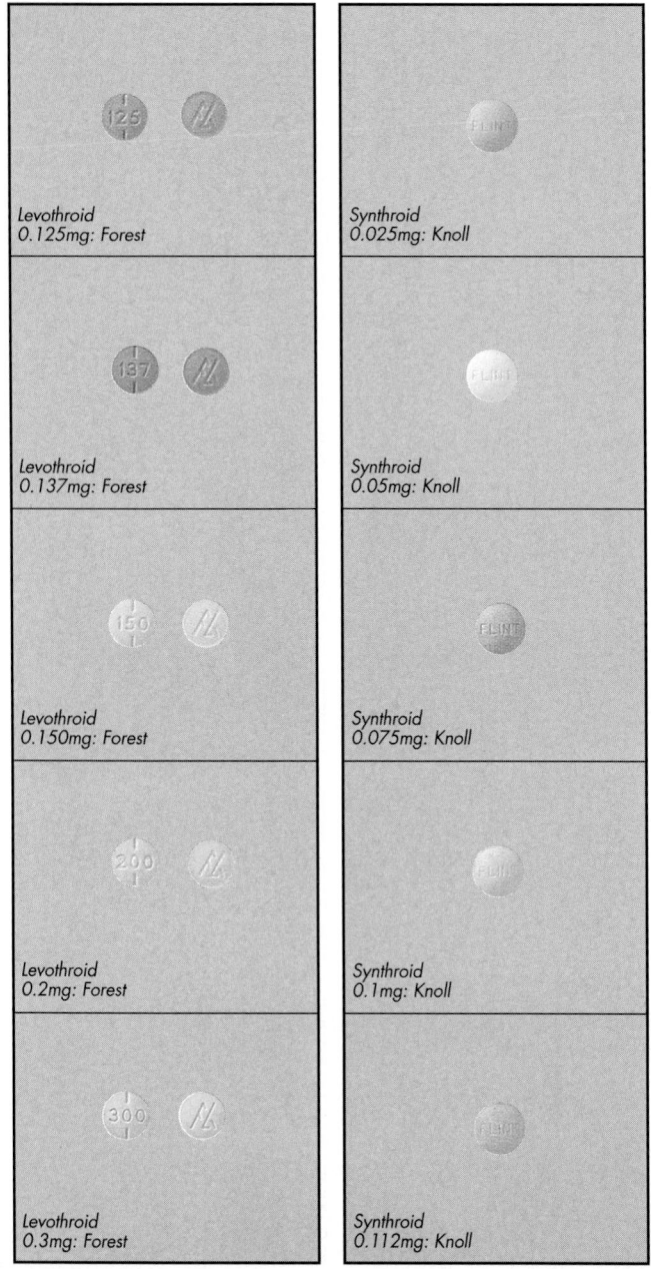

Levothroid
0.125mg: Forest

Synthroid
0.025mg: Knoll

Levothroid
0.137mg: Forest

Synthroid
0.05mg: Knoll

Levothroid
0.150mg: Forest

Synthroid
0.075mg: Knoll

Levothroid
0.2mg: Forest

Synthroid
0.1mg: Knoll

Levothroid
0.3mg: Forest

Synthroid
0.112mg: Knoll

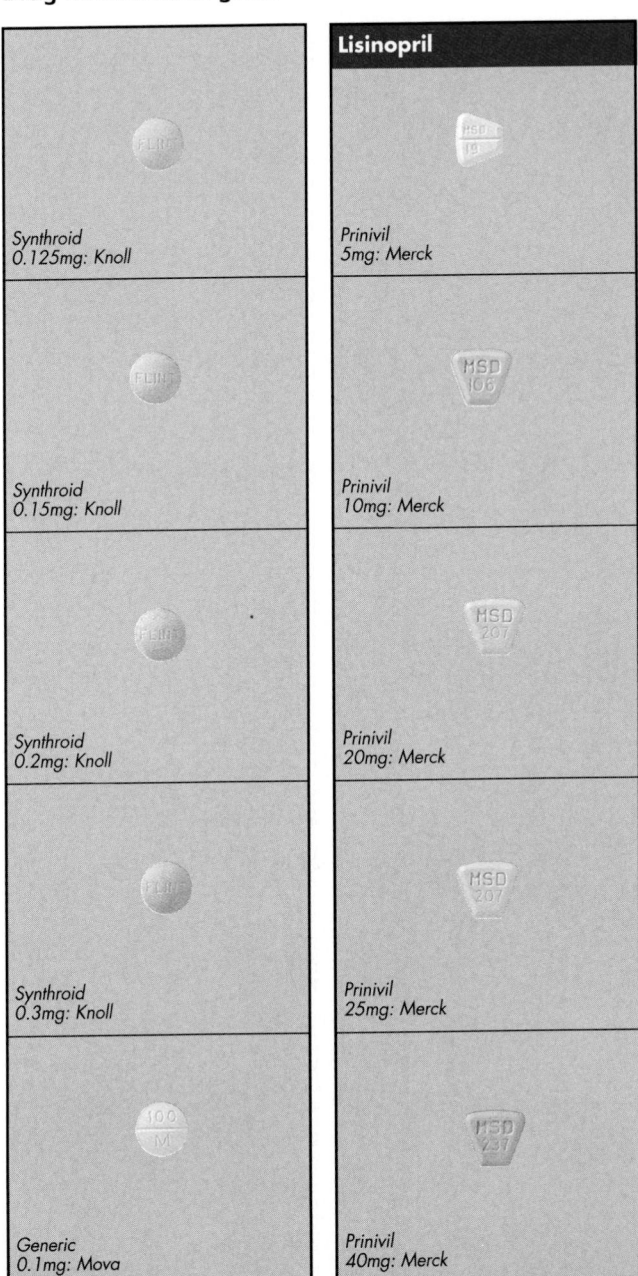

Lisinopril

Synthroid
0.125mg: Knoll

Prinivil
5mg: Merck

Synthroid
0.15mg: Knoll

Prinivil
10mg: Merck

Synthroid
0.2mg: Knoll

Prinivil
20mg: Merck

Synthroid
0.3mg: Knoll

Prinivil
25mg: Merck

Generic
0.1mg: Mova

Prinivil
40mg: Merck

Drug identification guide

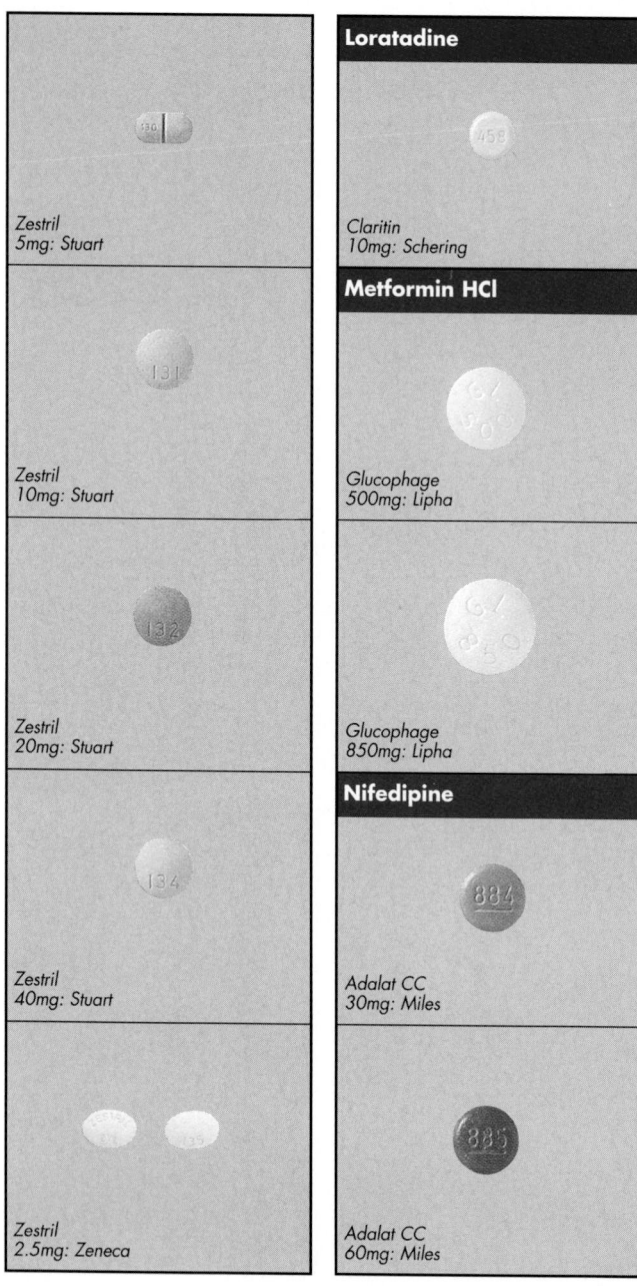

Zestril
5mg: Stuart

Zestril
10mg: Stuart

Zestril
20mg: Stuart

Zestril
40mg: Stuart

Zestril
2.5mg: Zeneca

Loratadine

Claritin
10mg: Schering

Metformin HCl

Glucophage
500mg: Lipha

Glucophage
850mg: Lipha

Nifedipine

Adalat CC
30mg: Miles

Adalat CC
60mg: Miles

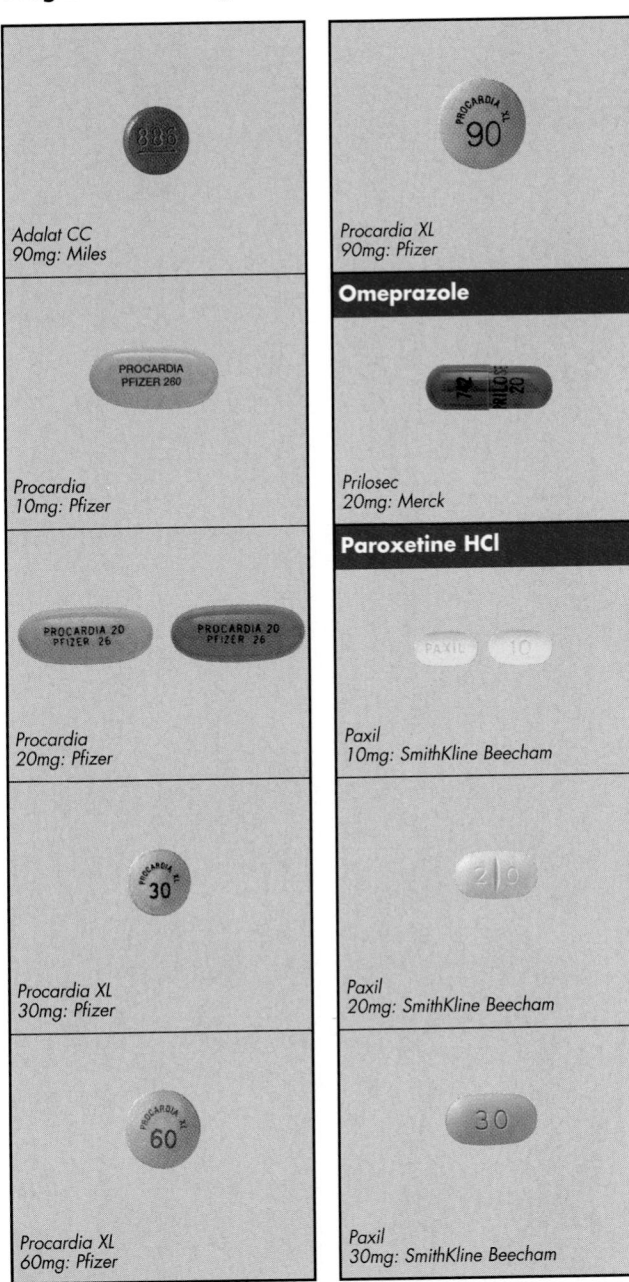

Adalat CC
90mg: Miles

Procardia
10mg: Pfizer

Procardia
20mg: Pfizer

Procardia XL
30mg: Pfizer

Procardia XL
60mg: Pfizer

Procardia XL
90mg: Pfizer

Omeprazole

Prilosec
20mg: Merck

Paroxetine HCl

Paxil
10mg: SmithKline Beecham

Paxil
20mg: SmithKline Beecham

Paxil
30mg: SmithKline Beecham

Drug identification guide

Paxil
40mg: SmithKline Beecham

Penicillin V Potassium

Veetids
250mg: Bristol-Myers Squibb

Veetids
500mg: Bristol-Myers Squibb

V-Cillin K
250mg: Lilly

V-Cillin K
500mg: Lilly

Beepen-VK
250mg: SmithKline Beecham

Beepen-VK
500mg: SmithKline Beecham

Potassium Chloride

Micro-K
600mg: A. H. Robins

Micro-K
750mg: A. H. Robins

K-Dur
750mg: Schering

K-Dur
1500mg: Schering

Klor-Con
600mg: Upsher-Smith

Klor-Con
750mg: Upsher-Smith

Pravastatin

Pravachol
10mg: Bristol-Myers Squibb

Pravachol
20mg: Bristol-Myers Squibb

Pravachol
40mg: Bristol-Myers Squibb

Quinapril HCl

Accupril
10mg: Parke-Davis

Accupril
20mg: Parke-Davis

Ranitidine HCl

Zantac
150mg: Glaxo Wellcome

Zantac
150mg: Glaxo Wellcome

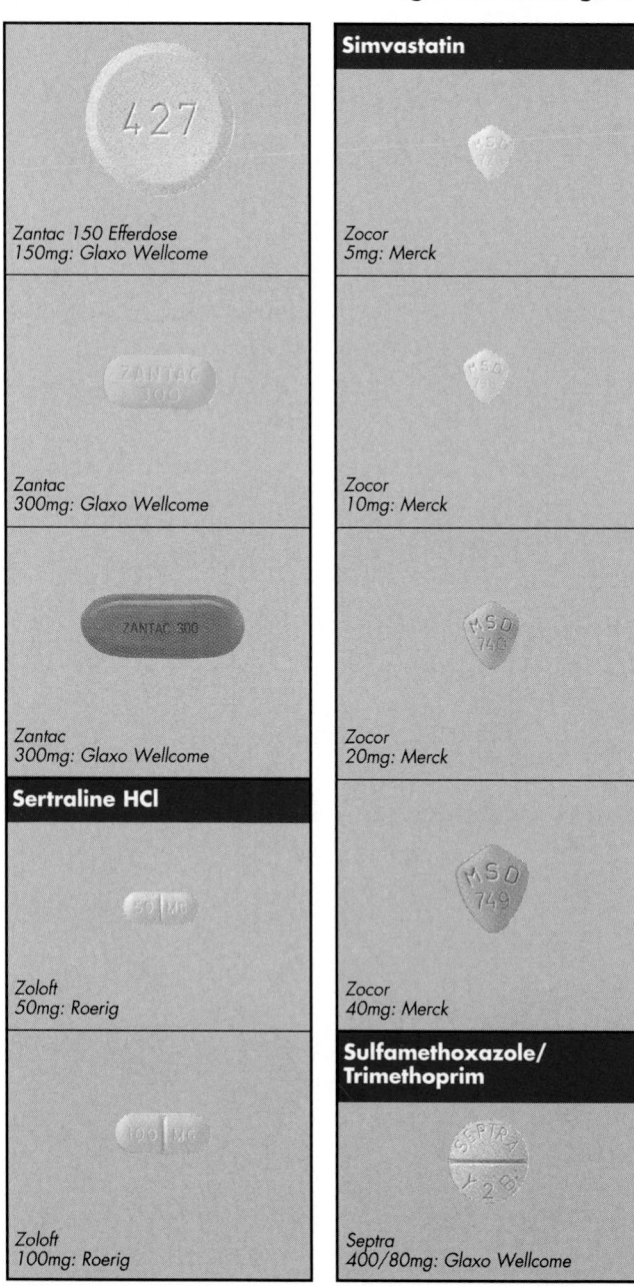

427

Zantac 150 Efferdose
150mg: Glaxo Wellcome

Zantac
300mg: Glaxo Wellcome

Zantac
300mg: Glaxo Wellcome

Sertraline HCl

Zoloft
50mg: Roerig

Zoloft
100mg: Roerig

Simvastatin

Zocor
5mg: Merck

Zocor
10mg: Merck

Zocor
20mg: Merck

Zocor
40mg: Merck

Sulfamethoxazole/
Trimethoprim

Septra
400/80mg: Glaxo Wellcome

Septra
800/160mg: Glaxo Wellcome

Cotrim
800/160mg: Lemmon

Generic
800/160mg: Mutual

Bactrim
400/80mg: Roche

Bactrim DS
800/160mg: Roche

Terazosin HCl

Hytrin
1mg: Abbott

Hytrin
2mg: Abbott

Hytrin
5mg: Abbott

Hytrin
10mg: Abbott

Tramadol HCl

Ultram
50mg: McNeil

Warfarin Sodium

Coumadin
1mg: DuPont

Coumadin
2mg: DuPont

Coumadin
2.5mg: DuPont

Coumadin
3mg: DuPont

Coumadin
4mg: DuPont

Coumadin
5mg: DuPont

Coumadin
7.5mg: DuPont

Coumadin
10mg: DuPont

Zolpidem

Ambien
5mg: Searle

Ambien
10mg: Searle

• That physical dependency may result from extended use

• That drowsiness, dizziness may occur; to call for assistance

• That withdrawal symptoms may occur: nausea, vomiting, cramps, fever, faintness, anorexia

• To make position changes slowly; orthostatic hypotension can occur

• To avoid OTC medications, alcohol unless directed by prescriber

Treatment of overdose: Naloxone (Narcan) 0.2-0.8 mg IV, O_2, IV fluids, vasopressors

---

meprobamate (R)

(me-proe-ba′mate)
Apo-Meprobamate*, Equanil, Meditran*, meprobamate, Meprospan, Miltown, Miltown 400, Miltown 600, Neo-Tran*, Tranhep

Func. class.: Antianxiety/sedative, hypnotic

Chem. class.: Propanediol carbamate derivative

Controlled Substance Schedule IV
Action: Produces widespread depression of the CNS
Uses: Anxiety
Dosage and routes:
• *Adult:* **PO** 1.2-1.6 g/day in 2-3 divided doses, not to exceed 2.4 g/day or 800-1600 mg/day in 2 divided doses (sus rel); max 2.4 g/day
• *Geriatric:* **PO** 200 mg bid-tid, adjust to lowest possible dose
• *Child 6-12 yr:* **PO** 100-200 mg bid-tid or 200 mg (sus rel) bid
Available forms: Tabs 200, 400, 600 mg; caps 400 mg; sus rel caps 200, 400 mg
Side effects/adverse reactions:
HEMA: ***Thrombocytopenia, leukopenia, eosinophilia***

CNS: Dizziness, drowsiness, headache, ***convulsions,*** ataxia
GI: Nausea, vomiting, anorexia, diarrhea, stomatitis
INTEG: Urticaria, pruritus, maculopapular rash
CV: Hypotension, tachycardia, palpitations, ***hyperthermia***
EENT: Blurred vision, tinnitus, mydriasis, slurred speech
Contraindications: Hypersensitivity, renal failure, porphyria, pregnancy (D), history of drug abuse or dependence
Precautions: Suicidal patients, severe depression, renal disease, hepatic disease, elderly
Pharmacokinetics:
PO: Onset 1 hr; metabolized by liver; excreted in urine, in feces, breast milk; crosses placenta; half-life 6-16 hr
Interactions:
• Increased effects of meprobamate: CNS depressants, alcohol, tricyclic antidepressants
Lab test interferences:
False increase: 17-OHCS
False positive: Phentolamine test
NURSING CONSIDERATIONS
Assess:
• Sleep pattern; note sleep apnea, obstructed airway, pain/discomfort, urinary frequency, other circumstances that interrupt sleep
• B/P (lying, standing), pulse; if systolic B/P drops 20 mm Hg, hold drug, notify prescriber
• Blood studies: CBC during long-term therapy; blood dyscrasias have occurred rarely
• Therapeutic blood levels 0.5-2 mg/100 ml
• Hepatic studies: AST, ALT, bilirubin, creatinine, LDH, alk phosphatase
• Mental status: mood, sensorium, affect, drowsiness, dizziness; suicidal tendencies

M

◆ Tolerance, withdrawal symptoms: headache, nausea, vomiting, muscle pain, weakness, hyperthermia, death, convulsions after long-term use

Administer:

PO

• With food, milk for GI symptoms
• Crushed tabs if patient is unable to swallow medication whole
🚫 Do not break, crush, or chew sus rel cap
• Sugarless gum, hard candy, frequent sips of water for dry mouth

Perform/provide:

• Assistance with ambulation during beginning therapy, since drowsiness/dizziness occurs
• Safety measures, side rails
• Check to see if PO medication has been swallowed

Evaluate:

• Therapeutic response: decreased anxiety, restlessness, insomnia

Teach patient/family:

• That drug may be taken with food
• Not to be used for everyday stress or used longer than 4 mo unless directed by prescriber; not to take more than prescribed amount; may be habit forming
• To avoid OTC preparations (alcohol, cold, hay fever) unless approved by prescriber
• To avoid driving, activities that require alertness, since drowsiness may occur
• To avoid alcohol ingestion, other psychotropic medications unless directed by prescriber
• Not to discontinue medication abruptly after long-term use
• To rise slowly or fainting may occur, especially elderly
• That drowsiness may worsen at beginning of treatment

Treatment of overdose: Lavage, VS, supportive care

---

mercaptopurine (℞)

(mer-kap-toe-pyoor'een)

Purinethol, 6-MP

Func. class.: Antineoplastic-antimetabolite

Chem. class.: Purine analog

Action: Inhibits purine metabolism at multiple sites, which inhibits DNA and RNA synthesis, S phase of cell cycle specific

Uses: Chronic myelocytic leukemia, acute lymphoblastic leukemia in children, acute myelogenous leukemia

Investigational uses: Polycythemia vera, psoriatic arthritis, colitis, lymphoma

Dosage and routes:

• *Adult and child:* **PO** 2.5 mg/kg/day, not to exceed 5 mg/kg/day; maintenance 1.5-2.5 mg/kg/day
• *Child:* 70 mg/m^2/day

Available forms: Tabs 50 mg

Side effects/adverse reactions:

CNS: Fever, headache, weakness

*HEMA: **Thrombocytopenia, leukopenia, myelosuppression, anemia***

*GI: Nausea, vomiting, anorexia, diarrhea, stomatitis, **hepatotoxicity** (high doses), jaundice, gastritis*

*GU: **Renal failure,** hyperuricemia, **oliguria,** crystalluria, **hematuria***

INTEG: Rash, dry skin, urticaria

Contraindications: Patients with prior drug resistance, leukopenia (<2500/mm^3), thrombocytopenia (<100,000/mm^3), anemia, pregnancy (D)

Precautions: Renal disease

Pharmacokinetics: Incompletely absorbed when taken orally; metabolized in liver, excreted in urine

Interactions:

• Increased toxicity: radiation or other antineoplastics

◆ = Nursing alert   = Herb-drug interaction   🚫 = Do not crush

• Increased bone marrow depression: allopurinol
• Reversal of neuromuscular blockade: nondepolarizing muscle relaxants

NURSING CONSIDERATIONS
Assess:
• CBC, differential, platelet count qwk; withhold drug if WBC is <3500 or platelet count is <100,000; notify prescriber; drug should be discontinued
• Renal function studies: BUN, serum uric acid, urine CrCl, electrolytes before, during therapy
• I&O ratio; report fall in urine output to <30 ml/hr
• Monitor temp q4h; fever may indicate beginning infection; no rectal temps
• Liver function tests before, during therapy: bilirubin, alk phosphatase, AST, ALT, qwk during beginning therapy
• Bleeding: hematuria, guaiac, bruising, petechiae; mucosa or orifices q8h
• Buccal cavity q8h for dryness, sores, ulceration, white patches, oral pain, bleeding, dysphagia
◆ Symptoms indicating severe allergic reaction: rash, urticaria, itching, flushing
Administer:
• Antacid before oral agent; give drug after evening meal before bedtime
• Allopurinol or sodium bicarbonate to maintain uric acid levels, alkalinization of urine
Perform/provide:
• Strict medical asepsis, protective isolation if WBC levels are low
• Increase fluid intake to 2-3 L/day to prevent urate deposits, calculi formation, unless contraindicated
• Diet low in purines: absence of organ meats (kidney, liver), dried beans, peas to maintain alkaline urine

• Rinsing of mouth tid-qid with water, club soda; brushing of teeth bid-tid with soft brush or cotton-tipped applicators for stomatitis; use unwaxed dental floss
• Nutritious diet with iron, vitamin supplements as ordered
• Storage in tightly closed container in cool environment
Evaluate:
• Therapeutic response: decreased size of tumor, spread of malignancy
Teach patient/family:
• To avoid foods with citric acid, hot or rough texture for stomatitis
• To report stomatitis: any bleeding, white spots, ulcerations in mouth; tell patient to examine mouth qd, report symptoms
• That contraceptive measures are recommended during therapy; to avoid breastfeeding
• To drink 10-12 (8 oz) glasses of fluid/day
• To notify prescriber of fever, chills, sore throat, nausea, vomiting, anorexia, diarrhea, bleeding, bruising, which may indicate blood dyscrasias
• To report signs of infection: fever, sore throat, flulike symptoms
• To report signs of anemia: fatigue, headache, faintness, shortness of breath, irritability
• To report bleeding: avoid use of razors, commercial mouthwash
• To avoid use of aspirin products, NSAIDs

meropenem (℞)
(mer-oh-pen'em)
Merrem IV
Func. class.: Antiinfective-misc.
Chem. class.: Carbapenem

Action: Interferes with cell wall replication of susceptible organisms;

osmotically unstable cell wall swells, bursts from osmotic pressure

Uses: Serious infections caused by gram-positive bacteria: *Streptococcus pneumoniae,* group A β-hemolytic streptococci, enterococcus; gram-negative: *Klebsiella, Proteus, Escherichia coli, Pseudomonas aeruginosa;* appendicitis, peritonitis caused by *viridans* group streptococci; *Bacteroides fragilis, B. thetaiotamicron,* bacterial meningitis (≥3 mo)

Dosage and routes:

Renal disease

• CrCl 26-50 ml/min 1 g q12h; CrCl 10-25 ml/min 500 mg q12h; CrCl <10 ml/min 500 mg q24h

• *Adult:* **IV** 1 g q8h, given over 15-30 min or as an **IV BOL** 5-20 ml given over 3-5 min

• *Child ≥3 mo:* **IV** 20-40 mg/kg q8h (max 2g q8h meningitis)

• *Child >50 kg:* **IV** 1 g q8h (intraabdominal infection) or 2 g q8h (meningitis) given over 15-30 min or as an **IV BOL** 5-20 ml over 3-5 min

Available forms: Inj 500 mg, 1 g

Side effects/adverse reactions:

CNS: Fever, somnolence, *seizures,* dizziness, weakness, myoclonia, *headache*

GI: Diarrhea, nausea, vomiting, *pseudomembranous colitis, hepatitis,* glossitis

CV: Hypotension, palpitations

HEMA: Eosinophilia, neutropenia, decreased Hgb, Hct

INTEG: Rash, urticaria, *pruritus,* pain at injection site, phlebitis, erythema at injection site

SYST: Anaphylaxis

RESP: Chest discomfort, dyspnea, hyperventilation

Contraindications: Hypersensitivity to meropenem or imipenem

Precautions: Pregnancy (B), lactation, elderly, renal disease

Pharmacokinetics:

IV: Onset immediate, peak dose dependent, half-life 1 hr, hepatic metabolism

Interactions:

• Increased meropenem plasma levels: probenecid

Lab test interferences:

Increase: AST, ALT, LDH, BUN, alk phosphatase, bilirubin, creatinine

False positive: Direct Coombs' test

NURSING CONSIDERATIONS

Assess:

• Sensitivity to carbapenem antibiotics, penicillins

• Renal disease: lower dose may be required

• Bowel pattern qd; if severe diarrhea occurs, drug should be discontinued; may indicate pseudomembranous colitis

• For infection: temp, sputum, characteristics of wound, before, during, and after treatment

• Allergic reactions: rash, urticaria, pruritus; may occur few days after therapy begins

• Overgrowth of infection: perineal itching, fever, malaise, redness, pain, swelling, drainage, rash, diarrhea, change in cough, sputum

Administer:

• By IV INF or IV BOL

• After C&S is taken

• Reconstitute with 0.9% NaCl, D₅W, LR, dilute in 5-20 ml comp sol, give by direct IV over 3-5 min; give by intermittent inf, dilute in 5-20 ml of comp sol, give over 15-30 min

Additive compatibilities: Aminophylline, atropine, cimetidine, dexamethasone, dobutamine, dopamine, enalaprilat, fluconazole, furosemide, gentamicin, heparin, insulin (regular), magnesium sulfate, metoclopramide, morphine, norepi-

---

 = Nursing alert   / = Herb-drug interaction   ⊘ = Do not crush nephrine, phenobarbital, ranitidine, vancomycin

Y-site compatibilities: Aminophylline, atenolol, atropine, cimetidine, dexamethasone, digoxin, diphenhydramine, enalaprilat, fluconazole, furosemide, gentamicin, heparin, insulin (regular), metoclopramide, morphine, norepinephrine, phenobarbital, vancomycin

Evaluate:

• Therapeutic response: negative C&S; absence of symptoms and signs of infection

Teach patient/family:

• To report severe diarrhea; may indicate pseudomembranous colitis

• To report sore throat, bruising, bleeding, joint pain; may indicate blood dyscrasias (rare)

• To report overgrowth of infection: black, furry tongue, vaginal itching, foul-smelling stools

Treatment of overdose: Epinephrine, antihistamines; resuscitate if needed (anaphylaxis)

---

mesalamine (℞)

(mez-al'a-meen)
Asacol, Pentasa, Rowasa
Salofalk*

Func. class.: GI antiinflammatory

Chem. class.: 5-aminosalicylic acid

Action: May diminish inflammation by blocking cyclooxygenase, inhibiting prostaglandin production in colon; local action only

Uses: Mild to moderate active distal ulcerative colitis, proctosigmoiditis, proctitis

Dosage and routes:

• *Adult:* **RECT** 60 ml (4 g) hs, retained for 8 hr × 3-6 wk; **PO** 800 mg tid × 6 wk; **SUPP** 500 mg bid × 3-6 wk

Available forms: Rect susp 4 g/60 ml; supp 500 mg; tab del rel 400 mg; con rel cap 250 mg (Pentasa)

Side effects/adverse reactions:

CV: Pericarditis, myocarditis

GI: Cramps, gas, nausea, diarrhea, rectal pain, constipation

CNS: Headache, fever, dizziness, insomnia, asthenia, weakness, fatigue

INTEG: Rash, itching, acne

SYST: Flulike symptoms, malaise, back pain, peripheral edema, leg and joint pain, arthralgia, dysmenorrhea

EENT: Sore throat, cough, pharyngitis, rhinitis

Contraindications: Hypersensitivity to this drug or salicylates

Precautions: Renal disease, pregnancy (B), lactation, children, sulfite sensitivity

Pharmacokinetics:

RECT: Primarily excreted in feces but some in urine as metabolite; half-life 1 hr, metabolite half-life 5-10 hr

NURSING CONSIDERATIONS

Assess:

• GI symptoms: cramps, gas, nausea, diarrhea, rectal pain; if severe, drug should be discontinued

• Renal function prior to treatment

Administer:

• May give orally; tabs should be swallowed whole

• Rectally; drug should be given hs, retained until morning

Perform/provide:

• Storage at room temp

Evaluate:

• Therapeutic response: absence of pain, bleeding from GI tract, decrease in number of diarrhea stools

Teach patient/family:

• That usual course of therapy is 3-6 wk

• To shake bottle well

• Method of rectal administration

• To inform prescriber of GI symptoms

🚫 Not to break, crush, or chew tabs

• To report abdominal cramping, pain, diarrhea with blood, headache, fever, rash, chest pain; drug should be discontinued

---

mesoridazine (℞)

(mez-oh-rid′a-zeen)
Serentil
Func. class.: Antipsychotic, neuroleptic
Chem. class.: Phenothiazine, piperidine

Action: Depresses cerebral cortex, hypothalamus, limbic system, which control activity, aggression; blocks neurotransmission produced by dopamine at synapse; exhibits strong α-adrenergic, anticholinergic blocking action; mechanism for antipsychotic effects is unclear

Uses: Psychotic disorders, schizophrenia, anxiety, alcoholism, behavioral problems in mental deficiency, chronic brain syndrome

Dosage and routes:
Schizophrenia
• *Adult:* **PO** 50 mg tid, optimum dose 100-400 mg/day; **IM** 25 mg may repeat ½-1 hr; dosage range 25-200 mg/day
Behavior problems
• *Adult:* **PO** 25 mg tid; optimum dose 75-300 mg/day
• *Geriatric:* **PO** 10 mg qd-bid, increase q3-7days by 10-25 mg to desired dose
Alcoholism
• *Adult:* **PO** 25 mg bid; optimum dose 50-200 mg/day
Schizoaffective disorders
• *Adult:* **PO** 10 mg tid; optimum dose 30-150 mg/day
Available forms: Tabs 10, 25, 50, 100 mg; conc 25 mg/ml; inj 25 mg/ml

Side effects/adverse reactions:
RESP: **Laryngospasm,** dyspnea, **respiratory depression**
CNS: EPS: pseudoparkinsonism, akathisia, dystonia, tardive dyskinesia, drowsiness, headache
HEMA: **Anemia, leukopenia, leukocytosis, agranulocytosis**
INTEG: **Rash,** photosensitivity, dermatitis
EENT: Blurred vision, glaucoma
GI: Dry mouth, nausea, vomiting, anorexia, constipation, diarrhea, jaundice, weight gain
GU: Urinary retention, urinary frequency, enuresis, impotence, amenorrhea, gynecomastia
CV: Orthostatic hypotension, hypertension, **cardiac arrest,** ECG changes, tachycardia
Contraindications: Hypersensitivity, circulatory collapse, liver damage, cerebral arteriosclerosis, coronary disease, severe hypertension/hypotension, blood dyscrasias, coma, brain damage, bone marrow depression, narrow-angle glaucoma
Precautions: Pregnancy (C), lactation, seizure disorders, hypertension, hepatic disease, cardiac disease, prostatic hypertrophy, intestinal obstruction, respiratory conditions
Pharmacokinetics:
PO: Onset erratic, peak 2 hr, duration 4-6 hr
IM: Onset 15-30 min, peak 30 min, duration 6-8 hr
Metabolized by liver, excreted in urine, crosses placenta, enters breast milk
Interactions:
• Oversedation: other CNS depressants, alcohol, barbiturate anesthetics
• Decreased absorption: aluminum hydroxide, magnesium hydroxide antacids

---

◆ = Nursing alert 🖋 = Herb-drug interaction 🚫 = Do not crush

• Increased anticholinergic effects: anticholinergics

🖋 Increased anticholinergic effect: henbane

Lab test interferences:

Increase: Liver function tests, cardiac enzymes, cholesterol, blood glucose, prolactin, bilirubin, PBI, cholinesterase, [131]I

Decrease: Hormones (blood, urine)

False positive: Pregnancy tests, PKU

False negative: Urinary steroids, 17-OHCS

NURSING CONSIDERATIONS
Assess:

• Mental status before initial administration

• Swallowing of PO medication; check for hoarding or giving to other patients

• I&O ratio; palpate bladder if low urinary output occurs

• Bilirubin, CBC, liver function studies monthly

• Urinalysis is recommended before, during prolonged therapy

• Affect, orientation, LOC, reflexes, gait, coordination, sleep pattern disturbances

• B/P standing and lying, pulse, respirations q4h during initial treatment; establish baseline before starting treatment; report drops of 30 mm Hg

• Dizziness, faintness, palpitations, tachycardia on rising

• EPS including akathisia (inability to sit still, no pattern to movements), tardive dyskinesia (bizarre movements of jaw, mouth, tongue, extremities), pseudoparkinsonism (rigidity, tremors, pill rolling, shuffling gait)

◆ For neuroleptic malignant syndrome: hyperthermia, altered mental status, muscle rigidity, increased CPK

• Constipation, urinary retention daily; if these occur, increase bulk, water in diet

Administer:

• Antiparkinsonian agent after securing order from prescriber for EPS

• Concentrate mixed in distilled water, orange, grape juice; do not prepare, store bulk dilutions

• IM inj into large muscle mass; do not use if precipitate present

• Lowest possible dose to elderly to minimize side effects

Perform/provide:

• Decreased sensory input by dimming lights, avoiding loud noises

• Supervised ambulation until stabilized on medication; do not involve in strenuous exercise program because fainting is possible; patient should not stand still for long periods

• Dose reduction in patients treated for behavior problems

• Increased fluids to prevent constipation

• Sips of water, candy, gum for dry mouth

• Storage in airtight, light-resistant container

Evaluate:

• Therapeutic response: decrease in emotional excitement, hallucinations, delusions, paranoia, and reorganization of patterns of thought, speech

Teach patient/family:

• That orthostatic hypotension is common and to rise from sitting or lying position gradually; to avoid hazardous activities until stabilized on medication

• To remain lying down for at least 30 min after IM injection

• To avoid hot tubs, hot showers, tub baths; hypotension may occur

• To avoid abrupt withdrawal of mesoridazine, or EPS may result; drug should be withdrawn slowly

• To avoid OTC preparations (cough,

M

hay fever, cold) unless approved by prescriber; serious drug interactions may occur; to avoid use with alcohol, CNS depressants; increased drowsiness may occur

• To use sunscreen during sun exposure to prevent burns

• Regarding compliance with drug regimen

• About necessity for meticulous oral hygiene, since oral candidiasis may occur

• To report sore throat, malaise, fever, bleeding, mouth sores; if these occur, a CBC should be drawn and drug discontinued

• That in hot weather heat stroke may occur; take extra precautions to stay cool

Treatment of overdose: Lavage if orally ingested; provide an airway; *do not induce vomiting*

---

metaproterenol (℞)
(met-a-proe-ter'e-nole)
Alupent, Arm-A-Med, Metaproterenol Sulfate, Metaprel
Func. class.: Bronchodilator-selective β_2-agonist

Action: Relaxes bronchial smooth muscle by direct action on β_2-adrenergic receptors with increased levels of cAMP with increased bronchodilation, diuresis, cardiac CNS stimulation

Uses: Bronchial asthma, bronchospasm

Dosage and routes:

• *Adult and child >12 yr:* **INH** 2-3 puffs; may repeat q3-4h, not to exceed 12 puffs/day

• *Adult:* **PO** 20 mg q6-8h

• *Geriatric:* **PO** 10 mg tid-qid, initially

• *Child >9 yr or >27 kg:* **PO** 20 mg q6-8h or 0.4-0.9 mg/kg tid

• *Child 6-9 yr or <27 kg:* **PO** 10 mg q6-8h or 0.4-0.9 mg/kg tid

• *Child 2-6 yr:* **PO** 1.3-2.6 mg/kg divided q6-8h

Available forms: Tabs 10, 20 mg; aerosol 0.65 mg/dose; syrup 10 mg/5 ml; sol for inh 0.4%, 0.6%, 5%

Side effects/adverse reactions:

CNS: Tremors, anxiety, insomnia, headache, dizziness, stimulation

CV: Palpitations, tachycardia, hypertension, dysrhythmias, *cardiac arrest*

GI: Nausea, vomiting

RESP: Paradoxical bronchospasm

Contraindications: Hypersensitivity to sympathomimetics, narrow-angle glaucoma

Precautions: Pregnancy (C), cardiac disorders, hyperthyroidism, diabetes mellitus, prostatic hypertrophy

Pharmacokinetics: Well absorbed (PO)

PO: Onset 15-30 min, peak 1 hr, duration 4 hr, excreted in urine as metabolites

INH: Onset 5 min, peak 1 hr, duration 4 hr

Interactions:

• Increased effects of both drugs: other sympathomimetics

• Decreased action of β-blockers, oral hypoglycemics

• Hypertensive crisis: MAOIs

🖋 Increased effect: ephedra

Lab test interferences:

Decrease: K

NURSING CONSIDERATIONS

Assess:

• Respiratory function: vital capacity, forced expiratory volume, ABGs; also B/P; lung sounds, secretions before and after treatment

• Tolerance over long-term therapy; dose may have to be changed; check for rebound bronchospasm

---

⬥ = Nursing alert   🖋 = Herb-drug interaction   🚫 = Do not crush

Administer:
• 2 hr before hs to avoid sleeplessness
• PO with food for GI upset

Perform/provide:
• Storage at room temp; do not use discolored sol
• Spacer device for elderly

Evaluate:
• Therapeutic response: absence of dyspnea, wheezing; improved ABGs

Teach patient/family:
• To increase fluid intake (2-3 L/day) to liquefy secretions
• Not to use OTC medications; excess stimulation may occur
• To notify prescriber of headaches, chest pain, weakness, dizziness, anxiety
• Use of inhaler; review package insert with patient
• To avoid getting aerosol in eyes
• To wash inhaler in warm water and dry qd
• All aspects of drug; avoid smoking, smoke-filled rooms, persons with respiratory infections

---

metformin (Ŗ)

(met-for′min)
Glucophage
Func. class.: Antidiabetic, oral
Chem. class.: Biguanide

Action: Inhibits hepatic glucose production and increases sensitivity of peripheral tissue to insulin

Uses: Stable adult-onset diabetes mellitus (NIDDM)

Dosage and routes:
• *Adult:* PO 500 mg bid initially, then increase to desired response 1-3 g; dosage adjustment q2-3wk or 850 mg qd with morning meal with dosage increased every other wk, max 2550 mg/day

Available forms: Tabs 500, 850 mg

Side effects/adverse reactions:
CNS: Headache, weakness, dizziness, drowsiness, tinnitus, fatigue, vertigo, *agitation*
GI: Nausea, vomiting, diarrhea, heartburn, anorexia, metallic taste
HEMA: **Thrombocytopenia,** decreased vit B$_{12}$ concentration
INTEG: Rash
ENDO: **Lactic acidosis,** hypoglycemia

Contraindications: Hypersensitivity, hepatic, renal disease, alcoholism, cardiopulmonary disease, history of lactic acidosis

Precautions: Previous hypersensitivity to phenformin or buformin, pregnancy (B), elderly, thyroid disease, CHF, renal disease

Pharmacokinetics: Excreted by the kidneys unchanged 35%-50%, half-life 1½-5 hr, terminal 9-17 hr, peak 1-3 hr

Interactions:
• Increased risk of lactic acidosis, ethanol, glucocorticoids
• Increased blood glucose levels: acetazolamide
• Increased hypoglycemia: cimetidine
• Do not give with iodinated contrast media; may cause renal failure

NURSING CONSIDERATIONS
Assess:
• For hypoglycemic reactions (sweating, weakness, dizziness, anxiety, tremors, hunger), hyperglycemic reactions soon after meals
• CBC (baseline, q3mo) during treatment; check liver function tests periodically AST, LDH, renal studies: BUN, creatinine during treatment
• For lactic acidosis: malaise, myalgia, abdominal distress; risk increases with age, poor renal function

Administer:
PO
• Twice a day given with meals to

M

Side effects: *italics* = common; **bold italics** = life-threatening

decrease GI upset and provide best absorption
• Tabs crushed and mixed with meal or fluids for patients with difficulty swallowing
Perform/provide:
• Conversion from other oral hypoglycemic agents; change may be made without gradual dosage change; monitor serum or urine glucose and ketones tid during conversion
• Storage in tight container in cool environment
Evaluate:
• Therapeutic response: decrease in polyuria, polydipsia, polyphagia; clear sensorium; absence of dizziness; stable gait, blood glucose at normal level
Teach patient/family:
• To use capillary glucose test or Chemstrip tid
• The symptoms of hypo/hyperglycemia, what to do about each
• That drug must be continued on daily basis; explain consequence of discontinuing drug abruptly
• To avoid OTC medications unless approved by prescriber
• That diabetes is a lifelong illness; that this drug is not a cure; only controls symptoms
• That all food included in diet plan must be eaten to prevent hypoglycemia
• To carry Medic Alert ID and glucagon emergency kit for emergencies
Treatment of overdose: Glucose 25 g IV via dextrose 50% sol, 50 ml or 1 mg glucagon

---

methadone (℞)
(meth′a-done)
Dolophine, methadone, Methadose
Func. class.: Opiate analgesic
Chem. class.: Synthetic diphenylheptane derivative

Controlled Substance Schedule II
Action: Depresses pain impulse transmission at the spinal cord level by interacting with opioid receptors, produce CNS depression
Uses: Severe pain, opiate withdrawal
Dosage and routes:
Pain
• *Adult:* **PO/SC/IM** 2.5-10 mg q4-12h prn
Opiate withdrawal
• *Adult:* **PO** 15-40 mg/day individualized initially, then 20-120 mg/day titrated to patient response
• *Child:* 0.05-0.1 mg/kg/dose q6-12h
Renal disease
• CrCl 10-50 ml/min dose q8h; CrCl <10 ml/min dose q8-12h
Available forms: Inj 10 mg/ml; tabs 5, 10 mg; oral sol 5, 10 mg/5 ml; dispersible tabs 40 mg; oral conc 10 mg/ml
Side effects/adverse reactions:
CNS: Drowsiness, dizziness, confusion, headache, sedation, euphoria
GI: Nausea, vomiting, anorexia, constipation, cramps, biliary tract spasm
GU: Increased urinary output, dysuria, urinary retention
INTEG: Rash, urticaria, bruising, flushing, diaphoresis, pruritus
EENT: Tinnitus, blurred vision, miosis, diplopia
CV: Palpitations, bradycardia, change in B/P
*RESP: **Respiratory depression***

◆ = Nursing alert   ⫽ = Herb-drug interaction   ⃠ = Do not crush

Contraindications: Hypersensitivity to this drug or chlorobutanol (inj), addiction (opiate)

Precautions: Addictive personality, pregnancy (B), lactation, increased intracranial pressure, MI (acute), severe heart disease, respiratory depression, hepatic disease, renal disease, children <18 yr, elderly

Pharmacokinetics:

PO: Onset 30-60 min, peak 1½-2 hr, duration 6-8 hr, cumulative 22-48hr

SC/IM: Onset 10-20 min, peak 1½-2 hr, duration 4-6 hr, cumulative 22-48 hr

Metabolized by liver; excreted by kidneys; crosses placenta; excreted in breast milk; half-life 15-30 hr, extended interval with continued dosing; 90% bound to plasma proteins

Interactions:

• Increased effects with other CNS depressants: alcohol, opiates, sedative/hypnotics, antipsychotics, skeletal muscle relaxants, rifampin, phenytoin

• Unpredictable reactions: MAOIs, do not use together

Lab test interferences:

Increase: Amylase

NURSING CONSIDERATIONS

Assess:

• For pain: type, location, intensity, grimacing before and 1½-2 hr after administration; use pain scoring

• I&O ratio; check for decreasing output; may indicate urinary retention

• CNS changes: dizziness, drowsiness, hallucinations, euphoria, LOC, pupil reaction

• Allergic reactions: rash, urticaria

• Respiratory dysfunction: respiratory depression, character, rate, rhythm; notify prescriber if respirations are <10/min

Administer:

• With antiemetic if nausea/vomiting occurs

• When pain is beginning to return; determine dosage interval by patient response

• Rotating inj sites, give deep in large muscle mass (IM)

Perform/provide:

• Storage in light-resistant container at room temp

• Assistance with ambulation

• Safety measures: night-light, call bell within easy reach

Evaluate:

• Therapeutic response: decrease in pain, successful opiate withdrawal

Teach patient/family:

• To report any symptoms of CNS changes, allergic reactions

• That physical dependency may result from extended use

◆ Withdrawal symptoms may occur: nausea, vomiting, cramps, fever, faintness, anorexia

Treatment of overdose: Naloxone (Narcan) 0.2-0.8 mg IV, O$_2$, IV fluids, vasopressors

M

---

methamphetamine (R)

(meth-am-fet'a-meen)

Desoxyn, Desoxyn Gradumet

Func. class.: Cerebral stimulant

Chem. class.: Amphetamine

Controlled Substance Schedule II

Action: Increases release of norepinephrine and dopamine in cerebral cortex to reticular activating system

Uses: Exogenous obesity, minimal brain dysfunction, attention deficit disorder with hyperactivity

Dosage and routes:

Attention deficit disorder

• *Child >6 yr:* **PO** 2.5-5 mg qd or bid increasing by 5 mg/wk

Obesity
• *Adult:* **PO** 2.5-5 mg, 30 min ac or 10-15 mg long-acting tab qd in AM
Available forms: Tabs 5 mg; tabs long-acting 5, 10, 15 mg
Side effects/adverse reactions:
CNS: Hyperactivity, insomnia, restlessness, talkativeness, dizziness, headache, chills, stimulation, dysphoria, irritability, aggressiveness, tremor
GI: Anorexia, dry mouth, diarrhea, constipation, weight loss, metallic taste, cramps
GU: Impotence, change in libido
CV: Palpitations, **tachycardia,** hypertension, decreased heart rate, **dysrhythmia**
INTEG: Urticaria
Contraindications: Hypersensitivity to sympathomimetic amines, hyperthyroidism, hypertension, glaucoma hypertrophy, severe arteriosclerosis, drug abuse, cardiovascular disease, anxiety
Precautions: Gilles de la Tourette's disorder, pregnancy (C), lactation, child <3 yr
Pharmacokinetics:
PO: Duration 3-6 hr, metabolized by liver, excreted by kidneys, crosses blood-brain barrier
Interactions:
• Hypertensive crisis: MAOIs or within 14 days of MAOIs
• Increased effect of methamphetamine: acetazolamide, antacids, sodium bicarbonate
• Decreased effects of methamphetamine: barbiturates, tricyclics, ascorbic acid, ammonium chloride
• Decreased effect of guanethidine
NURSING CONSIDERATIONS
Assess:
• VS, B/P; may reverse antihypertensives; check patients with cardiac disease more often

• CBC, urinalysis, in diabetes: blood sugar, urine sugar; insulin changes may have to be made, since eating will decrease
• Height, growth rate in children; growth rate may be decreased
• Mental status: mood, sensorium, affect, stimulation, insomnia, aggressiveness
• Physical dependency: should not be used for extended time; dose should be discontinued gradually; tolerance will occur (long-term use)
◆ Withdrawal symptoms: headache, nausea, vomiting, muscle pain, weakness
• Weight per regimen protocol
Administer:
• At least 6 hr before hs to avoid sleeplessness
• For obesity only if patient is on program including dietary changes, exercise; patient will develop tolerance; loss of weight won't occur without additional methods; give 2 hr before meals
• Gum, hard candy, or frequent sips of water for dry mouth
Evaluate:
• Therapeutic response: decreased weight, decreased hyperactivity
Teach patient/family:
• To decrease caffeine consumption (coffee, tea, cola, chocolate), which may increase irritability, stimulation
• To avoid OTC preparations unless approved by prescriber
• To taper off drug over several wk, or depression, increased sleeping, lethargy may ensue
• To avoid alcohol ingestion
• To avoid hazardous activities until patient is stabilized on medication
• To get needed rest; patients will feel more tired at end of day
🚫 Not to break, crush, or chew sus rel forms

◆ = Nursing alert   🌿 = Herb-drug interaction   🚫 = Do not crush

Treatment of overdose: Administer fluids, hemodialysis or peritoneal dialysis; antihypertensive for increased B/P; ammonium Cl for increased excretion

---

methantheline (R)

(meth-an'tha-leen)
Banthine
Func. class.: GI anticholinergic
Chem. class.: Synthetic quaternary ammonium antimuscarinic

Action: Inhibits muscarinic actions of acetylcholine at postganglionic parasympathetic neuroeffector sites

Uses: Treatment of peptic ulcer disease, irritable bowel syndrome, pancreatitis, gastritis, biliary dyskinesia, pylorospasm, reflex neurogenic bladder in children

Dosage and routes:
• *Adult:* **PO** 50-100 mg q6h
• *Child >1 yr:* **PO** 12.5-50 mg qid
• *Child <1 yr:* **PO** 12.5-25 mg qid
• *Neonate:* **PO** 12.5 mg bid-tid
Available forms: Tabs 50 mg

Side effects/adverse reactions:
CNS: Confusion, stimulation in elderly, headache, insomnia, dizziness, drowsiness, anxiety, weakness, hallucination
GI: Dry mouth, constipation, paralytic ileus, heartburn, nausea, vomiting, dysphagia, absence of taste
GU: Urinary hesitancy, retention, impotence
CV: Palpitations, tachycardia
EENT: Blurred vision, photophobia, mydriasis, cycloplegia, increased ocular tension
INTEG: Urticaria, rash, pruritus, anhidrosis, fever, allergic reactions

Contraindications: Hypersensitivity to anticholinergics, narrow-angle glaucoma, GI obstruction, myasthenia gravis, paralytic ileus, GI atony, toxic megacolon

Precautions: Hyperthyroidism, coronary artery disease, dysrhythmias, CHF, ulcerative colitis, hypertension, hiatal hernia, hepatic disease, renal disease, pregnancy (C), urinary retention, prostatic hypertrophy, elderly

Pharmacokinetics:
PO: Onset 30-45 min, duration 4-6 hr; metabolized by liver, excreted in urine, bile

Interactions:
• Increased anticholinergic effect: amantadine, tricyclic antidepressants, MAOIs, H_1-antihistamines
• Increased effect of nitrofurantoin
• Decreased effect of phenothiazines, levodopa

NURSING CONSIDERATIONS
Assess:
• VS, cardiac status: check for dysrhythmias, increased rate, palpitations
• I&O ratio; check for urinary retention, hesitancy
• GI complaints: pain, bleeding (frank or occult), nausea, vomiting, anorexia

Administer:
• ½-1 hr ac for better absorption
• Decreased dose to elderly patients; metabolism may be slowed
• Gum, hard candy, frequent rinsing of mouth for dryness of oral cavity

Perform/provide:
• Storage in tight container protected from light
• Increased fluids, bulk, exercise to decrease constipation

Evaluate:
• Therapeutic response: absence of epigastric pain, bleeding, nausea, vomiting

Teach patient/family:
• To avoid driving, other hazardous activities until stabilized on medication

M

• To avoid alcohol, other CNS depressants; will enhance sedating properties of this drug
• That drug may cause blurred vision

---

methazolamide (℞)
(meth-a-zoe′la-mide)
Neptazane
Func. class.: Carbonic anhydrase inhibitor diuretic
Chem. class.: Sulfonamide derivative

Action: Decreases production of aqueous humor in eye, which lowers intraocular pressure

Uses: Open-angle glaucoma or preoperatively in narrow-angle glaucoma; can be used with miotic, osmotic agents

Dosage and routes:
• *Adult:* **PO** 50-100 mg bid or tid
Available forms: Tabs 25, 50 mg

Side effects/adverse reactions:
GU: Urinary frequency, hypokalemia, polyuria, uremia, *glucosuria, hematuria,* dysuria, renal calculi
CNS: Drowsiness, paresthesia, anxiety, depression, headache, dizziness, confusion, stimulation, fatigue, *convulsions,* sedation, nervousness
GI: Nausea, vomiting, anorexia, constipation, diarrhea, melena, weight loss, *hepatic insufficiency,* metallic taste in mouth
EENT: Myopia
INTEG: Rash, pruritus, urticaria, fever, photosensitivity, *Stevens-Johnson syndrome*
ENDO: Hyperglycemia
HEMA: Aplastic anemia, hemolytic anemia, leukopenia, agranulocytosis, thrombocytopenia, purpura, pancytopenia

Contraindications: Hypersensitivity to sulfonamides, severe renal disease, severe hepatic disease, electrolyte imbalances (hyponatremia, hypokalemia), hyperchloremic acidosis, Addison's disease, COPD

Precautions: Hypercalciuria, pregnancy (C), diabetes mellitus

Pharmacokinetics:
PO: Onset 2-4 hr, peak 6-8 hr, duration 10-18 hr; excreted in urine, crosses placenta

Interactions:
• Decreased effectiveness of lithium, barbiturates
• Hypokalemia: with other diuretics, corticosteroids, amphotericin B
• Increased toxicity: salicylates, methazolamide

Lab test interferences:
False positive: Urinary protein

NURSING CONSIDERATIONS
Assess:
• Weight, I&O daily to determine fluid loss; effect of drug may be decreased if used qd
• Rate, depth, rhythm of respiration, effect of exertion
• B/P lying, standing; postural hypotension may occur
• Electrolytes: K, Na, Cl; include BUN, blood sugar, CBC, serum creatinine, blood pH, ABGs, liver function tests
• Signs of metabolic acidosis: drowsiness, restlessness
• Signs of hypokalemia: postural hypotension, malaise, fatigue, tachycardia, leg cramps, weakness
• Rashes, temp qd
• Confusion, especially in elderly; take safety precautions if needed

Administer:
• In AM to avoid sleeplessness
• K replacement if <3 mg/dl
• With food if nausea occurs; absorption may be decreased slightly

Evaluate:
• Therapeutic response: decrease in aqueous humor

◆ = Nursing alert   🖉 = Herb-drug interaction   🚫 = Do not crush

Teach patient/family:
• To increase fluid intake to 2-3 L/day unless contraindicated; to rise slowly from lying or sitting position
• To use sunscreen for photosensitivity
• To notify prescriber of sore throat, unusual bleeding, bruising, paresthesias, tremors, flank pain, or skin rash
• To avoid hazardous activities if drowsiness occurs

Treatment of overdose: Lavage if taken orally; monitor electrolytes; administer dextrose in saline; monitor hydration, CV, renal status

---

methimazole (℞)
(meth-im′a-zole)
Tapazole
Func. class.: Thyroid hormone antagonist (antithyroid)
Chem. class.: Thioamide

Action: Inhibits synthesis of thyroid hormones by decreasing iodine use in manufacture of thyroglobin and iodothyronine; does not affect already formed hormones

Uses: Hyperthyroidism, preparation for thyroidectomy, thyrotoxic crisis, thyroid storm

Dosage and routes:
Hyperthyroidism
• *Adult:* PO 5-20 mg tid depending on severity of condition; continue until euthyroid; maintenance dose 5-10 mg qd-tid, maximal dose 150 mg qd
• *Child:* PO 0.4 mg/kg/day in divided doses q8h; continue until euthyroid; maintenance dose 0.2 mg/kg/day in divided doses q8h
Preparation and thyroidectomy
• *Adult and child:* PO same as above; iodine may be added × 10 days before surgery

Thyrotoxic crisis
• *Adult and child:* PO same as hyperthyroidism with iodine and propranolol
Available forms: Tabs 5, 10 mg

Side effects/adverse reactions:
ENDO: Enlarged thyroid
INTEG: Rash, urticaria, pruritus, alopecia, hyperpigmentation, lupus-like syndrome
*GU: **Nephritis***
CNS: Drowsiness, headache, vertigo, fever, paresthesias, neuritis
*HEMA: **Agranulocytosis, leukopenia, thrombocytopenia, hypothrombinemia, lymphadenopathy,*** bleeding, vasculitis
*GI: Nausea, diarrhea, vomiting, **jaundice, hepatitis,*** loss of taste
MS: Myalgia, arthralgia, nocturnal muscle cramps

Contraindications: Hypersensitivity, pregnancy (D), lactation
Precautions: Infection, bone marrow depression, hepatic disease
Pharmacokinetics:
PO: Onset 1 wk, duration is up to 10 wk, half-life 1-2 hr; excreted in urine, breast milk; crosses placenta
Interactions:
• Increased bone marrow depression: radiation, antineoplastic agents
• Decreased effectiveness: amiodarone, potassium iodide
• Agranulocytosis: phenothiazines
• Altered response to digitalis, warfarin
Lab test interferences:
Increase: Pro-time, AST, ALT, alk phosphatase

NURSING CONSIDERATIONS
Assess:
• Pulse, B/P, temp
• I&O ratio; check for edema: puffy hands, feet, periorbits; indicate hypothyroidism
• Weight qd; same clothing, scale, time of day

M

• T_3, T_4, which are increased; serum TSH, which is decreased; free thyroxine index, which is increased if dosage is too low; discontinue drug 3-4 wk before RAIU

• Blood work: CBC for blood dyscrasias: leukopenia, thrombocytopenia, agranulocytosis; LFTs

⬥ Overdose: peripheral edema, heat intolerance, diaphoresis, palpitations, dysrhythmias, severe tachycardia, fever, delirium, CNS irritability

• Hypersensitivity: rash, enlarged cervical lymph nodes; drug may have to be discontinued

• Hypoprothrombinemia: bleeding, petechiae, ecchymosis

• Clinical response: after 3 wk should include increased weight, pulse; decreased T_4

• Bone marrow depression: sore throat, fever, fatigue

Administer:
• With meals to decrease GI upset
• At same time each day to maintain drug level
• Lowest dose that relieves symptoms; discontinue before RAIU

Perform/provide:
• Storage in light-resistant container
• Fluids to 3-4 L/day, unless contraindicated

Evaluate:
• Therapeutic response: weight gain, decreased pulse, decreased T_4, B/P

Teach patient/family:
• Not to breastfeed
• To take pulse daily
• To report redness, swelling, sore throat, mouth lesions, fever, which indicate blood dyscrasias
• To keep graph of weight, pulse, mood
• To avoid OTC products that contain iodine
• That seafood, other iodine products may be restricted
• Not to discontinue this medica-

tion abruptly; thyroid crisis may occur; stress patient response

• That response may take several mo if thyroid is large

• The symptoms and signs of overdose: periorbital edema, cold intolerance, mental depression

• The symptoms of inadequate dose: tachycardia, diarrhea, fever, irritability

---

methocarbamol (℞)

(meth-oh-kar′ba-mole)
Carbacot, methocarbamol,
Robaxin
Func. class.: Skeletal muscle relaxant, central acting
Chem. class.: Carbamate derivative

Action: Depresses multisynaptic pathways in the spinal cord, causing skeletal muscle relaxation

Uses: Adjunct for relief of spasm and pain in musculoskeletal conditions, tetanus management

Dosage and routes:

Pain
• *Adult:* **PO** 1.5 g × 2-3 days, then 1 g qid; **IM** 500 mg in each gluteal region, may repeat q8h; **IV BOL** 1-3 g/day at 3 ml/min; **IV INF** 1 g/ 250 ml D_5W or NS, not to exceed 3 g/day

• *Geriatric:* **PO** 500 mg qid, titrate to needed dose

Tetanus
• *Adult:* **IV INF** 1-3 g/L of solution q6h; **IV BOL** 1-2 g injected into running **IV**

• *Child:* **IV** 15 mg/kg q6h

Available forms: Tabs 500, 750 mg; inj 100 mg/ml

Side effects/adverse reactions:

CNS: Dizziness, weakness, drowsiness, headache, tremor, depression, insomnia, *seizures*

⬥ = Nursing alert   ⬗ = Herb-drug interaction   ⃠ = Do not crush

HEMA: Hemolysis, increased hemoglobin (IV only)

EENT: Diplopia, temporary loss of vision, blurred vision, nystagmus

CV: Postural hypotension, bradycardia

GI: Nausea, vomiting, hiccups, anorexia, metallic taste

GU: Brown, black, green urine

INTEG: Rash, pruritus, fever, facial flushing, urticaria

*SYST: **Anaphylaxis***

Contraindications: Hypersensitivity, child <12 yr, intermittent porphyria

Precautions: Renal disease, hepatic disease, addictive personalities, pregnancy (C), myasthenia gravis, epilepsy

Pharmacokinetics:

IM/IV: Onset rapid

PO: Onset ½ hr, peak 1-2 hr, half-life 1-2 hr

Metabolized in liver, excreted in urine unchanged, crosses placenta

Interactions:

• Increased CNS depression: alcohol, tricyclic antidepressants, narcotics, barbiturates, sedatives, hypnotics

• Considered incompatible with any drug in sol or syringe

Lab test interferences:

False increase: VMA, urinary 5-HIAA

NURSING CONSIDERATIONS

Assess:

• Blood studies: CBC, WBC, differential; blood dyscrasias may occur

• During and after injection: CNS effects, rash, conjunctivitis, nasal congestion may occur

• Liver function studies: AST, ALT, alk phosphatase; hepatitis may occur

• ECG in epileptic patients; poor seizure control has occurred

• Allergic reactions: rash, fever, respiratory distress

• Severe weakness, numbness in extremities

• Tolerance: increased need for medication, more frequent requests for medication, increased pain

• CNS depression: dizziness, drowsiness, psychiatric symptoms

Administer:

• With meals for GI symptoms

• IV undiluted over 1 min or more, give 300 mg or less/1 min or longer; may be diluted in 250 ml or less D$_5$ or isotonic NaCl sol

• By slow IV to prevent phlebitis; keep recumbent for 15 min to prevent orthostatic hypotension; check for extravasation

• IM deep in large muscle mass; rotate sites

Perform/provide:

• Storage in tight container at room temp

• Assistance with ambulation if dizziness/drowsiness occurs

• Recumbent position after IV administration

Evaluate:

• Therapeutic response: decreased pain, spasticity

Teach patient/family:

• Not to discontinue medication quickly; insomnia, nausea, headache, spasticity, tachycardia will occur; drug should be tapered off over 1-2 wk

• That urine may turn green, black, or brown

• Not to take with alcohol, other CNS depressants

• To avoid altering activities while taking this drug

• To avoid hazardous activities if drowsiness, dizziness occurs

• To avoid using OTC medication: cough preparations, antihistamines, unless directed by prescriber

M

Treatment of overdose: Induce emesis of conscious patient, lavage, dialysis; have epinephrine, antihistamines, and corticosteroids available

---

methotrexate (amethopterin, MTX) (℞)
(meth-oh-trex′ate)
Folex PFS, methotrexate, Methotrexate LPF, Rheumatrex Dose Pack
Func. class.: Antineoplastic-antimetabolite
Chem. class.: Folic acid antagonist

Action: Inhibits an enzyme that reduces folic acid, which is needed for nucleic acid synthesis in all cells; S phase of cell cycle specific; immunosuppressive

Uses: Acute lymphocytic leukemia, in combination for breast, lung, head, neck carcinoma; lymphosarcoma, gestational choriocarcinoma, hydatidiform mole, psoriasis, rheumatoid arthritis, mycosis fungoides

Investigational uses: Used investigationally to produce abortion

Dosage and routes:
Leukemia
• *Adult and child:* **PO** 3.3 mg/m^2/day with prednisone **IT** 12 mg/m^2, maintenance 30 mg/m^2/day 2 ×/wk; **IV** 2.5 mg/kg q2wk
Choriocarcinoma
• *Adult and child:* **PO** 15-30 mg/m^2 qd × 5 days, then off 1 wk; may repeat
Osteosarcoma
• *Adult and child:* **IV** 12 g/m^2 given over 4 hr, then leucovorin rescue
Mycosis fungoides
• *Adult:* **PO** 2.5-10 mg/day until cleared (may be many months); **IM** 50 mg qwk or 25 mg 2 ×/wk

Psoriasis
• *Adult:* **PO/IM/IV** 10 mg qwk, may increase to 25 mg qwk
Breast cancer
• *Adult:* **IV** 40 mg/m^2 on days 1 and 8 with other antineoplastics
Arthritis
• *Adults:* **PO** 7.5 mg/wk
Available forms: Tabs 2.5 mg; inj 25 mg/ml; powder for inj 20, 25, 50, 100, 250 mg, 1 g; sodium inj 2.5, 25 mg/ml

Side effects/adverse reactions:
*HEMA: **Leukopenia, thrombocytopenia, myelosuppression, anemia***
*GI: Nausea, vomiting, anorexia, diarrhea, stomatitis, **hepatotoxicity**, cramps, ulcer, gastritis, **GI hemorrhage**, abdominal pain, hematemesis*
*GU: Urinary retention, **renal failure**, menstrual irregularities, defective spermatogenesis, **hematuria, azotemia, uric acid nephropathy***
INTEG: Rash, alopecia, dry skin, urticaria, photosensitivity, folliculitis, vasculitis, petechiae, ecchymosis, acne, alopecia
*CNS: Dizziness, **convulsions,** headache, confusion, hemiparesis, malaise, fatigue, chills, fever*

Contraindications: Hypersensitivity, leukopenia (<3500/mm^3), thrombocytopenia (<100,000/mm^3), anemia, psoriatic patients with severe renal/hepatic disease, pregnancy (X), alcoholism, HIV

Precautions: Renal disease, lactation

Pharmacokinetics:
PO: Readily absorbed
PO/IM/IV: Onset 4-7 days; peak 1-2 wk; duration 3 wk
IT: Onset, peak, duration unknown
Not metabolized; excreted in urine (unchanged); crosses placenta, blood-brain barrier; 50% plasma protein bound

---

◆ = Nursing alert　　🖋 = Herb-drug interaction　　🚫 = Do not crush

Interactions:

• Increased toxicity: aspirin, sulfa drugs, other antineoplastics, radiation, alcohol, probenecid, phenytoin, phenylbutazone, pyrimethamine, penicillins, NSAIDs

• Decreased effect of oral digoxin

• Increased hypoprothrombinemia: oral anticoagulants

• Decreased effect of methotrexate: folic acid supplements

◆ Possible fatal interactions: nonsteroidal antiinflammatory drugs

NURSING CONSIDERATIONS
Assess:

• CBC, differential, platelet count weekly; withhold drug if WBC is <3500/mm^3 or platelet count is <100,000/mm^3; notify prescriber; drug should be discontinued

• Renal function studies: BUN, serum uric acid, urine CrCl, electrolytes before, during therapy

• I&O ratio; report fall in urine output to <30 ml/hr

• Monitor temp q4h; fever may indicate beginning infection; no rectal temps

• Liver function tests before and during therapy: bilirubin, alk phosphatase, AST, ALT; liver biopsy should be done before start of therapy (psoriasis patients)

• Bleeding time, coagulation time during treatment; bleeding: hematuria, guaiac, bruising or petechiae, mucosa or orifices q8h

• Effects of alopecia on body image; discuss feelings about body changes

◆ Hepatotoxicity: jaundiced skin and sclera, dark urine, clay-colored stools, pruritus, abdominal pain, fever, diarrhea

• Buccal cavity q8h for dryness, sores, ulceration, white patches, oral pain, bleeding, dysphagia

• Symptoms indicating severe allergic reaction: rash, urticaria, itching, flushing

Administer:

• Antacid before oral agent; give drug after evening meal before bedtime

• Antiemetic 30-60 min before giving drug

• Allopurinol or sodium bicarbonate to maintain uric acid levels, alkalinization of urine, adequate fluids

IV

• After diluting 5 mg/2 ml of sterile H$_2$O for inj; give through Y-tube or 3-way stopcock at 10 mg or less/min

◆ Leucovorin Ca within 12 hr of this drug to prevent tissue damage; check agency policy

Additive compatibilities: Cephalothin, cyclophosphamide, cytarabine, fluorouracil, hydroxyzine, mercaptopurine, ondansetron, sodium bicarbonate, vincristine

Solution compatibilities: Amino acids, 4.25%/D$_{25}$, D$_5$W, sodium bicarbonate 0.05 mol/L, sodium chloride 0.9%

Syringe compatibilities: Bleomycin, cisplatin, cyclophosphamide, doxapram, doxorubicin, fluorouracil, furosemide, heparin, leucovorin, mitomycin, vinblastine, vincristine

Y-site compatibilities: Allopurinol, amifostine, amphotericin B cholesteryl, asparaginase, aztreonam, bleomycin, cefepime, ceftriaxone, cimetidine, cisplatin, cyclophosphamide, cytarabine, daunorubicin, dexchlorpheniramine, diphenhydramine, doxorubicin, doxorubicin liposome, etoposide, famotidine, filgrastim, fludarabine, fluorouracil, furosemide, gallium, ganciclovir, granisetron, heparin, hydromorphone, imipenem/cilastatin, leucovorin, lorazepam, melphalan, mesna, methylprednisolone, metoclopramide, mitomycin, morphine, ondansetron, oxacillin, paclitaxel, piperacillin/tazobactam, prochlorperazine, ranitidine, sargramostim, teniposide, thiotepa, vinblastine, vincristine, vinorelbine

Perform/provide:

• Strict medical asepsis and protective isolation if WBC levels are low

• Liquid diet: carbonated beverage, Jell-O; dry toast, crackers may be added when patient is not nauseated or vomiting

• Increased fluid intake to 2-3 L/day to prevent urate deposits, calculi formation, unless contraindicated

• Diet low in purines: absence of organ meats (kidney, liver), dried beans, peas to maintain alkaline urine

• Rinsing of mouth tid-qid with water, club soda; brushing of teeth bid-tid with soft brush or cotton-tipped applicators for stomatitis; use unwaxed dental floss

• Nutritious diet with iron, vitamin supplements

• Storage in tightly closed container in cool environment; store injection, powder for injection in dark, dry area

Evaluate:

• Therapeutic response: decreased tumor size, spread of malignancy

Teach patient/family:

• To report any complaints, side effects to nurse or prescriber: black tarry stools, chills, fever, sore throat, bleeding, bruising, cough, shortness of breath, dark or bloody urine

• That hair may be lost during treatment; wig or hairpiece may make patient feel better; tell patient that new hair may be different in color, texture (alopecia is rare)

• To avoid foods with citric acid, hot or rough texture if stomatitis is present

• To report stomatitis: any bleeding, white spots, ulcerations in mouth to prescriber; tell patient to examine mouth qd, report symptoms to nurse

• That contraceptive measures are recommended during therapy and for at least 8 wk following cessation of therapy

• To drink 10-12 glasses of fluid/day

• To avoid alcohol, salicylates, live vaccines

• To avoid use of razors, commercial mouthwash

---

methylcellulose (OTC)

(meth-ill-sell'yoo-lose)

Citrucel

Func. class.: Laxative, bulk

Chem. class.: Hydrophilic semi-synthetic cellulose derivative

Action: Attracts water, expands in intestine to increase peristalsis; also absorbs excess water in stool; decreases diarrhea

Uses: Constipation

Dosage and routes:

• *Adult:* **PO** 5-20 ml tid with 8 oz H_2O

• *Child:* **PO** 5-10 ml qd or bid with H_2O or 500 mg tid with 8 oz H_2O

Available forms: Powder 105 mg/g; sol 450 mg/5 ml; tab 500 mg

Side effects/adverse reactions:

*GI: **Obstruction**,* abdominal distention

Contraindications: Hypersensitivity, GI obstruction, hepatitis

Pharmacokinetics:

PO: Onset 12-24 hr, peak 1-3 days

Interactions:

• Decreased absorption: antibiotics, digitalis, nitrofurantoin, salicylates, tetracyclines, oral anticoagulants

---

◆ = Nursing alert   🖊 = Herb-drug interaction   🚫 = Do not crush

NURSING CONSIDERATIONS
Assess:

• Blood, urine electrolytes if used often
• I&O ratio to identify fluid loss
• Cause of constipation; lack of fluids, bulk, exercise
• Cramping, rectal bleeding, nausea, vomiting; drug should be discontinued

Administer:

PO

• Alone for better absorption; do not take within 1 hr of other drugs
• In morning or evening (oral dose)

Evaluate:

• Therapeutic response: decrease in constipation

Teach patient/family:

🚫 To swallow tabs whole; do not break, crush, or chew
• To increase fluid intake
• That normal bowel movements do not always occur daily
• Not to use in presence of abdominal pain, nausea, vomiting
• To notify prescriber if constipation unrelieved or if symptoms of electrolyte imbalance occur: muscle cramps, pain, weakness, dizziness, excessive thirst

---

methyldopa/methyldopate (Ɍ)

(meth-ill-doe′pa)
Aldomet, Apo-Methyldopa*, Dopamet*, methyldopa/ methyldopate, Nova-medopa*, Nu-Medopa*

Func. class.: Antihypertensive
Chem. class.: Centrally acting α-adrenergic inhibitor

Action: Stimulates central inhibitory α-adrenergic receptors or acts as false transmitter, resulting in reduction of arterial pressure
Uses: Hypertension

Dosage and routes:

• *Adult:* **PO** 250-500 mg bid or tid, then adjusted q2d as needed, 0.5-2 g qd in 2-4 divided doses (maintenance), not to exceed 3 g/day; **IV** 250-500 mg in 100 ml D_5W q6h, run over 30-60 min, not to exceed 1 g q6h
• *Geriatric:* **PO** 125 mg bid-tid, increase q2d as needed, max 3 g/day
• *Child:* **PO** 10 mg/kg/day in 2-4 divided doses, not to exceed 65 mg/kg or 3 g/day, whichever is less; **IV** 20-40 mg/kg/day in 4 divided doses, not to exceed 65 mg/kg or 3 g, whichever is less

Available forms: Methyldopa: Tabs 125, 250, 500 mg; oral susp 50 mg/ml; methyldopate: inj 50 mg/ml

Side effects/adverse reactions:

ENDO: Breast enlargement, gynecomastia, lactation, amenorrhea
GI: Nausea, vomiting, diarrhea, constipation, ***hepatic dysfunction,*** sore or "black" tongue, ***pancreatitis***
CV: Bradycardia, ***myocarditis,*** orthostatic hypotension, angina, edema, weight gain, ***CHF***
CNS: Drowsiness, weakness, dizziness, sedation, headache, depression, psychosis paresthesias, parkinsonism, Bell's palsy, nightmares
EENT: Nasal congestion
HEMA: ***Leukopenia, thrombocytopenia, hemolytic anemia, granulocytopenia,*** positive Coombs' test
INTEG: Rash, ***toxic epidermal necrolysis,*** lupuslike syndrome, eczema
GU: Impotence, failure to ejaculate
Contraindications: Active hepatic disease, hypersensitivity, blood dyscrasias
Precautions: Pregnancy (C), liver disease, eclampsia, severe cardiac disease
Pharmacokinetics:
PO: Peak 2-4 hr, duration 12-24 hr
IV: Peak 2 hr, duration 10-16 hr

M

Metabolized by liver, excreted in urine

Interactions:

• Increased pressor effect: sympathomimetic amines (norepinephrine, phenylpropanolamine), MAOIs

• Increased hypotension: levodopa

• Increased psychosis: haloperidol

• Lithium toxicity: lithium

• Increased B/P: phenothiazines, β-blockers, amphetamines, NSAIDs, tricyclics, barbiturates

⚜ Decreased effect, increased EPS: Indian snakeroot

Lab test interferences:

Interference: Urinary uric acid, serum creatinine, AST

False increase: Urinary catecholamines

NURSING CONSIDERATIONS

Assess:

• Blood studies: neutrophils, decreased platelets

• Baselines in renal, liver function tests before therapy begins

• B/P when beginning treatment, periodically thereafter

• Allergic reaction: rash, fever, pruritus, urticaria; drug should be discontinued if antihistamines fail to help

• CNS symptoms, especially in the elderly

• Symptoms of CHF: edema, dyspnea, wet rales, B/P

• Renal symptoms: polyuria, oliguria, urinary frequency; I & O ratio, weight

Administer:

IV route

• After diluting with 100-200 ml D_5W; run over ½-1 hr

Additive compatibilities: Aminophylline, ascorbic acid, chloramphenicol, diphenhydramine, heparin, magnesium sulfate, multivitamins, netilmicin, potassium chloride, promazine, sodium bicarbonate, succinylcholine, verapamil, vit B/C

Solution compatibilities: D_5W, D_5/0.9% NaCl, Ringer's, sodium bicarbonate 5%, 0.9% NaCl, amino acids 4.25%/D_{25}, Dextran$_6$/0.9% NaCl, Normosol R, Normosol M/D_5W

Y-site compatibilities: Esmolol, heparin, meperidine, morphine, theophylline

Perform/provide:

• Storage of tabs in tight container

Evaluate:

• Therapeutic response: decrease in B/P in hypertension

Teach patient/family:

• To avoid hazardous activities

• To administer 1 hr before meals

• Not to discontinue drug abruptly, or withdrawal symptoms may occur: anxiety, increased B/P, headache, insomnia, increased pulse, tremors, nausea, sweating

• Not to use OTC (cough, cold, allergy) products unless directed by prescriber

• To avoid sunlight or wear sunscreen; photosensitivity may occur

• To comply with dosage schedule even if feeling better

• To rise slowly to sitting or standing position to minimize orthostatic hypotension

• To notify prescriber of mouth sores, sore throat, fever, swelling of hands or feet, irregular heartbeat, chest pain, signs of angioedema

• That excessive perspiration, dehydration, vomiting, diarrhea may lead to fall in blood pressure; consult prescriber

• That dizziness, fainting, lightheadedness may occur during first few days of therapy

• That compliance is necessary; not to skip or stop drug unless directed by prescriber

• That drug may cause skin rash or impaired perspiration

Treatment of overdose: Gastric evacuation, sympathomimetics may be indicated; if severe, hemodialysis

---

methylergonovine (℞)
(meth-ill-er-goe-noe′veen)
Methergine, methylergonovine
Func. class.: Oxytocic
Chem. class.: Ergot alkaloid

Action: Stimulates uterine, vascular, smooth muscle, causing contractions; decreases bleeding

Uses: Treatment of hemorrhage postpartum or postabortion, uterine contractions

Dosage and routes:
• *Adult:* **IM** 0.2 mg q2-5h, not to exceed 5 doses; **IV** 0.2 mg given over 1 min; **PO** 0.2-0.4 mg q6-12h × 2-7 days after initial **IM** or **IV** dose

Available forms: Inj 0.2 mg/ml; tabs 0.2 mg

Side effects/adverse reactions:
RESP: Dyspnea
GU: Cramping
CNS: Headache, dizziness
GI: Nausea, vomiting
CV: Chest pain, palpitation, *hypertension,* ***dysrhythmias***
EENT: Tinnitus
INTEG: Sweating, rash, allergic reactions

Contraindications: Hypersensitivity to ergot preparations, indication of labor, before delivery of placenta, hypertension, pelvic inflammatory disease, respiratory disease, cardiac disease, peripheral vascular disease

Precautions: Pregnancy (C), severe hepatic disease, severe renal disease, jaundice, diabetes mellitus, convulsive disorders, sepsis

Pharmacokinetics:
PO: Onset 5-25 min, duration 3 hr
IM: Onset 2-5 min, duration 3 hr
IV: Onset immediate, duration 45 min
Metabolized in liver, excreted in urine

Interactions:
• Increase vasoconstriction: vasopressors, nicotine

NURSING CONSIDERATIONS
Assess:
• B/P, pulse, character and amount of vaginal bleeding; watch for indications of hemorrhage
• Respiratory rate, rhythm, depth; notify prescriber of abnormalities
• For uterine relaxation; observe for severe cramping
◆ Ergot toxicity: tinnitus, hypertension, palpitations, chest pain, nausea, vomiting, weakness; cold, numb extremities

Administer:
• Only during fourth stage of labor; not to be used to augment labor
• IM in deep muscle mass; rotate injection sites of additional doses
IV
• Undiluted through Y-tube or 3-way stopcock; give 0.2 mg or less/min or diluted in 5 ml 0.9% NaCl given through Y-site
• With crash cart available on unit; IV route used only in emergencies
Y-site compatibilities: Heparin, hydrocortisone sodium succinate, potassium chloride, vit B/C
Evaluate:
• Therapeutic response: absence of hemorrhage
Teach patient/family:
• To report increased blood loss, severe abdominal cramps, fever or foul-smelling lochia
• To avoid smoking

M

Side effects: *italics* = common; ***bold italics*** = life-threatening

---

methylphenidate (R)
(meth-ill-fen'i-date)
Methidate, Ritalin, Ritalin SR
Func. class.: Cerebral stimulant
Chem. class.: Piperidine derivative

Controlled Substance Schedule II

Action: Increases release of norepinephrine, dopamine in cerebral cortex to reticular activating system; exact action not known

Uses: Attention deficit hyperactivity disorder, narcolepsy

Investigational uses: Depression in the elderly; cancer, stroke patients

Dosage and routes:

Attention deficit hyperactivity disorder
• *Child >6 yr:* **PO** 5 mg before breakfast and lunch, increasing by 5-10 mg/wk, not to exceed 60 mg/day; sus rel 20 mg qd-tid

Narcolepsy
• *Adult:* **PO** 10 mg bid-tid, 30-45 min before meals, may increase up to 40-60 mg/day

Depression (elderly)
• *Geriatric:* **PO** 2.5 mg qAM, increase q 3rd day by 2.5 mg to desired dose, max 20 mg/day

Available forms: Tabs 5, 10, 20 mg; tabs sus rel 20 mg

Side effects/adverse reactions:

MISC: Fever, arthralgia, scalp hair loss

CNS: Hyperactivity, insomnia, restlessness, talkativeness, dizziness, headache, akathisia, dyskinesia, masking or worsening of Gilles de la Tourette's syndrome

GI: Nausea, anorexia, dry mouth, weight loss, abdominal pain

CV: Palpitations, tachycardia, B/P changes, angina, ***dysrhythmias, thrombocytopenic purpura***

*INTEG: **Exfoliative dermatitis,*** urticaria, rash, erythema multiforme

ENDO: Growth retardation

*GU: **Uremia***

*HEMA: **Leukopenia, anemia***

Contraindications: Hypersensitivity, anxiety, history of Gilles de la Tourette's syndrome; children <6 yr, glaucoma

Precautions: Hypertension, depression, pregnancy (C), seizures, lactation, drug abuse

Pharmacokinetics:

PO: Onset ½-1 hr, duration 4-6 hr, metabolized by liver, excreted by kidneys

Interactions:

• Hypertensive crisis: MAOIs or within 14 days of MAOIs, vasopressors

• Increased sympathomimetic effect: decongestants, vasoconstrictors

• Decreased effects of: warfarin, tricyclics, anticonvulsants

• Drug/food: increased stimulation: caffeine

NURSING CONSIDERATIONS

Assess:

• VS, B/P; may reverse antihypertensives; check patients with cardiac disease more often for increased B/P

• CBC, urinalysis, in diabetes: blood sugar, urine sugar; insulin changes may have to be made, since eating will decrease

• Height, growth rate q3mo in children; growth rate may be decreased

• Mental status: mood, sensorium, affect, stimulation, insomnia, aggressiveness

◆ Withdrawal symptoms: headache, nausea, vomiting, muscle pain, weakness

• Appetite, sleep, speech patterns

• For attention span, decreased hyperactivity in ADHD persons

---

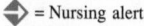 = Nursing alert   ∥ = Herb-drug interaction   ⊘ = Do not crush

Administer:

• At least 6 hr before hs to avoid sleeplessness

• Gum, hard candy, frequent sips of water for dry mouth

Evaluate:

• Therapeutic response: decreased hyperactivity or ability to stay awake

Teach patient/family:

• To decrease caffeine consumption (coffee, tea, cola, chocolate); may increase irritability, stimulation

🚫 Not to break, crush, or chew time-released medication

• To avoid OTC preparations unless approved by prescriber

• To taper off drug over several wk, or depression, increased sleeping, lethargy will occur

• To avoid alcohol ingestion

• To avoid hazardous activities until stabilized on medication

• To get needed rest; patients will feel more tired at end of day

Treatment of overdose: Administer fluids; hemodialysis or peritoneal dialysis; antihypertensive for increased B/P; administer short-acting barbiturate before lavage

---

methylprednisolone/ methylprednisolone acetate/methylprednisolone sodium succinate (℞)

(meth-il-pred-niss'oh-lone)

Medrol/Depo-Medrol, Duralone, Medralone, Rep-Pred/ A-Methapred, Solu-Medrol

Func. class.: Corticosteroid

Chem. class.: Glucocorticoid, immediate acting

Action: Decreases inflammation by suppression of migration of polymorphonuclear leukocytes, fibroblasts; reversal of increased capillary permeability and lysosomal stabilization

Uses: Severe inflammation, shock, adrenal insufficiency, collagen disorders

Dosage and routes:

Adrenal insufficiency/inflammation

• *Adult:* **PO** 2-60 mg in 4 divided doses; **IM** 40-80 mg (acetate); **IM/IV** 10-250 mg (succinate); intraarticular 4-30 mg (acetate)

• *Child:* **IV** 117 μg-1.66 mg/kg in 3-4 divided doses (succinate)

Shock

• *Adult:* **IV** 100-250 mg q2-6h (succinate)

Available forms: Tabs 2, 4, 6, 8, 16, 24, 32 mg; inj 20, 40, 80 mg/ml acetate; inj 40, 125, 500, 1000 mg/ vial succinate; dose pack 4 mg tabs

Side effects/adverse reactions:

CNS: Depression, flushing, sweating, headache, mood changes

CV: Hypertension, *circulatory collapse, thrombophlebitis, embolism,* tachycardia

EENT: Fungal infections, increased intraocular pressure, blurred vision, cataracts

GI: Diarrhea, nausea, abdominal distention, *GI hemorrhage,* increased appetite, pancreatitis

HEMA: Thrombocytopenia

INTEG: Acne, poor wound healing, ecchymosis, petechiae

MS: Fractures, osteoporosis, weakness

Contraindications: Psychosis, hypersensitivity, idiopathic thrombocytopenia, acute glomerulonephritis, amebiasis, fungal infections, nonasthmatic bronchial disease, child <2 yr, AIDS, TB

Precautions: Pregnancy (C), lactation, diabetes mellitus, glaucoma, osteoporosis, seizure disorders, ulcerative colitis, CHF, myasthenia

M

Side effects: *italics* = common; **bold italics** = life-threatening

gravis, renal disease, esophagitis, peptic ulcer

Pharmacokinetics: Well absorbed PO, IM

PO: Peak 1-2 hr, duration 1½ days
IM: Peak 4-8 days, duration 1-4 wk
Intraarticular: Peak 1 wk

Half-life >3½ hr; crosses placenta, enters breast milk in small amounts; metabolized in liver, excreted by kidneys (unchanged)

Interactions:

• Decreased action of methylprednisolone: cholestyramine, colestipol, barbiturates, rifampin, ephedrine, phenytoin, theophylline

• Decreased effects of anticoagulants, anticonvulsants, antidiabetics, ambenonium, neostigmine, isoniazid, toxoids, vaccines, anticholinesterases, salicylates, somatrem

• Increased side effects: alcohol, salicylates, indomethacin, amphotericin B, digitalis, cyclosporine, diuretics

• Increased action of methylprednisolone: salicylates, estrogens, indomethacin, oral contraceptives, ketoconazole, macrolide antibiotics

🍃 Potassium deficiency: aloe, cascara sagrada, buckthorn, rhubarb root, senna

Lab test interferences:

Increase: Cholesterol, Na, blood glucose, uric acid, Ca, urine glucose
Decrease: Ca, K, T_4, T_3, thyroid ^{131}I uptake test, urine 17-OHCS, 17-KS

False negative: Skin allergy tests

NURSING CONSIDERATIONS
Assess:

• K depletion: parethesias, fatigue, nausea, vomiting, depression, polyuria, dysrhythmias, weakness

• Edema, hypertension, cardiac symptoms

• Mental status: affect, mood, behavioral changes, aggression

• K, blood sugar, urine glucose while on long-term therapy; hypokalemia and hyperglycemia

• Joint mobility, pain, edema if given intraarticularly

• Weight daily; notify prescriber of weekly gain >5 lb

• B/P q4h, pulse; notify prescriber of chest pain, rales

• I&O ratio; be alert for decreasing urinary output, increasing edema

• Adrenal insufficiency: weight loss, nausea, vomiting, confusion, anxiety, hypotension, weakness

• Plasma cortisol levels during long-term therapy (normal level: 138-635 nmol/L SI units when drawn at 8 AM)

• Growth in children on long-term treatment

Administer:

• Titrated dose; use lowest effective dose

• IM inj deep in large muscle mass; rotate sites; avoid deltoid; use 21G needle; after shaking suspension (parenteral)

• In one dose in AM to prevent adrenal suppression; avoid SC administration; may damage tissue

• With food or milk to decrease GI symptoms (PO)

IV

• After diluting with diluent provided; agitate slowly; give 500 mg or less/1 min or longer; may be given as IV infusion in its own diluent over 10-20 min

Additive compatibilities: Chloramphenicol, cimetidine, clindamycin, dopamine, granisetron, heparin, norepinephrine, penicillin G potassium, ranitidine, theophylline, verapamil

Syringe compatibilities: Granisetron, metoclopramide

Y-site compatibilities: Acyclovir, amifostine, amphotericin B cholesteryl, amrinone, aztreonam, cefe-

---

⬥ = Nursing alert   🍃 = Herb-drug interaction   🚫 = Do not crush

pime, cisplatin, cladribine, cyclophosphamide, cytarabine, dopamine,
doxorubicin, enalaprilat, famotidine,
fludarabine, granisetron, heparin,
melphalan, meperidine, methotrexate, metronidazole, midazolam, morphine, piperacillin/tazobactam, remifentanil, sodium bicarbonate, tacrolimus, teniposide, theophylline,
thiotepa

Perform/provide:
• Assistance with ambulation in patient with bone tissue disease to prevent fractures

Evaluate:
• Therapeutic response: ease of respirations, decreased inflammation;
decreased symptoms of adrenal insufficiency
• Infection: increased temp, WBC,
even after withdrawal of medication; drug masks infection

Teach patient/family:
• To increase intake of K, Ca, protein
• That ID as steroid user should be
carried
• To notify prescriber if therapeutic
response decreases; dosage adjustment may be needed
• Not to discontinue abruptly, or adrenal crisis can result
• To avoid OTC products: salicylates, alcohol in cough products, cold
preparations unless directed by prescriber; to avoid vaccinations, since
immunosuppression occurs
• About cushingoid symptoms
• To recognize the symptoms of adrenal insufficiency: nausea, anorexia,
fatigue, dizziness, dyspnea, weakness, joint pain

methysergide (R̶x)
(meth-i-ser′jide)
Sansert
Func. class.: Adrenergic blocker,
serotonin antagonist
Chem. class.: Ergot derivative

Action: Competitively blocks serotonin HT receptors in CNS and periphery; potent vasoconstrictor
Uses: Prophylaxis for migraine and
other vascular headaches. If no improvement is noted in 3 wk, drug is
unlikely to be beneficial
Dosage and routes:
• *Adult:* **PO** 2 mg bid with meals
Available forms: Tabs 2 mg
Side effects/adverse reactions:
CNS: Tremors, anxiety, insomnia,
headache, dizziness, euphoria, confusion, depersonalization, hallucination, paresthesias, drowsiness
*CV: **Retroperitoneal fibrosis,*** valvular thickening, palpitations, tachycardia, postural hypertension, angina, ***thrombophlebitis,*** ECG
changes, ***cardiac fibrosis***
GI: Nausea, vomiting, weight gain
MS: Arthralgia, myalgia
INTEG: Flushing, rash, alopecia
*HEMA: **Blood dyscrasias***
Contraindications: Hypersensitivity to ergot, tartrazine, occlusion (peripheral, vascular), CAD, hepatic
disease, renal disease, peptic ulcer,
hypertension, connective tissue disease, fibrotic pulmonary disease
Precautions: Pregnancy (C), lactation, children
Pharmacokinetics:
PO: Half-life 10 hr, metabolized by
liver, excreted in urine (metabolites/
unchanged drug)
Interactions:
• Increased vasoconstriction: β-
blockers

• Decreased effect of narcotic analgesics

NURSING CONSIDERATIONS
Assess:

• Weight daily; check for peripheral edema in feet, legs; B/P

• For stress, activity, recreation, coping mechanisms

• Neurologic status: LOC, blurring vision, nausea, vomiting, tingling in extremities that precedes headache

• Ingestion of tyramine foods (pickled products, beer, wine, aged cheese), food additives, preservatives, colorings, artificial sweeteners, chocolate, caffeine may precipitate these types of headaches

Administer:

PO

• Give with or after meals to avoid GI symptoms

• Only to women who are not pregnant; harm to fetus may occur

• For less than 6 mo continuously, a 3-4 wk drug-free period must follow each 6 mo period

Perform/provide:

• Storage in dark area

• Quiet, calm environment with decreased stimulation such as noise, bright light, or excessive talking

Evaluate:

• Therapeutic response: decrease in frequency, severity of headache

Teach patient/family:

• Not to use OTC medications; serious drug interactions may occur

• To maintain dose at approved level, not to increase even if drug does not relieve headache

• To report side effects: increased vasoconstriction starting with cold extremities, then paresthesia, weakness

• That headaches may increase when drug discontinued after long-term use

◆ To keep drug out of reach of children; death may occur

• To report at once: dyspnea, paresthesias, urinary problems, pain in abdomen, chest, back, legs

• To use drug for less than 6 mo unless a 3-4 wk rest period has been taken

• That drug may cause drowsiness

---

metoclopramide (℞)

(met-oh-kloe-pra′mide)
Apo-Metoclop*, Clopra, Emex*, Maxeran*, Maxolon, metoclopramide, Octamide, Octamide PFS, Reclomide, Reglan

Func. class.: Cholinergic
Chem. class.: Central dopamine receptor antagonist

Action: Enhances response to acetylcholine of tissue in upper GI tract, which causes contraction of gastric muscle; relaxes pyloric, duodenal segments; increases peristalsis without stimulating secretions, blocks dopamine in chemoreceptor trigger zone of CNS

Uses: Prevention of nausea, vomiting induced by chemotherapy, radiation, delayed gastric emptying, gastroesophageal reflux

Investigational uses: Hiccups, migraines

Dosage and routes:
Renal dose

• CrCl <40 ml/min 50% of dose

Nausea/vomiting

• *Adult:* **IV** 2 mg/kg q2h × 5 doses 30 min before administration of chemotherapy

• *Child:* **IV** 0.1-0.2 mg/kg/dose

Delayed gastric emptying

• *Adult:* **PO** 10 mg 30 min ac, hs × 2-8 wk

• *Geriatric:* **PO** 5 mg ½ hr ac hs, increase to 10 mg if needed

Gastroesophageal reflux

• *Adult:* **PO** 10-15 mg qid 30 min ac
• *Child:* 0.4-0.8 mg/kg/day divided in 4 doses

Available forms: Tabs 5, 10 mg; syr 5 mg/5 ml; inj 5 mg/ml

Side effects/adverse reactions:

CNS: Sedation, fatigue, restlessness, headache, sleeplessness, dystonia, dizziness, drowsiness

GI: Dry mouth, constipation, nausea, anorexia, vomiting, diarrhea

GU: Decreased libido, prolactin secretion, amenorrhea, galactorrhea

CV: Hypotension, supraventricular tachycardia

INTEG: Urticaria, rash

HEMA: Neutropenia, leukopenia

Contraindications: Hypersensitivity to this drug or procaine or procainamide, seizure disorder, pheochromocytoma, breast cancer (prolactin dependent), GI obstruction

Precautions: Pregnancy (B), lactation, GI hemorrhage, CHF, Parkinson's disease

Pharmacokinetics:

IV: Onset 1-3 min, duration 1-2 hr
PO: Onset ½-1 hr, duration 1-2 hr
IM: Onset 10-15 min, duration 1-2 hr

Metabolized by liver, excreted in urine, half-life 4 hr

Interactions:

• Decreased action of metoclopramide: anticholinergics, opiates
• Increased sedation: alcohol, other CNS depressants
• Increased risk of EPS: haloperidol, phenothiazines
• Increased risk of toxicity: cyclosporine
• Avoid use with MAOIs

Lab test interferences:

Increase: Prolactin, aldosterone, thyrotropin

NURSING CONSIDERATIONS

Assess:

• For EPS and tardive dyskinesia, more likely to occur in elderly patient
• Mental status: depression, anxiety, irritability
• GI complaints: nausea, vomiting, anorexia, constipation

Administer:

• ½-1 hr before meals for better absorption
• Gum, hard candy, frequent rinsing of mouth for dry oral cavity

IV

• Undiluted if dose is <10 mg; give over 2 min; 10 mg or more may be diluted in 50 ml or more D_5W, NaCl, Ringer's, LR and given over 15 min or more

Additive compatibilities: Clindamycin, meropenem, morphine, multivitamins, potassium acetate, potassium chloride, potassium phosphate, verapamil

Syringe compatibilities: Aminophylline, ascorbic acid, atropine, benztropine, bleomycin, butorphanol, chlorpromazine, cisplatin, cyclophosphamide, cytarabine, dexamethasone, dimenhydrinate, diphenhydramine, doxorubicin, droperidol, fentanyl, fluorouracil, heparin, hydrocortisone, hydroxyzine, insulin (regular), leucovorin, lidocaine, magnesium sulfate, meperidine, methotrimeprazine, methylprednisolone, midazolam, mitomycin, morphine, pentazocine, perphenazine, prochlorperazine, promazine, promethazine, ranitidine, scopolamine, sufentanil, vinblastine, vincristine, vit B/C

Y-site compatibilities: Acyclovir, aldesleukin, amifostine, aztreonam, bleomycin, ciprofloxacin, cisatracurium, cisplatin, cladribine, cyclophosphamide, cytarabine, diltiazem, doxorubicin, droperidol, famotidine,

M

---

* = Canada only   Side effects: *italics* = common; **bold italics** = life-threatening

filgrastim, fluconazole, fludarabine, fluorouracil, foscarnate, gallium, granisetron, heparin, idarubicin, leucovorin, melphalan, meperidine, meropenum, methotrexate, mitomycin, morphine, ondansetron, paclitaxel, piperacillin/tazobactam, propofol, remifentanil, sargramostim, sufentanil, tacrolimus, teniposide, thiotepa, vinblastine, vincristine, vinorelbine, zidovudine

Perform/provide:
• Protect from light with aluminum foil during infusion
• Discard open ampules

Evaluate:
• Therapeutic response: absence of nausea, vomiting, anorexia, fullness

Teach patient/family:
• To avoid driving, other hazardous activities until patient is stabilized on this medication
• To avoid alcohol, other CNS depressants that will enhance sedating properties of this drug

---

metolazone (R)

(me-tole′a-zone)
Mykrox, Zaroxolyn
Func. class.: Diuretic
Chem. class.: Thiazide-like quinazoline derivative

Action: Acts on distal tubule and cortical thick ascending limb of the loop of Henle by increasing excretion of water, sodium, chloride, potassium, magnesium, bicarbonate

Uses: Edema, hypertension, CHF

Dosage and routes:

Edema
• *Adult:* **PO** 5-20 mg/day

Hypertension
• *Adult:* **PO** 2.5-5 mg/day (Zaroxolyn)

• *Child:* **PO** 0.2-0.4 mg/kg/day divided q12-24h
• *Adult:* **PO** 0.5 mg (Mykrox) qd in AM, may increase to 1 mg

Available forms: Tabs 0.5 (Mykrox), 2.5, 5, 10 mg

Side effects/adverse reactions:

GU: Urinary frequency, polyuria, **uremia, glucosuria**

CNS: Drowsiness, paresthesia, anxiety, depression, headache, *dizziness, fatigue, weakness*

GI: Nausea, vomiting, anorexia, constipation, diarrhea, cramps, pancreatitis, GI irritation, **hepatitis**

EENT: Blurred vision

INTEG: Rash, urticaria, purpura, photosensitivity, fever

META: Hyperglycemia, increased creatinine, BUN

HEMA: **Aplastic anemia, hemolytic anemia, leukopenia, agranulocytosis, neutropenia**

CV: Irregular pulse, orthostatic hypotension, palpitations, volume depletion

ELECT: Hypokalemia, hypomagnesemia, hypercalcemia, hyponatremia, hypochloremia, hypophosphatemia

Contraindications: Hypersensitivity to thiazides or sulfonamides, anuria, lactation

Precautions: Hypokalemia, renal disease, hepatic disease, gout, COPD, lupus erythematosus, diabetes mellitus, pregnancy (B)

Pharmacokinetics:
PO: Onset 1 hr, peak 2 hr, duration 12-24 hr; excreted unchanged by kidneys; crosses placenta; enters breast milk; half-life 8 hr

Interactions:
• Increased hypokalemia: mezlocillin, piperacillin, amphotericin B, glucocorticoids, digoxin
• Increased hypotension: alcohol (large amounts), nitrates, antihypertensives

---

• Increased toxicity: lithium

🖉 Potassium deficiency: aloe, cascara sagrada, buckthorn, rhubarb root, senna

Lab test interferences:

Increase: BSP retention, Ca, amylase, parathyroid test

Decrease: PBI, PSP

NURSING CONSIDERATIONS
Assess:

• Weight, I&O daily to determine fluid loss; effect of drug may be decreased if used qd

• Rate, depth, rhythm of respiration, effect of exertion

• B/P lying, standing; postural hypotension may occur

• Electrolytes: K, Mg, Na, Cl; include BUN, blood sugar, CBC, serum creatinine, blood pH, ABGs, uric acid, Ca

• Improvement in edema of feet, legs, sacral area daily if medication is being used in CHF

• Improvement in CVP q8h

• Signs of metabolic alkalosis: drowsiness, restlessness

• Signs of hypokalemia: postural hypotension, malaise, fatigue, tachycardia, leg cramps, weakness

• Rashes, fever qd

• Confusion, especially in elderly; take safety precautions if needed

Administer:

• In AM to avoid interference with sleep if using drug as a diuretic

• K replacement if K <3 mg/dl

• With food, if nausea occurs; absorption may be decreased slightly

• Extended product is Zaroxolyn; prompt product is Mykrox

Evaluate:

• Therapeutic response: decreased edema, B/P

Teach patient/family:

• To increase fluid intake to 2-3 L/day unless contraindicated, to rise slowly from lying or sitting position

• To notify prescriber of muscle weakness, cramps, nausea, dizziness

• That drug may be taken with food or milk

• To use sunscreen for photosensitivity

• That blood sugar may be increased in diabetics

• To take early in day to avoid nocturia

Treatment of overdose: Lavage if taken orally; monitor electrolytes; administer dextrose in saline; monitor hydration, CV, renal status

---

metoprolol (℞)

(meh-toe′proe-lole)
Apo-Metoprolol*, Betaloc*, Betaloc Durules*, Lopresor*, Lopressor, Lopressor SR*, Novometoprol*, Toprol XL

Func. class.: Antihypertensive, antianginal

Chem. class.: β₁-blocker

Action: Lowers B/P by β-blocking effects; elevated plasma renins are reduced; blocks β_2-adrenergic receptors in bronchial, vascular smooth muscle only at high doses

Uses: Mild to moderate hypertension, acute MI to reduce cardiovascular mortality, angina pectoris

Investigational uses: Dysrhythmias, hypertrophic cardiomyopathy, mitral valve prolapse, pheochromocytoma, tremors, prevention of vascular headaches, aggression

Dosage and routes:

Hypertension

• *Adult:* **PO** 50 mg bid, or 100 mg qd; may give up to 200-450 mg in divided doses; **SUS REL** give qd

• *Geriatric:* **PO** 25 mg/day initially, increase weekly as needed

Myocardial infarction

• *Adult:* (early treatment) **IV BOL** 5 mg q2min × 3, then 50 mg **PO** 15

M

---

min after last dose and q6h × 48 hr; (late treatment) **PO** maintenance 100 mg bid for 3 mo

Available forms: Tabs 50, 100 mg; inj 1 mg/ml; sus rel tab 50, 100, 200 mg

Side effects/adverse reactions:

CV: Hypotension, *bradycardia*

CHF: Palpitations, dysrhythmias, *cardiac arrest, AV block*

CNS: Insomnia, dizziness, mental changes, hallucinations, *depression,* anxiety, headaches, nightmares, confusion, fatigue

GI: Nausea, vomiting, colitis, cramps, *diarrhea,* constipation, flatulence, dry mouth, *hiccups*

INTEG: Rash, purpura, alopecia, dry skin, urticaria, pruritus

HEMA: Agranulocytosis, eosinophilia, thrombocytopenia, purpura

EENT: Sore throat; dry, burning eyes

GU: Impotence

RESP: Bronchospasm, dyspnea, wheezing

Contraindications: Hypersensitivity to β-blockers, cardiogenic shock, heart block (2nd, 3rd degree), sinus bradycardia, bronchial asthma

Precautions: Major surgery, pregnancy (C), lactation, diabetes mellitus, renal disease, thyroid disease, COPD, heart failure, CAD, nonallergic bronchospasm, hepatic disease, CHF

Pharmacokinetics:

PO: Peak 2-4 hr, duration 13-19 hr; half-life 3-4 hr; metabolized in liver (metabolites); excreted in urine; crosses placenta; enters breast milk

Interactions:

• Increased hypotension, bradycardia: reserpine, hydralazine, methyldopa, prazosin, amphetamines, ephedrine, epinephrine, norepinephrine

• Increased hypoglycemic effects: insulin oral antiglycemics

• Do not use with MAOIs

• Decreased effects of dopamine, dobutamine, xanthines

Lab test interferences:

Increase: Liver function tests, renal function tests

NURSING CONSIDERATIONS

Assess:

• ECG directly when giving IV during initial treatment

• I&O, weight daily

• B/P during initial treatment, periodically thereafter; pulse q4h; note rate, rhythm, quality

• Apical/radial pulse before administration; notify prescriber of any significant changes or pulse <50 bpm

• Baselines in renal, liver function tests before therapy begins

• Edema in feet, legs daily

• Skin turgor, dryness of mucous membranes for hydration status

Administer:

• PO ac, hs, tab may be crushed or swallowed whole, except for sus rel tab

IV

• IV, undiluted, give over 1 min, keep patient recumbent for 3 hr

Y-site compatibilities: Alteplase, meperidine, morphine

Perform/provide:

• Storage in dry area at room temp, do not freeze

Evaluate:

• Therapeutic response: decreased B/P after 1-2 wk

Teach patient/family:

• To take with or immediately after meals

• Not to discontinue drug abruptly; taper over 2 wk; may cause precipitate angina

• Not to use OTC products containing α-adrenergic stimulants (nasal decongestants, OTC cold preparations) unless directed by prescriber

• To report bradycardia, dizziness, confusion, depression, fever, sore

---

⬥ = Nursing alert   ▮ = Herb-drug interaction   ⊘ = Do not crush

throat, shortness of breath to prescriber
• To take pulse at home; advise when to notify prescriber
• To avoid alcohol, smoking, Na intake
• To comply with weight control, dietary adjustments, modified exercise program
• To carry Medic Alert ID to identify drug, allergies
• To avoid hazardous activities if dizziness is present
• To report symptoms of CHF: difficult breathing, especially on exertion or when lying down, night cough, swelling of extremities
• To take medication hs to prevent effect of orthostatic hypotension
• To wear support hose to minimize effects of orthostatic hypotension

Treatment of overdose: Lavage, IV atropine for bradycardia, IV theophylline for bronchospasm, digitalis, O_2, diuretic for cardiac failure, hemodialysis, hypotension administer vasopressor (norepinephrine)

---

metronidazole (℞)

(me-troe-ni′da-zole)
Apo-Metronidazole*, Femazole, Flagyl, Flagyl IV, Flagyl IV RTU, Metro IV, metronidazole, Metronidazole Redi-Infusion, Metryl, Neo-Metric*, Novonidazole*, PMS-Metronidazole*, Protostat, Satric, Trikacide*

Func. class.: Antiinfective—misc

Chem. class.: Nitroimidazole derivative

Action: Direct-acting amebicide/trichomonacide binds, degrades DNA in organism

Uses: Intestinal amebiasis, amebic abscess, trichomoniasis, refractory trichomoniasis, bacterial anaerobic infections, giardiasis, septicemia, endocarditis, bone, joint infections, lower respiratory tract infections

Dosage and routes:
Trichomoniasis
• *Adult:* **PO** 250 mg tid × 7 days or 2 g in single dose; do not repeat treatment for 4-6 wk
Refractory trichomoniasis
• *Adult:* **PO** 250 mg bid × 10 days
Amebic abscess
• *Adult:* **PO** 500-750 mg tid × 5-10 days
• *Child:* **PO** 35-50 mg/kg/day in 3 divided doses × 10 days
Intestinal amebiasis
• *Adult:* **PO** 750 mg tid × 5-10 days
• *Child:* **PO** 35-50 mg/kg/day in 3 divided doses × 10 days; then oral iodoquinol
Anaerobic bacterial infections
• *Adult:* **IV INF** 15 mg/kg over 1 hr, then 7.5 mg/kg **IV** or **PO** q6h, not to exceed 4 g/day; first maintenance dose should be administered 6 hr following loading dose
Giardiasis
• *Adult:* **PO** 250 mg tid × 5 days
• *Child:* **PO** 5 mg/kg tid × 5 days
Antibiotic-associated pseudomembranous colitis
• *Adult:* **PO** 250-500 mg 3-4 ×/day × 10-14 days
• *Child:* **PO** 20 mg/kg/day (max 2 g) divided q6h
Available forms: Tabs 250, 500 mg; film-coated tabs 250, 1500 mg; inj 5 mg/vial; HCl inj 500 mg

Side effects/adverse reactions:
CV: Flat T waves
CNS: Headache, dizziness, confusion, irritability, restlessness, ataxia, depression, fatigue, drowsiness, insomnia, paresthesia, peripheral neuropathy, ***convulsions,*** incoordination, depression

M

EENT: Blurred vision, sore throat, retinal edema, dry mouth, metallic taste, furry tongue, glossitis, stomatitis

GI: Nausea, vomiting, diarrhea, epigastric distress, *anorexia,* constipation, *abdominal cramps,* metallic taste, ***pseudomembranous colitis***

GU: Darkened urine, vaginal dryness, polyuria, ***albuminuria,*** dysuria, cystitis, decreased libido, ***neurotoxicity,*** incontinence, dyspareunia

HEMA: ***Leukopenia, bone marrow, depression, aplasia***

INTEG: Rash, pruritus, urticaria, flushing

Contraindications: Hypersensitivity to this drug, renal disease, hepatic disease, contracted visual or color fields, blood dyscrasias, pregnancy (1st trimester), lactation, CNS disorders

Precautions: *Candida* infections, pregnancy (B) (2nd, 3rd trimesters)

Pharmacokinetics:
IV: Onset immediate, peak end of inf
PO: Peak 1-2 hr, half-life 6-11 hr
Crosses placenta, enters breast milk, excreted in feces; absorbed PO (80%-85%)

Interactions:
• Disulfiram reaction: alcohol
• May increase action of warfarin
• Decreased action of metronidazole: phenobarbital, phenytoin

Lab test interferences:
Decrease: AST, ALT

NURSING CONSIDERATIONS
Assess:
• For infection: WBC, wound symptoms, fever, skin or vaginal secretions; start treatment after C&S
• Stools during entire treatment; should be clear at end of therapy; stools should be free of parasites for 1 yr before patient is considered cured (amebiasis)
• Vision by ophthalmic exam during, after therapy; vision problems often occur
• I&O; weight daily; stools for number, frequency, character
 Neurotoxicity: peripheral neuropathy, seizures, dizziness, uncoordination, pruritus, joint pains; drug may be discontinued
• Allergic reaction: fever, rash, itching, chills; drug should be discontinued if these symptoms occur
• Superinfection: fever, monilial growth, fatigue, malaise
• Renal and reproductive dysfunction: dysuria, polyuria, impotence, dyspareunia, decreased libido

Administer:
• PO with or after meals to avoid GI symptoms, metallic taste; crush tabs if needed
IV
• Prediluted; metronidazole IV, dilute with 4.4 ml sterile H_2O or 0.9% NaCl; must be diluted further with 8 mg/ml or more 0.9% NaCl, D_5W, or LR; must neutralize with 5 mEq Na_2CO_3/500 mg; CO_2 gas will be generated and may require venting; run over 1 hr; primary IV must be discontinued; may be given as continuous infusion; do not use aluminum products; IV may require venting

Additive compatibilities: Amikacin, aminophylline, cefazolin, cefotaxime, cefotiam, ceftazidime, ceftizoxime, ceftriaxone, cefuroxime, chloramphenicol, ciprofloxacin, clindamycin, disopyramide, floxacillin, fluconazole, gentamicin, heparin, moxalactam, multielectrolyte concentrate, multivitamins, netilmicin, penicillin G potassium, tobramycin

Y-site compatibilities: Acyclovir, allopurinol, amifostine, amiodarone, cefepime, cisatracurium, cyclophosphamide, diltiazem, dopamine, doxorubicin liposome, enalaprilat, esmolol, fluconazole, foscarnet, granisetron, heparin, hydromorphone, labetalol, lorazepam, magnesium sulfate, melphalan, meperidine, methylprednisolone, midazolam, morphine, perphenazine, piperacillin/tazobactam, remifentanil, sargramostim, tacrolimus, teniposide, theophylline, thiotepa, vinorelbine

Perform/provide:

• Storage in light-resistant container; do not refrigerate

Evaluate:

• Therapeutic response: decreased symptoms of infection

Teach patient/family:

• That urine may turn dark-reddish brown, drug may cause metallic taste

• Proper hygiene after BM; handwashing technique

• To notify physician for numbness or tingling of extremities

• To avoid hazardous activities, since dizziness can occur

• Need for compliance with dosage schedule, duration of treatment

• To use condoms if treatment for trichomoniasis, or cross-contamination may occur

• To use frequent sips of water, sugarless gum for dry mouth

• That treatment of both partners is necessary in trichomoniasis

• Not to drink alcohol or use preparations containing alcohol; disulfiram-like reaction can occur

---

mexiletine (℞)

(mex-il'e-teen)

Mexitil

Func. class.: Antidysrhythmic (Class IB)

Chem. class.: Lidocaine analog

Action: Increases electrical stimulation threshold of ventricle, His-Purkinje system, which stabilizes cardiac membrane

Uses: Ventricular tachycardia, ventricular dysrhythmias during cardiac surgery, MI

Dosage and routes:

• *Adult:* **PO** 400 mg (loading dose), then 200 mg q8h, then 200-400 mg q8h

Available forms: Caps 150, 200, 250 mg

Side effects/adverse reactions:

CNS: Headache, dizziness, confusion, *convulsions,* tremors, psychosis, nervousness, paresthesias, weakness, fatigue, coordination difficulties, change in sleep habits

EENT: Blurred vision, hearing loss, tinnitus

GI: Nausea, vomiting, anorexia, diarrhea, abdominal pain, *hepatitis,* dry mouth, peptic ulcer, altered taste, *GI bleeding*

CV: Hypotension, bradycardia, angina, PVCs, *heart block, cardiovascular collapse or arrest,* sinus node slowing, *left ventricular failure,* syncope, *cardiogenic shock*

RESP: Dyspnea, *fibrosis, embolism, pneumonia*

INTEG: Rash, alopecia, dry skin

HEMA: Thrombocytopenia, leukopenia, agranulocytosis, hypoplastic anemia, systemic lupus erythematosus syndrome

GU: Urinary hesitancy, decreased libido

MISC: Edema, arthralgia, fever

Contraindications: Hypersensitivity to amides, cardiogenic shock, blood dyscrasias, severe heart block

Precautions: Pregnancy (C), lactation, children, renal disease, liver disease, CHF, respiratory depression, myasthenia gravis

Pharmacokinetics:

PO: Peak 2-3 hr; half-life 12 hr, metabolized by liver, excreted unchanged by kidneys (10%), excreted in breast milk

---

M

Interactions:
• Decreased or increased effects of mexiletine: cimetidine
• Decreased levels of mexiletine: phenytoin, phenobarbital, rifampin, urinary acidifiers, aluminum/magnesium hydroxide, atropine, opiates
• Increased effects of mexiletine: metoclopramide, urinary alkalinizers
• Increased levels of: caffeine, theophylline
• Drug/smoking: decreased drug effect

⚱ Increased potassium loss, increased antidysrhythmic action: aloe, cascara sagrada, buckthorn, rhubarb, senna

Lab test interferences:
Increase: CPK

NURSING CONSIDERATIONS
Assess:
• ECG continuously for increased PR or QRS segments; discontinue or reduce rate; watch for increased ventricular ectopic beats; may have to rebolus
• Blood levels (therapeutic level 0.5-2 µg/ml)
• B/P continuously for fluctuations in cardiac rate
• I&O ratio, electrolytes (K, Na, Cl), liver enzymes
◆ Malignant hyperthermia: tachypnea, tachycardia, changes in B/P, fever
• Respiratory status: rate, rhythm, lung fields for rales, watch for respiratory depression
• CNS effects: dizziness, confusion, psychosis, paresthesias, convulsions; drug should be discontinued
• Lung fields, bilateral rales may occur in CHF patient
• Increased respiration, increased pulse; drug should be discontinued
Administer:
• With food for GI upset

Evaluate:
• Therapeutic response: decreased dysrhythmias
Treatment of overdose: O_2, artificial ventilation, ECG; administer dopamine for circulatory depression, diazepam or thiopental for convulsions, to acidify urine

---

mezlocillin (℞)
(mez-loe-sill'in)
Mezlin
Func. class.: Antiinfective, broad-spectrum
Chem. class.: Extended-spectrum penicillin

Action: Interferes with cell wall replication of susceptible organisms; osmotically unstable cell wall swells, bursts from osmotic pressure
Uses: Effective for gram-positive cocci *(Staphylococcus aureus, Streptococcus viridans, S. faecalis, S. pneumoniae),* gram-negative cocci *(Neisseria gonorrhoeae),* gram-positive bacilli *(Clostridium perfringens, C. tetani),* gram-negative bacilli *(Bacteroides, Escherichia coli, Haemophilus influenzae, Klebsiella, Proteus mirabilis, P. vulgaris, P. rettgeri, Peptococcus, Peptostreptococcus, Morganella morganii, Enterobacter, Serratia, Pseudomonas, Shigella, Citrobacter, Veillonella)*
Dosage and routes:
• Dose reduction indicated in renal impairment (CrCl <30 ml/min)
• Hepatic dose give 50% of dose
• *Adult:* **IM/IV** 3-4 g q4-6h or **IV** 500 mg q8h, may give up to 24 g/day for severe infections
• *Child:* **IM/IV** 50 mg/kg q4-6h
• *Infant >8 days (>2000 g):* 75 mg/kg q6h; *<2000 g:* 75 mg/kg q8h
• *Infant <8 days:* 75 mg/kg q12h

◆ = Nursing alert   *⚱* = Herb-drug interaction   ⊘ = Do not crush

Available forms: Powder for inj 1, 2, 3, 4, 20 g

Side effects/adverse reactions:

HEMA: Anemia, increased bleeding time, **bone marrow depression, granulocytopenia**

GI: Nausea, vomiting, diarrhea; increased AST, ALT; abdominal pain, glossitis, colitis, abnormal taste

GU: Oliguria, proteinuria, hematuria, (vaginitis, moniliasis), **glomerulonephritis,** increased BUN, creatinine

CNS: Lethargy, hallucinations, anxiety, depression, twitching, **coma, convulsions**

META: Hyperkalemia, hypokalemia, alkalosis, hypernatremia

Contraindications: Hypersensitivity to penicillins

Precautions: Pregnancy (B), lactation, hypersensitivity to cephalosporins, neonates, renal disease

Pharmacokinetics:

IM: Peak 45 min

IV: Peak 5 min

Half-life 50-55 min; partially metabolized in liver; excreted in urine, bile, breast milk (small amount); crosses placenta

Interactions:

• Decreased excretion of lithium

• Increased hypokalemia: diuretics, digoxin

• Increased mezlocillin concentrations: aspirin, probenecid

🖉 Delayed/reduced absorption: khat, separate by ≥2 hr

Lab test interferences:

False positive: Urine glucose, urine protein

NURSING CONSIDERATIONS

Assess:

• I&O ratio; report hematuria, oliguria, since penicillin in high doses is nephrotoxic

• Any patient with compromised renal system, since drug is excreted slowly in poor renal system function; toxicity may occur rapidly

• Liver studies: AST, ALT

• Blood studies: WBC, RBC, Hct, Hgb, bleeding time

• Renal studies: urinalysis, protein, blood, BUN, creatinine

• C&S before drug therapy; drug may be given as soon as culture is taken

• Bowel pattern before and during treatment

• Skin eruptions after administration of penicillin to 1 wk after discontinuing drug

• Respiratory status: rate, character, wheezing, and tightness in chest

• Check IV site for thrombophlebitis

• WBC, differential, liver, renal studies periodically for patients on long-term therapy

• Allergies before initiation of treatment, and reaction of each medication; highlight allergies on chart

Administer:

• Drug after C&S completed

IV

• After diluting 1 g or less/10 ml of sterile H_2O, D_5, or 0.9% NaCl for inj; shake, dilute further with D_5W or 0.45 NaCl, and give over 3-5 min; may be given by intermittent inf over ½ hr

Solution compatibilities: $D_{10}W$, D_5W, 0.9% NaCl

Syringe compatibilities: Heparin

Y-site compatibilities: Amifostine, aztreonam, cyclophosphamide, doxorubicin liposome, famotidine, fludarabine, granisetron, hydromorphone, morphine, perphenazine, propofol, remifentanil, sargramostim, tacrolimus, teniposide, thiotepa

Perform/provide:

• Adrenaline, suction, tracheostomy set, endotracheal intubation equipment

M

• Adequate fluid intake (2 L) during diarrhea episodes

• Scratch test to assess allergy after securing order from prescriber; usually done when penicillin is only drug of choice

• Storage at room temp; reconstituted sol is stable for 24 hr refrigerated

Evaluate:

• Therapeutic response: absence of fever, draining wounds

Teach patient/family:

• That culture may be taken after completed course of medication

• To report sore throat, fever, fatigue (may indicate superinfection)

• To wear or carry Medic Alert ID if allergic to penicillins

• To report diarrhea, symptoms of *Candida* vaginitis

Treatment of anaphylaxis: Withdraw drug, maintain airway, administer epinephrine, aminophylline, O₂, IV corticosteroids

---

miconazole (℞)

(mi-kon′a-zole)
Monistat, Monistat I.V.
Func. class.: Antifungal
Chem. class.: Imidazole

Action: Alters cell membranes, inhibits fungal enzymes

Uses: Coccidioidomycosis, candidiasis, cryptococcoses, paracoccidioidomycosis, chronic mucocutaneous candidiasis, fungal meningitis; IV for severe infections only

Dosage and routes:

• *Adult:* IV INF 200-3600 mg/day; may be divided in 3 infusions 200-1200 mg/infusion; may have to repeat course; **INTRATHECAL** 20 mg given simultaneously with **IV** for fungal meningitis q1-2d

• *Child:* IV 20-40 mg/kg/day, not to exceed 15 mg/kg/dose

Available forms: Inj 10 mg/ml; aerosol 2%

Side effects/adverse reactions:

CV: Tachycardia, dysrhythmias (rapid IV)

CNS: Drowsiness, headache, laziness

GI: Nausea, vomiting, anorexia, diarrhea, cramps

GU: Vulvovaginal burning, itching, hyponatremia, pelvic cramps (topical forms)

*HEMA: **Decreased Hct, thrombocytopenia, hyperlipidemia***

INTEG: Pruritus, rash, fever, flushing, ***anaphylaxis,*** hives

Contraindications: Hypersensitivity

Precautions: Renal disease, hepatic disease, pregnancy (C)

Pharmacokinetics:

IV: Onset immediate; peak end of inf; half-life triphasic 0.4, 2.1, 24.1 hr; metabolized in liver; excreted in feces, urine (inactive metabolites); >90% protein binding

Interactions:

• Increased effect: warfarin, sulfonylureas, phenytoin

Lab test interferences:

False positive: Urine glucose, urine protein

NURSING CONSIDERATIONS
Assess:

• Cardiac system: B/P, pulse, ECG; watch for increasing pulse, cardiac dysrhythmias; drug should be discontinued

• Blood studies: WBC, RBC, Hct, Hgb, bleeding time

• Renal studies: urinalysis, protein, blood

• C&S before drug therapy; drug may be given as soon as culture is taken; monitor signs of infection prior to and throughout treatment

---

◆ = Nursing alert 🖋 = Herb-drug interaction 🚫 = Do not crush

• Bowel pattern before and during treatment; diarrhea is common
• Skin eruptions after administration of drug to 1 wk after discontinuing drug
• Respiratory status: rate, character, wheezing, tightness in chest
• IV site for thrombophlebitis
• WBC and differential liver and renal studies periodically for patients on long-term therapy
• Allergies before initiation of treatment, and reaction of each medication; highlight allergies on chart

Administer:
• Drug after C&S completed

IV
• 200 mg initially to prevent severe hypersensitive reaction
• IV after diluting 1 g or less/10 ml of sterile H_2O, D_5W, or 0.45% NaCl; give over 3-5 min; may be given by intermittent inf over 2 hr

Y-site compatibilities: Allopurinol, filgrastim, foscarnet, granisetron, melphalan, ondansetron, propofol, sargramostim, teniposide, thiotepa, vinorelbine

Perform/provide:
• Adrenaline, suction, tracheostomy set, endotracheal intubation equipment
• Adequate fluid intake (2 L) during diarrhea episodes
• Scratch test to assess allergy after securing order from prescriber; usually done when penicillin is only drug of choice
• Storage at room temp; reconstituted sol stable for 24 hr refrigerated

Evaluate:
• Therapeutic response: absence of fever, draining wounds

Teach patient/family:
• That culture may be taken after completed course of medication
• To report sore throat, fever, fatigue (may indicate superinfection)
• To wear or carry Medic Alert ID if allergic to drug
• To report diarrhea, symptoms of *Candida* vaginitis

Treatment of overdose: Withdraw drug; maintain airway; administer epinephrine, aminophylline, O_2, IV corticosteroids for anaphylaxis

---

midazolam (℞)
(mid′ay-zoe-lam)
Versed
Func. class.: Sedative, hypnotic
Chem. class.: Benzodiazepine, short-acting

Controlled Substance Schedule IV

Action: Depresses subcortical levels in CNS; may act on limbic system, reticular formation; may potentiate γ-aminobutyric acid (GABA) by binding to specific benzodiazepine receptors

Uses: Preoperative sedation, general anesthesia induction, sedation for diagnostic endoscopic procedures, intubation

Investigational uses: Epileptic seizures, refractory status epilepticus

Dosage and routes:

Preoperative sedation
• *Adult:* **IM** 0.07-0.08 mg/kg ½-1 hr before general anesthesia
• *Child:* **IM** 0.1-0.15 mg/kg, may give up to 0.5 mg/kg if needed

Induction of general anesthesia
• *Adult and child 12-16 yr:* **IV** (unpremedicated patients) 0.3-0.35 mg/kg over 30 sec, wait 2 min, follow with 25% of initial dose if needed; (premedicated patients) 0.15-0.35 mg/kg over 20-30 sec, allow 2 min for effect
• *Child 6-12 yr:* **IV** 0.025-0.05 mg/kg, total dose up to 0.4 mg/kg may be needed
• *Child 6 mo-5 yr:* **IV** 0.05-0.1 mg/

kg, total dose up to 0.6 mg/kg may be needed

• *Child <6 mo:* Titrate with small increments

Available forms: Inj 1, 5 mg/ml, syrup

Side effects/adverse reactions:

CNS: Retrograde amnesia, euphoria, confusion, headache, anxiety, insomnia, slurred speech, paresthesia, tremors, weakness, chills

RESP: Coughing, *apnea, bronchospasm, laryngospasm,* dyspnea

CV: Hypotension, PVCs, tachycardia, bigeminy, nodal rhythm

EENT: Blurred vision, nystagmus, diplopia, blocked ears, loss of balance

GI: Nausea, vomiting, increased salivation, hiccups

INTEG: Urticaria, pain, swelling at injection site, rash, pruritus

Contraindications: Pregnancy (D), hypersensitivity to benzodiazepines, shock, coma, alcohol intoxication, acute narrow-angle glaucoma

Precautions: COPD, CHF, chronic renal failure, chills, elderly, debilitated, children, lactation

Pharmacokinetics:

IM: Onset 15 min, peak ½-1 hr

IV: Onset 3-5 min, onset of anesthesia 1½-2½ min; protein binding 97%; half-life 1.2-12.3 hr

Metabolized in liver; metabolites excreted in urine; crosses placenta, blood-brain barrier

Interactions:

• Prolonged respiratory depression: other CNS depressants, alcohol, barbiturates, opiate analgesics, verapamil, ritonavir, indinavir, fluvoxamine

NURSING CONSIDERATIONS

Assess:

• Injection site for redness, pain, swelling

• Degree of amnesia in elderly; may be increased

• Anterograde amnesia

• Vital signs for recovery period in obese patient, since half-life may be extended

• Apnea, respiratory depression that may be increased in the elderly

Administer:

• IM deep into large muscle mass

IV

• After diluting with D₅W or 0.9% NaCl to 0.25 mg/ml; give over 2 min (conscious sedation) or over 30 sec (anesthesia induction)

Additive compatibility: Hydromorphone

Syringe compatibilities: Atracurium, atropine, benzquinamide, buprenorphine, butorphanol, chlorpromazine, cimetidine, cisatracurium, diphenhydramine, droperidol, fentanyl, glycopyrrolate, hydromorphone, hydroxyzine, meperidine, metoclopramide, morphine, nalbuphine, promazine, promethazine, remifentanil, scopolamine, sufentanil, thiethylperazine, trimethobenzamide

Y-site compatibilities: Amikacin, amiodarone, atracurium, calcium gluconate, cefazolin, cefmetazole, cefotaxime, cimetidine, ciprofloxacin, clindamycin, digoxin, diltiazem, dopamine, epinephrine, erythromycin, esmolol, etomidate, famotidine, fentanyl, fluconazole, gentamicin, haloperidol, heparin, hydromorphone, insulin (regular), labetalol, lorazepam, methylprednisolone, metronidazole, milrinone, morphine, nicardipine, nitroglycerin, norepinephrine, pancuronium, piperacillin, potassium chloride, ranitidine, sodium nitroprusside, sufentanil, theophylline, tobramycin, vancomycin, vecuronium

Perform/provide:

• Assistance with ambulation until drowsy period relieved

• Storage at room temp

 = Nursing alert   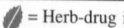 = Herb-drug interaction $\bigcirc$ = Do not crush

• Immediate availability of resuscitation equipment, O_2 to support airway; do not give by rapid bolus
Evaluate:
• Therapeutic response: induction of sedation, general anesthesia
Teach patient/family:
• That amnesia occurs; events may not be remembered
Treatment of overdose: O_2, vasopressors, physostigmine, resuscitation

---

midodrine (℞)
(mye'doh-dreen)
ProAmatine
Func. class.: Vasopressor

Action: Activates α-adrenergic receptors of arteriolar venous vasculature
Uses: Orthostatic hypotension
Dosage and routes:
• *Adult:* **PO** 10 mg tid
Renal dose
• *Adult:* **PO** 2.5 mg tid
Available forms: Tabs 2.5, 5 mg
Side effects/adverse reactions:
CNS: Drowsiness, restlessness, headache, *paresthesia, pain,* chills
GI: Nausea, anorexia
EENT: Dry mouth, blurred vision
INTEG: Pruritus, piloerection, rash
GU: Urinary urgency
CV: Supine hypertension
Contraindications: Hypersensitivity, severe organic heart disease, acute renal disease, urinary retention, pheochromocytoma, thyrotoxicosis, persistent/excessive supine hypertension
Precautions: Children, urinary retention, lactation, prostatic hypertrophy, pregnancy (C)
Pharmacokinetics:
PO: Peak 1-2 hr, half-life 3-4 hr

Interactions:
• Increased bradycardia: β-blockers, psychopharmacologics, cardiac glycosides
• Increased pressor effects: α-agonist
• Increased intraocular pressure: steroids
NURSING CONSIDERATIONS
Assess:
• VS, B/P (standing, supine)
• Observe for drowsiness, dizziness, LOC
Administer:
• Tablets may be swallowed whole, chewed, or allowed to dissolve
• Upon arising, midday, and late afternoon (no later than 6 PM)
• Avoid administering if patient is to be supine during day
Evaluate:
• Therapeutic response: decreased orthostatic hypotension
Teach patient/family:
• To avoid hazardous activities, activities requiring alertness; dizziness may occur; instruct patient to request assistance with ambulation
• To avoid alcohol, other depressants

---

miglitol (℞)
(mig'lih-tol)
Glyset
Func. class.: Oral hypoglycemic
Chem. class.: α-glucosidase inhibitor

Action: Delays digestion of ingested carbohydrates, results in smaller rise in blood glucose after meals; does not increase insulin production
Uses: Non–insulin-dependent diabetes mellitus (NIDDM) Type II
Dosage and routes:
• *Adult:* **PO** 25 mg tid initially, with first bite of meal; maintenance dose

may be increased to 50 mg tid; may be increased to 100 mg tid if needed (only in patients >60 kg) with dosage adjustment at 4-8 wk intervals
Available forms: Tabs 25, 50, 100 mg
Side effects/adverse reactions:
*GI: Abdominal pain, diarrhea, flatulence, **hepatotoxicity***
HEMA: Low iron
INTEG: Rash
Contraindications: Hypersensitivity, diabetic ketoacidosis, cirrhosis, inflammatory bowel disease, colonic ulceration, partial intestinal obstruction, chronic intestinal disease
Precautions: Pregnancy (B), renal disease, lactation, children, hepatic disease
Pharmacokinetics: Not metabolized, excreted in urine as unchanged drug, half-life 2 hr
Interactions:
• Increased hypoglycemia: sulfonylureas, insulin
• Decreased levels of: digoxin, propranolol, ranitidine
• Decreased levels of miglitol: digestive enzymes, intestinal adsorbents; do not use together
⬗ Decreased hypoglycemic effect: broom, buchu, dandelion, juniper
⬗ Increased or decreased hypoglycemic effect: chromium, fenugreek, ginseng
⬗ Improved glucose tolerance: karela
NURSING CONSIDERATIONS
Assess:
• Hypoglycemia, hyperglycemia; even though drug does not cause hypoglycemia, if patient is on sulfonylureas or insulin, hypoglycemia may be additive
• Blood glucose levels, glycosylated hemoglobin, LFTs
Administer:
• tid with first bite of each meal

Perform/provide:
• Storage in tight container in cool environment
Evaluate:
• Therapeutic response: decreased signs/symptoms of diabetes mellitus (polyuria, polydipsia, polyphagia, clear sensorium, absence of dizziness, stable gait)
Teach patient/family:
• The symptoms of hypo/hyperglycemia, what to do about each, that during periods of stress, infection, surgery, insulin may be required
• That medication must be taken as prescribed; explain consequences of discontinuing medication abruptly
• To avoid OTC medications unless approved by health-care provider
• That diabetes is lifelong illness; that this drug is not a cure
• To carry a Medic Alert ID for emergency purposes
• That diet and exercise regimen must be followed

milrinone (R)
(mill′rih-nohn)
Primacor
Func. class.: Inotropic/vasodilator agent with phosphodiesterase activity
Chem. class.: Bipyridine derivative

Action: Positive inotropic agent with vasodilator properties; reduces preload and afterload by direct relaxation on vascular smooth muscle
Uses: Short-term management of CHF that has not responded to other medication; can be used with digitalis
Dosage and routes:
• *Adult:* IV BOL 50 µg/kg given over 10 min; start infusion of 0.375-

◆ = Nursing alert ⬗ = Herb-drug interaction 🚫 = Do not crush

0.75 µg/kg/min; reduce dose in renal impairment

Available forms: Inj 1 mg/ml

Side effects/adverse reactions:

HEMA: **Thrombocytopenia**

MISC: Headache, hypokalemia, tremor

CV: **Dysrhythmias,** hypotension, chest pain

GI: Nausea, vomiting, anorexia, abdominal pain, **hepatotoxicity, jaundice**

Contraindications: Hypersensitivity to this drug, severe aortic disease, severe pulmonic valvular disease, acute myocardial infarction

Precautions: Lactation, pregnancy (C), children, renal disease, hepatic disease, atrial flutter/fibrillation, elderly

Pharmacokinetics:

IV: Onset 2-5 min, peak 10 min, duration variable; half-life 4-6 hr; metabolized in liver; excreted in urine as drug and metabolites 60%-90%

NURSING CONSIDERATIONS

Assess:

• B/P and pulse q5min during infusion; if B/P drops 30 mm Hg, stop infusion and call prescriber

• Electrolytes: K, Na, Cl, Ca; renal function studies: BUN, creatinine; blood studies: platelet count

• ALT, AST, bilirubin qd

• I&O ratio and weight qd; diuresis should increase with continuing therapy

• If platelets are <150,000/mm^3, drug is usually discontinued and another drug started

• Extravasation; change site q48h

Administer:

• K supplements if ordered for K levels <3 mg/dl

IV

• Into running dextrose infusion through Y-connector or directly into tubing; dilute with 0.9% NaCl to

1-3 mg/ml; do not mix with glucose for long-term infusion

• By infusion pump for doses other than bolus

Additive compatibilities: Quinidine

Syringe compatibilities: Atropine, calcium chloride, digoxin, epinephrine, lidocaine, morphine, propranolol, sodium bicarbonate, verapamil

Y-site compatibilities: Digoxin, diltiazem, dobutamine, dopamine, epinephrine, fentanyl, heparin, hydromorphone, labetalol, lorazepam, midazolam, morphine, nicardipine, nitroglycerin, norepinephrine, propranolol, quinidine, ranitidine, thiopental, vecuronium

Evaluate:

• Therapeutic response: increased cardiac output, decreased PCWP, adequate CVP, decreased dyspnea, fatigue, edema, ECG

Treatment of overdose: Discontinue drug, support circulation

M

---

mineral oil (OTC)

Agoral Plain, Fleet Mineral Oil Enema, Kondremul*, Kondremul Plain, Liqui-doss, Lansoyl*, Milkinol, Neo-Cultol, Nujol, Petrogalar Plain, Zymenol

Func. class.: Laxative-lubricant

Chem. class.: Petroleum hydrocarbon

Action: Eases passage of stool by increasing water retention in feces; acts as lubricant

Uses: Constipation, preparation for bowel surgery or exam

Dosage and routes:

• *Adult:* **PO** 15-30 ml hs; **ENEMA** 4 oz

• *Child 6-12 yr:* **PO** 5-15 ml hs; **ENEMA** 1-2 oz

• *Child 2-11 yr:* **ENEMA** 1-2 oz

Available forms: Oil, enema; jelly 55%; susp 1.4, 2.5, 2.75 mg/5 ml

Side effects/adverse reactions:

CNS: Muscle weakness

GI: Nausea, vomiting, anorexia, diarrhea, pruritus ani, hepatic infiltration

*META: **Hypoprothrombinemia***

RESP: Lipid pneumonia

Contraindications: Hypersensitivity, intestinal obstruction, abdominal pain, nausea/vomiting

Precautions: Pregnancy (UK), swallowing difficulty

Pharmacokinetics: Excreted in feces

Interactions:

• Increased effect of oral anticoagulants

• Decreased absorption: fat-soluble vitamins (A, D, E, K) if used for prolonged time

NURSING CONSIDERATIONS

Assess:

• Stool for color, consistency, amount

• Blood, urine electrolytes if drug is used often by patient

• I&O ratio to identify fluid loss

• Cause of constipation; lack of fluids, bulk, exercise

• Cramping, rectal bleeding, nausea, vomiting; drug should be discontinued

Administer:

• Alone for better absorption

• In morning or evening (oral dose)

• Cautiously in elderly to prevent aspiration

Evaluate:

• Therapeutic response: decrease in constipation

Teach patient/family:

• Not to use laxatives for long-term therapy; bowel tone will be lost

• That normal bowel movements do not always occur daily

• Not to use in presence of abdominal pain, nausea, vomiting

• To notify prescriber if constipation unrelieved or if symptoms of electrolyte imbalance occur: muscle cramps, pain, weakness, dizziness, excessive thirst

• Not to use with food or vitamin preparations; delays digestion and absorption of fat-soluble vitamins

---

minocycline (Ŗ)
(min-oh-sye′kleen)
Minocin, Minocin IV
Func. class.: Broad-spectrum antiinfective
Chem. class.: Tetracycline

Action: Inhibits protein synthesis, phosphorylation in microorganisms by binding to 30S ribosomal subunits, reversibly binding to 50S ribosomal subunits; bacteriostatic

Uses: Syphilis, *Chlamydia trachomatis,* gonorrhea, lymphogranuloma venereum, rickettsial infections, inflammatory acne, *Neisseria meningitidis, N. gonorrheae, Treponema pallidum, Chlamydia trachomatis, Ureaplasma urealyticum, Mycoplasma pneumoniae, Nocardia*

Dosage and routes:

• *Adult:* **PO/IV** 200 mg, then 100 mg q12h or 50 mg q6h, not to exceed 400 mg/24 hr **IV**

• *Child >8 yr:* **PO/IV** 4 mg/kg then 4 mg/kg/day **PO** in divided doses q12h

Gonorrhea

• *Adult:* **PO** 200 mg, then 100 mg q12h × 4 days

Chlamydia trachomatis

• *Adult:* **PO** 100 mg bid × 7 days

Syphilis

• *Adult:* **PO** 200 mg, then 100 mg q12h × 10-15 days

⬥ = Nursing alert   ✒ = Herb-drug interaction   ⊘ = Do not crush

Available forms: Tabs 50, 100 mg; caps 50, 100 mg; oral susp 50 mg/5 ml; powder for inj 100 mg/vial

Side effects/adverse reactions:

CNS: Dizziness, fever, light-headedness, vertigo

*HEMA: **Eosinophilia, neutropenia, thrombocytopenia, hemolytic anemia***

EENT: Dysphagia, glossitis, decreased calcification of deciduous teeth, permanent discoloration of teeth, oral candidiasis

GI: Nausea, abdominal pain, *vomiting, diarrhea,* anorexia, enterocolitis, ***hepatotoxicity,*** flatulence, abdominal cramps, epigastric burning, stomatitis

CV: Pericarditis

GU: Increased BUN, polyuria, polydipsia, ***renal failure, nephrotoxicity***

INTEG: Rash, urticaria, *photosensitivity, increased pigmentation, **exfoliative dermatitis,*** pruritus, angioedema, blue-gray color of skin, mucous membranes

Contraindications: Hypersensitivity to tetracyclines, children <8 yr, pregnancy (D)

Precautions: Hepatic disease, lactation

Pharmacokinetics:

PO: Peak 2-3 hr, half-life 11-17 hr; excreted in urine, feces, breast milk; crosses placenta; 70%-75% protein bound

Interactions:

• Decreased effect of minocycline: antacids, $NaHCO_3$, alkali products, iron, kaolin/pectin, cimetidine

• Increased effect: warfarin

• Decreased effect of barbiturates, carbamazepine, phenytoin, penicillins, oral contraceptives

• Nephrotoxicity: methoxyflurane

Lab test interferences:

False negative: Urine glucose with Clinistix or Tes-Tape

NURSING CONSIDERATIONS

Assess:

• I&O ratio

• Blood studies: PT, CBC, AST, ALT, BUN, creatinine

• Signs of anemia: Hct, Hgb, fatigue

• Allergic reactions: rash, itching, pruritus, angioedema

• Nausea, vomiting, diarrhea; administer antiemetic, antacids as ordered

• Overgrowth of infection: fever, malaise, redness, pain, swelling, drainage, perineal itching, diarrhea, changes in cough or sputum, black, furry tongue

Administer:

• After C&S obtained

• 2 hr before or after laxative or ferrous products; 3 hr after antacid or kaolin-pectin product (PO)

IV

• After diluting 100 mg/5 ml sterile H_2O for inj; further dilute in 500-1000 ml of NaCl, dextrose sol, LR, Ringer's sol; run 100 mg/6 hr

Y-site compatibilities: Aztreonam, cisatracurium, cyclophosphamide, filgrastim, fludarabine, granisetron, heparin, hydrocortisone, magnesium sulfate, melphalan, perphenazine, potassium chloride, remifentanil, sargramostim, teniposide, vinorelbine, vit B/C

Perform/provide:

• Storage in airtight, light-resistant container at room temp

Evaluate:

• Therapeutic response: decreased temp, absence of lesions, negative C&S

Teach patient/family:

• To avoid sunlight; sunscreen does not seem to decrease photosensitivity

• That all prescribed medication must be taken to prevent superinfection

M

• To take with a full glass of water; may take with food for GI symptoms

---

minoxidil (R)
(mi-nox'i-dill)
Loniten, Minodyl, minoxidil, Rogaine
Func. class.: Antihypertensive
Chem. class.: Vasodilator—peripheral

Action: Directly relaxes arteriolar smooth muscle, causing vasodilation

Uses: Severe hypertension unresponsive to other therapy (use with diuretic); topically to treat alopecia

Dosage and routes:
Severe hypertension
• *Adult:* **PO** 5 mg/day not to exceed 100 mg daily, usual range 10-40 mg/day in single doses
• *Geriatric:* **PO** 2.5 mg qd, may be increased gradually
• *Child <12 yr:* **PO** (initial) 0.2 mg/kg/day; (effective range) 0.25-1 mg/kg/day; (max) 50 mg/day
Alopecia
• *Adult:* Apply topically, rub into scalp daily

Available forms: Tabs 2.5, 10 mg; top 20, 50 mg/ml

Side effects/adverse reactions:
CV: Severe rebound hypertension, tachycardia, angina, increased T wave, **CHF, pulmonary edema, pericardial effusion,** edema, sodium, water retention
CNS: Drowsiness, dizziness, sedation, headache, depression, fatigue
GI: Nausea, vomiting
GU: Gynecomastia, breast tenderness
INTEG: Pruritus, **Stevens-Johnson syndrome,** rash, hirsutism

HEMA: Hct, Hgb, erythrocyte count may decrease initially

Contraindications: Acute MI, dissecting aortic aneurysm, hypersensitivity, pheochromocytoma

Precautions: Pregnancy (C) (PO), lactation, children, renal disease, CAD, CHF

Pharmacokinetics:
PO: Onset 30 min, peak 2-3 hr, duration 75 hr; half-life 4.2 hr; metabolized in liver; metabolites excreted in urine, feces

Interactions:
• Orthostatic hypotension: guanethidine

Lab test interferences:
Increase: Renal function studies
Decrease: Hgb/Hct/RBC

NURSING CONSIDERATIONS
Assess:
• Nausea, edema in feet, legs daily
• Skin turgor, dryness of mucous membranes for hydration status
• Rales, dyspnea, orthopnea
• Electrolytes: K, Na, Cl, CO_2
• Renal function studies: catecholamines, BUN, creatinine
• Hepatic function studies: AST, ALT, alk phosphatase
• B/P, pulse
• Weight daily, I&O
Administer:
TOP
• 1 ml no matter how much balding has occurred; increasing dosage does not speed growth
PO
• With meals for better absorption, to decrease GI symptoms
• With β-blocker and/or diuretic for hypertension
Perform/provide:
• Storage protected from light and heat
Evaluate:
• Therapeutic response: decreased B/P or increased hair growth

---

◆ = Nursing alert   🥢 = Herb-drug interaction   🚫 = Do not crush

Teach patient/family:

• That body hair will increase but is reversible after discontinuing treatment
• Not to discontinue drug abruptly
• To report pitting edema, dizziness, weight gain >5 lb, shortness of breath, bruising or bleeding, heart rate >20 beats/min over normal, severe indigestion, dizziness, lightheadedness, panting, new or aggravated symptoms of angina
• To take drug exactly as prescribed, or serious side effects may occur
• That for topical use, treatment must continue long-term or new hair will be lost
• Not to use except on scalp
Treatment of overdose: Administer normal saline IV, vasopressors

---

mirtazapine (R)

(mer-ta'za-peen)
Remeron
Func. class.: Antidepressant
Chem. class.: Tetracyclic

Action: Blocks reuptake of norepinephrine, serotonin into nerve endings, increasing action of norepinephrine, serotonin in nerve cells
Uses: Depression, dysthymic disorder, bipolar disorder—depressed, agitated depression
Dosage and routes:
• *Adult:* PO 15 mg/day at hs, maintenance to continue for 6 mo
• *Geriatric:* PO 7.5 mg q hs, increase by 7.5 mg q1-2wk to desired dose, max 45 mg/day
Available forms: Tabs 15, 30 mg
Side effects/adverse reactions:
*HEMA: **Agranulocytosis, thrombocytopenia, eosinophilia, leukopenia***
CNS: Dizziness, drowsiness, confusion, headache, anxiety, tremors, stimulation, weakness, insomnia, nightmares, EPS (elderly), increased psychiatric symptoms, *seizures*
GI: Diarrhea, dry mouth, nausea, vomiting, ***paralytic ileus,*** increased appetite, cramps, epigastric distress, ***jaundice, hepatitis,*** stomatitis
*GU: Urinary retention, **acute renal failure***
INTEG: Rash, urticaria, sweating, pruritus, photosensitivity
*CV: Orthostatic hypotension, ECG changes, tachycardia, **hypertension,*** palpitations
EENT: Blurred vision, tinnitus, mydriasis
Contraindications: Hypersensitivity to tricyclic antidepressants, recovery phase of MI, convulsive disorders, prostatic hypertrophy
Precautions: Suicidal patients, severe depression, increased intraocular pressure, narrow-angle glaucoma, urinary retention, cardiac disease, hepatic disease, hypothyroidism, hyperthyroidism, electroshock therapy, elective surgery, elderly, pregnancy (C)
Pharmacokinetics:
PO: Peak 12 hr, metabolized by liver; excreted in urine, feces; crosses placenta; half-life 20-40 hr
Interactions:
• Decreased effects of guanethidine, clonidine, indirect-acting sympathomimetics (ephedrine)
• Increased CNS depression, alcohol, barbiturates, benzodiazepines, CNS depressants
◆Hyperpyretic crisis, convulsions, hypertensive episode: MAOIs
⚕ Increased anticholinergic effect: belladonna, henbane
⚕ Increased antidepressant action: scopolia
Lab test interferences:
Increase: Serum bilirubin, blood glucose, alk phosphatase
False increase: Urinary catecholamines

Decrease: VMA, 5-HIAA

NURSING CONSIDERATIONS
Assess:

• B/P (lying, standing), pulse q4h; if systolic B/P drops 20 mm Hg, hold drug, notify prescriber; take vital signs q4h in patients with cardiovascular disease

• Blood studies: CBC, leukocytes, differential, cardiac enzymes if patient is receiving long-term therapy

• Hepatic studies: AST, ALT, bilirubin, creatinine

• Weight qwk; appetite may increase with drug

• ECG for flattening of T wave, bundle branch block, AV block, dysrhythmias in cardiac patients

• EPS primarily in elderly: rigidity, dystonia, akathisia

• Mental status: mood, sensorium, affect, suicidal tendencies, increase in psychiatric symptoms: depression, panic

• Urinary retention, constipation; constipation is more likely to occur in children

• Withdrawal symptoms: headache, nausea, vomiting, muscle pain, weakness; do not usually occur unless drug was discontinued abruptly

• Alcohol consumption; if alcohol is consumed, hold dose until morning

Administer:

• Increased fluids, bulk in diet for constipation, especially elderly

• With food, milk for GI symptoms

• Dosage hs if oversedation occurs during day; may take entire dose hs; elderly may not tolerate once/day dosing

• Gum, hard candy, or frequent sips of water for dry mouth

• Concentrate with fruit juice, water, or milk to disguise taste

Perform/provide:

• Storage in tight container at room temp; do not freeze

• Assistance with ambulation during beginning therapy, since drowsiness/dizziness occurs

• Safety measures, including side rails, primarily in elderly

• Checking to see PO medication swallowed

Evaluate:

• Therapeutic response: decreased depression

Teach patient/family:

• That therapeutic effects may take 2-3 wk

• To use caution in driving, other activities requiring alertness, because of drowsiness, dizziness, blurred vision

• To avoid alcohol ingestion, other CNS depressants

• Not to discontinue medication quickly after long-term use; may cause nausea, headache, malaise

• To wear sunscreen or large hat, since photosensitivity occurs

Treatment of overdose: ECG monitoring, induce emesis; lavage, activated charcoal; administer anticonvulsant

---

misoprostol (℞)
(mye-soe-prost′ole)
Cytotec

Func. class.: Gastric mucosa protectant

Chem. class.: Prostaglandin E$_1$-analog

Action: Inhibits gastric acid secretion; may protect gastric mucosa; can increase bicarbonate, mucus production

Uses: Prevention of nonsteroidal antiinflammatory drug-induced gastric ulcers

Investigational uses: Used investigationally with methotrexate to produce abortion

---

◆ = Nursing alert 🍃 = Herb-drug interaction 🚫 = Do not crush

Dosage and routes:
• *Adult:* **PO** 200 µg qid with food for duration of nonsteroidal anti-inflammatory therapy; if 200 µg is not tolerated, 100 µg may be given
Available forms: Tabs 100, 200 µg
Side effects/adverse reactions:
GI: Diarrhea, nausea, vomiting, flatulence, constipation, dyspepsia, abdominal pain
GU: Spotting, cramps, hypermenorrhea, menstrual disorders
Contraindications: Hypersensitivity, pregnancy (X)
Precautions: Lactation, children, elderly, renal disease
Pharmacokinetics:
PO: Peak 12 min, plasma steady state achieved within 2 days, excreted in urine
NURSING CONSIDERATIONS
Assess:
• GI symptoms: hematemesis, occult or frank blood in stools, gastric aspirate, cramping, severe diarrhea
• Obtain a negative pregnancy test; miscarriages are common
• Gastric pH (>5 should be maintained)
Administer:
• PO with meals for prolonged drug effect; avoid use of magnesium antacids
Perform/provide:
• Storage at room temp
Evaluate:
• Therapeutic response: absence of pain or GI complaints; prevention of ulcers
Teach patient/family:
• To take only as directed
• Not to take if pregnant (can cause miscarriage) and not to become pregnant while taking this medication; if pregnancy occurs during therapy, discontinue drug, notify prescriber; not to administer to nursing mothers
• Not to give drug to anyone else or

take for more than 4 wk unless directed by prescriber
• To avoid OTC preparations: aspirin, cough, cold products; condition may worsen

---

mitomycin ($\mathbf{R}$)
(mye-toe-mye'sin)
Mitomycin, Mutamycin
Func. class.: Antineoplastic, antibiotic

Action: Inhibits DNA synthesis, primarily; derived from *Streptomyces caespitosus;* appears to cause cross-linking of DNA, a vesicant
Uses: Pancreas, stomach cancer, head and neck or breast cancer
Investigational uses: Palliative treatment of head, neck, colon, breast, biliary, cervical, lung malignancies
Dosage and routes:
• *Adult:* 10-20 mg/m^2 q6-8wk
Available forms: Inj 5, 20, 40 mg/vial
Side effects/adverse reactions:
*HEMA: **Thrombocytopenia, leukopenia, anemia***
*GI: Nausea, vomiting, anorexia, stomatitis, **hepatotoxicity,** diarrhea*
GU: Urinary retention, ***renal failure,*** edema
INTEG: Rash, alopecia, ***extravasation***
*RESP: **Fibrosis, pulmonary infiltrate,** dyspnea*
CNS: Fever, headache, confusion, drowsiness, syncope, fatigue
EENT: Blurred vision, drowsiness, syncope
Contraindications: Hypersensitivity, pregnancy (D) (1st trimester), as a single agent, thrombocytopenia, coagulation disorders
Precautions: Renal disease, bone marrow depression
Pharmacokinetics: Half-life 1 hr,

M

metabolized in liver, 10% excreted in urine (unchanged)

Interactions:

• Increased toxicity: other antineoplastics (vinca alkaloids), radiation

NURSING CONSIDERATIONS
Assess:

• CBC, differential, platelet count weekly; withhold drug if WBC is <4000/mm^3 or platelet count is <75,000/mm^3; notify prescriber

• Pulmonary function tests, chest x-ray before, during therapy; chest x-ray should be obtained q2wk during treatment

• Renal function studies: BUN, serum uric acid, urine CrCl, electrolytes before, during therapy

• I&O ratio; report fall in urine output to <30 ml/hr

• Monitor temp q4h; fever may indicate beginning infection

• Liver function tests before, during therapy: bilirubin, AST, ALT, alk phosphatase as needed or monthly; check for jaundiced skin and sclera, dark urine, clay-colored stools, itchy skin, abdominal pain, fever, diarrhea

• Alkalosis if severe vomiting is present

• Bleeding: hematuria, guaiac, bruising, petechiae, mucosa or orifices q8h

• Dyspnea, rales, unproductive cough, chest pain, tachypnea, fatigue, increased pulse, pallor, lethargy

• Effects of alopecia on body image; discuss feelings about body changes

• Inflammation of mucosa, breaks in skin

• Buccal cavity q8h for dryness, sores, ulceration, white patches, oral pain, bleeding, dysphagia

• Local irritation, pain, burning at injection site

• GI symptoms: frequency of stools, cramping

• Acidosis, signs of dehydration: rapid respirations, poor skin turgor, decreased urine output, dry skin, restlessness, weakness

Administer:

• Apply ice compress for extravasation; stop infusion

• Antiemetic 30-60 min before giving drug to prevent vomiting

• IV after diluting 5 mg/10 ml sterile H$_2$O for inj; allow to stand, give through Y-tube or 3-way stopcock; give over 5-10 min

• Transfusion for anemia

• Antispasmodic for GI symptoms

Additive compatibilities: Dexamethasone, hydrocortisone

Solution compatibilities: LR, 0.3% NaCl, 0.5% NaCl

Syringe compatibilities: Bleomycin, cisplatin, cyclophosphamide, doxorubicin, droperidol, fluorouracil, furosemide, heparin, leucovorin, methotrexate, metoclopramide, vinblastine, vincristine

Y-site compatibilities: Allopurinol, amifostine, bleomycin, cisplatin, cyclophosphamide, doxorubicin, droperidol, fluorouracil, furosemide, granisetron, heparin, leucovorin, melphalan, methotrexate, metoclopramide, ondansetron, teniposide, thiotepa, vinblastine, vincristine

Perform/provide:

• Liquid diet: carbonated beverages, gelatin may be added if patient is not nauseated or vomiting

• Rinsing of mouth tid-qid with water; brushing of teeth with baking soda bid-tid with soft brush or cotton-tipped applicators for stomatitis; use unwaxed dental floss

• Storage at room temp 1 wk after reconstituting or 2 wk refrigerated

Evaluate:

• Therapeutic response: decreased tumor size, spread of malignancy

---

◆ = Nursing alert   🌿 = Herb-drug interaction   🚫 = Do not crush

Teach patient/family:

• To report any complaints, side effects to nurse or prescriber

• That hair may be lost during treatment and wig or hairpiece may make the patient feel better; tell patient that new hair may be different in color, texture

• To avoid foods with citric acid, hot or rough texture

• To report any bleeding, white spots, ulcerations in mouth; tell patient to examine mouth qd

• To avoid crowds, people with infections if granulocyte count is low

---

mitoxantrone (Ⓡ)

(mye-toe-zan'trone)

Novantrone

Func. class.: Antineoplastic, antibiotic

Chem. class.: Synthetic anthraquinone

Action: DNA reactive agent, cytocidal effect on both proliferating and nonproliferating cells, suggesting lack of cell cycle phase specificity (vesicant)

Uses: Acute nonlymphocytic leukemia (adult), relapsed leukemia, breast cancer; used with steroids to treat bone pain (advanced prostate cancer)

Investigational uses: Breast and liver malignancies, non-Hodgkin's lymphoma

Dosage and routes:

• *Adult:* **IV INF** 12 mg/m^2/day on days 1-3, and 100 mg/m^2 cytosine arabinoside × 7 days as a continuous 24 hr infusion

Available forms: Inj 2 mg/ml

Side effects/adverse reactions:

GI: Nausea, vomiting, diarrhea, anorexia, mucositis, **hepatotoxicity**

HEMA: **Thrombocytopenia, leuko-**

penia, myelosuppression, anemia

INTEG: Rash, necrosis at injection site, dermatitis, thrombophlebitis at injection site, alopecia

CV: **CHF, cardiopathy, dysrhythmias**

MISC: Fever

RESP: Cough, dyspnea

Contraindications: Hypersensitivity, pregnancy (D)

Precautions: Myelosuppression, lactation, cardiac disease, children; renal, hepatic disease; gout

Pharmacokinetics: Highly bound to plasma proteins, metabolized in liver, excreted via renal, hepatobiliary systems; half-life 24-72 hr

Interactions:

• Do not mix with heparin; precipitate will form

NURSING CONSIDERATIONS

Assess:

• CBC, differential, platelet count qwk; withhold drug if WBC is <4000/mm^3 or platelet count is <75,000/mm^3; notify prescriber of these results

• Liver function tests before, during therapy: bilirubin, AST, ALT, alk phosphatase prn or qmo

• Renal function studies: BUN, serum uric acid, urine CrCl, electrolytes before, during therapy

• Bleeding, hematuria, guaiac, bruising or petechiae, mucosa or orifices q8h

• Jaundiced skin and sclera, dark urine, clay-colored stools, itchy skin, abdominal pain, fever, diarrhea

• Acidosis, signs of dehydration: rapid respirations, poor skin turgor, decreased urine output, dry skin, restlessness, weakness

Administer:

• Medications by oral route if possible; avoid IM, SC, IV routes to prevent infections

• Antiemetic 30-60 min before giving drug to prevent vomiting

M

• IV after diluting with 50 ml or more normal saline or D_5W; give over 3-5 min, running IV of D_5W or NS; may be diluted further in D_5W, NS and run over 15-30 min; check for extravasation

Additive compatibilities: Cyclophosphamide, cytarabine, fluorouracil, hydrocortisone, potassium chloride

Solution compatibilities: D_5/0.9 NaCl, D_5W, 0.9% NaCl

Y-site compatibilities: Allopurinol, amifostine, cladribine, filgrastim, fludarabine, granisetron, melphalan, ondansetron, sargramostim, teniposide, thiotepa, vinorelbine

Perform/provide:

• Liquid diet: carbonated beverages, Jell-O; dry toast, crackers may be added if patient is not nauseated or vomiting

• Rinsing of mouth tid-qid with water, club soda; brushing of teeth bid-qid with soft brush or cotton-tipped applicators for stomatitis; use unwaxed dental floss

Evaluate:

• Therapeutic response: decreased tumor size, spread of malignancy

Teach patient/family:

• To report side effects to nurse or physician

• To avoid foods with citric acid, rough texture, or hot

• To report any bleeding, white spots, ulcerations in mouth; tell patient to examine mouth qd

---

mivacurium (R)
(miv-a-kure'ee-um)
Mivacron
Func. class.: Nondepolarizing neuromuscular blocker

Action: Inhibits transmission of nerve impulses by binding competitively with cholinergic receptor sites, antagonizing action of acetylcholine

Uses: Facilitation of endotracheal intubation, skeletal muscle relaxation during mechanical ventilation, surgery, or general anesthesia

Dosage and routes:

• *Adult:* **IV** 0.15 mg/kg; maintenance q15min

• *Child 2-12 yr:* **IV** 0.2 mg/kg for a 10 min block

Available forms: 5, 10 ml single-use vial (2 mg/ml); premixed infusion in D_5W 50-ml flex container

Side effects/adverse reactions:

CV: Decreased B/P, bradycardia, tachycardia

*RESP: **Prolonged apnea, bronchospasm, wheezing, respiratory depression***

EENT: Diplopia

MS: Weakness, prolonged skeletal muscle relaxation, *paralysis*

INTEG: Rash, urticaria

Contraindications: Hypersensitivity

Precautions: Pregnancy (C), renal or hepatic disease, lactation, children <3 mo, fluid and electrolyte imbalances, neuromuscular disease, respiratory disease, obesity, elderly

Pharmacokinetics: Rapidly hydrolyzed by plasma cholinesterases, peak 2-3 min, reversal within 15-30 min

Interactions:

• Increased neuromuscular blockade: aminoglycosides, quinidine, local anesthetics, polymyxin antibiotics, enflurane, isoflurane, tetracyclines, halothane, Mg, colistin, procainamide, bacitracin, lincomycin, clindamycin, lithium

NURSING CONSIDERATIONS
Assess:

• For electrolyte imbalances (K, Mg); may lead to increased action of this drug

---

◆ = Nursing alert　　🖉 = Herb-drug interaction　　🚫 = Do not crush

• Vital signs (B/P, pulse, respirations, airway) until fully recovered; rate, depth, pattern of respirations, strength of hand grip
• I&O ratio; check for urinary retention, frequency, hesitancy
• Recovery: decreased paralysis of face, diaphragm, leg, arm, rest of body
• Allergic reactions: rash, fever, respiratory distress, pruritus; drug should be discontinued

Administer:
• Using nerve stimulator by anesthesiologist to determine neuromuscular blockade
• Anticholinesterase to reverse neuromuscular blockade
• By slow IV over 1-2 min (only by qualified persons, usually an anesthesiologist)
• Only fresh sol

Y-site compatibilities: Etomidate, thiopental

Perform/provide:
• Storage at room temp; do not freeze
• Reassurance if communication is difficult during recovery from neuromuscular blockade
• Frequent (q2h) instillation of artificial tears and covering eyes to prevent drying of cornea

Evaluate:
• Therapeutic response: paralysis of jaw, eyelid, head, neck, rest of body

Treatment of overdose: Neostigmine, monitor VS; may require mechanical ventilation

---

modafinil
See appendix a—selected new drugs

---

moexipril (℞)
(moe-ex'ih-prill)
Univasc
Func. class.: Antihypertensive
Chem. class.: Angiotensin-converting enzyme inhibitor

Action: Selectively suppresses renin-angiotensin-aldosterone system; inhibits ACE; prevents conversion of angiotensin I to angiotensin II; results in dilation of arterial, venous vessels

Uses: Hypertension, alone or in combination with thiazide diuretics

Dosage and routes:
Renal dose
• CrCl <40 ml/min 3.75 mg/day titrate to desired dose
• *Adult:* **PO** 7.5 mg 1 hr ac initially, may be increased or divided depending on B/P response; maintenance dosage; 7.5-30 mg qd in 1-2 divided doses 1 hr ac

Available forms: Tabs 7.5, 15 mg

Side effects/adverse reactions:
CV: Hypotension, postural hypotension
GU: Impotence, dysuria, nocturia, proteinuria, nephrotic syndrome, acute reversible renal failure, polyuria, oliguria, frequency
HEMA: **Neutropenia**
INTEG: Rash
RESP: **Bronchospasm,** dyspnea, dry cough
META: Hypokalemia
GI: Loss of taste
CNS: Fever, chills
SYST: **Angioedema**

Contraindications: Hypersensitivity, children, lactation, heart block, bilateral renal stenosis, K-sparing diuretics

Precautions: Dialysis patients, hypovolemia, leukemia, scleroderma, lupus erythematosus, blood dyscra-

M

---

sias, CHF, diabetes mellitus, renal disease, thyroid disease, COPD, asthma, pregnancy (C)

Pharmacokinetics: Metabolized by liver (metabolites), excreted in urine; crosses placenta; excreted in breast milk

Interactions:

• Increased hypotension: diuretics, other antihypertensives, ganglionic blockers, adrenergic blockers

• Do not use with potassium-sparing diuretics, sympathomimetics, potassium supplements

Lab test interferences:

False positive: Urine acetone

NURSING CONSIDERATIONS
Assess:

• Blood studies: neutrophils, decreased platelets

• B/P

• Renal studies: protein, BUN, creatinine; watch for increased levels that may indicate nephrotic syndrome

• Baselines in renal, liver function tests before therapy begins

• K levels, although hyperkalemia rarely occurs

• Edema in feet, legs daily

• Allergic reaction: rash, fever, pruritus, urticaria; drug should be discontinued if antihistamines fail to help

• Symptoms of CHF; edema, dyspnea, wet rales, B/P

• Renal symptoms: polyuria, oliguria, frequency

Administer:

• PO 1 hr before meals

Perform/provide:

• Storage in tight container at 86° F (30° C) or less

Evaluate:

• Therapeutic response: decrease in B/P in hypertension

Teach patient/family:

• To take 1 hr ac

• Not to discontinue drug abruptly

• Not to use OTC (cough, cold, or allergy) products unless directed by prescriber

• To comply with dosage schedule, even if feeling better

• To rise slowly to sitting or standing position to minimize orthostatic hypotension

• To notify prescriber of mouth sores, sore throat, fever, swelling of hands or feet, irregular heartbeat, chest pain, signs of angioedema

• That excessive perspiration, dehydration, vomiting, diarrhea may lead to fall in blood pressure; consult prescriber if these occur

• That dizziness, fainting, lightheadedness may occur during first few days of therapy

• That skin rash or impaired perspiration may occur

• How to take B/P

Treatment of overdose: 0.9% NaCl IV inf, hemodialysis

---

montelukast (℞)
(mon-teh-loo'kast)
Singulair
Func. class.: Leukotriene receptor
Chem. class.: Cysteinyl

Action: Inhibits leukotriene (LTD$_4$) formation; leukotrienes exert their effects by increasing neutrophil, eosinophil migration; aggregation of neutrophils, monocytes; smooth muscle contraction, capillary permeability; these actions further lead to bronchoconstriction, inflammation, edema

Uses: Chronic asthma

Dosage and routes:

Asthma

• *Adult and child ≥15 yr:* **PO** 10 mg qd PM

◆ = Nursing alert   ⫰ = Herb-drug interaction   ⊘ = Do not crush

• *Child 6-14 yr:* **PO** 5 mg chew tab qd PM

Available forms: Tabs 10 mg; tabs, chew 5 mg

Side effects/adverse reactions:

CNS: Dizziness, fatigue, headache

GI: Abdominal pain, dyspepsia, LFT abnormalities

INTEG: Rash

MS: Asthenia

RESP: Influenza, cough, nasal congestion

Contraindications: Hypersensitivity

Precautions: Acute attacks of asthma, alcohol consumption, pregnancy (B), lactation, child <6 yr, aspirin sensitivity

Pharmacokinetics: Rapidly absorbed, peak 3-4 hr, half-life 2.7-5.5 hr; protein binding 99%; metabolized by liver, excreted via bile

Interactions:

• Decreased montelukast levels: phenobarbital, rifampin

• Increased stimulation: ephedrine

NURSING CONSIDERATIONS

Assess:

◆Adult patients carefully for symptoms of Churg-Strauss syndrome (rare), including eosinophilia, vasculitic rash, worsening pulmonary symptoms, cardiac complications, and/or neuropathy

• CBC, blood chemistry, during treatment

• LFTs before and qmo × 3 mo, then q2-3mo during treatment (ALT; AST)

• Respiratory rate, rhythm, depth; auscultate lung fields bilaterally; notify prescriber of abnormalities

• Allergic reactions: rash, urticaria; drug should be discontinued

Administer:

PO

• In PM qd

Evaluate:

• Therapeutic response: ability to breathe more easily

Teach patient/family:

• To check OTC medications, current prescription medications for ephedrine, which will increase stimulation; to avoid alcohol

• To avoid hazardous activities; dizziness may occur

• That drug is not to be used for acute asthma attacks

---

moricizine (℞)

(more-i'siz-een)

Ethmozine

Func. class.: Antidysrhythmic, group I

Chem. class.: Phenothiazine

Action: Decreased rate of rise of action potential, prolonging refractory period and shortening the action potential duration; depression of inward influx if sodium mediates the effects; drug may slow atrial and AV nodal conduction

Uses: Life-threatening dysrhythmias

Dosage and routes:

• *Adult:* **PO** 10-15 mg/kg/day or 600-900 mg/day in 2-3 divided doses

Available forms: Film-coated tabs 200, 250, 300 mg

Side effects/adverse reactions:

GI: Nausea, abdominal pain, vomiting, diarrhea

CNS: Dizziness, headache, fatigue, perioral numbness, euphoria, nervousness, sleep disorders, depression, tinnitus, fatigue

RESP: Dyspnea, hyperventilation, *apnea,* asthma, pharyngitis, cough

GU: Sexual dysfunction, difficult urination, dysuria, incontinence

CV: Palpitations, chest pain, *CHF,* hypertension, syncope, dysrhythmias, bradycardia, *MI, thrombophlebitis*

MISC: Sweating, musculoskeletal pain

Contraindications: 2nd or 3rd degree AV block, right bundle branch block, cardiogenic shock, hypersensitivity

Precautions: CHF, hypokalemia, hyperkalemia, sick sinus syndrome, pregnancy (B), lactation, children, impaired hepatic and renal function, cardiac dysfunction

Pharmacokinetics: Half-life 1.5-3.5 hr; peak 0.5-2.2 hr; metabolized by the liver; metabolites excreted in feces and urine, protein binding >90%

Interactions:
• Increased plasma levels of moricizine: cimetidine
• Digoxin or propranolol may enhance some cardiac effects of moricizine; moricizine may decrease effects of theophylline
⧸ Increased anticholinergic effect: henbane
⧸ Increased potassium loss, increased antidysrhythmic action: aloe, cascara sagrada, buckthorn, rhubarb, senna

Lab test interferences:
Increase: CPK

NURSING CONSIDERATIONS
Assess:
• GI status: bowel pattern, number of stools
• Cardiac status: rate, rhythm, quality
• Chest x-ray, pulmonary function test during treatment
• I&O ratio; check for decreasing output
• B/P for fluctuations
• Lung fields: bilateral rales may occur in CHF patient
• Increased respiration, increased pulse; drug should be discontinued
◆ Toxicity: fine tremors, dizziness
• Cardiac status: respiration, rate, rhythm, character continuously

Evaluate:
• Therapeutic response: absence of dysrhythmias
Teach patient/family:
• To report side effects to prescriber
Treatment of overdose: O_2 artificial ventilation, ECG; administer dopamine for circulatory depression, diazepam or thiopental for convulsions

---

morphine (℞)
(mor'feen)
Astramorph PF, Duramorph, Epimorph*, Kadian, Infumorph 200, Infumorph 500, morphine sulfate, Morphitec*, M.O.S.*, M.O.S.-S.R.*, MS Contin, MSIR, OMS Concentrate, Oramorph SR, RMS, Roxanol, Roxanol 100, Roxanol Rescudose, Roxanol SR, UltraJect
Func. class.: Opiate analgesic
Chem. class.: Opiate

Controlled Substance Schedule II
Action: Depresses pain impulse transmission at the spinal cord level by interacting with opioid receptors
Uses: Severe pain
Dosage and routes:
• *Adult:* **SC/IM** 4-15 mg q4h prn; **PO** 10-30 mg q4h prn; **EXT REL** q8-12h; **RECT** 10-20 mg q4h prn; **IV** 4-10 mg diluted in 4-5 ml H_2O for injection, over 5 min
• *Child:* **SC/IV** 0.1-0.2 mg/kg, not to exceed 15 mg; **PO** 0.2-0.5 mg/kg q4-6h (reg rel), q12h (sus rel)
Available forms: Inj 2, 4, 5, 8, 10, 15 mg/ml; sol tabs 10, 15, 30 mg; oral sol 10, 20 mg/5 ml, 20 mg/10 ml, 20 mg/ml; oral tabs 15, 30 mg; rect supp 5, 10, 20, 30 mg; ext rel tabs 15, 30, 60, 100, 200 mg; caps 15, 30 mg

---

◆ = Nursing alert ⧸ = Herb-drug interaction Ⓝ = Do not crush

Side effects/adverse reactions:

CNS: Drowsiness, dizziness, confusion, headache, sedation, euphoria

CV: Palpitations, bradycardia, change in B/P

EENT: Tinnitus, blurred vision, miosis, diplopia

GI: Nausea, vomiting, anorexia, constipation, cramps, biliary tract pressure

GU: Urinary retention

INTEG: Rash, urticaria, bruising, flushing, diaphoresis, pruritus

*RESP: **Respiratory depression***

Contraindications: Hypersensitivity, addiction (narcotic), hemorrhage, bronchial asthma, increased intracranial pressure

Precautions: Addictive personality, pregnancy (B), lactation, acute MI, severe heart disease, elderly, respiratory depression, hepatic disease, renal disease, child <18 yr

Pharmacokinetics:

PO: Onset variable, peak variable, duration variable

IM: Onset ½ hr, peak ½-1 hr, duration 3-7 hr

SC: Onset 15-20 min, peak 50-90 min, duration 3-5 hr

IV: Peak 20 min

RECT: Peak ½-1 hr, duration 4-5 hr

Intrathecal: Onset rapid, duration up to 24 hr

Metabolized by liver, crosses placenta; excreted in urine, breast milk; half-life 1½-2 hr

Interactions:

• Unpredictable reaction, avoid use: MAOIs

• Increased effects with other CNS depressants: alcohol, narcotics, sedative/hypnotics, antipsychotics, skeletal muscle relaxants

• Decreased morphine action: rifampin

Lab test interferences:

Increase: Amylase

NURSING CONSIDERATIONS

Assess:

• Pain: location, type, character; give dose before pain becomes severe

• Bowel status; constipation common

• I&O ratio; check for decreasing output; may indicate urinary retention

• B/P, pulse, respirations (character, depth, rate)

• CNS changes: dizziness, drowsiness, hallucinations, euphoria, LOC, pupil reaction

• Allergic reactions: rash, urticaria

• Respiratory dysfunction: depression, character, rate, rhythm; notify prescriber if respirations are <12/ min

Administer:

• With antiemetic for nausea, vomiting

• When pain is beginning to return; determine dosage interval by response; continuous dosing is more effective than prn

• May be given by patient: controlled analgesia

• Epidural cautiously in the elderly

IV

• After diluting with 5 ml or more sterile H_2O or NS; give 15 mg or less over 4-5 min; give through Y-tube or 3-way stopcock; may be added to IV sol, each 0.1-1 mg diluted in 1 ml D_5W, $D_{10}W$, 0.9% NaCl, 0.45% NaCl, Ringer's, LR, given with inf pump titrated to patient response

Additive compatibilities: Alteplase, atracurium, baclofen, bupivacaine, dobutamine, fluconazole, furosemide, meropenem, metoclopramide, ondansetron, succinylcholine, verapamil

Syringe compatibilities: Atropine, benzquinamide, bupivacaine, butorphanol, cimetidine, dimenhydrinate, diphenhydramine, droperidol, fentanyl, glycopyrrolate, hydroxyzine, ketamine, metoclopramide, midazolam, milrinone, pentazocine, perphenazine, promazine, ranitidine, scopolamine

Y-site compatibilities: Allopurinol, amifostine, amikacin, aminophylline, amiodarone, ampicillin, ampicillin/sulbactam, amsacrine, atenolol, atracurium, aztreonam, bumetanide, calcium chloride, cefamandole, cefazolin, cefmetazole, cefoperazone, cefotaxime, cefotetan, cefoxitin, ceftazidime, ceftizoxime, ceftriaxone, cefuroxime, cephalothin, cephapirin, chloramphenicol, cisatracurium, cisplatin, cladribine, clindamycin, cyclophosphamide, cytarabine, dexamethasone, digoxin, diltiazem, dobutamine, dopamine, doxycycline, enalaprilat, epinephrine, erythromycin, esmolol, etomidate, famotidine, fentanyl, filgrastim, fluconazole, fludarabine, foscarnet, gentamicin, granisetron, heparin, hydrocortisone, hydromorphone, IL-2, insulin (regular), kanamycin, labetalol, lidocaine, lorazepam, magnesium sulfate, melphalan, meropenem, methotrexate, methyldopa, methylprednisolone, metoclopramide, metoprolol, metronidazole, mezlocillin, midazolam, milrinone, moxalactam, nafcillin, nicardipine, nitroglycerin, norepinephrine, ondansetron, oxacillin, oxytocin, paclitaxel, pancuronium, penicillin G potassium, piperacillin, piperacillin/tazobactam, potassium chloride, propofol, propranolol, ranitidine, remifentanil, sodium bicarbonate, sodium nitroprusside, teniposide, thiotepa, ticarcillin, ticarcillin/clavulanate, tobramycin, trimethoprim-sulfamethoxazole, vancomycin, vecuronium, vinorelbine, vit B/C, warfarin, zidovudine

Perform/provide:
• Storage in light-resistant container at room temp
• Assistance with ambulation
• Safety measures: side rails, nightlight, call bell within easy reach
• Gradual withdrawal after long-term use

Evaluate:
• Therapeutic response; decrease in pain intensity

Teach patient/family:
• To change position slowly; orthostatic hypotension may occur
• To report any symptoms of CNS changes, allergic reactions
• That physical dependency may result from long-term use
• To avoid use of alcohol, CNS depressants
• That withdrawal symptoms may occur: nausea, vomiting, cramps, fever, faintness, anorexia

Treatment of overdose: Naloxone (Narcan) 0.2-0.8 mg IV, O_2, IV fluids, vasopressors

---

moxalactam
See cephalosporins—3rd generation

---

moxifloxacin
See appendix a—selected new drugs

---

multivitamins (OTC, ℞)

Adavite, Dayalets, LKV
Drops, Multi-75, Multiday,
One-A-Day, Optilets, Poly-Vi-
sol, Quin tabs, Ru-Lets,
Sesame Street Vitamins, Tab-
A-Vite, Therabid, Theragram,
Unicaps, Vita-Bob, Vita-Kid,
many other brands

Func. class.: Vitamins, multiple

Action: Needed for adequate metabolism

Uses: Prevention and treatment of vitamin deficiencies

Dosage and routes:
• *Adult and child:* **PO/IV**—depends on brand

Available forms: Many

Side effects/adverse reactions:
None known at recommended dosage

Precautions: Pregnancy (A)

NURSING CONSIDERATIONS

Assess:
• Vitamin deficiency: usually more than one vitamin is deficient

Administer:
• Liquid multivitamins diluted or dropped into patient's mouth using dropper provided with some brands
• Chew tabs should be chewed, not swallowed whole
• Give by cont IV inf only after diluting 5-10 ml multivitamins/500-1000 ml of D_5W, $D_{10}W$, $D_{20}W$, LR, D_5/LR, $D_5/0.9\%$ NaCl, 0.9% NaCl, 3% NaCl
• Do not use sol with crystals, precipate, or color other than bright yellow

Additive compatibilities: Cefoxitin, isoproterenol, methyldopa, metoclopramide, metronidazole, netilmicin, norepinephrine, sodium bicarbonate, verapamil

Y-site compatibilities: Acyclovir, ampicillin, cefazolin, cephalothin, cephapirin, diltiazem, erythromycin, fludarabine, gentamicin, tacrolimus

Evaluate:
• Therapeutic response: check each individual vitamin for guidelines

Teach patient/family:
• That adequate nutrition must be maintained to prevent further deficiencies
• The drug interactions that should be avoided
• To comply with regimen
• To avoid presenting flavored multivitamins as candy; child may overdose
• To store out of children's reach

muromonab-CD3 (℞)

(mur-oo-mone'ab)
Orthoclone OKT3

Func. class.: Immunosuppressant

Chem. class.: Murine monoclonal antibody

M

Action: Reverses graft rejection by blocking T-cell function

Uses: Acute allograft rejection in renal, cardiac/hepatic transplant patients

Dosage and routes:
• *Adult:* **IV BOL** 5 mg/day × 10-14 days
• *Child:* **IV** 100 µg/kg/day × 10-14 days

Cardiac/hepatic allograft rejection, steroid resistant
• *Adult:* **IV BOL** 5 mg/day × 10-14 days; begin when it is known that rejection has not been reversed by steroids

Available forms: Inj 5 mg/5 ml

Side effects/adverse reactions:
*CNS: Pyrexia, chills, tremors, **aseptic meningitis***

RESP: Dyspnea, wheezing, ***pulmonary edema***
CV: Chest pain
GI: Vomiting, nausea, diarrhea
MISC: ***Infection, cytokine release syndrome***
Contraindications: Hypersensitivity to murine origin, fluid overload
Precautions: Pregnancy (C), child <2 yr, fever
Pharmacokinetics: Trough level steady state 3-14 days
Interactions:

• Increased immunosuppression: immunosuppressants
• Increased risk of infection: cyclosporine, corticosteroids, azathioprine
• Increased CNS symptoms: indomethacin
• Decreased immune response: vaccines

NURSING CONSIDERATIONS
Assess:
◆ For cytokine release syndrome (CRS): nausea, vomiting, chills, fever, joint pain, weakness, dizziness, diarrhea, tremors, abdominal pain
• For hypersensitivity: dyspnea, bronchospasm, urticaria, tachycardia, angioedema; emergency equipment must be available
• Blood studies: Hgb, WBC, platelets during treatment qmo; if leukocytes are <3000/mm^3, drug should be discontinued; CD3, CD4, CD8, CD3 ≤25 cells/mm^3
• Liver function studies: alk phosphatase, AST, ALT, bilirubin
• Hepatotoxicity: dark urine, jaundice, itching, light-colored stools; drug should be discontinued
• For infection: sore throat, fever, chills, temp, notify prescriber immediately
• For aseptic meningitis: fever, headache, photophobia
• For fluid overload: increased weight, I&O, edema, rales

Administer:
• For several days before transplant surgery
• All medications PO if possible; avoid IM injection, since infection may occur
IV
• IV undiluted; withdraw with a 0.2-0.22 low protein-binding μm filter, discard and use new needle for administration; give over 1 min
• Incompatible with any drug in syringe or sol
Evaluate:
• Therapeutic response: absence of graft rejection
Teach patient/family:
• To report fever, chills, sore throat, fatigue, since serious infection may occur
• To use contraceptive measures during treatment
• To report cytokine release syndrome
• To avoid vaccinations during treatment

---

mycophenolate mofetil (℞)
(mye-koe-phen'oh-late)
CellCept
Func. class.: Immunosuppressant

Action: Inhibits inflammatory responses that are mediated by the immune system; prolongs the survival of allogenic transplants
Uses: Organ transplants (to prevent rejection); prophylaxis of organ rejection in allogenic cardiac transplants
Dosage and routes:
• *Adult:* **PO** give initial dose 72 hr prior to transplantation; 1 g bid given to renal transplant patients in combination with corticosteroids, cyclosporine

---

◆ = Nursing alert   🖋 = Herb-drug interaction   🚫 = Do not crush

Available forms: Caps 250 mg; tabs 500 mg; inj (powder) 500 mg

Side effects/adverse reactions:

GI: Diarrhea, constipation, nausea, vomiting, stomatitis

HEMA: **Leukopenia, thrombocytopenia, anemia, pancytopenia**

INTEG: Rash

MS: Arthralgia, muscle wasting

RESP: Dyspnea, respiratory infection, increased cough, pharyngitis, bronchitis, pneumonia

CNS: Tremor, dizziness, insomnia, headache, fever

META: Peripheral edema, hypercholesterolemia, hypophosphatemia, edema, hyperkalemia, hypokalemia, hyperglycemia

GU: UTI, hematuria, **renal tubular necrosis**

CV: Hypertension, chest pain

SYST: **Lymphoma,** *nonmelanoma skin carcinoma*

Contraindications: Hypersensitivity to this drug or mycophenolic acid

Precautions: Lymphomas, malignancies, neutropenia, renal disease, pregnancy (C), lactation

Pharmacokinetics: Rapidly and completely absorbed, metabolized to active metabolite (MPA), excreted in urine, feces

Interactions:

• Increased concentration of both drugs: acyclovir, ganciclovir

• Increased levels of mycophenolate: probenecid, salicylate

• Decreased levels of mycophenolate: antacids, cholestyramine

• Decreased protein binding of phenytoin, theophylline

• Avoid administration with azathioprine

NURSING CONSIDERATIONS

Assess:

• Blood studies: CBC during treatment monthly

• Liver function studies: alk phosphatase, AST, ALT, bilirubin

Administer:

• 72 hr prior to transplantation; may be given in combination with corticosteroids, cyclosporine

• Give alone for better absorption (PO)

IV

• Do not give by rapid or bolus inj; reconstitute and dilute to 6 mg/ml with D_5W, give over ≥2 hr

• Do not admix with mycophenolate IV in infusion catheter or with other IV drugs or infusion admixtures

Evaluate:

• Therapeutic response: absence of graft rejection

Teach patient/family:

• To report fever, rash, severe diarrhea, chills, sore throat, fatigue, since serious infections may occur

• To reduce risk of infection by avoiding crowds

Ⓝ Not to break, crush, or chew tabs, do not open caps

• The need for repeated lab tests

• To limit exposure to sunlight/UV light

• To use contraception before, during, and 6 wk after therapy

---

nabumetone (℞)

(na-byoo′me-tone)

Relafen

Func. class.: Nonsteroidal antiinflammatory

Chem. class.: Acetic acid derivative

Action: Inhibits prostaglandin synthesis by decreasing enzyme needed for biosynthesis; analgesic, antiinflammatory

Uses: Osteoarthritis, rheumatoid arthritis, acute or chronic treatment

Dosage and routes:

• *Adult:* **PO** 1 g as a single dose; may increase to 1.5-2 g/day if needed; may give qd or bid as a divided dose

Available forms: Tabs 500, 750 mg

Side effects/adverse reactions:

CNS: Dizziness, headache, drowsiness, fatigue, tremors, confusion, insomnia, anxiety, depression, nervousness

*GU: **Nephrotoxicity, dysuria, hematuria, oliguria, azotemia,** cystitis*

GI: Nausea, anorexia, vomiting, diarrhea, jaundice, ***cholestatic hepatitis,*** constipation, flatulence, cramps, dry mouth, peptic ulcer, gastritis, ***ulceration, perforation***

CV: Tachycardia, peripheral edema, palpitations, dysrhythmias, ***CHF***

INTEG: Purpura, rash, pruritus, sweating, photosensitivity

*HEMA: **Blood dyscrasias***

EENT: Tinnitus, hearing loss, blurred vision

RESP: Dyspnea, pharyngitis, ***bronchospasm***

Contraindications: Hypersensitivity to this drug or aspirin, iodides, NSAIDs, asthma, severe renal disease, severe hepatic disease

Precautions: Pregnancy (B) 1st and 2nd trimester, lactation, children, bleeding disorders, GI disorders, cardiac disorders, renal disorders, hepatic dysfunction, elderly

Pharmacokinetics:

PO: Peak 2½-4 hr, plasma protein binding >90%, half-life 22-30 hr; metabolized in liver to active metabolite; excreted in urine (metabolites), breast milk

Interactions:

• Decreased effect of: diuretics, antihypertensives

• Increased adverse reactions: warfarin

• Increased risk of bleeding: anticoagulants, thrombolytics, valproic acid, cefamandole, cefotetan, cefoperazone

• Increased risk of hematologic reactions: antineoplastics, radiation

• Increased GI reactions: salicylates, NSAIDs, alcohol, potassium, corticosteroids

NURSING CONSIDERATIONS

Assess:

• Pain: frequency, intensity, characteristics; relief of pain after med

• Asthma, aspirin sensitivity or nasal polyps; increased hypersensitivity reactions

• Renal, liver, blood studies: BUN, creatinine, AST, ALT, Hgb, LDH, blood glucose, WBC, platelets, CrCl before treatment, periodically thereafter

• Audiometric, ophthalmic exam before, during, after treatment

• For eye, ear problems: blurred vision, tinnitus; may indicate toxicity

Administer:

• With food for GI symptoms

Perform/provide:

• Storage at room temp

Evaluate:

• Therapeutic response: decreased pain and stiffness in joints

Teach patient/family:

• To avoid alcoholic beverages and aspirin

• To report blurred vision, ringing, roaring in ears; may indicate toxicity

• To avoid driving, other hazardous activities if dizziness, drowsiness occur

• To report change in urine pattern, increased weight, edema, increased pain in joints, fever, blood in urine; indicates nephrotoxicity

• That therapeutic effects may take up to 1 mo

• To take with a full glass of water to enhance absorption

• To report dark stools; may indicate GI bleeding

◆ = Nursing alert   ⫸ = Herb-drug interaction   ⊘ = Do not crush

nadolol (R)

(nay-doe'lole)

Corgard, Syn-Nadolol*

Func. class.: Antihypertensive, antianginal

Chem. class.: β-adrenergic receptor blocker

Action: Long-acting, nonselective β-adrenergic receptor blocking agent; mechanism is similar to that of propranolol

Uses: Chronic stable angina pectoris, mild to moderate hypertension, prophylaxis of migraine headaches

Investigational uses: Tachydysrhythmias, aggression, anxiety, tremors, esophageal varices (rebleeding only)

Dosage and routes:

• *Adult:* **PO** 40 mg qd, increase by 40-80 mg q3-7d; maintenance 40-240 mg/day for angina, 40-320 mg/day for hypertension

• *Geriatric:* **PO** 20 mg/day, may increase by 20 mg until desired dose

Renal dose

• CrCl 31-50 ml/min give q24-36h; CrCl 10-30 ml/min give q24-48h

Available forms: Tabs 20, 40, 80, 120, 160 mg

Side effects/adverse reactions:

RESP: Dyspnea, respiratory dysfunction, ***bronchospasm,*** cough, wheezing, nasal stuffiness, pharyngitis, ***laryngospasm***

CV: Bradycardia, hypotension, ***CHF,*** palpitations, ***AV block,*** chest pain, peripheral ischemia, flushing, edema, vasodilation, conduction disturbances

HEMA: ***Agranulocytosis, thrombocytopenia***

GI: Nausea, vomiting, diarrhea, colitis, constipation, cramps, dry mouth, flatulence, hepatomegaly, ***pancreatitis,*** taste distortion

INTEG: Rash, pruritus, fever

CNS: Depression, hallucinations, dizziness, fatigue, lethargy, paresthesias, headache

EENT: Sore throat

Contraindications: Hypersensitivity to this drug, cardiac failure, cardiogenic shock, 2nd or 3rd degree heart block, bronchospastic disease, sinus bradycardia, CHF, COPD

Precautions: Diabetes mellitus, pregnancy (C), renal disease, lactation, hyperthyroidism, peripheral vascular disease, myasthenia gravis

Pharmacokinetics:

PO: Onset variable, peak 3-4 hr, duration 17-24 hr; half-life 16-20 hr; not metabolized; excreted in urine (unchanged), bile, breast milk

Interactions:

• Decreased antihypertensive effect: NSAIDs

• Increased bradycardia: digoxin

• Increased hypotension, bradycardia: amphetamines, clonidine, ephedrine, epinephrine

• Do not use with MAOIs

• Increased hypotensive effects: other hypotensive agents, diuretics, phenothiazines

• Decreased effects of xanthines, thyroid

Lab test interferences:

Increase: Serum K, serum uric acid, ALT, AST, alk phosphatase, LDH, blood glucose, cholesterol

NURSING CONSIDERATIONS

Assess:

• B/P, pulse, respirations during beginning therapy

• Weight qd; report gain of 5 lb

• I&O ratio, CrCl if kidney damage is diagnosed

• qd, note need to be administered more often

• Pain: duration, time started, activity being performed, character

N

• Headache, light-headedness, decreased B/P; may indicate a need for decreased dosage

Administer:

PO

• With 8 oz water

Evaluate:

• Therapeutic response: decreased B/P, symptoms of angina

Teach patient/family:

• That drug may mask signs of hypoglycemia or alter blood glucose in diabetics

• Not to discontinue abruptly

• To avoid OTC drugs unless prescriber approves

• To avoid hazardous activities if dizziness occurs

• To comply with complete medical regimen

• To rise slowly to prevent orthostatic hypotension

---

nafarelin (℞)

(naf-ah-rell'in)

Synarel

Func. class.: Gonadotropin

Chem. class.: Analog of gonadotropin-releasing hormone

Action: Stimulates the release of LH and FSH, which increases ovarian steroid production; repeated dosing prevents stimulation of the pituitary gland

Uses: Endometriosis, gonadotropin-dependent precocious puberty

Dosage and routes:

• *Adult:* **NASAL** 400 µg/day as one spray (200 µg) into one nostril in morning and one spray into other nostril in evening; start treatment between days 2 and 4 of menstrual cycle; may increase to 800 µg/day (one spray into each nostril twice a day); recommended duration of treatment is 6 mo

Available forms: Nasal sol 2 mg/ml

Side effects/adverse reactions:

GU: Decreased libido, vaginal dryness, breast tenderness, increased pubic hair

CNS: Headache, flushing, depression, insomnia, emotional lability, hot flashes

INTEG: Nasal irritation, acne

MISC: Body odor, seborrhea, rhinitis

SENSITIVITY: Shortness of breath, chest pain, urticaria, pruritus

Contraindications: Hypersensitivity, pregnancy (X), lactation, undiagnosed abnormal vaginal bleeding

Precautions: Children

Pharmacokinetics: Rapidly absorbed, peak 10-40 min, half-life 3 hr; 80% bound to plasma proteins

NURSING CONSIDERATIONS

Assess:

• Test results: pituitary/hypothalamus dysfunction (decreased LH); postmenopausal (increased LH)

Administer:

NASAL

• Repeated doses may be necessary to elevate pituitary gonadotropin reserve

Perform/provide:

• Storage at room temp; protect from light

Evaluate:

• Therapeutic response: decreased symptoms of endometriosis

Teach patient/family:

• To use nonhormonal contraception

• About correct nasal use, one spray in right nostril AM, one in left nostril PM

• That medication may cause hot flashes, decreased libido, vaginal dryness

---

nafcillin (℞)

(naf-sill'in)
Nafcil, nafcillin sodium,
Nallpen, Unipen
Func. class.: Antiinfective,
broad-spectrum
Chem. class.: Penicillinase-
resistant penicillin

Action: Interferes with cell wall replication of susceptible organisms; osmotically unstable cell wall swells, bursts from osmotic pressure

Uses: Effective for gram-positive cocci *(Staphylococcus aureus, Streptococcus viridans, S. pneumoniae),* infections caused by penicillinase-producing *Staphylococcus*

Dosage and routes:
• *Adult:* PO 250-1000 mg q4-6h; **IM** 500 mg q4-6h; **IV** 500-1500 mg q4-6h
• *Child and infants, most infections:* **PO** 6.25-12.5 mg/kg q6h; pharyngitis **PO** 250 mg q8h; **IM** 25 mg/kg q12h; **IV** most infections 10-20 mg/kg q4h or 20-40 mg/kg q8h, max 200 mg/kg/day
• *Neonates:* **PO** 10 mg/kg q6-8h; **IM** 10 mg/kg q12h; **IV:** most infections 10-20 mg/kg q4h or 20-40 mg/kg q8h, max 200 mg/kg/day
Meningitis
• *Neonates ≥2 kg:* 50 mg/kg q8h × 1 wk of life, then 50 mg/kg q6h
• *Neonates <2 kg:* 25-50 mg/kg q12h × 1 wk of life, then 50 mg/kg q8h
Available forms: Caps 250 mg; tabs 500 mg; powder for oral susp 250 mg/5 ml; powder for inj 500 mg, 1, 2, 10 g; inj 1, 1.5, 2, 4 g

Side effects/adverse reactions:
HEMA: Anemia, increased bleeding time, *bone marrow depression, granulocytopenia*
GI: Nausea, *vomiting, diarrhea,* increased AST, ALT, abdominal pain, glossitis, *pseudomembranous colitis*
GU: Oliguria, *proteinuria, hematuria,* vaginitis, moniliasis, *glomerulonephritis,* interstitial nephritis
CNS: Lethargy, hallucinations, anxiety, depression, twitching, *coma, convulsions*

Contraindications: Hypersensitivity to penicillins
Precautions: Pregnancy (B), hypersensitivity to cephalosporins, neonates

Pharmacokinetics:
IM/PO: Peak 30-60 min, duration 4-6 hr, half-life 1 hr, metabolized by liver, excreted in bile, urine

Interactions:
• Increased risk of bleeding: anticoagulants
• Decreased effect of oral contraceptives
• Increased nafcillin concentrations: aspirin, probenecid, disulfiram
• Drug/food: decreased absorption: food, carbonated drinks, citrus juice
⬛ Delayed/reduced absorption: khat, separate by ≥2 hr

Lab test interferences:
False positive: Urine glucose, urine protein

NURSING CONSIDERATIONS
Assess:
• I&O ratio; report hematuria, oliguria, since penicillin in high doses is nephrotoxic
◆ Any patient with compromised renal system, since drug is excreted slowly in poor renal system function; toxicity may occur rapidly
• Liver studies: AST, ALT
• Blood studies: WBC, RBC, H&H, bleeding time
• Renal studies: urinalysis, protein, blood, BUN, creatinine
• C&S before drug therapy; drug

Side effects: *italics* = common; ***bold italics*** = life-threatening

may be given as soon as culture is taken

• Bowel pattern before and during treatment

• Skin eruptions after administration of penicillin to 1 wk after discontinuing drug

• Respiratory status: rate, character, wheezing, and tightness in chest

• Allergies before initiation of treatment and reaction of each medication; highlight allergies on chart, Kardex

• Differential WBC in patients on long-term therapy

Administer:

• IM deep in gluteal muscle

• Drug after C&S has been completed

• Divided oral doses on empty stomach before meals; oral absorption is erratic

IV

• After diluting 500 mg/1.7 ml of sterile H_2O for inj; further dilute each 500 mg/15-30 ml sterile H_2O or NS sol; give through Y-tube or 3-way stopcock; 500 mg or less/5-10 min; may be further diluted and run over 24 hr

Additive compatibilities: Chloramphenicol, chlorothiazide, dexamethasone, diphenhydramine, ephedrine, heparin, hydroxyzine, lidocaine, potassium chloride, prochlorperazine, sodium bicarbonate, sodium lactate

Syringe compatibilities: Cimetidine, heparin

Y-site compatibilities: Acyclovir, atropine, cyclophosphamide, diazepam, enalaprilat, esmolol, famotidine, fentanyl, fluconazole, foscarnet, hydromorphone, magnesium sulfate, morphine, perphenazine, propofol, theophylline, zidovudine

Perform/provide:

• Adrenalin, suction, tracheostomy set, endotracheal intubation equipment

• Adequate fluid intake (2 L) during diarrhea episodes

• Scratch test to assess allergy after securing order from prescriber; usually done when penicillin is only drug of choice

• Storage in tight container; refrigerate reconstituted sol

Evaluate:

• Therapeutic response: absence of fever, draining wounds

Teach patient/family:

• All aspects of drug therapy, including need to complete course of medication to ensure organism death (10-14 days); culture may be taken after completed course

• To report sore throat, fever, fatigue (may indicate superinfection)

• To wear or carry Medic Alert ID if allergic to penicillins

• To notify nurse of diarrhea

🚫 Not to break, crush, or chew caps

Treatment of anaphylaxis: Withdraw drug; maintain airway; administer epinephrine, aminophylline, O_2, IV corticosteroids

---

nalbuphine (℞)

(nal'byoo-feen)
Nubain, nalbuphine HCl
Func. class.: Opioid analgesic
Chem. class.: Synthetic opioid agonist, antagonist

Action: Depresses pain impulse transmission at the spinal cord level by interacting with opioid receptors

Uses: Moderate to severe pain

Dosage and routes:

Analgesic

• *Adult:* **SC/IM/IV** 10-20 mg q3-6h prn, not to exceed 160 mg/day

Balanced anesthesia supplement

• *Adult:* **IV** 0.3-3 mg/kg given over

10-15 min, may give 0.25-0.5 mg/kg as needed for maintenance

Available forms: Inj 10, 20 mg/ml

Side effects/adverse reactions:

CNS: Drowsiness, dizziness, confusion, headache, sedation, euphoria, dysphoria (high doses), hallucinations, dreaming, tolerance, physical, psychological dependency

GI: Nausea, vomiting, anorexia, constipation, cramps

GU: Increased urinary output, dysuria, urinary retention, urgency

INTEG: Rash, urticaria, bruising, flushing, diaphoresis, pruritus

EENT: Tinnitus, blurred vision, miosis, diplopia

CV: Palpitations, bradycardia, change in B/P, orthostatic hypotension

RESP: Respiratory depression

Contraindications: Hypersensitivity, addiction (opiate)

Precautions: Addictive personality, pregnancy (C), lactation, increased intracranial pressure, MI (acute), severe heart disease, respiratory depression, hepatic disease, renal disease

Pharmacokinetics:

SC/IM/IV: Duration 3-6 hr; metabolized by liver, excreted by kidneys, half-life 5 hr

Interactions:

• Increased effects with other CNS depressants: alcohol, narcotics, sedative/hypnotics, antipsychotics, skeletal muscle relaxants

Lab test interferences:

Increase: Amylase

NURSING CONSIDERATIONS

Assess:

• I&O ratio; check for decreasing output; may indicate urinary retention

◆ For withdrawal reactions in opiate-dependent individuals: pulmonary embolus, vascular occlusion; abscesses, ulcerations, nausea, vomiting, convulsions

• CNS changes: dizziness, drowsiness, hallucinations, euphoria, LOC, pupil reaction

• Allergic reactions: rash, urticaria

• Respiratory dysfunction: respiratory depression, character, rate, rhythm; notify prescriber if respirations are <10/min

• Need for pain medication by pain sedation scoring, physical dependency

Administer:

• With antiemetic if nausea, vomiting occur

• When pain is beginning to return; determine dosage interval by response

• IM deep in large muscle mass, rotate injection sites

IV

• Undiluted 10 mg or less over 3-5 min

Syringe compatibilities: Atropine, cimetidine, diphenhydramine, droperidol, glycopyrrolate, hydroxyzine, lidocaine, midazolam, prochlorperazine, ranitidine, scopolamine, trimethobenzamide

Y-site compatibilities: Amifostine, aztreonam, cefmetazole, cisatracurium, cladribine, filgrastim, fludarabine, granisetron, melphalan, paclitaxel, propofol, remifentanil, teniposide, thiotepa, vinorelbine

Perform/provide:

• Storage in light-resistant area at room temp

• Assistance with ambulation

• Safety measures: night-light, call bell within easy reach

Evaluate:

• Therapeutic response: decrease in pain

Teach patient/family:

• To report any symptoms of CNS changes, allergic reactions

• That physical dependency may result from long-term use

• That withdrawal symptoms may

N

occur: nausea, vomiting, cramps, fever, faintness, anorexia

Treatment of overdose: Naloxone (Narcan) 0.2-0.8 mg IV, O_2, IV fluids, vasopressors

---

nalidixic acid (Ŗ)
(nal-i-dix′ik)
NegGram, NegGram Caplets
Func. class.: Urinary tract anti-infective
Chem. class.: Fluoroquinolone

Action: Appears to inhibit DNA polymerization, primary target being single-stranded DNA precursors in late stages of chromosomal replication

Uses: UTIs (acute/chronic) caused by *Escherichia coli, Klebsiella, Enterobacter, Proteus mirabilis, P. vulgaris, P. morganii*

Dosage and routes:
Renal dose
• CrCl <50 ml/min avoid use
• *Adult:* **PO** 1 g qid × 1-2 wk, 2 g/day for long-term treatment
• *Child >3 mo:* **PO** 55 mg/kg/day in 4 divided doses for 1-2 wk; 33 mg/kg/day in 4 divided doses for long-term treatment
Available forms: Tabs 250, 500 mg, 1 g; susp 250 mg/5 ml

Side effects/adverse reactions:
INTEG: Pruritus, rash, urticaria, photosensitivity
CNS: Dizziness, headache, drowsiness, insomnia, ***convulsions***
GI: Nausea, vomiting, abdominal pain, diarrhea
EENT: Sensitivity to light, blurred vision, change in color perception
Contraindications: Hypersensitivity, CNS damage, liver failure, infants <3 mo
Precautions: Elderly, renal disease,

hepatic disease, pregnancy (B), lactation

Pharmacokinetics:
PO: Peak 1-2 hr, metabolized in liver, excreted in urine (unchanged/conjugates), crosses placenta, enters breast milk

Interactions:
• Increased effects of oral coagulants, check for bleeding
• Decreased effect: nitrofurantoin

Lab test interferences:
False positive: Urinary glucose
False increase: 17-OHCS, VMA

NURSING CONSIDERATIONS
Assess:
• Blood count for patients on chronic therapy
• I&O ratio; urine pH <5.5 is ideal
• Renal, hepatic function
• Photosensitivity: drug should be discontinued
• CNS symptoms: insomnia, vertigo, headache, drowsiness, convulsions
• Allergy: fever, flushing, rash, urticaria, pruritus

Administer:
PO
• After clean-catch urine for C&S
• Two daily doses if urine output is high or if patient has diabetes
• 2 hr before or 2 hr after antacids

Perform/provide:
• Protection from freezing

Evaluate:
• Therapeutic response: decreased dysuria, negative culture

Teach patient/family:
• That photosensitivity occurs; that patient should avoid sunlight or use sunscreen to prevent burns
• To take medication with food or milk to decrease GI irritation; take 2 hr before or 2 hr after antacids
• To protect suspension from freezing, shake well before taking
• That drug may cause drowsiness; instruct client to seek aid in walk-

---

◆ = Nursing alert   ▮ = Herb-drug interaction   ⊘ = Do not crush

ing, other activities; advise client not to drive or operate machinery while on medication

• That diabetics should monitor blood glucose

---

naloxone (R)

(nal-oks'one)
naloxone HCl, Narcan
Func. class.: Opioid antagonist
Chem. class.: Thebaine derivative

Action: Competes with opioids at opiate receptor sites

Uses: Respiratory depression induced by opioids, pentazocine, propoxyphene; refractory circulatory shock, asphyxia neonatorum

Dosage and routes:

Opioid-induced respiratory depression

• *Adult:* **IV/SC/IM** 0.4-2 mg; repeat q2-3min if needed

• *Child:* **IV/SC/IM** 0.5-2 µg/kg as small frequent, q/min **BOL** or as **INF** titrated to response

Postoperative respiratory depression

• *Adult:* **IV** 0.1-0.2 mg q2-3min prn

• *Child:* **IV/IM/SC** 0.01 mg/kg q2-3min prn

Asphyxia neonatorum

• *Neonate:* **IV** 0.01 mg/kg given into umbilical vein after delivery; may repeat q2-3min × 3 doses

Available forms: Inj 0.02, 0.4, 1 mg/ml

Side effects/adverse reactions:

CNS: Drowsiness, nervousness

CV: Rapid pulse, increased systolic B/P (high doses), ***ventricular tachycardia, fibrillation***

GI: Nausea, vomiting

RESP: Hyperpnea

Contraindications: Hypersensitivity, respiratory depression

Precautions: Pregnancy (B), children, cardiovascular disease, opioid dependency, lactation

Pharmacokinetics: Well absorbed IM, SC; metabolized by liver, crosses placenta; excreted in urine, breast milk; half-life 1 hr

IV: Onset 1 min, duration 45 min

IM/SC: Onset 2-5 min, duration 45-60 min

Interactions:

• Decreased effect of opioid analgesics

Lab test interferences:

Interference: Urine VMA, 5-HIAA, urine glucose

NURSING CONSIDERATIONS

Assess:

• Withdrawal: cramping, hypertension, anxiety, vomiting, signs of withdrawal in drug-dependent individuals may occur up to 2 hr after administration

• VS q3-5min

• ABGs including Po_2, Pco_2

• Cardiac status: tachycardia, hypertension; monitor ECG

• Respiratory dysfunction: respiratory depression, character, rate, rhythm; if respirations are <10/min, administer naloxone; probably due to opioid overdose; monitor LOC

• For pain: duration, intensity, location, before and after administration; may be used for respiratory depression

Administer:

• Only with resuscitative equipment, O_2 nearby

• Only sol prepared within 24 hr

IV

• Undiluted with sterile H_2O for inj; may be further diluted with NS or D_5 and given as an inf; give 0.4 mg or less over 15 sec or titrate inf to response

Additive compatibilities: Verapamil

Syringe compatibilities: Benzquinamide, heparin
Y-site compatibilities: Propofol
Perform/provide:
• Dark storage at room temp
Evaluate:
• Therapeutic response: reversal of respiratory depression; LOC-alert

---

naltrexone (℞)

(nal-trex'one)
Trexan
Func. class.: Opioid antagonist
Chem. class.: Thebaine derivative

Action: Competes with narcotics at narcotic receptor sites
Uses: Blockage of opioid analgesics, used in treatment of opiate addiction
Dosage and routes:
• *Adult:* **PO** 25 mg, may give 25 mg after 1 hr if no withdrawal symptoms; 50-150 mg may be given qd depending on need, maintenance 50 mg q24h; 100-150 mg may be given on alternate days or 3 days per wk
Available forms: Tabs 50 mg
Side effects/adverse reactions:
MISC: Increased thirst, chills, fever
MS: Joint and muscle pain
GU: Delayed ejaculation, decreased potency
CNS: Stimulation, drowsiness, dizziness, confusion, ***convulsion,*** headache, flushing, hallucinations, nervousness, irritability
GI: Nausea, vomiting, diarrhea, heartburn, anorexia, ***hepatitis,*** constipation
INTEG: Rash, urticaria, bruising, oily skin, acne, pruritus
EENT: Tinnitus, hearing loss, blurred vision
CV: Rapid pulse, ***pulmonary edema,*** hypertension
RESP: Wheezing, hyperpnea, nasal congestion, rhinorrhea, sneezing, sore throat
Contraindications: Hypersensitivity, opioid dependence, hepatic failure, hepatitis
Precautions: Pregnancy (C), hepatic disease, lactation, children
Pharmacokinetics:
PO: Onset 15-30 min, peak 1-2 hr, duration is dose dependent
Metabolized by liver, excreted by kidneys; crosses placenta, excreted in breast milk; half-life 4 hr; extensive first-pass metabolism

NURSING CONSIDERATIONS
Assess:
• VS q3-5min
• ABGs including Po_2, Pco_2
• Signs of withdrawal in drug-dependent individuals
• Cardiac status: tachycardia, hypertension
• Respiratory dysfunction: respiratory depression, character, rate, rhythm; if respirations are <10/min, respiratory stimulant should be administered
Administer:
• Only if resuscitative equipment is nearby
Perform/provide:
• Storage in tight container
Evaluate:
• Therapeutic response: blocking opiate ingestion
Teach patient/family:
• That they must be drug-free to start treatment
• That using opioid while taking this drug could prove fatal because high dose is needed to overcome this antagonist
• To carry MedicAlert ID stating med used
• If surgery is needed, all involved should be aware of this drug

---

 = Nursing alert   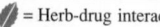 = Herb-drug interaction   Ⓢ = Do not crush

nandrolone (℞)

(nan'droe-lone)

Androlone-D 200, Deca-Durabolin, Durabolin, Hybolin Decanoate-50, Hybolin Decanoate-100, Hybolin Improved, Nandrobolic, nandrolone decanoate, nandrolone phenpropionate, Neo-Durabolic

Func. class.: Androgenic anabolic steroid

Chem. class.: Halogenated testosterone derivative

Action: Increases weight by building body tissue, increases potassium, phosphorus, chloride, nitrogen levels, increases bone development

Uses: Tissue building, severe disease, refractory anemias, metastatic breast cancer

Dosage and routes:

Tissue building (possibly effective)

• *Adult:* **IM** 50-100 mg q3-4wk (decanoate)

• *Child 2-13 yr:* **IM** 25-50 mg q3-4wk (decanoate)

Severe disease/refractory anemias

• *Adult:* **IM** 100-200 mg qwk (decanoate)

Breast cancer

• *Adult:* **IM** 50-100 mg qwk (phenpropionate)

Available forms: Phenpropionate inj 25, 50 mg/ml; decanoate inj 50, 100, 200 mg/ml

Side effects/adverse reactions:

INTEG: Rash, acneiform lesions, oily hair, skin, flushing, sweating, acne vulgaris, alopecia, hirsutism

CNS: Dizziness, headache, fatigue, tremors, paresthesias, flushing, sweating, anxiety, lability, insomnia, carpal tunnel syndrome

MS: Cramps, spasms

CV: Increased B/P

GU: ***Hematuria,*** amenorrhea, vaginitis, decreased libido, decreased breast size, clitoral hypertrophy, testicular atrophy

GI: Nausea, vomiting, constipation, weight gain, ***cholestatic jaundice***

EENT: Conjunctival edema, nasal congestion

ENDO: Abnormal GTT

Contraindications: Severe renal, severe cardiac, severe hepatic disease, hypersensitivity, pregnancy (X), lactation, abnormal genital bleeding, males with cancer of breast, prostate

Precautions: Diabetes mellitus, CV disease, MI

Pharmacokinetics:

IM: Metabolized in liver, crosses placenta, excreted in breast milk, urine

Interactions:

• Increased effects of oral antidiabetics, oxyphenbutazone

• Increased PT: anticoagulants

• Edema: ACTH, adrenal steroids

• Decreased effects of insulin

Lab test interferences:

Increase: Serum cholesterol, blood glucose, urine glucose

Decrease: Serum Ca, serum K, T_4, T_3, thyroid ^{131}I uptake test, urine 17-OHCS, 17-KS, PBI, BSP

NURSING CONSIDERATIONS

Assess:

• Weight daily; notify prescriber if weekly weight gain is >5 lb

• B/P q4h

• I&O ratio; be alert for decreasing urinary output, increasing edema

• Growth rate in children, since growth rate may be uneven (linear/bone growth) with extended use

• Electrolytes: K, Na, Cl, Ca; cholesterol

• Liver function studies: ALT, AST, bilirubin

• Edema, hypertension, cardiac symptoms, jaundice

N

• Mental status: affect, mood, behavioral changes, aggression

• Signs of masculinization in female: increased libido, deepening of voice, decreased breast tissue, enlarged clitoris, menstrual irregularities; male: gynecomastia, impotence, testicular atrophy

• Hypercalcemia: lethargy, polyuria, polydipsia, nausea, vomiting, constipation, drug may have to be decreased

• Hypoglycemia in diabetics, since oral antidiabetic action is increased

Administer:

• Titrated dose; use lowest effective dose

Perform/provide:

• Diet with increased calories, protein; decrease Na if edema occurs

Evaluate:

• Therapeutic response: increased appetite, increased stamina

Teach patient/family:

• That drug must be combined with complete health plan: diet, rest, exercise

• To notify prescriber if therapeutic response decreases

• Not to discontinue abruptly

• About changes in sex characteristics

• That females should report menstrual irregularities

• That 1-3 mo course is necessary for response in breast cancer

---

naproxen (OTC, ℞)
(na-prox′en)
Apo-Naproxen*, EC-Naprosyn, Naprelan, Napron X, Naprosyn, Naprosyn-E*, Naprosyn-SR*, Naxen*, Novo-Naprox*, Nu-Naprox*
naproxen sodium
Aleve, Anaprox, Anaprox DS, Apo-Napro-Na*, Apo-Napro-Na DS, Naprelan, Novo-Naprox Sodium*, Novo-Naprox Sodium DS*, Synflex*, Synflex DS*
Func. class.: Nonsteroidal antiinflammatory, nonopioid analgesic
Chem. class.: Propionic acid derivative

Action: Inhibits prostaglandin synthesis by decreasing an enzyme needed for biosynthesis; analgesic, antiinflammatory, antipyretic

Uses: Mild to moderate pain, osteoarthritis, rheumatoid, gouty arthritis, juvenile arthritis, primary dysmenorrhea

Dosage and routes:

• *Adult:* **PO** 250-500 mg bid, not to exceed 1 g/day (base); 525 mg, then 275 mg q6-8h prn, not to exceed 1475 mg (sodium)

• *Child:* **PO** 10 mg/kg in 2 divided doses

Available forms: Tabs, naproxen: 250, 375, 500 mg; DR 375, 500 mg; oral susp 125 mg/5 ml; naproxen sodium tabs 220, 275, 550 mg

Side effects/adverse reactions:

GI: Nausea, anorexia, vomiting, diarrhea, jaundice, *cholestatic hepatitis,* constipation, flatulence, cramps, dry mouth, peptic ulcer, *GI ulceration, bleeding, perforation*

CNS: Dizziness, drowsiness, fatigue,

---

tremors, confusion, insomnia, anxiety, depression

CV: Tachycardia, peripheral edema, palpitations, dysrhythmias

INTEG: Purpura, rash, pruritus, sweating

*GU: **Nephrotoxicity: dysuria, hematuria, oliguria, azotemia***

*HEMA: **Blood dyscrasias***

EENT: Tinnitus, hearing loss, blurred vision

Contraindications: Hypersensitivity, asthma, severe renal disease, severe hepatic disease, ulcer disease

Precautions: Pregnancy (B) 1st trimester, lactation, children <2 yr, bleeding disorders, GI disorders, cardiac disorders, hypersensitivity to other antiinflammatory agents, elderly, CrCl <25 ml/min

Pharmacokinetics:

PO: Peak 2-4 hr, half-life 3-3½ hr; metabolized in liver; excreted in urine (metabolites), breast milk; 99% protein binding

Interactions:

• Increased toxicity: methotrexate, oral anticoagulants, sulfonylureas, probenecid

• Decreased effect of: antihypertensives, diuretics

• Increased risk of GI side effects: aspirin, corticosteroids, alcohol

• Possible renal impairment: ACE inhibitors

Lab test interferences:

Increase: BUN, alk phosphatase

False increase: 5-HIAA, 17KGS

NURSING CONSIDERATIONS

Assess:

• Pain: frequency, characteristics, intensity; relief prior to and 1-2 hr after med

• Asthma, aspirin hypersensitivity or nasal polyps, increased risk of hypersensitivity

• Renal, liver, blood studies: BUN, creatinine, AST, ALT, Hgb, LDH, blood glucose, Hct, WBC, platelets CrCl before treatment, periodically thereafter

• Audiometric, ophthalmic exam before, during, after treatment

• For eye, ear problems: blurred vision, tinnitus (may indicate toxicity)

Administer:

• With food to decrease GI symptoms; best to take on empty stomach to facilitate absorption

Perform/provide:

• Storage at room temp

Evaluate:

• Therapeutic response: decreased pain, stiffness, swelling in joints, ability to move more easily

Teach patient/family:

• To use sunscreen to prevent photosensitivity

• To report blurred vision, ringing, roaring in ears (may indicate toxicity)

• To avoid driving, other hazardous activities if dizziness or drowsiness occurs

• To report change in urine pattern, weight increase, edema (face, lower extremities), pain increase in joints, fever, blood in urine (indicates nephrotoxicity); black stools, flulike symptoms

• That therapeutic effects may take up to 1 mo

• To avoid ASA, alcohol, steroids

---

naratriptan (℞)

(nair'ah-trip-tan)

Amerge

Func. class.: Antimigraine agent

Chem. class.: 5-HT₁ receptor agonist

Action: Binds selectively to the vascular 5-HT₁ receptor subtype, exerts antimigraine effect; causes vasoconstriction in cranial arteries

Uses: Acute treatment of migraine with or without aura

Dosage and routes:

• *Adult:* **PO** 1 or 2.5 mg with fluids, if headache returns, repeat once after 4 hr, max 5 mg/24 hr

Hepatic/renal dose

Max 2.5 mg/24 hr

Available forms: Tab 1, 2.5 mg

Side effects/adverse reactions:

GI: Nausea, vomiting

MS: Weakness, neck stiffness, myalgia

CNS: Dizziness, sedation, fatigue

CV: Increased B/P, palpitations, ***tachydysrhythmias, PR, QTc prolongation, ST/T wave changes, PVCs, atrial flutter/fibrillation, coronary vasospasm***

EENT: EENT infections, photophobia

MISC: Temperature change sensations; tightness, pressure sensations

Contraindications: Angina pectoris, history of MI, documented silent ischemia, ischemic heart disease, concurrent ergotamine-containing preparations, uncontrolled hypertension, hypersensitivity, severe renal disease (CrCl <15 ml/min); severe hepatic disease (child-Pugh grade C)

Precautions: Postmenopausal women, men >40 yr, risk factors for CAD, hypercholesterolemia, obesity, diabetes, impaired hepatic or renal function, pregnancy (C), lactation, children, elderly, peripheral vascular disease

Pharmacokinetics: Peak 2-3 hr, 28%-31% plasma protein binding, half-life 6 hr, metabolized in the liver (metabolite), excreted in urine, feces; may be excreted in breast milk

Interactions:

• Extended vasospastic effects: ergot, ergot derivatives, other 5-HT$_1$ agonists

• Weakness, hyperreflexia, incoordination: SSRIs (fluoxetine, fluvoxamine, paroxetine, sertraline)

• Increased naratriptan levels: oral contraceptives

• Increases clearance of naratriptan: smoking

NURSING CONSIDERATIONS

Assess:

• For stress level, activity, recreation, coping mechanisms

• Neurologic status: LOC blurred vision, nausea, vomiting, tingling in extremities preceding headache

Administer:

• With fluids

Perform/provide:

• Quiet, calm environment with decreased stimulation for noise, bright light, excessive talking

Evaluate:

• Therapeutic response: decrease in frequency, severity of headache

Teach patient/family:

• To report any side effects to prescriber

• Not to use if another 5-HT$_1$ agonist or an ergot preparation has been used in the past 24 hr

---

nedocromil inhaler (R)
(ned-o-kroe'mill)
Tilade
Func. class.: Antiasthmatic
Chem. class.: Mast cell stabilizer

Action: Stabilizes the membrane of the sensitized mast cell, preventing release of chemical mediators after an antigen-IgE interaction

Uses: Severe perennial bronchial asthma, exercise-induced bronchospasm (prevention), prevention of acute bronchospasm induced by en-

---

◆ = Nursing alert   🖋 = Herb-drug interaction   ⊘ = Do not crush

vironmental pollutants; *not* for treatment of acute asthma attacks

Dosage and routes:

Bronchospasm, bronchial asthma

• *Adult and child >12 yr:* **INH** 2 inhalations 2-4 ×/day at regular intervals to provide 14 g/day

Available forms: 1.75 mg nedocromil Na per activation in 16.2 g canisters providing at least 112 metered inhalations

Side effects/adverse reactions:

EENT: Throat irritation, cough, nasal congestion, burning eyes, rhinitis

CNS: Headache, dizziness, neuritis, dysphonia

GI: Nausea, vomiting, anorexia, dry mouth, bitter taste

Contraindications: Hypersensitivity to this drug or lactose, status asthmaticus

Precautions: Pregnancy (B), lactation, children

Pharmacokinetics:

INH: Peak 15 min, duration 4-6 hr; excreted unchanged in urine; half-life 80 min

NURSING CONSIDERATIONS

Assess:

• Pulmonary function testing baseline

• Respiratory status: rate, rhythm, characteristics, cough, wheezing, dyspnea

Administer:

• By inhalation only, with spacer device if needed

• Gargle, sip of water to decrease irritation in throat

Evaluate:

• Therapeutic response: decrease in asthmatic symptoms, congested, runny nose

Teach patient/family:

• To clear mucus before using

• The proper technique: exhale; using inhaler, inhale deeply with head tipped back to open airway; remove, hold breath, exhale

• That therapeutic effect may take up to 4 wk

• That drug is preventive only, not restorative

---

nefazodone (℞)

(ne-faz′o-done)

Serzone

Func. class.: Antidepressant—misc

Chem. class.: Phenylpiperazine

Action: Selectively inhibits serotonin uptake by brain, potentiates behavioral changes, occupies central S-H$_2$ receptors

Uses: Major depression

Dosage and routes:

• *Adult:* **PO** 200 mg/day (100 mg bid); dose may be increased to 300 mg/day (150 mg bid), max 600 mg/day

• *Elderly:* 100 mg/day (50 mg bid); increase to 100 mg bid after 2 wk to desired dose

Available forms: Tabs 100, 150, 200, 250 mg

Side effects/adverse reactions:

CNS: Somnolence, dizziness, *headache, insomnia*

GI: Nausea, constipation, dry mouth

GU: Urinary frequency, retention, UTI

CV: Postural hypotension

RESP: Pharyngitis, cough

EENT: Blurred vision, abnormal vision

Contraindications: Hypersensitivity to this drug or phenylpiperazines

Precautions: Pregnancy (C), lactation, children, elderly, cardiovascular disease, seizure disorder

Pharmacokinetics: Metabolized in liver extensively to metabolites; excreted in urine, breast milk; peak 1-3 hr; half-life triphasic 2-4 hr

N

Interactions:
• Increased effect: CNS depressants, alcohol

◆ *Fatal reaction:* antihistamines, nonsedating

• Increased plasma concentrations: benzodiazepines
• Hypertensive crisis: MAOIs
• Increased toxicity: triazolam, alprazolam, midazolam, phenytoin, MAOI

NURSING CONSIDERATIONS
Assess:
• B/P (lying, standing), pulse q4h; if systolic B/P drops 20 mm Hg, hold drug, notify prescriber; take vital signs q4h in patients with cardiovascular disease
• Blood studies: CBC, leukocytes, differential, cardiac enzymes (long-term therapy)
• Hepatic studies: AST, ALT, bilirubin
• Mental status: mood, sensorium, affect, suicidal tendencies; increase in psychiatric symptoms: depression, panic
• Urinary retention, constipation; constipation is more likely in children, elderly

◆ For withdrawal symptoms: headache, nausea, vomiting, muscle pain, weakness; unusual unless drug discontinued abruptly

• Alcohol consumption; hold dose until morning
Administer:
• With food, milk for GI symptoms
• Crushed if patient cannot swallow whole
Perform/provide:
• Storage at room temp; do not freeze
Evaluate:
• Therapeutic response: decrease in depression; absence of suicidal thoughts
Teach patient/family:
• That therapeutic effects may take 3-4 wk

• To use caution in driving, other activities requiring alertness because of drowsiness, dizziness; to avoid rising quickly from sitting to standing, especially elderly
• To avoid alcohol ingestion, other CNS depressants, benzodiazepines
• Not to discontinue medication quickly after long-term use; may cause nausea, headache, malaise
• To increase bulk in diet for constipation, especially elderly
• To take gum, hard sugarless candy, frequents sips of water for dry mouth
Treatment of overdose: ECG monitoring; induce emesis; lavage, activated charcoal; administer anticonvulsant

---

nelfinavir (℞)
(nell-fin'a-ver)
Viracept
Func. class.: Antiviral
Chem. chass.: HIV protease inhibitor

Action: Inhibits human immunodeficiency virus (HIV) protease, which prevents maturation of the infectious virus
Uses: HIV alone or in combination
Dosage and routes:
• *Adult:* **PO** 750 mg tid
• *Child 2-13 yr:* **PO** 20-30 mg/kg tid
Available forms: Tabs 250 mg; powder, oral 50 mg/g
Side effects/adverse reactions:
*HEMA: **Anemia, leukopenia, thrombocytopenia, Hgb abnormalities***
GI: Diarrhea, anorexia, dyspepsia, *nausea, flatulence*
CNS: Headache, asthenia, poor concentration, *seizures*
INTEG: Rash, dermatitis
MS: Pain
CV: Bleeding

ENDO: Hypoglycemia, hyperlipidemia

Contraindications: Hypersensitivity to protease inhibitors

Precautions: Liver disease, pregnancy (B), lactation, renal disease, hemophilia, PKU

Pharmacokinetics: Half-life 3½-5 hr

Interactions:

◆Serious dysrhythmias: ergots, midazolam, triazolam

• Decreased effect of oral contraceptives

• Increased effect: rifabutin

• Increased nelfinavir levels: ketoconazole, indinavir, ritonavir

• Decreased nelfinavir levels: rifamycins, nevirapine, phenobarbital, phenytoin, carbamazepine

NURSING CONSIDERATIONS
Assess:

• Signs of infection, anemia

• Liver function studies: ALT, AST

• C&S before drug therapy; drug may be taken as soon as culture is taken; repeat C&S after treatment; determine the presence of other sexually transmitted diseases

• Bowel pattern before, during treatment; if severe abdominal pain with bleeding occurs, drug should be discontinued; monitor hydration

• Skin eruptions, rash, urticaria, itching

• Allergies before treatment, reaction of each medication; place allergies on chart

Administer:

• With food

• Oral powder mixed with fluids if desired, do not mix with juice or acidic fluids, stable mixed for 6 hr

Teach patient/family:

• To avoid taking with other medications unless directed by prescriber

• That drug does not cure, but does manage symptoms

• To use a nonhormonal form of birth control while taking this drug

• If dose is missed, to take as soon as remembered up to 1 hr before next dose; do not double dose

• To take with food

---

neomycin (℞)
(nee-oh-mye′sin)
Mycifradin, Myciguent
Func. class.: Antiinfective
Chem. class.: Aminoglycoside

Action: Interferes with protein synthesis in bacterial cell by binding to 30S ribosomal subunit, causing inaccurate peptide sequence to form in protein chain, causing bacterial death

Uses: Severe systemic infections of CNS, respiratory, GI, urinary tract, eye, bone, skin, soft tissues caused by *Pseudomonas aeruginosa, Escherichia coli, Enterobacter, Klebsiella pneumoniae, Proteus vulgaris;* also used for hepatic coma, preoperatively to sterilize bowel, infectious diarrhea caused by enteropathogenic *E. coli*

Dosage and routes:

Hepatic coma

• *Adult:* **PO** 4-12 g/day in divided doses × 5-6 days

• *Child:* 50-100 mg/kg/day in divided doses

Preoperative bowel sterilization

• *Adult:* **PO** on 3rd day of a 3-day regimen, give 1 g early PM, repeat in 1 hr, repeat at hs (given with erythromycin); give saline cathartic before giving this drug

Available forms: Tabs 500 mg; oral sol 125 mg/5 ml

Side effects/adverse reactions:

GU: Oliguria, hematuria, renal damage, azotemia, renal failure, nephrotoxicity

N

CNS: Confusion, depression, numbness, tremors, **convulsions,** muscle twitching, **neurotoxicity,** dizziness, vertigo

EENT: **Ototoxicity,** deafness, visual disturbances, tinnitus

HEMA: **Agranulocytosis, thrombocytopenia,** leukopenia, eosinophilia, anemia

GI: *Nausea, vomiting, anorexia;* increased ALT, AST, bilirubin; hepatomegaly, *hepatic necrosis,* splenomegaly

CV: Hypotension, hypertension, palpitation

INTEG: *Rash,* burning, urticaria, photosensitivity, dermatitis, alopecia

Contraindications: Bowel obstruction (oral use), severe renal disease, hypersensitivity, infants, children

Precautions: Mild renal disease, pregnancy (C), hearing deficits, lactation, myasthenia gravis, Parkinson's disease

Pharmacokinetics:

PO: Onset rapid, peak 1-2 hr
Plasma half-life 2-3 hr; not metabolized, excreted unchanged in feces, crosses placenta

Interactions:

• Increased ototoxicity, neurotoxicity, nephrotoxicity: other aminoglycosides, amphotericin B, polymyxin, vancomycin, ethacrynic acid, furosemide, mannitol, methoxyflurane, cisplatin, cephalosporins, bacitracin

• Increased effects: nondepolarizing muscle relaxants, succinylcholine, oral anticoagulants when given with oral neomycin

• Decreased effects of digoxin, penicillin V when given with oral neomycin

NURSING CONSIDERATIONS

Assess:

• Weight before treatment; calculation of dosage is usually based on ideal body weight, but may be calculated on actual body weight

• I&O ratio, urinalysis qd for proteinuria, cells, casts; report sudden change in urine output

• Urine pH if drug is used for UTI; urine should be kept alkaline

• Renal impairment by securing urine for CrCl testing, BUN, serum creatinine; lower dosage should be given in renal impairment

• Deafness by audiometric testing, ringing, roaring in ears, vertigo; assess hearing before, during, after treatment

• Dehydration: high specific gravity, decrease in skin turgor, dry mucous membranes, dark urine

• Overgrowth of infection: fever, malaise, redness, pain, swelling, perineal itching, diarrhea, stomatitis, change in cough, sputum

• C&S before starting treatment to identify infecting organism

• Vestibular dysfunction: nausea, vomiting, dizziness, headache; drug should be discontinued if severe

• Injection sites for redness, swelling, abscesses; use warm compresses at site

Administer:

• Drug in evenly spaced doses to maintain blood level

• Bicarbonate to alkalinize urine if ordered in treating UTI, as drug is most active in alkaline environment

Perform/provide:

• Adequate fluids of 2-3 L/day unless contraindicated to prevent irritation of tubules

• Supervised ambulation, other safety measures, with vestibular dysfunction

Evaluate:

• Therapeutic response: absence of fever, draining wounds, negative C&S after treatment

---

⬥ = Nursing alert   🌿 = Herb-drug interaction   🚫 = Do not crush

Teach patient/family:
• To report headache, dizziness, symptoms of overgrowth of infection, renal impairment
• To report loss of hearing, ringing, roaring in ears or a feeling of fullness in head
• To take all of medication, to take a missed dose as soon as remembered, do not double doses
Treatment of overdose: Hemodialysis; monitor serum levels of drug

---

neostigmine (R)
(nee-oh-stig′meen)
neostigmine, Prostigmin
Func. class.: Cholinergic stimulant; anticholinesterase
Chem. class.: Quaternary compound

Action: Inhibits destruction of acetylcholine, which increases concentration at sites where acetylcholine is released; this facilitates transmission of impulses across myoneural junction

Uses: Myasthenia gravis, nondepolarizing neuromuscular blocker antagonist, bladder distention, postoperative ileus

Dosage and routes:
Renal dose
• CrCl 10-50 ml/min 50% of dose; CrCl <10 ml/min 25% of dose
Myasthenia gravis
• *Adult:* **PO** 15-375 mg/day; **IM/IV** 0.5-2 mg q1-3h
• *Child:* **PO** 2 mg/kg/day q3-4h
Nondepolarizing neuromuscular blocker antagonist
• *Adult:* **IV** 0.5-2 mg slowly, may repeat if needed (give 0.6-1.2 mg atropine before this drug)
• *Infant/child:* **IV** 0.025-0.1 mg/kg/dose

Abdominal distention/postoperative ileus
• *Adult:* **IM/SC** 0.25-1 mg (1:4000) q4-6h depending on condition × 2-3 days
Available forms: Tabs 15 mg; inj 1:1000, 1:2000, 1:4000
Side effects/adverse reactions:
INTEG: Rash, urticaria, flushing
CNS: Dizziness, headache, sweating, weakness, *convulsions,* incoordination, *paralysis,* drowsiness, loss of consciousness
GI: Nausea, diarrhea, vomiting, cramps, increased peristalsis, salivary and gastric secretions
CV: Tachycardia, dysrhythmias, bradycardia, hypotension, AV block, ECG changes, *cardiac arrest,* syncope
GU: Urinary frequency, incontinence, urgency
RESP: Respiratory depression, bronchospasm, constriction, laryngospasm, respiratory arrest, dyspnea
EENT: Miosis, blurred vision, lacrimation, visual changes
Contraindications: Obstruction of intestine, renal system, bromide sensitivity, peritonitis
Precautions: Bradycardia, pregnancy (C), hypotension, seizure disorders, bronchial asthma, coronary occlusion, hyperthyroidism, dysrhythmias, peptic ulcer, megacolon, poor GI motility, lactation, children
Pharmacokinetics:
PO: Onset 45-75 min, duration 2½-4 hr
IM/SC: Onset 10-30 min, duration 2½-4 hr
IV: Onset 4-8 min; duration 2-4 hr; metabolized in liver, excreted in urine
Interactions:
• Decreased action of gallamine, metocurine, pancuronium, tubocurarine, atropine

N

• Increased action of decamethonium, succinylcholine

• Decreased action of neostigmine: aminoglycosides, anesthetics, procainamide, quinidine, mecamylamine, polymyxin, magnesium

NURSING CONSIDERATIONS
Assess:

• VS, respiration q8h

• I&O ratio; check for urinary retention or incontinence

◆ For bradycardia, hypotension, bronchospasm, headache, dizziness, convulsions, respiratory depression; drug should be discontinued if toxicity occurs

Administer:

• Only with atropine sulfate available for cholinergic crisis

• Only after all other cholinergics have been discontinued

• Increased doses if tolerance occurs

• Larger doses after exercise or fatigue

PO

• On empty stomach for better absorption

IV

• Undiluted, give through Y-tube or 3-way stopcock; give 0.5 mg or less over 1 min

Additive compatibilities: Netilmicin

Syringe compatibilities: Glycopyrrolate, heparin, pentobarbital, thiopental

Y-site compatibilities: Heparin, hydrocortisone, potassium chloride, vit B/C

Perform/provide:

• Storage at room temp

Evaluate:

• Therapeutic response: increased muscle strength, hand grasp, improved gait, absence of labored breathing (if severe)

Teach patient/family:

• That drug is not a cure; it only relieves symptoms

• To wear Medic Alert ID specifying myasthenia gravis, drugs taken

Treatment of overdose: Respiratory support, atropine 1-4 mg (IV)

---

nevirapine
(ne-veer′a-peen)
Viramune

Func. class.: Antiviral

Chem. class.: Non-nucleoside reverse transcriptase inhibitor (NNRTI)

Action: Binds directly to reverse transcriptase and blocks RNA, DNA, causing a disruption of the enzyme's site

Uses: HIV-1 in combination with nucleoside analogs in those experiencing deterioration

Dosage and routes:

• *Adult:* **PO** 200 mg qd × 2 wk, then 200 mg bid in combination with nucleoside analogs

Available forms: Tabs 200 mg

Side effects/adverse reactions:

GI: Diarrhea, abdominal pain, *nausea, stomatitis,* **hepatitis**

CNS: Paresthesia, headache, fever, peripheral neuropathy

INTEG: Rash

MS: Pain, myalgia

HEMA: **Neutropenia, anemia, thrombocytopenia**

Contraindications: Hypersensitivity

Precautions: Liver disease, pregnancy (C), lactation, children, renal disease

Pharmacokinetics: Rapidly absorbed, 60% bound to plasma proteins, metabolized by liver

Interactions:

• Decreased nevirapine levels: rifamycins

◆ = Nursing alert   🌿 = Herb-drug interaction   ⊘ = Do not crush

• Decreased effects of protease inhibitors, oral contraceptives

NURSING CONSIDERATIONS
Assess:
• Signs of infection, anemia
• Liver, blood studies during treatment: ALT, AST, viral load, CD4; renal studies
• C&S before drug therapy; drug may be taken as soon as culture is taken; repeat C&S after treatment; determine the presence of other sexually transmitted disease
• Bowel pattern before, during treatment; if severe abdominal pain with bleeding occurs, drug should be discontinued; monitor hydration
• Skin eruptions; rash, urticaria, itching
• Allergies before treatment, reaction to each medication; place allergies on chart

Administer:
• Without regard to meals

Teach patient/family:
• To report any right quadrant pain, jaundice, rash immediately
• That drug may be taken with food, antacids, didanosine
• To take as prescribed; if dose is missed, take as soon as remembered up to 1 hr before next dose; do not double dose
• That drug is not a cure, controls symptoms of HIV
• To avoid OTC agents unless approved by prescriber
• To use a nonhormonal form of contraception during treatment
• That drug must be taken in equal intervals around the clock to maintain blood levels for duration of therapy

---

niacin (nicotinic acid)/ niacinamide (OTC, ℞)
(nye′a-sin)/(nye-a-sin′a-mide)
Nia-Bid, Niac, Niacels, Niacin TD, Niacin TR Niacor, Niaspan, Nico-400, Nicobid, Nicolar, Nicotinex, Nicotinic Acid, Novaniacin*, Slo-Niacin, SpaN Niacin, Tri-B*, vitamin B₃

Func. class.: Vit B₃
Chem. class.: Water-soluble vitamin

Action: Needed for conversion of fats, protein, carbohydrates, by oxidation reduction; acts directly on vascular smooth muscle, causing vasodilation; high doses decrease serum lipids

Uses: Pellagra, hyperlipidemias, peripheral vascular disease

Dosage and routes:
Adjunct in hyperlipidemia
• *Adult:* **PO** 500 mg qd in 3 divided doses after meals, may be increased to 4 g/day
Pellagra
• *Adult:* **PO** 300-500 mg qd in divided doses
• *Child:* **PO** 100-300 mg qd in divided doses
Peripheral vascular disease
• *Adult:* **PO** 250-800 mg qd in divided doses

Available forms: Niacin tabs 25, 50, 100, 125, 250, 500 mg; caps, time rel 125, 250, 300, 400, 500 mg; tabs, ext rel 125, 250, 400, 500, 750, 1000 mg; cap, ext rel 125, 250, 300, 400, 500 mg; elix 50 mg/5 ml; nicotinamide—tabs 50, 100, 125, 250, 500 mg

Side effects/adverse reactions:
CNS: Paresthesias, headache, dizziness, anxiety
GI: Nausea, vomiting, anorexia, flat-

ulence, xerostomia, *jaundice,* diarrhea, peptic ulcer

GU: Hyperuricemia, *glycosuria, hypoalbuminemia*

CV: Postural hypotension, vasovagal attacks, dysrhythmias, vasodilation

EENT: Blurred vision, ptosis

INTEG: Flushing, dry skin, rash, pruritus

RESP: Wheezing

Contraindications: Hypersensitivity, peptic ulcer, hepatic disease, lactation, hemorrhage, severe hypotension

Precautions: Glaucoma, cardiovascular disease, CAD, diabetes mellitus, gout, schizophrenia, pregnancy (C)

Pharmacokinetics:

PO: Peak 30-70 min, half-life 45 min; metabolized in liver; 30% excreted unchanged in urine

Interactions:

• Increased action of ganglionic blockers

Lab test interferences:

Increase: Bilirubin, alk phosphatase, liver enzymes, LDH, uric acid

Decrease: Cholesterol

False increase: Urinary catecholamines

False positive: Urine glucose

NURSING CONSIDERATIONS
Assess:

• Liver function studies: AST, ALT, bilirubin, uric acid, alk phosphatase; blood glucose before and during treatment

• Cardiac status: rate, rhythm, quality; postural hypotension, dysrhythmias

• Nutritional status: liver, yeast, legumes, organ meat, lean poultry; fat in diet

• Liver dysfunction: clay-colored stools, itching, dark urine, jaundice

• CNS symptoms: headache, paresthesias, blurred vision

• For symptoms of niacin deficiency: nausea, vomiting, anemia, poor memory, confusion, dermatitis

• For lipid, triglyceride, cholesterol level, if using for hyperlipidemia

Administer:

• With meals for GI symptoms, and 325 mg aspirin ½ hr before dose to decrease flushing

Evaluate:

• Therapeutic response: decreased lipids, warm extremities, absence of numbness in extremities

Teach patient/family:

• That flushing and increase in feelings of warmth will occur several hr after taking drug (PO); after 2 wk of therapy, these side effects diminish

• To remain recumbent if postural hypotension occurs; to rise slowly to prevent orthostatic hypotension

• To abstain from alcohol if drug is prescribed for hyperlipidemia

• To avoid sunlight if skin lesions are present

🚫 Not to break, crush, or chew ext rel tabs, caps

---

nicardipine (℞)
(nye-card′i-peen)
Cardene, Cardene IV,
Cardene SR

Func. class.: Calcium channel blocker, antianginal, antihypertensive

Chem. class.: Dihydropyridine

Action: Inhibits calcium ion influx across cell membrane during cardiac depolarization; produces relaxation of coronary vascular smooth muscle, peripheral vascular smooth muscle; dilates coronary vascular arteries; increases myocardial oxygen delivery in patients with vasospastic angina

---

◆ = Nursing alert   🖋 = Herb-drug interaction   🚫 = Do not crush

Uses: Chronic stable angina pectoris, hypertension

Dosage and routes:

• *Adult:* **PO** 20 mg tid initially, may increase after 3 days (range 20-40 mg tid); **IV** 0.5-2.2 mg/hr

Available forms: Caps 20, 30 mg; caps sus rel 30, 45, 60 mg; inj 2.5 mg/ml

Side effects/adverse reactions:

CV: **Dysrhythmia,** edema, **CHF,** bradycardia, hypotension, palpitations, **MI, pulmonary edema**

GI: Nausea, vomiting, diarrhea, gastric upset, constipation, **hepatitis,** abdominal cramps

GU: Nocturia, polyuria, **acute renal failure**

INTEG: Rash, pruritus, urticaria, photosensitivity, hair loss

CNS: Headache, fatigue, drowsiness, dizziness, anxiety, depression, weakness, insomnia, confusion, paresthesia, somnolence

OTHER: Blurred vision, flushing, nasal congestion, sweating, shortness of breath, gynecomastia, hyperglycemia, sexual difficulties, **Stevens-Johnson syndrome**

Contraindications: Sick sinus syndrome, 2nd- or 3rd-degree heart block, hypotension <90 mm Hg systolic, hypersensitivity

Precautions: CHF, hypotension, hepatic injury, pregnancy (C), lactation, children, renal disease, elderly

Pharmacokinetics:

PO: Onset 30 min, peak 1-2 hr, duration 8 hr

PO-SR: Onset unknown, peak 2-6 hr, duration 10-12 hr, half-life 2-5 hr

Metabolized by liver, excreted in urine (98% as metabolites)

Interactions:

• Increased effects of digitalis, neuromuscular blocking agents, theophylline, other antihypertensives, nitrates, alcohol, quinidine

• Increased effects of nicardipine: cimetidine

• Decreased antihypertensive effect: NSAIDs

• Increased risk of toxicity: cyclosporine, prazosin, carbamazepine, quinidine, cimetidine, propranolol

• Food/drug: increased hypotensive effect: grapefruit

NURSING CONSIDERATIONS

Assess:

• Cardiac status: B/P, pulse, respiration, ECG

• Anginal pain: intensity, location, duration, alleviating factors

• Potassium, LFTs, renal studies, periodically

Administer:

• Without regard to meals

IV

• Dilute each 25 mg/240 ml of compatible sol (0.1 mg/ml), give slowly

• Stable at room temp 24 hr

Y-site compatibilities: Diltiazem, dobutamine, dopamine, epinephrine, fentanyl, hydromorphone, labetalol, lorazepam, midazolam, milrinone, morphine, nitroglycerin, norepinephrine, ranitidine, vecuronium

Evaluate:

• Therapeutic response: decreased anginal pain, decreased B/P

Teach patient/family:

• To avoid hazardous activities until stabilized on drug, dizziness is no longer a problem

• To limit caffeine consumption, take no alcohol products

• To avoid OTC drugs unless directed by prescriber

• To comply in all areas of medical regimen: diet, exercise, stress reduction, drug therapy

• To notify prescriber of irregular heartbeat, shortness of breath, swelling of feet and hands, pronounced dizziness, constipation, nausea, hypotension

Treatment of overdose: Defibrillation, β-agonists, IV Ca, diuretics, atropine for AV block, vasopressor for hypotension

---

nicotine resin complex (OTC, ℞)
(nik'o-teen)
Nicorette, Nicorette DS
Func. class.: Smoking deterrent
Chem. class.: Ganglionic cholinergic agonist

Action: Agonist at nicotinic receptors in peripheral, central nervous systems; acts at sympathetic ganglia, on chemoreceptors of aorta, carotid bodies; also affects adrenalin-releasing catecholamines

Uses: Deter cigarette smoking

Dosage and routes:
• *Adult:* Gum 1 piece chewed × ½ hr as needed to abstain from smoking, not to exceed 30/day

Available forms: Gum 2 mg/piece

Side effects/adverse reactions:
RESP: Breathing difficulty, cough, hoarseness, sneezing, wheezing
EENT: Jaw ache, irritation in buccal cavity
CNS: Dizziness, vertigo, insomnia, headache, confusion, convulsions, depression, euphoria, numbness, tinnitus
GI: Nausea, vomiting, anorexia, indigestion, diarrhea, abdominal pain, constipation, eructation
CV: Dysrhythmias, tachycardia, palpitations, edema, flushing, hypertension

Contraindications: Hypersensitivity, immediate post MI recovery period, severe angina pectoris, pregnancy (D)

Precautions: Vasospastic disease, dysrhythmias, diabetes mellitus, hyperthyroidism, pheochromocytoma, coronary disease, esophagitis, peptic ulcer, lactation, hepatic/renal disease

Pharmacokinetics: Onset 15-30 min, metabolized in liver, excreted in urine, half-life 2-3 hr, 30-120 hr (terminal)

Interactions:
• Decreased absorption: glutethimide
• Increased absorption: SC insulin
• Decreased metabolism of propoxyphene
• Smoking cessation increases diuretic effects of furosemide
• Increased blood levels with cessation of smoking: caffeine, theophylline, pentazocine, imipramine, oxazepam, propranolol, acetaminophen

NURSING CONSIDERATIONS
Assess:
• Adverse reaction: irritation of buccal cavity, dislike of taste, jaw ache
Evaluate:
• Therapeutic response: decrease in urge to smoke, decreased need for gum after 3-6 mo
Teach patient/family:
• To chew gum slowly for 30 min to promote buccal absorption of the drug; do not chew over 45 min
• To begin drug withdrawal after 3 mo use; not to exceed 6 mo
• All aspects of drug use; give package insert to patient and explain
• That gum will not stick to dentures, dental appliances
• That gum is as toxic as cigarette; to be used only to deter smoking
• Not to use during pregnancy; birth defects may occur

◆ = Nursing alert   ∥ = Herb-drug interaction   ⊘ = Do not crush

nicotine transdermal/ inhaler system
(OTC, ℞)
(nik′o-teen)

Habitrol, Nicoderm, Nicotrol, Prostep

Func. class.: Smoking deterrent

Chem. class.: Ganglionic cholinergic agonist

Action: Agonist at nicotinic receptors in peripheral, central nervous systems; acts at sympathetic ganglia, on chemoreceptors of aorta, carotid bodies; also affects adrenalin-releasing catecholamines

Uses: Deter cigarette smoking

Dosage and routes:

• *Habitrol, Nicoderm:* 21 mg/day × 4-8 wk; 14 mg/day × 2-4 wk; 7 mg/day × 2-4 wk

• *Nicotrol:* 15 mg/day × 12 wk; 10 mg/day × 2 wk; 5 mg/day × 2 wk

• *Nicotrol Inhaler:* delivers 30% of what a smoker receives from an actual cigarette

• *Prostep:* 22 mg/day × 4-8 wk; 11 mg/day × 2-4 wk; nicotine inhaler

Available forms: Transdermal patch delivering 7, 14, 21 mg/day (Habitrol, Nicoderm); 5, 10, 15 mg/day (Nicoderm); nicotine inhaler 11, 22 mg/day (Prostep)

Side effects/adverse reactions:

RESP: Cough, pharyngitis, sinusitis

MISC: Back pain, chest pain

INTEG: Erythema, pruritus, burning at application site, cutaneous hypersensitivity, sweating, rash

GI: Diarrhea, dyspepsia, constipation, nausea, abdominal pain, vomiting

MS: Arthralgia, myalgia

EENT: Dry mouth, abnormal taste

CNS: Abnormal dreams, insomnia, nervousness, headache, dizziness, paresthesia

Contraindications: Hypersensitivity, children, pregnancy (D), nonsmokers, immediate post MI period, life-threatening dysrhythmias, severe or worsening angina pectoris

Precautions: Skin disease, angina pectoris, MI, renal or hepatic insufficiency, peptic ulcer, accelerated hypertension, serious cardiac dysrhythmias, hyperthyroidism, pheochromocytoma, insulin-dependent diabetes, elderly

Pharmacokinetics: Half-life 3-4 hr, protein binding <5%, 30% is excreted unchanged in urine

Interactions:

• Decreased absorption: glutethimide

• Decreased dose needed with cessation of smoking: acetaminophen, caffeine, imipramine, oxazepam, pentazocine, propranolol, theophylline, insulin, adrenergic antagonists

• Increased dose with cessation of smoking: adrenergic agonists

• Decreased metabolism of propoxyphene

• Increased diuretic effects of furosemide

• Increased requirements of insulin

NURSING CONSIDERATIONS

Assess:

• Adverse reactions: irritation, pruritus, burning at patch site

Perform/provide:

• Storage below 86° F (30° C)

Evaluate:

• Therapeutic response: decrease in urge to smoke, absence of nicotine withdrawal symptoms

Teach patient/family:

• All aspects of drug use; give package insert to patient and explain

Transdermal patch

• That patch is as toxic as cigarettes; to be used only to deter smoking

• Not to use during pregnancy; birth defects may occur

N

• To keep used and unused system out of reach of children and pets
• To apply once a day to a nonhairy, clean, dry area of skin on upper body or upper outer arm; to rotate sites to prevent skin irritation
• To stop smoking immediately when beginning patch treatment
• To apply promptly after removing from protective patch; system may lose strength

Inhaler

• That puffing on mouthpiece delivers nicotine through the mouth lining

---

nifedipine (R)

(nye-fed'i-peen)
Adalat, Adalat CC, Adalat
P.A.*, Apo-Nifed*, nifedipine,
Novo-Nifedin*, Nu N. Sed*,
Procardia, Procardia XL
Func. class.: Calcium-channel blocker, antianginal
Chem. class.: Dihydropyridine

Action: Inhibits calcium ion influx across cell membrane during cardiac depolarization; relaxes coronary vascular smooth muscle; dilates coronary arteries; increases myocardial oxygen delivery in patients with vasospastic angina; dilates peripheral arteries

Uses: Chronic stable angina pectoris, vasospastic angina, hypertension

Investigational uses: Hypertension (acute), migraines, CHF, Raynaud's disease

Dosage and routes:

• *Adult:* PO immediate release 10 mg tid, increase in 10 mg increments q4-6h, not to exceed 180 mg/24 hr or single dose of 30 mg; sus rel 30-60 mg/qd, may increase q7-14d, doses >120 mg not recommended
• *Child:* PO 0.25-0.5 mg/kg/dose q4-6h, max 1-2 mg/kg/day

Available forms: Caps 5*, 10, 20 mg; tabs, ext rel 10*, 20*, 30, 60, 90 mg; tabs 10 mg*

Side effects/adverse reactions:
CNS: Headache, fatigue, drowsiness, dizziness, anxiety, depression, weakness, insomnia, light-headedness, paresthesia, tinnitus, blurred vision, nervousness
CV: Dysrhythmias, edema, *CHF,* hypotension, palpitations, *MI, pulmonary edema,* tachycardia
GI: Nausea, vomiting, diarrhea, gastric upset, constipation, increased liver function studies, dry mouth
GU: Nocturia, polyuria
INTEG: Rash, pruritus, flushing, photosensitivity, hair loss
MISC: Flushing, sexual difficulties, cough, fever, chills

Contraindications: Hypersensitivity

Precautions: CHF, hypotension, sick sinus syndrome, 2nd or 3rd degree heart block, hypotension less than 90 mm Hg systolic, hepatic injury, pregnancy (C), lactation, children, renal disease

Pharmacokinetics:
Well absorbed PO
PO-ER: Duration 24 hr
PO: Onset 20 min, peak 0.5-6 hr, duration 6-8 hr, half-life 2-5 hr
Metabolized by liver, excreted in urine (98% as metabolites)

Interactions:
• Decreased antihypertensive effect: NSAIDs
• Increased risk of toxicity: cimetidine, propranolol, cyclosporine, prazosin, carbamazepine, quinidine, digoxin
• Increased effects of theophylline, β-blockers, antihypertensives

---

◆ = Nursing alert   ∥ = Herb-drug interaction   ⊘ = Do not crush

• Food/drug: increased nifedipine level: grapefruit juice
• Decreased effects: quinidine
Lab test interferences:
Positive: ANA, direct Coombs' test
NURSING CONSIDERATIONS
Assess:
• Anginal pain: location, intensity, duration, character, alleviating, aggravating factors
• Cardiac status: B/P, pulse, respiration, ECG
• Potassium, LFTs, renal studies periodically during treatment
Administer:
• Without regard to meals
Evaluate:
• Therapeutic response: decreased anginal pain, B/P, activity tolerance
Teach patient/family:
• To avoid hazardous activities until stabilized on drug, dizziness is no longer a problem
• To limit caffeine consumption; take no alcohol products
• To avoid OTC drugs unless directed by a prescriber
• That ext rel nonabsorbable shell may appear in stools
• To comply with all areas of medical regimen: diet, exercise, stress reduction, drug therapy
• To change position slowly; orthostatic hypotension is common
🚫 Not to break, crush, or chew ext rel tabs
• To notify prescriber of dyspnea, edema of extremities, nausea, vomiting, severe ataxia
Treatment of overdose: Defibrillation, atropine for AV block, vasopressor for hypotension

nilutamide
(nye-loo'ta-mide)
Anandron*, Nilandron
Func. class.: Antineoplastic-hormone
Chem. class.: Antiandrogen

Action: Interferes with testosterone uptake in the nucleus or testosterone activity in target tissues; arrests tumor growth in androgen-sensitive tissue (e.g., prostate gland); prostatic carcinoma is androgen-sensitive, so tumor growth is arrested
Uses: Metastatic prostatic carcinoma, stage D2 in combination with surgical castration
Dosage and routes:
• *Adult:* **PO** 300 mg qd × 30 days, then 150 mg qd
Available forms: Tabs 50, 100 mg*
Side effects/adverse reactions:
CNS: Hot flashes, drowsiness, insomnia, dizziness, hyperthesia, depression
GU: Decreased libido, impotence, testicular atrophy, UTI, hematuria, nocturia, gynecomastia
GI: Diarrhea, nausea, vomiting, increased liver function studies, constipation, dyspepsia, ***hepatotoxicity***
INTEG: Rash, sweating, alopecia, dry skin
RESP: Dyspnea, URI, pneumonia, ***interstitial pneumonitis***
HEMA: Anemia
EENT: Delay in adaptation to dark
MISC: Edema
Contraindications: Hypersensitivity, severe hepatic impairment, severe respiratory disease
Precautions: Pregnancy (C)
Pharmacokinetics: Rapidly and completely absorbed; excreted in urine and feces as metabolites
Interactions:
• Increased toxicity of vit K, phenytoin, theophylline

NURSING CONSIDERATIONS
Assess:

- Liver function studies: AST, ALT, alk phosphatase, which may be elevated
- For CNS symptoms: drowsiness, insomnia, dizziness
- Chest x-rays, routinely; dyspnea, cough, which may indicate interstitial pneumonitis; discontinue treatment if this condition is suspected

Administer:

- Without regard to meals

Evaluate:

- Therapeutic response: decrease in prostatic tumor size, decrease in spread of cancer

Teach patient/family:

- To report side effects: decreased libido, impotence, breast enlargement, hot flashes, diarrhea, dyspnea, cough
- To report signs of hepatotoxicity
- To wear tinted lens to alleviate delay in adapting to the dark

Treatment of overdose: Induce vomiting, provide supportive care

---

nisoldipine
(nye-sole'dih-peen)
Sular
Func. class.: Antihypertensive, calcium channel blocker
Chem. class.: Dihydropyridine

Action: Inhibits calcium ion influx across cell membrane, resulting in dilation of peripheral arteries

Uses: Essential hypertension, alone or with other antihypertensives

Dosage and routes:

- *Adult:* PO 20 mg qd initially, may increase by 10 mg/wk, usual dose 20-40 mg qd
- *Geriatric:* PO 10 mg/day, increase by 10 mg/wk

Available forms: Tabs, ext rel 10, 20, 30, 40 mg

Side effects/adverse reactions:

CV: Dysrhythmia, edema, CHF, hypotension, palpitations, *MI, pulmonary edema,* tachycardia, syncope, AV block, angina

GI: Nausea, vomiting, diarrhea, gastric upset, constipation, increased liver function studies, dry mouth

GU: Nocturia, polyuria

INTEG: Rash, pruritus

MISC: Flushing, sexual difficulties, cough, nasal congestion, shortness of breath, wheezing, epistaxis, respiratory infection, chest pain

CNS: Headache, fatigue, drowsiness, dizziness, anxiety, depression, nervousness, insomnia, lightheadedness, paresthesia, tinnitus, psychosis, somnolence

HEMA: Anemia

Contraindications: Hypersensitivity, sick sinus syndrome, 2nd or 3rd degree heart block

Precautions: CHF, hypotension <90 mm Hg systolic, hepatic injury, pregnancy (C), lactation, children, renal disease, elderly

Pharmacokinetics: Metabolized by liver, excreted in urine

Interactions:

- Increased effects of β-blockers, antihypertensives, digitalis
- Increased felodipine level: cimetidine, ranitidine
- Drug/food: increased nisoldipine level: high-fat foods; increased hypotensive effect: grapefruit

NURSING CONSIDERATIONS
Assess:

- Cardiac status: B/P, pulse, respiration, ECG
- I&O ratios, weight qd
- For CHF: weight gain, jugular vein distention, edema, rales

Administer:

- Once daily as whole tablet; avoid high-fat foods, grapefruit

---

 = Nursing alert   ⫘ = Herb-drug interaction   ⊘ = Do not crush

Evaluate:

• Therapeutic response: decreased B/P

Teach patient/family:

🚫 To swallow whole; not to break, crush, or chew

• To avoid hazardous activities until stabilized on drug, dizziness is no longer a problem

• To report nausea, dizziness, edema, shortness of breath, palpitations

• To limit caffeine consumption

• To avoid OTC drugs unless directed by a prescriber

• The importance of complying with all areas of medical regimen: diet, exercise, stress reduction, drug therapy

• To rise slowly to prevent orthostatic hypotension

Treatment of overdose: Defibrillation, atropine for AV block, vasopressor for hypotension

---

nitric oxide
See appendix a—selected new drugs

---

nitrofurantoin (℞)
(nye-troe-fyoor′an-toyn)
Apo-Nitrofurantoin*, Furadantin*, Furalan, Macpac, Macrobid, Macrodantin, Nephronex*, Nitrofuracot, Nitrofurantoin, Novofuran*

Func. class.: Urinary tract anti-infective

Chem. class.: Synthetic nitrofuran derivative

Action: Appears to inhibit bacterial enzymes

Uses: Urinary tract infections caused by *Escherichia coli, Klebsiella, Pseudomonas, Proteus vulgaris, P. morganii, Serratia, Citrobacter, Staphylococcus aureus, S. epidermidis, Enterococcus, Salmonella, Shigella*

Dosage and routes:

• *Adult and child >12 yr:* **PO** 50-100 mg qid pc or 50-100 mg hs for long-term treatment

• *Child 1 mo-3 yr:* **PO** 5-7 mg/kg/day in 4 divided doses; 1-3 mg/kg/day for long-term treatment

Available forms: Caps 25, 50, 100 mg; tabs 50, 100 mg; susp 25 mg/5 ml; ext rel caps 100 mg; macrocrystal caps (Macrodantin) 25, 50, 100 mg

Side effects/adverse reactions:

INTEG: Pruritus, rash, urticaria, angioedema, alopecia, tooth staining

CNS: Dizziness, headache, drowsiness, peripheral neuropathy

*GI: Nausea, vomiting, abdominal pain, diarrhea, **cholestatic jaundice***

Contraindications: Hypersensitivity, anuria, severe renal disease, infants <1 mo

Precautions: Pregnancy (B), lactation, G-6-PD deficiency, elderly

Pharmacokinetics:

PO: Half-life 20-60 min; crosses blood-brain barrier, placenta; enters breast milk; excreted as inactive metabolites in liver, unchanged in urine

Interactions:

• Increased levels of nitrofurantoin: probenecid

• Antagonistic effect: nalidixic acid

• Decreased absorption of Mg trisilicate antacid

NURSING CONSIDERATIONS

Assess:

• Blood count during chronic therapy

• I&O ratio; urine pH <5.5 is ideal; C&S before treatment, after completion; symptoms of UTI

• CNS symptoms: insomnia, vertigo, headache, drowsiness, convulsions

• Allergy: fever, flushing, rash, urticaria, pruritus

Administer:

PO

• After clean-catch urine for C&S

• Two daily doses if urine output is high or if patient has diabetes

Evaluate:

• Therapeutic response: decreased dysuria, fever; neg C&S

Teach patient/family:

• To take with food or milk; avoid alcohol

• To protect susp from freezing and shake well before taking

• That drug may cause drowsiness; instruct client to seek aid in walking and other activities; advise client not to drive or operate machinery while on medication

• That diabetics should monitor blood glucose level

🚫 Not to crush tabs, open caps

• That drug may turn urine rust-yellow to brown

---

nitroglycerin (℞)

(nye-troe-gli′ser-in)

Deponit, Minitran, Nitrek, Nitro-Bid, Nitro-Bid IV, Nitro-Bid Plateau Caps, Nitrocine, Nitrocine Timecaps, Nitro-disc, Nitro-Dur, Nitrogard, nitroglycerin, nitroglycerin transdermal, Nitroglyn, Nitrol, Nitrolingual, Nitrong, Nitrostat, Transderm-Nitro, Tridil

Func. class.: Coronary vasodilator, antianginal

Chem. class.: Nitrate

Action: Decreases preload, afterload, which is responsible for decreasing left ventricular end-diastolic pressure, systemic vascular resistance; dilates coronary arteries, improves blood flow

Uses: Chronic stable angina pectoris, prophylaxis of angina pain, CHF associated with acute MI, controlled hypotension in surgical procedures

Dosage and routes:

• *Adult:* **SL** dissolve tab under tongue when pain begins; may repeat q5min until relief occurs; take no more than 3 tabs/15 min; use 1 tab prophylactically 5-10 min before activities; **SUS CAP** q6-12h on empty stomach; **TOP** 1-2 in q8h, increase to 4 in q4h as needed; **IV** 5 µg/min, then increase by 5 µg/min q3-5min; if no response after 20 µg/min, increase by 10-20 µg/min until desired response; **TRANS** apply a pad qd to a site free of hair; remove patch hs to provide 10-12h nitrate-free interval to avoid tolerance

• *Child:* **IV** initial: 0.25-0.5 µg/kg/min, titrate to patient response, usual dose 1-3 µg/kg/min

Available forms: Buccal tabs 1, 2, 3 mg; aero 0.4 mg/metered spray; sus rel caps 2.5, 6.5, 9, 13 mg; tabs, sus rel 2.6, 6.5, 9 mg; inj 0.5, 5, mg/ml; SL tabs 0.15, 0.3, 0.4, 0.6 mg; trans oint 2%; trans syst 0.1, 0.2, 0.3, 0.4, 0.6 mg/24 hr; inj sol 25 mg/250 ml, 50 mg/250 ml, 50 mg/500 ml, 100 mg/500 ml, 200 mg/500 ml; patch 22.4, 44.8, 67.2 mg

Side effects/adverse reactions:

CV: *Postural hypotension,* tachycardia, ***collapse,*** syncope

GI: Nausea, vomiting

INTEG: Pallor, sweating, rash

CNS: Headache, flushing, dizziness

Contraindications: Hypersensitivity to this drug or nitrites, severe anemia, increased intracranial pressure, cerebral hemorrhage

Precautions: Postural hypotension, pregnancy (C), lactation

⬥ = Nursing alert　　🥢 = Herb-drug interaction　　🚫 = Do not crush

Pharmacokinetics:

SUS REL: Onset 20-45 min, duration 3-8 hr

SL: Onset 1-3 min, duration 30 min

TRANS: Onset ½-1 hr, duration 12-24 hr

IV: Onset 1-2 min, duration 3-5 min

TRANSMUC: Onset 3 min, duration 3-5 hr

AEROSOL: Onset 2 min, duration 30-60 min

TOP OINT: Onset 30-60 min, duration 2-12 hr

Metabolized by liver, excreted in urine, half-life 1-4 min

Interactions:

• Increased effects: β-blockers, diuretics, antihypertensives, anticoagulants, alcohol

• Decreased heparin: IV nitroglycerin

NURSING CONSIDERATIONS
Assess:

• Orthostatic B/P, pulse

• Pain: duration, time started, activity being performed, character

• Tolerance if taken over long period

• Headache, light-headedness, decreased B/P; may indicate a need for decreased dosage

Administer:

• With 8 oz H_2O on empty stomach (oral tablet) 1 hr before or 2 hr after meals

• Trans tab should be placed between cheek and gum line

• Topical ointment should be measured on papers supplied

• Apply a new TD patch qd and remove after 12-14 hr to prevent tolerance

IV

• Diluted in amount specified D_5, D_5W, 0.9% NaCl for infusion; use glass infusion bottles, non–polyvinyl chloride infusion tubing; titrate to patient response; do not use filters

Additive compatibilities: Alteplase, aminophylline, dobutamine, dopamine, enalaprilat, furosemide, lidocaine, verapamil

Syringe compatibilities: Heparin

Y-site compatibilities: Amiodarone, amphotericin B cholesteryl, amrinone, atracurium, cefmetazole, cisatracurium, diltiazem, dobutamine, dopamine, epinephrine, esmolol, famotidine, fentanyl, fluconazole, furosemide, haloperidol, heparin, hydromorphone, insulin (regular), labetalol, lidocaine, lorazepam, midazolam, milrinone, morphine, nicardipine, norepinephrine, pancuronium, propofol, ranitidine, remifentanil, sodium nitroprusside, streptokinase, tacrolimus, theophylline, thiopental, vecuronium, warfarin

Evaluate:

• Therapeutic response: decrease, prevention of anginal pain

Teach patient/family:

• To place buccal tab between lip and gum above incisors or between cheek and gum

🚫 That sus rel must be swallowed whole, not chewed

• That SL should be dissolved under tongue, not swallowed

• That aerosol should be sprayed under tongue, not inhaled

• To use inhaler only when lying down

• Not to inhale spray

• To keep tabs in original container

• If 3 SL tabs in 15 min do not relieve pain, to seek immediate medical attention

• To avoid alcohol

• That drug may cause headache; tolerance usually develops; use non-narcotic analgesic

• That drug may be taken before stressful activity: exercise, sexual activity

---

Side effects: *italics* = common; ***bold italics*** = life-threatening

• That SL may sting when drug comes in contact with mucous membranes
• To avoid hazardous activities if dizziness occurs
• To comply with complete medical regimen
• To make position changes slowly to prevent fainting

---

nitroprusside (Ŗ)

(nye-troe-pruss'ide)
Nitropress, sodium nitroprusside
Func. class.: Antihypertensive
Chem. class.: Peripheral vasodilator

Action: Directly relaxes arteriolar, venous smooth muscle, resulting in reduction in cardiac preload, afterload

Uses: Hypertensive crisis, to decrease bleeding by creating hypotension during surgery, acute CHF, cardiogenic shock

Dosage and routes:
• *Adult:* IV INF dissolve 50 mg in 2-3 ml of D_5W, then dilute in 250-1000 ml of D_5W; run at 0.5-8 μg/kg/min
• *Child:* IV 0.3-0.5 μg/kg/min, titrate to response

Available forms: Inj 50 mg

Side effects/adverse reactions:
GI: Nausea, vomiting, abdominal pain
CNS: Dizziness, headache, agitation, twitching, decreased reflexes, *LOC,* restlessness
EENT: Tinnitus, blurred vision
GU: Impotence
INTEG: Pain, irritation at injection site, sweating
CV: Palpitation, severe hypotension, dyspnea
MISC: **Cyanide, thiocyanate toxicity**

Contraindications: Hypersensitivity, hypertension (compensatory)

Precautions: Pregnancy (C), lactation, children, fluid, electrolyte imbalances, hepatic disease, renal disease, hypothyroidism, elderly

Pharmacokinetics:
IV: Onset 1-2 min, duration 1-10 min, half-life 4 days in patients with abnormal renal function; metabolized in liver, excreted in urine

Interactions:
• Severe hypotension: ganglionic blockers, volatile liquid anesthetics, halothane, enflurane, circulatory depressants

NURSING CONSIDERATIONS
Assess:
• Electrolytes: K, Na, Cl, CO_2, CBC, serum glucose, serum methemoglobin if pulmonary O_2 levels are decreased
• Renal function studies: catecholamines, BUN, creatinine
• Hepatic function studies: AST, ALT, alk phosphatase
• B/P by direct means if possible; check ECG continuously; pulse, jugular vein distention; PCWP
• Weight qd, I&O
• Thiocyanate, lactate, cyanide levels if on long-term treatment
• Nausea, vomiting, diarrhea
• Edema in feet, legs daily; skin turgor, dryness of mucous membranes for hydration status
• Rales, dyspnea, orthopnea q30min
• For decrease in bicarbonate, P_{CO_2} blood pH, acidosis

Administer:
IV
• Depending on B/P reading q15min
• IV after diluting 50 mg/2-3 ml of D_5W, further dilute in 250 ml of D_5W; use an infusion pump only; wrap bottle with aluminum foil to protect from light; observe for color change in the infusion; discard if

---

◆ = Nursing alert   🌿 = Herb-drug interaction   ⊘ = Do not crush

highly discolored (blue, green, dark red); titrate to patient response

Syringe compatibilities: Heparin

Y-site compatibilities: Amrinone, atracurium, diltiazem, dobutamine, dopamine, enalaprilat, famotidine, lidocaine, nitroglycerin, pancuronium, tacrolimus, theophylline, vecuronium

Evaluate:
• Therapeutic response: decreased B/P, absence of bleeding

Teach patient/family:
• To report headache, dizziness, loss of hearing, blurred vision, dyspnea, faintness

Treatment of overdose: Administer amyl nitrite inhalation until 3% sodium nitrate solution can be prepared for IV administration, then inject sodium thiosulfate IV, correct drop in B/P with vasopressor

---

nizatidine

(ni-za′ti-deen)

Axid, Axid AR

Func. class.: H₂-receptor antagonist

Chem. class.: Substituted thiazole

Action: Blocks H₂-receptors, thereby reducing gastric acid output

Uses: Benign gastric and duodenal ulceration, prevention of duodenal ulcer recurrence, symptomatic relief of gastroesophageal reflux, heartburn prevention

Dosage and routes:
Renal dose
• CrCl 20-50 ml/min give 150 mg/day; CrCl <20 ml/min give 150 mg qod

Gastric and duodenal ulcer
• *Adult:* **PO** 300 mg at night or 150 mg bid for 4-8 wk; maintenance 150 mg at night

Gastroesophageal reflux
• *Adult:* **PO** 150 mg bid

Available forms: Caps 75, 150 mg, 300 mg

Side effects/adverse reactions:

CNS: Headache, somnolence, confusion, abnormal dreams, dizziness

ENDO: Gynecomastia

HEMA: **Thrombocytopenia**

INTEG: Pruritus, sweating, urticaria, **exfoliative dermatitis**

MS: Myalgia

RESP: **Bronchospasm, laryngeal edema**

METAB: Hyperuricemia

GI: Elevated liver enzymes, **hepatitis**, jaundice, nausea

CV: Cardiac dysrhythmias, **cardiac arrest**

Contraindications: Hypersensitivity

Precautions: Renal or hepatic impairment (reduce dose in renal impairment), pregnancy (C), lactation

Pharmacokinetics: Partially metabolized by liver, excreted by kidneys, plasma half-life 1½ hr, 70% absorbed orally, small amount (0.1% of plasma concentration) enters breast milk, 35% bound to plasma proteins

NURSING CONSIDERATIONS
Assess:
• Gastric pH (>5 should be maintained)
• Fluid balance, I&O

Administer:
PO
• With meals for prolonged drug effect; antacids 1 hr before or 1 hr after drug

Evaluate:
• Mental status, confusion, dizziness, depression, anxiety, weakness, tremors, psychosis, diarrhea, jaundice, report immediately
• For GI symptoms: nausea, vomiting, diarrhea, cramps

N

Teach patient/family:
• That gynecomastia, impotence may occur, are reversible
• To avoid driving or other hazardous activities until patient is stabilized on this medication; dizziness may occur
• To avoid black pepper, caffeine, alcohol, harsh spices, extremes in temp of food
• To avoid OTC preparations: aspirin, cough, cold preparations

Treatment of overdose: Symptomatic and supportive therapy is recommended; activated charcoal, emesis or lavage may reduce absorption

---

norepinephrine (R)

(nor-ep-i-nef′rin)
Levophed
Func. class.: Adrenergic
Chem. class.: Catecholamine

Action: Causes increased contractility and heart rate by acting on β-receptors in heart; also acts on α-receptors, causing vasoconstriction in blood vessels; B/P is elevated, coronary blood flow improves, cardiac output increases

Uses: Acute hypotension, shock

Dosage and routes:
• *Adult:* IV INF 8-12 μg/min titrated to B/P
• *Child:* IV INF 0.05-0.1 μg/kg/min titrated to B/P

Available forms: Inj 1 mg/ml

Side effects/adverse reactions:
CNS: Headache, anxiety, dizziness, insomnia, restlessness, tremor
CV: Palpitations, tachycardia, hypertension, ectopic beats, angina
GI: Nausea, vomiting
INTEG: Necrosis, tissue sloughing with extravasation, *gangrene*
RESP: Dyspnea
GU: Decreased urine output

Contraindications: Hypersensitivity, ventricular fibrillation, tachydysrhythmias, pheochromocytoma

Precautions: Lactation, arterial embolism, peripheral vascular disease, hypertension, hyperthyroidism, elderly, heart disease, pregnancy (C)

Pharmacokinetics:
IV: Onset 1-2 min; metabolized in liver; excreted in urine (inactive metabolites); crosses placenta

Interactions:
• Severe hypertension: guanethidine
◆Do not use within 2 wk of MAOIs, or hypertensive crisis may result
• Dysrhythmias: general anesthetics, bretylium
• Decreased action of norepinephrine: α-blockers
• Increased B/P: oxytocics
• Increased pressor effect: tricyclic antidepressant, MAOIs
• Incompatible with alkaline solutions: Na, HCO_3

NURSING CONSIDERATIONS
Assess:
• I&O ratio; notify prescriber if output <30 ml/hr
• ECG during administration continuously; if B/P increases, drug is decreased
• B/P and pulse q2-3min after parenteral route
• CVP or PWP during infusion if possible
• For paresthesias and coldness of extremities; peripheral blood flow may decrease
• Injection site: tissue sloughing; administer phentolamine mixed with 0.9% NaCl
• Sulfite sensitivity, which may be life-threatening

Administer:
• Plasma expanders for hypovolemia
• IV after diluting with 500-1000 ml D_5W or D_5/0.9% NaCl; average

dilution is 4 mg/1000 ml diluent (4 µg base/ml); give as infusion 2-3 ml/min; titrate to response

• Using 2-bottle setup so drug may be discontinued while IV is still running; use infusion pump

Additive compatibilities: Amikacin, calcium chloride, calcium gluconate, cimetidine, corticotropin, dimenhydrinate, dobutamine, heparin, hydrocortisone, magnesium sulfate, meropenem, methylprednisolone, multivitamins, netilmicin, potassium chloride, succinylcholine, verapamil, vit B/C

Syringe compatibilities: Heparin

Y-site compatibilities: Amiodarone, amrinone, cisatracurium, diltiazem, dobutamine, dopamine, epinephrine, esmolol, famotidine, fentanyl, furosemide, haloperidol, heparin, hydrocortisone, hydromorphone, labetalol, lorazepam, meropenem, midazolam, milrinone, morphine, nicardipine, nitroglycerin, potassium chloride, propofol, ranitidine, remifentanil, vecuronium, vit B/C

Perform/provide:

• Storage of reconstituted sol if refrigerated no longer than 24 hr
• Do not use discolored sol

Evaluate:

• Therapeutic response: increased B/P with stabilization

Teach patient/family:

• The reason for drug administration and to report dyspnea, dizziness, chest pain

Treatment of overdose: Administer fluids, electrolyte replacement

---

norethindrone (℞)

(nor-eth-in′drone)

Micronor, Norlutin, Nor-QD

Func. class.: Progestogen

Chem. class.: Progesterone derivative

Action: Inhibits secretion of pituitary gonadotropins, which prevents follicular maturation, ovulation; stimulates growth of mammary tissue; antineoplastic action against endometrial cancer

Uses: Uterine bleeding (abnormal), amenorrhea, endometriosis

Dosage and routes:

• *Adult:* **PO** 5-20 mg qd days 5-25 of menstrual cycle

Endometriosis

• *Adult:* **PO** 10 mg qd × 2 wk, then increased by 5 mg qd × 2 wk, up to 30 mg qd

Available forms: Tabs 5 mg

Side effects/adverse reactions:

CNS: Dizziness, headache, migraines, depression, fatigue

CV: Hypotension, ***thrombophlebitis,*** edema, ***thromboembolism, stroke, pulmonary embolism, MI***

GI: Nausea, vomiting, anorexia, cramps, increased weight, ***cholestatic jaundice***

EENT: Diplopia

GU: Amenorrhea, cervical erosion, breakthrough bleeding, dysmenorrhea, vaginal candidiasis, breast changes, (gynecomastia, testicular atrophy, impotence), endometriosis, ***spontaneous abortion***

INTEG: Rash, urticaria, acne, hirsutism, alopecia, oily skin, seborrhea, purpura, melasma

META: Hyperglycemia

Contraindications: Breast cancer, hypersensitivity, thromboembolic disorders, reproductive cancer, genital bleeding (abnormal, undiagnosed), pregnancy (X)

Precautions: Lactation, hypertension, asthma, blood dyscrasias, gallbladder disease, CHF, diabetes mellitus, bone disease, depression, migraine headache, convulsive disorders, hepatic disease, renal disease, family history of breast or reproductive tract cancer

Pharmacokinetics:

PO: Duration 24 hr, excreted in urine, feces, metabolized in liver

Lab test interferences:

Increase: Alk phosphatase, nitrogen (urine), pregnanediol, amino acids, factors VII, VIII, IX, X

Decrease: GTT, HDL

NURSING CONSIDERATIONS
Assess:

• Weight qd: notify prescriber of weekly weight gain >5 lb
• B/P at beginning of treatment and periodically
• I&O ratio; be alert for decreasing urinary output, increasing edema
• Liver function studies: ALT, AST, bilirubin, periodically during long-term therapy
• Edema, hypertension, cardiac symptoms, jaundice
• Mental status: affect, mood, behavioral changes, depression
• Hypercalcemia

Administer:

• Titrated dose; use lowest effective dose
• In one dose in AM
• With food or milk to decrease GI symptoms

Perform/provide:

• Storage in dark area

Evaluate:

• Therapeutic response: decreased abnormal uterine bleeding, absence of amenorrhea

Teach patient/family:

• About cushingoid symptoms

• To report breast lumps, vaginal bleeding, edema, jaundice, dark urine, clay-colored stools, dyspnea, headache, blurred vision, abdominal pain, numbness or stiffness in legs, chest pain; male to report impotence or gynecomastia
• To report suspected pregnancy

---

norfloxacin (R)

(nor-flox'-a-sin)
Chibroxin, Noroxin
Func. class.: Urinary antiinfective
Chem. class.: Fluoroquinolone

Action: Interferes with conversion of intermediate DNA fragments into high-molecular-weight DNA in bacteria, inhibits DNA gyrase

Uses: Adult urinary tract infections (including complicated) caused by *Escherichia coli, Enterobacter cloacae, Proteus mirabilis, Klebsiella pneumoniae,* group D strep, indole-positive *Proteus, Citrobacter freundii, Staphylococcus aureus;* uncomplicated gonorrhea, ocular infection

Dosage and routes:

Renal dose
• CrCl ≤30 ml/min 400 mg **PO** qd

Uncomplicated infections
• *Adult:* **PO** 400 mg bid × 3-10 days 1 hr before or 2 hr after meals

Complicated infections
• *Adult:* **PO** 400 mg bid × 10-21 days; 400 mg qd × 7-10 days in impaired renal function

Uncomplicated gonorrhea
• *Adult:* **PO** 800 mg as a single dose

Ocular infection
• *Adult and child:* **OPHTH** 1 gtt qid, may increase to 1 gtt q2h for severe infections

Prostatitis
• *Adult:* **PO** 400 mg bid × 4 wk

Available forms: Tabs 400 mg; ophth sol 3 mg/ml

Side effects/adverse reactions:
CNS: Headache, dizziness, fatigue, somnolence, depression, insomnia
GI: Nausea, constipation, increased ALT, AST, flatulence, heartburn, vomiting, diarrhea, dry mouth
INTEG: Rash
EENT: Visual disturbances
Contraindications: Hypersensitivity to quinolones
Precautions: Pregnancy (C), lactation, children, renal disease, seizure disorders
Pharmacokinetics: Peak 1 hr, half-life 3-4 hr; steady state 2 days; excreted in urine as active drug, metabolites
Interactions:
• Decreased effect of norfloxacin: antacids, iron products, sucralfate; give 2 hr apart
• Increased serum concentrations of: cyclosporine, probenecid
• Antagonizes effects of norfloxacin: nitrofurantoin, monitor closely
• Increased anticoagulation: oral anticoagulants
• Possible increased levels, toxicity: theophylline
Lab test interferences:
Increase: AST, ALT, BUN, creatinine, alk phosphatase
NURSING CONSIDERATIONS
Assess:
• Kidney, liver function studies: BUN, creatinine, AST, ALT
• I&O ratio; urine pH, <5.5 is ideal
• CNS symptoms: insomnia, vertigo, headache, agitation, confusion
• Allergic reactions: fever, flushing, rash, urticaria, pruritus
Administer:
PO
• After clean-catch urine for C&S
• Two daily doses if urine output is high or if patient has diabetes
Evaluate:
• Therapeutic response: decreased pain, frequency, urgency, C&S, absence of infection
Teach patient/family:
• That fluid intake must be 3 L/day to avoid crystallization in kidneys
• That if dizziness occurs, to walk, perform activities with assistance
• To complete full course of drug therapy
• To contact prescriber if adverse reaction occurs
• To take 1 hr before or 2 hr after meals; not to take antacids with or within 2 hr of this drug; to sip water or use hard candy for dry mouth

---

norgestrel (℞)
(nor-jess'trel)
Ovral*, Ovrette
Func. class.: Progestogen
Chem. class.: Progesterone derivative

Action: Inhibits secretion of pituitary gonadotropins, which prevents follicular maturation, ovulation, stimulates growth of mammary tissue, antineoplastic action against endometrial cancer
Uses: Female contraception
Dosage and routes:
• *Adult:* **PO** 1 tab qd
Available forms: Tabs 0.35, 0.075 mg
Side effects/adverse reactions:
CNS: Dizziness, headache, migraines, depression, fatigue
CV: Hypotension, ***thrombophlebitis,*** edema, ***thromboembolism, stroke, pulmonary embolism, myocardial infarction***
GI: Nausea, vomiting, anorexia, cramps, increased weight, ***cholestatic jaundice***
EENT: Diplopia
GU: Amenorrhea, cervical erosion, breakthrough bleeding, dysmenor-

rhea, vaginal candidiasis, breast changes, *gynecomastia, testicular atrophy, impotence,* endometriosis, ***spontaneous abortion***
INTEG: Rash, urticaria, acne, hirsutism, alopecia, oily skin, seborrhea, purpura, melasma
META: Hyperglycemia
Contraindications: Breast cancer, hypersensitivity, thromboembolic disorders, reproductive cancer, genital bleeding (abnormal, undiagnosed), cerebral hemorrhage, pregnancy (X)
Precautions: Lactation, hypertension, asthma, blood dyscrasias, gallbladder disease, CHF, diabetes mellitus, bone disease, depression, migraine headache, convulsive disorders, hepatic disease, renal disease, family history of breast or reproductive tract cancer
Pharmacokinetics:
PO: Duration 24 hr; excreted in urine, feces; metabolized in liver
Lab test interferences:
Increase: Alk phosphatase, nitrogen (urine), pregnanediol, amino acids, factors VII, VIII, IX, X
Decrease: GTT, HDL
NURSING CONSIDERATIONS
Assess:
• Weight qd; notify prescriber of weekly weight gain >5 lb
• B/P at beginning of treatment and periodically
• I&O ratio; be alert for decreasing urinary output, increasing edema
• Liver function studies: ALT, AST, bilirubin, periodically during long-term therapy
• Edema, hypertension, cardiac symptoms, jaundice
• Mental status: affect, mood, behavioral changes, depression
• Hypercalcemia
Administer:
• Titrated dose; use lowest effective dose

• In one dose in AM
• With food or milk to decrease GI symptoms
• After warming to dissolve crystals
Perform/provide:
• Storage in dark area
Evaluate:
• Therapeutic response: absence of pregnancy
Teach patient/family:
• About cushingoid symptoms
• To report breast lumps, vaginal-bleeding, edema, jaundice, dark urine, clay-colored stools, dyspnea, headache, blurred vision, abdominal pain, numbness or stiffness in legs, chest pain
• To report suspected pregnancy
• To monitor blood sugar if diabetic

---

nortriptyline (℞)

(nor-trip'ti-leen)
Aventyl, Pamelor
Func. class.: Antidepressant—tricyclic
Chem. class.: Dibenzocycloheptene—secondary amine

Action: Blocks reuptake of norepinephrine, serotonin into nerve endings, increasing action of norepinephrine, serotonin in nerve cells
Uses: Major depression
Investigational uses: Chronic pain management
Dosage and routes:
• *Adult:* **PO** 25 mg tid or qid; may increase to 150 mg/day; may give daily dose hs
• *Geriatric:* **PO** 10-25 mg q hs, increase by 10-25 mg at weekly intervals to desired dose; usual maintenance 30-50 mg
Available forms: Caps 10, 25, 50, 75 mg; sol 10 mg/5 ml

Side effects/adverse reactions:

HEMA: **Agranulocytosis, thrombocytopenia, eosinophilia, leukopenia**

CNS: Dizziness, drowsiness, confusion, headache, anxiety, tremors, stimulation, weakness, insomnia, nightmares, EPS (elderly), increased psychiatric symptoms

GI: Constipation, dry mouth, nausea, vomiting, ***paralytic ileus,*** increased appetite, cramps, epigastric distress, jaundice, ***hepatitis,*** stomatitis

GU: Urinary retention, ***acute renal failure***

INTEG: Rash, urticaria, sweating, pruritus, photosensitivity

CV: Orthostatic hypotension, ECG changes, tachycardia, ***hypertension,*** palpitations

EENT: Blurred vision, tinnitus, mydriasis

Contraindications: Hypersensitivity to tricyclic antidepressants, recovery phase of MI, convulsive disorders, prostatic hypertrophy

Precautions: Suicidal patients, severe depression, increased intraocular pressure, narrow-angle glaucoma, urinary retention, cardiac disease, hepatic disease, hyperthyroidism, electroshock therapy, elective surgery, pregnancy (C), lactation

Pharmacokinetics:

PO: Steady state 4-19 days; metabolized by liver; excreted by kidneys; crosses placenta; excreted in breast milk; half-life 18-28 hr

Interactions:

• Decreased effects of guanethidine, clonidine, indirect-acting sympathomimetics (ephedrine)

• Increased effects of direct-acting sympathomimetics (epinephrine), alcohol, barbiturates, benzodiazepines, CNS depressants

◆Hyperpyretic crisis, convulsions, hypertensive episode: MAOI

🖋 Increased anticholinergic effect: belladonna, henbane

🖋 Increased antidepressant action: scopolia

Lab test interferences:

Increase: Serum bilirubin, blood glucose, alk phosphatase

False increase: Urinary catecholamines

Decrease: VMA, 5-HIAA

NURSING CONSIDERATIONS

Assess:

• B/P (lying, standing), pulse q4h; if systolic B/P drops 20 mm Hg, hold drug, notify prescriber; take vital signs q4h in patients with cardiovascular disease

• Blood studies: CBC, leukocytes, differential, cardiac enzymes if patient is receiving long-term therapy

• Hepatic studies: AST, ALT, bilirubin

• Weight qwk; appetite may increase with drug

• ECG for flattening of T wave, bundle branch block, AV block, dysrhythmias in cardiac patients

• EPS primarily in elderly: rigidity, dystonia, akathisia

• Mental status changes: mood, sensorium, affect, suicidal tendencies, increase in psychiatric symptoms, depression, panic

• Urinary retention, constipation; constipation is more likely to occur in children

◆Withdrawal symptoms: headache, nausea, vomiting, muscle pain, weakness; do not usually occur unless drug was discontinued abruptly

• Alcohol intake; if alcohol is consumed, hold dose until AM

Administer:

• Increased fluids, bulk in diet if constipation occurs

• With food, milk for GI symptoms

• Dosage hs for oversedation during day; may take entire dose hs;

N

elderly may not tolerate once/day dosing

• Gum, hard candy, frequent sips of water for dry mouth

• Concentrate with fruit juice, water, or milk to disguise taste

Perform/provide:

• Storage in tight, light-resistant container at room temp

• Assistance with ambulation during beginning therapy, since drowsiness/dizziness occurs

• Safety measures including side rails, primarily for elderly

• Checking to see if PO medication swallowed

Evaluate:

• Therapeutic response: decreased depression

Teach patient/family:

• That therapeutic effects may take 2-3 wk

• To use caution in driving, other activities requiring alertness because of drowsiness, dizziness, blurred vision

• To avoid alcohol ingestion, other CNS depressants

• Not to discontinue medication quickly after long-term use; may cause nausea, headache, malaise

• To wear sunscreen or large hat, since photosensitivity occurs

Treatment of overdose: ECG monitoring; induce emesis; lavage, activated charcoal; administer anticonvulsant

---

nystatin (℞)

(nye-stat'in)

Mycostatin, Mycostatin Pastilles, Nadostine*, nystatin

Func. class.: Antifungal

Chem.class.: Amphotericpolyene

Action: Interferes with fungal DNA replication; binds sterols in fungal cell membrane, which increases permeability, leaking of cell nutrients

Uses: *Candida* species causing oral, vaginal, intestinal infections

Dosage and routes:

Oral infection

• *Adult:* **SUSP** 400,000-600,000 U qid, use ½ dose in each side of mouth, swish and swallow

Infants: 200,000 U qid (100,000 U in each side of mouth)

• *Newborn and premature infant:* **SUSP** 100,000 U qid

• *Adult and child:* Troches 200,000-400,000 U qid × up to 2 wk

GI infection

• *Adult:* **PO** 500,000-1,000,000 U tid

Available forms: Tabs 500,000 U; powder 50 million, 150 million, 500 million, 1 billion, 2 billion, 5 billion U; susp 100,000 U per ml; troches 200,000 U

Side effects/adverse reactions:

INTEG: Rash, urticaria (rare)

GI: Nausea, vomiting, anorexia, diarrhea, cramps

Contraindications: Hypersensitivity

Precautions: Pregnancy (B)

Pharmacokinetics:

PO: Little absorption, excreted in feces

NURSING CONSIDERATIONS

Assess:

• For allergic reaction: rash, urticaria; drug may have to be discontinued

---

⬥ = Nursing alert   🍃 = Herb-drug interaction   ⊘ = Do not crush

• For predisposing factors: antibiotic therapy, pregnancy, diabetes mellitus, sexual partner infection (vaginal infections)
Administer:
• Oral susp dose by placing ½ in each cheek, then swallow
• Topical dose after cleansing area; mouth may be swabbed
Perform/provide:
• Storage in refrigerator for oral susp; tabs in tight, light-resistant containers at room temp
Evaluate:
• Therapeutic response: culture negative for *Candida*
Teach patient/family:
• That long-term therapy may be needed to clear infection; to complete entire course of medication
• Proper hygiene: changing socks if feet are infected; using no commercial mouthwashes for mouth infection
• Shake susp before measuring each dose
• To avoid getting preparation on hands
• To wear light-day pad for vaginal preparations
• To avoid tight shoes, bandages when using on feet
• To avoid sexual contact during treatment to minimize reinfection
• To notify prescriber of irritation; drug may have to be discontinued
• That relief from itching may occur after 24-72 hr

---

octreotide
See appendix a—selected new drugs

---

ofloxacin (℞)
(o-flox′a-sin)
Floxin, Floxin IV, Occuflox
Func. class.: Antiinfective
Chem. class.: Fluoroquinolone

Action: Interferes with conversion of intermediate DNA fragments into high-molecular-weight DNA in bacteria, inhibits DNA gyrase
Uses: Treatment of lower respiratory tract infections (pneumonia, bronchitis), genitourinary infections (prostatitis, UTIs) caused by *Escherichia coli, Klebsiella pneumoniae, Chlamydia trachomatis, Neisseria gonorrhoeae;* skin and skin structure infections; conjunctivitis (ophth)
Dosage and routes:
Renal dose
• CrCl 10-50 ml/min give q24h; CrCl <10 ml/min give ½ of dose q24h
Lower respiratory tract infections/ skin and skin structure infections
• *Adult:* **PO, IV** 400 mg q12h × 10 days
Cervicitis, urethritis
• *Adult:* **PO, IV** 300 mg q12h × 7 days
Prostatitis
• *Adult:* **PO, IV** 300 mg q12h × 6 wk
Acute, uncomplicated gonorrhea
• *Adult:* **PO, IV** 400 mg as a single dose
Conjunctivitis
• *Adult and child:* **OPHTH** 1-2 gtt q2-4h × 2 days, then qid × 5 days
Urinary tract infection
• *Adult:* **PO, IV** 200-400 mg q12h × 3-10 days
Available forms: Tabs 200, 300, 400 mg; 200, 400 mg; ophth sol 0.3%
Side effects/adverse reactions:
CNS: Dizziness, headache, fatigue,

---

somnolence, depression, insomnia, lethargy, malaise

GI: Diarrhea, nausea, vomiting, anorexia, flatulence, heartburn, dry mouth, increased AST, ALT, abdominal pain, constipation

INTEG: Rash, pruritus

EENT: Visual disturbances

Contraindications: Hypersensitivity to quinolones

Precautions: Pregnancy (C), lactation, children, elderly, renal disease, seizure disorders, excessive sunlight

Pharmacokinetics:

PO: Peak 1-2 hr, half-life 9 hr, steady state 2 days; excreted in urine as active drug, metabolites; 90%-95% bioavailability

Interactions:

• May decrease absorption: antacids with aluminum, magnesium, iron products, sucralfate, zinc products; separate by 2 hr

• May alter blood glucose levels: antidiabetics

• May increase CNS stimulation, seizures: NSAIDs

• Increased anticoagulation: oral anticoagulants

• Possible theophylline toxicity: theophylline

• Drug/food: decreased absorption

NURSING CONSIDERATIONS

Assess:

• Kidney, liver function studies: BUN, creatinine, AST, ALT

• I&O ratio; urine pH <5.5 is ideal

• CNS symptoms: insomnia, vertigo, headache, agitation, confusion

• Allergic reactions: rash, flushing, urticaria, pruritus

Administer:

PO

• 2 hr before or 2 hr after antacids, calcium, iron, zinc products

• After clean-catch urine for C&S

IV

• Over 1 hr or more

Additive compatibilities: Amoxicillin, ceftazidime, clindamycin, gentamicin, piperacillin, tobramycin, vancomycin

Syringe compatibilities: Cefotaxime

Y-site compatibilities: Ampicillin, cisatracurium, granisetron, propofol, remifentanil, thiotepa

Perform/provide:

• Storage for 2 wk refrigerated or 6 mo frozen after reconstitution

Evaluate:

• Therapeutic response: negative C&S; absence of redness, swelling (ophth)

Teach patient/family:

• That fluid intake must be 3 L/day to avoid crystallization in kidneys

• That if dizziness or lightheadedness occurs, ambulate, perform activities with assistance

• To complete full course of therapy

• To notify prescriber of adverse reactions or tendon pain

• To avoid iron- or mineral-containing supplements within 2 hr before or after dose

• To prevent sun exposure, photosensitivity can occur

---

olanzapine

(oh-lanz′a-peen)

Zyprexa

Func. class.: Antipsychotic, neuroleptic

Chem. class.: Thienbenzodiazepine

Action: Unknown; may mediate antipsychotic activity by both dopamine and serotonin type 2 (5-HT2) antagonist; also, may antagonize muscarinic receptors, histaminic (H$_1$)- and α-adrenergic receptors

---

◆ = Nursing alert   ∥ = Herb-drug interaction   ⊘ = Do not crush

Uses: Psychotic disorders

Dosage and routes:

• *Adult:* **PO** 5-10 mg initially qd, may increase dosage by 5 mg at 1 wk or more intervals

• *Elderly:* **PO** 5 mg, may increase cautiously at 1 wk intervals

Available forms: Tab 2.5, 5, 7.5, 10 mg

Side effects/adverse reactions:

CV: Orthostatic hypotension, tachycardia, chest pain

EENT: Blurred vision

GI: Dry mouth, nausea, vomiting, anorexia, constipation, abdominal pain, weight gain

GU: Urinary retention, urinary frequency, enuresis, impotence, amenorrhea, gynecomastia, breast engorgement, premenstrual syndrome

INTEG: Rash

RESP: Dyspnea, rhinitis, cough, pharyngitis

CNS: EPS: pseudoparkinsonism, akathisia, dystonia, tardive dyskinesia, seizures, headache, *neuroleptic malignant syndrome (rare),* fever, insomnia, somnolence, agitation, nervousness, hostility, dizziness, hypertonia, tremor, euphoria

MS: Joint pain, twitching

Contraindications: Hypersensitivity

Precautions: Pregnancy (C), lactation, hypertension, hepatic disease, cardiac disease, elderly

Pharmacokinetics: Well absorbed, peak 6 hr, metabolized by liver, excreted in urine, 93% bound to plasma proteins

Interactions:

• Oversedation: other CNS depressants, alcohol, barbiturate anesthetics, antihistamines, sedatives/hypnotics, antidepressants

• Decreased levels of olanzapine: carbamazepine, omeprazole, rifampin

• Increased hypotension: antihypertensives

• Decreased antiparkinson activity: levodopa, bromocriptine, other dopamine agonists

• Increased anticholinergic effects: anticholinergics

Lab test interferences:

Increase: Liver function test, prolactin, CPK

NURSING CONSIDERATIONS

Assess:

• Mental status: orientation, mood, behavior, presence of hallucinations and type before initial administration and monthly

• Swallowing of PO medication: check for hoarding or giving of medication to other patients

• I&O ratio; palpate bladder if low urinary output occurs, especially in elderly

• Bilirubin, CBC, liver function studies monthly

• Urinalysis recommended before, during prolonged therapy

• Affect, orientation, LOC, reflexes, gait, coordination, sleep pattern disturbances

• B/P sitting, standing, lying: take pulse and respirations q4h during initial treatment; establish baseline before starting treatment; report drops of 30 mm Hg; obtain baseline ECG

• Dizziness, faintness, palpitations, tachycardia on rising

◆ For neuroleptic malignant syndrome: hyperpyrexia, muscle rigidity, increased CPK, altered mental status, for acute dystonia (check chewing, swallowing, eyes, pill rolling)

• EPS, including akathisia (inability to sit still, no pattern to movements), tardive dyskinesia (bizarre movements of the jaw, mouth, tongue, extremities), pseudoparkin-

sonism (rigidity, tremors, pill rolling, shuffling gait)
• Skin turgor daily
• Constipation, urinary retention daily; increase bulk, H_2O in diet
Administer:
• Antiparkinsonian agent for EPS
• Decreased dose in elderly
• PO with full glass of water, milk; or with food to decrease GI upset
Perform/provide:
• Decreased stimuli by dimming light, avoiding loud noises
• Supervised ambulation until stabilized on medication; do not involve in strenuous exercise program because fainting is possible; patient should not stand still for long periods
• Increased fluids to prevent constipation
• Sips of water, candy, gum for dry mouth
• Storage in tight, light-resistant container
Evaluate:
• Therapeutic response: decrease in emotional excitement, hallucinations, delusion, paranoia, reorganization of patterns of thought, speech
Teach patient/family:
• To use good oral hygiene; frequent rinsing of mouth, sugarless gum for dry mouth
• To avoid hazardous activities until drug response is determined
• That orthostatic hypotension occurs often and to rise from sitting or lying position gradually
• To avoid hot tubs, hot showers, tub baths, since hypotension may occur
• To avoid abrupt withdrawal of this drug, or EPS may result; drug should be withdrawn slowly
• To avoid OTC preparations (cough, hay fever, cold) unless approved by prescriber, since serious drug interactions may occur; avoid use with

alcohol, CNS depressants; increased drowsiness may occur
• That in hot weather, heat stroke may occur; take extra precautions to stay cool
Treatment of overdose: Lavage if orally ingested; provide airway; do not induce vomiting or use epinephrine

---

olsalazine (R)

(ohl-sal'ah-zeen)
Dipentum
Func. class.: Antiinflammatory
Chem. class.: Salicylate derivative

Action: Bioconverted to 5-aminosalicylic acid, which decreases inflammation
Uses: Maintenance of remission of ulcerative colitis in patients intolerant to sulfasalazine
Dosage and routes:
• *Adult:* **PO** 1 g/day in 2 divided doses
Available forms: Caps 250 mg
Side effects/adverse reactions:
EENT: Dry mouth, dry eyes, watery eyes, blurred vision
SYST: **Anaphylaxis**
GI: Nausea, vomiting, abdominal pain, stomatitis, ***hepatitis,*** pancreatitis, diarrhea, bloating
CNS: Headache, insomnia, hallucinations, depression, vertigo, fatigue, ***drug fever,*** chills, dizziness, drowsiness, tremors
HEMA: **Leukopenia, neutropenia, thrombocytopenia, agranulocytosis, anemia**
INTEG: Rash, dermatitis, urticaria, ***Stevens-Johnson syndrome,*** erythema, photosensitivity, alopecia
GU: Urinary frequency, dysuria, hematuria, impotence
CV: **Allergic myocarditis,** 2nd degree heart block, hypertension, pe-

---

➤ = Nursing alert   🦋 = Herb-drug interaction   ⊘ = Do not crush ripheral edema, chest pain, palpitations

RESP: **Bronchospasm,** shortness of breath

Contraindications: Hypersensitivity to salicylates

Precautions: Pregnancy (C), child <14 yr, lactation; impaired hepatic, renal function, severe allergy, bronchial asthma

Pharmacokinetics:

PO: Partially absorbed, peak 1½ hr, half-life 5-10 hr, excreted in urine as 5-aminosalicylic acid and metabolites, crosses placenta

Lab test interferences:

False positive: Urinary glucose test

NURSING CONSIDERATIONS

Assess:

• I&O ratio: note color, character, pH of urine in treatment for UTIs; output should be 800 ml less than intake; if urine is highly acidic, alkalization may be needed

• Kidney function studies: BUN, creatinine, urinalysis (long-term therapy)

• Blood dyscrasias: skin rash, fever, sore throat, bruising, bleeding, fatigue, joint pain

• Allergic reaction: rash, dermatitis, urticaria, pruritus, dyspnea, bronchospasm

Administer:

• With food in evenly divided doses

• Medication after C&S; repeat C&S after full course of medication

• With resuscitative equipment available; severe allergic reactions may occur

• Total daily dose evenly spaced to minimize GI intolerance

Perform/provide:

• Storage in tight, light-resistant container at room temp

Evaluate:

• Therapeutic response: absence of fever, mucus in stools

---

omeprazole (℞)

(oh-mep′ray-zole)

Losec*, Prilosec

Func. class.: Proton pump inhibitor

Chem. class.: Benzimidazole

Action: Suppresses gastric secretion by inhibiting hydrogen/potassium ATPase enzyme system in gastric parietal cell; characterized as gastric acid pump inhibitor, since it blocks final step of acid production

Uses: Gastroesophageal reflux disease (GERD), severe erosive esophagitis, poorly responsive systemic GERD, pathologic hypersecretory conditions (Zollinger-Ellison syndrome, systemic mastocytosis, multiple endocrine adenomas); treatment of active duodenal ulcers with or without antiinfectives for *Helicobacter pylori*

Investigational uses: Posterior laryngitis, enhancing pancreatin

Dosage and routes:

Active duodenal ulcers

• *Adult:* **PO** 20 mg qd × 4-8 wk; associated with *Helicobacter pylori* 40 mg q AM and clarithromycin 500 mg tid on day 1-14, then 20 mg qd day 15-28

Severe erosive esophagitis/poorly responsive GERD

• *Adult:* **PO** 20 mg qd × 4-8 wk

Pathologic hypersecretory conditions

• *Adult:* **PO** 60 mg/day; may increase to 120 mg tid; daily doses >80 mg should be divided

Gastric ulcer

• *Adult:* **PO** 40 mg qd 4-8 wk

Available forms: Caps, delayed rel 10, 20 mg

Side effects/adverse reactions:

CNS: Headache, dizziness, asthenia

GI: Diarrhea, abdominal pain, vomiting, nausea, constipation, flatulence, acid regurgitation, abdominal swelling, anorexia, irritable colon, esophageal candidiasis, dry mouth

RESP: Upper respiratory infections, cough, epistaxis

INTEG: Rash, dry skin, urticaria, pruritus, alopecia

META: Hypoglycemia, increased hepatic enzymes, weight gain

EENT: Tinnitus, taste perversion

CV: Chest pain, angina, tachycardia, bradycardia, palpitations, peripheral edema

GU: UTI, urinary frequency, increased creatinine, *proteinuria, hematuria,* testicular pain, glycosuria

HEMA: Pancytopenia, thrombocytopenia, neutropenia, leukocytosis, anemia

MISC: Back pain, fever, fatigue, malaise

Contraindications: Hypersensitivity

Precautions: Pregnancy (C), lactation, children

Pharmacokinetics: Peak ½-3½ hr, half-life ½-1 hr, protein binding 95%, eliminated in urine as metabolites and in feces; in elderly elimination rate decreased, bioavailability increased

Interactions:
• Increased serum levels of omeprazole: diazepam, phenytoin, flurazepam, triazolam, clarithromycin
• Possible increased bleeding: warfarin
• Delayed absorption: sucralfate

NURSING CONSIDERATIONS

Assess:
• GI system: bowel sounds q8h, abdomen for pain, swelling, anorexia
• Hepatic enzymes: AST, ALT, alk phosphatase during treatment

Administer:
🚫 Before eating; swallow capsule whole; do not break, crush, or chew

Evaluate:
• Therapeutic response: absence of epigastric pain, swelling, fullness

Teach patient/family:
• To report severe diarrhea; drug may have to be discontinued
• That diabetic patient should know hypoglycemia may occur
• To avoid hazardous activities; dizziness may occur
• To avoid alcohol, salicylates, ibuprofen; may cause GI irritation

---

ondansetron (℞)
(on-dan-seh'tron)
Zofran
Func. class.: Antiemetic
Chem. class.: 5-HT3 receptor antagonist

Action: Prevents nausea, vomiting by blocking serotonin peripherally, centrally, and in the small intestine

Uses: Prevention of nausea, vomiting associated with cancer chemotherapy, radiotherapy, and prevention of postoperative nausea, vomiting

Dosage and routes:

Hepatic dose
• Max dose 8 mg qd

Prevention of nausea/vomiting of cancer chemotherapy
• *Adult and child 4-18 yr:* **IV** 0.15 mg/kg infused over 15 min, 30 min before start of cancer chemotherapy; 0.15 mg/kg given 4 hr and 8 hr after first dose or 32 mg as a single dose; dilute in 50 ml of D_5 or 0.9% NaCl before giving

Prevention of nausea/vomiting of radiotherapy
• *Adult:* **PO** 8 mg tid

Prevention of postoperative nausea/vomiting

• *Adult:* **IV** 4 mg undiluted over >30 sec

• *Child 2-12 yr:* **IV** 0.1 mg/kg (≤40 kg); **IV** 4 mg (≥40 kg) give ≥30 sec

Available forms: Inj 2 mg/ml, 32 mg/50 ml (premixed); tabs 4, 8 mg; oral sol 4 mg/5 ml

Side effects/adverse reactions:

GI: Diarrhea, constipation, abdominal pain

CNS: Headache, dizziness, drowsiness, fatigue, extrapyramidal syndrome

MISC: Rash, **bronchospasm** (rare), *MS pain, wound problems, shivering, fever, hypoxia, urinary retention*

Contraindications: Hypersensitivity

Precautions: Pregnancy (B), lactation, children, elderly

Pharmacokinetics:

IV: Mean elimination half-life 3.5-4.7 hr, plasma protein binding 70%-76%; extensively metabolized in the liver

NURSING CONSIDERATIONS
Assess:

• For absence of nausea, vomiting during chemotherapy

• Hypersensitivity reaction: rash, bronchospasm

• For EPS: shuffling gait, tremors, grimacing, rigidity

Administer:

IV

• After diluting a single dose in 50 ml NS or D₅W, 0.45% or NS and given over 15 min

Additive compatibilities: Cisplatin, cyclophosphamide, cytarabine, dacarbazine, dexamethasone, doxorubicin, etoposide, fluconazole, hydromorphone, meperidine, methotrexate, morphine

Solution compatibilities: May also be diluted with D₅W, lactated Ringer's, D₅/0.9% NaCl, D₅/0.45% NaCl

Y-site compatibilities: Aldesleukin, amifostine, amikacin, aztreonam, bleomycin, carboplatin, carmustine, cefazolin, cefmetazole, cefotaxime, cefoxitin, ceftazidime, ceftizoxime, cefuroxime, chlorpromazine, cimetidine, cisatracurium, cisplatin, cladribine, clindamycin, cyclophosphamide, cytarabine, dacarbazine, dactinomycin, daunorubicin, dexamethasone, diphenhydramine, dopamine, doxorubicin, doxorubicin liposome, doxycycline, droperidol, etoposide, famotidine, filgrastim, floxuridine, fluconazole, fludarabine, gallium, gentamicin, haloperidol, heparin, hydrocortisone, hydromorphone, hydroxyzine, ifosfamide, imipenem/cilastatin, magnesium sulfate, mannitol, mechlorethamine, melphalan, meperidine, mesna, methotrexate, metoclopramide, miconazole, mitomycin, mitoxantrone, morphine, paclitaxel, pentostatin, piperacillin/tazobactam, potassium chloride, prochlorperazine, promethazine, ranitidine, remifentanil, streptozocin, teniposide, thiotepa, ticarcillin, ticarcillin/clavulanate, vancomycin, vinblastine, vincristine, vinorelbine, zidovudine

Perform/provide:

• Storage at room temp 48 hr after dilution

Evaluate:

• Therapeutic response: absence of nausea, vomiting during cancer chemotherapy

Teach patient/family:

• To report diarrhea, constipation, rash, or changes in respirations

Side effects: *italics* = common; **bold italics** = life-threatening

opium tincture/ camphorated opium tincture

(oh'pee-um)

Opium Tincture Deodorized, Pantopan, Paregoric, Parego-rique*

Func. class.: Antidiarrheal

Chem. class.: Opium, opium and morphine

Controlled Substance Schedule III/II (depending on amount of opium)

Action: Antiperistaltic activity

Uses: Diarrhea (cause undetermined); withdrawal symptoms in infants born to addicted mothers

Dosage and routes:

• *Adult:* **PO** 0.3-1 ml qid, not to exceed 6 ml/day (tincture) or 5-10 ml qd-qid (camphorated)

• *Child:* **PO** 0.25-0.5 ml/kg qd-qid (camphorated)

Withdrawal

• *Neonate:* **PO** 1:25 dilution, 3-6 gtt q3-6h (tincture), dosage adjustment to control symptoms

Available forms: Liq 2 mg morphine equivalent per 5 ml

Side effects/adverse reactions:

CNS: Dizziness, drowsiness, fainting, flushing, physical dependency, *CNS depression*

GI: Nausea, vomiting, constipation, abdominal pain

Contraindications: Hypersensitivity, severe ulcerative colitis, pseudomembranous colitis

Precautions: Liver disease, addiction proneness, prostatic hypertrophy (severe), pregnancy (B)

Pharmacokinetics:

PO: Duration 4 hr, half-life 2-3 hr; metabolized in liver; excreted in urine

Interactions:

• Increased action of both drugs: other CNS depressants

• Increased CNS toxicity: cimetidine

NURSING CONSIDERATIONS

Assess:

• Electrolytes (K, Na, Cl) if on long-term therapy

• Skin turgor q8h if dehydration is suspected

• Bowel pattern before; for rebound constipation

• Response after 48 hr; if no response, drug should be discontinued

• Dehydration in children

• Abdominal distention; toxic megacolon may occur in ulcerative colitis

Administer:

• Undiluted with water

• For 48 hr only

Evaluate:

• Therapeutic response: decreased diarrhea

Teach patient/family:

• To avoid OTC products (cough, cold, hay fever preparations) unless directed by prescriber

• Not to exceed recommended dose

• That drug may be habit-forming

• To avoid hazardous activities; drowsiness may occur

oral contraceptives (℞)

Func. class.: Hormone

Chem. class.: Estrogen, progestin combinations

Action: Prevents ovulation by suppressing FSH, LH; *monophasic:* estrogen/progestin (fixed dose) used during a 21-day cycle; ovulation is inhibited by suppression of FSH and LH; thickness of cervical mucus and endometrial lining prevents pregnancy; *biphasic:* ovulation is inhibited by suppression of FSH and LH; alteration of cervical mucus, endometrial lining prevents pregnancy; *triphasic:* ovulation is inhibited by suppression of FSH and LH; change of cervical mucus, endometrial lining prevents pregnancy; variable doses of estrogen/progestin combinations may be similar to natural hormonal fluctuations; *progestin-only pill and implant:* change of cervical mucus and endometrial lining prevents pregnancy; ovulation may be suppressed

Uses: To prevent pregnancy, endometriosis, hypermenorrhea

Dosage and routes:
• *Adult:* PO 1 qd starting on day 5 of menstrual cycle; day 1 is 1st day of period

21 tablet packs
• *Adult:* PO 1 qd starting on day 7 of menstrual cycle; day 1 is 1st day of period, then on 20 or 21 days, off 7 days

28 tablet packs
• *Adult:* PO 1 qd continuously

Biphasic
• *Adult:* 1 qd × 10 days, then next color 1 qd × 11 days

Triphasic
• *Adult:* 1 qd; check package insert

Endometriosis
• *Adult:* PO 1 qd × 20 days from day 5 to 24 of cycle

Available forms: Check specific brand

Side effects/adverse reactions:
GI: Nausea, vomiting, cramps, diarrhea, bloating, constipation, change in appetite, ***cholestatic jaundice***

INTEG: Chloasma, melasma, acne, rash, urticaria, erythema, pruritus, hirsutism, alopecia, photosensitivity

CV: Increased B/P, ***cerebral hemorrhage, thrombosis, pulmonary embolism,*** fluid retention, edema

ENDO: Decreased glucose tolerance, increased TBG, PBI, T_4, T_3

GU: Breakthrough bleeding, amenorrhea, spotting, dysmenorrhea, galactorrhea, endocervical hyperplasia, vaginitis, cystitis-like syndrome, breast change

CNS: Depression, fatigue, dizziness, nervousness, anxiety, headache

EENT: Optic neuritis, retinal thrombosis, cataracts

HEMA: Increased fibrinogen, clotting factor

Contraindications: Pregnancy (X), lactation, reproductive cancer, thrombophlebitis, MI, hepatic tumors, hepatic disease, CAD, women 40 and over, CVA

Precautions: Depression, hypertension, renal disease, seizure disorders, lupus erythematosus, rheumatic disease, migraine headache, amenorrhea, irregular menses, breast cancer (fibrocystic), gallbladder disease, diabetes mellitus, heavy smoking, acute mononucleosis, sickle cell disease

Pharmacokinetics: Excreted in breast milk

Interactions:
• Decreased effectiveness of oral contraceptives: anticonvulsants, rifampin, analgesics, antibiotics, antihistamines, chenodiol, griseofulvin
• Decreased action of oral anticoagulants
• Increased clotting: aminocaproic acid
• Drug/food: increased peak level: grapefruit
⬛ Decreased effect of oral contraceptives: St. John's wort

Lab test interferences:
Increase: Pro-time; clotting factors VII, VIII, IX, X; TBG, PBI, T_4,

platelet aggregability, BSP, triglycerides, bilirubin, AST, ALT
Decrease: T_3, antithrombin III, folate, metyrapone test, GTT, 17-OHCS

NURSING CONSIDERATIONS
Assess:
• Glucose, thyroid function, liver function tests
• Reproductive changes: change in breasts, tumors, positive Pap smear; drug should be discontinued
Administer:
• PO with food for GI symptoms; give at same time each day
• Subdermal implant of 6 caps effective for 5 yr; then should be removed
• IM inj deep in large muscle mass after shaking suspension; ensure patient not pregnant if injections are 2 wk or more apart
Evaluate:
• Therapeutic response: absence of pregnancy, endometriosis, hypermenorrhea
Teach patient/family:
• About detection of clots using Homan's sign
• To use sunscreen or avoid sunlight; photosensitivity can occur
• To take at same time each day to ensure equal drug level
• To report GI symptoms that occur after 4 mo
• To use another birth control method during 1st week of oral contraceptive use
• To take another tablet as soon as possible if one is missed
• That after drug is discontinued, pregnancy may not occur for several months
• To report abdominal pain, change in vision, shortness of breath, change in menstrual flow, spotting, breakthrough bleeding, breast lumps, swelling, headache, severe leg pain
• That continuing medical care is needed: Pap smear and gynecologic examinations q6mo
• To notify health care providers and dentists of oral contraceptive use

---

orlistat
See appendix a—selected new drugs

---

oseltamivir
See appendix a—selected new drugs

---

oxacillin (℞)
(ox-a-sill'in)
Bactocill, oxacillin sodium, Prostaphilin
Func. class.: Broad-spectrum antiinfective
Chem. class.: Penicillinase-resistant penicillin

Action: Interferes with cell wall replication of susceptible organisms; osmotically unstable cell wall swells, bursts from osmotic pressure
Uses: Effective for gram-positive cocci *(Staphylococcus aureus, Streptococcus pneumoniae)*, infections caused by penicillinase-producing *Staphylococcus*
Dosage and routes:
• *Adult:* **PO** 2-6 g/day in divided doses q4-6h; **IM/IV** 2-12 g/day in divided doses q4-6h
• *Child:* **PO** 50-100 mg/kg/day in divided doses q6h; **IM/IV** 50-100 mg/kg/day in divided doses q4-6h
Available forms: Caps 250, 500 mg; powder for oral susp 250 mg/5 ml; powder for inj 250, 500 mg, 1, 2, 4, 10 g
Side effects/adverse reactions:
HEMA: Anemia, increased bleeding time, *bone marrow depression, granulocytopenia*

◆ = Nursing alert   ∥ = Herb-drug interaction   🚫 = Do not crush

GI: Nausea, vomiting, diarrhea, increased AST, ALT, abdominal pain, glossitis, colitis

*GU: **Oliguria, proteinuria, hematuria,** vaginitis, moniliasis, **glomerulonephritis***

CNS: Lethargy, hallucinations, anxiety, depression, twitching, *coma, convulsions*

Contraindications: Hypersensitivity to penicillins

Precautions: Pregnancy (B), hypersensitivity to cephalosporins, neonates

Pharmacokinetics:

PO/IM: Peak 30-60 min, duration 4-6 hr

IV: Peak 5 min, duration 4-6 hr, half-life 30-60 min

Metabolized in the liver; excreted in urine, bile, breast milk; crosses placenta

Interactions:

• Decreased antimicrobial effectiveness of oxacillin: tetracyclines

• Decreased effect of oral contraceptives

• Increased oxacillin concentrations: aspirin, probenecid, disulfiram

🍴 Delayed/reduced absorption: khat, separate by ≥2 hr

Lab test interferences:

False positive: Urine glucose, urine protein

NURSING CONSIDERATIONS
Assess:

• I&O ratio; report hematuria, oliguria, since penicillin in high doses is nephrotoxic

◆ Any patient with compromised renal system, since drug is excreted slowly in poor renal system function; toxicity may occur rapidly

• Liver studies: AST, ALT

• Blood studies: WBC, RBC, Hct/Hgb, bleeding time

• Renal studies: urinalysis, protein

• C&S before therapy; drug may be given as soon as culture is taken

• Bowel pattern before and during treatment

• Skin eruptions after administration of penicillin to 1 wk after discontinuing drug

• Respiratory status: rate, character, wheezing, tightness in chest

• Allergies before initiation of treatment, and reaction of each medication; highlight allergies on chart

Administer:

• Drug after C&S completed

• PO with full glass of water 1 hr before or 2 hr after meals

• IM inj deep in gluteal muscle

IV

• After diluting 500 mg or less/5 ml sterile H_2O or NaCl for inj; may dilute further in D_5W, NS, LR and give 1 g over 10 min; may be given as infusion over 6 hr

Additive compatibilities: Cephapirin, chloramphenicol, dopamine, potassium chloride, sodium bicarbonate

Y-site compatibilities: Acyclovir, cyclophosphamide, diltiazem, famotidine, fluconazole, foscarnet, heparin, hydrocortisone, hydromorphone, labetalol, magnesium sulfate, meperidine, methotrexate, morphine, perphenazine, potassium chloride, tacrolimus, vit B/C, zidovudine

Perform/provide:

• Adrenalin, suction, tracheostomy set, endotracheal intubation equipment

• Scratch test to assess allergy, after securing order from prescriber; usually done when penicillin is only drug of choice

• Storage in airtight container; refrigerate reconstituted sol up to 2 wk

Evaluate:

• Therapeutic response: absence of fever, draining wounds

Teach patient/family:
• All aspects of drug therapy, including need to complete course of medication to ensure organism death (10-14 days); culture may be taken after completed course
• To report sore throat, fever, fatigue (may indicate superinfection); persistent diarrhea
• To wear or carry Medic Alert ID if allergic to penicillins
• To take on empty stomach with a full glass of water
Treatment of anaphylaxis: Withdraw drug, maintain airway, administer epinephrine, aminophylline, O_2, IV corticosteroids

---

oxaprozin (R)
(ox-a-proe′zin)
Daypro
Func. class.: Nonsteroidal antiinflammatory
Chem. class.: Propionic acid derivative

Action: May inhibit prostaglandin synthesis by decreasing enzyme needed for biosynthesis; analgesic, antiinflammatory
Uses: Acute and long-term management of osteoarthritis, rheumatoid arthritis
Dosage and routes:
• *Adult:* **PO** 1200 mg qd; maximum dose 1800 mg/day or 26 mg/kg, whichever is lower
Available forms: Tabs 600 mg
Side effects/adverse reactions:
*MISC: **Anaphylaxis, angioneurotic edema***
GI: Nausea, anorexia, vomiting, diarrhea, jaundice, *cholestatic hepatitis,* constipation, flatulence, cramps, dry mouth, peptic ulcer, *GI bleeding*
CNS: Dizziness, headache, drowsi-

ness, fatigue, tremors, confusion, insomnia, anxiety, depression
CV: Tachycardia, peripheral edema, palpitations, dysrhythmias
INTEG: Purpura, rash, pruritus, sweating
*GU: **Nephrotoxicity: dysuria, hematuria, oliguria, azotemia***
*HEMA: **Increased bleeding time***
EENT: Tinnitus, hearing loss, blurred vision
Contraindications: Hypersensitivity, asthma, patients in whom aspirin and iodides have induced symptoms of allergic reactions or asthma
Precautions: Pregnancy (C), lactation, children, bleeding disorders, GI disorders, cardiac disorders, hypersensitivity to other antiinflammatory agents, severe renal and hepatic disease, elderly, CHF
Pharmacokinetics:
PO: Onset 1 wk, peak unknown, duration unknown, half-life 40-50 hr; metabolized in liver; excreted in urine (metabolites), breast milk; 99% plasma protein binding
Interactions:
• Increased toxicity: aspirin, cyclosporine, methotrexate
• Possible risk of bleeding: oral anticoagulants
• Increased levels of phenytoin, lithium, avoid concomitant use
• Decreased effect: antihypertensives, diuretics
• Increased GI side effects: aspirin, corticosteroids
NURSING CONSIDERATIONS
Assess:
• Pain: frequency, intensity, characteristics; relief of pain after med
• Asthma, aspirin hypersensitivity, oronasal polyps; increased hypersensitivity reactions
• Renal, liver, blood studies: BUN, creatinine, AST, ALT, Hgb, before treatment, periodically thereafter

---

◆ = Nursing alert   ∥ = Herb-drug interaction   ⊘ = Do not crush

- Audiometric, ophthalmic exam before, during, after treatment
- For eye, ear problems: blurred vision, tinnitus; may indicate toxicity

Administer:
- With food to decrease GI symptoms

Perform/provide:
- Storage at room temp

Evaluate:
- Therapeutic response: decreased pain, stiffness in joints, decreased swelling in joints, ability to move more easily

Teach patient/family:
- To report blurred vision, ringing, roaring in ears; may indicate toxicity
- To avoid driving, other hazardous activities if dizziness/drowsiness occurs
- To report change in urine pattern, increased weight, edema, increased pain in joints, fever, blood in urine; indicates nephrotoxicity
- That therapeutic effects may take up to 1 mo
- To take with a full glass of water to enhance absorption

---

oxazepam (R)
(ox-ay′ze-pam)
Apo-Oxazepam*, Novoxa-pam*, oxazepam, Ox-Pam*, Serax, Zapex*
Func. class.: Sedative/hypnotic; antianxiety
Chem. class.: Benzodiazepine

Controlled Substance Schedule IV
Action: Potentiates the actions of GABA, especially in limbic system and reticular formation
Uses: Anxiety, alcohol withdrawal
Dosage and routes:
Anxiety
- *Adult:* **PO** 10-30 mg tid-qid

Alcohol withdrawal
- *Adult:* **PO** 15-30 mg tid-qid
Available forms: Caps 10, 15, 30 mg; tabs 15 mg
Side effects/adverse reactions:
CNS: Dizziness, drowsiness, confusion, headache, anxiety, tremors, fatigue, depression, insomnia, hallucinations, paradoxical excitement, transient amnesia
GI: Nausea, vomiting, anorexia
INTEG: Rash, dermatitis, itching
CV: Orthostatic hypotension, ***ECG changes, tachycardia,*** hypotension
EENT: Blurred vision, tinnitus, mydriasis
Contraindications: Hypersensitivity to benzodiazepines, narrow-angle glaucoma, psychosis, pregnancy (D), lactation, child <12 yr
Precautions: Elderly, debilitated, hepatic disease, renal disease
Pharmacokinetics:
PO: Peak 2-4 hr, metabolized by liver, excreted by kidneys, half-life 5-15 hr
Interactions:
- Decreased effects of oxazepam: oral contraceptives, valproic acid
- Increased effects of oxazepam: CNS depressants, alcohol, disulfiram, oral contraceptives
Lab test interferences:
Increase: AST, ALT, serum bilirubin
Decrease: RAIU
False increase: 17-OHCS
NURSING CONSIDERATIONS
Assess:
- B/P (lying, standing), pulse; if systolic B/P drops 20 mm Hg, hold drug, notify prescriber
- Blood studies: CBC during long-term therapy; blood dyscrasias have occurred rarely
- Hepatic studies: AST, ALT, bilirubin, creatinine, LDH, alk phosphatase

---

• Mental status: mood, sensorium, affect, sleeping pattern, drowsiness, dizziness

◆ Physical dependency, withdrawal symptoms: headache, nausea, vomiting, muscle pain, weakness, tremors, convulsions (long-term use)

• Suicidal tendencies

Administer:

PO

• With food, milk for GI symptoms

• Sugarless gum, hard candy, frequent sips of water for dry mouth

Perform/provide:

• Assistance with ambulation during beginning therapy; drowsiness/dizziness occurs

• Safety measures, including side rails

• Check to see if PO medication has been swallowed

Evaluate:

• Therapeutic response: decreased anxiety, restlessness, insomnia

Teach patient/family:

• That drug may be taken with food

• That medication is not to be used for everyday stress or used longer than 4 mo unless directed by prescriber; not to take more than prescribed dose; may be habit forming

• To avoid OTC preparations (cough, cold, hay fever) unless approved by prescriber

• To avoid driving, activities that require alertness, since drowsiness may occur

• To avoid alcohol ingestion, other psychotropic medications unless directed by prescriber

• Not to discontinue medication abruptly after long-term use

• To rise slowly, or fainting may occur, especially elderly

• That drowsiness may worsen at beginning of treatment

Treatment of overdose: Lavage, VS, supportive care, flumazenil

oxtriphylline (Ŗ)

(ox-trye'fi-lin)

Apo-Oxtriphylline*, Choledyl*, Choledyl SA, Novotriphyl*, oxtriphylline

Func. class.: Bronchodilator, spasmolytic

Chem. class.: Choline salt of theophylline

Action: Relaxes smooth muscle of respiratory system by blocking phosphodiesterase, which increases cyclic AMP; 64% theophylline

Uses: Acute bronchial asthma, reversible bronchospasm in chronic bronchitis and COPD

Dosage and routes:

• *Adult and child >12 yr:* **PO** 4.7 mg/kg q8h or sus action q12h

• *Child 9-16 yr and smokers (adult):* 4.7 mg/kg q6h

• *Child 1-9 yr:* 6.2 mg/kg q6h

Available forms: Elix 100 mg/5 ml*; syr 50 mg/5 ml; tabs 100, 200 mg; ext rel tabs 400, 600 mg

Side effects/adverse reactions:

CNS: Anxiety, restlessness, insomnia, dizziness, **convulsions,** headache, light-headedness

CV: Palpitations, **sinus tachycardia,** hypotension

GI: Nausea, vomiting, anorexia, diarrhea, bitter taste, dyspepsia

RESP: Increased rate, **respiratory arrest**

INTEG: Flushing, urticaria, alopecia

Contraindications: Hypersensitivity to xanthines, tachydysrhythmias

Precautions: Elderly, CHF, cor pulmonale, hepatic disease, active peptic ulcer disease, diabetes mellitus, hyperthyroidism, hypertension, children, pregnancy (C), glaucoma, prostatic hypertrophy

Pharmacokinetics:

ELIXIR: Peak 1 hr

◆ = Nursing alert   ⫸ = Herb-drug interaction   ⊘ = Do not crush

PO-ER: Peak 4-7 hr, duration 8-12 hr
Metabolized in liver; excreted in urine, breast milk; crosses placenta

Interactions:

• Toxicity: fluoroquinolones, β-blockers, cimetidine, oral contraceptives, corticosteroids, fluvoxamine

• May increase effects of: ephedrine, anticoagulants, coffee (caffeine items)

• Decreased effect of lithium

• Decreased theophylline level: rifampin, phenytoin

• Drug/food: caffeine: increased effect

⚠ Increased action of both: ephedra

NURSING CONSIDERATIONS

Assess:

• Therapeutic blood levels; toxicity may occur with small increase above therapeutic level; therapeutic theophylline levels: 11-20 µg/ml

• Smoking: reduces effects of theophyllines, requiring larger doses

• Respiratory rate, rhythm, depth; auscultate lung fields bilaterally; notify prescriber of abnormalities

• Allergic reactions: rash, urticaria; drug should be discontinued

Administer:

• PO after meals to decrease GI symptoms; absorption may be affected

• After meals, hs

Perform/provide:

• Storage in closed container away from heat; protect elixir from light

Evaluate:

• Therapeutic response: absence of dyspnea, wheezing

Teach patient/family:

🚫 Not to break, crush, or chew tab

• To check OTC medications, prescription medications for ephedrine, which will increase stimulation

• To avoid hazardous activities; dizziness may occur

• If GI upset occurs, to take drug with 8 oz water; avoid food; absorption may be decreased

• To notify prescriber of toxicity: nausea, vomiting, anxiety, convulsions, insomnia, rapid pulse

• To notify prescriber of change in smoking habit; may need to change dose; encourage not to smoke

---

oxybutynin (℞)

(ox-i-byoo'ti-nin)
Ditropan, Ditropan XL, oxybutynin
Func. class.: Spasmolytic
Chem. class.: Synthetic tertiary amine

Action: Relaxes smooth muscles in urinary tract by inhibiting acetylcholine at postganglionic sites

Uses: Antispasmodic for neurogenic bladder

Dosage and routes:

• *Adult:* PO 5 mg bid-tid, not to exceed 5 mg qid

• *Geriatric:* PO 2.5-5 mg tid, increase by 2.5 mg q several days

• *Child >5 yr:* PO 5 mg bid, not to exceed 5 mg tid

• *Child 1-5 yr:* PO 0.2 mg/kg/dose 2-4 ×/day

Available forms: Syr 5 mg/5 ml; tabs 5 mg; tabs ext rel 5, 10 mg

Side effects/adverse reactions:

CNS: Anxiety, restlessness, dizziness, **convulsions,** headache, drowsiness, confusion

CV: Palpitations, sinus tachycardia, hypotension

GI: Nausea, vomiting, anorexia, abdominal pain, constipation

GU: Dysuria, urinary retention, hesitancy

EENT: Blurred vision, increased intraocular tension, dry mouth, throat

Contraindications: Hypersensitivity, GI obstruction, GI hemorrhage,

---

GU obstruction, glaucoma, severe colitis, myasthenia gravis, unstable CV status in acute hemorrhage

Precautions: Pregnancy (B), lactation, suspected glaucoma, children <12 yr, elderly

Pharmacokinetics: Onset ½-1 hr, peak 3-4 hr, duration 6-10 hr; metabolized by liver, excreted in urine

Interactions:
• Increased levels of atenolol, digoxin, nitrofurantoin, oxybutynin
• Decreased levels of acetaminophen, haloperidol, levodopa
• Increased or decreased levels of phenothiazines

NURSING CONSIDERATIONS
Assess:
• Urinary patterns: distention, nocturia, frequency, urgency, incontinence
• Allergic reactions: rash, urticaria; if these occur, drug should be discontinued
• CNS effects: confusion, anxiety; anticholinergic effects in the elderly

Administer:
• Without regard to meals

Evaluate:
• Urinary status: dysuria, frequency, nocturia, incontinence

Teach patient/family:
• To avoid hazardous activities; dizziness may occur
• To avoid OTC medications with alcohol, other CNS depressants
• To prevent photophobia by wearing sunglasses
• Avoid hot weather, strenuous activity, drug decreases perspiration

oxycodone (℞)
(ox-i-koe'done)
Roxicodone Supeudol*, OxyFast

oxycodone/aspirin
Endodan*, Oxycodan*, Percodan, Percodan-Demi, Roxiprin

oxycodone/ acetaminophen
Endocet*, Oxycocet*, OxyIR, Percocet, Roxicet, Roxilox, Tylox
Func. class.: Opiate analgesic
Chem. class.: Semisynthetic derivative

Controlled Substance Schedule II
Action: Inhibits ascending pain pathways in CNS, increases pain threshold, alters pain perception

Uses:
Moderate to severe pain

Dosage and routes:
• *Adult:* **PO** 10-30 mg q4hr (5 mg q6h for OxyIR, OxyFast) **OxyFast Conc. Sol is extremely concentrated; do not use interchangeably**
• *Child:* **PO** 0.05-0.15 mg/kg/dose up to 5 mg/dose q4-6h; not recommended in children

Available forms: Oxycodone supp 10, 20 mg; tabs 5 mg; caps, immediate rel 5 mg; oral sol conc 20 mg/ml; oxycodone with acetaminophen tabs 5 mg/325 mg; cap 5 mg/ 500 mg; oral sol 5 mg/325 mg/5 ml; oxycodone with aspirin 2.44 mg/ 325 mg, 4.88/325 mg

Side effects/adverse reactions:
CNS: Drowsiness, dizziness, confusion, headache, sedation, euphoria
GI: Nausea, vomiting, anorexia, constipation, cramps
GU: Increased urinary output, dysuria, urinary retention

 = Nursing alert   = Herb-drug interaction   🚫 = Do not crush

INTEG: Rash, urticaria, bruising, flushing, diaphoresis, pruritus
EENT: Tinnitus, blurred vision, miosis, diplopia
CV: Palpitations, bradycardia, change in B/P
*RESP: **Respiratory depression***
Contraindications: Hypersensitivity, addiction (opiate)
Precautions: Addictive personality, pregnancy (B), lactation, increased intracranial pressure, MI (acute), severe heart disease, respiratory depression, hepatic disease, renal disease, child <18 yr
Pharmacokinetics:
PO: Onset 15-30 min, peak 1 hr, duration 4-6 hr; detoxified by liver, excreted in urine, crosses placenta, excreted in breast milk
Interactions:
• Increased effects with other CNS depressants: alcohol, narcotics, sedative/hypnotics, antipsychotics, skeletal muscle relaxants
Lab test interferences:
Increase: Amylase
NURSING CONSIDERATIONS
Assess:
• I&O ratio; check for decreasing output; may indicate urinary retention
• CNS changes: dizziness, drowsiness, hallucinations, euphoria, LOC, pupil reaction
• Allergic reactions: rash, urticaria
• Respiratory dysfunction: respiratory depression, character, rate, rhythm; notify prescriber if respirations are <10/min
• Need for pain medication by pain, sedation scoring; physical dependence
Administer:
• With antiemetic if nausea, vomiting occur
• When pain is beginning to return; determine dosage interval by response

Perform/provide:
• Storage in light-resistant area at room temp
• Assistance with ambulation
• Safety measures: night-light, call bell within easy reach
Evaluate:
• Therapeutic response: decrease in pain
Teach patient/family:
• To report any symptoms of CNS changes, allergic reactions
• That physical dependency may result from extended use
• That withdrawal symptoms may occur: nausea, vomiting, cramps, fever, faintness, anorexia
Treatment of overdose: Naloxone (Narcan) 0.2-0.8 mg IV, O₂, IV fluids, vasopressors

---

oxymorphone (℞)
(ox-i-mor'fone)
Numorphan
Func. class.: Opiate analgesic
Chem. class.: Semisynthetic phenanthrene derivative

Controlled Substance Schedule II
Action: Inhibits ascending pain pathways in CNS, increases pain threshold, alters pain perception
Uses: Moderate to severe pain
Dosage and routes:
• *Adult:* **IM/SC** 1-1.5 mg q4-6h prn; **IV** 0.5 mg q4-6h prn; **RECT** 5 mg q4-6h prn
Labor analgesia
• *Adult:* **IM:** 0.5-1 mg
Available forms: Inj 1, 1.5 mg/ml; supp 5 mg
Side effects/adverse reactions:
CNS: Drowsiness, dizziness, confusion, headache, sedation, euphoria (elderly)
GI: Nausea, vomiting, anorexia, constipation, cramps

GU: Increased urinary output, dysuria, urinary retention

INTEG: Rash, urticaria, bruising, flushing, diaphoresis, pruritus

EENT: Tinnitus, blurred vision, miosis, diplopia

CV: Palpitations, bradycardia, change in B/P

*RESP: **Respiratory depression***

Contraindications: Hypersensitivity, addiction (opiate)

Precautions: Addictive personality, pregnancy (B) (short-term), lactation, increased intracranial pressure, MI (acute), severe heart disease, respiratory depression, hepatic disease, renal disease, child <18 yr

Pharmacokinetics:

SC/IM: Onset 10-15 min, peak 1½ hr, duration, 3-6 hr

IV: Onset 5-10 min, peak 15-30 min, duration 3-6 hr

RECT: Onset 15-30 min, duration 3-6 hr

Metabolized by liver, excreted in urine, crosses placenta

Interactions:

• Increased effects with other CNS depressants: alcohol, narcotics, sedative/hypnotics, antipsychotics, skeletal muscle relaxants

Lab test interferences:

Increase: Amylase

NURSING CONSIDERATIONS

Assess:

• I&O ratio for decreasing output; may indicate urinary retention

• CNS changes: dizziness, drowsiness, hallucinations, euphoria, LOC, pupil reaction

• Allergic reactions: rash, urticaria

• Respiratory dysfunction: respiratory depression, character, rate, rhythm; notify prescriber if respirations are <10/min

• Need for pain medication, physical dependence

Administer:

• With antiemetic for nausea, vomiting

• When pain is beginning to return; determine interval by response

IV

• After diluting with 5 ml sterile H_2O or NS for inj; give over 2-5 min through Y-tube or 3-way stopcock

Syringe compatibilities: Glycopyrrolate, hydroxyzine, ranitidine

Perform/provide:

• Storage in light-resistant area at room temp

• Assistance with ambulation

• Safety measures: night-light, call bell within easy reach

Evaluate:

• Therapeutic response: decrease in pain

Teach patient/family:

• To report any symptoms of CNS changes, allergic reactions

• That physical dependency may result from extended use

• That withdrawal symptoms may occur: nausea, vomiting, cramps, fever, faintness, anorexia

Treatment of overdose: Naloxone (Narcan) 0.2-0.8 mg IV, O_2, IV fluids, vasopressors

---

oxytocin, injection (R)

(ox-i-toe'sin)

Pitocin, Syntocinon

Func. class.: Oxytocic

Chem. class.: Hormone

Action: Acts directly on myofibrils, producing uterine contraction; stimulates milk ejection by the breast

Uses: Stimulation, induction of labor; missed or incomplete abortion; postpartum bleeding

⬥ = Nursing alert   🌿 = Herb-drug interaction   🚫 = Do not crush

Dosage and routes:

Postpartum hemorrhage

• *Adult:* IV 10 U infused at 20-40 μU/min

• *Adult:* IM 10 U after delivery of placenta

Fetal stress test

• *Adult:* IV 0.5 μU/min, increase q20min until 3 contractions within 10 min

Stimulation of labor

• *Adult:* IV 1-2 μU/min, increase by 1-2 μU q15-60min until contractions occur; then decrease dose

Incomplete abortion

• *Adult:* IV INF 10 U/500 ml D_5W or 0.9% NaCl at 20-40 μU/min

Available forms: Inj 10 U/ml

Side effects/adverse reactions:

CNS: **Convulsions, tetanic contractions**

CV: Hypotension, hypertension, dysrhythmias, increased pulse, bradycardia, tachycardia, PVC

FETUS: Dysrhythmias, jaundice, hypoxia, **intracranial hemorrhage**

GI: Anorexia, nausea, vomiting, constipation

GU: **Abruptio placentae, decreased uterine blood flow**

HEMA: Increased hyperbilirubinemia

INTEG: Rash

RESP: **Asphyxia**

Contraindications: Hypersensitivity, serum toxemia, cephalopelvic disproportion, fetal distress, hypertonic uterus

Precautions: Cervical/uterine surgery, uterine sepsis, primipara >35 yr, 1st, 2nd stage of labor

Pharmacokinetics:

IM: Onset 3-7 min, duration 1 hr, half-life 12-17 min

IV: Onset 1 min, duration 30 min, half-life 12-17 min

Interactions:

• Hypertension: vasopressors

🍃 Hypertension: ephedra

NURSING CONSIDERATIONS

Assess:

• I&O ratio

• Respiration

• B/P, pulse; watch for changes that may indicate hemorrhage

• Respiratory rate, rhythm, depth; notify prescriber of abnormalities

• Length, intensity, duration of contraction; notify prescriber of contractions lasting over 1 min or absence of contractions; turn patient on her side

• FHTs, fetal distress; watch for acceleration, deceleration; notify prescriber if problems occur; fetal presentation, pelvic dimensions; turn patient on left side if FHT change in rate

◆ For signs and symptoms of water intoxication; confusion, anuria, drowsiness, headache

Administer:

Labor induction

• After diluting 10 U/L of 0.9% NS or D_5 NS run at 1-2 μU/min at 15-30 min intervals to begin normal labor; dilute 10-40 μU/min, titrate to control postpartum bleeding; dilute 10 U/500 ml sol; run 10 U-20 μU/ml; administer by only 1 route at a time; use inf pump; rotate inf to provide mixing; do not shake

Control of postpartum bleeding

• Dilute 10-40 U/1 L of sol, run at 10-20 μU/min; adjust rate as needed

• With crash cart available on unit (Mg^+SO_4 at bedside)

Additive compatibilities: Chloramphenicol, metaraminol, netilmicin, sodium bicarbonate, thiopental, verapamil

Y-site compatibilities: Heparin, hydrocortisone, insulin (regular), meperidine, morphine, potassium chloride, vit B/C, warfarin

Evaluate:

• Therapeutic response: stimulation

Side effects: *italics* = common; **bold italics** = life-threatening

of labor, control of postpartum bleeding

Teach patient/family:

• To report increased blood loss, abdominal cramps, fever, foul-smelling lochia

• That contractions will be similar to menstrual cramps, gradually increasing in intensity

---

paclitaxel (℞)
(pa-kli-tax′el)
Taxol
Func. class.: Misc. antineoplastic
Chem. class.: Antimicrotubule, natural diterpene

Action: Inhibits reorganization of microtubule network needed for interphase and mitotic cellular functions; also causes abnormal bundles of microtubules during cell cycle and multiple esters of microtubules during mitosis

Uses: Metastatic carcinoma of the ovary, breast; AIDS-related Kaposi's sarcoma (2nd-line), non–small cell lung cancer (1st-line)

Investigational uses: Advanced head, neck, small cell lung cancer; non-Hodgkin's lymphoma, adenocarcinoma of the upper GI tract, hormone-refractory prostate cancer

Dosage and routes:

Ovarian carcinoma

• *Adult:* **IV INF** 135 mg/m^2 given over 24 hr q3wk or 175 mg/m^2 over 3 hr q3wk

Breast carcinoma

• *Adult:* **IV INF** 175 mg/m^2 over 3 hr q3wk

AIDS-related Kaposi's sarcoma

• *Adult:* **IV INF** 135 mg/m^2 over 3 hr q3wk or 100 mg/m^2 over 3 hr q2wk

1st-line non–small cell lung cancer

• *Adult:* **IV INF** 135 mg/m^2/24 hr inf with cisplatin

Available forms: Inj 30 mg/5 ml vial

Side effects/adverse reactions:

*HEMA: **Neutropenia, leukopenia, thrombocytopenia, anemia,** bleeding, infections*

SYST: Hypersensitivity reactions, anaphylaxis

CV: Bradycardia, *hypotension,* abnormal ECG

NEURO: Peripheral neuropathy

MS: Arthralgia, myalgia

GI: Nausea, vomiting, diarrhea, mucositis, increased bilirubin, alk phosphatase, AST

INTEG: Alopecia

Contraindications: Hypersensitivity to paclitaxel or other drugs with polyoxyethylated castor oil, neutropenia of <1500/mm^3, pregnancy (D)

Precautions: Children, lactation; hepatic, cardiovascular disease; CNS disorder

Pharmacokinetics: 89%-98% of drug is serum protein bound, metabolized in liver, excreted in bile and urine; terminal half-life 5.3-17.4 hr

Interactions:

• Increased myelosuppression: other antineoplastics, radiation

• Decreased metabolism of paclitaxel: ketoconazole, verapamil, diazepam, cyclosporine, teniposide, etoposide, quinidine, dexamethasone, vincristine, testosterone

• Increased doxorubicin levels: doxorubicin

• Decreased immune response: live virus vaccines

NURSING CONSIDERATIONS
Assess:

• CBC, differential, platelet count prior to and qwk; withhold drug if WBC is <1500/mm^3 or platelet

---

◆ = Nursing alert   *✐* = Herb-drug interaction   ⊘ = Do not crush count is <100,000/mm^3, notify prescriber

• Monitor temp q4h (may indicate beginning infection)

• Liver function tests before, during therapy (bilirubin, AST, ALT, LDH, bilirubin) prn or qmo, check for jaundiced skin and sclera, dark urine, clay-colored stool, itchy skin, abdominal pain, fever, diarrhea

• VS during 1st hr of infusion, check IV site for signs of infiltration

• Hypersensitive reactions including hypotension, dyspnea, angioedema, generalized urticaria; discontinue infusion immediately

• Bleeding: hematuria, guaiac, bruising or petechiae, mucosa or orifices q8h; obtain prescription for viscous lidocaine (Xylocaine)

• Effects of alopecia on body image; discuss feelings about body changes

Administer:

• Antiemetic 30-60 min before giving drug and prn

IV

• After diluting in 0.9% NaCl, D$_5$, D$_5$ and 0.9% NaCl, D$_5$LR to a concentration of 0.3-1.2 mg/ml

• Using an in-line filter ≤0.22 μm

• After premedicating with dexamethasone 20 mg PO 12 hr and 6 hr before paclitaxel, diphenhydramine 50 mg IV ½-1 hr before paclitaxel and cimetidine 300 mg or ranitidine 50 mg IV ½-1 hr before paclitaxel

• Using only glass bottles, polypropylene, polyolefin bags and administration sets; do not use PVC infusion bags or sets

• Using gloves and cytotoxic handling precautions

Y-site compatibilities: Acyclovir, amikacin, aminophylline, ampicillin/sulbactam, bleomycin, butorphanol, calcium chloride, carboplatin, cefepime, cefotetan, ceftazidime, ceftriaxone, cimetidine, cisplatin, cladribine, cyclophosphamide, cytarabine, dacarbazine, dexamethasone, diphenhydramine, doxorubicin, droperidol, etoposide, famotidine, floxuridine, fluconazole, fluorouracil, furosemide, ganciclovir, gentamicin, granisetron, haloperidol, heparin, hydrocortisone, hydromorphone, ifosfamide, lorazepam, magnesium sulfate, mannitol, meperidine, mesna, methotrexate, metoclopramide, morphine, nalbuphine, ondansetron, pentostatin, potassium chloride, prochlorperazine, propofol, ranitidine, sodium bicarbonate, thiotepa, vancomycin, vinblastine, vincristine, zidovudine

Perform/provide:

• Confirmation that dexamethasone was given 12 hr and 6 hr before infusion begins

• Storage of prepared sol up to 27 hr in refrigeration

Evaluate:

• Therapeutic response: decreased tumor size, spread of malignancy

Teach patient/family:

• To report signs of infection: fever, sore throat, flulike symptoms

• To report signs of anemia: fatigue, headache, faintness, shortness of breath, irritability

• To report bleeding; avoid use of razors, commercial mouthwash

• To avoid use of aspirin, ibuprofen

• To report any complaints or side effects to nurse or prescriber

• That hair may be lost during treatment; a wig or hairpiece may make patient feel better; new hair may be different in color, texture

• That pain in muscles and joints 2-5 days after infusion is common

palivizumab (Ŗ)

(pal-ih-viz'uh-mab)
Synagis
Func. class.: Monoclonal antibody

Action: A humanized monoclonal antibody that exhibits neutralizing and fusion-inhibitory activity against respiratory syncytial virus (RSV)

Uses: Prevention of serious lower respiratory tract disease caused by RSV in pediatric patients

Dosage and routes:
• *Child:* **IM** 15 mg/kg, those patient who develop RSV should receive monthly doses during RSV season

Available forms: Lyophilized inj 100 mg

Side effects/adverse reactions:
GI: Nausea, vomiting, diarrhea, increased AST
RESP: URI, **apnea**
EENT: Otitis media, rhinitis, pharyngitis
INTEG: Rash, inj site reaction

Contraindications: Hypersensitivity, adults, cyanotic congenital heart disease

Precautions: Thrombocytopenia, coagulation disorders, established RSV, congenital heart disease, chronic lung disease, systemic allergic reactions, pregnancy (C)

Pharmacokinetics: Mean half-life 20 days

NURSING CONSIDERATIONS
Assess:
• For presence of RSV infection, drug is given to prevent infection For side effects; report if allergic reaction is evident

Administer:
• IM only
• After adding 1 ml of sterile water for inj per 100 mg vial, gently swirl, let stand at room temp for 20 min until sol clarifies; given within 6 hr of reconstitution

Teach patient/family:
• To report upper respiratory infections, earaches, rash, sore throat

pamidronate (Ŗ)

(pam-i-drone'ate)
Aredia
Func. class.: Bone-resorption inhibitor
Chem. class.: Bisphosphonate

Action: Absorbs calcium phosphate crystals in bone and may directly block dissolution of hydroxyapatite crystals of bone; inhibits bone resorption, apparently without inhibiting bone formation and mineralization

Uses: Moderate to severe hypercalcemia associated with malignancy with or without bone metastases, osteolytic lesions in breast cancer patients

Dosage and routes:
• *Adult:* **IV INF** 60-90 mg in moderate hypercalcemia, 90 mg in severe hypercalcemia over 24 hr

Available forms: Inj 30, 60, 90 mg/vial

Side effects/adverse reactions:
INTEG: Redness, swelling, induration, pain on palpation at site of catheter insertion
META: Anemia, hypokalemia, hypomagnesemia, hypophosphatemia
GI: Abdominal pain, anorexia, constipation, nausea, vomiting
MS: Bone pain
CV: Hypertension
GU: UTI, fluid overload

Contraindications: Hypersensitivity to bisphosphonates

Precautions: Children, nursing mothers, pregnancy (C), renal dysfunction

---

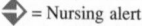 = Nursing alert   = Herb-drug interaction   Ⓢ = Do not crush

Pharmacokinetics: Rapidly cleared from circulation and taken up mainly by bones, eliminated primarily by kidneys

Interactions:

• Do not mix with Ca-containing infusion sol such as Ringer's sol

NURSING CONSIDERATIONS
Assess:

• Renal studies and Ca, P, Mg, K
• For hypercalcemia: paresthesia, twitching, laryngospasm, Chvostek's, Trousseau's signs

Administer:
IV

• After reconstituting by adding 10 ml of sterile water for inj to each vial (30 mg/10 ml, or 60 mg/10 ml, or 90 mg/10 ml depending on vial used), then add to 1000 ml of sterile 0.45%, 0.9% NaCl, D_5W, run over 24 hr for hypercalcemia or 60 mg ≥4 hr, 90 mg over 24 hr

Perform/provide:

• Storage of infusion sol up to 24 hr at room temp
• Reconstituted sol with sterile water may be stored under refrigeration for up to 24 hr

Evaluate:

• Therapeutic response: decreased Ca levels

---

pancreatin (℞)
(pan'kree-a-tin)
Elzyme 303 Enseals
Func. class.: Digestant
Chem. class.: Pancreatic enzyme concentrate—bovine\porcine

Action: Pancreatic enzyme needed for breakdown of substances released from the pancreas

Uses: Exocrine pancreatic secretion insufficiency, cystic fibrosis (digestive aid)

Dosage and routes:
• *Adult:* **PO** 8000-24,000 USP U with meals

Available forms: Tabs 650, 2000, 12,000 U

Side effects/adverse reactions:

GI: Anorexia, nausea, vomiting, diarrhea, glossitis, anal soreness
GU: Hyperuricuria, hyperuricemia
INTEG: Rash, hypersensitivity
EENT: Buccal soreness

Contraindications: Hypersensitivity to pork, chronic pancreatic disease

Precautions: Pregnancy (C), lactation

• Decreased absorption: cimetidine, antacids, oral iron

NURSING CONSIDERATIONS
Assess:

• I&O ratio; watch for increasing urinary output
• Fecal fat, nitrogen, pro-time, Ca during treatment
• For polyuria, polydipsia, polyphagia (may indicate diabetes mellitus)
• For allergy to pork

Administer:
PO

• After antacid or H_2-blockers; decreased pH inactivates drug
🚫 Whole; do not break, crush, or chew (enteric coated)
• Low-fat diet for GI symptoms

Perform/provide:

• Storage in tight container at room temp

Evaluate:

• Therapeutic response: relief of GI symptoms

P

---

pancrelipase (℞)

(pan-kre-li'pase)

Cotazym, Cotazym Capsules, Cotazym-S Capsules, Creon Capsules, Festal II Tablets, Ilozyme, Ku-Zyme HP Capsules, Pancrease Capsules, Pancrease MT 4, Pancrease MT 10, Pancrease MT 16, Ultrase MT 12, Ultrase MT 20, Ultrase MT 24, Viokase Powder, Viokase Tablets, Zymase

Func. class.: Digestant

Chem. class.: Pancreatic enzyme—bovine/porcine

Action: Pancreatic enzyme needed for breakdown of substances released from the pancreas

Uses: Exocrine pancreatic secretion insufficiency, cystic fibrosis (digestive aid), steatorrhea, pancreatic enzyme deficiency

Dosage and routes:

• *Adult and child:* **PO** 1-3 caps/tabs ac or with meals, or 1 cap/tab with snack or 1-2 powder pkt ac

Available forms: Powder: 16,800 U lipase/70,000 U protease and amylase; caps: 8000 U lipase/30,000 U protease and amylase; cap, delayed rel 4000 U lipase/12,000 U protease and amylase, 4000 U lipase/25,000 U protease/ 20,000 U amylase, 5000 U lipase/20,000 U protease and amylase, 10,000 U lipase/30,000 U protease and amylase, 12,000 U lipase/ 24,000 U protease and amylase, 12,000 U lipase/39,000 U protease and amylase, 16,000 U lipase/48,000 U protease and amylase, 20,000 U lipase/65,000 U protease and amylase, 24,000 U lipase/78,000 U protease and amylase

Side effects/adverse reactions:

GI: Anorexia, nausea, vomiting, diarrhea

GU: Hyperuricuria, hyperuricemia

Contraindications: Allergy to pork, chronic pancreatic disease

Precautions: Pregnancy (C)

Interactions:

• Decreased absorption: cimetidine, antacids, oral iron

NURSING CONSIDERATIONS

Assess:

• For appropriate height, weight development; may be delayed

• I&O ratio; watch for increasing urinary output

• Fecal fat, nitrogen, pro-time during treatment

• For polyuria, polydipsia, polyphagia (may indicate diabetes mellitus)

• For pork sensitivity, cross-sensitivity may occur

Administer:

• After antacid or cimetidine; decreased pH inactivates drug

• Powder mixed in prepared fruit juice for infants, children

• Low-fat diet for GI symptoms

Perform/provide:

• Storage in tight container at room temp

Evaluate:

• Therapeutic response: improved digestion of carbohydrates, protein, fat; absence of steatorrhea

Teach patient/family:

• Not to inhale powder; may be very irritating to mucous membranes; some powder may irritate skin

• To take with 8 oz water or more, not to allow to sit in mouth, have patient sit up during administration

• To notify prescriber of allergic reactions, abdominal pain, cramping, or blood in the urine

pancuronium (℞)

(pan-kyoo-roe′nee-um)
pancuronium bromide,
Pavulon

Func. class.: Neuromuscular
blocker (nondepolarizing)
Chem. class.: Synthetic curariform

Action: Inhibits transmission of
nerve impulses by binding with cholinergic receptor sites, antagonizing
action of acetylcholine
Uses: Facilitation of endotracheal
intubation, skeletal muscle relaxation during mechanical ventilation,
surgery, or general anesthesia
Dosage and routes:
• *Adult:* IV 0.04-0.1 mg/kg, then
0.01 mg/kg q½-1h
• *Child >10 yr:* IV 0.04-0.1 mg/kg,
then ⅕ initial dose q½-1h
Available forms: Inj 1, 2 mg/ml
Side effects/adverse reactions:
CV: Bradycardia; tachycardia; increased, decreased B/P; ventricular
extrasystoles
RESP: **Prolonged apnea, bronchospasm, cyanosis, respiratory depression**
EENT: Increased secretions
MS: Weakness to prolonged skeletal
muscle relaxation
INTEG: Rash, flushing, pruritus, urticaria, sweating, salivation
Contraindications: Hypersensitivity to bromide ion
Precautions: Pregnancy (C), renal
disease, cardiac disease, lactation,
children <2 yr, electrolyte imbalances, dehydration, neuromuscular
disease, respiratory disease
Pharmacokinetics:
IV: Onset 30-45 sec, peak 3-5 min;
metabolized (small amounts), excreted in urine (unchanged), crosses
placenta

Interactions:
• Increased neuromuscular blockade: aminoglycosides, clindamy-
cin, enflurane, isoflurane, lincomycin, lithium, local anesthetics,
narcotic analgesics, polymyxin antibiotics, quinidine, thiazides
• Dysrhythmias: theophylline
Lab test interferences:
Decrease: Cholinesterase
NURSING CONSIDERATIONS
Assess:
• For electrolyte imbalances (K,
Mg); may lead to increased action
of this drug
• Vital signs (B/P, pulse, respirations, airway) until fully recovered;
rate, depth, pattern of respirations,
strength of hand grip
• I&O ratio; check for urinary retention, frequency, hesitancy
• Recovery: decreased paralysis of
face, diaphragm, leg, arm, rest of
body; allow to recover fully before
neuro assessment
• Allergic reactions: rash, fever, respiratory distress, pruritus; drug
should be discontinued
Administer:
IV, direct
• With diazepam or morphine when
used for therapeutic paralysis; this
drug provides no sedation
• Using nerve stimulator by anesthesiologist to determine neuromuscular blockade
• Atropine to counteract muscarinic
effects
• After succinylcholine effects subside
• Anticholinesterase to reverse neuromuscular blockade
• IV undiluted, give over 1-2 min
(only by qualified persons)
Additive compatibilities: Verapamil
Syringe compatibilities: Heparin
Y-site compatibilities: Aminophy-
ylline, cefazolin, cefuroxime, ci-

P

Side effects: *italics* = common; **bold italics** = life-threatening

metidine, dobutamine, dopamine, epinephrine, esmolol, fentanyl, fluconazole, gentamicin, heparin, hydrocortisone, isoproterenol, lorazepam, midazolam, morphine, nitroglycerin, nitroprusside, ranitidine, sulfamethoxazole-trimethoprim, vancomycin

Perform/provide:

• Storage in refrigerator; do not store in plastic; use only fresh sol

• Reassurance if communication is difficult during recovery from neuromuscular blockade

• Frequent (q2h) instillation of artificial tears and covering eyes to prevent drying of cornea

Evaluate:

• Therapeutic response: paralysis of jaw, eyelid, head, neck, rest of body

Treatment of overdose: Edrophonium or neostigmine, atropine, monitor VS; may require mechanical ventilation

---

paricalcitol (Ŗ)

(par-ih-cal′sih-tol)

Zemplar

Func. class.: Vit D analong

Chem. class.: Fat-soluble vitamin

Action: Reduces parathyroid hormone (PTH) levels; suppresses PTH levels in patients with chronic renal failure with absence of hypercalcemia/hyperphosphatemia. Serum PO_4, Ca, CaXP may increase

Uses: Hypoparathyroidism

Dosage and routes:

• *Adult:* **IV BOL** 0.04-0.1 µg/kg (2.8-7 µg) no more than qod during dialysis; may increase by 2-4 µg q2-4wk

Available forms: Inj µg/ml

Side effects/adverse reactions:

GI: Nausea, vomiting, anorexia, dry mouth

CNS: Lightheadedness

CV: Palpitations

OTHER: Pneumonia, edema, chills, fever, flu, *sepsis*

Contraindications: Hypersensitivity, hypercalcemia

Precautions: Cardiovascular disease, renal calculi, pregnancy (C), elderly, lactation, children

Interactions:

• Digitalis toxicity: digitalis

NURSING CONSIDERATIONS

Assess:

• Ca, PO_4, q2×/wk during initial therapy; after dose is established take calcium and phosphorus qmo

Administer:

IV

• By IV bolus only

Evaluate:

• Decreased hypoparathyroidism in chronic renal disease

Teach patient/family:

• To report weakness, lethargy, headache, anorexia, loss of weight

• To report nausea, vomiting, palpitations

---

paroxetine (Ŗ)

(par-ox′e-teen)

Paxil, Paxil CR

Func. class.: Antidepressant, SSRI

Chem. class.: Phenylpiperidine derivative

Action: Inhibits CNS neuron uptake of serotonin but not of norepinephrine or dopamine

Uses: Major depressive disorder, obsessive-compulsive disorder, panic disorder

Investigational uses: Diabetic neuropathy, headaches, premature ejaculation

---

◆ = Nursing alert 🖉 = Herb-drug interaction 🚫 = Do not crush

Dosage and routes:

Depression

• *Adult:* **PO** 20 mg qd in AM; after 4 wk if no clinical improvement is noted, dose may be increased by 10 mg/day qwk to desired response, not to exceed 50 mg/day

• *Geriatric:* **PO** 10 mg qd, increase by 10 mg to desired dose, max 40 mg/day

Renal dose

• *Adult:* **PO** 10 mg qd in AM, may increase by 10 mg/day qwk, max 40 mg qd

Obsessive-compulsive disorder

• *Adult:* **PO** 40 mg/day in AM, start with 20 mg/day, increase 10 mg/day increments, max 60 mg/day

Panic disorder

• *Adult:* **PO** 40 mg/day, start with 10 mg/day and increase in 10 mg/day increments, max 60 mg/day

Available forms: Tabs 10, 20, 30, 40 mg; susp 10 mg/15 ml; con rel tabs 12.5, 25 mg

Side effects/adverse reactions:

CNS: Headache, nervousness, insomnia, drowsiness, anxiety, tremor, dizziness, fatigue, sedation, abnormal dreams, agitation, apathy, euphoria, hallucinations, delusions, psychosis

GI: Nausea, diarrhea, dry mouth, anorexia, dyspepsia, constipation, cramps, vomiting, taste changes, flatulence, decreased appetite

INTEG: Sweating, rash

RESP: Infection, pharyngitis, nasal congestion, sinus headache, sinusitis, cough, dyspnea

CV: Vasodilation, postural hypotension, palpitations

MS: Pain, arthritis, myalgia, myopathy, myosthenia

GU: Dysmenorrhea, decreased libido, urinary frequency, UTI, amenorrhea, cystitis, impotence, abnormal ejaculation

EENT: Visual changes

SYST: Asthenia, fever

Contraindications: Hypersensitivity, patients taking MAOIs

Precautions: Pregnancy (B), lactation, children, elderly, seizure history, patients with history of mania, renal and hepatic disease

Pharmacokinetics:

PO: Peak 5.2 hr; metabolized in liver, unchanged drugs and metabolites excreted in feces and urine; half-life 21 hr; protein binding 95%

Interactions:

• Increased bleeding: warfarin

• Do not use with MAOIs

• Cimetidine increases paroxetine plasma levels

• Increased agitation: L-tryptophan

• Phenobarbital and phenytoin decrease paroxetine levels

• Increased side effects: highly protein-bound drugs

• Paroxetine may decrease digoxin levels

• Increased theophylline levels: theophylline

Lab test interferences:

Increase: Serum bilirubin, blood glucose, alk phosphatase

Decrease: VMA, 5-HIAA

False increase: Urinary catecholamines

NURSING CONSIDERATIONS

Assess:

• Mental status: mood, sensorium, affect, suicidal tendencies, increase in psychiatric symptoms, depression, panic

• B/P (lying/standing), pulse q4h; if systolic B/P drops 20 mm Hg, hold drug, notify prescriber; take vital signs q4h in patients with cardiovascular disease

• Blood studies: CBC, leukocytes, differential, cardiac enzymes if patient is receiving long-term therapy

• Hepatic studies: AST, ALT, bilirubin, creatinine

P

• Weight qwk; appetite may decrease with drug
• ECG for flattening of T wave, bundle branch, AV block, dysrhythmias in cardiac patients
• EPS primarily in elderly: rigidity, dystonia, akathisia
• Urinary retention, constipation
• Withdrawal symptoms: headache, nausea, vomiting, muscle pain, weakness; not usual unless drug discontinued abruptly
• Alcohol intake; if alcohol is consumed, hold dose until morning

Administer:
• Increased fluids, bulk in diet for constipation, urinary retention
• With food, milk for GI symptoms
• Crushed if patient is unable to swallow medication whole
• Dosage hs for oversedation during day; may take entire dose hs; elderly may not tolerate once/day dosing
• Gum, hard candy, frequent sips of water for dry mouth

Perform/provide:
• Storage at room temp; do not freeze
• Assistance with ambulation during therapy, since drowsiness, dizziness occur
• Safety measures primarily in elderly
• Checking to see if PO medication swallowed

Evaluate:
• Therapeutic response: decreased depression

Teach patient/family:
• That therapeutic effect may take 1-4 wk
• To use caution in driving, other activities requiring alertness because of drowsiness, dizziness, blurred vision
• Not to discontinue medication quickly after long-term use; may cause nausea, headache, malaise

• To avoid alcohol ingestion, other CNS depressants

Treatment of overdose: Airway, for seizures give diazepam, symptomatic treatment

---

pegaspargase (℞)
(peg-as'per-gase)
Oncaspar, PEG-L-asparaginase
Func. class.: Antineoplastic
Chem. class.: E. coli enzyme

Action: Indirectly inhibits protein synthesis in tumor cells; without amino acid, DNA, RNA synthesis is halted; asparagine, protein synthesis is halted; G_1 phase; cell-cycle specific; a nonvesicant; a modified version of L-asparaginase

Uses: Acute lymphocytic leukemia in combination with other antineoplastics

Dosage and routes:
In combination
• *Adult and child with BSA ≥0.6 m²:* **IV/IM** 2500 IU/m² q14 days, run **IV** over 1-2 hr in 100 ml of NaCl or D_5 through a running **IV**; **IM** should be no more than 2 ml in one inj site
• *Child with BSA <0.6 m²:* **IV/IM** 82.5 IU/kg q14 days

Sole induction
• *Adult:* **IV** 2500 IU/m² q14 days

Available forms: Inj 750 IU/ml in a phosphate buffered saline sol

Side effects/adverse reactions:
*SYST: **Anaphylaxis, hypersensitivity***

*HEMA: **Thrombocytopenia, leukopenia, myelosuppression, anemia, decreased clotting factors, pancytopenia***

*GI: Nausea, vomiting, anorexia, cramps, stomatitis, **hepatotoxicity, pancreatitis**, diarrhea*

*GU: Urinary retention, **renal failure**, glycosuria, polyuria, azotemia, uric acid neuropathy*

⬦ = Nursing alert   ✇ = Herb-drug interaction   ⃠ = Do not crush

INTEG: Rash, urticaria, chills, fever
ENDO: Hyperglycemia
*RESP: **Fibrosis, pulmonary infil-trate, severe bronchospasm***
CV: Chest pain, ***hypertension***
CNS: Neuritis, dizziness, headache, ***coma,*** depression, fatigue, confusion, hallucinations, ***seizures***

Contraindications: Hypersensitivity, infant, lactation, pancreatitis

Precautions: Renal disease, hepatic disease, pregnancy (C), CNS disease

Pharmacokinetics: Half-life 5½ days, onset rapid, duration 2 wk, metabolized in reticuloendothelial system

Interactions:
• Decreased action of methotrexate
• Do not use with radiation
• Coagulation factor imbalances: heparin, warfarin, aspirin, NSAIDs

NURSING CONSIDERATIONS
Assess:
◆ For signs and symptoms of pancreatitis (nausea, vomiting, severe abdominal pain), anaphylaxis (bronchospasm, dyspnea), cyanosis
• CBC, differential, platelet count qwk; withhold drug if WBC count is <4000 or platelet count is <75,000; notify prescriber of results
• Pulmonary function tests, chest x-ray studies before and during therapy; chest x-ray film should be obtained q2wk during treatment, watch for severe bronchospasm, fibrosis, pulmonary infiltrate
• Renal function studies: BUN, serum uric acid, ammonia, urine CrCl, electrolytes before and during therapy
• I&O ratio; report fall in urine output of 30 ml/hr, may indicate renal failure
• Temp q4h (may indicate beginning infection)

• Liver function tests before and during therapy (bilirubin, AST, ALT, LDH) as needed or monthly; hepatotoxicity can occur; check for jaundiced skin, sclera; dark urine, clay-colored stools, itchy skin, abdominal pain, fever, diarrhea
• RBC, Hct, Hgb; may be decreased
• Serum, urine glucose levels, glycosuria can occur
• Bleeding: hematuria, stool guaiac, bruising or petechiae, mucosa or orifices q8h
• Dyspnea, rales, nonproductive cough, chest pain, tachypnea, fatigue, increased pulse, pallor, lethargy, swelling around eyes or lips; anaphylaxis may occur
• B/P, since hypertension can occur
• Local irritation, pain, burning, discoloration at injection site
• Symptoms of severe allergic reaction: rash, pruritus, urticaria, purpuric skin lesions, itching, flushing, dyspnea
• Frequency of stools, characteristics; cramping, acidosis; signs of dehydration: rapid respirations, poor skin turgor, decreased urine output, dry skin, restlessness, weakness

Administer:
• Antispasmodic if GI symptoms occur
• Allopurinol or sodium bicarbonate to reduce uric acid levels, alkalinization of urine

IV infusion
• Using 21, 23, 25G needle; administer by slow IV infusion via Y-tube or 3-way stopcock of flowing D_5W or NS infusion over 2 hr after diluting
• Considered incompatible with other drugs in syringe or sol

Perform/provide:
• Deep-breathing exercises with patient tid-qid; place in semi-Fowler's position

• Increase fluid intake to 2-3 L/day to prevent urate deposits, calculi formation

• Diet low in purines: no organ meats (kidney, liver), dried beans, peas to maintain alkaline urine

• Rinsing of mouth tid-qid with water, club soda; brushing of teeth bid-tid with soft brush or cotton-tipped applicator for stomatitis; use unwaxed dental floss

• Warm compresses at injection site for inflammation

• Nutritious diet with iron, vitamin supplements

• HOB raised to facilitate breathing

Evaluate:

• Therapeutic response: decreased exacerbations in acute lymphocytic leukemia

Teach patient/family:

• To report nausea, vomiting, bruising, bleeding, stomatitis, severe diarrhea, jaundice, chest pain, abdominal pain, trouble breathing, rash

• To avoid vaccinations without advice of prescriber

• Not to use hard-bristled toothbrush, razors

• To avoid OTC medications, alcohol

Treatment of anaphylaxis: Administer epinephrine, diphenhydramine, IV corticosteroids

---

pemoline (℞)

(pem'oh-leen)
Cylert, Cylert Chewable
Func. class.: Cerebral stimulant
Chem. class.: Oxazolidinone derivative

Controlled Substance Schedule IV
Action: Exact mechanism unknown; may act through dopaminergic mechanisms; produces CNS stimu-lation and a paradoxic effect in ADHD

Uses: Attention deficit hyperactivity disorder

Investigational uses: Schizophrenia, fatigue, depression

Dosage and routes:

• *Child >6 yr:* **PO** 37.5 mg in AM, increasing by 18.75 mg/wk, not to exceed 112.5 mg/day

Available forms: Tabs 18.75, 37.5, 75 mg; chewable tabs 37.5 mg

Side effects/adverse reactions:

MISC: Rashes, growth suppression in children

CNS: Hyperactivity, insomnia, restlessness, dizziness, depression, headache, stimulation, irritability, aggressiveness, hallucinations, *seizures, masking or worsening of Gilles de la Tourette's syndrome,* drowsiness, dyskinetic movements

GI: Nausea, anorexia, diarrhea, abdominal pain, increased liver enzymes, *hepatitis,* jaundice, weight loss

CV: Tachycardia

Contraindications: Hypersensitivity, hepatic insufficiency

Precautions: Renal disease, pregnancy (B), lactation, drug abuse, child <6 yr, psychosis, tics, seizure disorder

Pharmacokinetics:

PO: Peak 2-4 hr, duration 8 hr, metabolized (50%) by liver, excreted (40%) by kidneys, half-life 10-30 hr

Interactions:

• Increased CNS stimulation: other CNS stimulants

NURSING CONSIDERATIONS
Assess:

• For attention span, decreased hyperactivity in ADHD persons

• Hepatic function studies: ALT, AST, bilirubin; renal, creatinine, prior to treatment and periodically thereafter

---

• Height, growth rate q3mo in child; growth rate may be decreased
• Mental status: mood, sensorium, affect, stimulation, insomnia, aggressiveness

PO
• At least 6 hr before hs

Evaluate:
• Therapeutic response: decreased hyperactivity

Teach patient/family:
• To decrease caffeine consumption (coffee, tea, cola, chocolate); may increase irritability, stimulation
• To avoid OTC preparations unless approved by prescriber
• To withdraw over several wk
• To avoid alcohol ingestion
• To avoid hazardous activities until patient is stabilized
• That therapeutic effect may take 2-4 wk
• To notify prescriber if tremors, insomnia, palpitations, restlessness, jaundice, bleeding occur

PENICILLINS

penicillin G benzathine (R)
(pen-i-sill'in)
Bicillin L-A, Permapen

penicillin G potassium (R)
Megacillin*, Pfizerpen

penicillin G procaine (R)
Ayercillin*, Wycillin

penicillin G sodium (R)
Crystapen*

penicillin V potassium (R)
Apo-Pen-VK*, Betapen-VK, Ledercillin-VK, Novopen-VK*, Penapar-VK, Pen-Vee K*, PVFK*, Robicillin-VK, Uticillin-VK, V-Cillin K, Veetids

Func. class.: Broad-spectrum antiinfective
Chem. class.: Natural penicillin

Action: Interferes with cell wall replication of susceptible organisms; osmotically unstable cell wall swells, bursts from osmotic pressure, results in cell death

Uses: Respiratory infections, scarlet fever, erysipelas, otitis media, pneumonia, skin and soft tissue infections, gonorrhea; effective for gram-positive cocci *(Staphylococcus, Streptococcus pyogenes, S. viridans, S. faecalis, S. bovis, S. pneumoniae),* gram-negative cocci *(Neisseria gonorrhoeae),* gram-positive bacilli *(Actinomyces, Bacillus anthracis, Clostridium perfringens, C. tetani, Corynebacterium diphtheriae, Listeria monocytogenes),* gram-negative bacilli *(Escherichia coli, Proteus mirabilis, Salmonella, Shi-*

P

gella, Enterobacter, Streptobacillus moniliformis), spirochetes (Treponema pallidum)

Dosage and routes:
Penicillin G benzathine
Early syphilis
• *Adult:* **IM** 2.4 million U in single dose
Congenital syphilis
• *Child <2 yr:* **IM** 50,000 U/kg in single dose
Prophylaxis of rheumatic fever, glomerulonephritis
• *Adult and child >27 kg:* **IM** 1.2 million U in single dose qmo or 600,000 U q2wk
• *Child <27 kg:* **IM** 600,000 U in single dose qmo
Upper respiratory infections (group A streptococcal)
• *Adult:* **IM** 1.2 million U in single dose
• *Child >27 kg:* **IM** 900,000 U in single dose
• *Child <27 kg:* **IM** 300,000-600,000 g in single dose
Available forms: Inj 300,000 U/ml; 600,000; 1,200,000; 2,400,000 U/dose
Penicillin G potassium
• Dosage reduction indicated in renal impairment (CrCl <50 ml/min)
Pneumococcal/streptococcal infections (mild to moderate)
• *Adult:* **IM/IV** 1.2-24 million U in divided doses q4h
• *Child <12 yr:* **IV** 100,000-400,000 U/kg/day in 4-6 divided doses
Available forms: Tabs 500,000 U*, oral susp 250,000, 500,000 U*; powder for inj 1, 5, 10, 20 million U/vial
Penicillin G procaine
Renal dose
• CrCl 10-30 ml/min give q8-12h; CrCl <10 ml/min give q12-18h
Moderate to severe infections
• *Adult and child:* **IM** 600,000-1.2 million U in 1 or 2 doses/day for 10 days to 2 wk

• *Newborn:* 50,000 U/kg **IM** once daily (avoid use in newborns)
Gonorrhea
• *Adult and child >12 yr:* **IM** 4.8 million U in two injections given 30 min after probenecid 1 g
Pneumococcal pneumonia
• *Adult and child >12 yr:* **IM** 600,000-1.2 million U/day × 7-10 days
Available forms: INJ 600,000, 1,200,000, 2,400,000 U/unit dose
Penicillin G sodium
• Dosage reduction indicated in renal impairment (CrCl <50 ml/min)
Moderate to severe infections
• *Adult:* **IM/IV** 2 million-24 million U/day in divided doses q4h
• *Child:* **IM/IV** 50,000-400,000 U/kg/day in divided doses q4-12h
Dental surgery prophylaxis for endocarditis
• *Adult:* **IM/IV** 2 million U ½-1 hr before procedure, then 1 million U 6 hr after procedure
Available forms: Inj 5 million U/vial
Penicillin V potassium
• Dosage reduction indicated in renal impairment (CrCl <50 ml/min)
Pneumococcal/staphylococcal infections
• *Adult:* **PO** 250-500 mg q6h
• *Child <12 yr:* **PO** 25-50 mg/kg/day in divided doses q6-8h
Streptococcal infections
• *Adult:* **PO** 125-250 mg q6-8h × 10 days
Prevention of recurrence of rheumatic fever/chorea
• *Adult:* **PO** 125 mg bid continuously
• *Child <5 yr:* **PO** 125 mg bid
• *Child >5 yr:* **PO** 250 mg bid
Vincent's gingivitis/pharyngitis
• *Adult:* **PO** 250 mg q6-8h
Available forms: Tabs 250, 500 mg; powder for oral sol 125, 250 mg/5 ml

◆ = Nursing alert   ⫟ = Herb-drug interaction   ⊘ = Do not crush

Side effects/adverse reactions:
HEMA: Anemia; increased bleeding time; ***bone marrow depression, granulocytopenia***
GI: Nausea, vomiting, diarrhea, increased AST, ALT, abdominal pain, glossitis, colitis
GU: ***Oliguria, proteinuria, hematuria,*** *vaginitis, moniliasis,* ***glomerulonephritis***
CNS: Lethargy, hallucinations, anxiety, depression, twitching, ***coma, convulsions***
META: Hyperkalemia, hypokalemia, alkalosis, hypernatremia
MISC: ***Anaphylaxis,*** *local pain,* tenderness and fever with IM injection
Contraindications: Hypersensitivity to penicillins; neonates
Precautions: Hypersensitivity to cephalosporins, pregnancy (B), lactation, severe renal disease
Pharmacokinetics:
Penicillin G benzathine
IM: Very slow absorption, duration 21-28 days, half-life 30-60 min; excreted in urine, feces, breast milk; crosses placenta
Penicillin G potassium
IV: Peak immediate
IM: Peak ¼-½ hr
PO: Peak 1 hr, duration 6 hr
Excreted in urine unchanged, excreted in breast milk, crosses placenta, half-life 30-60 min
Penicillin G procaine
IM: Peak 1-4 hr, duration 15 hr, excreted in urine
Penicillin G sodium
IM: Peak 1-3 hr, duration 6 hr; excreted in urine
Penicillin V potassium
PO: Peak 30-60 min, duration 6-8 hr, half-life 30 min, excreted in urine, breast milk
Interactions:
• Decreased antimicrobial effect of penicillin: tetracyclines

• Increased penicillin concentrations: aspirin, probenecid
• Decreased effect of oral contraceptives
• Increased effect of heparin
⬤ Delayed, reduced absorption of penicillin: khat, separate doses by 2 or more hr
Lab test interferences:
False positive: Urine glucose, urine protein

NURSING CONSIDERATIONS
Assess:
• For infection: temp, characteristics of sputum, wounds, urine, stools before, during, and after treatment
• I&O ratio; report hematuria, oliguria, since penicillin in high doses is nephrotoxic
◆ Any patient with compromised renal system, since drug is excreted slowly in poor renal system function; toxicity may occur rapidly
• Liver studies: AST, ALT
• Blood studies: WBC, RBC, Hct, Hgb, bleeding time
• Renal studies: urinalysis, protein, blood
• C&S before therapy; drug may be given as soon as culture is taken
• Bowel pattern before and during treatment
• Skin eruptions after administration of penicillin to 1 wk after discontinuing drug
• Respiratory status: rate, character, wheezing, tightness in chest
• Allergies before initiation of treatment, reaction of each medication; highlight allergies on chart; because of prolonged action, allergic reaction may be prolonged and severe
Administer:
Penicillin G benzathine
• Drug after C&S completed
• After shaking well, deep IM inj in large muscle mass; avoid intravascular inj, aspirate

P

Side effects: *italics* = common; ***bold italics*** = life-threatening

Penicillin G potassium

• Drug after C&S

Solution compatibility: Sterile H_2O for inj

Additive compatibilities: Ascorbic acid, calcium chloride, calcium gluconate, cephapirin, chloramphenicol, cimetidine, clindamycin, colistimethate, corticotropin, dimenhydrinate, diphenhydramine, ephedrine, erythromycin, furosemide, hydrocortisone, kanamycin, lidocaine, magnesium sulfate, methicillin, methylprednisolone, metronidazole, polymyxin B, prednisolone, potassium chloride, procaine, prochlorperazine, ranitidine, verapamil

Syringe compatibilities: Heparin

Y-site compatibilities: Acyclovir, amiodarone, cyclophosphamide, diltiazem, enalaprilat, esmolol, fluconazole, foscarnet, heparin, hydromorphone, labetalol, magnesium sulfate, meperidine, morphine, perphenazine, potassium chloride, tacrolimus, theophylline, verapamil, vit B/C

Penicillin G procaine

• Drug after C&S

• Deep IM inj avoid intravascular inj, aspirate

Penicillin G sodium

• IV after diluting with sterile H_2O; shake; follow manufacturer's instructions for dilution; may be added to 0.9% NaCl; give by continuous inf, usually over 12 hr

• Drug after C&S

Solution compatibility: Sterile H_2O for inj

Additive compatibilities: Calcium chloride, calcium gluconate, chloramphenicol, clindamycin, colistimethate, diphenhydramine, erythromycin, furosemide, gentamicin, hydrocortisone, kanamycin, methicillin, polymyxin B, prednisolone, procaine, ranitidine, verapamil, vit B/C

Syringe compatibilities: Aminoglycosides, chloramphenicol, cimetidine, colistimethate, gentamicin, heparin, kanamycin, lincomycin, polymyxin B, streptomycin

Penicillin V potassium

• Orally on empty stomach for best absorption

• Drug after C&S

Perform/provide:

• Adrenaline, suction, tracheostomy set, endotracheal intubation equipment

• Adequate fluid intake (2 L) during diarrhea episodes

• Scratch test to assess allergy after securing order from prescriber; usually done when penicillin is only drug of choice

• Storage in dry, tight container; oral susp refrigerated 2 wk, 1 wk at room temp

Evaluate:

• Therapeutic response: absence of fever, draining wounds

• Allergies before initiation of treatment, reaction of each medication; highlight allergies on chart; hypersensitivity reaction may be delayed

Teach patient/family:

• To report sore throat, fever, fatigue; may indicate superinfection

• To wear or carry Medic Alert ID if allergic to penicillins

• To report diarrhea, prevent dehydration

• To shake susp well before each dose; store in refrigerator for up to 2 wk

• To use all medication prescribed

• To use additional contraception if using any of these drugs

Treatment of anaphylaxis: Withdraw drug; maintain airway; administer epinephrine, aminophylline, O_2, IV corticosteroids

---

◆ = Nursing alert   ⫻ = Herb-drug interaction   ⊘ = Do not crush

pentamidine (R)

(pen-tam′i-deen)
Nebupent, Pentam 300,
Pentacarinat*, Pneumopent*
Func. class.: Antiprotozoal
Chem. class.: Aromatic diamide
derivative

Action: Interferes with DNA/RNA synthesis in protozoa

Uses: Treatment/prevention of *Pneumocystis carinii* infections

Dosage and routes:
• *Adult and child:* **IV/IM** 4 mg/kg/day × 2-3 wk; **NEB** 300 mg via specific nebulizer given q4wk for prevention

Available forms: Inj, aerosol 300 mg/vial; sol for aerosol 60 mg/vial*

Side effects/adverse reactions:
CV: Hypotension, ventricular tachycardia, ECG abnormalities, *dysrhythmias*
HEMA: Anemia, *leukopenia, thrombocytopenia*
INTEG: Sterile abscess, pain at injection site, pruritus, urticaria, *rash*
GU: Acute renal failure, increased serum creatinine, renal toxicity
GI: Nausea, vomiting, anorexia; increased AST, ALT; *acute pancreatitis,* metallic taste
CNS: Disorientation, hallucinations, *dizziness,* confusion
RESP: Cough, shortness of breath, *bronchospasm* (with aerosol)
MISC: Fatigue, chills, night sweats, *anaphylaxis, Stevens-Johnson syndrome*
META: Hyperkalemia, hypocalcemia, hypoglycemia

Precautions: Blood dyscrasias, hepatic disease, renal disease, diabetes mellitus, cardiac disease, hypocalcemia, pregnancy (C), hypertension, hypotension, lactation, children

Pharmacokinetics: Excreted unchanged in urine (66%)

Interactions:
• Nephrotoxicity: aminoglycosides, amphotericin B, colistin, cisplatin, foscarnet, methoxyflurane, polymyxin B, vancomycin
◆ Fatal dysrhythmias: erythromycin IV
• Increased myelosuppression: antineoplastics, radiation

NURSING CONSIDERATIONS
Assess:
• Blood studies, blood glucose, CBC, platelets, calcium, magnesium
• I&O ratio; report hematuria, oliguria
• ECG for cardiac dysrhythmias
• Patient should be lying down when receiving drug; severe hypotension may develop; monitor B/P during administration and until B/P stable
◆ Any patient with compromised renal system; drug is excreted slowly in poor renal system function; toxicity may occur rapidly
• Liver studies: AST, ALT
• Renal studies: urinalysis, BUN, creatinine; nephrotoxicity may occur
• Signs of infection, anemia
• Bowel pattern before, during treatment
• Sterile abscess, pain at injection site
• Respiratory status: rate, character, wheezing, dyspnea
• Dizziness, confusion, hallucination
• Allergies before treatment, reaction of each medication; place allergies on chart in bright red letters; notify all people giving drugs

Administer:
INH
• Through nebulizer; mix contents in 6 ml of sterile H_2O; do not use low pressure (<20 psi); flow rate

Side effects: *italics* = common; **bold italics** = life-threatening

should be 5-7 L/min (40-50 psi) air or O_2 source over 30-45 min until chamber is empty

IM
• 300 mg diluted in 3 ml sterile H_2O; give deep IM by Z-track; painful by this route

IV
• Reconstitute 300 mg/3-5 ml of sterile water for inj, D_5W, withdraw dose and further dilute in 50-250 ml D_5W, give over 1-2 hr

Y-site compatibilities: Diltiazem, zidovudine

Perform/provide:
• Storage in refrigerator protected from light

Evaluate:
• Therapeutic response: decreased temp, increased ability to breathe

Teach patient/family:
• To report sore throat, fever, fatigue (may indicate superinfection)
• To maintain adequate fluid intake

---

pentazocine (℞)
(pen-taz'oh-seen)
Fortral*, Talwin, Talwin NX
Func. class.: Opiate analgesic, antagonist
Chem. class.: Synthetic benzomorphan

Controlled Substance Schedule IV
Action: Inhibits ascending pain pathways in CNS, increases pain threshold, alters pain perception
Uses: Moderate to severe pain
Dosage and routes:
Renal dose
• CrCl 10-50 ml/min give q24-36h; CrCl <10 ml/min give q48h
• *Adult:* **PO** 50-100 mg q3-4h prn, not to exceed 600 mg/day; **IV/ IM/SC** 30 mg q3-4h prn, not to exceed 360 mg/day

Labor
• *Adult:* **IM** 60 mg; **IV** 30 mg q2-3h when contractions are regular
Available forms: Inj 30 mg/ml; tabs 50 mg
Side effects/adverse reactions:
CNS: Drowsiness, dizziness, confusion, headache, sedation, euphoria, hallucinations, dreaming
GI: Nausea, vomiting, anorexia, constipation, *cramps*
GU: Increased urinary output, dysuria, urinary retention
INTEG: Rash, urticaria, bruising, flushing, diaphoresis, pruritus, severe irritation at injection sites
EENT: Tinnitus, blurred vision, miosis, diplopia
CV: Palpitations, bradycardia, change in B/P, tachycardia, increased B/P (high doses)
RESP: Respiratory depression
Contraindications: Hypersensitivity, addiction (opiate)
Precautions: Addictive personality, pregnancy (C), lactation, increased intracranial pressure, MI (acute), severe heart disease, respiratory depression, hepatic disease, renal disease, seizure disorder, child <18 yr, head trauma
Pharmacokinetics:
SC/IM: Onset 15-30 min, peak 1-2 hr, duration 2-4 hr
IV: Onset 2-3 min, duration 4-6 hr
Metabolized by liver, excreted by kidneys, crosses placenta, half-life 2-3 hr, extensive first-pass metabolism with less than 20% entering circulation
Interactions:
• Unpredictable reactions: MAOIs
• Increased effects: CNS depressants; alcohol, sedative/hypnotics, antipsychotics, skeletal muscle relaxants
• Decreased effects: opiates
Lab test interferences:
Increase: Amylase

NURSING CONSIDERATIONS

Assess:

- For pain: intensity, duration, location prior to and 1 hr after dose
- I&O ratio; check for decreasing output; may indicate urinary retention
- For withdrawal symptoms in opiate-dependent patients
- Pulmonary embolism, abscesses, ulcerations, vascular occlusion, WBC
- CNS changes: dizziness, drowsiness, hallucinations, euphoria, LOC, pupil reaction
- Allergic reactions: rash, urticaria
- Respiratory dysfunction: respiratory depression, character, rate, rhythm; notify prescriber if respirations are <10/min
- Need for pain medication, physical dependence

Administer:

- With antiemetic if nausea, vomiting occur
- When pain is beginning to return; determine dosage interval by patient response

IV

- Undiluted or diluted 5 mg/ml of sterile H_2O for inj; give 5 mg or less over 1 min

Syringe compatibilities: Atropine, benzquinamide, butorphanol, chlorpromazine, cimetidine, dimenhydrinate, diphenhydramine, droperidol, fentanyl, hydromorphone, hydroxyzine, meperidine, metoclopramide, morphine, perphenazine, prochlorperazine, promazine, promethazine, ranitidine, scopolamine

Y-site compatibilities: Heparin, hydrocortisone, potassium chloride, vit B/C

Perform/provide:

- Storage in light-resistant area at room temp
- Assistance with ambulation
- Safety measures: night-light, call bell within easy reach

Evaluate:

- Therapeutic response: decrease in pain

Teach patient/family:

- To report any symptoms of CNS changes, allergic reactions
- That physical dependency may result from extended use
- That withdrawal symptoms may occur: nausea, vomiting, cramps, fever, faintness, anorexia

Treatment of overdose: Naloxone (Narcan) 0.2-0.8 mg IV, O_2, IV fluids, vasopressors

---

pentobarbital (℞)

(pen-toe-bar′bi-tal)
Nembutal, Nova-Rectal*, pentobarbital sodium, Pentogen*
Func. class.: Sedative/hypnotic barbiturate
Chem. class.: Barbitone, short acting

Controlled Substance Schedule II (USA), Schedule G (Canada)

Action: Depresses activity in brain cells, primarily in reticular activating system in brain stem; selectively depresses neurons in posterior hypothalamus, limbic structures

Uses: Insomnia, sedation, preoperative medication, increased intracranial pressure, dental anesthetic

Dosage and routes:

Insomnia

- *Adult:* **PO** 100-200 mg hs; **IM** 150-200 mg hs; **IV** 100 mg initially, then up to 500 mg; **RECT** 120-200 mg hs
- *Child:* **IM** 2-6 mg/kg, not to exceed 100 mg; **PO** 2-6 mg/kg/day in divided doses; **PO** preoperatively 2-6 mg/kg, max 100 mg/dose; **IV** 100 mg (hypnotic/anticonvulsant)

Side effects: *italics* = common; ***bold italics*** = life-threatening

Available forms: Caps 50, 100 mg; elix 18.2 mg/5 ml; rect supp 25*, 30, 50*, 60, 120, 200 mg; inj 50 mg/ml

Side effects/adverse reactions:

CNS: Lethargy, drowsiness, hangover, dizziness, paradoxical stimulation in elderly and children, lightheadedness, dependence, *CNS depression,* mental depression, slurred speech

GI: Nausea, vomiting, diarrhea, constipation

INTEG: Rash, urticaria, pain, abscesses at injection site, angioedema, thrombophlebitis, *Stevens-Johnson syndrome*

CV: Hypotension, bradycardia

RESP: Respiratory depression, apnea, laryngospasm, bronchospasm

HEMA: Agranulocytosis, thrombocytopenia, megaloblastic anemia (long-term treatment)

Contraindications: Hypersensitivity to barbiturates, pregnancy (D), respiratory depression, addiction to barbiturates; severe liver, renal impairment; porphyria, uncontrolled pain

Precautions: Anemia, lactation, hepatic disease, renal disease, hypertension, elderly, acute/chronic pain

Pharmacokinetics:

PO: Onset 15-30 min, duration 4-6 hr

RECT: Onset slow, duration 4-6 hr Metabolized by liver, excreted by kidneys (metabolites); half-life 15-48 hr

Interactions:

• Increased CNS depression: alcohol, MAOIs, sedatives, other CNS depressants, antihistamines, opiates

• Decreased effect of oral anticoagulants, corticosteroids, griseofulvin, quinidine

• Increased half-life of doxycycline

🍃 Elevated pentobarbital levels: quinine

Lab test interferences:

False increase: Sulfobromophthalein

NURSING CONSIDERATIONS

Assess:

• VS q30min after parenteral route for 2 hr

• Blood studies: Hct, Hgb, RBCs, serum folate, vit D (long-term therapy); pro-time in patients receiving anticoagulants

• Hepatic studies: AST, ALT, bilirubin; if increased, drug is usually discontinued

• Mental status: mood, sensorium, affect, memory (long, short)

• Physical dependency: more frequent requests for medication, shakes, anxiety

◆ Barbiturate toxicity: hypotension; pupillary constriction; cold, clammy skin; cyanosis of lips; insomnia; nausea; vomiting; hallucinations; delirium; weakness; coma; mild symptoms may occur in 8-12 hr without drug

• Respiratory changes: respiratory depression, character, rate, rhythm; hold drug if respirations are <10/min or if pupils are dilated

• Blood dyscrasias: fever, sore throat, bruising, rash, jaundice, epistaxis

Administer:

• For <14 days, since not effective after that; tolerance develops

• After removal of cigarettes to prevent fires

• After trying conservative measures for insomnia

PO

• Use elixir alone or diluted in fluids

• ½-1 hr before hs for sleeplessness

• On empty stomach for best absorption

• Crushed or whole

◆ = Nursing alert   🍃 = Herb-drug interaction   🚫 = Do not crush

• Alone; do not mix with other drugs or inject if there is precipitate

IM

• Inj deep in large muscle mass to prevent tissue sloughing and abscesses; do not inject more than 5 ml in one site

IV

• IV undiluted or dilute in sterile H_2O, LR, NaCl, give 50 mg or less/min; titrate to patient response; use only clear sol; avoid extravasation

• IV only with resuscitative equipment available; administer at <100 mg/min (only by qualified personnel)

Additive compatibilities: Amikacin, aminophylline, calcium chloride, cephapirin, chloramphenicol, dimenhydrinate, erythromycin lactobionate, lidocaine, thiopental, verapamil

Syringe compatibilities: Aminophylline, ephedrine, hydromorphone, neostigmine, scopolamine, sodium bicarbonate, thiopental

Y-site compatibilities: Acyclovir, insulin (regular), propofol

Perform/provide:

• Assistance with ambulation after receiving dose

• Safety measures: night-light, call bell within easy reach

• Checking to see if PO medication has been swallowed

• Storage of suppositories in refrigerator; do not use aqueous solutions that contain precipitate

Evaluate:

• Therapeutic response: ability to sleep at night, less early morning awakening if taking drug for insomnia, or decrease in number, severity of seizures if taking drug for seizure disorder

Teach patient/family:

• That hangover is common

• That drug is indicated only for short-term treatment of insomnia; probably ineffective after 2 wk

• That physical dependency may result from extended use (45-90 days depending on dose)

• To avoid driving, other activities requiring alertness

• To avoid alcohol ingestion, CNS depressants; serious CNS depression may result

• Not to discontinue medication quickly after long-term use; drug should be tapered over 1-2 wk

• To tell all prescribers that a barbiturate is being taken

• That withdrawal insomnia may occur after short-term use; not to start using drug again; insomnia will improve in 1-3 nights

• That effects may take 2 nights for benefits to be noticed

• Alternative measures to improve sleep (reading, exercise several hr before hs, warm bath, warm milk, TV, self-hypnosis, deep breathing)

Treatment of overdose: Lavage, activated charcoal, warming blanket, vital signs, hemodialysis, I&O ratio

pentostatin (R)

(pen-toh-stat'in)

Nipent

Func. class.: Antineoplastic, enzyme inhibitor

Chem. class.: Streptomyces antibioticus derivative

Action: Inhibits the enzyme adenosine deaminase (ADA), which is able to block DNA synthesis and some RNA synthesis

Uses: α-Interferon-refractory hairy cell leukemia, chronic lymphocytic leukemia

Dosage and routes:

• *Adult:* **IV** 4 mg/m^2 every other wk; may be given **IV BOL,** or diluted in a larger volume and given over 20-30 min

Available forms: Inj 10 mg/vial

Side effects/adverse reactions:

CNS: Headache, anxiety, confusion, depression, dizziness, insomnia, nervousness, paresthesia

RESP: Cough, upper respiratory infection, bronchitis, dyspnea, epistaxis, pneumonia, pharyngitis, rhinitis, sinusitis

SYST: Fever, infection, fatigue, pain, allergic reaction, chills, ***death, sepsis,*** chest pain, flu syndrome

HEMA: ***Leukopenia, anemia, thrombocytopenia,*** *ecchymosis,* ***lymphadenopathy,*** petechiae

GI: Nausea, vomiting, anorexia, diarrhea, constipation, flatulence, stomatitis, elevated liver function tests

INTEG: Rash, eczema, dry skin, pruritus, sweating, herpes simplex/zoster

GU: ***Hematuria,*** dysuria, increased BUN/creatinine

Contraindications: Hypersensitivity to this drug or mannitol, pregnancy (D)

Precautions: Renal disease, lactation, children, bone marrow depression

Pharmacokinetics:

IV: Elimination half-life 5.7 hr, low protein binding, 90% excreted in urine unchanged or as metabolites

Interactions:

◆ Fatal pulmonary toxicity: fludarabine

• Increased adverse reactions: vidarabine

Lab test interferences:

Increase: Uric acid

NURSING CONSIDERATIONS

Assess:

• CBC, differential, platelet count qwk; withhold drug if WBC is <2000/mm^3 or platelet count is <75,000/mm^3; notify prescriber

• Renal function studies; BUN, serum uric acid, urine CrCl, electrolytes before, during therapy

• I&O ratio; report fall in urine output to <30 ml/hr

• Monitor temp q4h; fever may indicate beginning infection

• Liver function tests before, during therapy: bilirubin, AST, ALT, alk phosphatase, prn or qmo; check for jaundiced skin and sclera, dark urine, clay-colored stools, itchy skin, abdominal pain, fever, diarrhea

• Bleeding: hematuria, guaiac stools, bruising, petechiae, mucosa or orifices q8h

• Effects of alopecia on body image; discuss feelings about body changes

• Inflammation of mucosa, breaks in skin

• Buccal cavity q8h for dryness, sores, ulceration, white patches, oral pain, bleeding, dysphagia

• Local irritation, pain, burning at injection site

• Symptoms of severe allergic reaction: rash, pruritus, urticaria, purpuric skin lesions, itching, flushing

• GI symptoms: frequency of stools, cramping

• Acidosis, signs of dehydration; rapid respiration, poor skin turgor, decreased urine output, dry skin, restlessness, weakness

Administer:

• Antiemetic 30-60 min before giving drug to prevent vomiting

• Antibiotics as ordered for prophylaxis of infection

IV

• After diluting, use with 5 ml sterile H$_2$O for injection and mix thoroughly (2 mg/ml); may be given by bolus or diluted in 25-50 ml 5% dextrose, or 0.9% NaCl (0.33 or 0.18 mg/ml)

Solution compatibilities: D$_5$W, 0.9% NaCl, LR

◆ = Nursing alert   *▯* = Herb-drug interaction   ⊘ = Do not crush

Y-site compatibilities: Fludarabine, melphalan, ondansetron, paclitaxel, sargramostim
Perform/provide:
• Hydrocortisone, sodium thiosulfate to infiltration area, and ice compress after stopping infusion
• Strict hand-washing technique, gloves, protective covering
• Liquid diet: carbonated beverages; gelatin may be added if patient is not nauseated or vomiting
• Rinsing of mouth tid-qid with water, club soda; brushing of teeth bid-qid with soft brush or cotton-tipped applicators for stomatitis; use unwaxed dental floss
• Storage in refrigerator; reconstituted or diluted sol may be stored at room temp up to 8 hr
Evaluate:
• Therapeutic response: decrease in tumor size, spread of malignancy
Teach patient/family:
• To report any complaints, side effects to nurse or prescriber
• That hair may be lost during treatment and wig or hairpiece may make patient feel better; tell patient that new hair may be different in color, texture
• To avoid foods with citric acid, hot or rough texture
• To report any bleeding, white spots, ulcerations in mouth to prescriber; tell patient to examine mouth qd
• To avoid crowds and sources of infection when granulocyte count is low

pentoxifylline (℞)

(pen-tox'ih-fill-in)
Trental
Func. class.: Hemorrheologic agent
Chem. class.: Dimethylxanthine derivative

Action: Decreases blood viscosity, stimulates prostacyclin formation, increases blood flow by increasing flexibility of RBCs; decreases RBC hyperaggregation; reduces platelet aggregation, decreases fibrinogen concentration

Uses: Intermittent claudication related to chronic occlusive vascular disease

Investigational uses: Cerebrovascular insufficiency, diabetic neuropathies, TIAs, leg ulcers, strokes

Dosage and routes:
• *Adult:* **PO** 400 mg tid with meals
Available forms: Tabs, extended release 400 mg

Side effects/adverse reactions:
MISC: Epistaxis, flulike symptoms, laryngitis, nasal congestion, *leukopenia,* malaise, weight changes
EENT: Blurred vision, earache, increased salivation, sore throat, conjunctivitis
CNS: Headache, anxiety, *tremors,* confusion, *dizziness*
GI: Dyspepsia, nausea, vomiting, anorexia, bloating, belching, constipation, cholecystitis, dry mouth, thirst, bad taste
INTEG: Rash, pruritus, urticaria, brittle fingernails
CV: Angina, dysrhythmias, palpitation, hypotension, chest pain, dyspnea, edema

Contraindications: Hypersensitivity to this drug or xanthines, retinal/cerebral hemorrhage

Precautions: Pregnancy (C), an-

P

gina pectoris, cardiac disease, lactation, children, impaired renal function, recent surgery, peptic ulceration

Pharmacokinetics:
PO: Peak 1 hr, half-life ½-1 hr, degradation in liver, excreted in urine

Interactions:
• Increased risk of bleeding: warfarin, salicylates, NSAIDs, thrombolytics, plicamycin, valproic acid
• Increased theophylline level: theophylline
• Increased hypotension: antihypertensives, nitrates

NURSING CONSIDERATIONS
Assess:
• B/P, respirations of patient also taking antihypertensives

Administer:
• With meals to prevent GI upset
🚫 Do not break, crush, or chew ext rel tabs

Evaluate:
• Therapeutic response: decreased pain, cramping, increased ambulation

Teach patient/family:
• That therapeutic response may take 2-4 wk
• That decreased fats, increased cholesterol, increased exercise, decreased smoking are necessary to correct condition
• To observe feet for arterial insufficiency
• To use cotton socks, well-fitted shoes; not to go barefoot
• To watch for bleeding, bruises, petechiae, epistaxis

---

perindopril
See appendix a—selected new drugs

---

perphenazine (℞)
(per-fen'a-zeen)
Apo-Perphenazine*, perphenazine, PMS Perphenazine*, Trilafon

Func. class.: Antipsychotic, neuroleptic

Chem. class.: Phenothiazine piperidine

Action: Depresses cerebral cortex, hypothalamus, limbic system, which control activity, aggression; blocks neurotransmission produced by dopamine at synapse; exhibits strong α-adrenergic, anticholinergic blocking action; as antiemetic inhibits medullary chemoreceptor trigger zone; mechanism for antipsychotic effects is unclear

Uses: Psychotic disorders, schizophrenia, nausea, vomiting

Dosage and routes:
• *Geriatric:* **PO** 2-4 mg qd-bid, increase by 2-4 mg/wk to desired dose
Nausea/vomiting
• *Adult and child >12 yr:* **IM** 5-10 mg prn, max 15 mg in ambulatory patients, 30 mg in hospitalized patients; **PO** 8-16 mg/day in divided doses, up to 24 mg; **IV** not to exceed 5 mg, give diluted or slow **IV** drip
Psychiatric use in hospitalized patients
• *Adult:* **PO** 8-16 mg bid-qid, gradually increased to desired dose, not to exceed 64 mg/day; **IM** 5 mg q6h, not to exceed 30 mg/day
• *Child >12 yr:* **PO** 6-12 mg in divided doses
Nonhospitalized patients
• *Adult:* **PO** 4-8 mg tid

Available forms: Tabs 2, 4, 8, 16 mg; oral sol 16 mg/5 ml; inj 5 mg/ml; syr 2 mg/5 ml*

Side effects/adverse reactions:
*RESP: **Laryngospasm**,* dyspnea, ***respiratory depression***

◆ = Nursing alert   🌿 = Herb-drug interaction   🚫 = Do not crush

CNS: EPS: pseudoparkinsonism, akathisia, dystonia, tardive dyskinesia, seizures, headache, neuroleptic malignant syndrome
HEMA: Anemia, *leukopenia, leukocytosis, agranulocytosis*
INTEG: Rash, photosensitivity, dermatitis
EENT: Blurred vision, glaucoma
GI: Dry mouth, nausea, vomiting, anorexia, constipation, diarrhea, jaundice, weight gain
GU: Urinary retention, urinary frequency, enuresis, impotence, amenorrhea, gynecomastia
CV: Orthostatic hypotension (elderly), *cardiac arrest,* ECG changes, *tachycardia*

Contraindications: Hypersensitivity, blood dyscrasias, coma, child <12 yr, brain damage, bone marrow depression

Precautions: Pregnancy (C), lactation, seizure disorders, hypertension, hepatic disease, cardiac disease, elderly

Pharmacokinetics:
Metabolized by liver; excreted in urine, breast milk; crosses placenta
PO: Onset erratic, peak 2-4 hr
IM: Onset 10 min, peak 1-2 hr; duration 6 hr, occasionally 12-24 hr

Interactions:
• Oversedation: other CNS depressants, alcohol, barbiturate anesthetics
• Toxicity: epinephrine
• Decreased absorption: aluminum hydroxide or magnesium hydroxide antacids
• Increased risk of EPS: lithium
• Increased effects of both drugs: β-adrenergic blockers, alcohol
• Increased anticholinergic effects: anticholinergics
• Decreased antiparkinson effect: levodopa
✐ Increased anticholinergic effect: henbane leaf

Lab test interferences:
Increase: Liver function tests, cardiac enzymes, cholesterol, blood glucose, prolactin, bilirubin, PBI, cholinesterase, ^{131}I
Decrease: Hormones (blood, urine)
False positive: Pregnancy tests, PKU
False negative: Urinary steroids, 17-OHCS

NURSING CONSIDERATIONS
Assess:
• Mental status before initial administration
• Swallowing of PO medication; check for hoarding or giving of medication to other patients
• I&O ratio; palpate bladder if urinary output is low
• Bilirubin, CBC, liver function studies qmo
• Urinalysis is recommended before and during prolonged therapy
• Affect, orientation, LOC, reflexes, gait, coordination, sleep pattern disturbances
• B/P standing and lying; also include pulse, respirations q4h during initial treatment; establish baseline before starting treatment; report drops of 30 mm Hg
• Dizziness, faintness, palpitations, tachycardia on rising
• EPS including akathisia (inability to sit still, no pattern to movements), tardive dyskinesia (bizarre movements of jaw, mouth, tongue, extremities), pseudoparkinsonism (rigidity, tremors, pill rolling, shuffling gait)
• Skin turgor daily
➧ For neuroleptic malignant syndrome: hyperthermia, altered mental status, increased CPK, muscle rigidity
• Constipation, urinary retention daily; increase bulk, water in diet
Administer:
• Antiparkinsonian agent on order from prescriber for EPS

P

Side effects: *italics* = common; **bold italics** = life-threatening

- Concentrate mixed in water, orange, pineapple, apricot, prune, tomato, grapefruit juice; do not mix with caffeine beverages (coffee, cola), tannics (tea), or pectinates (apple juice), since incompatibility may result; use 60 ml diluent for each 5 ml of concentrate
- IM inj into large muscle mass

IV

- After diluting each 5 mg/9 ml of NaCl, shake, give 0.5 mg or less (1 ml = 0.5 mg) over 1 min; may be further diluted and infused

Additive compatibilities: Ascorbic acid, ethacrynate, netilmicin

Syringe compatibilities: Atropine, benztropine, butorphanol, chlorpromazine, cimetidine, dimenhydrinate, diphenhydramine, droperidol, fentanyl, hydroxyzine, meperidine, methotrimeprazine, metoclopramide, morphine, pentazocine, prochlorperazine, promethazine, ranitidine, scopolamine

Y-site compatibilities: Acyclovir, amikacin, ampicillin, azlocillin, cefamandole, cefazolin, cefotaxime, cefoxitin, cefuroxime, cephalothin, cephapirin, chloramphenicol, clindamycin, doxycycline, erythromycin, famotidine, gentamicin, kanamycin, metronidazole, mezlocillin, minocycline, moxalactam, nafcillin, oxacillin, penicillin G potassium, piperacillin, tacrolimus, ticarcillin, ticarcillin/clavulanate, tobramycin, trimethoprim/sulfamethoxazole, vancomycin

Perform/provide:

- Decreased sensory input by dimming lights, avoiding loud noises
- Supervised ambulation until stabilized on medication; do not involve in strenuous exercise program because fainting is possible; patient should not stand still for long periods
- Increased fluids to prevent constipation
- Sips of water, candy, gum for dry mouth
- Storage in tight, light-resistant container

Evaluate:

- Therapeutic response: decrease in emotional excitement, hallucinations, delusions, paranoia, reorganization of patterns of thought, speech

Teach patient/family:

- That orthostatic hypotension occurs frequently and to rise from sitting or lying position gradually; to avoid hazardous activities until stabilized on medication
- To remain lying down after IM inj for at least 30 min
- To avoid hot tubs, hot showers, tub baths, since hypotension may occur
- To avoid abrupt withdrawal of this drug, or EPS may result; drug should be withdrawn slowly
- To avoid OTC preparations (cough, hay fever, cold) unless approved by prescriber, since serious drug interactions may occur; avoid use with alcohol or CNS depressants; increased drowsiness may occur
- To use a sunscreen
- About compliance with drug regimen
- About necessity for meticulous oral hygiene, since oral candidiasis may occur
- To report sore throat, malaise, fever, bleeding, mouth sores; if these occur, CBC should be drawn and drug discontinued
- In hot weather, that heat stroke may occur; to take extra precautions to stay cool

Treatment of overdose: Lavage if orally ingested; provide an airway; *do not induce vomiting*

 = Nursing alert   ⫰ = Herb-drug interaction   ⊘ = Do not crush

phenazopyridine (R, OTC)

(fen-az-oh-peer'i-deen)
Azo-Standard, Baridium,
Geridium, Phenazo*,
phenazopyridine, Prodium,
Pyridiate, Pyridium, Urodine,
Urogesic
Func. class.: Nonopioid analgesic
Chem. class.: Azodye

Action: Exerts analgesic, anesthetic action on the urinary tract mucosa

Uses: Urinary tract irritation, infection used with a urinary antiinfective

Dosage and routes:
• *Adult:* **PO** 200 mg tid × 2 days or less when used with antibacterial for UTI
• *Child 6-12 yr:* **PO** 4 mg/kg tid × 2 days

Renal dose
• Do not use in CrCl <50 ml/min

Available forms: Tabs 100, 200 mg

Side effects/adverse reactions:

*HEMA: **Thrombocytopenia, agranulocytosis, leukopenia, neutropenia, hemolytic anemia, methemoglobinemia***

CNS: Headache

GI: Nausea, vomiting, diarrhea, heartburn, anorexia, **hepatic toxicity**

INTEG: Rash, skin pigmentation, pruritus

GU: **Renal toxicity,** orange-red urine

Contraindications: Hypersensitivity, renal insufficiency

Precautions: Pregnancy (B), lactation, children <12 yr

Pharmacokinetics:
Metabolized by liver, excreted by kidneys, crosses placenta, duration 6-8 hr

Lab test interferences:
Interference: Urinalysis

NURSING CONSIDERATIONS
Assess:
• Urinary status: burning, pain, itching, urgency, frequency, hematuria, before/after treatment completed
• Liver function studies: AST, ALT, bilirubin if patient is on long-term therapy
◆ Hepatotoxicity: dark urine, clay-colored stools, jaundiced skin and sclera, itching, abdominal pain, fever, diarrhea if patient is on long-term therapy
• Allergic reactions: rash, urticaria; drug may have to be discontinued

Administer:
PO
• To patient crushed or whole; chewable tablets may be chewed
• With food or milk to decrease gastric symptoms

Evaluate:
• Therapeutic response: decrease in urinary pain

Teach patient/family:
• Not to exceed recommended dosage and to take with meals
• To discontinue after pain is relieved but continue to take concurrent prescribed antiinfective until finished
• That urine may turn red-orange; may stain clothing or contact lenses

Treatment of overdose: Methylene blue 1-2 mg/kg IV or 100-200 mg vit C PO

phenelzine (R)

(fen'el-zeen)
Nardil
Func. class.: Antidepressant, MAOI
Chem. class.: Hydrazine

Action: Increases concentrations of endogenous epinephrine, norepi-

P

nephrine, serotonin, dopamine in storage sites in CNS by inhibition of MAO; increased concentration reduces depression

Uses: Depression, when uncontrolled by other means

Investigational uses: Bulimia, cocaine addiction, migraines, seasonal affective disorder, panic disorder

Dosage and routes:
• *Adult:* **PO** 45 mg/day in divided doses; may increase to 60 mg/day; dose should be reduced to 15 mg/day, not to exceed 90 mg/day
• *Geriatric:* **PO** 7.5 mg qd, increase by 7.5-15 mg q3-4 days

Available forms: Tabs 15 mg

Side effects/adverse reactions:
*HEMA: **Anemia***
CNS: Dizziness, drowsiness, confusion, headache, anxiety, tremors, stimulation, weakness, hyperreflexia, mania, insomnia, fatigue, weight gain
GI: Constipation, dry mouth, nausea, vomiting, *anorexia,* diarrhea, weight gain
GU: Change in libido, urinary frequency
INTEG: Rash, flushing, increased perspiration
*CV: Orthostatic hypotension, hypertension, dysrhythmias, **hypertensive crisis***
EENT: Blurred vision
*ENDO: **SIADH-like syndrome***

Contraindications: Hypersensitivity to MAOIs, hypertension, CHF, severe hepatic disease, pheochromocytoma, severe renal disease, severe cardiac disease

Precautions: Suicidal patients, convulsive disorders, severe depression, schizophrenia, hyperactivity, diabetes mellitus, pregnancy (C)

Pharmacokinetics: Metabolized by liver, excreted by kidneys

Interactions:
• Increased hypotension: thiazide diuretics
• Confusion, shivering, hyperreflexia: L-tryptophan
• Toxicity: sumatriptan, sulfonamides
• Decreased serotonin, norepinephrine: rauwolfia alkaloids
• Increased pressor effects: guanethidine, clonidine, indirect-acting or mixed sympathomimetics (ephedrine)
• Increased effects of direct-acting sympathomimetics (epinephrine): alcohol, barbiturates, benzodiazepines, CNS depressants, levodopa
◆ Hyperpyretic crisis, convulsions, hypertensive episode: tricyclic antidepressants, SSRIs, meperidine, methylphenidate
• Increased hypoglycemic effect: antidiabetics
• Drug/food: avoid tyramine foods, caffeine
⫸ Increased sympathomimetic action: ephedra
⫸ Hypertension: brewer's yeast
⫸ Tension headaches, irritability, visual hallucinations: ginseng

NURSING CONSIDERATIONS
Assess:
• B/P (lying, standing), pulse; if systolic B/P drops 20 mm Hg, hold drug, notify prescriber
• Blood studies: CBC, leukocytes, cardiac enzymes (long-term therapy)
• Hepatic studies: ALT, AST, bilirubin; hepatotoxicity may occur
◆ Toxicity: increased headache, palpitation; discontinue drug immediately; prodromal signs of hypertensive crisis
• Mental status changes: mood, sensorium, affect, memory (long, short); increase in psychiatric symptoms
• Urinary retention, constipation, edema; take weight qwk

◆ = Nursing alert   ⫸ = Herb-drug interaction   ⊘ = Do not crush

• Withdrawal symptoms: headache, nausea, vomiting, muscle pain, weakness

Administer:

PO

• Increased fluids, bulk in diet for constipation
• With food, milk for GI symptoms
• Crushed if patient cannot swallow medication whole
• Dosage hs for oversedation during day
• Gum, hard candy, or frequent sips of water for dry mouth
• Phentolamine for severe hypertension

Perform/provide:

• Storage in tight container in cool environment
• Ambulation assistance at start of therapy, since drowsiness/dizziness occurs, especially elderly
• Safety measures including side rails
• Checking to see if PO medication swallowed

Evalute:

• Therapeutic response: decreased depression

Teach patient/family:

• That therapeutic effects may take 1-4 wk
• To avoid driving, other activities requiring alertness
• To avoid alcohol ingestion, CNS depressants, OTC medications: cold, weight loss, hay fever, cough syrup
• Not to discontinue medication quickly after long-term use
• To avoid high-tyramine foods: cheese (aged), sour cream, beer, wine, pickled products, liver, raisins, bananas, figs, avocados, meat tenderizers, chocolate, yogurt; increased caffeine
• To report headache, palpitation, neck stiffness, dizziness, constriction in chest, throat

Treatment of overdose: Lavage, activated charcoal, monitor electrolytes, vital signs, diazepam IV, $NaHCO_3$

---

phenobarbital (℞)
(fee-noe-bar′bi-tal)
Ancalixir*, Barbita, Luminal, phenobarbital sodium, solfoton
Func. class.: Anticonvulsant
Chem. class.: Barbiturate

Controlled Substance Schedule IV

Action: Decreases impulse transmission; increases seizure threshold at cerebral cortex level

Uses: All forms of epilepsy, status epilepticus, febrile seizures in children, sedation, insomnia

Investigational uses: Hyperbilirubinemia, chronic cholestasis

Dosage and routes:

Seizures

• *Adult:* **PO** 60-200 mg/day in divided doses tid or total dose hs
• *Child:* **PO** 4-6 mg/kg/day in divided doses q12h; may be given as single dose

Status epilepticus

• *Adult:* **IV INF** 10 mg/kg; run no faster than 50 mg/min; may give up to 20 mg/kg
• *Child:* **IV INF** 5-10 mg/kg; may repeat q10-15min up to 20 mg/kg; run no faster than 50 mg/min

Insomnia

• *Adult:* **PO/IM** 100-320 mg
• *Child:* **PO/IM** 3-5 mg/kg

Sedation

• *Adult:* **PO** 30-120 mg/day in 2-3 divided doses
• *Child:* **PO** 3-5 mg/kg/day in 3 divided doses

Preoperative sedation

• *Adult:* **IM** 100-200 mg 1-1½ hr before surgery

P

• *Child:* **IM** 16-100 mg or **PO/ IM/IV** 1-3 mg/kg 1-1½ hr before surgery

Available forms: Caps 16 mg; elix 15*, 20 mg/5 ml; tabs 15, 30, 60, 100 mg; inj 30, 60, 65, 130 mg/ml

Side effects/adverse reactions:

CNS: Paradoxic excitement (elderly), drowsiness, lethargy, hangover headache, flushing, hallucinations, *coma*

GI: Nausea, vomiting, diarrhea, constipation

INTEG: Rash, urticaria, *Stevens-Johnson syndrome, angioedema,* local pain, swelling, necrosis, *thrombophlebitis*

Contraindications: Hypersensitivity to barbiturates, porphyria, hepatic disease, respiratory disease, nephritis, hyperthyroidism, diabetes mellitus, elderly, lactation, pregnancy (D)

Precautions: Anemia

Pharmacokinetics:

IV: Onset 5 min, peak 30 min, duration 4-6 hr

IM/SC: Onset 10-30 min, duration 4-6 hr

PO: Onset 20-60 min, peak 8-12 hr, duration 6-10 hr

Metabolized by liver; crosses placenta; excreted in urine, breast milk; half-life 53-118 hr

Interactions:

• Increased effects: CNS depression, alcohol, chloramphenicol, valproic acid, disulfiram, nondepolarizing skeletal muscle relaxants, sulfonamides

• Decreased effects: theophylline, oral anticoagulants, corticosteroids, metronidazole, doxycycline, quinidine

• Increased orthostatic hypotension: furosemide

🌿 Increased phenobarbital levels: quinine

NURSING CONSIDERATIONS

Assess:

• Mental status: mood, sensorium, affect, memory (long, short)

• For respiratory depression

• Blood dyscrasias: fever, sore throat, bruising, rash, jaundice

• Convulsion activity: type, duration, precipitating factors

• Blood studies, liver function tests during long-term treatment

• Therapeutic blood level periodically: 15-40 µg/ml

• Respiratory status: rate, rhythm, depth

Administer:

• IM inj deep in large muscle mass to prevent tissue sloughing; use <5 ml in each site

IV

• Slow IV after dilution with at least 10 ml sterile H_2O for inj regardless of dose; give 65 mg or less/min; titrate to patient response

Additive compatibilities: Amikacin, aminophylline, calcium chloride, calcium gluconate, cephapirin, colistimethate, dimenhydrinate, meropenem, polymyxin B, sodium bicarbonate, thiopental, verapamil

Solution compatibilities: D_5W, $D_{10}W$, 0.45% NaCl, 0.9% NaCl, Ringer's, dextrose/saline combinations, dextrose/Ringer's, dextrose/ LR combinations, sodium lactate

Syringe compatibilities: Heparin

Y-site compatibilities: Enalaprilat, meropenem, propofol, sufentanil

Perform/provide:

• Supervision of ambulation for dizziness, drowsiness

Evaluate:

• Therapeutic response: decreased seizures, increased sedation

Teach patient/family:

• To use exactly as ordered

• To avoid other CNS depressants, including alcohol

• To avoid hazardous activities until stabilized on drug; drowsiness may occur

• Never to withdraw drug abruptly; withdrawal symptoms may occur

• That therapeutic effects (PO) may not be seen for 2-3 wk

Treatment of overdose: Calcium gluconate IV

---

phentolamine (℞)

(fen-tole'a-meen)
Regitine, Rogitine*
Func. class.: Antihypertensive
Chem. class.: α-adrenergic blocker

Action: α-adrenergic blocker, binds to α-adrenergic receptors, dilating peripheral blood vessels, lowering peripheral resistances, lowering blood pressure

Uses: Hypertension, pheochromocytoma, prevention, treatment of dermal necrosis following extravasation of norepinephrine or dopamine, impotence

Dosage and routes:

Treatment of hypertensive episodes in pheochromocytoma

• *Adult:* **IV/IM,** 5 mg, repeat if necessary

• *Child:* **IV/IM,** 1 mg, repeat if necessary

Prevention, treatment of necrosis

• *Adult:* 5-10 mg/10 ml **NS** injected into area of norepinephrine extravasation within 12 hr

• *Child:* 0.1-0.2 mg/kg, max 10 mg

Impotence (adjunct)

• *Adult:* **INTRACAVERNOSAL** 0.5-1 mg with 30 mg papaverine given 1, 2, or 3 treatments/wk

Available forms: Inj 5 mg/ml

Side effects/adverse reactions:

GI: Dry mouth, nausea, vomiting, diarrhea, abdominal pain

CV: Hypotension, tachycardia, angina, dysrhythmias, **MI**

CNS: Dizziness, flushing, weakness, **cerebrovascular spasm**

EENT: Nasal congestion

Contraindications: Hypersensitivity, MI, coronary insufficiency, angina

Precautions: Pregnancy (C), lactation

Pharmacokinetics:

IV: Peak 2 min, duration 10-15 min

IM: Peak 15-20 min, duration 3-4 hr

Metabolized in liver, excreted in urine

Interactions:

• Increased effects of epinephrine, antihypertensives

NURSING CONSIDERATIONS

Assess:

• Electrolytes: K, Na, Cl, CO_2; weight qd, I&O

• B/P lying, standing before starting treatment, q4h after

• Nausea, vomiting, diarrhea, edema in feet, legs daily; skin turgor, dryness of mucous membranes for hydration status, postural hypotension, cardiac system: pulse, ECG

Administer:

• Gum, frequent rinsing of mouth, or hard candy for dry mouth

• With vasopressor available

• After discontinuing all medication for 24 hr

IV

• After diluting 5 mg/1 ml sterile H_2O for inj; give 5 mg or less/min; patient to remain recumbent during administration

Cont Inf

• Dilute 5-10 mg/500 ml D_5W, titrate to patient response

• 10 mg/L may be added to norepinephrine in IV sol for prevention of dermal necrosis

Additive compatibilities: Dobutamine, verapamil

Syringe compatibilities: Papaverine

Y-site compatibilities: Amiodarone

P

Evaluate:
• Therapeutic response: decreased B/P
Teach patient/family:
• That bed rest is required during treatment, 1 hr after
Treatment of overdose: Administer norepinephrine; discontinue drug

---

phenylephrine (R)

(fen-ill-ef'rin)
Neo-Synephrine
Func. class.: Adrenergic, direct-acting
Chem. class.: Substituted phenylethylamine

Action: Powerful and selective (α_1) receptor agonist causing contraction of blood vessels
Uses: Hypotension, paroxysmal supraventricular tachycardia, shock, maintain B/P for spinal anesthesia
Dosage and routes:
Hypotension
• *Adult:* **SC/IM** 2-5 mg, may repeat q10-15 min if needed, do not exceed initial dose; **IV** 0.1-0.5 mg, may repeat q10-15 min if needed, do not exceed initial dose
• *Child:* **IM/SC** 0.1 mg/kg/dose q1-2h prn
PVCs
• *Adult:* **IV BOL** 0.5 mg given rapidly, not to exceed prior dose by >0.1 mg, total dose >1 mg
Shock
• *Adult:* **IV INF** 10 mg/500 ml D_5W given 100-180 µg/min (if 20 gtt/ml inf device), then maint of 40-60 µg/min (if 20 gtt/ml inf device)
• *Child:* **IV BOL** 5-20 µg/kg/dose q10-15 min; **IV INF** 0.1-0.5 µg/kg/min
Available forms: Inj 1% (10 mg/ml)
Side effects/adverse reactions:
CNS: Headache, anxiety, tremor, insomnia, dizziness

CV: Palpitations, tachycardia, hypertension, ectopic beats, angina, reflex bradycardia, *dysrhythmias*
GI: Nausea, vomiting
INTEG: Necrosis, tissue sloughing with extravasation, *gangrene*
SYST: Anaphylaxis
Contraindications: Hypersensitivity, ventricular fibrillation, tachydysrhythmias, pheochromocytoma, narrow-angle glaucoma
Precautions: Pregnancy (C), lactation, arterial embolism, peripheral vascular disease, elderly, hyperthyroidism, bradycardia, myocardial disease, severe arteriosclerosis
Pharmacokinetics:
IV: Duration 20-30 min
IM/SC: Duration 45-60 min
Interactions:
• Do not use within 2 wk of MAOIs, or hypertensive crisis may result
• Dysrhythmias: general anesthetics, bretylium
• Decreased action of phenylephrine: α-blockers
• Increase in B/P: oxytocics
• Increased pressor effect: tricyclic antidepressants, MAOIs, guanethidine
NURSING CONSIDERATIONS
Assess:
• I&O ratio; notify prescriber if output <30 ml/hr
• ECG during administration continuously; if B/P increases, drug is decreased
• B/P and pulse q5min after parenteral route
• CVP or PWP during inf if possible
• For paresthesias and coldness of extremities; peripheral blood flow may decrease
Administer:
IV
• Plasma expanders for hypovolemia
• IV after diluting 1 mg/9 ml sterile H_2O for inj; give dose over ½-1

---

min; may be diluted 10 mg/500 ml of D_5W or NS; titrate to response (normal B/P); check for extravasation, check site for infiltration, use infusion pump

Additive compatibilities: Chloramphenicol, dobutamine, lidocaine, potassium chloride, sodium bicarbonate

Y-site compatibilities: Amiodarone, amrinone, cisatracurium, famotidine, haloperidol, remifentanil, zidovudine

Perform/provide:
• Storage of reconstituted sol if refrigerated for no longer than 24 hr
• Discard discolored sol

Evaluate:
• Therapeutic response: increased B/P with stabilization

Teach patient/family:
• The reason for administration
• To report pain at infusion site or other adverse reactions immediately

Treatment of overdose: Administer an α-blocker

---

phenytoin (℞)
(fen'i-toh-in)
Dilantin, Dilantin Infatab, Dilantin Kapseals, Dilantin-125, diphenylhydantoin, Phenytex
Func. class.: Anticonvulsant; antidysrhythmic (IB)
Chem. class.: Hydantoin

Action: Inhibits spread of seizure activity in motor cortex by altering ion transport; increases AV conduction

Uses: Generalized tonic-clonic seizures; status epilepticus; nonepileptic seizures associated with Reye's syndrome or after head trauma; migraines, trigeminal neuralgia, Bell's palsy, ventricular dysrhythmias uncontrolled by antidysrhythmics

Dosage and routes:
Renal dose
• Do not use loading dose CrCl <10 ml/min or hepatic failure
Seizures
• *Adult:* **PO** 1 g or 20 mg/kg (ext rel) in 3-4 divided doses given q2h, or 400 mg, then 300 mg q2h × 2 doses, maintenance 300-400 mg/day, max 600 mg/day; **IV** 15-20 mg/kg, max 25-50 mg/min, then 100 mg q6-8h
• *Child:* **PO** 5 mg/kg/day in 2-3 divided doses, maintenance 4-8 mg/kg/day in 2-3 divided doses, max 300 mg/day; **IV** 15-20 mg/kg at 1-3 mg/kg/min
Status epilepticus
• *Adult:* **IV** 10-15 mg/kg, max 25-50 mg/min, may give 100 mg q6-8h thereafter
• *Child:* **IV** 15-20 mg/kg, max in divided doses 1-3 mg/kg/min
Neuritic pain
• *Adult:* **PO** 200-600 mg/day in divided doses
Ventricular dysrhythmias
• *Adult:* **PO** loading dose 1 g divided over 24 hr, then 500 mg/day × 2 days; **IV** 250 mg over 5 min until dysrhythmias subside or until 1 g is given, or 100 mg q15min until dysrhythmias subside or until 1 g given
• *Child:* **PO** 3-8 mg/kg or 250 mg/m^2/day as single dose or 2 divided doses; **IV** 3-8 mg/kg over several min, or 250 mg/m^2/day as single dose or 2 divided doses
Available forms: Susp 125 mg/5 ml; tabs, chewable 50 mg; inj 50 mg/ml; caps ext rel 30, 100 mg; caps prompt 100 mg

Side effects/adverse reactions:
CNS: Drowsiness, dizziness, insomnia, paresthesias, depression, suicidal tendencies, aggression, headache, confusion, slurred speech

P

CV: Hypotension, *ventricular fibrillation*

EENT: Nystagmus, diplopia, blurred vision

GI: Nausea, vomiting, constipation, anorexia, weight loss, *hepatitis,* jaundice, gingival hyperplasia

GU: Nephritis, urine discoloration

HEMA: Agranulocytosis, leukopenia, aplastic anemia, thrombocytopenia, megaloblastic anemia

INTEG: Rash, *lupus erythematosus, Stevens-Johnson syndrome,* hirsutism

SYST: Hypocalcemia

Contraindications: Hypersensitivity, psychiatric condition, pregnancy (D), bradycardia, SA and AV block, Stokes-Adams syndrome, hepatic failure

Precautions: Allergies, hepatic disease, renal disease, elderly, petit mal seizures

Pharmacokinetics:

PO-ER: Onset 2-24 hr, peak 4-12 hr, duration 12-36 hr

IV: Onset 1-2 hr, duration 12-24 hr

PO: Onset 2-24 hr, peak 1½-2½ hr, duration 6-12 hr

Metabolized by liver, excreted by kidneys; highly protein-bound, half-life 22 hr

Interactions:

• Decreased effects of phenytoin: alcohol (chronic use), antihistamines, antacids, antineoplastics, CNS depressants, rifampin, folic acid

• Increased effect of phenytoin: low plasma albumin levels

🔌 Increased potassium loss, increased antidysrhythmic action: aloe, buckthorn, cascara sagrada, senna

Lab test interferences:

Decrease: Dexamethasone, metyrapone test serum, PBI, urinary steroids

Increase: Glucose, alk phosphatase, BSP

NURSING CONSIDERATIONS
Assess:

• For phenytoin hypersensitivity syndrome 3-12 wk after start of treatment: rash, temp, lymphadenopathy

• Drug level: toxic level 30-50 μg/ml, ther level: 7.5-20 μg/ml, wait ≥1 wk to draw levels

• For seizures: duration, type, intensity precipitating factors

• Blood studies: CBC, platelets q2wk until stabilized, then qmo × 12, then q3mo; discontinue drug if neutrophils <1600/mm^3; renal function: albumin conc

• Mental status: mood, sensorium, affect, memory (long, short)

• Respiratory depression; rate, depth, character

• Blood dyscrasias: fever, sore throat, bruising, rash, jaundice

Administer:

• Do not interchange chewable product with caps, not equivalent

• Shake susp well before each dose G tube/NG tube: dilute susp prior to administration, flush tube with 20 ml H_2O after dose

IV

• After diluting with diluent provided (2.2 ml/100 mg, 5.2 ml/250 mg) (1 ml/50 mg); shake; place vial in warm water to dissolve powder; give through Y-tube or 3-way stopcock; inject slowly <50 mg/min; clear IV tubing first with NS sol; use in-line filter; discard 4 hr after preparation; inject into large veins to prevent purple glove syndrome

Additive compatibilities: Bleomycin, sodium bicarbonate, verapamil

Y-site compatibilities: Esmolol, famotidine, fluconazole, foscarnet, tacrolimus

Evaluate:

• Therapeutic response; decrease in severity of seizures, ventricular dysrhythmias

---

◆ = Nursing alert   🔌 = Herb-drug interaction   🚫 = Do not crush

Teach patient/family:

• To take PO doses divided with or after meals to decrease adverse effects

• That if diabetic, urine glucose should be monitored

• That urine may turn pink

• Not to discontinue drug abruptly; seizures may occur

• Proper brushing of teeth using a soft toothbrush, flossing to prevent gingival hyperplasia; need to see dentist frequently

• To avoid hazardous activities until stabilized on drug

• To carry Medic Alert ID stating drug use

• That heavy use of alcohol may diminish effect of drug; to avoid OTC medications

• Not to change brands or forms once stabilized on therapy; brands may vary

---

phytonadione (vit K₁) (℞)
(fye-toe-na-dye′one)
AquaMEPHYTON, Konakion, Mephyton
Func. class.: Vit K₁, fat-soluble vitamin

Action: Needed for adequate blood clotting (factors II, VII, IX, X)

Uses: Vit K malabsorption, hypoprothrombinemia, prevention of hypoprothrombinemia caused by oral anticoagulants, prevention of hemorrhagic disease of the newborn

Dosage and routes:

Hypoprothrombinemia caused by vit K malabsorption

• *Adult:* **PO/IM** 2.5-25 mg, may repeat or increase to 50 mg

• *Child:* **PO/IM** 5-10 mg

• *Infant:* **PO/IM** 2 mg

Prevention of hemorrhagic disease of the newborn

• *Neonate:* **IM** 0.5-1 mg within 1 hr after birth, repeat in 2-3 wk if required

Hypoprothrombinemia caused by oral anticoagulants

• *Adult and child:* **PO/SC/IM** 2.5-10 mg, may repeat 12-48 hr after **PO** dose or 6-8 hr after **SC/IM** dose, based on PT

Available forms: Tabs 5 mg; inj 2 mg, 10 ml aqueous colloidal; inj aqueous dispersion 10 mg/ml, (IM)

Side effects/adverse reactions:

CNS: Headache, ***brain damage*** (large doses)

GI: Nausea, decreased liver function tests

HEMA: ***Hemolytic anemia, hemoglobinuria, hyperbilirubinemia***

INTEG: Rash, urticaria

Contraindications: Hypersensitivity, severe hepatic disease, last few wk of pregnancy

Precautions: Pregnancy (C), neonates

Pharmacokinetics:

PO/INJ: Metabolized, crosses placenta

Interactions:

• Decreased action of phytonadione: cholestyramine, mineral oil

• Decreased action of oral anticoagulants

NURSING CONSIDERATIONS
Assess:

• For bleeding: emesis, stools, urine

• Pro-time during treatment (2-sec deviation from control time, bleeding time, and clotting time); monitor for bleeding, pulse, and B/P

• Nutritional status: liver (beef), spinach, tomatoes, coffee, asparagus, broccoli, cabbage, lettuce, greens

---

Administer:

IV

• After diluting with D_5NS 10 ml or more; give 1 mg/min or more

◆ IV only when other routes not possible (deaths have occurred)

Additive compatibilities: Amikacin, calcium gluceptate, cephapirin, chloramphenicol, cimetidine, netilmicin, sodium bicarbonate

Syringe compatibilities: Doxapram

Y-site compatibilities: Ampicillin, epinephrine, famotidine, heparin, hydrocortisone, potassium chloride, tolazoline, vit B/C

Perform/provide:

• Storage in tight, light-resistant container

Evaluate:

• Therapeutic response: decreased bleeding tendencies, decreased protime, decreased clotting time

Teach patient/family:

• Not to take other supplements unless directed by prescriber

• The necessary foods for diet

• To avoid IM injections, use soft toothbrush, don't floss, use electric razor until coagulation defect corrected

• To report symptoms of bleeding

• Not to use OTC medications unless approved by prescriber

• The importance of frequent lab tests to monitor coagulation factors

---

pindolol (R)

(pin'doe-lole)

Novo-Pindol*, Syn-Pindolol*, Visken

Func. class.: Antihypertensive

Chem. class.: Nonselective β-blocker

Action: Competitively blocks stimulation of β-adrenergic receptor within vascular smooth muscle; (decreases rate of SA node discharge, increases recovery time), slows conduction of AV node, decreases heart rate, which decreases O_2 consumption in myocardium; also decreases renin-aldosterone-angiotensin system, at high doses inhibits β-2 receptors in bronchial system

Uses: Mild to moderate hypertension

Investigational uses: Mitral valve prolapse, hypertrophic cardiomyopathy, angina pectoris, ventricular dysrhythmias, anxiety

Dosage and routes:

• *Adult:* **PO** 5 mg bid, usual dose 15 mg/day (5 mg tid), may increase by 10 mg/day q3-4wk to a max of 60 mg/day

• *Geriatric:* **PO** 5 mg qd, increase by 5 mg q3-4wk

Available forms: Tabs 5, 10 mg

Side effects/adverse reactions:

CV: Hypotension, bradycardia, **CHF,** edema, chest pain, palpitation, claudication, tachycardia, **AV block**

CNS: Insomnia, dizziness, hallucinations, anxiety, fatigue

GI: Nausea, vomiting, **ischemic colitis,** diarrhea, *abdominal pain,* **mesenteric arterial thrombosis**

INTEG: Rash, alopecia, pruritus, fever

HEMA: **Agranulocytosis, thrombocytopenia, purpura**

EENT: Visual changes, sore throat, *double vision;* dry, burning eyes

GU: Impotence, urinary frequency

RESP: **Bronchospasm,** *dyspnea,* cough, rales

MISC: Joint pain, muscle pain

Contraindications: Hypersensitivity to β-blockers, cardiogenic shock; 2nd, 3rd degree heart block; sinus bradycardia, CHF, cardiac failure, bronchial asthma

Precautions: Major surgery, pregnancy (B), lactation, diabetes mellitus, renal disease, thyroid disease,

---

◆ = Nursing alert   ▱ = Herb-drug interaction   ○ = Do not crush

COPD, well-compensated heart failure, CAD, nonallergic bronchospasm

Pharmacokinetics:

PO: Peak 2-4 wk; half-life 3-4 hr, excreted 30%-45% unchanged; 60%-65% metabolized by liver; excreted in breast milk

Interactions:

• Increased hypotension, bradycardia: reserpine, hydralazine, methyldopa, prazosin, anticholinergics

• Decreased antihypertensive effects: NSAIDs, sympathomimetics, thyroid

• Increased hypoglycemic effect: insulin, oral hypoglycemics

• Decreased bronchodilation: theophyllines, β_2-agonists

Lab test interferences:

Increase: Liver function tests, renal function tests

NURSING CONSIDERATIONS

Assess:

• I&O, weight qd

• B/P during initial treatment, periodically thereafter; pulse q4h, note rate, rhythm, quality; apical, radial pulse before administration; notify prescriber of any significant changes

• Baselines in renal, liver function tests before therapy begins

• Skin turgor, dryness of mucous membranes for hydration status; edema in feet, legs qd

Administer:

• PO ac, hs; tablet may be crushed or swallowed whole

• Reduced dosage in renal dysfunction

Perform/provide:

• Storage in dry area at room temp; do not freeze

Evaluate:

• Therapeutic response: decreased B/P after 1-2 wk

Teach patient/family:

• To take with or immediately after meals

• Not to discontinue drug abruptly; taper over 2 wk; may cause precipitate angina

• Not to use OTC products containing α-adrenergic stimulants (nasal decongestants, OTC cold preparations) unless directed by prescriber

• To report bradycardia, dizziness, confusion, depression, fever, sore throat, shortness of breath to prescriber

• To take pulse at home; to notify prescriber if pulse <60 BPM

• To avoid alcohol, smoking, Na

• To comply with weight control, dietary adjustments, modified exercise program

• To carry Medic Alert ID to identify drug, allergies

• To avoid hazardous activities if dizziness is present

• To report symptoms of CHF: difficult breathing, especially on exertion or when lying down, night cough, swelling of extremities

• To take medication at bedtime to prevent orthostatic hypotension

• To wear support hose to minimize effects of orthostatic hypotension

Treatment of overdose: Lavage, IV atropine for bradycardia, IV theophylline for bronchospasm, digitalis, O_2, diuretic for cardiac failure, hemodialysis, hypotension; give vasopressor (norepinephrine)

---

pioglitazone
See appendix a—selected new drugs

---

pipecuronium (R)

(pip-e-kyoor-oh'nee-um)

Arduran

Func. class.: Neuromuscular blocker (nondepolarizing)

Chem. class.: Synthetic curariform

Action: Inhibits transmission of nerve impulses by binding with cholinergic receptor sites, antagonizing action of acetylcholine

Uses: Facilitation of endotracheal intubation; skeletal muscle relaxation during mechanical ventilation, surgery, or general anesthesia

Dosage and routes:

• *Adult:* **IV** dosage is individualized; in patients with normal renal function who are not obese, initial dose is 70-85 µg/kg; maintenance dose ranges from 10-15 µg/kg

• *Child 1-14 yr:* **IV** 57 µg/kg

• *Child 3 mo-1 yr:* **IV** 40 µg/kg

Available forms: Inj 10 mg vials

Side effects/adverse reactions:

CV: Bradycardia, tachycardia, increased or decreased B/P, ventricular extrasystole, *myocardial ischemia, cardiovascular accident, thrombosis, atrial fibrillation*

RESP: Prolonged apnea, bronchospasm, cyanosis, respiratory depression

GU: Anuria

EENT: Increased secretions

CNS: Hypesthesia, CNS depression

MS: Weakness to prolonged skeletal muscle relaxation

INTEG: Rash, urticaria

META: Hypoglycemia, hyperkalemia, increased creatinine

Contraindications: Hypersensitivity to bromide ion

Precautions: Pregnancy (C), renal disease, cardiac disease, lactation, children <3 mo, fluid and electrolyte imbalances, neuromuscular diseases, respiratory disease, obesity

Pharmacokinetics:

IV: Onset 30-45 sec, peak 3-5 min: metabolized (small amounts), excreted in urine (unchanged), crosses placenta

Interactions:

• Increased neuromuscular blockade: aminoglycosides, quinidine, local anesthetics, polymyxin antibiotics, enflurane, isoflurane, tetracyclines, halothane, magnesium, colistin

NURSING CONSIDERATIONS

Assess:

• For electrolyte imbalances (K, Mg); may lead to increased action of this drug

• Vital signs (B/P, pulse, respirations, airway) until fully recovered; rate, depth, pattern of respirations; strength of hand grip

• I&O ratio; check for urinary retention, frequency, hesitancy

• Recovery: decreased paralysis of face, diaphragm, leg, arm, rest of body

• Allergic reactions: rash, fever, respiratory distress, pruritus; drug should be discontinued

Administer:

• Using nerve stimulator by anesthesiologist to determine neuromuscular blockade

• Atropine to counteract muscarinic effects

• After succinylcholine effects subside

• Anticholinesterase to reverse neuromuscular blockade

IV

• By slow IV over 1-2 min (only by qualified persons, usually an anesthesiologist)

• Only fresh sol

Perform/provide:

• Storage in refrigerator; do not store in plastic container or syringe

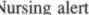 = Nursing alert   // = Herb-drug interaction   ⃠ = Do not crush

• Reassurance if communication is difficult during recovery from neuromuscular blockade
• Use of reconstituted sol within 24 hr or discard
• Frequent (q2h) instillation of artificial tears and covering eyes to prevent drying of cornea

Evaluate:
• Therapeutic response: paralysis of jaw, eyelid, head, neck, rest of body

Treatment of overdose: Neostigmine, atropine; monitor VS; may require mechanical ventilation

---

piperacillin (R)

(pip′er-ah-sill′in)
Pipracil
Func. class.: Broad-spectrum antiinfective
Chem. class.: Extended-spectrum penicillin

Action: Interferes with cell wall replication of susceptible organisms; osmotically unstable cell wall swells and bursts from osmotic pressure

Uses: Respiratory, skin, urinary tract, bone infections; gonorrhea; pneumonia; effective for gram-positive cocci *(Staphylococcus aureus, Streptococcus pyogenes, S. viridans, S. faecalis, S. bovis, S. pneumoniae),* gram-negative cocci *(Neisseria gonorrhoeae, Neisseria meningitidis),* gram-positive bacilli *(Acinetobacter, Clostridium perfringens, C. tetani),* gram-negative bacilli *(Bacteroides, Citrobacter, Enterobacter, Escherichia coli, Eubacterium, Fusobacterium nucleatum, Klebsiella, Morganella morganii, Peptococcus, Peptostreptococcus, Proteus mirabilis, P. vulgaris, P. rettgeri, Pseudomonas aeruginosa, Serratia)*

Dosage and routes:
Renal dose
• CrCl 20-40 ml/min give q8h; CrCl <20 ml/min give q12h
Urinary tract infections
• *Adult:* **IV** 8-16 g/day (125-200 mg/kg/day) in divided doses q6-8h
Serious systemic infections
• *Adult and child >12 yr:* **IM/IV** 2-4 g q4-6h (2 g/site **IM**)
• *Child< 12 yr:* **IM/IV** 200-300 mg/kg/day in divided doses q4-6h
• *Neonates < 36 wk:* **IV** 75 mg/kg q12h in the 1st wk of life, then q8h in 2nd wk
• *Full-term infants:* **IV** 75 mg/kg q8h in 1st wk of life, then q6h thereafter
Prophylaxis of surgical infections
• *Adult:* **IV** 2 g ½-1 hr before procedure; may be repeated during surgery or after surgery
Available forms: Powder for inj 2, 3, 4, 40 g

Side effects/adverse reactions:
HEMA: Anemia, increased bleeding time, ***bone marrow depression,*** thrombocytopenia
GI: Nausea, vomiting, diarrhea; increased AST, ALT; abdominal pain, glossitis, colitis
GU: ***Oliguria, proteinuria, hematuria,*** *vaginitis, moniliasis,* ***glomerulonephritis***
CNS: Lethargy, hallucinations, anxiety, depression, twitching, ***coma, convulsions***
META: Hypokalemia, hypernatremia

Contraindications: Hypersensitivity to penicillins

Precautions: Pregnancy (B), lactation, hypersensitivity to cephalosporins; CHF, renal disease

Pharmacokinetics:
IM: Peak 30-50 min
IV: Peak 20-30 min
Half-life 0.7-1.33 hr; excreted in

P

---

urine, bile, breast milk; crosses placenta

Interactions:

• Decreased antimicrobial effect of piperacillin: tetracyclines (with high concentrations of piperacillin), aminoglycosides

• Increased piperacillin concentrations: aspirin, probenecid

⚕ Delayed/reduced absorption: khat, separate by ≥2 hr

Lab test interferences:

False positive: Urine glucose, urine protein, Coombs' test

NURSING CONSIDERATIONS
Assess:

• For infection: temp, WBC, sputum, stools, urine, wounds

• I&O ratio; report hematuria, oliguria, since penicillin in high doses is nephrotoxic

◆ Any patient with compromised renal system, since drug is excreted slowly in poor renal system function; toxicity may occur rapidly

• Liver studies: AST, ALT

• Blood studies: WBC, RBC, Hgb, Hct, bleeding time prior to and periodically during treatment

• Renal studies: urinalysis, protein, blood, BUN, creatinine prior to and periodically during treatment

• C&S before drug therapy; drug may be taken as soon as culture is taken

• Bowel pattern before and during treatment

• Skin eruptions after administration of penicillin to 1 wk after discontinuing drug

• Respiratory status: rate, character, wheezing, tightness in chest

• Allergies before initiation of treatment, reaction of each medication; highlight allergies on chart

Administer:

• Drug after C&S completed

IM

• 2 g/4 ml, 3 g/6 ml, 4 g/8 ml of sterile water, 0.9% NaCl max 2 g/site

IV

• After diluting 1 g or less/5 ml or more sterile H_2O or 0.9% NaCl; shake; give dose over 3-5 min; may further dilute to 50-100 ml with D_5W, 0.9% NS, and give over ½ hr; discontinue primary IV

Additive compatibilities: Ciprofloxacin, clindamycin, flucloxacillin, fluconazole, hydrocortisone, ofloxacin, potassium chloride, verapamil

Syringe compatibilities: Heparin

Y-site compatibilities: Acyclovir, allopurinol, amifostine, aztreonam, ciprofloxacin, cyclophosphamide, diltiazem, doxorubicin liposome, enalaprilat, esmolol, famotidine, fludarabine, foscarnet, gallium, granisetron, heparin, hydromorphone, IL-2, labetalol, lorazepam, magnesium sulfate, melphalan, meperidine, midazolam, morphine, perphenazine, propofol, ranitidine, remifentanil, tacrolimus, teniposide, theophylline, thiotepa, verapamil, zidovudine

Perform/provide:

• Adrenaline, suction, tracheostomy set, endotracheal intubation equipment on unit

• Adequate intake of fluids (2 L) during diarrhea episodes

• Scratch test to assess allergy after securing order from prescriber; usually done when penicillin is only drug of choice

• Storage of reconstituted sol 24 hr at room temp or 7 days refrigerated

Evaluate:

• Therapeutic response: absence of fever, purulent drainage, redness, inflammation

Teach patient/family:

• That culture may be taken after completed course of medication

◆ = Nursing alert   ⚕ = Herb-drug interaction   ⊘ = Do not crush

- To report sore throat, fever, fatigue; may indicate superinfection
- To wear or carry Medic Alert ID if allergic to penicillins
- To notify nurse of diarrhea

Treatment of anaphylaxis: Withdraw drug, maintain airway, administer epinephrine, aminophylline, O₂, IV corticosteroids

piperacillin and tazobactam (℞)

(pip′er-ah-sill′in & ta-zoe-bak′tam)
Zosyn

Func. class.: Antiinfective, broad-spectrum

Chem. class.: Extended-spectrum penicillin, β-lactamase inhibitor

Action: Interferes with cell wall replication of susceptible organisms; osmotically unstable cell wall swells and bursts from osmotic pressure

Uses: Moderate to severe infections: piperacillin-resistant, β-lactamase-producing strains causing infections in respiratory, skin, urinary tract, bone, gonorrhea, pneumonia; effective for resistant *Staphylococcus aureus,* resistant *Escherichia coli, Bacteroides fragilis, B. ovatus, B. thetaiotaomicron, B. vulgatus, Haemophilus influenzae*

Dosage and routes:

Renal dose
- CrCl 20-40 ml/min give 2.25 g q6h; CrCl <20 ml/min give 2.25 g q8h

Nosocomial pneumonia
- *Adult:* 3.375g q4h with an aminoglycoside × 1-2 wk; continue aminoglycoside only if *P. aeruginosa* is isolated

Other infections
- *Adult:* **IV INF** 6-12 g/day given

2.25 g q8h to 3.375 g q6h over 30 min × 7-10 days

Available forms: Powder for inj 2 g piperacillin/0.25 g tazobactam, 3 g piperacillin/0.375 g tazobactam, 4 g piperacillin/0.5 g tazobactam, 36 g piperacillin/4.5 g tazobactam

Side effects/adverse reactions:

CNS: Lethargy, hallucinations, anxiety, depression, twitching, ***coma, convulsions,*** insomnia, headache, fever, dizziness

GI: *Nausea, vomiting, diarrhea;* increased AST, ALT; abdominal pain, glossitis, colitis, constipation

GU: ***Oliguria, proteinuria, hematuria,*** *vaginitis, moniliasis,* ***glomerulonephritis***

HEMA: Anemia, increased bleeding time, ***bone marrow depression***

META: Hypokalemia, hypernatremia

CV: Hypertension

INTEG: Rash, pruritus

Contraindications: Hypersensitivity to penicillins, neonates

Precautions: Pregnancy (B), lactation, hypersensitivity to cephalosporins, CHF

Pharmacokinetics:

IV: Peak completion of IV, duration 6 hr

Half-life 0.7-1.2 hr; excreted in urine, bile, breast milk; crosses placenta; 33% bound to plasma proteins

Interactions:
- Increased effect of neuromuscular blockers, heparin
- Decreased antimicrobial effect of piperacillin: tetracyclines, aminoglycosides IV
- Increased piperacillin concentrations: aspirin, probenecid

⚠ Delayed/reduced absorption: khat, separate by ≥2 hr

Lab test interferences:

False positive: Urine glucose, urine protein, Coombs' test

Decrease: Hct, Hgb, electrolytes

Increase: Platelet count, eosinophilia, neutropenia, leukopenia, serum creatinine, PTT, AST, ALT, alk phosphatase, bilirubin, BUN, electrolytes

NURSING CONSIDERATIONS

Assess:

• For infection: temp, stools, urine, sputum, wounds
• I&O ratio; report hematuria, oliguria, since penicillin in high doses is nephrotoxic

◆ Any patient with compromised renal system, since drug is excreted slowly in poor renal system function; toxicity may occur rapidly

• Liver studies: AST, ALT prior to and periodically thereafter
• Blood studies: WBC, RBC, Hct, Hgb, bleeding time prior to and periodically thereafter
• Renal studies: urinalysis, protein, blood, BUN, creatinine prior to and periodically thereafter
• C&S before drug therapy; drug may be given as soon as culture is taken
• Bowel pattern before and during treatment
• Skin eruptions after administration of penicillin to 1 wk after discontinuing drug
• Respiratory status: rate, character, wheezing, tightness in chest
• Allergies before initiation of treatment, reaction of each medication; highlight allergies on chart

Administer:

• Drug after C&S is complete

IV

• After diluting 5 ml 0.9% NaCl for injection or sterile H_2O for injection, dextran 6% in NS, dextrose 5%, KCl 40 mEq, bacteriostatic saline/parabens, bacteriostatic saline/benzyl alcohol, bacteriostatic H_2O/benzyl alcohol per 1 g piperacillin; shake well; further dilute in at least 50 ml compatible IV sol and run as int inf over at least 30 min

Y-site compatibilities: Aminophylline, aztreonam, bleomycin, bumetanide, buprenorphine, butorphanol, calcium gluconate, carboplatin, carmustine, cefepime, cimetidine, clindamycin, cyclophosphamide, cytarabine, dexamethasone, diphenhydramine, dopamine, enalaprilat, etoposide, floxuridine, fluconazole, fludarabine, fluorouracil, furosemide, gallium, granisetron, heparin, hydrocortisone, hydromorphone, ifosfamide, leucovorin, lorazepam, magnesium sulfate, mannitol, meperidine, mesna, methotrexate, methylprednisolone, metoclopramide, metronidazole, morphine, ondansetron, plicamycin, potassium chloride, ranitidine, remifentanil, sargramostim, sodium bicarbonate, thiotepa, trimethoprim-sulfamethoxazole, vinblastine, vincristine, zidovudine

Perform/provide:

• Adrenaline, suction, tracheostomy set, endotracheal intubation equipment on unit
• Adequate intake of fluids (2 L) during diarrhea episodes
• Scratch test to assess allergy on order from prescriber; usually when penicillin is only drug of choice
• Discard after 24 hr if stored at room temp or after 48 hr if refrigerated; use single-dose vials immediately after reconstitution; stable in ambulatory IV pump for 12 hr

Evaluate:

• Therapeutic response: absence of fever, purulent drainage, redness, inflammation; culture shows decreased organisms

Teach patient/family:

• That culture may be taken after completed course of medication
• To report sore throat, fever, fatigue (may indicate superinfection)

◆ = Nursing alert   ⦅/⦆ = Herb-drug interaction   ⊘ = Do not crush

• To wear or carry Medic Alert ID if allergic to penicillins
• To notify nurse of diarrhea
Treatment of overdose: Withdraw drug, maintain airway, administer epinephrine, aminophylline, O_2, IV corticosteroids for anaphylaxis

---

pirbuterol (℞)
(peer-byoo'ter-ole)
Maxair
Func. class.: Bronchodilator
Chem. class.: β-adrenergic agonist

Action: Causes bronchodilation with little effect on heart rate by action on β-receptors, causing increased cAMP and relaxation of smooth muscle
Uses: Reversible bronchospasm (prevention, treatment) including asthma; may be given with theophylline or steroids
Dosage and routes:
• *Adult and child >12 yr:* **INH** 1-2 puffs (0.4 mg) q4-6h; max 12 **INH**/day
Available forms: Aerosol delivery 0.2 mg pirbuterol/actuation
Side effects/adverse reactions:
CNS: Tremors, anxiety, insomnia, headache, dizziness, stimulation, restlessness, hallucinations, drowsiness, irritability
EENT: Dry nose and mouth, irritation of nose, throat
CV: Palpitations, tachycardia, hypertension, angina, hypotension, dysrhythmias
GI: Gastritis, nausea, vomiting, anorexia
MS: Muscle cramps
RESP: **Paradoxical bronchospasm,** dyspnea, coughing
Contraindications: Hypersensitivity to sympathomimetics, tachycardia

Precautions: Lactation, pregnancy (C), cardiac disorders, hyperthyroidism, diabetes mellitus, prostatic hypertrophy
Pharmacokinetics:
INH: Onset 3 min, peak ½-1 hr, duration 5 hr
Interactions:
• Increased action of other aerosol bronchodilators
• Increased action of pirbuterol: tricyclic antidepressants, antihistamines, levothyroxine
• Decreased action of pirbuterol: β-blockers
◆ Hypertensive crisis: MAOIs
✎ Increased action of both: ephedra
NURSING CONSIDERATIONS
Assess:
• Respiratory function: vital capacity, forced expiratory volume, ABGs, B/P, lung sounds, pulse, characteristics of sputum
Administer:
• After shaking; exhale, place mouthpiece in mouth, inhale slowly, hold breath, remove, exhale slowly
• Gum, sips of water for dry mouth
Perform/provide:
• Storage in light-resistant container; do not expose to temps over 86° F (30° C)
Evaluate:
• Therapeutic response: absence of dyspnea, wheezing over 1 hr
Teach patient/family:
• Not to use OTC medications; extra stimulation may occur
• Use of inhaler; review package insert with patient
• To avoid getting aerosol in eyes
• To wash inhaler in warm water and dry qd, rinse mouth after use; if used with inhalers containing glucocorticosteroids, wait 5 min before using steroid inhaler
• About all aspects of drug; avoid smoking, smoke-filled rooms, persons with respiratory infections

• To keep fluid intake >2 L/day to liquefy thick secretions

Treatment of overdose: Administer a β-adrenergic blocker

---

piroxicam (R)

(peer-ox′i-kam)

Apo-Piroxicam*, Feldene, Novopirocam*, Nu-Pirox

Func. class.: Nonsteroidal antiinflammatory

Chem. class.: Oxicam derivative

Action: Inhibits prostaglandin synthesis by decreasing an enzyme needed for biosynthesis; has analgesic, antiinflammatory, antipyretic properties

Uses: Mild to moderate pain, osteoarthritis, rheumatoid arthritis

Dosage and routes:

• *Adult:* **PO** 20 mg qd or 10 mg bid

Available forms: Caps 10, 20 mg

Side effects/adverse reactions:

GI: Nausea, anorexia, vomiting, diarrhea, jaundice, **cholestatic hepatitis,** constipation, flatulence, cramps, dry mouth, peptic ulcer, **bleeding, ulceration, perforation**

CNS: Dizziness, *drowsiness,* fatigue, tremors, confusion, insomnia, anxiety, depression, *headache*

CV: Tachycardia, peripheral edema, palpitations, dysrhythmias

INTEG: Purpura, rash, pruritus, sweating, photosensitivity

GU: **Nephrotoxicity: dysuria, hematuria, oliguria, azotemia**

HEMA: **Blood dyscrasias**

EENT: Tinnitus, hearing loss, blurred vision

Contraindications: Hypersensitivity, asthma, severe renal disease, severe hepatic disease, ulcer disease, cardiac disease

Precautions: Pregnancy (C), lactation, children, bleeding disorders, GI disorders, cardiac disorders, hypersensitivity to other antiinflammatory agents, CHF

Pharmacokinetics:

PO: Peak 2 hr; duration 48-72 hr; half-life 30-80 hr; metabolized in liver; excreted in urine (metabolites), breast milk; 99% protein binding

Interactions:

• Increased toxicity: cyclosporine, methotrexate, lithium, alcohol, oral anticoagulants, aspirin, corticosteroids

• Decreased effects of: antihypertensives, diuretics

• Hypoglycemia: oral antidiabetics

NURSING CONSIDERATIONS

Assess:

• For pain: location, duration, type, ROM before and 1-2 hr after administration

• Renal, liver, blood studies: BUN, creatinine, AST, ALT, Hgb, before treatment, periodically thereafter

• Audiometric, ophthalmic exam before, during, after treatment

• For eye, ear problems: blurred vision, tinnitus (may indicate toxicity)

• Those with aspirin sensitivity, asthma, nasal polyps may develop allergic reactions

Administer:

• With food to decrease GI symptoms; best to take on empty stomach to facilitate absorption; take drug same time qd

Perform/provide:

• Storage at room temp

Evaluate:

• Therapeutic response: decreased pain, stiffness, swelling in joints; ability to move more easily

Teach patient/family:

🚫 Not to break, crush, or chew caps

• To report blurred vision or ring-

◆ = Nursing alert   ∅ = Herb-drug interaction   🚫 = Do not crush

ing, roaring in ears (may indicate toxicity)
• To avoid driving, other hazardous activities if dizzy or drowsy
• That patient should drink at least 6-8 glasses of water/day
• To report change in urine pattern, weight increase, edema, pain increase in joints, fever, blood in urine (indicates nephrotoxicity)
• That therapeutic effects may take up to 1 mo
• To avoid ASA, other OTC meds, alcohol; advise patient to use sunscreen

---

plasma protein fraction (℞)

Plasmanate, Plasma Plex, Plasmatein, Protenate
Func. class.: Blood derivative
Chem. class.: Human plasma in NaCl

Action: Exerts similar oncotic pressure as human plasma, expands blood volume
Uses: Hypovolemic shock, hypoproteinemia, ARDS, preoperative cardiopulmonary bypass, acute liver failure, nephrotic syndrome
Dosage and routes:

Hypovolemia
• *Adult:* **IV INF** 250-500 ml (12.5-25 g protein), not to exceed 10 ml/min
• *Child:* **IV INF** 22-33 ml/kg at 5-10 ml/min

Hypoproteinemia
• *Adult:* **IV INF** 1000-1500 ml qd, not to exceed 8 ml/min
Available forms: Inj 5%
Side effects/adverse reactions:

GI: Nausea, vomiting, increased salivation
INTEG: Rash, urticaria, cyanosis

CNS: Fever, chills, headache, paresthesias, flushing
RESP: Altered respirations, dyspnea, ***pulmonary edema***
CV: ***Fluid overload,*** hypotension, erratic pulse
Contraindications: Hypersensitivity, CHF, severe anemia, renal insufficiency
Precautions: Decreased salt intake, decreased cardiac reserve, lack of albumin deficiency, hepatic disease, renal disease, pregnancy (C)
Pharmacokinetics: Metabolized as a protein/energy source
Lab test interferences:

False increase: Alk phosphatase
NURSING CONSIDERATIONS
Assess:
• Blood studies: Hct, Hgb, electrolytes, serum protein; if serum protein declines, dyspnea, hypoxemia can result
• B/P (decreased), pulse (erratic), respiration during infusion
• I&O ratio; urinary output may decrease
• CVP, pulmonary wedge pressure (increases if overload occurs), jugular vein distention
• Allergy: fever, rash, itching, chills, flushing, urticaria, nausea, vomiting, or hypotension requires discontinuation of infusion; use new lot if therapy reinstituted
⬧ Increased CVP reading: distended neck veins indicate circulatory overload; SOB, anxiety, insomnia, expiratory rales, frothy blood-tinged cough, cyanosis indicate pulmonary overload
Administer:
IV
• No dilution required; use infusion pump, use large-gauge needle (≥20G), discard unused portion, infuse slowly
• Within 4 hr of opening

P

Additive compatibilities: Carbohydrate and electrolyte sol, whole blood, packed red blood cells, chloramphenicol, tetracycline
Perform/provide:

• Adequate hydration before administration

• Storage—check type of albumin, date; may have to refrigerate
Evaluate:

• Therapeutic response: increased B/P, decreased edema, increased serum albumin

---

plicamycin (℞)

(ply-ka-my'sin)
Mithramycin, Mithracin
Func. class.: Antineoplastic, antibiotic; hypocalcemic
Chem. class.: Crystalline aglycone

Action: Inhibits DNA, RNA, protein synthesis; derived from *Streptomyces plicatus;* replication is decreased by binding to DNA; demonstrates calcium-lowering effect not related to its tumoricidal activity; also acts on osteoclasts and blocks action of parathyroid hormone; a vesicant

Uses: Testicular cancer, hypercalcemia, hypercalciuria, symptomatic treatment of advanced neoplasms
Dosage and routes:
Testicular tumors

• *Adult:* **IV** 25-30 µg/kg/day × 8-10 days, not to exceed 30 µg/kg/day
Hypercalcemia/hypercalciuria

• *Adult:* **IV** 25 µg/kg/day × 3-4 days, repeat at intervals of 1 wk
Available forms: Inj 2500 µg/vial powder
Side effects/adverse reactions:
META: Decreased serum Ca, P, K
HEMA: **Hemorrhage, thrombocyto-**

penia, decreased pro-time, WBC count
GI: Nausea, vomiting, anorexia, diarrhea, stomatitis, increased liver enzymes
GU: Increased BUN, creatinine; **proteinuria**
INTEG: Rash, cellulitis, **extravasation,** facial flushing
CNS: Drowsiness, weakness, lethargy, headache, flushing, fever, depression
Contraindications: Hypersensitivity, thrombocytopenia, bone marrow depression, bleeding disorders, pregnancy (X), lactation
Precautions: Renal disease, hepatic disease, electrolyte imbalances
Pharmacokinetics: Crosses blood-brain barrier, excreted in urine; little known about pharmacokinetics
Interactions:

• Increased toxicity: other antineoplastics or radiation
NURSING CONSIDERATIONS
Assess:

• CBC, differential, platelet count qwk; withhold drug if WBC is <4000/mm^3 or platelet count is <50,000/mm^3; notify prescriber

• Renal function studies: BUN, serum uric acid, urine CrCl, electrolytes before, during therapy

• I&O ratio; report urine output <30 ml/hr

• Monitor temp q4h; fever may indicate beginning infection

• Liver function tests before, during therapy: bilirubin, AST, ALT, alk phosphatase prn or qmo; jaundiced skin, sclera; dark urine, clay-colored stools; itchy skin, abdominal pain, fever, diarrhea

• Alkalosis if severe vomiting is present

◆ Toxicity: facial flushing, epistaxis, increased pro-time, thrombocytopenia; drug should be discontinued

---

◆ = Nursing alert   🖉 = Herb-drug interaction   ⊘ = Do not crush

• Bleeding: hematuria, guaiac stools, bruising or petechiae, mucosa or orifices q8h
• Inflammation of mucosa, breaks in skin
• Buccal cavity q8h for dryness, sores, ulceration, white patches, oral pain, bleeding, dysphagia
• Local irritation, pain, burning at injection site
• Frequency of stools, characteristics, cramping
• Acidosis, signs of dehydration: rapid respirations, poor skin turgor, decreased urine output, dry skin, restlessness, weakness

Administer:
• Antiemetic 30-60 min before giving drug and 4-10 hr after treatment to prevent vomiting
• Transfusion for anemia
• Antispasmodic for diarrhea, phenothiazine for nausea and vomiting
IV
• Dilute 2.5 mg/4.9 ml of sterile H_2O; (500 µg/ml) dilute single dose in 1000 ml of D_5W run over 4-6 hr
• EDTA for extravasation, apply ice compress
• Slow IV infusion using 20G, 21G needle

Y-site compatibilities: Allopurinol, amifostine, aztreonam, filgrastim, granisetron, melphalan, piperacillin/tazobactam, teniposide, thiotepa, vinorelbine

Perform/provide:
• Liquid diet: carbonated beverages; gelatin may be added if patient is not nauseated or vomiting
• Rinsing of mouth tid-qid with water; brushing of teeth with baking soda bid-tid with soft brush or cotton-tipped applicator for stomatitis; unwaxed dental floss
• Usage immediately after mixing

Evaluate:
• Therapeutic response: decreased tumor size, spread of malignancy

Teach patient/family:
• To report any complaints or side effects to nurse or prescriber
• To avoid foods with citric acid, hot or rough texture
• To report to prescriber any bleeding, white spots, ulcerations in the mouth; tell patient to examine mouth qd
• To avoid driving, activities requiring alertness; drowsiness may occur
• To report leg cramps, tingling of fingertips, weakness; may indicate hypocalcemia
• To avoid crowds, persons with infections when granulocyte count is low

---

poliovirus vaccine, live, oral, trivalent (TOPV) (R)
Orimune
poliovirus vaccine, (IPV) (R)
IPOL
Func. class.: Vaccine

Action: Produces specific antibodies for poliomyelitis

Uses: Prevention of polio

Dosage and routes:
• *Adult and child >2 yr:* **PO** 0.5 ml, given q8wk × 2 doses, then 0.5 ml ½-1 yr after dose 2
• *Infant:* **PO** 0.5 ml at 2, 4, 18 mo; booster at 4-6 yr; may also be given: **IPV** at 2, 4 mo, then **OPV** at 12-18 mo, booster at 4-6 yr

Available forms: Oral vaccine; 0.5 ml single dose; Dispettes; inactivated inj 0.5 ml prefilled syringes

Side effects/adverse reactions:
*SYST: **Paralysis***

Contraindications: Hypersensitivity, active infection, allergy to neomycin/streptomycin, immunosuppression, vomiting, or diarrhea

P

Precautions: Pregnancy (C)
Interactions:

• Do not use TB skin test or other live virus vaccines within 6 wk of vaccine

• Do not use within 3 mo of transfusion of whole blood, plasma, or use with immune serum globulin

NURSING CONSIDERATIONS
Assess:

• For anaphylaxis: inability to breathe, bronchospasm

• For allergies to immunizations; immunodeficiency syndrome; do not give (TOPV)

Administer:

• Only PO (TOPV)

• Do not administer within 1 mo of other live virus vaccines

Perform/provide:

• Storage at 7° F (−13° C)

• Written record of immunization

Evalute:

• For history of allergies, skin conditions (eczema, psoriasis, dermatitis), reactions to vaccinations

---

poractant alfa
See appendix a—selected new drugs

---

porfimer (℞)
(pour′fih-mur)
Photofrin
Func. class.: Antineoplastic-miscellaneous

Action: Used in photodynamic treatment of tumors (PDT); antitumor and cytotoxic actions are light and O_2 dependent; used with 630 nm laser light

Uses: Esophageal cancer (completely obstructing), endobronchial non–small cell lung cancer

Dosage and routes:

• Refer to Optiguide for complete instructions

• *Adult:* IV 2 mg/kg, then illumination with laser light 40-50 hr after inj; a second laser light application may be given 96-120 hr after inj; may repeat q30 days × 3

Endobronchial cancer

• *Adult:* 200 joules/cm of tumor length

Available forms: Cake/powder for inj 75 mg

Side effects/adverse reactions:

*CV: Hypotension, hypertension, atrial fibrillation, **cardiac failure,** tachycardia*

GI: Abdominal pain, constipation, diarrhea, dyspepsia, dysphagia, eructation, esophageal edema/bleeding, hematemesis, melena, nausea, vomiting, anorexia

CNS: Anxiety, confusion, insomnia

*RESP: **Pleural effusion,** pneumonia, dyspnea, respiratory insufficiency, **tracheoesophageal fistula***

MISC: Dehydration, weight decrease, anemia, photosensitivity reaction, UTI, moniliasis

Contraindications: Porphyria, porphyrin allergy (porfimer); tracheoesophageal, bronchoesophageal fistula; major blood vessels with eroding tumors (PDT)

Precautions: Elderly, pregnancy (C), lactation, children

Pharmacokinetics: Half-life 250 hr, 90% protein bound

Interactions:

• Increased photosensitivity: tetracyclines, sulfonamides, phenothiazines, sulfonylureas, thiazides, griseofulvin

NURSING CONSIDERATIONS
Assess:

• Ocular sensitivity: sensitivity to sun, bright lights, car headlights, patients should wear dark sunglasses

---

with an average light transmittance of <4%

• Chest pain: may be so severe as to necessitate opiate analgesics

• For extravasation at inj site: take care to protect from light

Administer:

• As a single slow IV inj over 3-5 min at 2 mg/kg; reconstitute each vial with 31.8 ml D$_5$ or 0.9% NaCl (2.5 mg/ml), shake well; do not mix with other drugs or sol; protect from light and use immediately

• Laser light is initiated 630 nm wave length laser light

Perform/provide:

• Wiping of spills with damp cloth, avoid skin/eye contact, use rubber gloves, eye protection, dispose of material in polyethylene bag according to policy

Teach patient/family:

• To report chest pain, eye sensitivity

• To wear sunglasses with average white light transmittance of <4%

potassium acetate
potassium bicarbonate (OTC, ℞)
K+ Care ET, K-Electrolyte, K-Ide, Klor-Con EF, K-Lyte, K-Vescent
potassium bicarbonate and potassium chloride (OTC, ℞)
Klorvess, Klorvess Effervescent Granules, K-Lyte/Cl, Neo-K*
potassium bicarbonate and potassium citrate (OTC, ℞)
Effer-K, K-Lyte DS
potassium chloride (OTC, ℞)
Apo-K*, Cena-K, Gen-K, K+ Care, K+ 10, Kalium Durules*, Kaochlor, Kaochlor S-F, Kaon-Cl, Kay Ciel, KCl, K-Dur, K-Lease, K-Long*, K-Lor, Klor-Con, Klorvess, Klotrix, K-Lyte/C1 powder, K-med, K-Norm, K-Sol, K-tab, Micro-K, Micro-LS, Potasalan, Roychlor, Rum-K, Slow-K, Ten-K
potassium chloride/ potassium bicarbonate/ potassium citrate (OTC, ℞)
Kaochlor Eff
potassium gluconate (OTC, ℞)
Kaon, Kaylixir, K-G Elixir, Potassium-Rougier*
potassium gluconate/ potassium chloride (OTC, ℞)
Kolyum
potassium gluconate/ potassium citrate (OTC, ℞)
Twin-K
Func. class.: Electrolyte
Chem. class.: Potassium

P

Action: Needed for adequate transmission of nerve impulses and cardiac contraction, renal function, intracellular ion maintenance

Uses: Prevention and treatment of hypokalemia

Dosage and routes:

Potassium bicarbonate

• *Adult:* PO dissolve 25-50 mEq in water qd-qid

Potassium acetate—hypokalemia

• *Adult and child:* PO 40-100 mEq/day in divided doses 2-4 days

Hypokalemia (prevention)

• *Adult and child:* PO 20 mEq/day in 2-4 divided doses

Potassium chloride

• *Adult:* PO 40-100 mEq in divided doses tid-qid; IV 20 mEq/hr when diluted as 40 mEq/1000 ml, not to exceed 150 mEq/day

• *Child:* PO 2-4 mEq/kg/day

Potassium gluconate

• *Adult:* PO 40-100 mEq in divided doses tid-qid

Potassium phosphate

• *Adult:* IV 1 mEq/hr in sol of 60 mEq/L, not to exceed 150 mEq/day; PO 40-100 mEq/day in divided doses

• *Child:* IV max rate of inf 1 mEq/kg/hr

Available forms: Tabs for sol 6.5, 25 mEq; caps, ext rel 8, 10 mEq; powder for sol 3.3, 5, 6.7, 10, 13.3 mEq/5 ml; tabs 2, 4, 5, 13.4 mEq; tabs, ext rel 6.7, 8, 10 mEq; elix 6.7 mEq/5 ml; oral sol 2.375 mEq/5 ml; inj for prep of IV 1.5, 2, 2.4, 3, 3.2, 4.4, 4.7 mEq/ml

Side effects/adverse reactions:

CNS: Confusion

CV: Bradycardia, *cardiac depression, dysrhythmias, arrest, peaking T waves, lowered R and depressed RST, prolonged P-R interval, widened QRS complex*

GI: Nausea, vomiting, cramps, pain, *diarrhea,* ulceration of small bowel

GU: Oliguria

INTEG: Cold extremities, rash

Contraindications: Renal disease (severe), severe hemolytic disease, Addison's disease, hyperkalemia, acute dehydration, extensive tissue breakdown

Precautions: Cardiac disease, K-sparing diuretic therapy, systemic acidosis, pregnancy (A)

Pharmacokinetics:

PO: Excreted by kidneys and in feces; onset of action ≈30 min

IV: Immediate onset of action

Interactions:

• Hyperkalemia: potassium phosphate IV and products containing Ca or Mg; K-sparing, diuretic, or other K products

NURSING CONSIDERATIONS

Assess:

• ECG for peaking T waves, lowered R, depressed RST, prolonged P-R interval, widening QRS complex, hyperkalemia; drug should be reduced or discontinued

• K level during treatment (3.5-5 mg/dl is normal level)

• I&O ratio; watch for decreased urinary output; notify prescriber immediately

• Cardiac status: rate, rhythm, CVP, PWP, PAWP, if being monitored directly

Administer:

PO

• With meal or pc; dissolve effervescent tabs, powder in 8 oz cold water or juice; do not give IM, SC

IV

• Through large-bore needle to decrease vein inflammation; check for extravasation

• In large vein, avoiding scalp vein in child (IV)

• IV after diluting in large volume of IV sol and give as an inf, slowly by IV inf to prevent toxicity; never give IV bolus or IM

◆ = Nursing alert   ▮ = Herb-drug interaction   ⊘ = Do not crush

Potassium acetate

Additive compatibilities: Metoclopramide

Y-site compatibilities: Ciprofloxacin

Potassium chloride

Additive compatibilities: Aminophylline, amiodarone, atracurium, bretylium, calcium gluconate, cefepime, cephalothin, cephapirin, chloramphenicol, cimetidine, ciprofloxacin, cisatracurium, clindamycin, cloxacillin, corticotropin, cytarabine, dimenhydrinate, dopamine, doxorubicin liposome, enalaprilat, erythromycin, floxacillin, fluconazole, fosphenytoin, furosemide, heparin, hydrocortisone, isoproterenol, lidocaine, metaraminol, methicillin, methyldopate, metoclopramide, mitoxantrone, nafcillin, netilmicin, norepinephrine, oxacillin, penicillin G potassium, phenylephrine, piperacillin, ranitidine, sodium bicarbonate, thiopental, vancomycin, verapamil, vit B/C

Y-site compatibilities: Acyclovir, aldesleukin, allopurinol, amifostine, aminophylline, amiodarone, ampicillin, amrinone, atropine, aztreonam, betamethasone, calcium gluconate, cefmetazole, cephalothin, cephapirin, chlordiazepoxide, chlorpromazine, ciprofloxacin, cladribine, cyanocobalamin, dexamethasone, digoxin, diltiazem, diphenhydramine, dobutamine, dopamine, droperidol, edrophonium, enalaprilat, epinephrine, esmolol, estrogens, ethacrynate, famotidine, fentanyl, filgrastim, fludarabine, fluorouracil, furosemide, gallium, granisetron, heparin, hydralazine, idarubicin, indomethacin, insulin (regular), isoproterenol, kanamycin, labetalol, lidocaine, lorazepam, magnesium sulfate, melphalan, meperidine, methicillin, methoxamine, methylergonovine, midazolam, minocycline, morphine, neostigmine, norepinephrine, ondansetron, oxacillin, oxytocin, paclitaxel, penicillin G potassium, pentazocine, phytonadione, piperacillin/tazobactam, prednisolone, procainamide, prochlorperazine, propofol, propranolol, pyridostigmine, remifentanil, sargramostim, scopolamine, sodium bicarbonate, succinylcholine, tacrolimus, teniposide, theophylline, thiotepa, trimethaphan, trimethobenzamide, vinorelbine, warfarin, zidovudine

Perform/provide:
• Storage at room temp

Evaluate:
• Therapeutic response: absence of fatigue, muscle weakness; decreased thirst and urinary output; cardiac changes

Teach patient/family:
• To add potassium-rich foods to diet: bananas, orange juice, avocados; whole grains, broccoli, carrots, prunes, cocoa after this medication is discontinued
• To avoid OTC products: antacids, salt substitutes, analgesics, vitamin preparations, unless specifically directed by prescriber
• To report hyperkalemia symptoms (lethargy, confusion, diarrhea, nausea, vomiting, fainting, decreased output) or continued hypokalemia symptoms (fatigue, weakness, polyuria, polydipsia, cardiac changes)
• To take capsules with full glass of liquid
• To dissolve powder or tablet completely in at least 120 ml water or juice
🚫 Not to chew time-rel or ext-rel preparations
• Importance of regular follow-up visits

P

potassium iodide (Ŗ)
Pima, potassium iodide solution, SSKI, Thyro-Block

Func. class.: Thyroid hormone antagonist
Chem. class.: Iodine product

Action: Inhibits secretion of thyroid hormone, fosters colloid accumulation in thyroid follicles, decreases vascularity of gland

Uses: Preparation for thyroidectomy, thyrotoxic crisis, neonatal thyrotoxicosis, radiation protectant, thyroid storm

Dosage and routes:
Thyrotoxic crisis
• *Adult and child:* **PO** 1 ml in water tid after meals (strong iodine sol)
Preparation for thyroidectomy
• *Adult and child:* **PO** 0.1-0.3 ml tid (strong iodine sol) or 5 gtt in water tid pc × 2-3 wk before surgery (potassium iodide sol)

Available forms: Sol 5%, 10%, 21 mg/gtt; tabs 130, 300 mg; inj 10%, 20%; oral syr 325 mg/5 ml; tabs 130 mg*

Side effects/adverse reactions:
ENDO: Hypothyroidism, hyperthyroid adenoma
INTEG: Rash, urticaria, ***angineurotic edema***, acne, mucosal hemorrhage, fever
CNS: Headache, confusion, paresthesias
GI: Nausea, diarrhea, vomiting, small-bowel lesions, upper gastric pain
MS: Myalgia, arthralgia, weakness
EENT: Metallic taste, stomatitis, salivation, periorbital edema, sore teeth and gums, cold symptoms

Contraindications: Hypersensitivity to iodine, pulmonary edema, pulmonary TB, pregnancy (D)
Precautions: Lactation, children

Pharmacokinetics:
PO: Onset 24-48 hr, peak 10-15 days after continuous therapy, uptake by thyroid gland or excreted in urine; crosses placenta
Interactions:
• Hypothyroidism: lithium, other antithyroid agents
Lab test interferences:
Interference: Urinary 17-OHCS
NURSING CONSIDERATIONS
Assess:
• Pulse, B/P, temp
• I&O ratio; check for edema: puffy hands, feet, periorbit; indicate hypothyroidism
• Weight qd; same clothing, scale, time of day
• T_3, T_4, which is increased; serum TSH, which is decreased; free thyroxine index, which is increased if dosage is too low; discontinue drug 3-4 wk before RAIU
◆ Overdose: peripheral edema, heat intolerance, diaphoresis, palpitations, dysrhythmias, severe tachycardia, fever, delirium, CNS irritability
• Hypersensitivity: rash; enlarged cervical lymph nodes may indicate drug should be discontinued
• Hypoprothrombinemia: bleeding, petechiae, ecchymosis
• Clinical response: after 3 wk should include increased weight, pulse; decreased T_4
Administer:
• Strong iodine solution after diluting with water or juice to improve taste
• Through straw to prevent tooth discoloration
• With meals to decrease GI upset
• At same time each day to maintain drug level
• Lowest dose that relieves symptoms, discontinue before RAIU

◆ = Nursing alert   🖋 = Herb-drug interaction   🚫 = Do not crush

Perform/provide:
• Fluids to 3-4 L/day, unless contraindicated

Evaluate:
• Therapeutic response: weight gain, decreased pulse, T_4, size of thyroid gland

Teach patient/family:
• To abstain from breastfeeding after delivery
• To keep graph of weight, pulse, mood
• To avoid OTC products that contain iodine
• That seafood, other iodine products may be restricted
• Not to discontinue this medication abruptly; thyroid crisis may occur; stress response
• That response may take several mo if thyroid is large
• To discontinue drug, notify prescriber of fever, rash, metallic taste, swelling of throat; burning of mouth, throat; sore gums, teeth; severe GI distress, enlargement of thyroid, cold symptoms

---

pramipexole (℞)
(pra-mi-pex'ol)
Mirapex
Func. class.: Antiparkinson agent
Chem. class.: Dopamine-receptor agonist, non-ergot

Action: Selective agonist for D_2 receptors (presynaptic/postsynaptic sites); binding at D_3 receptor contributes to antiparkinson effects
Uses: Parkinsonism
Dosage and routes:
Initial treatment
• *Adult:* PO from a starting dose of 0.375 mg/day given in 3 divided doses; increase gradually at 5-7 day intervals until total daily dose of 4.5 mg is reached

Maintenance treatment
• *Adult:* PO 1.5-4.5 mg qd in 3 divided doses
Available forms: Tabs 0.125, 0.25, 1.5 mg
Side effects/adverse reactions:
HEMA: **Hemolytic anemia, leukopenia, agranulocytosis**
CNS: Agitation, insomnia, psychosis, hallucination, depression, dizziness
GI: Nausea, anorexia, constipation
CV: Orthostatic hypotension
GU: Impotence
EENT: Blurred vision
Contraindications: Hypersensitivity
Precautions: Renal disease, cardiac disease, MI with dysrhythmias, affective disorders, psychosis, pregnancy (C)
Pharmacokinetics: Minimally metabolized
Interactions:
• Increased pramipexole levels: levodopa, cimetidine, ranitidine, diltiazem, triamterene, verapamil, quinidine
• Decreased pramipexole levels: dopamine antagonists, phenothiazines, metoclopramide, butyrophenones
⊘ Decreased effect of pramipexole: chaste tree fruit
NURSING CONSIDERATIONS
Assess:
• Renal function studies
• Involuntary movements in parkinsonism: akinesia, tremors, staggering gait, muscle rigidity, drooling
• B/P, respiration during initial treatment; hypo/hypertension should be reported
• Mental status: affect, mood, behavioral changes, depression; complete suicide assessment
Administer:
• Drug until NPO before surgery
• Adjust dosage to patient response
• With meals

Perform/provide:

• Assistance with ambulation during beginning therapy

• Testing for diabetes mellitus, acromegaly if on long-term therapy

Evaluate:

• Therapeutic response: decrease in akathisia, increased mood

Teach patient/family:

• That therapeutic effects may take several wk to a few mo

• To change positions slowly to prevent orthostatic hypotension

• To use drug exactly as prescribed: if drug is discontinued abruptly, parkinsonian crisis may occur

---

pravastatin (℞)

(pra′va-sta-tin)
Pravachol
Func. class.: Antilipidemic

Action: Inhibits HMG-CoA reductase enzyme, which reduces cholesterol synthesis

Uses: As an adjunct in primary hypercholesterolemia (types IIa, IIb), to reduce the risk of recurrent MI, atherosclerosis

Dosage and routes:

• *Adult:* **PO** 10-20 mg qd at hs (range 10-40 mg qd)

• *Elderly/renal hepatic disease:* **PO** 10 mg/day

Available forms: Tabs 10, 20, 40 mg

Side effects/adverse reactions:

INTEG: Rash, pruritus

GI: Nausea, constipation, diarrhea, dyspepsia, flatus, abdominal pain, heartburn, *liver dysfunction,* pancreatitis, *hepatitis*

EENT: Lens opacities, common cold, rhinitis, cough

MS: Muscle cramps, myalgia, *myositis, rhabdomyolysis*

CNS: Headache, dizziness, psychic disturbances

Contraindications: Hypersensitivity, pregnancy (X), lactation, active liver disease

Precautions: Past liver disease, alcoholism, severe acute infections, trauma, hypotension, uncontrolled seizure disorders, severe metabolic disorders, electrolyte imbalances

Pharmacokinetics: Peak 1-1½ hr; metabolized by the liver, highly protein bound; excreted in urine, feces, breast milk; crosses placenta

Interactions:

• Increased risk for myopathy: erythromycin, niacin, cyclosporine, gemfibrozil, clofibrate, clarithromycin, itraconazole, protease inhibitors

• Increased effects of warfarin

• Decreased bioavailability of pravastatin: bile acid sequestrants

Lab test interferences:

Increase: CPK, liver function tests

NURSING CONSIDERATIONS

Assess:

• Whether patient is pregnant

• Fasting lipid profile: LDL, HDL, TG, cholesterol q8wk, then q3-6mo when stable

• Liver function studies: baseline, q6wk during the first 3 mo, q8wk for remainder of yr, then q6mo; AST, ALT, liver function tests may increase

• Renal studies in patients with compromised renal system: BUN, I&O ratio, creatinine

Administer:

• Without regard to meals, hs

Perform/provide:

• Storage in cool environment in tight container protected from light

Evaluate:

• Therapeutic response: decrease in cholesterol to desired level after 8 wk

Teach patient/family:

• That blood work will be necessary during treatment

• To report blurred vision, severe

◆ = Nursing alert   ⫽ = Herb-drug interaction   ⊘ = Do not crush

GI symptoms, dizziness, headache, muscle pain, fever

• That regimen will continue: low-cholesterol diet, exercise program

• To report suspected pregnancy, not to use during pregnancy

prazosin (R)

(pray'zoe-sin)

Minipress, Prazosin

Func. class.: Antihypertensive

Chem. class.: α_1-adrenergic blocker

Action: Peripheral blood vessels dilate, peripheral resistance drops; reduction in blood pressure results from α-adrenergic receptors being blocked

Uses: Hypertension, refractory CHF, Raynaud's vasospasm

Investigational uses: Benign prostatic hypertrophy to decrease urine outflow obstruction

Dosage and routes:

• *Adult:* **PO** 1 mg bid or tid, increasing to 20 mg qd in divided doses if required; usual range 6-15 mg/day, not to exceed 1 mg initially; max 20-40 mg/day

• *Child:* **PO** 0.5-7 mg tid

Available forms: Caps 1, 2, 5 mg

Side effects/adverse reactions:

CV: Palpitations, orthostatic hypotension, tachycardia, edema, rebound hypertension

CNS: Dizziness, headache, drowsiness, anxiety, depression, vertigo, weakness, fatigue

GI: Nausea, vomiting, diarrhea, constipation, abdominal pain

GU: Urinary frequency, incontinence, impotence, priapism, H_2O, sodium retention

EENT: Blurred vision, epistaxis, tinnitus, dry mouth, red sclera

Contraindications: Hypersensitivity

Precautions: Pregnancy (C), children

Pharmacokinetics:

PO: Onset 2 hr, peak 1-3 hr, duration 6-12 hr; half-life 2-3 hr, metabolized in liver, excreted via bile, feces (>90%), in urine (<10%)

Interactions:

• Increased hypotensive effects: β-blockers, nitroglycerin

• Decreased effect: indomethacin

Lab test interferences:

Increase: Urinary norepinephrine, VMA

NURSING CONSIDERATIONS

Assess:

• B/P (sitting, standing) during initial treatment, periodically thereafter; pulse, jugular venous distention q4h

• BUN, uric acid if on long-term therapy

• Weight qd, I&O; edema in feet, legs qd

• Skin turgor, dryness of mucous membranes for hydration status

• Rales, dyspnea, orthopnea q30min

Perform/provide:

• Storage in tight container in cool environment

Evaluate:

• Therapeutic response: decreased B/P

Teach patient/family:

• That fainting occasionally occurs after 1st dose; do not drive or operate machinery for 4 hr after 1st dose, or take 1st dose at bedtime

• To change positions slowly, to prevent orthostatic hypotension

• To avoid OTC medications unless approved by prescriber

Treatment of overdose: Administer volume expanders or vasopressors, discontinue drug, place in supine position

prednisolone (℞)

(pred-niss'oh-lone)

Articulose-50, Delta-Cortef, Hydeltrasol, Hydeltra-T.B.A., Key-Pred 25, Key-Pred 50, Key-Pred-SP, Pediapred, Predaject-50, Predalone 50, Predalone-T.B.A., Predcor-25, Predcor-50, prednisolone, Prednisolone Acetate, Prednisol TBA, Prelone

Func. class.: Corticosteroid

Chem. class.: Glucocorticoid, immediate acting

Action: Decreases inflammation by suppression of migration of polymorphonuclear leukocytes, fibroblasts; reversal to increase capillary permeability and lysosomal stabilization

Uses: Severe inflammation, immunosuppression, neoplasms

Dosage and routes:

• *Adult:* **PO** 2.5-15 mg bid-qid; **IM** 2-30 mg (acetate, phosphate) q12h; **IV** 2-30 mg (phosphate) q12h; 2-30 mg in joint or soft tissue (phosphate), 4-40 mg in joint of lesion (tebutate)

Asthma/antiinflammatory

• *Child:* **PO** 1-2 mg/kg/day; **IV** 2-4 mg/kg/day

Available forms: Prednisolone Tabs 5 mg; syrup 5 mg/5 ml 15 mg/15 ml; acetate: inj 25, 50 mg/ml; tebutate: inj 20 mg/ml; phosphate: inj 20 mg/ml, oral liquid 5 mg/ml, tabs 1, 2.5, 5, 10, 20, 50 mg, oral sol 5 mg/ml, 5 mg/5 ml, syrup 5 mg/5 ml

Side effects/adverse reactions:

INTEG: Acne, poor wound healing, ecchymosis, petechiae

CNS: Depression, flushing, sweating, headache, mood changes

CV: Hypertension, **circulatory collapse, thrombophlebitis, embolism,** tachycardia

HEMA: **Thrombocytopenia**

MS: Fractures, osteoporosis, weakness

GI: Diarrhea, nausea, abdominal distention, **GI hemorrhage,** increased appetite, *pancreatitis*

EENT: Fungal infections, increased intraocular pressure, blurred vision

Contraindications: Psychosis, hypersensitivity, idiopathic thrombocytopenia, acute glomerulonephritis, amebiasis, fungal infections, nonasthmatic bronchial disease, child <2 yr

Precautions: Pregnancy (C), diabetes mellitus, glaucoma, osteoporosis, seizure disorders, ulcerative colitis, CHF, myasthenia gravis

Pharmacokinetics:

PO: Peak 1-2 hr, duration 2 days

IM: Peak 3-45 hr

Interactions:

• Decreased action of prednisolone: cholestyramine, colestipol, barbiturates, rifampin, ephedrine, phenytoin, theophylline

• Decreased effects of anticoagulants, anticonvulsants, antidiabetics, ambenonium, neostigmine, isoniazid, toxoids, vaccines, anticholinesterases, salicylates, somatrem

• Increased side effects: alcohol, salicylates, indomethacin, amphotericin B, digitalis, cyclosporine, diuretics

• Increased action of prednisolone: salicylates, estrogens, indomethacin, oral contraceptives, ketoconazole, macrolide antibiotics

𝄞 Potassium deficiency: aloe, buckthorn, cascara sagrada, senna

Lab test interferences:

Increase: Cholesterol, Na, blood glucose, uric acid, Ca, urine glucose

Decrease: Ca, K, T_4, T_3, thyroid ^{131}I uptake test, urine 17-OHCS, 17-KS, PBI

False negative: Skin allergy tests

◆ = Nursing alert   𝄞 = Herb-drug interaction   ⊘ = Do not crush

NURSING CONSIDERATIONS
Assess:

• K, blood sugar, urine glucose while on long-term therapy; hypokalemia and hyperglycemia

• Weight qd; notify prescriber if weekly gain >5 lb

• B/P q4h, pulse; notify prescriber if chest pain occurs

• I&O ratio; be alert for decreasing urinary output, increasing edema

• Plasma cortisol levels (long-term therapy) (normal level: 138-635 nmol/L SI units when drawn at 8 AM)

• Infection: increased temp, WBC, even after withdrawal of medication; drug masks infection

• K depletion: paresthesias, fatigue, nausea, vomiting, depression, polyuria, dysrhythmias, weakness

• Edema, hypertension, cardiac symptoms

• Mental status: affect, mood, behavioral changes, aggression

Administer:

• After shaking suspension (parenteral)

• Titrated dose; use lowest effective dose

• IM inj deep in large muscle mass; rotate sites; avoid deltoid; use 21G needle

• In 1 dose in AM to prevent adrenal suppression; avoid SC administration; may damage tissue

• With food or milk to decrease GI symptoms

IV

• Undiluted or added to NaCl or D_5 and given by IV inf; give 10 mg or less/1 min; decrease rate if burning occurs

Additive compatibilities: Ascorbic acid, cephalothin, cytarabine, erythromycin, fluorouracil, heparin, methicillin, penicillin G potassium, penicillin G sodium, vit B/C

Y-site compatibilities: Ciprofloxacin, heparin/hydrocortisone, potassium chloride, vit B/C

Perform/provide:

• Assistance with ambulation to patient with bone tissue disease to prevent fractures

Evaluate:

• Therapeutic response: ease of respirations, decreased inflammation

Teach patient/family:

• That ID as steroid user should be carried

• To notify prescriber if therapeutic response decreases; dosage adjustment may be needed

• Not to discontinue abruptly; adrenal crisis can result

• To avoid OTC products: salicylates, alcohol in cough products, cold preparations unless directed by prescriber

• About cushingoid symptoms

• The symptoms of adrenal insufficiency: nausea, anorexia, fatigue, dizziness, dyspnea, weakness, joint pain

---

prednisone (℞)
(pred'ni-sone)
Apo-Prednisone*, Deltasone*, Liquid Pred, Meticorten, Orasone, Panasol-S, Prednicen-M, Prednisone, Sterapred, Winpred

Func. class.: Corticosteroid
Chem. class.: Intermediate-acting glucocorticoid

Action: Decreases inflammation by suppression of migration of polymorphonuclear leukocytes, fibroblasts, reversal to increase capillary permeability, and lysosomal stabilization

Uses: Severe inflammation, immunosuppression, neoplasms, multiple sclerosis, collagen disorders, dermatologic disorders

---

Dosage and routes:
• *Adult:* **PO** 1.5-2.5 mg bid-qid, then qd or qod; maintenance up to 250 mg/day
• *Child:* **PO** 0.05-2 mg/kg/day divided 1-4 ×/day
Nephrosis
• *Child 18 mo-4 yr:* 7.5-10 mg qid initially
• *Child 4-10 yr:* 15 mg qid initially
• *Child >10 yr:* 20 mg qid initially
Multiple sclerosis
• *Adult:* **PO** 200 mg/day × 1 wk, then 80 mg qod × 1 mo
Available forms: Tabs 1, 2.5, 5, 10, 20, 50 mg; oral sol 5 mg/5 ml; syr 5 mg/5 ml
Side effects/adverse reactions:
CNS: Depression, flushing, sweating, headache, mood changes
CV: Hypertension, *circulatory collapse, thrombophlebitis, embolism,* tachycardia
EENT: Fungal infections, increased intraocular pressure, blurred vision
GI: Diarrhea, nausea, abdominal distention, *GI hemorrhage,* increased appetite, pancreatitis
HEMA: **Thrombocytopenia**
INTEG: Acne, poor wound healing, ecchymosis, petechiae
MS: Fractures, osteoporosis, weakness
Contraindications: Psychosis, hypersensitivity, idiopathic thrombocytopenia, acute glomerulonephritis, amebiasis, fungal infections, nonasthmatic bronchial disease, child <2 yr, AIDS, TB
Precautions: Pregnancy (C), diabetes mellitus, glaucoma, osteoporosis, seizure disorders, ulcerative colitis, CHF, myasthenia gravis, renal disease, esophagitis, peptic ulcer
Pharmacokinetics:
PO: Well absorbed PO, peak 1-2 hr, duration 1-1½ days, half-life 3½-4 hr

Crosses placenta, enters breast milk, metabolized by liver after conversion
Interactions:
• Decreased action of prednisone: cholestyramine, colestipol, barbiturates, rifampin, ephedrine, phenytoin, theophylline
• Decreased effects of anticoagulants, anticonvulsants, antidiabetics, ambenonium, neostigmine, isoniazid, toxoids, vaccines, anticholinesterases, salicylates, somatrem
• Increased side effects: alcohol, salicylates, indomethacin, amphotericin B, digitalis, cyclosporine, diuretics
• Increased action of prednisone: salicylates, estrogens, indomethacin, oral contraceptives, ketoconazole, macrolide antibiotics
🌿 Potassium deficiency: aloe, buckthorn, rhubarb, senna
Lab test interferences:
Increase: Cholesterol, Na, blood glucose, uric acid, Ca, urine glucose
Decrease: Ca, K, T_4, T_3, thyroid ^{131}I uptake test, urine 17-OHCS, 17-KS, PBI
False negative: Skin allergy tests
NURSING CONSIDERATIONS
Assess:
• Adrenal insufficiency: nausea, vomiting, anorexia, confusion, hypotension
• K, blood sugar, urine glucose while on long-term therapy; hypokalemia and hyperglycemia
• Weight qd; notify prescriber of weekly gain >5 lb
• B/P q4h, pulse; notify prescriber of chest pain; monitor for rales, crackles, dyspnea if edema is present
• I&O ratio; be alert for decreasing urinary output, increasing edema
• Plasma cortisol (long-term therapy) (normal: 138-635 nmol/L SI units drawn at 8 AM)

◆ = Nursing alert   🌿 = Herb-drug interaction   🚫 = Do not crush

• Infection: increased temp, WBC, even after withdrawal of medication; drug masks infection

• K depletion: paresthesias, fatigue, nausea, vomiting, depression, polyuria, dysrhythmias, weakness

• Edema, hypertension, cardiac symptoms

• Mental status: affect, mood, behavioral changes, aggression

Administer:

• Titrated dose; use lowest effective dose

• With food or milk to decrease GI symptoms

Perform/provide:

• Assistance with ambulation to patient with bone tissue disease to prevent fractures

Evaluate:

• Therapeutic response: ease of respirations, decreased inflammation

Teach patient/family:

• That ID as steroid user should be carried; information on drug being taken and condition

• To notify prescriber if therapeutic response decreases; dosage adjustment may be needed

• To avoid vaccinations

• Not to discontinue abruptly, or adrenal crisis can result

• To avoid OTC products: salicylates, alcohol in cough products, cold preparations unless directed by prescriber

• About cushingoid symptoms: moon face, weight gain

• That drug causes immunosuppression; to report any symptoms of infection (fever, sore throat, cough)

• The symptoms of adrenal insufficiency: nausea, anorexia, fatigue, dizziness, dyspnea, weakness, joint pain

---

primaquine (R̪)
(prim′a-kween)

Func. class.: Antimalarial
Chem. class.: Synthetic 8-aminoquinolone

Action: Unknown; thought to destroy exoerythrocytic forms by gametocidal action

Uses: Malaria caused by *P. vivax,* in combination with clindamycin for *Pneumocystis carinii* pneumonia

Dosage and routes:

• *Adult:* **PO** 15 mg (base) qd × 2 wk; 26.3-mg tab is 15-mg base

• *Child:* **PO** 0.5 mg/kg (0.3 mg/base/day) qd × 2 wk

Available forms: Tabs 26.3 mg, powder

Side effects/adverse reactions:

INTEG: Pruritus, skin eruptions

CNS: Headache

EENT: Blurred vision, difficulty focusing

GI: Nausea, vomiting, anorexia, cramps

CV: Hypertension

*HEMA: **Agranulocytosis, granulocytopenia, leukopenia, hemolytic anemia, leukocytosis,** mild anemia, **methemoglobinemia***

Contraindications: Hypersensitivity, anemia, lupus erythematosus, methemoglobinemia, porphyria, rheumatoid arthritis, methemoglobin reductase deficiency, G6PD deficiency

Precautions: Pregnancy (C)

Pharmacokinetics:

PO: Metabolized by liver (metabolites), half-life 3.7-9.6 hr

Interactions:

• Toxicity: quinacrine

NURSING CONSIDERATIONS

Assess:

• Ophthalmic test if long-term treatment or drug dosage >150 mg/day

P

- Liver studies qwk: AST, ALT, bilirubin, if on long-term therapy
- Blood studies: CBC; blood dyscrasias occur
- Allergic reactions: pruritus, rash, urticaria
- Blood dyscrasias: malaise, fever, bruising, bleeding (rare)
- For renal status: dark urine, hematuria, decreased output

◆ For hemolytic reaction: chills, fever, chest pain, cyanosis; drug should be discontinued immediately

Administer:
PO
- Before or after meals at same time each day to maintain drug level

Evaluate:
- Therapeutic response: decreased symptoms of malaria

Teach patient/family:
- To report visual problems, fever, fatigue, dark urine, bruising, bleeding; may indicate blood dyscrasias
- To complete full course of therapy

---

primidone (℞)
(pri'mi-done)
Apo-Primidone*, Mysoline, PMS-Primidone*, primidone, Sertan*

Func. class.: Anticonvulsant
Chem. class.: Barbiturate derivative

Action: Raises seizure threshold by conversion of drug to phenobarbital, decreases neuron firing
Uses: Generalized tonic-clonic (grand mal), complex-partial psychomotor seizures
Dosage and routes:
- *Adult and child >8 yr:* **PO** 100-125 mg hs on days 1, 2, 3; then 100-125 mg bid on days 4, 5, 6; then 100-125 mg tid on days 7, 8, 9, then maintenance 250 mg tid-qid, max 2 g/day in divided doses

- *Child <8 yr:* **PO** 50 mg hs on days 1, 2, 3; then 50 mg bid on days 4, 5, 6; then 100 mg bid on days 7, 8, 9, maintenance 125-250 mg tid
Available forms: Tabs 50, 250 mg; susp 250 mg/5 ml; chew tabs 125 mg*
Side effects/adverse reactions:
*HEMA: **Thrombocytopenia, leukopenia, neutropenia, eosinophilia, megaloblastic anemia,*** decreased serum folate level, lymphadenopathy
CNS: Stimulation, drowsiness, dizziness, confusion, sedation, headache, flushing, hallucinations, *coma,* psychosis, ataxia, vertigo
*GI: Nausea, vomiting, anorexia, **hepatitis***
INTEG: Rash, edema, alopecia, lupuslike syndrome
*EENT: Diplopia, nystagmus, edema of eyelids
GU: Impotence
Contraindications: Hypersensitivity, porphyria, pregnancy (D)
Precautions: COPD, hepatic disease, renal disease, hyperactive children
Pharmacokinetics:
PO: Peak 4 hr; excreted by kidneys, in breast milk; half-life 3-24 hr
Interactions:
- Primidone levels are decreased by acetazolamide, succinimides, carbamazepine
- Primidone levels are increased by: isoniazid, nicotinamide, hydantoins
- Increased blood levels: alcohol, heparin, CNS depressants, isoniazid, phenytoin, phenobarbital
- May decrease effect of: oral contraceptives, acebutolol, metoprolol, propranolol, tricyclics, phenothiazines

NURSING CONSIDERATIONS
Assess:
- For seizures: location, duration, type; folic acid deficiency; fatigue, weakness, neuropathy, depression

---

◆ = Nursing alert   ∥ = Herb-drug interaction   ⊘ = Do not crush

• Drug level: therapeutic level 5-12 μg/ml; CBC should be done q6mo
• Mental status: mood, sensorium, affect, memory (long, short)
• Respiratory depression, wheezing
• Blood dyscrasias: fever, sore throat, bruising, rash, jaundice

Administer:

PO

• After shaking liquid susp well
• With food for GI upset
• Tablets crushed and mixed with food or fluid for swallowing difficulties

Evaluate:

• Therapeutic response: decreased seizures

Teach patient/family:

• Not to withdraw drug quickly; withdrawal symptoms may occur
• To avoid hazardous activities until stabilized on drug; drowsiness, dizziness may occur
• To carry Medic Alert ID with condition and medication
• To recognize the signs of blood dyscrasias; when to notify prescriber
• To avoid alcohol, CNS depressants

---

probenecid (℞)
(proe-ben'e-sid)
Benemid, Benuryl*, probenecid
Func. class.: Uricosuric
Chem. class.: Sulfonamide derivative

Action: Inhibits tubular reabsorption of urates, with increased excretion of uric acids

Uses: Hyperuricemia in gout, gouty arthritis, adjunct to cephalosporin or penicillin treatment

Dosage and routes:

Renal dose

• Avoid use if CrCl <30 ml/min

Gonorrhea

• *Adult:* **PO** 1 g with 3.5 g ampicillin or 1 g ½ hr before 4.8 million U of aqueous penicillin G procaine injected into 2 sites **IM**

Gout/gouty arthritis

• *Adult:* **PO** 250 mg bid for 1 wk, then 500 mg bid, not to exceed 2 g/day; maintenance: 500 mg/day × 6 mo

Adjunct in penicillin/cephalosporin treatment

• *Adult and child >50 kg:* **PO** 500 mg qid
• *Child <50 kg:* **PO** 25 mg/kg, then 40 mg/kg in divided doses qid

Available forms: Tabs 0.5 g

Side effects/adverse reactions:
CNS: Drowsiness, headache
CV: Bradycardia
GU: Glycosuria, thirst, frequency, ***nephrotic syndrome***
GI: Gastric irritation, nausea, vomiting, anorexia, ***hepatic necrosis***
INTEG: Rash, dermatitis, pruritus, fever
META: Acidosis, hypokalemia, hyperchloremia, hyperglycemia
RESP: ***Apnea,*** irregular respirations

Contraindications: Hypersensitivity, severe hepatic disease, severe renal disease, CrCl <50 mg/min, history of uric acid calculus

Precautions: Pregnancy (B), child <2 yr

Pharmacokinetics:
PO: Peak 2-4 hr, duration 8 hr, half-life 5-8 hr; metabolized by liver; excreted in urine

Interactions:

• Increased effect of acyclovir, barbiturates, allopurinol, benzodiazepines, dyphylline, zidovudine
• Increased toxicity: sulfa drugs, dapsone, clofibrate, indomethacin, rifampin, naproxen, methotrexate, pantothenic acid

P

Side effects: *italics* = common; ***bold italics*** = life-threatening

• Decreased action of probenecid: salicylates

Lab test interferences:
False positive: Urine glucose with copper sulfate test (Clinitest)
Increase: BSP/urinary PSP, theophylline levels

NURSING CONSIDERATIONS
Assess:
• Uric acid levels (3-7 mg/dl); mobility, joint pain, swelling
• Respiratory rate, rhythm, depth; notify prescriber of abnormalities
• Electrolytes, CO_2 before, during treatment
• Urine pH, output, glucose during beginning treatment
◆ For CNS symptoms: confusion, twitching, hyperreflexia, stimulation, headache; may indicate overdose

Administer:
• After meals or with milk if GI symptoms occur
• Increase fluid intake to 2-3 L/day to prevent urinary calculi

Evaluate:
• Therapeutic response: absence of pain, stiffness in joints

Teach patient/family:
• To avoid OTC preparations (aspirin) unless directed by prescriber

---

procainamide (℞)
(proe-kane-ah'mide)
procainamide, Procanbid,
Promine, Pronestyl,
Pronestyl-SR
Func. class.: Antidysrhythmic (Class IA)
Chem. class.: Procaine HCl amide analog

Action: Depresses excitability of cardiac muscle to electrical stimulation and slows conduction in atrium, bundle of His, and ventricle
Uses: Ventricular dysrhythmias

Dosage and routes:
Renal dose
• CrCl 10-50 ml/min give q6-12h; CrCl <10 ml/min give q8-24h
• *Adult:* **IV BOL** 100 mg q5min, given 25-50 mg/min, not to exceed 500 mg; or 17 mg/kg total then **IV INF** 2-6 mg/min
Available forms: Caps 250, 375, 500 mg; tabs 250, 375, 500 mg; tabs sus rel 250, 500, 750, 1000 mg; inj 100, 500 mg/ml

Side effects/adverse reactions:
CNS: Headache, dizziness, confusion, psychosis, restlessness, irritability, weakness
GI: Nausea, vomiting, anorexia, diarrhea, hepatomegaly
*CV: Hypotension, **heart block, cardiovascular collapse, arrest***
HEMA: SLE syndrome, ***agranulocytosis, thrombocytopenia, neutropenia, hemolytic anemia***
INTEG: Rash, urticaria, edema, swelling (rare), pruritus

Contraindications: Hypersensitivity, myasthenia gravis, severe heart block

Precautions: Pregnancy (C), lactation, children, renal disease, liver disease, CHF, respiratory depression

Pharmacokinetics:
PO: Peak 1-2 hr, duration 3 hr (8 hr extended)
IM: Peak 10-60 min, duration 3 hr; half-life 3 hr
Metabolized in liver to active metabolites, excreted unchanged by kidneys (60%)

Interactions:
• Increased effects of neuromuscular blockers, anticholinergics, antihypertensives
• Increased procainamide effects: cimetidine
• Decreased effects of procainamide: barbiturates

◆ = Nursing alert   🖋 = Herb-drug interaction   ⊘ = Do not crush

• Increased toxicity: other antidysrhythmics

🖋 Increased anticholinergic effect: henbane

NURSING CONSIDERATIONS
Assess:

• ECG continuously if using IV to determine increased PR or QRS segments; discontinue immediately; watch for increased ventricular ectopic beats, maximum need to rebolus

• Blood levels, 3-10 µg/ml or NAPA levels

• CBC q2wk × 3 mo

• B/P continuously for fluctuations

• I&O ratio; electrolytes (K, Na, Cl)

• Malignant hyperthermia: tachypnea, tachycardia, changes in B/P, fever

• Cardiac rate, rhythm, character

• Respiratory status: rate, rhythm, character, lung fields; bilateral rales may occur in CHF patient; watch for respiratory depression

• CNS effects: dizziness, confusion, psychosis, paresthesias, convulsions; drug should be discontinued

• Increased respiration, increased pulse; drug should be discontinued

Administer:
IM

• IM injection in deltoid; aspirate to avoid intravascular administration
IV

• After diluting 100 mg/ml of D₅W or sterile H₂O for inj; give 20 mg or less/1 min; may dilute 1 g/250-500 ml D₅W, run at 2-6 mg/min

• Check IV site q8h for infiltration or extravasation

Additive compatibilities: Amiodarone, atracurium, dobutamine, flumazenil, lidocaine, netilmicin, verapamil

Solution compatibilities: D₅W, D₅/0.9% NaCl, 0.45% NaCl, 0.9% NaCl, water for inj

Y-site compatibilities: Amiodarone, cisatracurium, famotidine, heparin, hydrocortisone, potassium chloride, ranitidine, remifentanil, vit B/C

Evaluate:

• Therapeutic response: decreased dysrhythmias

Teach patient/family:

• That wax matrix may appear in stools

• Not to discontinue without healthcare provider's advice

---

procaine (℞)
(proe′kane)
Novocain, Unicaine
Func. class.: Local anesthetic
Chem. class.: Ester

Action: Competes with calcium for sites in nerve membrane that control sodium transport across cell membrane; decreases rise of depolarization phase of action potential

Uses: Spinal anesthesia, epidural, peripheral nerve block, perineum, lower extremities, infiltration

Dosage and routes:
Vary by route of anesthesia

Available forms: Inj 1%, 2%, 10%

Side effects/adverse reactions:
CNS: Anxiety, restlessness, ***convulsions, loss of consciousness,*** drowsiness, disorientation, tremors, shivering

CV: ***Myocardial depression, cardiac arrest, dysrhythmias,*** bradycardia, hypotension, hypertension, fetal bradycardia

GI: Nausea, vomiting

EENT: Blurred vision, tinnitus, pupil constriction

INTEG: Rash, urticaria, allergic reactions, edema, burning, skin discoloration at injection site, tissue necrosis

RESP: ***Status asthmaticus, respiratory arrest, anaphylaxis***

Contraindications: Hypersensitivity, child <12 yr, severe liver disease

Precautions: Elderly, severe drug allergies, pregnancy (C)

Pharmacokinetics: Onset 2-5 min, duration 1 hr; metabolized by liver, excreted in urine (metabolites)

Interactions:
• Dysrhythmias: epinephrine, halothane, enflurane
• Hypertension: MAOIs, tricyclic antidepressants, phenothiazines
• Decreased action of procaine: chloroprocaine

NURSING CONSIDERATIONS
Assess:
• B/P, pulse, respiration during treatment
• Fetal heart tones if drug is used during labor
• Allergic reactions: rash, urticaria, itching
• Cardiac status: ECG for dysrhythmias, pulse, B/P during anesthesia

Administer:
• Only drugs that are not cloudy, do not contain precipitate
• Only with crash cart, resuscitative equipment nearby
• Only drugs without preservatives for epidural or caudal anesthesia

Additive compatibilities: Ascorbic acid, cephalothin, hydrocortisone, methicillin, penicillin G potassium, penicillin G sodium, vit B/C

Syringe compatibilities: Ampicillin, cloxacillin, glycopyrrolate, hydroxyzine, methicillin

Perform/provide:
• Use of new sol; discard unused portions

Evaluate:
• Therapeutic response: anesthesia necessary for procedure

Treatment of overdose: Airway, O₂, vasopressor, IV fluids, anticonvulsants for seizures

---

procarbazine (R)
(proe-kar′ba-zeen)
Matulane, Natulan*
Func. class.: Antineoplastic, alkylating agent
Chem. class.: Hydrazine derivative

Action: Inhibits DNA, RNA, protein synthesis; has multiple sites of action; a nonvesicant

Uses: Lymphoma, Hodgkin's disease, cancers resistant to other therapy

Investigational uses: Brain, lung malignancies, other lymphomas, multiple myeloma, malignant melanoma, polycythemia vera
• *Adult:* **PO** 2-4 mg/kg/day for first wk; maintain dosage of 4-6 mg/kg/day until platelets and WBC fall; after recovery, 1-2 mg/kg/day
• *Child:* **PO** 50 mg/m²/day for 7 days, then 100 mg/m² until desired response, leukopenia, or thrombocytopenia occurs; 50 mg/day is maintenance after bone marrow recovery

Available forms: Caps 50 mg

Side effects/adverse reactions:
HEMA: **Thrombocytopenia, anemia, leukopenia, myelosuppression, bleeding tendencies,** purpura, petechiae, epistaxis
GI: **Nausea, vomiting,** anorexia, diarrhea, constipation, dry mouth, stomatitis
EENT: Retinal hemorrhage, nystagmus, photophobia, diplopia
INTEG: Rash, pruritus, dermatitis, alopecia, herpes, hyperpigmentation
CNS: Headache, dizziness, insomnia, hallucinations, confusion, *coma,* pain, chills, fever, sweating, paresthesias, *seizures*
RESP: Cough, pneumonitis

◆ = Nursing alert   ∥ = Herb-drug interaction   ⊘ = Do not crush

MS: Arthralgias, myalgias

GU: Azoospermia, cessation of menses

Contraindications: Hypersensitivity, pregnancy (D), thrombocytopenia, bone marrow depression

Precautions: Renal disease, hepatic disease, radiation therapy

Pharmacokinetics: Half-life 1 hr; concentrates in liver, kidney, skin; metabolized in liver, excreted in urine

Interactions:

• Increased CNS depression: barbiturates, antihistamines, opioids, hypotensive agents, phenothiazines

• Disulfiram-like reaction: ethyl alcohol, MAOIs, tricyclic antidepressants, tyramine foods, sympathomimetic drugs

• Hypertension: guanethidine, levodopa, methyldopa, reserpine

• Increased hypoglycemia: insulin, oral hypoglycemics

NURSING CONSIDERATIONS

Assess:

• CBC, differential, platelet count qwk; withhold drug if WBC is <4000/mm^3 or platelet count is <100,000/mm^3; notify prescriber

• Renal function studies: BUN, serum uric acid, urine CrCl, electrolytes before, during therapy

• I&O ratio, report fall in urine output to <30 ml/hr

• Monitor temp q4h; fever may indicate beginning infection

• Liver function tests before, during therapy: bilirubin, AST, ALT, alk phosphatase prn or qmo

• CNS changes: confusion, paresthesias, neuropathies, drug should be discontinued

◆ For tyramine foods in diet, hypertensive crisis can occur

◆ Toxicity: facial flushing, epistaxis, increased pro-time, thrombocytopenia; drug should be discontinued

• Bleeding: hematuria, guaiac stools, bruising or petechiae, mucosa or orifices q8h

• Effects of alopecia on body image; discuss feelings about body changes

• Jaundiced skin, sclera; dark urine, clay-colored stools, itchy skin, abdominal pain, fever, diarrhea

• Buccal cavity q8h for dryness, sores or ulceration, white patches, oral pain, bleeding, dysphagia

• Alkalosis if vomiting is severe

• GI symptoms: frequency of stools, cramping

• Acidosis, signs of dehydration: rapid respirations, poor skin turgor, decreased urine output, dry skin, restlessness, weakness

Administer:

• In divided doses and at hs to minimize nausea and vomiting

• Nonphenothiazine antiemetic 30-60 min before giving drug and 4-10 hr after treatment to prevent vomiting

• Transfusion for anemia

• Antispasmodic for GI symptoms

Perform/provide:

• Liquid diet: carbonated beverages; gelatin may be added if patient is not nauseated or vomiting

• Storage in tight, light-resistant container in cool environment

Evaluate:

• Therapeutic response: decreased tumor size, spread of malignancy

Teach patient/family:

• To report any complaints, side effects to nurse or prescriber; cough, shortness of breath, fever, chills, sore throat, bleeding, bruising, vomiting blood; black, tarry stools

• That hair may be lost during treatment and wig or hairpiece may make patient feel better; tell patient that new hair may be different in color, texture

P

• To avoid foods with citric acid, hot or rough texture

• To report any bleeding, white spots, ulcerations in mouth to prescriber; tell patient to examine mouth qd

• To avoid driving, activities requiring alertness; dizziness may occur

• That contraceptive measures are recommended during therapy

• To avoid ingestion of alcohol, tyramine-containing foods; cold, hay fever, weight-reducing products may cause serious drug interactions

• To avoid crowds, persons with infections if granulocytes are low

---

prochlorperazine (℞)

(proe-klor-pair′a-zeen)
Chlorpazine, Compa-Z, Compazine, Contranzine, Provacin*, Stemetil*, Ultrazine
Func. class.: Antiemetic, antipsychotic
Chem. class.: Phenothiazine, piperazine derivative

Action: Acts centrally by blocking chemoreceptor trigger zone, which in turn acts on vomiting center
Uses: Nausea, vomiting
Dosage and routes:
Postoperative nausea/vomiting
• *Adult:* **IM** 5-10 mg 1-2 hr before anesthesia; may repeat in 30 min; **IV** 5-10 mg 15-30 min before anesthesia; **IV INF** 20 mg/L D_5W or NS 15-30 min before anesthesia, not to exceed 40 mg/day
Severe nausea/vomiting
• *Adult:* **PO** 5-10 mg tid-qid; **SUS REL** 15 mg qd in AM or 10 mg q12h; **RECT** 25 mg/bid; **IM** 5-10 mg; may repeat q4h, not to exceed 40 mg/day
• *Child 18-39 kg:* **PO** 2.5 mg tid or 5 mg bid, not to exceed 15 mg/day; **IM** 0.132 mg/kg

• *Child 14-17 kg:* **PO/RECT** 2.5 mg bid-tid, not to exceed 10 mg/day; **IM** 0.132 mg/kg
• *Child 9-13 kg:* **PO/RECT** 2.5 mg qd-bid, not to exceed 7.5 mg/day; **IM** 0.132 mg/kg
Antipsychotic
• *Adult and child ≥12 yr:* **PO** 5-10 mg tid-qid; may increase q2-3day, max 150 mg/day; **IM** 10-20 mg q2-4hr up to 4 doses, then 10-20 mg q4-6h, max 200 mg/day; **RECT** 10 mg tid-qid, may increase by 5-10 mg q2-3 days as needed
• *Child 2-12 yr:* **PO** 2.5 mg bid-tid; **IM** 132 μg/kg, max 10 mg/dose
Antianxiety
• *Adult and child ≥12 yr:* 5 mg tid-qid, max 20 mg/day or >12 wk; **IM** 5-10 mg q3-4hr, max 40 mg/day; **IV** 2.5-10 mg; max 40 mg/day
• *Child 2-12 yr:* **IM** 132 μg/kg
Available forms: Syr 5 mg/ml; inj 5 mg/ml; tabs 5, 10, 25 mg; caps, sus rel 10, 15 mg; supp 2.5, 5, 25 mg
Side effects/adverse reactions:
CNS: **Neuroleptic malignant syndrome,** *extrapyramidal reactions, tardive dyskinesia, euphoria,* **depression,** *EPS,* restlessness, tremor, dizziness
GI: Nausea, vomiting, anorexia, dry mouth, diarrhea, constipation, weight loss, metallic taste, cramps
CV: **Circulatory failure, tachycardia**
RESP: **Respiratory depression**
Contraindications: Hypersensitivity to phenothiazines, coma, seizure, encephalopathy, bone marrow depression
Precautions: Children <2 yr, pregnancy (C), elderly, lactation
Pharmacokinetics:
PO: Onset 30-40 min, duration 3-4 hr
SUS REL: Onset 30-40 min, duration 10-12 hr

◆ = Nursing alert   ⫻ = Herb-drug interaction   ⊘ = Do not crush

RECT: Onset 60 min, duration 3-4 hr
IM: Onset 10-20 min, duration 12 hr
Metabolized by liver; excreted in urine, breast milk; crosses placenta

Interactions:

• Decreased effect of prochlorperazine: barbiturates, antacids
• Increased anticholinergic action: anticholinergics, antiparkinson drugs, antidepressants
⬗ Increased anticholinergic effect: henbane

Lab test interferences:

Increase: Liver function tests, cardiac enzymes, cholesterol, blood glucose, prolactin, bilirubin, PBI, ^{131}I, alk phosphatase, leukocytes, granulocytes, platelets

Decrease: Hormones (blood and urine)

False positive: Pregnancy tests, PKU, urine bilirubin

False negative: Urinary steroids, 17-OHCS, pregnancy tests

NURSING CONSIDERATIONS
Assess:

• EPS: abnormal movement, tardive dyskinesia, akathisia
• VS, B/P; check patients with cardiac disease more often
• Respiratory status before, during, after administration of emetic; check rate, rhythm, character; respiratory depression can occur rapidly with elderly or debilitated patients

Administer:

IM

• IM injection in large muscle mass; aspirate to avoid IV administration
• Keep patient recumbent for ½ hr

IV

• IV after diluting 5 mg/9 ml of NaCl for inj (0.5 mg/ml); give 5 mg or less/min; may dilute 10-20 mg/L NaCl and give as infusion; can cause contact dermatitis

Additive compatibilities: Amikacin, ascorbic acid, dexamethasone, dimenhydrinate, erythromycin, ethacrynate, lidocaine, nafcillin, sodium bicarbonate, vit B/C

Syringe compatibilities: Atropine, butorphanol, chlorpromazine, cimetidine, diamorphine, diphenhydramine, droperidol, fentanyl, glycopyrrolate, hydroxyzine, meperidine, metoclopramide, nalbuphine, pentazocine, perphenazine, promazine, promethazine, ranitidine, scopolamine, sufentanil

Y-site compatibilities: Amsacrine, calcium gluconate, cisatracurium, cisplatin, cladribine, cyclophosphamide, cytarabine, doxorubicin, doxorubicin liposome, fluconazole, granisetron, heparin, hydrocortisone, melphalan, methotrexate, ondansetron, paclitaxel, potassium chloride, propofol, remifentanil, sargramostim, sufentanil, teniposide, thiotepa, vinorelbine, vit B/C

Evaluate:

• Therapeutic response: absence of nausea, vomiting

Teach patient/family:

• To avoid hazardous activities, activities requiring alertness; dizziness may occur
• To avoid alcohol
• Not to double or skip doses
• That urine may be pink to reddish brown
• To report dark urine, clay-colored stools, bleeding, bruising, rash, blurred vision

P

progesterone (℞)

(proe-jess′ter-one)
Crinone, progesterone,
Progesterone in Oil
Func. class.: Progestogen
Chem. class.: Progesterone derivative

Action: Inhibits secretion of pituitary gonadotropins, which prevents follicular maturation, ovulation; stimulates growth of mammary tissue; antineoplastic action against endometrial cancer

Uses: Contraception, amenorrhea, premenstrual syndrome, abnormal uterine bleeding

Dosage and routes:
Infertility
• *Adult:* **VAG** 90 mg qd
Amenorrhea/uterine bleeding
• *Adult:* **IM** 5-10 mg qd × 6-8 doses
Available forms: Inj 50 mg/ml; powder micronized, vag gel 8%; caps 100 mg

Side effects/adverse reactions:
CNS: Dizziness, headache, migraines, depression, fatigue
CV: Hypotension, *thrombophlebitis,* edema, *thromboembolism, stroke, pulmonary embolism, MI*
GI: *Nausea,* vomiting, anorexia, cramps, increased weight, *cholestatic jaundice*
EENT: Diplopia
GU: Amenorrhea, cervical erosion, breakthrough bleeding, dysmenorrhea, vaginal candidiasis, breast changes, *gynecomastia, testicular atrophy, impotence,* endometriosis, *spontaneous abortion*
INTEG: Rash, urticaria, acne, hirsutism, alopecia, oily skin, seborrhea, purpura, melasma
META: Hyperglycemia

Contraindications: Breast cancer, hypersensitivity, thromboembolic disorders, reproductive cancer, genital bleeding (abnormal, undiagnosed), cerebral hemorrhage, pregnancy (X)

Precautions: Lactation, hypertension, asthma, blood dyscrasias, gallbladder disease, CHF, diabetes mellitus, bone disease, depression, migraine headache, convulsive disorders, hepatic disease, renal disease, family history of breast or reproductive tract cancer

Pharmacokinetics:
IM, Rect, Vag: Duration 24 hr
Excreted in urine, feces; metabolized in liver

Lab test interferences:
Increase: Alk phosphatase, nitrogen (urine), pregnanediol, amino acids, factors VII, VIII, IX, X
Decrease: GTT, HDL

NURSING CONSIDERATIONS
Assess:
• Weight qd; notify prescriber of weekly weight gain >5 lb
• B/P at beginning of treatment and periodically
• I&O ratio; be alert for decreasing urinary output, increasing edema
• Liver function studies: ALT, AST, bilirubin periodically during long-term therapy
• Edema, hypertension, cardiac symptoms, jaundice
• Mental status: affect, mood, behavioral changes, depression
• Hypercalcemia

Administer:
• Titrated dose; use lowest effective dose
• Oil solution deep in large muscle mass IM; rotate sites
• After warming to dissolve crystals
• In one dose in AM
• With food or milk to decrease GI symptoms

Perform/provide:
• Storage in dark area

 = Nursing alert   = Herb-drug interaction   🚫 = Do not crush

Evaluate:
• Therapeutic response: decreased abnormal uterine bleeding, absence of amenorrhea

Teach patient/family:
• To report breast lumps, vaginal bleeding, edema, jaundice, dark urine, clay-colored stools, dyspnea, headache, blurred vision, abdominal pain, numbness or stiffness in legs, chest pain
• To report suspected pregnancy
• To monitor blood sugar if diabetic

promazine (℞)

(proe′ma-zeen)
promazine, Sparine
Func. class.: Antipsychotic, neuroleptic
Chem. class.: Phenothiazine, aliphatic

Action: Depresses cerebral cortex, hypothalamus, limbic system, which control activity, aggression; blocks neurotransmission produced by dopamine at synapse; exhibits a strong α-adrenergic, anticholinergic blocking action; as antiemetic, inhibits medullary chemoreceptor trigger zone; mechanism for antipsychotic effects is unclear

Uses: Psychotic disorders, schizophrenia, nausea, vomiting, alcohol withdrawal

Dosage and routes:
Psychosis
• *Adult:* **PO** 10-200 mg q4-6h, max dose 1 g/day; **IM** 50-150 mg, followed in 30 min with additional dose up to a total dose of 300 mg
• *Geriatric:* **PO** 25 mg qd-bid, increase by 25 mg q4-7 days
• *Child >12 yr:* **PO** 10-25 mg q4-6h
Available forms: Tabs 25, 50 mg; inj 25, 50 mg/ml

Side effects/adverse reactions:
RESP: ***Laryngospasm,*** dyspnea, ***respiratory depression***
*CNS: EPS: pseudoparkinsonism, akathisia, dystonia, tardive dyskinesia, drowsiness, headache, **seizures***
HEMA: Anemia, ***leukopenia, leukocytosis, agranulocytosis***
INTEG: Rash, photosensitivity, dermatitis
EENT: Blurred vision, glaucoma, dry eyes
GI: Dry mouth, nausea, vomiting, anorexia, constipation, diarrhea, jaundice, weight gain
GU: Urinary retention, urinary frequency, enuresis, impotence, amenorrhea, gynecomastia
*CV: Orthostatic hypotension, **cardiac arrest,*** ECG changes, ***tachycardia***

Contraindications: Hypersensitivity, blood dyscrasias, coma, child <12 yr, brain damage, bone marrow depression, glaucoma

Precautions: Pregnancy (C), lactation, seizure disorders, hypertension, hepatic or cardiac disease

Pharmacokinetics:
PO: Onset erratic, peak 2-4 hr
IM: Onset 15 min, peak 1 hr, duration 4-6 hr; metabolized by liver; excreted in urine, breast milk; crosses placenta

Interactions:
• Oversedation: other CNS depressants, alcohol, barbiturate anesthetics
• Toxicity: epinephrine
• Decreased absorption: aluminum hydroxide, magnesium hydroxide antacids
• Decreased effects of lithium, levodopa
• Increased effects of both drugs: β-adrenergic blockers, alcohol
• Increased anticholinergic effects: anticholinergics

P

🌿 Increased anticholinergic effect: henbane

Lab test interferences:

Increase: Liver function tests, cardiac enzymes, cholesterol, blood glucose, prolactin, bilirubin, PBI, cholinesterase, ^{131}I

Decrease: Hormones (blood and urine)

False positive: Pregnancy tests, PKU

False negative: Urinary steroids, 17-OHCS, pregnancy tests

NURSING CONSIDERATIONS
Assess:

• Mental status before initial administration

• Swallowing of PO medication; check for hoarding or giving of medication to other patients

• I&O ratio; palpate bladder if urinary output is low

• Bilirubin, CBC, liver function studies qmo

• Urinalysis is recommended before and during prolonged therapy

• Affect, orientation, LOC, reflexes, gait, coordination, sleep pattern disturbances

• B/P standing and lying; also include pulse, respirations, q4h during initial treatment; establish baseline before starting treatment; report drops of 30 mm Hg

• Dizziness, faintness, palpitations, tachycardia on rising

• EPS including akathisia (inability to sit still, no pattern to movements), tardive dyskinesia (bizarre movements of jaw, mouth, tongue, extremities), pseudoparkinsonism (rigidity, tremors, pill rolling, shuffling gait)

🔷 For neuroleptic malignant syndrome: muscle rigidity, altered mental status, hyperthermia, increased CPK

• Skin turgor qd

• Constipation, urinary retention qd; increase bulk, water in diet

Administer:

• Reduced dose in elderly

• Antiparkinsonian agent on order from prescriber for EPS

• Syrup mixed in citrus- or chocolate-flavored drinks

• IM inj into large muscle mass

IV

• IV undiluted; give at 25 mg/min or less over 1 min; may dilute 25-60 mg/9 ml NaCl for inj

Additive compatibilities: Chloramphenicol, erythromycin, ethacrynate, heparin, lidocaine, metaraminol, methyldopa

Syringe compatibilities: Atropine, chlorpromazine, cimetidine, diphenhydramine, droperidol, fentanyl, glycopyrrolate, hydroxyzine, meperidine, metoclopramide, midazolam, morphine, pentazocine, prochlorperazine, promethazine, scopolamine

Perform/provide:

• Decreased sensory input by dimming lights, avoiding loud noises

• Supervised ambulation until stabilized on medication; do not involve in strenuous exercise program because fainting is possible; patient should not stand still for long periods

• Increased fluids to prevent constipation

• Sips of water, candy, gum for dry mouth

• Storage in airtight, light-resistant container; avoid contact with hands

Evaluate:

• Therapeutic response: decrease in emotional excitement, hallucinations, delusions, paranoia; reorganization of patterns of thought, speech

Teach patient/family:

• That orthostatic hypotension commonly occurs and to rise from sitting or lying position gradually, to

---

🔷 = Nursing alert   🌿 = Herb-drug interaction   🚫 = Do not crush avoid hazardous activities until stabilized on medication

• To remain lying down for at least 30 min after IM injection

• To avoid hot tubs, hot showers, tub baths; hypotension may occur

• To avoid abrupt withdrawal of this drug, or EPS may result; drug should be withdrawn slowly

• To avoid OTC preparations (cough, hay fever, cold) unless approved by prescriber, since serious drug interactions may occur; avoid use with alcohol, CNS depressants; increased drowsiness may occur

• To use a sunscreen

• About compliance with drug regimen

• About EPS and necessity for meticulous oral hygiene, since oral candidiasis may occur

• To report sore throat, malaise, fever, bleeding, mouth sores; CBC should be drawn and drug discontinued

• That in hot weather, heat stroke may occur; take extra precautions to stay cool

Treatment of overdose: Lavage if orally ingested; provide an airway; do not induce vomiting

---

promethazine (℞)

(proe-meth′a-zeen)

Anergan 50, Phenergan, Phenergan Fortis, Phenergan Plain, promethazine HCl

Func. class.: Antihistamine, H$_1$-receptor antagonist

Chem. class.: Phenothiazine derivative

Action: Acts on blood vessels, GI, respiratory system by competing with histamine for H$_1$-receptor site; decreases allergic response by blocking histamine

Uses: Motion sickness, rhinitis, allergy symptoms, sedation, nausea, preoperative and postoperative sedation

Dosage and routes:

Nausea

• *Adult:* **PO/IM/IV** 10-25 mg; may repeat 12.5-25 mg q4-6h

• *Child >2 yr:* **PO/IM** 0.25-0.5 mg/kg q4-6h

Motion sickness

• *Adult:* **PO** 25 mg bid, give ½-1 hr before departure

• *Child >2 yr:* **PO/IM/RECT** 12.5-25 mg bid, give ½-1 hr before departure

Allergy/rhinitis

• *Adult:* **PO** 12.5 mg qid, or 25 mg hs

• *Child >2 yr:* **PO** 6.25-12.5 mg tid or 25 mg hs

Sedation

• *Adult:* **PO/IM** 25-50 mg hs

• *Child >2 yr:* **PO/IM/RECT** 12.5-25 mg hs

Sedation (preoperative/postoperative)

• *Adult:* **PO/IM/IV** 25-50 mg

• *Child >2 yr:* **PO/IM/IV** 12.5-25 mg

Available forms: Tabs 12.5, 25, 50 mg; supp 12.5, 25, 50 mg; inj 25, 50 mg/ml, syrup 6.25 mg/5 ml, 10 mg/5 ml*, 25 mg/5 ml

Side effects/adverse reactions:

CNS: Dizziness, drowsiness, poor coordination, fatigue, anxiety, euphoria, confusion, paresthesia, neuritis, EPS

CV: Hypotension, palpitations, tachycardia

RESP: Increased thick secretions, wheezing, chest tightness, ***apnea in neonates, infants, young children***

*HEMA: **Thrombocytopenia, agranulocytosis, hemolytic anemia***

GI: Constipation, dry mouth, nausea, vomiting, anorexia, diarrhea

P

INTEG: Rash, urticaria, photosensitivity

GU: Urinary retention, dysuria, frequency

EENT: Blurred vision, dilated pupils, tinnitus, nasal stuffiness; dry nose, throat, mouth; photosensitivity

Contraindications: Hypersensitivity to H_1-receptor antagonist, acute asthma attack, lower respiratory tract disease

Precautions: Increased intraocular pressure, renal disease, cardiac disease, hypertension, bronchial asthma, seizure disorder, stenosed peptic ulcers, hyperthyroidism, prostatic hypertrophy, bladder neck obstruction, pregnancy (C)

Pharmacokinetics:

PO: Onset 20 min, duration 4-6 hr; metabolized in liver; excreted by kidneys, GI tract (inactive metabolites)

Interactions:

• Increased CNS depression: barbiturates, narcotics, hypnotics, tricyclic antidepressants, alcohol

• Decreased effect of oral anticoagulants, heparin

• Increased effect of promethazine: MAOIs

🍃 Increased anticholinergic effect: henbane

Lab test interferences:

False negative: Skin allergy test

False positive: Urine pregnancy test

NURSING CONSIDERATIONS
Assess:

• I&O ratio; be alert for urinary retention, frequency, dysuria; drug should be discontinued

• CBC during long-term therapy; blood dyscrasias

• Respiratory status: rate, rhythm, increase in bronchial secretions, wheezing, chest tightness

• Cardiac status: palpitations, increased pulse, hypotension

Administer:

• With meals for GI symptoms; absorption may slightly decrease

• When used for motion sickness, 30 min before travel

IM

• IM inj deep in large muscle; rotate site

IV

• After diluting each 25-50 mg/9 ml of NaCl for inj; give 25 mg or less/2 min

Additive compatibilities: Amikacin, ascorbic acid, chloroquine, hydromorphone, netilmicin, vit B/C

Syringe compatibilities: Atropine, butorphanol, chlorpromazine, cimetidine, diphenhydramine, droperidol, fentanyl, glycopyrrolate, hydromorphone, hydroxyzine, meperidine, metoclopramide, midazolam, pentazocine, perphenazine, prochlorperazine, promazine, ranitidine, scopolamine

Y-site compatibilities: Amifostine, amsacrine, aztreonam, ciprofloxacin, cisatracurium, cisplatin, cladribine, cyclophosphamide, cytarabine, doxorubicin, filgrastim, fluconazole, fludarabine, granisetron, melphalan, ondansetron, remifentanil, sargramostim, teniposide, thiotepa, vinorelbine

Perform/provide:

• Hard candy, gum, frequent rinsing of mouth for dryness

• Storage in tight, light-resistant container

Evaluate:

• Therapeutic response: absence of running, congested nose, rashes, absence of motion sickness, nausea; sedation

Teach patient/family:

• That drug may cause photosensitivity; to avoid prolonged sunlight

◆ = Nursing alert   🍃 = Herb-drug interaction   🚫 = Do not crush

• To notify prescriber of confusion, sedation, hypotension
• To avoid driving, other hazardous activity if drowsy
• To avoid concurrent use of alcohol, other CNS depressants

Treatment of overdose: Administer ipecac syrup or lavage, diazepam, vasopressors, barbiturates (short-acting)

---

propafenone (℞)

(pro-pah-fen'ohn)

Rythmol

Func. class.: Antidysrhythmic, (Class Ic)

Action: Slows conduction velocity; reduces membrane responsiveness; inhibits automaticity; increases ratio of effective refractory period to action potential duration; β-blocking activity

Uses: Life-threatening dysrhythmias, sustained ventricular tachycardia

Dosage and routes:
• *Adult:* **PO** 300-900 mg/day in divided doses, 150 mg q8h; allow a 3-4 day interval before increasing dose

Available forms: Tabs 150, 225, 300 mg

Side effects/adverse reactions:
INTEG: Rash
CV: Dysrhythmias, bradycardia, prodysrhythmia, palpitations, AV block, intraventricular conduction delay, AV dissociation, *CHF, sudden death, atrial flutter*
HEMA: Leukopenia, agranulocytosis, granulocytopenia, thrombocytopenia, anemia
CNS: Headache, dizziness, abnormal dreams, syncope, confusion, *seizures*
GI: Nausea, vomiting, constipation, dyspepsia, cholestasis, *hepatitis,* ab-

normal liver function studies, dry mouth
RESP: Dyspnea
EENT: Blurred vision, altered taste, tinnitus

Contraindications: 2nd- or 3rd-degree AV block, right bundle branch block, cardiogenic shock, hypersensitivity, bradycardia, uncontrolled CHF, sick-sinus syndrome, marked hypotension, bronchospastic disorders

Precautions: CHF, hypokalemia, hyperkalemia, recent MI, nonallergic bronchospasm, pregnancy (C), lactation, children, hepatic or renal disease

Pharmacokinetics: Peak 3-5 hr, half-life 2-10 hr; metabolized in liver; excreted in urine (metabolite)

Interactions:
• Increased effect of propafenone: cimetidine, quinidine
• Increased anticoagulation: warfarin
• Increased digoxin level: digoxin
• Increased β-blocker effect: propranolol, metoprolol
• Increased cyclosporine levels: cyclosporine
• Decreased propafenone effect: rifampin
🍃 Decreased potassium, increased antidysrhythmic action: aloe, buckthorn, cascara sagrada, senna pod/leaf

Lab test interferences:
Increase: CPK

NURSING CONSIDERATIONS
Assess:
• GI status: bowel pattern, number of stools
• Cardiac status: rate, rhythm, quality
• Chest x-ray film, pulmonary function test during treatment
• I&O ratio; check for decreasing output
• B/P for fluctuations

• Lung fields; bilateral rales may occur in CHF patient
• Increased respiration, increased pulse; drug should be discontinued
◆ Toxicity: fine tremors, dizziness
• Cardiac function: respiratory rate, rhythm, character continuously

Evaluate:
• Therapeutic response: absence of dysrhythmias

Treatment of overdose: O_2, artificial ventilation, ECG; administer dopamine for circulatory depression, diazepam or thiopental for convulsions

---

propantheline (R)
(proe-pan'the-leen)
Pro-Banthine, Propanthel*,
propantheline bromide
Func. class.: GI anticholinergic
Chem. class.: Synthetic quaternary ammonium compound

Action: Inhibits muscarinic actions of acetylcholine at postganglionic parasympathetic neuroeffector sites

Uses: Treatment of peptic ulcer disease, irritable bowel syndrome, duodenography, urinary incontinence

Investigational uses: Antispasmodic uses

Dosage and routes:
• *Adult:* **PO** 15 mg tid ac, 30 mg hs
• *Elderly:* **PO** 7.5 mg tid ac
• *Child:* 1.5 mg/kg/day divided in 3-4 doses (antisecretory); 2-3 mg/kg/day divided q4-6hr and hs (antispasmodic)

Available forms: Tabs 7.5, 15 mg

Side effects/adverse reactions:
CNS: Confusion, stimulation in elderly, headache, insomnia, dizziness, drowsiness, anxiety, weakness, hallucinations
*GI: Dry mouth, constipation, **paralytic ileus,** heartburn, nausea, vomiting, dysphagia, absence of taste

GU: Urinary hesitancy, retention, impotence
CV: Palpitations, tachycardia, orthostatic hypotension (elderly)
EENT: Blurred vision, photophobia, mydriasis, cycloplegia, increased ocular tension
INTEG: Urticaria, rash, pruritus, anhidrosis, fever, allergic reactions

Contraindications: Hypersensitivity to anticholinergics, narrow-angle glaucoma, GI obstruction, myasthenia gravis, paralytic ileus, GI atony, toxic megacolon

Precautions: Hyperthyroidism, coronary artery disease, dysrhythmias, CHF, ulcerative colitis, hypertension, hiatal hernia, hepatic disease, renal disease, pregnancy (C), urinary retention, prostatic hypertrophy, elderly

Pharmacokinetics:
PO: Onset 30-45 min, duration 6 hr; metabolized by liver, GI system; excreted in urine, bile

Interactions:
• Increased anticholinergic effect: amantadine, tricyclic antidepressants, MAOIs, H_1-antihistamines
• Decreased effect of phenothiazines, levodopa, ketoconazole

NURSING CONSIDERATIONS
Assess:
• VS, cardiac status: checking for dysrhythmias, increased rate, palpitations
• I&O ratio; check for urinary retention or hesitancy
• GI complaints: pain, bleeding (frank or occult), nausea, vomiting, anorexia

Administer:
• ½-1 hr ac for better absorption
• Decreased dose to elderly patients; metabolism may be slowed
• Gum, hard candy, frequent rinsing for dry mouth

◆ = Nursing alert   �herb = Herb-drug interaction   ⊘ = Do not crush

Perform/provide:

• Storage in tight container protected from light

• Increased fluids, bulk, exercise to decrease constipation

Evaluate:

• Therapeutic response: absence of epigastric pain, bleeding, nausea, vomiting

Teach patient/family:

• To avoid driving, other hazardous activities until stabilized on medication; may cause blurred vision; to use caution when standing due to orthostatic hypotension

• To avoid alcohol, other CNS depressants; will enhance sedating properties of this drug

• To drink plenty of fluids

• To report dysphagia

---

propofol (℞)

(pro'poh-fole)

Diprivan, Disoprofol

Func. class.: General anesthetic

Action: Produces dose-dependent CNS depression; action is unknown

Uses: Induction or maintenance of anesthesia as part of balanced anesthetic technique; sedation in mechanically ventilated patients

Dosage and routes:

Induction

• *Adult:* **IV** 2-2.5 mg/kg, approximately 40 mg q10sec until induction onset

• *Child ≥3 yr:* **IV** 2.5-3.5 mg/kg over 20-30 sec

• *Elderly:* **IV** 1-1.5 mg/kg, approximately 20 mg q10sec until induction onset

Maintenance

• *Adult:* **IV** 0.1-0.2 mg/kg/min (6-12 mg/kg/hr)

• *Child ≥3 yr:* **IV** 0.125-0.3 mg/kg/min (7.5-18 mg/kg/hr)

• *Elderly:* **IV** 0.05-0.1 mg/kg/min (3-6 mg/kg/hr)

ICU sedation

• *Adult:* **IV** 5 µg/kg/min over 5 min; may give 5-10 µg/kg/min over 5-10 min until desired response

Available forms: Inj 10 mg/ml in 20 ml ampule, 50-cc and 100-cc vials

Side effects/adverse reactions:

CNS: Movement, headache, jerking, fever, dizziness, shivering, tremor, confusion, somnolence, paresthesia, agitation, abnormal dreams, euphoria, fatigue

GI: Nausea, vomiting, abdominal cramping, dry mouth, swallowing, hypersalivation

MS: Myalgia

GU: Urine retention, green urine

EENT: Blurred vision, tinnitus, eye pain, strange taste

CV: Bradycardia, hypotension, hypertension, PVC, PAC, tachycardia, abnormal ECG, ST segment depression, ***asystole***

RESP: ***Apnea,*** *cough, hiccups,* dyspnea, hypoventilation, sneezing, wheezing, tachypnea, hypoxia

INTEG: Flushing, phlebitis, hives, burning/stinging at injection site

Contraindications: Hypersensitivity, hyperlipidemia

Precautions: Elderly, respiratory depression, severe respiratory disorders, cardiac dysrhythmias, pregnancy (B), labor and delivery, lactation, children

Pharmacokinetics: Onset 40 sec, rapid distribution, half-life 1-8 min, terminal elimination half-life 5-10 hr; 70% excreted in urine; metabolized in liver by conjugation to inactive metabolites

Interactions:

• Increased CNS depression: alcohol, narcotics, sedative/hypnotics, antipsychotics, skeletal muscle relaxants, inhalational anesthetics

• Do not administer with other drugs

P

NURSING CONSIDERATIONS
Assess:
• Injection site: phlebitis, burning, stinging
• ECG for changes: PVC, PAC, ST segment changes
• CNS changes: movement, jerking, tremors, dizziness, LOC, pupil reaction
• Allergic reactions: hives
• Respiratory dysfunction: respiratory depression, character, rate, rhythm; notify prescriber if respirations are <10/min
Administer:
IV
• After diluting with D_5W mixed in lipid base; use only glass containers when mixing, not stable in plastic
• Alone; do not mix with other agents before using
• Only with resuscitative equipment available
• Only by qualified persons trained in anesthesia
Syringe compatibilities: Thiopental
Y-site compatibilities: Acyclovir, alfentanil, amikacin, aminophylline, ampicillin, amrinone, aztreonam, bumetanide, buprenorphine, butorphanol, calcium gluconate, carboplatin, cefazolin, cefonicid, cefoperazone, cefotaxime, cefotetan, cefoxitin, ceftazidime, ceftizoxime, ceftriaxone, cefuroxime, chlorpromazine, cimetidine, ciprofloxacin, cisplatin, clindamycin, cyclophosphamide, cyclosporine, cytarabine, dexamethasone, digoxin, diphenhydramine, dobutamine, dopamine, doxorubicin, doxycycline, droperidol, enalaprilat, ephedrine, epinephrine, esmolol, famotidine, fentanyl, fluconazole, fluorouracil, furosemide, ganciclovir, glycopyrrolate, granisetron, haloperidol, heparin, hydrocortisone, hydromorphone, hydroxyzine, ifosfamide, imipenem/cilastatin, insulin, isoproterenol, ketamine, labetalol, levorphanol, lidocaine, lorazepam, magnesium sulfate, mannitol, meperidine, metoclopramide, mezlocillin, miconazole, morphine, nafcillin, nalbuphine, naloxone, nitroglycerin, norepinephrine, ofloxacin, paclitaxel, pentobarbital, phenobarbital, piperacillin, potassium chloride, prochlorperazine, propranolol, ranitidine, scopolamine, sodium bicarbonate, sodium nitroprusside, succinylcholine, sufentanil, ticarcillin, ticarcillin/clavulanate, vancomycin, vecuronium, verapamil
Perform/provide:
• Storage in light-resistant area at room temp
• Safety measures: night-light, call bell within easy reach
Evaluate:
• Therapeutic response: induction of anesthesia
Treatment of overdose: Discontinue drug; administer vasopressor agents or anticholinergics, artificial ventilation

---

propoxyphene (℞)
(proe-pox'i-feen)
Darvon, Darvon-N, Dolene, Novapropoxyn*
Func. class.: Opiate analgesic
Chem. class.: Synthetic opiate

Controlled Substance Schedule IV
Action: Depresses pain impulse transmission at the spinal cord level by interacting with opioid receptors
Uses: Mild to moderate pain
Dosage and routes:
• *Adult:* **PO** 65 mg q4h prn (HCl)
• *Adult:* **PO** 100 mg q4h prn (napsylate)
Available forms: Propoxyphene HCl Caps 32, 65 mg; propoxyphene

---

napsylate tabs 100 mg; oral susp 50 mg/5 ml

Side effects/adverse reactions:

CNS: Drowsiness, dizziness, confusion, headache, sedation, euphoria, **convulsions, hyperthermia** (elderly)

GI: Nausea, vomiting, anorexia, constipation, cramps

GU: Urinary retention, dysuria

INTEG: Rash, urticaria, bruising, flushing, diaphoresis, pruritus

EENT: Tinnitus, blurred vision, miosis, diplopia

CV: Palpitations, bradycardia, change in B/P, **dysrhythmias**

*RESP: **Respiratory depression***

Contraindications: Hypersensitivity to ASA products (some preparations), addiction (opioid)

Precautions: Addictive personality, pregnancy (C), lactation, increased intracranial pressure, MI (acute), severe heart disease, respiratory depression, hepatic disease, renal disease, child <18 yr, elderly

Pharmacokinetics:

PO: Onset ½-1 hr, peak 2-2½ hr, duration 4-6 hr

Metabolized by liver, excreted by kidneys (as metabolites), crosses placenta, excreted in breast milk, half-life 6-12 hr (metabolites)

Interactions:

• Increased effects with other CNS depressants: alcohol, narcotics, sedative/hypnotics, antipsychotics, skeletal muscle relaxants

Lab test interferences:

Increase: Amylase

NURSING CONSIDERATIONS

Assess:

• For pain: duration, location, type

• I&O ratio; check for decreasing output; may indicate retention

• CNS changes: dizziness, drowsiness, hallucinations, euphoria, loss of consciousness, pupil reaction

• Allergic reactions: rash, urticaria

• Respiratory dysfunction: respiratory depression, character, rate, rhythm; notify prescriber if respirations are <10/min

• Need for pain medication; physical dependence

Administer:

• With antiemetic for nausea, vomiting

• When pain is beginning to return; determine dosage interval by response

Perform/provide:

• Storage in light-resistant area at room temp

• Assistance with ambulation

• Safety measures: night-light, call bell within easy reach

Evaluate:

• Therapeutic response: decrease in pain

Teach patient/family:

• To report any symptoms of CNS changes, allergic reactions

• That physical dependency may result when used for extended periods; not to exceed dose

• That withdrawal symptoms may occur: nausea, vomiting, cramps, fever, faintness, anorexia

Treatment of overdose: Naloxone (Narcan) 0.2-0.8 mg IV, O$_2$, IV fluids, vasopressors

P

---

propranolol (℞)

(proe-pran′oh-lole)

Apo-Propranolol*, Detensol*, Inderal, Inderal LA, propranolol HCl, Propranolol Intensol, Novo-Pranol*

Func. class.: Antihypertensive, antianginal

Chem. class.: β-Adrenergic blocker

Action: Nonselective β-blocker with negative inotropic, chronotropic, dromotropic properties

Uses: Chronic stable angina pectoris, hypertension, supraventricular dysrhythmias, migraine, prophylaxis, MI, pheochromocytoma, essential tremor, tetralogy of Fallot, cyanotic spells

Investigational uses: Mitral valve prolapse, anxiety, dysrhythmias associated with thyrotoxicosis

Dosage and routes:
Dysrhythmias
• *Adult:* **PO** 10-30 mg tid-qid; **IV BOL** 0.5-3 mg give 1 mg/min; may repeat in 2 min, may repeat q4h thereafter
• *Child:* **PO** 0.5-1 mg/kg/day divided q6-8h; **IV** 0.01-0.1 mg/kg

Hypertension
• *Adult:* **PO** 40 mg bid or 80 mg qd (ext rel) initially; usual dose 120-240 mg/day bid-tid or 120-160 mg qd (ext rel)
• *Child:* **PO** 0.5-1 mg/kg/day divided q6-12h

Angina
• *Adult:* **PO** 80-320 mg in divided doses bid-qid or 80 mg qd (ext rel); usual dose 160 mg qd (ext rel)

MI prophylaxis
• *Adult:* **PO** 180-240 mg/day tid-qid starting 5 day to 2 wk after MI

Pheochromocytoma
• *Adult:* **PO** 60 mg/day × 3 days preoperatively in divided doses or 30 mg/day in divided doses (inoperable tumor)

Migraine
• *Adult:* **PO** 80 mg/day (ext rel) or in divided doses; may increase to 160-240 mg/day in divided doses
• *Child:* **PO** 0.6-1.5 mg/kg/day divided q8h **PO**

Essential tremor
• *Adult:* **PO** 40 mg bid; usual dose 120 mg/day

Tetralogy of Fallot
• *Child:* **PO** 1-2 mg/kg/dose q6h
Available forms: Caps, sus rel 60, 80, 120, 160 mg; caps ext rel 60 mg; tabs 10, 20, 40, 60, 80, 90 mg; inj 1 mg/ml; oral sol 4 mg/ml, 8 mg/ml; conc oral sol 80 mg/ml

Side effects/adverse reactions:
RESP: Dyspnea, respiratory dysfunction, *bronchospasm*
CV: Bradycardia, hypotension, ***CHF,*** palpitations, AV block, peripheral vascular insufficiency, vasodilation
HEMA: **Agranulocytosis, thrombocytopenia**
GI: Nausea, vomiting, diarrhea, colitis, constipation, cramps, dry mouth, hepatomegaly, gastric pain, acute pancreatitis
GU: Impotence, decreased libido, UTIs
MS: Joint pain, arthralgia, muscle cramps, pain
MISC: Facial swelling, weight change, Raynaud's phenomenon
INTEG: Rash, pruritus, fever
CNS: Depression, hallucinations, dizziness, fatigue, lethargy, paresthesias, bizarre dreams, disorientation
EENT: Sore throat, *laryngospasm,* blurred vision, dry eyes
META: Hyperglycemia, hypoglycemia

Contraindications: Hypersensitivity to this drug, cardiac failure, cardiogenic shock, 2nd- or 3rd-degree heart block, bronchospastic disease, sinus bradycardia, CHF

Precautions: Diabetes mellitus, pregnancy (C), renal disease, lactation, hyperthyroidism, COPD, hepatic disease, children, myasthenia gravis, peripheral vascular disease, hypotension, CHF

Pharmacokinetics:
PO: Onset 30 min, peak 1-1½ hr, duration 6-12 hr
PO-ER: Peak 6 hr, duration 24 hr
IV: Onset 2 min, peak 15 min, duration 3-6 hr; immediate rel half-life 3-5 hr; ext rel half-life 8-11 hr; metabolized by liver; crosses placenta,

---

◆ = Nursing alert   ✔ = Herb-drug interaction   ⊘ = Do not crush

blood-brain barrier; excreted in breast milk

Interactions:

• AV block: digitalis, calcium channel blockers

• Increased negative inotropic effects: verapamil, disopyramide

• Increased effects of reserpine, digitalis, neuromuscular blocking agents

• Decreased β-blocking effects: norepinephrine, isoproterenol, barbiturates, rifampin, dopamine, dobutamine, smoking

• Increased β-blocking effect: cimetidine

• Increased hypotension: quinidine, haloperidol, hydralazine

Lab test interferences:

Increase: Serum K, serum uric acid, ALT, AST, alk phosphatase, LDH

Decrease: Blood glucose

NURSING CONSIDERATIONS

Assess:

• B/P, pulse, respirations during beginning therapy; notify prescriber if pulse <50 BPM

• Weight qd; report gain of 5 lb

• I&O ratio, CrCl if kidney damage is diagnosed

• ECG if using as antidysrhythmic

• Hepatic enzymes: AST, ALT, bilirubin

• Angina pain: duration, time started, activity being performed, character

• Tolerance (long-term use)

• Headache, light-headedness, decreased B/P; may indicate a need for decreased dosage

Administer:

• With 8 oz water on empty stomach

• Do not give with aluminum-containing antacid; may decrease GI absorption

IV

• IV undiluted or diluted 10 ml D_5W for inj; give 1 mg or less/min; may be diluted in 50 ml NaCl and run 1 mg over 10-15 min

Additive compatibilities: Dobutamine, verapamil

Solution compatibilities: 0.9% NaCl, 0.45 NaCl, Ringer's, D_5W, D_5/0.9% NaCl, D_5/0.45% NaCl

Syringe compatibilities: Amrinone, benzquinamide, milrinone

Y-site compatibilities: Alteplase, amrinone, heparin, hydrocortisone, meperidine, milrinone, morphine, potassium chloride, propofol, tacrolimus, vit B/C

Perform/provide:

• Protection from light (injection)

Evaluate:

• Therapeutic response: decreased B/P, dysrhythmias

Teach patient/family:

• Not to discontinue abruptly, to take drug at same time each day; to decrease dosage over 2 wk to prevent cardiac damage

• To avoid OTC drugs unless approved by prescriber

• To avoid hazardous activities if dizzy

• The importance of compliance with complete medical regimen

• To make position changes slowly to prevent fainting

---

propylthiouracil (R)

(proe-pill-thye-oh-yoor'a-sill)
propylthiouracil, Propyl-Thyracil*, PTU

Func. class.: Thyroid hormone antagonist (antithyroid)

Chem. class.: Thioamide

Action: Blocks synthesis peripherally of T_3, T_4 (triiodothyronine, thyroxine), inhibits organification of iodine

Uses: Preparation for thyroidectomy, thyrotoxic crisis, hyperthyroidism, thyroid storm

---

Dosage and routes:

Thyrotoxic crisis

• *Adult and child:* PO same as hyperthyroidism with iodine and propranolol

Preparation for thyroidectomy

• *Adult:* 600-1200 mg/day

• *Child:* 10 mg/kg/day in divided doses

Hyperthyroidism

• *Adult:* PO 100 mg tid increasing to 300 mg q8h if condition is severe; continue to euthyroid state, then 100 mg qd-tid

• *Child >10 yr:* PO 100 mg tid; continue to euthyroid state, then 25 mg tid to 100 mg bid

• *Child 6-10 yr:* PO 50-150 mg in divided doses q8h

• *Neonate:* PO 10 mg/kg/day in divided doses

Available forms: Tabs 50 mg

Side effects/adverse reactions:

INTEG: Rash, urticaria, pruritus, alopecia, hyperpigmentation, lupus-like syndrome

*GU: **Nephritis***

CNS: Drowsiness, headache, vertigo, fever, paresthesias, neuritis

*HEMA: **Agranulocytosis, leukopenia, thrombocytopenia, hypothrombinemia, lymphadenopathy,*** bleeding, vasculitis, periarteritis

*GI: Nausea, diarrhea, vomiting, **jaundice, hepatitis,*** loss of taste

MS: Myalgia, arthralgia, nocturnal muscle cramps, osteoporosis

Contraindications: Hypersensitivity, pregnancy (D), lactation

Precautions: Infection, bone marrow depression, hepatic disease

Pharmacokinetics:

PO: Onset up to 3 wk, peak 6-10 wk, duration 1 wk to 1 mo, half-life 1-2 hr; excreted in urine, bile, breast milk; crosses placenta; concentration in thyroid gland

Interactions:

• Increased anticoagulant effect: heparin, oral anticoagulants

• Bone marrow depression: radiation, antineoplastics

• Additive effects: potassium/sodium iodide, lithium

• Agranulocytosis: phenothiazines

Lab test interferences:

Increase: Pro-time, AST, ALT, alk phosphatase

NURSING CONSIDERATIONS

Assess:

• Pulse, B/P, temp

• I&O ratio; check for edema: puffy hands, feet, periorbits; indicates hypothyroidism

• Weight qd; same clothing, scale, time of day

• T_3, T_4, which are increased; serum TSH, which is decreased; free thyroxine index, which is increased if dosage is too low; discontinue drug 3-4 wk before RAIU

• Blood work: CBC for blood dyscrasias: leukopenia, thrombocytopenia, agranulocytosis; LFTs

◆ Overdose: peripheral edema, heat intolerance, diaphoresis, palpitations, dysrhythmias, severe tachycardia, increased temp, delirium, CNS irritability

• Hypersensitivity: rash, enlarged cervical lymph nodes; drug may have to be discontinued

• Hypoprothrombinemia: bleeding, petechiae, ecchymosis

• Clinical response: after 3 wk should include increased weight, pulse; decreased T_4

• Bone marrow depression: sore throat, fever, fatigue

Administer:

• With meals to decrease GI upset

• At same time each day to maintain drug level

• Lowest dose that relieves symptoms

◆ = Nursing alert   🖊 = Herb-drug interaction   🚫 = Do not crush

Perform/provide:

• Storage in light-resistant container
• Fluids to 3-4 L/day, unless contraindicated

Evaluate:

• Therapeutic response: weight gain, decreased pulse, decreased T_4, decreased B/P

Teach patient/family:

• To abstain from breastfeeding after delivery
• To take pulse qd
• To report redness, swelling, sore throat, mouth lesions, which indicate blood dyscrasias
• To keep graph of weight, pulse, mood
• To avoid OTC products that contain iodine
• That seafood, other iodine products may be restricted
• Not to discontinue this medication abruptly; thyroid crisis may occur; stress response
• That response may take several months if thyroid is large
• The symptoms/signs of overdose: periorbital edema, cold intolerance, mental depression
• The symptoms of inadequate dose: tachycardia, diarrhea, fever, irritability
• To take medication as prescribed; not to skip or double dose; missed doses should be taken when remembered up to 1 hr before next dose
• To carry Medic Alert ID listing condition, medication

---

protamine (℞)

(proe'ta-meen)

Func. class.: Heparin antagonist

Chem. class.: Low-molecular-weight protein

Action: Binds heparin, making it ineffective

Uses: Heparin overdose

Dosage and routes:

• *Adult and child:* IV 1 mg of protamine/90-115 U heparin given; administer slowly 1-3 min; not to exceed 50 mg/10 min

Available forms: Inj 10 mg/ml

Side effects/adverse reactions:

CV: Hypotension, bradycardia, *circulatory collapse*

GI: Nausea, vomiting, anorexia

INTEG: Rash, dermatitis, urticaria

CNS: Lassitude

HEMA: Bleeding, *anaphylaxis*

RESP: Dyspnea, *pulmonary edema, severe respiratory distress*

Contraindications: Hypersensitivity

Precautions: Pregnancy (C), lactation, children, allergy to fish

Pharmacokinetics:

IV: Onset 5 min, duration 2 hr

NURSING CONSIDERATIONS

Assess:

• Blood studies (Hct, platelets, occult blood in stools) q3mo
• Coagulation tests (APTT, ACT) 15 min after dose, then in several hours
• VS, B/P, pulse after 30 min; plus 3 hr after dose
• Skin rash, urticaria, dermatitis
• Allergy to fish; use with caution

Administer:

IV

• After diluting 50 mg/5 ml sterile bacteriostatic H_2O for inj; shake, give 20 mg or less over 1-3 min; may further dilute with equal volume of NaCl or D_5W and run over 2-3 hr; titrate to APTT, ACT; use infusion pump

Additive compatibilities: Cimetidine, ranitidine, verapamil

Perform/provide:

• Storage at 36°-46° F (2°-8° C)

Evaluate:

• Therapeutic response: reversal of heparin overdose

P

Side effects: *italics* = common; ***bold italics*** = life-threatening

protriptyline (℞)

(proe-trip′tih-leen)
Triptil*, Vivactil
Func. class.: Tricyclic antidepressant

Chem. class.: Dibenzocycloheptene—secondary amine

Action: Blocks reuptake of norepinephrine, serotonin into nerve endings, increasing action of norepinephrine, serotonin in nerve cells

Uses: Depression

Dosage and routes:
• *Adult:* **PO** 15-40 mg/day in divided doses; may increase to 60 mg/day
• *Geriatric:* **PO** 5-10 mg/day, increase q3-7 days by 5-10 mg

Available forms: Tabs 5, 10 mg

Side effects/adverse reactions:

*HEMA: **Agranulocytosis, thrombocytopenia, eosinophilia, leukopenia***

CNS: Dizziness, drowsiness, confusion, headache, anxiety, tremors, stimulation, weakness, insomnia, nightmares, EPS (elderly), increased psychiatric symptoms, paresthesia, **seizures**

GI: Diarrhea, dry mouth, nausea, vomiting, **paralytic ileus,** increased appetite, cramps, epigastric distress, jaundice, **hepatitis,** stomatitis, constipation

*GU: Urinary retention, **acute renal failure***

INTEG: Rash, urticaria, sweating, pruritus, photosensitivity

CV: Orthostatic hypotension, ECG changes, tachycardia, **hypertension,** palpitations

EENT: Blurred vision, tinnitus, mydriasis

Contraindications: Hypersensitivity to tricyclic antidepressants, recovery phase of MI, convulsive disorders, prostatic hypertrophy

Precautions: Suicidal patients, severe depression, increased intraocular pressure, narrow-angle glaucoma, urinary retention, cardiac disease, hepatic disease, hyperthyroidism, electroshock therapy, elective surgery, pregnancy (C), elderly

Pharmacokinetics:

PO: Onset 15-30 min, peak 24-30 hr, duration 4-6 hr; therapeutic effect 2-3 wk; metabolized by liver, excreted by kidneys, crosses placenta, half-life 54-98 hr

Interactions:
• Decreased effects of guanethidine, clonidine, indirect-acting sympathomimetics (ephedrine)
• Increased effects of direct-acting sympathomimetics (epinephrine), alcohol, barbiturates, benzodiazepines, CNS depressants
• Hyperpyretic crisis, convulsions, hypertensive episode: MAOI (pargyline [Eutonyl])
🌿 Increased anticholinergic effect: belladonna, henbane
🌿 Increased antidepressant action: scopolia

Lab test interferences:

Increase: Serum bilirubin, blood glucose, alk phosphatase

False increase: Urinary catecholamines

Decrease: VMA, 5-HIAA

NURSING CONSIDERATIONS

Assess:
• B/P (lying, standing), pulse q4h; if systolic B/P drops 20 mm Hg, hold drug, notify prescriber; take vital signs q4h in patients with cardiovascular disease
• Blood studies: CBC, leukocytes, differential, cardiac enzymes (long-term therapy)
• Hepatic studies: AST, ALT, bilirubin
• Weight qwk; appetite may increase with drug

◆ = Nursing alert　　🌿 = Herb-drug interaction　　🚫 = Do not crush

• ECG for flattening of T wave, bundle branch block, AV block, dysrhythmias in cardiac patients
• EPS primarily in elderly: rigidity, dystonia, akathisia
• Mental status changes: mood, sensorium, affect, suicidal tendencies, increase in psychiatric symptoms: depression, panic
• Urinary retention, constipation; constipation most likely in children/ elderly
• Withdrawal symptoms: headache, nausea, vomiting, muscle pain, weakness; not usual unless discontinued abruptly
• Alcohol consumption; hold dose until morning

Administer:

PO

• Increased fluids, bulk in diet if constipation occurs
• With food, milk for GI symptoms
• Dosage hs if oversedation occurs during day; may take entire dose hs; elderly may not tolerate once/day dosing
• Gum, hard candy, or frequent sips of water for dry mouth

Perform/provide:

• Storage in tight, light-resistant container at room temp
• Assistance with ambulation during beginning therapy for drowsiness/dizziness
• Safety measures primarily in elderly
• Checking to see if PO medication swallowed

Evaluate:

• Therapeutic response: decreased depression

Teach patient/family:

• That therapeutic effects may take 2-3 wk
• To use caution in driving, other activities requiring alertness because of drowsiness, dizziness, blurred vision

• To avoid alcohol ingestion, other CNS depressants
• Not to discontinue medication quickly after long-term use; may cause nausea, headache, malaise
• To wear sunscreen or large hat

Treatment of overdose: ECG monitoring; induce emesis; lavage, activated charcoal; administer anticonvulsant

---

pseudoephedrine
(OTC, ℞)

(soo-doh-eh-fed′rin)

Afrin, Allermed, Canafed, Cenafed, Children's Congestion Relief, Children's Silfedrine, Congestion Relief, Decofed Syrup, DeFed-60, Dorcol Children's Decongestant, Drixoral Non-Drowsy Formula, Dynafed, Efidac/24, Eltor*, Genaphed, Halofed, Mini Thin Pseudo, PediaCare Infant's Decongestant, Pseudo, pseudoephedrine HCl, Pseudogest, Seudotabs, Sinustop Pro, Sudafed, Sudafed 12 Hour, Sudex, Triaminic AM Decongestant Formula

Func. class.: Adrenergic
Chem. class.: Substituted phenylethylamine

Action: Primary activity through α-effects on respiratory mucosal membranes reducing congestion hyperemia, edema; minimal bronchodilation secondary to β-effects

Uses: Nasal decongestant, adjunct in otitis media; with antihistamines

Dosage and routes:

• *Adult:* **PO** 60 mg q6h; ext rel 60-120 mg q12h or q24h
• *Geriatric:* **PO** 30-60 mg q6h prn
• *Child 6-12 yr:* **PO** 30 mg q6h, not to exceed 120 mg/day

---

Side effects: *italics* = common; ***bold italics*** = life-threatening

• *Child 2-6 yr:* **PO** 15 mg q6h, not to exceed 60 mg/day

Available forms: Caps, ext rel 120, 240 mg; oral sol 15 mg, 30 mg/5 ml; drops 7.5 mg/0.8 ml; tabs 30, 60 mg; caps 60 mg; tabs, ext rel 120 mg

Side effects/adverse reactions:

CNS: Tremors, anxiety, insomnia, headache, dizziness, hallucinations, *seizures* (elderly)

EENT: Dry nose, irritation of nose and throat

CV: Palpitations, tachycardia, hypertension, chest pain, *dysrhythmias*

GI: Anorexia, nausea, vomiting, dry mouth

GU: Dysuria

Contraindications: Hypersensitivity to sympathomimetics, narrow-angle glaucoma

Precautions: Pregnancy (C), cardiac disorders, hyperthyroidism, diabetes mellitus, prostatic hypertrophy, lactation, hypertension

Pharmacokinetics:

PO: Onset 15-30 min, duration 4-6 hr, 8-12 hr (ext rel); metabolized in liver, excreted in feces and breast milk

Interactions:

◆ Do not use with MAOIs or tricyclic antidepressants; hypertensive crisis may occur

• Decreased effect of this drug: methyldopa, urinary acidifiers, rauwolfia alkaloids

• Increased effect of this drug: urinary alkalizers

NURSING CONSIDERATIONS

Assess:

• For nasal congestion; auscultate lung sounds; check for tenacious bronchial secretions

• B/P, pulse throughout treatment

• For CNS side effects in the elderly: excitation, seizures, hallucinations

Perform/provide:

• Storage at room temp

Evaluate:

• Therapeutic response: decreased nasal congestion

Teach patient/family:

• The reason for drug administration

• Not to use continuously, or more than recommended dose; rebound congestion may occur

• To check with prescriber before using other drugs, as drug interactions may occur

• To avoid taking near hs; stimulation can occur

• Not to use if stimulation, restlessness, or tremors occur

• That use in children may cause excessive agitation

---

psyllium (OTC, ℞)

(sill'ee-um)

Alramucil, Fiberall, Fiberall Natural Flavor and Orange Flavor, Genifiber, Hydrocil Instant, Karacil*, Konsyl, Konsyl Orange, Maalox Daily Fiber Therapy, Metamucil, Metamucil Lemon Lime, Metamucil Orange Flavor, Metamucil Sugar Free, Metamucil Sugar Free Orange Flavor, Modane Bulk, Mylanta Natural Fiber Supplement, Natural Fiber Laxative, Natural Fiber Laxative Sugar Free, Natural Vegetable Reguloid, Perdiem, Prodiem Plain*, Reguloid Natural, Reguloid Orange, Reguloid Sugar Free Orange, Reguloid Sugar Free Regular, Restore, Restore Sugar Free, Serutan, Syllact, V-Lax

Func. class.: Bulk laxative

Chem. class.: Psyllium colloid

Action: Bulk-forming laxative

Uses: Chronic constipation, ulcer-

◆ = Nursing alert　　🍥 = Herb-drug interaction　　🚫 = Do not crush ative colitis, irritable bowel syndrome

Dosage and routes:

• *Adult:* **PO** 1-2 tsp in 8 oz H_2O bid or tid, then 8 oz H_2O or 1 premeasured packet in 8 oz H_2O bid or tid, then 8 oz H_2O

• *Child >6 yr:* **PO** 1 tsp in 4 oz H_2O hs

Available forms: Chew pieces 1.7, 3.4 g/piece; effervescent powder 3.4, 3.7 g/packet; powder 3.3, 3.4, 3.5, 4.94 g/tsp; granules 2.5, 4.03 g/tsp; wafers 3.4 g/wafer

Side effects/adverse reactions:

GI: Nausea, vomiting, anorexia, diarrhea, cramps

Contraindications: Hypersensitivity, intestinal obstruction, abdominal pain, nausea/vomiting, fecal impaction

Precautions: Pregnancy (C)

Pharmacokinetics: Excreted in feces, not absorbed in GI tract

NURSING CONSIDERATIONS

Assess:

• Blood, urine electrolytes if used often

• I&O ratio to identify fluid loss

• Cause of constipation; fluids, bulk, exercise missing

• Cramping, rectal bleeding, nausea, vomiting; drug should be discontinued

Administer:

PO

• Alone for better absorption

• In morning or evening (oral dose)

• Immediately after mixing with H_2O

• With 8 oz H_2O or juice followed by another 8 oz of fluid

Evaluate:

• Therapeutic response: decrease in constipation or decreased diarrhea in colitis

Teach patient/family:

• To maintain adequate fluid consumption

• That normal bowel movements do not always occur daily

• Not to use in presence of abdominal pain, nausea, vomiting

• To notify prescriber if constipation unrelieved or if symptoms of electrolyte imbalance occur: muscle cramps, pain, weakness, dizziness, excessive thirst

---

pyrantel (℞)

(pie-ran'tel)

Antiminth, Combantrin*, Pin-Rid, Pin-X, Reese's Pinworm

Func. class.: Anthelmintic

Chem. class.: Pyrimidine derivative

Action: Causes paralysis in worm by neuroblockade via stimulation of ganglionic receptors; worms expelled by normal peristalsis

Uses: Pinworms, roundworms, hookworms

Dosage and routes:

• *Adult and child >2 yr:* **PO** 11 mg/kg as single dose, not to exceed 1 g; repeat in 2 wk for pinworms

Available forms: Oral susp 50 mg/ml; liquid 50 mg/ml; caps, soft gel 180 mg

Side effects/adverse reactions:

INTEG: Rash

CNS: Dizziness, headache, drowsiness, insomnia, fever, weakness

GI: Nausea, vomiting, anorexia, diarrhea, distention, abdominal cramps

Contraindications: Hypersensitivity

Precautions: Seizure disorders, hepatic disease, dehydration, anemia, child <2 yr, pregnancy (C)

Pharmacokinetics:

PO: Peak 1-3 hr; metabolized in liver; excreted in feces, urine (unchanged/metabolites)

Interactions:
• Antagonizes effect of pyrantel: piperazine
NURSING CONSIDERATIONS
Assess:
• Stools during entire treatment; specimens must be sent to lab while still warm
• For allergic reaction: rash
• For diarrhea during expulsion of worms
Administer:
PO
• After meals to avoid GI symptoms
• After shaking suspension
Perform/provide:
• Storage in tight, light-resistant container in cool environment
Evaluate:
• Therapeutic response: expulsion of worms, 3 negative stool cultures after completion of treatment
Teach patient/family:
• Proper hygiene after BM, including hand-washing technique; tell patient not to put fingers in mouth
• That infected person should sleep alone; not to shake bed linen; to change bed linen qd, wash in hot water
• To clean toilet qd with disinfectant (green soap solution)
• The need for compliance with dosage schedule, duration of treatment
• To drink fruit juice to help expel worms
• To wear shoes, wash all fruits, vegetables well before eating

---

pyrazinamide (R)
(peer-a-zin'a-mide)
PMS Pyrazinamide*, pyrazinamide, Tebrazid*
Func. class.: Antitubercular agent
Chem. class.: Pyrazinoic acid amine, nicoturimide analog

Action: Bactericidal interference with lipid, nucleic acid biosynthesis
Uses: Tuberculosis, as an adjunct when other drugs are not feasible
Dosage and routes:
• *Adult and child:* **PO** 15-30 mg/kg/day not to exceed 3 g/day
Available forms: Tabs 500 mg
Side effects/adverse reactions:
INTEG: Photosensitivity, urticaria
CNS: Headache
GI: **Hepatotoxicity,** abnormal liver function tests, peptic ulcer
GU: Urinary difficulty, increased uric acid, nausea, vomiting, anorexia
HEMA: **Hemolytic anemia**
Contraindications: Hypersensitivity, severe hepatic damage
Precautions: Pregnancy (C), child <13 yr
Pharmacokinetics:
PO: Peak 2 hr, half-life 9-10 hr; metabolized in liver, excreted in urine (metabolites/unchanged drug)
Lab test interferences:
Increase: PBI
Decrease: 17-KS
NURSING CONSIDERATIONS
Assess:
• Signs of anemia: Hct, Hgb, fatigue
• Temp; if >101° F (38° C), drug should be reduced
• Liver studies qwk: ALT, AST, bilirubin
• Renal status before, qmo: BUN, creatinine, output, sp gr, urinalysis, uric acid

---

◆ = Nursing alert   / = Herb-drug interaction   ⊘ = Do not crush

• Hepatic status: decreased appetite, jaundice, dark urine, fatigue
Administer:
PO
• With meals for GI symptoms
• After C&S is completed; qmo to detect resistance
Evaluate:
• Therapeutic response: decreased symptoms of TB, culture negative
Teach patient/family:
• That compliance with dosage schedule, length is necessary
• To avoid alcohol
• To report fever, loss of appetite, malaise, nausea, vomiting, darkened urine, pale stools

---

pyridostigmine (℞)

(peer-id-oh-stig'meen)
Regonol
Func. class.: Cholinergic; anticholinesterase
Chem. class.: Tertiary amine carbamate

Action: Inhibits destruction of acetylcholine, which increases concentration at sites where acetylcholine is released; this facilitates transmission of impulses across myoneural junction
Uses: Nondepolarizing muscle relaxant antagonist, myasthenia gravis
Dosage and routes:
Myasthenia gravis
• *Adult:* **PO** 60-180 mg bid-qid, not to exceed 1.5 g/day; **IM/IV** 2 mg or ¹/₃₀ of **PO** dose; **SUS REL** 180-540 mg qd or bid at intervals of at least 6 hr
• *Child:* 7 mg/kg/day in 5-6 divided doses

Nondepolarizing neuromuscular blocker antagonist
• *Adult:* 0.6-1.2 mg **IV** atropine, then 10-30 mg
• *Child:* **IV** 0.1-0.25 mg/kg/dose
Available forms: Tabs 60 mg; tabs, sus rel 180 mg; syr 60 mg/5 ml; inj 5 mg/ml
Side effects/adverse reactions:
INTEG: Rash, urticaria, flushing
CNS: Dizziness, headache, sweating, weakness, ***convulsions,*** incoordination, ***paralysis,*** drowsiness, LOC
GI: *Nausea, diarrhea, vomiting, cramps, increased salivary and gastric secretions, peristalsis*
CV: Tachycardia, dysrhythmias, bradycardia, AV block, hypotension, ECG changes, ***cardiac arrest,*** syncope
GU: Urinary frequency, incontinence, urgency
RESP: ***Respiratory depression, bronchospasm, constriction, laryngospasm, respiratory arrest***
EENT: Miosis, blurred vision, lacrimation, visual changes
Contraindications: Bradycardia; hypotension; obstruction of intestine, renal system; bromide sensitivity
Precautions: Seizure disorders, bronchial asthma, coronary occlusion, hyperthyroidism, dysrhythmias, peptic ulcer, megacolon, poor GI motility, pregnancy (C)
Pharmacokinetics:
PO: Onset 20-30 min, duration 3-6 hr
IM/IV/SC: Onset 2-15 min, duration 2½-4 hr; metabolized in liver, excreted in urine
Interactions:
• Decreased action: gallamine, metocurine, pancuronium, tubocurarine, atropine
• Increased action: decamethonium, succinylcholine

P

• Decreased action of pyridostigmine: aminoglycosides, anesthetics, procainamide, quinidine, mecamylamine, polymyxin, magnesium, corticosteroids, antidysrhythmics

NURSING CONSIDERATIONS
Assess:
• VS, respiration q8h
• I&O ratio; check for urinary retention or incontinence
• Bradycardia, hypotension, bronchospasm, headache, dizziness, convulsions, respiratory depression; drug should be discontinued if toxicity occurs
Administer:
• Only with atropine sulfate available for cholinergic crisis
• Only after all other cholinergics have been discontinued
• Increased doses for tolerance
• Larger doses after exercise or fatigue
• On empty stomach for better absorption
IV
• Undiluted, give through Y-tube or 3-way stopcock, give 0.5 mg or less/min
Syringe compatibilities: Glycopyrrolate
Y-site compatibilities: Heparin, hydrocortisone, potassium chloride, vit B/C
Perform/provide:
• Storage at room temp
Evaluate:
• Therapeutic response: increased muscle strength, hand grasp, improved gait, absence of labored breathing (if severe)
Teach patient/family:
🚫 Not to break, crush, or chew sus rel tabs
• That drug is not a cure, only relieves symptoms

• To wear Medic Alert ID specifying myasthenia gravis, drugs taken
Treatment of overdose: Discontinue drug, atropine 1-4 mg IV

---

pyridoxine (vit B$_6$)
(R, OTC)
(peer-i-dox'een)
Nestrex, pyridoxine HCl, vitamin B$_6$
Func. class.: Vit B$_6$, water soluble

Action: Needed for fat, protein, carbohydrate metabolism; enhances glycogen release from liver and muscle tissue; needed as coenzyme for metabolic transformations of a variety of amino acids
Uses: Vit B$_6$ deficiency of inborn errors of metabolism, seizures, isoniazid therapy, oral contraceptives, alcoholic polyneuritis
Dosage and routes:
RDA
• *Adult:* Male 1.7-2 mg; female 1.4-1.6 mg
Vit B$_6$ deficiency
• *Adult:* **PO/IM/IV** 10-20 mg qd × 3wk
• *Child:* **PO/IM/IV** 100 mg until desired response
Deficiency caused by isoniazid
• *Adult:* **PO** 6-100 mg qd
• *Child:* **PO** 5-25 mg/day
Prevention of deficiency caused by isoniazid
• *Adult:* **PO** 6-50 mg qd
• *Child:* **PO** 0.5-1.5 mg qd
• *Infant:* **PO** 0.1-0.5 mg qd
Available forms: Tabs 10, 25, 50, 100 mg; tabs, time rel 100 mg; inj 100 mg/ml
Side effects/adverse reactions:
CNS: Paresthesia, flushing, warmth, lethargy (rare with normal renal function)
INTEG: Pain at injection site

◆ = Nursing alert   ▨ = Herb-drug interaction   🚫 = Do not crush

Contraindications: Hypersensitivity

Precautions: Pregnancy (A), lactation, children, Parkinson's disease

Pharmacokinetics:

PO/Inj: Half-life 2-3 wk, metabolized in liver, excreted in urine

Interactions:

• Decreased effects of levodopa

• Decreased effects of pyridoxine: oral contraceptives, isoniazid, cycloserine, hydralazine, penicillamine

NURSING CONSIDERATIONS
Assess:

• Pyridoxine levels throughout treatment

• Nutritional status: yeast, liver, legumes, bananas, green vegetables, whole grains

Administer:

IM

• Rotate sites; burning or stinging at site may occur

• Z-track to minimize pain

IV

• Undiluted or added to most IV sol; give 50 mg or less/1 min if undiluted

Syringe compatibilities: Doxapram

Perform/provide:

• Storage in tight, light-resistant container

Evaluate:

• Therapeutic response: absence of nausea, vomiting, anorexia, skin lesions, glossitis, stomatitis, edema, convulsions, restlessness, paresthesia

Teach patient/family:

• To avoid vitamin supplements unless directed by prescriber

• To keep out of children's reach

• To increase meat, bananas, potatoes, lima beans, whole grain cereals in diet

• To discuss birth control status with prescriber

---

pyrimethamine (℞)

(peer-i-meth'a-meen)
Daraprim, Fansidar (with sulfadoxine)

Func. class.: Antimalarial
Chem. class.: Folic acid antagonist

Action: Inhibits folic acid metabolism in parasite, prevents transmission by stopping growth of fertilized gametes

Uses: Malaria prophylaxis, *P. vivax*

Investigational uses: *Pneumocystis carinii* pneumonia as an adjunct

Dosage and routes:

Prophylaxis of malaria

• *Adult and child >10 yr:* **PO** 25 mg qwk

• *Child 4-10 yr:* **PO** 12.5 mg qwk

• *Child <4 yr:* **PO** 6.25 mg qwk

Toxoplasmosis

• *Adult:* **PO** 100 mg, then 25 mg qd × 4-5 wk, with 1 g sulfadoxine q6h

• *Child:* **PO** 1 mg/kg/day in 2 divided doses or 2 mg/kg/day × 3 days, then 1 mg/kg/day or divided twice qd × 4 wk, max 25 mg/day

Toxoplasmosis in AIDS patients

• *Adult:* **PO** 100-200 mg/day × 1-2 days, then 50-100 mg/day × 3-6 wk, then 25-50 mg/day for life (given with clindamycin or sulfadiazine)

Available forms: Tabs 25 mg; combo tabs 500 mg sulfadoxine/25 mg pyrimethamine

Side effects/adverse reactions:

*RESP: **Respiratory failure***

INTEG: Skin eruptions, photosensitivity

CNS: Stimulation, irritability, ***convulsions,*** tremors, ataxia, fatigue

GI: Nausea, vomiting, cramps, anorexia, diarrhea, atrophic glossitis, gastritis

*HEMA: **Thrombocytopenia, leuko-***

---

penia, pancytopenia, megaloblastic anemia, decreased folic acid, *agranulocytosis*

Contraindications: Hypersensitivity, chloroquine-resistant malaria, megaloblastic anemia caused by folate deficiency

Precautions: Blood dyscrasias, seizure disorder, pregnancy (C), lactation, G6PD disease, renal, hepatic disease

Pharmacokinetics:

PO: Peak 2 hr, half-life 111 hr; metabolized in liver, highly protein bound, excreted in urine (metabolites)

Interactions:

• Synergistic action: paraaminobenzoic acid or folic acid

• Increased bone marrow suppression: antibiotics

NURSING CONSIDERATIONS
Assess:

• Folic acid level; megaloblastic anemia occurs

• Blood studies, CBC, platelets, since blood dyscrasias occur; twice weekly if dosage is increased

◆ For toxicity: vomiting, anorexia, seizure, blood dyscrasia, glossitis; drug should be discontinued immediately

Administer:

• Leucovorin IM 3-9 mg/day × 3 days if folic acid deficiency occurs

• Before or after meals at same time each day to maintain drug level, to decrease GI symptoms

Perform/provide:

• Storage in tight, light-resistant container

Evaluate:

• Therapeutic response: decreased symptoms of malaria

Teach patient/family:

• To report visual problems, fever, fatigue, bruising, bleeding; may indicate blood dyscrasias

Treatment of overdose: Gastric lavage, short-acting barbiturate, leucovorin, respiratory support if needed

---

quetiapine (℞)
(kwe-tie'a-peen)
Seroquel
Func. class.: Antipsychotic/neuroleptic

Action: Functions as an antagonist at multiple neurotransmitter receptors in the brain including $5HT_{1A}$, $5HT_2$, dopamine D_1, D_2, H_1, and adrenergic alpha$_1$, alpha$_2$ receptors

Uses: Psychotic disorders

Dosage and routes:

• *Adult:* **PO** 25 mg bid, with incremental increases of 25 mg bid-tid on days 2 and 3 to a dose of 300-400 mg qd given bid-tid

Available forms: Tabs 25, 100, 200 mg

Side effects/adverse reactions:

CNS: EPS, pseudoparkinsonism, akathisia, dystonia, tardive dyskinesia; drowsiness, insomnia, agitation, anxiety, *headache, seizures, neuroleptic malignant syndrome, dizziness*

CV: Orthostatic hypotension, *tachycardia*

GI: Nausea, anorexia, constipation, abdominal pain, dry mouth

RESP: Rhinitis

INTEG: Rash

MISC: Asthenia, back pain, fever, ear pain

Contraindications: Hypersensitivity

Precautions: Children, pregnancy (C), hepatic disease, elderly, breast cancer, lactation, long-term use, seizures, dementia

Pharmacokinetics:

PO: Extensively metabolized by liver half-life ≥6 hr; peak 1½ hr

---

◆ = Nursing alert   ◢ = Herb-drug interaction   Ⓝ = Do not crush

Interactions:

• Decreased clearance of quetiapine: cimetidine

• Increased clearance of quetiapine: phenytoin, thioridazine, barbiturates, glucocorticoids

• Decreased clearance of lorazepam: lorazepam

• Decreased clearance of levodopa: levodopa

• Decreased effects of dopamine agonists: dopamine agonists

NURSING CONSIDERATIONS
Assess:

• Mental status before initial administration

• Swallowing of PO medication: check for hoarding or giving of medication to other patients

• I&O ratio; palpate bladder if urinary output is low

• Bilirubin, CBC, liver function studies qmo

• Urinalysis before, during prolonged therapy

• Affect, orientation, LOC, reflexes, gait, coordination, sleep pattern disturbances

• B/P standing and lying; also pulse, respirations; take these q4h during initial treatment; establish baseline before starting treatment; report drops of 30 mm Hg; watch for ECG changes

• Dizziness, faintness, palpitations, tachycardia on rising

• EPS, including akathisia (inability to sit still, no pattern to movements), tardive dyskinesia (bizarre movements of the jaw, mouth, tongue, extremities), pseudoparkinsonism (rigidit/y, tremors, pill rolling, shuffling gait)

◆ For neuroleptic malignant syndrome: hyperthermia, increased CPK, altered mental status, muscle rigidity

• Skin turgor qd

• Constipation, urinary retention qd; if these occur, increase bulk and water in the diet

Administer:

• Reduced dose in elderly

• Antiparkinsonian agent on order from prescriber, to be used for EPS

Perform/provide:

• Decreased stimulus by dimming lights, avoiding loud noises

• Supervised ambulation until patient is stabilized on medication; do not involve in strenuous exercise program because fainting is possible; patient should not stand still for a long time

• Increased fluids to prevent constipation

• Sips of water, candy, gum for dry mouth

• Storage in tight, light-resistant container

Evaluate:

• Therapeutic response: decrease in emotional excitement, hallucinations, delusions, paranoia; reorganization of patterns of thought, speech

---

quinapril (℞)
(kwin′a-pril)
Accupril
Func. class.: Antihypertensive
Chem. class.: Angiotensin-converting enzyme (ACE) inhibitor

Action: Selectively suppresses renin-angiotensin-aldosterone system; inhibits ACE, prevents conversion of angiotensin I to angiotensin II; results in dilation of arterial, venous vessels

Uses: Hypertension, alone or in combination with thiazide diuretics; systolic CHF

Side effects: *italics* = common; ***bold italics*** = life-threatening

Dosage and routes:
Renal dose
• CrCl 30-60 ml/min 5 mg/day initially; CrCl <30 ml/min 2.5 mg/day initially
Hypertension (alone)
• *Adult:* **PO** 10-20 mg qd initially, then 20-80 mg/day divided bid or qd
• *Geriatric:* **PO** 10 mg qd, titrate to desired response
Congestive heart failure
• *Adult:* **PO** 2.5 mg initially, then 5-40 mg/day maintenance qd or in 2 divided doses
Available forms: Tabs 5, 10, 20, 40 mg

Side effects/adverse reactions:
CV: Hypotension, postural hypotension, syncope, palpitations, angina pectoris, *MI, tachycardia,* vasodilation
GU: Increased BUN, creatinine, decreased libido, impotence, urinary tract infection
HEMA: **Thrombocytopenia, agranulocytosis**
INTEG: **Angioedema,** rash, sweating, photosensitivity, pruritus
RESP: Cough, bronchitis
META: Hyperkalemia
GI: Nausea, constipation, vomiting, gastritis, *GI hemorrhage,* dry mouth
CNS: Headache, dizziness, fatigue, somnolence, depression, malaise, nervousness, vertigo
MISC: Back pain, amblyopia, pharyngitis
MS: Arthralgia, arthritis, myalgia

Contraindications: Hypersensitivity to ACE inhibitors, pregnancy (D) 2nd/3rd trimester, children
Precautions: Impaired renal, liver function, dialysis patients, hypovolemia, blood dyscrasias, COPD, asthma, elderly, lactation
Pharmacokinetics:
PO: Peak ½-1 hr, serum protein binding 97%, half-life 2 hr, metabolized by liver (metabolites), metabolites excreted in urine

Interactions:
• Increased hypotension: diuretics, other antihypertensives, ganglionic blockers, adrenergic blockers, phenothiazines
• Use caution with vasodilators, hydralazine, prazosin, potassium-sparing diuretics, sympathomimetics, K supplements
• Decreased absorption of tetracycline
• Reduced hypotensive effect of quinapril: indomethacin
• Increased toxicity: lithium, digoxin

Lab test interferences:
False positive: Urine acetone

NURSING CONSIDERATIONS
Assess:
• Blood studies: neutrophils, decreased platelets
• B/P, orthostatic hypotension, syncope
• Renal studies: protein, BUN, creatinine; watch for increased levels; may indicate nephrotic syndrome
• Baselines in renal, liver function tests before therapy begins
• K levels; hyperkalemia is rare
• Edema in feet, legs qd
• Allergic reactions: rash, fever, pruritus, urticaria; drug should be discontinued if antihistamines fail to help
• Renal symptoms: polyuria, oliguria, urinary frequency, dysuria
Administer:
• IV infusion of 0.9% NaCl (as ordered) to expand fluid volume if severe hypotension occurs
Perform/provide:
• Supine or Trendelenburg position for severe hypotension
Evaluate:
• Therapeutic response: decrease in B/P

◆ = Nursing alert   ∥ = Herb-drug interaction   ⊘ = Do not crush

Teach patient/family:
• To take 1 hr before meals; not to take antacids within 1-2 hr of quinapril
• Not to discontinue drug abruptly
• Not to use OTC products (cough, cold, allergy); not to use salt substitutes containing potassium unless directed by prescriber
• To comply with dosage schedule, even if feeling better
• To rise slowly to sitting or standing position to minimize orthostatic hypotension
• To notify prescriber of mouth sores, sore throat, fever, swelling of hands or feet, irregular heartbeat, chest pain, persistent dry cough
• To report excessive perspiration, dehydration, vomiting, diarrhea; may lead to fall in B/P
• That drug may cause dizziness, fainting, light-headedness; may occur during first few days of therapy
• That drug may cause skin rash or impaired taste perception
• How to take B/P, and normal readings for age group

Treatment of overdose: 0.9% NaCl IV inf

---

quinidine (℞)
(kwin'i-deen)
Apo-Quinidine*, Cardioquin; Cin-Quin*, Novoquinidin*, Quinaglute, Quinalan, Quinidex Extentabs, quinidine gluconate; quinidine sulfate
Func. class.: Antidysrhythmic (Class Ia)
Chem. class.: Quinine dextroisomer

Action: Prolongs duration of action potential and effective refractory period, thus decreasing myocardial excitability; anticholinergic properties

Uses: PVCs, atrial fibrillation, PAT, ventricular tachycardia, atrial dysrhythmias

Investigational uses: Malaria/IV quinidine gluconate

Dosage and routes:
Quinidine sulfate
Atrial fibrillation/flutter
• *Adult:* PO 200 mg q2-3h × 5-8 doses; may increase qd until sinus rhythm is restored; max 4 g/day given only after digitalization
Paroxysmal supraventricular tachycardia
• *Adult:* PO 400-600 mg q2-3h, then 200-300 mg q6-8h or 300-600 mg q8-12h (sus rel)
Premature atrial/ventricular contraction
• *Adult:* PO 200-300 mg q6-8h or 300-600 mg (sus rel) q8-12h; max 4 g/day
• *Child:* PO 30 mg/kg/day or 900 mg/m^2/day in 5 divided doses
Quinidine gluconate
• *Adult:* PO 324-660 mg q6-12h (sus rel); IM 600 mg, then 400 mg q2h; IV give 16 mg/min
Quinidine polygalacturonate
• *Adult:* PO 275-825 mg q3-4h × 4 doses, then increase by 137.5-275 mg; repeat up to 4× until dysrhythmias decreased
• *Child:* PO 8.25 mg/kg (247.5 mg/m^2) 5×/day
Available forms: Gluconate tabs sus rel 324, 330 mg; inj gluconate 80 mg/ml; sulfate tabs 200, 300 mg; tabs sus rel 300 mg; polygalacturonate tabs 275 mg

Side effects/adverse reactions:
CNS: Headache, dizziness, involuntary movement, confusion, psychosis, restlessness, irritability, syncope, excitement
EENT: Cinchonism: tinnitus, blurred

vision, hearing loss, mydriasis, disturbed color vision

GI: Nausea, vomiting, anorexia, *diarrhea, hepatotoxicity*

CV: Hypotension, bradycardia, PVCs, *heart block, cardiovascular collapse, arrest,* torsades de pointes

HEMA: Thrombocytopenia, hemolytic anemia, agranulocytosis, hypoprothrombinemia

RESP: Dyspnea, *respiratory depression*

INTEG: Rash, urticaria, angioedema, swelling, photosensitivity

Contraindications: Hypersensitivity, blood dyscrasias, severe heart block, myasthenia gravis

Precautions: Pregnancy (C), lactation, children, renal disease, K imbalance, liver disease, CHF, respiratory depression

Pharmacokinetics:

PO: Peak 0.5-6 hr, duration 6-8 hr; half-life 6-7 hr, metabolized in liver, excreted unchanged by kidneys

Interactions:

• Increased effects of neuromuscular blockers, digoxin, warfarin

• Increased effects of quinidine: cimetidine, propranolol, thiazides, sodium bicarbonate, carbonic anhydrase inhibitors, antacids, hydroxide suspensions, amiodarone

• May decrease effects of quinidine: barbiturates, phenytoin, rifampin, nifedipine

• Additive vagolytic effect: anticholinergic blockers

• Additive cardiac depression: other antidysrhythmics, phenothiazines, reserpine

🌿 Potassium deficiency, increased antidysrhythmic action: aloe, buckthorn, cascara sagrada, senna

• Food/drug: delayed absorption, decreased metabolism: grapefruit

Lab test interferences:

Increase: CPK

NURSING CONSIDERATIONS

Assess:

• ECG continuously to determine increased PR or QRS segments, QT interval; discontinue or reduce dose

• Blood levels (therapeutic level 2-6 μg/ml)

• B/P continuously for fluctuations

• For cinchonism: tinnitus, headache, nausea, dizziness, fever, vertigo, tremor; may lead to hearing loss

• Cardiac status: rate, rhythm, character, continuously

• Respiratory status: rate, rhythm, lung fields for rales; increased respiration, increased pulse; drug should be discontinued

• CNS effects: dizziness, confusion, psychosis, paresthesias, convulsions; drug should be discontinued

Administer:

• AV node blocker (digoxin, verapamil) before starting quinidine to avoid increased ventricular rate

IM

• IM inj in deltoid; aspirate to avoid intravascular administration

IV

• After diluting 800 mg/40 ml or more D_5; give 16 mg or less over 1 min as inf; use inf pump

Additive compatibilities: Bretylium, cimetidine, milrinone, ranitidine, verapamil

Y-site compatibilities: Diazepam, milrinone

Evaluate:

• Therapeutic response: decreased dysrhythmias

Treatment of overdose: O_2, artificial ventilation, ECG, administer dopamine for circulatory depression, diazepam or thiopental for convulsions

---

◆ = Nursing alert   🌿 = Herb-drug interaction   ⊘ = Do not crush

quinine (OTC, ℞)

(kwye'nine)
Novoquine*, quinine sulfate
Func. class.: Antimalarial
Chem. class.: Cinchona tree alkaloid

Action: Inhibits parasite replications, transcription of DNA to RNA by forming complexes with DNA of parasite

Uses: *Plasmodium falciparum,* malaria, nocturnal leg cramps

Dosage and routes:
• *Adult:* **PO** 650 mg q8h × 10 days, given with pyrimethamine 25 mg q12h × 3 days, with sulfadiazine 500 mg qid × 5 days
• *Child:* **PO** 25 mg/kg/day divided q8h for 3-7 days

Leg cramps
• *Adult:* **PO** 250-300 mg hs

Available forms: Caps 200, 260, 325 mg; tabs 260 mg

Side effects/adverse reactions:
RESP: Dyspnea
INTEG: Pruritus, pigmentary changes, skin eruptions, lichen planuslike eruptions, flushing, facial edema, sweating
HEMA: ***Thrombocytopenia, purpura, hypothrombinemia, hemolysis***
CNS: Headache, stimulation, fatigue, irritability, ***convulsions,*** bad dreams, dizziness, fever, confusion, anxiety
EENT: Blurred vision, corneal changes, retinal changes, difficulty focusing, tinnitus, vertigo, deafness, photophobia, diplopia, night blindness
GU: Renal tubular damage, *anuria*
GI: Nausea, vomiting, anorexia, diarrhea, epigastric pain
CV: Angina, dysrhythmias, tachycardia, hypotension, ***acute circulatory failure***
ENDO: Hypoglycemia

Contraindications: Hypersensitivity, G6PD deficiency, retinal field changes, pregnancy (X)

Precautions: Blood dyscrasias, severe GI disease, neurologic disease, severe hepatic disease, psoriasis, cardiac dysrhythmias, tinnitus

Pharmacokinetics:
PO: Peak 1-3 hr, metabolized in liver, excreted in urine, half-life 4-5 hr

Interactions:
• Toxicity: $NaHCO_3$, acetazolamide
• Decreased absorption: magnesium or aluminum salts
• Increased levels of digoxin, digitoxin, neuromuscular blockers, other anticoagulants

Lab test interferences:
Increase: 17-KS
Interference: 17-OHCS

NURSING CONSIDERATIONS
Assess:
• B/P, pulse, watch for hypotension, tachycardia
• Liver studies qwk: ALT, AST, bilirubin
• Blood studies, CBC, since blood dyscrasias occur
• For cinchonism: nausea, blurred vision, tinnitus, headache, difficulty focusing

Administer:
• Before or after meals at same time each day to maintain level

Perform/provide:
• Storage in tight, light-resistant container

Evaluate:
• Therapeutic response: decreased symptoms of malaria

Teach patient/family:
• To avoid OTC preparations: cold preparations, tonic water

rabeprazole
See appendix a—selected new drugs

R

---

* = Canada only   Side effects: *italics* = common; ***bold italics*** = life-threatening

rabies immune globulin, human (℞)

Hyperab, Imogam
Func. class.: Immune serum
Chem. class.: IgG

Action: Provides passive immunity; given with HDCV; may be used regardless of time of bite, treatment
Uses: Exposure to rabies
Dosage and routes:
• *Adult and child:* **IM** 20 IU/kg given at same time as 1st rabies vaccine; infiltrate wound with ½ dose, then administer rest **IM**
Available forms: Inj 150 IU/ml
Side effects/adverse reactions:
INTEG: Pain at injection site, rash, pruritus
MS: Arthralgia
SYST: Lymphadenopathy, *anaphylaxis,* fever
CNS: Headache, fatigue, malaise
GI: Abdominal pain
Contraindications: Hypersensitivity to equine products and thimerosal
Interactions:
• Decreased action of rabies immune globulin: corticosteroids, immunosuppressants
NURSING CONSIDERATIONS
Administer:
• Test dose: dilute drug either with 1:100 or 1:1000 0.9% NaCl for inj, inj 0.1 ml 0.9% NaCl in other arm intradermally, check for wheal [dG]10 mm after 10 min; if present, drug should not be used
• Only with epinephrine 1:1000, resuscitative equipment available
• As soon as possible after exposure
Perform/provide:
• Storage at 36°-46°F (2°-8°C)
Evaluate:
• Allergic reactions: dyspnea, rash, pruritus, eruptions

Teach patient/family:
• That pain, swelling, itching may occur at injection site
• To take acetaminophen to alleviate headache, fever, and pain

radioactive iodine (sodium iodide) ^{131}I (℞)

Func. class.: Antithyroid
Chem. class.: Radiopharmaceutical

Action: Converted to protein-bound iodine by thyroid gland for use when needed
Uses:
High dose: Thyroid cancer, hyperthyroidism
Low dose: Visualization to determine thyroid cancer, diagnostic aid in thyroid function studies
Dosage and routes:
Thyroid cancer
• *Adult:* **PO** 50-150 mCi, may repeat depending on clinical status
Hyperthyroidism
• *Adult:* **PO** 4-10 mCi, depending on serum thyroxine level
Available forms: Caps 1-50, 0.8-100 mCi; oral sol 7.05 mCi/ml, 3.5-150 mCi/vial
Side effects/adverse reactions:
ENDO: Hypothyroidism, *hyperthyroid adenoma,* transient thyroiditis
INTEG: Alopecia
HEMA: Eosinophilia, lymphedema, leukemia, bone marrow depression, leukopenia, anemia
GI: Nausea, diarrhea, vomiting
EENT: Sore throat, cough
Contraindications: Recent MI, lactation, large nodular goiter, pregnancy (X), age <30 yr, vomiting/diarrhea, acute hyperthyroidism, use of thyroid drugs, lactation

◆ = Nursing alert   ⫽ = Herb-drug interaction   ◎ = Do not crush

Pharmacokinetics:

PO: Onset 3-6 days; excreted in urine, sweat, feces, breast milk; crosses placenta; excreted in 56 days

Interactions:

• Hypothyroidism: lithium

• Decreased uptake if recent intake of stable iodine, thyroid, antithyroid drugs

NURSING CONSIDERATIONS
Assess:

• Weight qd in same clothing, scale, time of day

• Blood work, including CBC for blood dyscrasias (leukopenia, thrombocytopenia, agranulocytosis)

• Overdose: peripheral edema, heat intolerance, diaphoresis, palpitations, dysrhythmias, severe tachycardia, increased temp, delirium, CNS irritability

• Hypersensitivity: rash, enlarged cervical lymph nodes; drug may have to be discontinued

• Hypoprothrombinemia: bleeding, petechiae, ecchymosis

• Clinical response: after 3 wk should include increased weight, pulse; decreased T_4

• Bone marrow depression: sore throat, fever, fatigue

Administer:

• Only after discontinuing all other antithyroid agents × 5-7 days

• After NPO overnight, food delays action

• During or within 10 days after menstruation

Perform/provide:

• Limited contact with patient ½ hr/day for each person

• Adequate rest after treatment

• Fluids to 3-4 L/day for 48 hr to remove agent from body

Evaluate:

• Therapeutic response: weight gain, decreased pulse, decreased T_4, B/P

Teach patient/family:

• To empty bladder often during treatment; avoid irradiation of gonads

• To report redness, swelling, sore throat, mouth lesions; indicate blood dyscrasias

• To avoid extended contact with children, spouse for 1 wk

• That bathroom may be used by entire family

• Not to take antithyroid agents but propranolol, which decreases hyperthyroid symptoms, until total effect of taking ^{131}I has occurred (about 6 wk)

• To avoid coughing, expectorating for 24 hr (saliva and vomitus are highly radioactive for 6-8 hr)

---

raloxifene (℞)

(ral-ox'ih-feen)

Evista

Func. class.: Selective estrogen receptor modulator (SERM)

Chem. class.: Benzthiophene

Action: Reduces resorption of bone and decreases bone turnover; mediated through estrogen receptor binding

Uses: Prevention of osteoporosis in postmenopausal women

Dosage and routes:

• *Adult:* **PO** 60 mg qd

Available forms: Tabs 60 mg

Side effects/adverse reactions:

CNS: Insomnia, migraines, depression

CV: Hot flashes

GI: Nausea, vomiting, diarrhea, anorexia, cramps

GU: Vaginitis, UTI, leukorrhea, endometrial disorder, breast pain

INTEG: Rash, sweating

META: Weight gain, peripheral edema

R

MS: Arthralgia, myalgia, leg cramps, arthritis

RESP: Sinusitis, pharyngitis, increased cough, pneumonia, laryngitis

Contraindications: Hypersensitivity, pregnancy (X), lactation

Precautions: Lactation, venous thromboembolic events, hepatic disease

Pharmacokinetics: Elimination half-life 28 hr; excreted in feces; excreted in breast milk; highly bound to plasma proteins

Interactions:

• Decreased action of anticoagulants

• Decreased action of raloxifene: ampicillin, cholestyramine

• Administer cautiously with other highly protein-bound drugs

Lab test interferences:

Increase: Apolipoprotein A_1, B, lipoprotein, fibrinogen, LDL cholesterol, total cholesterol, corticosteroid-binding globulin, thyroxine-binding globulin (TBG)

Decrease: Calcium, total protein, albumin, platelets

NURSING CONSIDERATIONS
Assess:

• Blood glucose of diabetic patient

• Weight daily, notify prescriber of weekly weight gain >5 lb

• B/P q4h, watch for increase caused by H_2O and Na retention

• I&O ratio; decreasing urinary output, increasing edema

• Liver function studies, including AST, ALT, bilirubin, alk phosphatase

Administer:
PO

• Without regard to meals

Evaluate:

• Therapeutic response: prevention of osteoporosis

Teach patient/family:

• To weigh weekly, report gain >5 lb

• To discontinue 72 hr before prolonged bedrest; advise to avoid one position for long periods

• To take calcium supplements, vit D if intake is inadequate

• To increase exercise using weights

• To stop smoking and to decrease alcohol consumption

• That this drug does not help control hot flashes

• To report fever, acute migraine, insomnia, emotional distress; urinary tract infection, or vaginal burning/itching; swelling, warmth, or pain in calves

---

ramipril (℞)

(ra-mi′pril)
Altace

Func. class.: Antihypertensive
Chem. class.: Angiotensin-converting enzyme inhibitor (ACE)

Action: Selectively suppresses renin-angiotensin-aldosterone system; inhibits ACE, prevents conversion of angiotensin I to angiotensin II; results in dilation of arterial, venous vessels

Uses: Hypertension, alone or in combination with thiazide diuretics; CHF (post MI)

Dosage and routes:

• *Adult:* **PO** 2.5 mg qd initially, then 2.5-20 mg/day divided bid or qd; *renal impairment:* 1.25 mg qd with CrCl <40 ml/min/1.73 m^2, increase as needed to max or 5 mg/day
CHF

• *Adult:* **PO** 1.25-2.5 mg bid; may increase to 5 mg bid

Available forms: Caps 1.25, 2.5, 5, 10 mg

Side effects/adverse reactions:

CV: Hypotension, chest pain, palpi-

◆ = Nursing alert   🌿 = Herb-drug interaction   🚫 = Do not crush

tations, angina, syncope, dysrhythmia

GU: **Proteinuria,** increased BUN, creatinine, impotence

HEMA: Decreased Hct, Hgb, *eosinophilia, leukopenia*

INTEG: **Angioedema,** rash, sweating, photosensitivity, pruritus

RESP: Cough, dyspnea

META: Hyperkalemia

GI: *Nausea,* constipation, vomiting, dyspepsia, dysphagia, anorexia, diarrhea, abdominal pain

CNS: *Headache, dizziness,* anxiety, insomnia, paresthesia, fatigue, depression, malaise, vertigo, ***convulsions,*** hearing loss

MS: Arthralgia, arthritis, myalgia

Contraindications: Hypersensitivity to ACE inhibitors, pregnancy (D), lactation, children

Precautions: Impaired renal, liver function; dialysis patients, hypovolemia, blood dyscrasias, CHF, COPD, asthma, elderly, renal artery stenosis

Pharmacokinetics:

PO: Peak ½-1 hr, serum protein binding 97%, half-life 1-2 hr, metabolized by liver (metabolites excreted in urine, feces)

Interactions:

• Increased hypotension: diuretics, other antihypertensives, ganglionic blockers, adrenergic blockers

• Increased toxicity: vasodilators, hydralazine, prazosin, K-sparing diuretics, sympathomimetics, K supplements

• Decreased absorption: antacids

• Decreased antihypertensive effect: indomethacin

• Increased serum levels of digoxin, lithium

• Increased hypersensitivity: allopurinol

Lab test interferences:

False positive: Urine acetone

NURSING CONSIDERATIONS
Assess:

• Blood studies: neutrophils, decreased platelets

• B/P, orthostatic hypotension, syncope

• Renal studies: protein, BUN, creatinine; increased levels may indicate nephrotic syndrome

• Baselines in renal, liver function tests before therapy begins

• K levels, although hyperkalemia rarely occurs

• Dipstick of urine for protein qd in first morning specimen; if protein is increased, a 24-hr urinary protein should be collected

• Edema in feet, legs qd

• Allergic reactions: rash, fever, pruritus, urticaria; drug should be discontinued if antihistamines fail to help

• Renal symptoms: polyuria, oliguria, urinary frequency, dysuria

Administer:

• Caps can be opened and added to food

Perform/provide:

• Storage in tight container at 86° F (30° C) or less

• Supine position for severe hypotension

Evaluate:

• Therapeutic response: decrease in B/P

Teach patient/family:

• Not to discontinue drug abruptly

• Not to use OTC products (cough, cold, allergy) unless directed by prescriber; not to use salt substitutes containing potassium without consulting prescriber

• To comply with dosage schedule, even if feeling better

• To rise slowly to sitting or standing position to minimize orthostatic hypotension

• To notify prescriber of mouth sores, sore throat, fever, swelling of

R

hands or feet, irregular heartbeat, chest pain
• To report excessive perspiration, dehydration, vomiting, diarrhea; may lead to fall in B/P
• That drug may cause dizziness, fainting, light-headedness; may occur during first few days of therapy
• That drug may cause skin rash or impaired perspiration
• How to take B/P, and normal readings for age group
Treatment of overdose: 0.9% NaCl IV inf, hemodialysis

---

ranitidine (℞, OTC)
(ra-nit'i-deen)
Apo-Ranitidine*, Zantac, Zantac C*, Zantac EFFER-dose, Zantac GELdose
Func. class.: H_2-histamine receptor antagonist

Action: Inhibits histamine at H_2-receptor site in parietal cells, which inhibits gastric acid secretion
Uses: Duodenal ulcer, Zollinger-Ellison syndrome, gastric ulcers, hypersecretory conditions, gastroesophageal reflux disease, stress ulcers, erosive esophagitis (maintenance), active duodenal ulcers with *Helicobacter pylori* in combination with clarithromycin
Investigational uses: Prevention of aspiration pneumonitis, stress ulcers, upper GI bleeding
Dosage and routes:
Renal dose
• CrCl <50 ml/min give **PO** q24h give **IM/IV** q8-24h
Duodenal ulcer
• *Adult:* **PO** 150 mg bid, maintenance 150 hs
Zollinger-Ellison syndrome
• *Adult:* **PO** 150 mg bid, may increase if needed

Gastric ulcer
• *Adult:* **PO** 150 mg bid × 6 wk, then 150 mg hs
GERD
• *Adult:* **PO** 150 mg bid
Erosive esophagitis
• *Adult:* **PO** 150 mg qid
• *Adult:* **PO** 150 mg bid, 300 mg hs; **IM** 50 mg q6-8h; **IV BOL** 50 mg diluted to 20 ml over 5 min q6-8h; **IV INT INF** 50 mg/100 ml D_5 over 15-20 min q6-8h
• *Child:* **PO** 4-5 mg/kg/day divided q8-12h, max 6 mg/kg/day or 300 mg; **IV** 2-4 mg/kg/day divided q6-8h
Available forms: Tabs 75, 150, 300 mg; tabs, effervescent 150 mg; inj 0.5, 25 mg/ml; caps 150, 300 mg; syr 15 mg/ml; granules, effervescent 150 mg
Side effects/adverse reactions:
CNS: Headache, sleeplessness, dizziness, confusion, agitation, depression, hallucination (elderly)
GI: Constipation, abdominal pain, diarrhea, nausea, vomiting, ***hepatotoxicity***
GU: Impotence, gynecomastia
CV: Tachycardia, bradycardia, PVCs
EENT: Blurred vision, increased ocular pressure
INTEG: Urticaria, rash, fever
Contraindications: Hypersensitivity
Precautions: Pregnancy (B), lactation, child <12 yr, hepatic disease, renal disease
Pharmacokinetics:
PO: Peak 2-3 hr, duration 8-12 hr; metabolized by liver; excreted in urine, breast milk; half-life 2-3 hr
Interactions:
• Increased absorption, toxicity: anticoagulants, sulfonylureas, procainamide
• Decreased absorption of ranitidine: antacids, diazepam, anticholinergics, metoclopramide

---

◆ = Nursing alert   ⬤ = Herb-drug interaction   🚫 = Do not crush

Lab test interferences:

Increase: AST, ALT, alk phosphatase, creatinine, LDH, bilirubin

False positive: Urine protein

NURSING CONSIDERATIONS

Assess:

• Gastric pH (>5 should be maintained)

• I&O ratio, BUN, creatinine

• Mental status: confusion, dizziness, depression, anxiety, weakness, tremors, psychosis, diarrhea, abdominal discomfort, jaundice; report immediately

• GI complaints: nausea, vomiting, diarrhea, cramps

Administer:

• With meals for prolonged effect

• Antacids 1 hr before or 1 hr after ranitidine

IV

• IV after diluting 50 mg/20 ml 0.9% NaCl, D_5W, $D_{10}W$, LR, $NaCO_3$ 5% and give 50 mg or less/5 min or more; may dilute 50 mg/50-100 ml of 0.9% NaCl, D_5W, $D_{10}W$, LR, $NaCO_3$ 5% and give over 15-20 min

Additive compatibilities: Acetazolamide, amikacin, aminophylline, chloramphenicol, chlorothiazide, ciprofloxacin, colistimethate, dexamethasone, digoxin, dobutamine, dopamine, doxycycline, epinephrine, erythromycin, floxacillin, fluconazole/ondansetron, flumazenil, furosemide, gentamicin, heparin, insulin (regular), isoproterenol, lidocaine, lincomycin, meropenem, methylprednisolone, moxalactam, penicillin G potassium, penicillin G sodium, polymyxin B, potassium chloride, protamine, quinidine, sodium nitroprusside, ticarcillin, tobramycin, vancomycin

Syringe compatibilities: Atropine, cyclizine, dexamethasone, dimenhydrinate, diphenhydramine, dobutamine, dopamine, fentanyl, glycopyrrolate, hydromorphone, isoproterenol, meperidine, metoclopramide, morphine, nalbuphine, oxymorphone, pentazocine, perphenazine, prochlorperazine, promethazine, scopolamine

Y-site compatibilities: Acyclovir, aldesleukin, allopurinol, amifostine, aminophylline, amsacrine, atracurium, aztreonam, bretylium, cefepime, cefmetazole, ceftazidime, ciprofloxacin, cisatracurium, cisplatin, cladribine, cyclophosphamide, cytarabine, diltiazem, dobutamine, dopamine, doxorubicin, doxorubicin liposome, enalaprilat, epinephrine, esmolol, fentanyl, filgrastim, fluconazole, fludarabine, foscarnet, furosemide, gallium, granisetron, heparin, hydromorphone, idarubicin, labetalol, lorazepam, melphalan, meperidine, methotrexate, midazolam, milrinone, morphine, nicardipine, nitroglycerin, norepinephrine, ondansetron, paclitaxel, pancuronium, piperacillin, piperacillin/tazobactam, procainamide, propofol, remifentanil, sargramostim, tacrolimus, teniposide, theophylline, thiopental, thiotepa, vecuronium, vinorelbine, warfarin, zidovudine

Perform/provide:

• Storage at room temp

Evaluate:

• Therapeutic response: decreased abdominal pain

Teach patient/family:

• That gynecomastia, impotence may occur but are reversible

• To avoid driving, other hazardous activities until stabilized on this medication

• To avoid black pepper, caffeine, alcohol, harsh spices, extremes in temp of food

• That drug must be continued for prescribed time to be effective

R

Side effects: *italics* = common; **_bold italics_** = life-threatening

rapacuronium

See appendix a—selected new drugs

remifentanil (℞)

(rem-ih-fin'ta-nill)
Ultiva

Func. class.: Opiate agonist analgesic

Chem. class.: Mu-opioid agonist

Controlled Substance Schedule II
Action: Inhibits ascending pain pathways in limbic system, thalamus, midbrain, hypothalamus

Uses: In combination with other drugs in general anesthesia, as a primary anesthetic in general surgery

Dosage and routes:
• *Adult:* Induction **IV** 0.5-1 µg/kg/min with a hypnotic or volative agent; maintenance with isoflurane (0.4-1.5 MAC) or propofol (100-200 µg/kg/min); cont inf 0.25 µg/kg/min

Available forms: Powder for inj-lyophilized 1 mg/ml after reconstitution

Side effects/adverse reactions:
CNS: Drowsiness, *dizziness,* confusion, *headache,* sedation, euphoria, delirium, agitation, anxiety
GI: Nausea, vomiting, anorexia, constipation, cramps, dry mouth
GU: Urinary retention, dysuria
INTEG: Rash, urticaria, bruising, flushing, diaphoresis, pruritus
EENT: Tinnitus, blurred vision, miosis, diplopia
CV: Palpitations, *bradycardia,* change in B/P, facial flushing, syncope, *asystole*
RESP: Respiratory depression, apnea

MS: Rigidity

Contraindications: Child <12 yr, hypersensitivity

Precautions: Pregnancy (C), lactation, increased intracranial pressure, acute MI, severe heart disease, renal disease, hepatic disease, asthma, respiratory conditions, convulsive disorders, elderly

Pharmacokinetics: Unknown

Interactions:
• Respiratory depression, hypotension, profound sedation: alcohol, sedatives, hypnotics, or other CNS depressants; antihistamines, phenothiazines

◢ Increased CNS depression: kava

NURSING CONSIDERATIONS
Assess:
• I&O ratio, check for decreasing output; may indicate urinary retention, especially in elderly
• CNS changes; dizziness, drowsiness, hallucinations, euphoria, LOC, pupil reaction
• Allergic reactions: rash, urticaria
• Respiratory dysfunction: respiratory depression, character, rate, rhythm; notify prescriber if respirations are <12/min; CV status; bradycardia, syncope
• Use pain scoring to determine pain perception

Administer:
• Direct IV over 1½-3 min; use tuberculin syringe

Y-site compatibilities: Acyclovir, alfentanil, amikacin, aminophylline, ampicillin, ampicillin/sulbactam, amrinone, aztreonam, bretylium, bumetanide, buprenorphine, butorphanol, calcium gluconate, cefazolin, cefotaxime, cefotetan, cefoxitin, ceftazidime, ceftizoxime, ceftriaxone, cefuroxime, cimetidine, ciprofloxacin, cisatracurium, clindamycin, dexamethasone, digoxin, diphenhydramine, dobutamine, do-

◆ = Nursing alert   *◢* = Herb-drug interaction   ⊘ = Do not crush pamine, doxycycline, droperidol, enalaprilat, epinephrine, esmolol, famotidine, fentanyl, fluconazole, furosemide, ganciclovir, gentamicin, haloperidol, heparin, hydrocortisone sodium succinate, hydromorphone, hydroxyzine, imipenem/cilastatin, isoproterenol, ketorolac, lidocaine, lorazepam, magnesium sulfate, mannitol, meperidine, methyl prednisolone, sodium succinate, metoclopramide, metronidazole, mezlocillin, midazolam, minocycline, morphine, nalbuphine, netilmicin, nitroglycerin, norepinephrine, ofloxacin, ondansetron

Perform/provide:

• Storage in light-resistant area at room temp

Evaluate:

• Therapeutic response: maintenance of anesthesia

Teach patient/family:

• To call for assistance when ambulating or smoking; drowsiness, dizziness may occur

• To make position changes slowly to prevent orthostatic hypotension

---

repaglinide (R)

(re-pag'lih'nide)
Prandin
Func. class.: Antidiabetic
Chem. class.: Meglitinide

Action: Causes functioning β-cells in pancreas to release insulin, leading to drop in blood glucose levels; closes ATP-dependent potassium channels in the β-cell membrane; this leads to opening of calcium channels; increased calcium influx induces insulin secretion

Uses: Stable adult-onset diabetes mellitus (type II) NIDDM

Dosage and routes:
• *Adult:* **PO** 0.5-4 mg
Available forms: Tabs 0.5, 1, 2 mg
Side effects/adverse reactions:
CNS: Headache, weakness, paresthesia
ENDO: **Hypoglycemia**
GI: Nausea, vomiting, diarrhea, constipation, dyspepsia
INTEG: Rash, allergic reactions
MS: Back pains, arthralgia
RESP: URI, sinusitis, rhinitis, bronchitis
Contraindications: Hypersensitivity to meglitinides, diabetic ketoacidosis, type I diabetes
Precautions: Pregnancy (C), elderly, cardiac disease, severe renal disease, severe hepatic disease, thyroid disease, severe hypoglycemic reactions, lactation, children
Pharmacokinetics:
PO: Competely absorbed by GI route; onset 2-4 hr, peak 2-8 hr, duration 24 hr; half-life 1 hr; metabolized in liver; excreted in urine, feces (metabolites); crosses placenta; 98% plasma protein bound
Interactions:
• Increased repaglinide metabolism: troglitazone, rifampin, barbiturates, carbamazepine
• Decreased repaglinide metabolism: antifungals (ketoconazole, miconazole), erythromycin
• Increased effect of repaglinide: NSAIDs, salicylates, sulfonamides, chloramphenicol, MAOIs, coumarins, β-blockers, probenecid
• Decreased action of repaglinide: calcium channel blockers, corticosteroids, oral contraceptives, thiazide diuretics, thyroid preparations, estrogens, phenothiazines, phenytoin, rifampin, isoniazid, phenobarbital, sympathomimetics
⚕ May decrease hypoglycemic effect: broom, buchu, dandelion, juniper

R

✏ May increase or decrease hypoglycemic effect: chromium, fenugreek, ginseng

✏ May improve glucose tolerance: karela

NURSING CONSIDERATIONS

Assess:

• Hypo/hyperglycemic reaction that can occur soon after meals

Administer:

• 15 min before meals; 2, 3, or 4×/day preprandially

• Skip dose if meal is skipped; add dose if meal is added

Perform/provide:

• Storage in tight container in cool environment

Evaluate:

• Therapeutic response: decrease in polyuria, polydipsia, polyphagia, clear sensorium, absence of dizziness, stable gait

Teach family/patient:

• To avoid alcohol; explain disulfiram-like reaction

• To use a capillary blood glucose test while on this drug

• The symptoms of hypo/hyperglycemia; what to do about each

• That drug must be continued on daily basis; explain consequences of discontinuing drug abruptly

• To avoid OTC medications unless ordered by prescriber

• That diabetes is a lifelong illness; drug will not cure disease

• That all food included in diet plan must be eaten to prevent hypoglycemia; to have glucagon emergency kit available

• To carry a MedicAlert ID for emergency purposes

Treatment of overdose: Glucose 25 g IV via dextrose 50% solution, 50 ml or 1 mg glucagon

---

reserpine (R)

(re-ser'peen)

Novoreserpine*, Reserfia*, reserpine

Func. class.: Antihypertensive

Chem. class.: Antiadrenergic agent, peripheral action

Action: Inhibits norepinephrine release, depleting norepinephrine stores in adrenergic nerve endings

Uses: Hypertension

Dosage and routes:

• *Adult:* **PO** 0.25-0.5 mg qd × 1-2 wk, then 0.1-0.25 mg qd maintenance

• *Geriatric:* **PO** 0.05 mg qd, increase by 0.05 weekly to desired dose

Available forms: Tabs 0.1, 0.25 mg

Side effects/adverse reactions:

CV: Bradycardia, chest pain, dysrhythmias, prolonged bleeding time, *thrombocytopenia,* purpura

CNS: Drowsiness, fatigue, lethargy, dizziness, depression, anxiety, headache, increased dreaming, nightmares, *convulsions,* parkinsonism, EPS (high doses)

GI: Nausea, vomiting, cramps, peptic ulcer, dry mouth, increased appetite, anorexia

INTEG: Rash, purpura, alopecia, flushing, warm feeling, pruritus, ecchymosis

EENT: Lacrimation, miosis, blurred vision, ptosis, dry mouth, epistaxis

GU: Impotence, dysuria, nocturia, Na and H_2O retention, edema, breast engorgement, galactorrhea, gynecomastia

RESP: Bronchospasm, dyspnea, cough, rales

Contraindications: Hypersensitivity, depression, suicidal patients, active peptic ulcer disease, ulcerative

---

◆ = Nursing alert   *✏* = Herb-drug interaction   Ⓝ = Do not crush colitis, pregnancy (D), Parkinson's disease

Precautions: Lactation, seizure disorders, renal disease

Pharmacokinetics:

PO: Peak 4 hr, duration 2-6 wk; half-life 50-100 hr; metabolized by liver; excreted in urine, feces, breast milk; crosses placenta; blood-brain barrier

Interactions:

• Increased hypotension: diuretics, hypotension, β-blockers, methotrimeprazine

• Dysrhythmias: cardiac glycosides

• Increased cardiac depression: quinidine, procainamide

• Excitation, hypertension: MAOIs, avoid use

• Increased CNS depression: barbiturates, alcohol, opioids

• Increased pressor effects: epinephrine, isoproterenol, norepinephrine

• Decreased pressor effects: ephedrine, amphetamine

Lab test interferences:

Increase: VMA excretion, 5-HIAA excretion

Interferences: 17-OHCS, 17-KS

NURSING CONSIDERATIONS

Assess:

• Renal function studies in renal impairment (BUN, creatinine)

• Bleeding time; check for ecchymosis, thrombocytopenia, purpura

• I&O in renal disease patient

• Cardiac status: B/P, pulse; watch for hypotension, bradycardia

• Edema in feet, legs qd; take weight qd

• Skin turgor, dryness of mucous membranes for hydration status

• Symptoms of CHF: edema, dyspnea, wet rales

Evaluate:

• Therapeutic response: decreased hypertension

Teach patient/family:

• To avoid driving, hazardous activities if drowsiness occurs

• Not to discontinue drug abruptly

• Not to use OTC products (cough, cold preparations) unless directed by prescriber

• To report bradycardia, dizziness, confusion, depression, fever, sore throat

• That impotence, gynecomastia may occur but are reversible

• To rise slowly to sitting or standing position to minimize orthostatic hypotension

• That therapeutic effect may take 2-4 wk

Treatment of overdose: Lavage, IV atropine for bradycardia, supportive therapy

---

respiratory syncytial virus immune globulin (RSV-IGIV) (℞)

RespiGam

Func. class.: Immune serums

Chem. class.: Immunoglobulin G (IgG)

Action: High titer of neutralizing antibody against RSV (respiratory syncytial virus)

Uses: Prevention of serious lower respiratory tract infection caused by RSV in children <2 yr with bronchopulmonary dysplasia, or premature birth

Dosage and routes:

• *Child:* <2 yr **IV INF** 1.5 ml/kg/hr × 15 min, then 3 ml/kg/hr 15-30 min; then 6 ml/kg/hr from 30 min to end of **INF,** given monthly

Available forms: Inj 2500 mg RSV immunoglobulin

Side effects/adverse reactions:

RESP: **Respiratory distress, hypoxia,** tachypnea, rales, wheezing

R

CNS: Fever

CV: Hypertension, tachycardia, fluid overload

GI: Diarrhea, gastroenteritis, vomiting

MISC.: Rash, overdose effect, inflammation at inj site, ***anaphylaxis, angioneurotic edema***

Contraindications: Hypersensitivity to this drug or other human immunoglobulin preparations, IgA deficiency

Precautions: Pregnancy (C), fluid overload

Pharmacokinetics: Unknown

Interactions:

• Interference with immune response in: MMR, DPT, *H. influenzae b*

NURSING CONSIDERATIONS

Assess:

• VS for increases in heart rate, respiratory rate, retractions, rales; a loop diuretic may be needed for fluid overload

• For aseptic meningitis syndrome (AMS): severe headache, drowsiness, photophobia, fever, painful eye movements, nausea, vomiting, muscle rigidity, discontinue RSV-IGIV if these occur

Administer:

IV inf

• Do not admix; begin inf within 6 hr and complete within 12 hr after the single-use vial is entered

Perform/provide:

• Refrigerated storage, do not freeze, do not shake vial, discard after use

• The reason for IV inf and expected results

Rh₀(D) immune globulin, human (℞)
Gamulin Rh, Hydro Rho-D, HypoRho-D, MICRhoGAM, Mini-Dose, Mini-Gamulin RH, Rhesonatre Rho-Gam
Rh₀(D) immune globulin intravenous, human (℞)
WinRho SD
Func. class.: Immunizing agent
Chem. class.: IgG

Action: Suppresses immune response of nonsensitized Rh₀ (D or Dᵘ)-negative patients who are exposed to Rh₀ (D or Dᵘ)-positive blood

Uses: Prevention of isoimmunization in Rh-negative women given Rh-positive blood after abortions, miscarriages, amniocentesis

Dosage and routes:

Rh₀(D) immune globulin, human

Prior delivery

• *Adult:* IM 1 vial (standard dose) at 26-28 wk, 1 vial (standard dose) 72 hr after delivery

Pregnancy termination <13 wk

• *Adult:* IM 1 vial (microdose) within 72 hr

Following delivery

• *Adult:* IM 1 vial if fetal-packed RBCs <15 ml, or 2 vials if fetal-packed RBCs >15 ml; given within 72 hr of delivery or miscarriage

Transfusion error

• *Adult:* IM give within 72 hr

Rh₀ (D) immune globulin IV, human

After 34 wk gestation

• *Adult:* IM/IV 120 μg given within 72 hr

Available forms: Inj single-dose vial (50 μg/vial-microdose; 300 μg/vial-

---

⬥ = Nursing alert   🖋 = Herb-drug interaction   🚫 = Do not crush

standard); inj 120, 300 µg Rh₀ (D) immune globulin IV, human

Side effects/adverse reactions:

INTEG: Irritation at inj site, fever

CNS: Lethargy

MS: Myalgia

Contraindications: Previous immunization with this drug, Rh₀ (O)-positive/Dᵘ-positive patient

NURSING CONSIDERATIONS

Assess:

• Allergies, reactions to immunizations; previous immunization with this drug

Administer:

IM

• After sending newborn's cord blood to lab after delivery for crossmatch, type; infant must be Rh-positive, with Rh-negative mother

• IM inj in deltoid; aspirate

• Only equal lot numbers of drug, cross-match

• Only MICRhoGAM for abortions or miscarriages <12 wk unless fetus or father is Rh negative; unless patient is Rh₀ (D)-positive, Dᵘ-positive, Rh antibodies are present

Perform/provide:

• Storage in refrigerator

Evaluate:

• Rh₀ (D) sensitivity in transfusion error, prevention of erythroblastosis fetalis

Teach patient/family:

• How drug works; that drug must be given after subsequent deliveries if subsequent babies are Rh positive

---

riboflavin (vit B₂)
(OTC)

(rye'boh-flay-vin)

Func. class.: Vit B₂, water soluble

Action: Needed for respiratory reactions by catalyzing proteins and for normal vision

Uses: Vit B₂ deficiency or polyneuritis; cheilosis adjunct with thiamine

Dosage and routes:

• *Adult and child >12 yr:* **PO** 5-25 mg qd

• *Child <12 yr:* **PO** 2-10 mg qd, then 0.6 mg/1000 calories ingested

RDA

• *Adult:* males 1.4-1.8 mg, females 1.2-1.3 mg

Available forms: Tabs 25, 50, 100 mg

Side effects/adverse reactions:

GU: Yellow discoloration of urine (large doses)

Contraindications: Child <12 yr

Precautions: Pregnancy (A)

Pharmacokinetics:

PO: Half-life 65-85 min, 60% protein bound, unused amounts excreted in urine (unchanged)

Interactions:

• Decreased action of tetracyclines

Lab test interferences:

• May cause false elevations of urinary catecholamines

NURSING CONSIDERATIONS

Assess:

• Nutritional status: liver, eggs, dairy products, yeast, whole grain, green vegetables

Administer:

• With food for better absorption

Perform/provide:

• Storage in airtight, light-resistant container

Evaluate:

• Therapeutic response: absence of headache, GI problems, cheilosis, skin lesions, depression, burning, itchy eyes, anemia

Teach patient/family:

• That urine may turn bright yellow

• About addition of needed foods that are rich in riboflavin

• To avoid alcohol

R

Side effects: *italics* = common; ***bold italics*** = life-threatening

rifabutin (R)

(riff'a-byoo-ten)
Mycobutin
Func. class.: Antimycobacterial agent
Chem. class.: Rifamycin S derivative

Action: Inhibits DNA-dependent RNA polymerase in susceptible strains of *Escherichia coli* and *Bacillus subtilis;* mechanism of action against *Mycobacterium avium* unknown

Uses: Prevention of *Mycobacterium avium* complex (MAC) in patients with advanced HIV infection

Dosage and routes:
• *Adult:* 300 mg qd (may take as 150 mg bid)

Available forms: Caps 150 mg

Side effects/adverse reactions:
INTEG: Rash
MS: Asthenia, arthralgia, myalgia
MISC: Flulike syndrome, shortness of breath, chest pressure
GI: Nausea, vomiting, anorexia, diarrhea, heartburn, **hepatitis**
GU: Hematuria, *discolored urine*
CNS: Headache, fatigue, anxiety, confusion, insomnia
*HEMA: **Hemolytic anemia, eosinophilia, thrombocytopenia, leukopenia***

Contraindications: Hypersensitivity, active TB, WBC <1000 or platelet count <50,000

Precautions: Pregnancy (B), lactation, hepatic disease, blood dyscrasias, children

Pharmacokinetics:
PO: Peak 2-3 hr, duration >24 hr, half-life 3 hr; metabolized in liver (active/inactive metabolites), excreted in urine primarily as metabolites

Interactions:
• Decreased action: barbiturates, clofibrate, corticosteroids, dapsone, anticoagulants, sulfonylureas, estrogens, digitoxin and digoxin, oral contraceptives, theophylline, β-blockers, verapamil, cyclosporine, zidovudine, ketoconazole
• Drug/food: high-fat diet decreases absorption

Lab test interferences:
Interference: Folate level, vit B$_{12}$, BSP, gallbladder studies

NURSING CONSIDERATIONS
Assess:
• CBC for neutropenia, thrombocytopenia, eosinophilia
• For acute TB: chest x-ray, sputum culture, blood culture, biopsy of lymph nodes, PPD; drug should not be given for acute TB
• Signs of anemia: Hct, Hgb, fatigue
• Liver studies qwk: ALT, AST, bilirubin
• Renal status before, qmo: BUN, creatinine, output, specific gravity, urinalysis
• Hepatic studies: decreased appetite, jaundice, dark urine, fatigue

Administer:
• With food if GI upset occurs; better to take on empty stomach 1 hr ac or 2 hr pc, high-fat foods slow absorption
• Antiemetic if vomiting occurs
• After C&S is completed; qmo to detect resistance

Evaluate:
• Therapeutic response: not used for active TB because of risk of development of resistance to rifampin; culture negative

Teach patient/family:
• That patients using oral contraceptives should consider using nonhormonal methods of birth control, since rifabutin may decrease their efficacy

---

◆ = Nursing alert   ▨ = Herb-drug interaction   ⊘ = Do not crush

• That compliance with dosage schedule, duration is necessary

• That scheduled appointments must be kept; relapse may occur

• That urine, feces, saliva, sputum, sweat, tears may be colored red-orange; soft contact lenses may be permanently stained

• To report flulike symptoms: excessive fatigue, anorexia, vomiting, sore throat; unusual bleeding, yellowish discoloration of skin, eyes

rifampin (Ⓡ)

(rif'am-pin)
Rifadin, Rimactane, Rofact*
Func. class.: Antitubercular
Chem. class.: Rifamycin B derivative

Action: Inhibits DNA-dependent polymerase, decreases tubercle bacilli replication

Uses: Pulmonary tuberculosis, meningococcal carriers (prevention)

Dosage and routes:

Tuberculosis

• *Adult:* **PO/IV** 600 mg/day as single dose 1 hr ac or 2 hr pc or 10 mg/kg/day

• *Child >5 yr:* **PO/IV** 10-20 mg/kg/day as single dose 1 hr ac or 2 hr pc, not to exceed 600 mg/day, with other antituberculars

• 6-mo regimen: 2 mo treatment of isoniazid, rifampin, pyrazinamide and possibly streptomycin or ethambutol; then rifampin and isoniazid × 4 mo

• 9-mo regimen: rifampin and isoniazid supplemented with pyrazinamide, or streptomycin or ethambutol

Meningococcal carriers

• *Adult:* **PO/IV** 600 mg bid × 2 days

• *Child >5 yr:* **PO/IV** 10-20 mg/kg not to exceed 600 mg/dose

• *Infant 3 mo-1 yr:* 5 mg/kg **PO** bid for 2 days

Available forms: Caps 150, 300 mg; powder for inj 600 mg/vial

Side effects/adverse reactions:

INTEG: Rash, pruritus, urticaria

EENT: Visual disturbances

MS: Atoxia, weakness

MISC: Flulike syndrome, menstrual disturbances, edema, shortness of breath

*GI: Nausea, vomiting, anorexia, diarrhea, **pseudomembranous colitis,** heartburn, sore mouth and tongue, **pancreatitis***

*GU: **Hematuria, acute renal failure, hemoglobinuria***

CNS: Headache, fatigue, anxiety, drowsiness, confusion

*HEMA: **Hemolytic anemia, eosinophilia, thrombocytopenia, leukopenia***

Contraindications: Hypersensitivity

Precautions: Pregnancy (C), lactation, hepatic disease, blood dyscrasias

Pharmacokinetics:

PO: Peak 2-3 hr, duration >24 hr, half-life 3 hr; metabolized in liver (active/inactive metabolites), excreted in urine as free drug (30% crosses placenta), excreted in breast milk

Interactions:

• Decreased action: barbiturates, clofibrate, corticosteroids, dapsone, anticoagulants, antidiabetics, hormones, digoxin, PAS, alcohol, oral contraceptives, verapamil, diltiazem, nifedipine, cyclosporine, haloperidol, theophylline, chloramphenicol, acetaminophen, benzodiazepines, phenytoin, sulfonamides, beta-blockers, doxycycline, fluoroquinolones, zidovudine

• Lithium toxicity: lithium

• Hepatotoxicity: isoniazid

• Incompatible with sodium lactate

Side effects: *italics* = common; **bold italics** = life-threatening

Lab test interferences:

Interference: Folate level, vit B$_{12}$, BSP, gallbladder studies

NURSING CONSIDERATIONS

Assess:

• For infection: sputum culture, lung sounds

• Signs of anemia: Hct, Hgb, fatigue

• Liver studies qwk: ALT, AST, bilirubin

• Renal status before, qmo: BUN, creatinine, output, specific gravity, urinalysis

• Hepatic status: decreased appetite, jaundice, dark urine, fatigue

Administer:

• After C&S is completed; qmo to detect resistance

PO

• On empty stomach, 1 hr ac or 2 hr pc

• Antiemetic if vomiting occurs

IV

• After diluting each 600 mg/10 ml of sterile water for inj (60 mg/ml), agitate, withdraw dose and dilute in 100 ml or 500 ml of D$_5$W or 0.9% NaCl given as an inf over 3 hr, or if diluted in 100 ml, give over ½ hr

Evaluate:

• Therapeutic response: decreased symptoms of TB, culture negative

Teach patient/family:

• That compliance with dosage schedule, duration is necessary

• That scheduled appointments must be kept; relapse may occur

• To avoid alcohol

• That urine, feces, saliva, sputum, sweat, tears may be colored redorange; soft contact lenses may be permanently stained

• To report flulike symptoms: excessive fatigue, anorexia, vomiting, sore throat; unusual bleeding, yellowish discoloration of skin, eyes

---

rifapentine (℞)

(riff′ah-pen-teen′)

Priftin

Func. class.: Antitubercular

Chem. class.: Rifamycin derivative

Action: Inhibits DNA-dependent polymerase, decreases tubercle bacilli replication

Uses: Pulmonary tuberculosis, must be used with at least one other antitubercular

Dosage and routes:

Intensive phase

• *Adult:* **PO** 600 mg (four 150 mg tabs 2×/wk), with an interval of 72 hr between doses × 2 mo; must be given with at least one other antitubercular

Continuation phase

• *Adult:* **PO** continue with 1×/wk × 4 mo in combination with isoniazid or other appropriate antitubercular

Available forms: Tabs 150 mg

Side effects/adverse reactions:

INTEG: Rash, pruritus, urticaria, acne

EENT: Visual disturbances

MS: Gout, arthrosis

MISC: Edema, aggressive reaction

GI: Nausea, vomiting, anorexia, diarrhea, bilirubinemia, hepatitis, increased ALT, AST, *heartburn, **pancreatitis***

*GU: **Hematuria,** pyuria, **proteinuria,** urinary casts*

CNS: Headache, fatigue, anxiety, dizziness

*HEMA: **Thrombocytopenia, leukopenia, neutropenia, lymphopenia,** anemia, **leukocytosis,** purpura, hematoma*

Contraindications: Hypersensitivity to rifamycins

Precautions: Pregnancy (C), lactation, hepatic disease, blood dyscrasias, children <12 yr

---

◆ = Nursing alert   ∅ = Herb-drug interaction   ⊘ = Do not crush

Pharmacokinetics:
PO: Peak 5-6 hr, half-life 13 hr; metabolized in liver (active/inactive metabolites), excreted in urine and feces, excreted in breast milk, protein binding 97%, steady state 10 days

Interactions:
• Use with extreme caution with protease inhibitors
• Decreased action of: amitriptyline, anticoagulants, antidiabetics, barbiturates, chloramphenicol, clarithromycin, clofibrate, corticosteroids, cyclosporine, dapsone, delavirdine, diazepam, digoxin, diltiazem, disopyramide, doxyclycline, fluconazole, fluoroquinolones, haloperidol, indinavir, itraconazole, ketoconazole, methadone, mexiletine, nelfinavir, nifedipine, nortriptyline, oral contraceptives, phenytoin, progestins, quinidine, quinine, ritonavir, saquinavir, sildenafil, tacrolimus, theophylline, thyroid preparations, tocainide, verapamil, zidovudine

Lab test interferences:
Interference: Folate level, vit B_{12}

NURSING CONSIDERATIONS
Assess:
• Baselines in CBC, AST, ALT, bilirubin, platelets
• For infection: sputum culture, lung sounds
• Signs of anemia: Hct, Hgb, fatigue
• Liver studies qmo: ALT, AST, bilirubin
• Renal status qmo: BUN, creatinine, output, specific gravity, urinalysis
• Hepatic status: decreased appetite, jaundice, dark urine, fatigue

Administer:
PO
• May give with food for GI upset
• Antiemetic if vomiting occurs
• After C&S is completed; qmo to detect resistance

Evaluate:
• Therapeutic response: decreased symptoms of TB, culture negative

Teach patient/family:
• That compliance with dosage schedule, duration is necessary
• That scheduled appointments must be kept; relapse may occur
• That urine, feces, saliva, sputum, sweat, tears may be colored red-orange; soft contact lenses may be permanently stained
• To use alternative method of contraception, oral contraceptive action may be decreased
• To report flulike symptoms: excessive fatigue, anorexia, vomiting, sore throat; unusual bleeding, yellowish discoloration of skin, eyes

---

riluzole (℞)

(rill'you-zole)
Rilutek
Func. class.: ALS agent
Chem. class.: Benzathiazole

Action: Unknown; may act by inhibiting glutamate, interfering with binding of amino acid receptors, and inactivating of voltage-dependent sodium channels

Uses: Amyotropic lateral sclerosis (ALS)

Dosage and routes:
• *Adult:* **PO** 50 mg q12h, take 1 hr ac or 2 hr pc

Available forms: Tabs 50 mg

Side effects/adverse reactions:
GI: Nausea, vomiting, dyspepsia, anorexia, diarrhea, flatulence, stomatitis, dry mouth
HEMA: **Neutropenia**
CNS: Hypertonia, depression, dizziness, insomnia, somnolence, vertigo
INTEG: Pruritus, eczema, alopecia, **exfoliative dermatitis**

R

RESP: Decreased lung function, rhinitis, increased cough

CV: Hypertension, tachycardia, phlebitis, palpitation, postural hypertension

GU: UTI, dysuria

Contraindications: Hypersensitivity

Precautions: Neutropenia, renal disease, hepatic disease, elderly, pregnancy (C), lactation, children

Pharmacokinetics: Well absorbed, extensively metabolized by the liver, excretion in urine/feces

Interactions:

• Decreased elimination of riluzole: caffeine, theophylline, amitriptyline, quinolones

• Increased elimination of riluzole: cigarette smoking, rifampin, omeprazole, charcoal-broiled food

NURSING CONSIDERATIONS

Assess:

• LFTs: AST, ALT, bilirubin, GGT, baseline and q mo × 3 mo, then q3mo; monitor liver chemistries

• For neutropenia <500/mm

Administer:

• 1 hr ac or 2 hr pc; a high-fat meal decreases absorption

Teach patient/family:

• To report febrile illness, which may indicate neutropenia

• The reason for drug and expected results

---

rimantadine (R)

(ri-man'tah-deen)
Flumadine

Func. class.: Synthetic antiviral
Chem. class.: Tricyclic amine

Action: Prevents uncoating of nucleic acid in viral cell, preventing penetration of virus to host; causes release of dopamine from neurons

Uses: Prophylaxis or treatment of influenza type A

Dosage and routes:

Renal/hepatic dose

• Reduce dose as needed

Influenza type A

Prophylaxis

• *Adult and child >10 yr:* **PO** 100 mg bid; in renal, hepatic disease, lower dose to 100 mg/day

• *Child <10 yr:* **PO** 5 mg/kg/day, not to exceed 150 mg

Treatment

• *Adult:* **PO** 100 mg bid; in renal or hepatic disease, lower dose to 100 mg/day; start treatment at onset of symptoms, continue for at least 1 wk

• *Geriatric:* **PO** 100 mg/day

Available forms: Tabs 100 mg; syr 50 mg/5 ml

Side effects/adverse reactions:

CNS: Headache, dizziness, fatigue, depression, hallucinations, tremors, ***convulsions,*** insomnia, *poor concentration,* asthenia, gait abnormalities, *anxiety, confusion*

CV: Pallor, palpitations, *hypotension,* edema

EENT: Tinnitus, taste abnormality, eye pain

GI: Nausea, vomiting, constipation, dry mouth, anorexia, abdominal pain, diarrhea, dyspepsia

INTEG: Rash

Contraindications: Hypersensitivity

Precautions: Epilepsy, hepatic disease, renal disease, pregnancy (C), lactation, children <1 yr

Pharmacokinetics:

PO: Peak 6 hr, elimination half-life 25½ hr, plasma protein binding (40%)

Interactions:

• Decreased peak concentration of rimantadine: acetaminophen, aspirin

• Increased rimantadine concentration: cimetidine

 = Nursing alert   = Herb-drug interaction   = Do not crush

NURSING CONSIDERATIONS
Assess:
• I&O ratio; report urinary frequency, hesitancy in renal disease
• Bowel pattern before, during treatment
• CNS effect in elderly or patients with severe hepatic/renal disease
• Skin eruptions, photosensitivity after administration of drug
• Respiratory status: rate, character, wheezing, tightness in chest
• Allergies before initiation of treatment, reaction of each medication; list allergies on chart in bright red letters
• Signs of infection

Administer:
• Within 48 hr of exposure to influenza; continue for 10 days after contact
• At least 4 hr before hs to prevent insomnia
• After meals for better absorption, to decrease GI symptoms
• In divided doses to prevent CNS disturbances: headache, dizziness, fatigue, drowsiness

Perform/provide:
• Storage in tight, dry container

Evaluate:
• Therapeutic response: absence of fever, malaise, cough, dyspnea in infection

Teach patient/family:
• About aspects of drug therapy: need to report dyspnea, dizziness, poor concentration, behavioral changes
• To avoid hazardous activities if dizziness occurs

Treatment of overdose: Withdraw drug, maintain airway, administer epinephrine, aminophylline, O_2, IV corticosteroids, physostigmine

risedronate (Ⓡ)
(rih-sed′roh-nate)
Actonel
Func. class.: Bone resorption inhibitor
Chem. class.: Biphosphonate

Action: Absorbs calcium phosphate crystal in bone and may directly block dissolution of hydroxyapatite crystals of bone; inhibits bone resorption, apparently without inhibiting bone formation, mineralization

Uses: Paget's disease

Investigational uses: Osteoporosis in postmenopausal women

Dosage and routes:
• *Adult:* **PO** 30 mg qd × 2 mo; patients with Paget's disease should receive calcium and vit D if dietary intake is lacking; if relapse occurs, retreatment is advised

Available forms: Tabs 30 mg

Side effects/adverse reactions:
CNS: Dizziness, heacache
GI: Abdominal pain, anorexia, diarrhea, nausea
MS: Bone pain, arthralgia
CV: Chest pain

Contraindications: Hypersensitivity to biphosphonates

Precautions: Children, lactation, pregnancy (C), renal disease

Pharmacokinetics: Rapidly cleared from circulation, taken up mainly by bones, eliminated primarily through kidneys

Interactions:
• Decreased absorption of risedronate: calcium supplements, antacids
• Drug/food: decreased bioavailability: take ½ hr before food or drinks

R

NURSING CONSIDERATIONS
Assess:

• Electrolytes: renal function studies; Ca, P, Mg, K
• For hypercalcemia: paresthesia, twitching, laryngospasm, Chvostek's, Trousseau's signs

Administer:

• PO for 2 months to be effective in Paget's disease
• With a full glass of water, patient should be in upright position
• Supplemental calcium and vit D in Paget's disease

Perform/provide:

• Storage in cool environment, out of direct sunlight

Evaluate:

• Therapeutic response: increased bone mass, absence of fractures

---

risperidone (℞)
(ris-pehr′ih-dohn)
Risperdal
Func. class.: Antipsychotic/neuroleptic
Chem. class.: Benzisoxazole derivative

Action: Unknown; may be mediated through both dopamine type 2 (D_2) and serotonin type 2 (5-HT_2) antagonism

Uses: Psychotic disorders

Dosage and routes:

• *Adult:* **PO** 1 mg bid, with incremental increases of 1 mg bid on days 2 and 3 to a dose of 3 mg bid by day 3; then do not increase dose for at least 1 wk
• *Geriatric:* **PO** 0.5 mg qd-bid, increase by 1 mg qwk

Available forms: Tabs 1, 2, 3, 4 mg; oral sol 1 mg/ml

Side effects/adverse reactions:

*CNS: EPS, pseudoparkinsonism, akathisia, dystonia, tardive dyskinesia; drowsiness, insomnia, agitation, anxiety, headache, **seizures, neuroleptic malignant syndrome***
CV: Orthostatic hypotension, ***tachycardia***
EENT: Blurred vision
GI: Nausea, vomiting, *anorexia, constipation,* jaundice, weight gain
RESP: Rhinitis

Contraindications: Hypersensitivity, lactation, seizure disorders

Precautions: Children, renal disease, pregnancy (C), hepatic disease, elderly, breast cancer

Pharmacokinetics:

PO: Extensively metabolized by liver to a major active metabolite, plasma protein binding 90%

Interactions:

• Increased sedation: other CNS depressants, alcohol
• Increased EPS: other antipsychotics, lithium
• Increased excretion of risperidone: carbamazepine
• Increased CNS depression: kava

Lab test interferences: Not known

NURSING CONSIDERATIONS
Assess:

• Mental status before initial administration
• Swallowing of PO medication; check for hoarding or giving of medication to other patients
• I&O ratio; palpate bladder if urinary output is low
• Bilirubin, CBC, liver function studies qmo
• Urinalysis before, during prolonged therapy
• Affect, orientation, LOC, reflexes, gait, coordination, sleep pattern disturbances
• B/P standing and lying; also pulse, respirations; take these q4h during initial treatment; establish baseline before starting treatment; report drops of 30 mm Hg; watch for ECG changes

---

◆ = Nursing alert   🖋 = Herb-drug interaction   Ⓝ = Do not crush

• Dizziness, faintness, palpitations, tachycardia on rising
• EPS, including akathisia (inability to sit still, no pattern to movements), tardive dyskinesia (bizarre movements of the jaw, mouth, tongue, extremities), pseudoparkinsonism (rigidity, tremors, pill rolling, shuffling gait)
◆ For neuroleptic malignant syndrome: hyperthermia, increased CPK, altered mental status, muscle rigidity
• Skin turgor qd
• Constipation, urinary retention qd; if these occur, increase bulk and water in diet
Administer:
• Reduced dose in elderly
• Antiparkinsonian agent on order from prescriber, to be used for EPS
Perform/provide:
• Decreased stimulus by dimming lights, avoiding loud noises
• Supervised ambulation until patient is stabilized on medication; do not involve in strenuous exercise program because fainting is possible; patient should not stand still for a long time
• Increased fluids to prevent constipation
• Sips of water, candy, gum for dry mouth
• Storage in tight, light-resistant container
Evaluate:
• Therapeutic response: decrease in emotional excitement, hallucinations, delusions, paranoia; reorganization of patterns of thought, speech
Teach patient/family:
• That orthostatic hypotension may occur and to rise from sitting or lying position gradually
• To avoid hot tubs, hot showers, tub baths; hypotension may occur
• To avoid abrupt withdrawal of this

drug; EPS may result; drug should be withdrawn slowly
• To avoid OTC preparations (cough, hay fever, cold) unless approved by prescriber, since serious drug interactions may occur; avoid use with alcohol, CNS depressants; increased drowsiness may occur
• To avoid hazardous activities if drowsy or dizzy
• Compliance with drug regimen
• To report impaired vision, tremors, muscle twitching
• In hot weather, that heat stroke may occur; take extra precautions to stay cool
Treatment of overdose: Lavage if orally ingested; provide airway; *do not induce vomiting*

ritodrine (℞)
(rih'toh-dreen)
ritodrine, Yutopar
Func. class.: Tocolytic, uterine relaxant
Chem. class.: β₂-adrenergic agonist

Action: Reduces frequency, intensity of uterine contractions by stimulation of the β₂-receptors in uterine smooth muscle
Uses: Management of preterm labor
Dosage and routes:
• *Adult:* **IV INF** 150 mg/500 ml (0.3 mg/ml) given 0.1 mg/min, increased gradually by 0.05 mg/min q10min until desired response
Available forms: Inj 10 mg/ml, 15 mg/ml
Side effects/adverse reactions:
MISC: Erythema, rash, dyspnea, hyperventilation, glycosuria, *lactic acidosis*
META: Hyperglycemia, hypokalemia
CNS: Headache, restlessness, anxi-

ety, nervousness, sweating, chills, drowsiness, tremor

GI: Nausea, vomiting, anorexia, malaise, bloating, constipation, diarrhea

CV: Altered maternal, fetal heart rate, B/P, dysrhythmias, palpitations, chest pain, maternal pulmonary edema

Contraindications: Hypersensitivity, eclampsia, hypertension, dysrhythmias, thyrotoxicosis, before 20th wk of pregnancy, antepartum hemorrhage, intrauterine fetal death, maternal cardiac disease, pulmonary hypertension, uncontrolled diabetes, pheochromocytoma, bronchial asthma

Precautions: Migraine, sulfite sensitivity, pregnancy-induced hypertension, diabetes, pregnancy (B)

Pharmacokinetics:

IV: Immediate, distribution half-life 6 min, 2nd phase 1½-2½ hr, elimination phase >10 hr; metabolized in liver; 90% excreted in urine; crosses placenta

Interactions:

• Pulmonary edema: corticosteroids
• Increased CV effects of ritodrine: magnesium sulfate, diazoxide, meperidine, potent general anesthetics
• Increased effects of sympathomimetic amines
• Systemic hypertension: atropine
• Decreased action of ritodrine: β-blockers

Lab test interferences:

Increase: Blood glucose, free fatty acids, insulin, GTT

Decrease: K

NURSING CONSIDERATIONS

Assess:

• Maternal, fetal heart tones during infusion; maternal ECG to determine CV disease
• Intensity, length of uterine contractions

• Fluid intake to prevent fluid overload; discontinue if this occurs
• Blood glucose in diabetics

Administer:

• Only clear sol
• After dilution: 150 mg/500 ml D_5W or NS, give at 0.3 mg/ml
• Using infusion pump
• Considered incompatible with any drug in sol or syringe

Perform/provide:

• Positioning of patient in left lateral recumbent position to decrease hypotension, increase renal blood flow

Evaluate:

• Therapeutic response: decreased intensity, length of contraction, absence of preterm labor, decreased B/P

Teach patient/family:

• To remain in bed during infusion

---

ritonavir (℞)

(ri-toe′na-veer)

Norvir

Func. class.: Antiviral

Chem. class.: Petidomimetic inhibitor

Action: Inhibits human immunodeficiency virus (HIV) protease and prevents maturation of the infectious virus

Uses: HIV in combination with zidovudine, ddc, or alone

Dosage and routes:

• *Adult:* **PO** 600 mg bid. If nausea occurs begin dose at ½ and gradually increase
• *Child:* **PO** 250 mg/m² bid, titrate upward to 400 mg/m² bid

Available forms: Caps 100 mg; oral sol 80 mg/ml

Side effects/adverse reactions:

GI: Diarrhea, buccal mucosa ulceration, abdominal pain, *nausea,* taste

---

◆ = Nursing alert   ▬ = Herb-drug interaction   ⊘ = Do not crush perversion, dry mouth, dizziness, insomnia, headache, vomiting

CNS: Paresthesia, *headache,* vomiting

INTEG: Rash

MS: Pain

MISC.: Asthenia

Contraindications: Hypersensitivity

Precautions: Liver disease, pregnancy (B), lactation, children

Pharmacokinetics: Well absorbed; 98% protein binding, hepatic metabolism

Interactions:

• Increased ritonavir levels: fluconazole

• Decreased ritonavir levels: rifamycins, nevirapine

• Increased level of both drugs: clarithromycin, ddI

• Toxicity: amiodarone, benzodiazepines, bepridil, bupropion, clozapine, desipramine, flecainide, meperidine, piroxicam, propafenone, propoxyphene, quinidine, saquinavir, terfenadine, zolpidem

• Decreased ethinyl estradiol, sulfamethoxazole, theophylline, zidovudine levels when used with ritonavir

Lab test interferences:

Increase: ALT, GGT, PT, triglycerides

Decrease: Hct, RBC

NURSING CONSIDERATIONS

Assess:

• Signs of infection, anemia

• Liver studies: ALT, AST

• C&S before drug therapy; drug may be taken as soon as culture is taken; repeat C&S after treatment; determine the presence of other sexually transmitted diseases

• Bowel pattern before, during treatment; if severe abdominal pain with bleeding occurs, drug should be discontinued; monitor hydration

• Skin eruptions; rash

• Allergies before treatment, reaction to each medication; place allergies on chart

Teach patient/family:

• To take as prescribed; if dose is missed, take as soon as remembered up to 1 hr before next dose; do not double dose

• That drug must be taken in equal intervals around the clock to maintain blood levels for duration of therapy

• To take with food; mix liquid formulation with chocolate milk or liquid nutritional supplement

---

rituximab

(rih-tuks′ih-mab)

Rituxan

Func. class.: Misc. antineoplastic

Chem. class.: Murine/human monoclonal antibody

Action: Directed against the CD20 antigen that is found on malignant B lymphocytes; CD20 regulates a portion of cell-cycle initiation/differentiation

Uses: Non-Hodgkin's lymphoma (CD20 positive, B-cell)

Dosage and routes:

• *Adult:* **IV INF** 375 mg/m^2 qwk × 4 doses; give at 50 mg/hr for 1st inf; if hypersensitivity does not occur, increase rate by 50 mg/hr q½h, max 400 mg/hr; slow/interrupt inf if hypersensitivity occurs; other inf can be given at 100 mg/hr and increased by 100 mg/hr, max 400 mg/hr

Available forms: Inj 10 mg/ml

Side effects/adverse reactions:

GI: Nausea, vomiting, anorexia

INTEG: Irritation at site, rash

HEMA: Leukopenia, neutropenia, thrombocytopenia

R

OTHER: Fever, chills, asthenia, headache, angioedema, hypotension, myalgia, ***bronchospasm***

Contraindications: Hypersensitivity, murine proteins

Precautions: Lactation, children, elderly, pregnancy (C)

Pharmacokinetics: Half-life 42-79 min

NURSING CONSIDERATIONS
Assess:

• CBC, differential, platelet count weekly; withhold drug if WBC is <3500/mm³, or platelet count <100,000/mm³; notify prescriber of these results; drug should be discontinued

• Food preferences: list likes, dislikes

• GI symptoms: frequency of stools

• Signs of dehydration: rapid respirations, poor skin turgor, decreased urine output, dry skin, restlessness, weakness

Administer:
IV inf

• After diluting to a final conc. of 1-4 mg/ml; use 0.9% NaCl, D₅W, gently invert bag to mix; do not mix with other drugs

Perform/provide:

• Increased fluid intake to 2-3 L/day to prevent dehydration, unless contraindicated

• Changing of IV site q48h

• Nutritious diet with iron, vitamin supplement, low fiber, few dairy products

• Storage of vials at 36°-40° F, protect vials from direct sunlight, inf sol is stable at 36°-46° F × 24 hr and room temp for another 12 hr

Evaluate:

• Therapeutic response: decrease in tumor size, decrease in spread of cancer

Teach patient/family:

• To report adverse reactions

---

rizatriptan (Ⴛ)
(rye-zah-trip′tan)
Maxalt, Maxalt-MLT
Func. class.: Migraine agent
Chem. class.: 5-HT₁ receptor agonist

Action: Binds selectively to the vascular 5-HT₁ receptor subtype, exerts antimigraine effect; causes vasoconstriction in cranial arteries

Uses: Acute treatment of migraine

Dosage and routes:

• *Adult:* **PO** 5-10 mg single dose, redosing separate by 2 hr or more; max 30 mg/24 hr

Available forms: Maxalt: tabs 5, 10 mg; Maxalt-MLT: tabs, orally disintegrating 5, 10 mg

Side effects/adverse reactions:

CNS: Dizziness, headache, fatigue
RESP: Chest tightness, pressure
GI: Nausea, dry mouth

Contraindications: Angina pectoris, history of MI, documented silent ischemia, Prinzmetal's angina, ischemic heart disease, concurrent ergotamine-containing preparations, uncontrolled hypertension, hypersensitivity, basilar or hemiplegic migraine

Precautions: Postmenopausal women, men >40 yr, risk factors for CAD, hypercholesterolemia, obesity, diabetes, impaired hepatic or renal function, pregnancy (C), lactation, children, elderly

Pharmacokinetics: Onset of pain relief 10 min-2 hr, 14% plasma protein binding, metabolized in the liver (metabolite), excreted in urine, feces, half-life 2-3 hr

Interactions:

• Extended vasospastic effects: ergot, ergot derivatives, other 5-HT receptor agonists

---

◆ = Nursing alert   ∥ = Herb-drug interaction   ⃠ = Do not crush

• Increased action of rizatriptan: cimetidine, oral contraceptives, MAOIs, nonselective MAOI (type A and B), isocarboxazide, pargyline, phenelzine, propranolol, tranylcypromine

• Weakness, hyperreflexia, incoordination: SSRIs

NURSING CONSIDERATIONS
Assess:
• Tingling, hot sensation, burning, feeling of pressure, numbness, flushing, injection site reaction
• For stress level, activity, recreation, coping mechanisms
• Neurologic status: LOC, blurring vision, nausea, vomiting, tingling in extremities preceding headache
• Ingestion of tyramine foods (pickled products, beer, wine, aged cheese), food additives, preservatives, colorings, artificial sweeteners, chocolate, caffeine, which may precipitate these types of headaches

Perform/provide:
• Quiet, calm environment with decreased stimulation for noise, bright light, excessive talking

Evaluate:
• Therapeutic response: decrease in frequency, severity of headache

Teach patient/family:
• Use of orally disintegrating tab: instruct patient not to open blister until use, to peel blister open with dry hands, to place tab on tongue, where it will dissolve, and to swallow with saliva (contains phenylalanine)
• To report any side effects to prescriber
• To use alternative contraception while taking drug if oral contraceptives are being used

rocuronium (℞)
(ro-kyur-oh′nium)
Zemuron
Func. class.: Neuromuscular blocker (nondepolarizing)
Chem. class.: Biquaternary ammonium ester

Action: Inhibits transmission of nerve impulses by binding with cholinergic receptor sites, antagonizing action of acetylcholine

Uses: Facilitation of endotracheal intubation, skeletal muscle relaxation during mechanical ventilation, surgery, or general anesthesia

Dosage and routes:
Intubation
• *Adult and child:* IV 0.6 mg/kg
Available forms: Inj 10 mg/ml

Side effects/adverse reactions:
CV: Bradycardia, tachycardia, change in B/P
RESP: ***Prolonged apnea, bronchospasm, cyanosis, respiratory depression***
GI: Nausea, vomiting
INTEG: Rash, flushing, pruritus, urticaria

Contraindications: Hypersensitivity

Precautions: Pregnancy (C), cardiac disease, lactation, child <2 yr, electrolyte imbalances, dehydration, neuromuscular disease, respiratory disease

Pharmacokinetics: Half-life 71-203 min, duration ½ hr

Interactions:
• Blocked action of rocuronium: phenylephrine
• Increased effect of rocuronium: anesthetics

NURSING CONSIDERATIONS
Assess:
• For electrolyte imbalances (K,

R

Mg), before drug is used; electrolyte imbalances may lead to increased action of this drug

• Vital signs (B/P, pulse, respirations, airway) until fully recovered; rate, depth, pattern of respirations, strength of hand grip; patient should be intubated before use

• Recovery: decreased paralysis of face, diaphragm, leg, arm, rest of body; residual weakness and respiratory problems may occur during recovery

• Allergic reactions: rash, fever, respiratory distress, pruritus; drug should be discontinued

Administer:

• Using peripheral nerve stimulator by anesthesiologist to determine neuromuscular blockade; deep tendon reflexes should be monitored during extended use

• Undiluted direct IV over 2 min (only by qualified person, usually anesthesiologist); do not administer IM

• Maintenance q20-45min after 1st dose; titrate to response

Perform/provide:

• Storage in light-resistant area

• Reassurance if communication is difficult during recovery from neuromuscular blockade

Evaluate:

• Therapeutic response: paralysis of jaw, eyelid, head, neck, rest of body as evaluated by peripheral nerve stimulator

Teach patient/family:

• About all procedures or treatments; patient will remain conscious if anesthesia is not given also

Treatment of overdose: Edrophonium or neostigmine, atropine, monitor VS; may require mechanical ventilation

rofecoxib

See appendix a—selected new drugs

ropinirole (℞)

(roh-pin'ih-role)

Requip

Func. class.: Antiparkinson agent

Chem. class.: Dopamine-receptor agonist, non-ergot

Action: Selective agonist for D_2 receptors (presynaptic/postsynaptic sites); binding at D_3 receptor contributes to antiparkinson effects

Uses: Parkinsonism

Dosage and routes:

• *Adult:* **PO** 0.25 mg tid, titrate weekly to a max of 24 mg/day

Available forms: Tabs 0.25, 0.5, 1, 2, 5 mg

Side effects/adverse reactions:

HEMA: **Hemolytic anemia, leukopenia, agranulocytosis**

CNS: Agitation, insomnia, psychosis, hallucination, dystonia, depression, dizziness

GI: Nausea, vomiting, anorexia, dry mouth, constipation, dyspepsia, flatulence

INTEG: Rash, sweating

CV: Orthostatic hypotension, tachycardia, hypertension, hypotension, syncope, palpitations

EENT: Blurred vision

GU: Impotence, urinary frequency

RESP: Pharyngitis, rhinitis, sinusitis, bronchitis, dyspnea

Contraindications: Hypersensitivity

Precautions: Renal disease, cardiac disease, dysrhythmias, affective disorder, psychosis, pregnancy (C)

Pharmacokinetics:

PO: Half-life 6 hr

◆ = Nursing alert   ⫸ = Herb-drug interaction   ⊘ = Do not crush

Interactions:
• Increased ropinirole effect: cimetidine, ciprofloxacin, diltiazem, enoxacin, erythromycin, fluvoxamine, mexiletine, norfloxacin, tacrine

🍃 Decreased ropinirole action: chaste tree fruit

NURSING CONSIDERATIONS
Assess:
• Involuntary movements in parkinsonism: akinesia, tremors, staggering gait, muscle rigidity, drooling
• B/P, respiration during initial treatment; hypo/hypertension should be reported
• Mental status: affect, mood, behavioral changes, depression; complete suicide assessment
Administer:
• Drug until NPO before surgery
• Adjust dosage to patient response
• With meals
Perform/provide:
• Assistance with ambulation during beginning therapy
• Testing for diabetes mellitus, acromegaly if on long-term therapy
Evaluate:
• Therapeutic response: decrease in akathisia, increased mood
Teach patient/family:
• That therapeutic effects may take several wk to a few mo
• To change positions slowly to prevent orthostatic hypotension
• To use drug exactly as prescribed; if drug is discontinued abruptly, parkinsonian crisis may occur

---

ropivacaine (℞)

(roe-pi′va-kane)
Naropin
Func. class.: Local anesthetic
Chem. class.: Amide

Action: Competes with calcium for sites in nerve membrane that control sodium transport across cell membrane; decreases rise of depolarization phase of action potential

Uses: Peripheral nerve block, caudal anesthesia, central neural block, vaginal block

Dosage and routes:
• Varies with route of anesthesia
Available forms: Inj 2, 5, 7.5 mg/ml

Side effects/adverse reactions:
CNS: Anxiety, restlessness, ***convulsions, loss of consciousness,*** drowsiness, disorientation, tremors, shivering
CV: ***Myocardial depression, cardiac arrest, dysrhythmias,*** bradycardia, hypotension, hypertension, ***fetal bradycardia***
GI: Nausea, vomiting
EENT: Blurred vision, tinnitus, pupil constriction
INTEG: Rash, urticaria, allergic reactions, edema, burning, skin discoloration at injection site, tissue necrosis
RESP: ***Status asthmaticus, respiratory arrest, anaphylaxis***

Contraindications: Hypersensitivity, child <12 yr, elderly, severe liver disease

Precautions: Severe drug allergies, pregnancy (B)

Pharmacokinetics: Onset 2-8 min, duration 3-6 hr; metabolized by liver, excreted in urine (metabolites)

Interactions:
• Dysrhythmias: epinephrine, halothane, enflurane
• Hypertension: MAOIs, tricyclic antidepressants, phenothiazines
• Decreased action of ropivacaine: chloroprocaine

NURSING CONSIDERATIONS
Assess:
• B/P, pulse, respiration during treatment
• Fetal heart tones during labor
• Allergic reactions: rash, urticaria, itching

R

• Cardiac status: ECG for dysrhythmias, pulse, B/P during anesthesia
Administer:
• Only with crash cart, resuscitative equipment nearby
• Only drugs without preservatives for epidural or caudal anesthesia
Perform/provide:
• Use of new sol; discard unused portions
Evaluate:
• Therapeutic response: anesthesia necessary for procedure
Treatment of overdose: Airway, O_2, vasopressor, IV fluids, anticonvulsants for seizures

---

rosiglitazone
See appendix a—selected new drugs

---

salmeterol (R)
(sal-met′er-ole)
Serevent
Func. class.: β₂-adrenergic agonist

Action: Causes bronchodilation by action on β₂ (pulmonary) receptors by increasing levels of cAMP, which relaxes smooth muscle; with very little effect on heart rate, maintains improvement in FEV from 3 to 12 hr; prevents nocturnal asthma symptoms
Uses: Prevention of exercise-induced asthma, bronchospasm, COPD
Dosage and routes:
• *Adult:* **INH** 2 puffs bid (AM and PM)
Available forms: Aerosol 25 μg/actuation; inhalation powder 50 μg
Side effects/adverse reactions:
CNS: Tremors, anxiety, insomnia, headache, dizziness, stimulation,

restlessness, hallucinations, flushing, irritability
CV: Palpitations, tachycardia, hypertension, angina, hypotension, dysrhythmias
EENT: Dry nose, irritation of nose and throat
GI: Heartburn, nausea, vomiting
MS: Muscle cramps
*RESP: **Bronchospasm***
Contraindications: Hypersensitivity to sympathomimetics, tachydysrhythmias, severe cardiac disease
Precautions: Lactation, pregnancy (C), cardiac disorders, hyperthyroidism, diabetes mellitus, hypertension, prostatic hypertrophy, narrow-angle glaucoma, seizures
Pharmacokinetics:
INH: Onset 5-15 min, peak 4 hr, duration 12 hr, metabolized in liver, excreted in urine, breast milk; crosses placenta; blood-brain barrier
Interactions:
• Increased action of aerosol bronchodilators
• Increased action of salmeterol: tricyclic antidepressants, MAOIs
• May inhibit action of salmeterol: other β-blockers
NURSING CONSIDERATIONS
Assess:
• Respiratory function: vital capacity, forced expiratory volume, ABGs, lung sounds, heart rate and rhythm
Administer:
• After shaking; exhale, place mouthpiece in mouth, inhale slowly, hold breath, remove, exhale slowly
• Gum, sips of water for dry mouth
• Using spacing device for pediatric/geriatric patients
Perform/provide:
• Storage in light-resistant container; do not expose to temps over 86° F (30° C)

◆ = Nursing alert   ∅ = Herb-drug interaction   Ⓢ = Do not crush

Evaluate:
• Therapeutic response: absence of dyspnea, wheezing
Teach patient/family:
• Not to use OTC medications; extra stimulation may occur
• Use of inhaler; review package insert with patient
• To avoid getting aerosol in eyes
• To wash inhaler in warm water qd and dry
• To avoid smoking, smoke-filled rooms, persons with respiratory infections
Treatment of overdose: β_2-adrenergic blocker

---

salsalate (R)

(sal′sah-late)
Amigesic, Argesic-SA, Arthra-G, Disalcid, Marthritic, Mono-Gesic, Salflex, salsalate, Salsitab
Func. class.: Nonnarcotic analgesic, nonsteroidal antiinflammatory
Chem. class.: Salicylate

Action: Blocks formation of peripheral prostaglandins, which cause pain and inflammation; antipyretic action results from inhibition of hypothalamic heat-regulating center; does not inhibit platelet aggregation
Uses: Mild to moderate pain or fever, including arthritis, juvenile rheumatoid arthritis
Dosage and routes:
• *Adult:* **PO** 3 g/day in divided doses
Available forms: Caps 500 mg; tabs 500, 750 mg
Side effects/adverse reactions:
HEMA: Thrombocytopenia, agranulocytosis, leukopenia, neutropenia, hemolytic anemia, increased pro-time
CNS: Stimulation, drowsiness, dizziness, confusion, *convulsions,*

headache, flushing, hallucinations, *coma*
GI: Nausea, vomiting, GI bleeding, diarrhea, heartburn, anorexia, *hepatotoxicity*
INTEG: Rash, urticaria, bruising
EENT: Tinnitus, hearing loss
CV: Rapid pulse, *pulmonary edema*
RESP: Wheezing, hyperpnea
ENDO: Hypoglycemia, hyponatremia, hypokalemia, alteration in acid-base balance
Contraindications: Hypersensitivity to salicylates, NSAIDs, GI bleeding, bleeding disorders, children <3 yr, vit K deficiency
Precautions: Anemia, hepatic disease, renal disease, Hodgkin's disease, pregnancy (C), lactation, elderly
Pharmacokinetics: Metabolized by liver; excreted by kidneys; half-life 1 hr; highly protein bound; crosses blood-brain barrier and placenta slowly
Interactions:
• Decreased effects of salsalate: antacids, steroids, urinary alkalizers
• Increased blood loss: alcohol, heparin, ibuprofen, warfarin
• Increased effects of anticoagulants, insulin, methotrexate, probenecid, penicillins, phenytoin
• Decreased effects of spironolactone, sulfinpyrazone, sulfonamides, loop diuretics
• Toxic effects: PABA
• Decreased blood sugar levels: salicylates
• Drug/food: foods that cause acidic urine, may increase salsalate levels
Lab test interferences:
Increase: Coagulation studies, liver function studies, serum uric acid, amylase, CO_2, urinary protein
Decrease: Serum K, PBI, cholesterol, blood glucose

Side effects: *italics* = common; ***bold italics*** = life-threatening

Interference: Urine catecholamines, pregnancy test

NURSING CONSIDERATIONS
Assess:

• Pain: frequency, intensity, characteristics; relief of pain after medication

• For asthma, aspirin hypersensitivity, nasal polyps; may develop hypersensitivity to this product

• Liver function studies: AST, ALT, bilirubin (long-term therapy)

• Renal function studies: BUN, urine creatinine (long-term therapy)

• Blood studies: CBC, Hct, Hgb, pro-time (long-term therapy)

• I&O ratio; decreasing output may indicate renal failure (long-term therapy)

• Hepatotoxicity: dark urine, clay-colored stools; jaundiced skin, sclera; itching, abdominal pain, fever, diarrhea (long-term therapy)

• Allergic reactions: rash, urticaria; drug may have to be discontinued

• Ototoxicity: tinnitus, ringing, roaring in ears; audiometric testing is needed before, after long-term therapy

• Visual changes: blurring, halos, corneal and retinal damage

• Edema in feet, ankles, legs

• Drug history; many interactions
Administer:

• To patient crushed or whole; chewable tablets may be chewed

• With food or milk to decrease gastric symptoms; give 30 min before or 2 hr after meals
Evaluate:

• Therapeutic response: decreased pain, fever
Teach patient/family:

• To report any symptoms of hepatotoxicity, renal toxicity, visual changes, ototoxicity, allergic reactions (long-term therapy)

• Not to exceed recommended dosage; acute poisoning may result

• To read label on other OTC drugs; many contain aspirin

• That therapeutic response takes 2 wk (arthritis)

• To avoid alcohol ingestion; GI bleeding may occur

• To watch for signs of bleeding: dark stools

Treatment of overdose: Lavage, activated charcoal, monitor electrolytes, VS

---

saquinavir (R̥)
(sa-quen'ah-veer)
Invirase, Fortovase
Func. class.: Antiviral
Chem. class.: Synthetic peptide-like substrate analog

Action: Inhibits human immunodeficiency virus (HIV) protease, which prevents maturation of the infectious virus

Uses: HIV in combination with AZT, zalcitabine, ddc

Dosage and routes:

• *Adult:* **PO** 600 mg (hard cap-Invirase) or 1200 mg (soft cap-Fortovase) tid within 2 hr after a full meal; given with either zalcitabine 0.75 mg tid or zidovudine 200 mg tid

Available forms: Caps 200 mg (soft); 200 mg (hard)

Side effects/adverse reactions:
GI: Diarrhea, buccal mucosa ulceration, *abdominal pain, nausea*
CNS: Paresthesia, headache
INTEG: Rash
MS: Pain
MISC.: Asthenia, hyperglycemia
Contraindications: Hypersensitivity

Precautions: Liver disease, pregnancy (B), lactation, children
Pharmacokinetics: Absorption increased with food, protein binding

---

◆ = Nursing alert   ⫽ = Herb-drug interaction   ⊘ = Do not crush

98%, extensive first-pass metabolism

• Toxicity: ergots, midazolam, triazolam, dapsone, quinidine, calcium channel blockers, clindamycin

Interactions:

• Increased saquinavir levels: ketoconazole

• Decreased saquinavir levels: rifamycins

• Drug/food: increased bioavailability after high-fat meal

Lab test interferences:

CPK, glucose (low)

NURSING CONSIDERATIONS

Assess:

• Signs of infection, anemia

• Liver function studies: ALT, AST

• C&S before drug therapy; drug may be taken as soon as culture is taken; repeat C&S after treatment; determine the presence of other sexually transmitted diseases

• Bowel pattern before, during treatment; if severe abdominal pain with bleeding occurs, drug should be discontinued; monitor hydration

• Skin eruptions, rash, urticaria, itching

• Allergies before treatment, reaction of each medication; place allergies on chart

Teach patient/family:

• To take as prescribed within 2 hr of a full meal; if dose is missed, take as soon as remembered up to 1 hr before next dose; do not double dose

• That drug must be taken in equal intervals around the clock to maintain blood levels for duration of therapy

---

sargramostim (℞)

(sar-gram′oh-stim)

Leukine, rhu GM-CSF recombinant human

Func. class.: Biologic modifier: cytokine

Action: Stimulates proliferation and differentiation of hematopoietic progenitor cells (granulocytes, macrophages)

Uses: Acceleration of myeloid recovery in patients with non-Hodgkin's lymphoma, acute lymphoblastic leukemia, autologous bone marrow transplantation in Hodgkin's disease; bone marrow transplantation failure or engraftment delay

Dosage and routes:

Myeloid reconstitution after autologous bone marrow transplantation

• *Adult:* **IV** 250 µg/m^2/day × 3 wk; give over 2 hr, 2-4 hr after autologous bone marrow infusion, not less than 24 hr after last dose of antineoplastics and 12 hr after last dose of radiotherapy, bone marrow transplantation failure, or engraftment delay

Acceleration of myeloid recovery

• *Adult:* **IV** 250 µg/m^2/day × 14 days; give over 2 hr; may repeat in 7 days, may repeat 500 µg/m^2/day × 14 days after another 7 days if no improvement

Available forms: Powder for inj lyophilized 250, 500 µg; liquid 500 µg/ml

Side effects/adverse reactions:

CNS: Fever, malaise, CNS disorder, weakness, chills

GI: Nausea, vomiting, diarrhea, anorexia, *GI hemorrhage,* stomatitis, *liver damage*

S

HEMA: **Blood dyscrasias, hemorrhage**

INTEG: Alopecia, rash, peripheral edema

GU: Urinary tract disorder, abnormal kidney function

RESP: Dyspnea

CV: **Supraventricular tachycardia,** peripheral edema, **pericardial effusion**

Contraindications: Hypersensitivity to GM-CSF, yeast products; excessive leukemic myeloid blast in bone marrow, peripheral blood

Precautions: Pregnancy (C), lactation, child; renal, hepatic, lung disease; cardiac disease; pleural, pericardial effusions

Pharmacokinetics: Half-life 2 hr, detected within 5 min after administration, peak 2 hr

Interactions:

• Do not use this drug concomitantly with antineoplastics

• Increased myeloproliferation: lithium, corticosteroids

NURSING CONSIDERATIONS
Assess:

• Blood studies: CBC, differential count before treatment and twice weekly; leukocytosis may occur (WBC >50,000 cells/mm^3, ANC >20,000 cells/mm^3)

• Renal and hepatic studies before treatment: BUN, creatinine, urinalysis; AST, ALT, alk phosphatase; twice weekly monitoring is needed in renal, hepatic disease

• For hypersensitivity, rashes, local inj site reactions; usually transient

• For increased fluid retention in cardiac disease

Administer:

IV

• After reconstituting with 1 ml sterile water for inj without preservative; do not reenter vial; discard un-used portion; direct reconstitution sol at side of vial; rotate contents; do not shake

• Dilute in 0.9% NaCl inj to prepare IV inf; if final concentration is <10 µg/ml, add human albumin to make a final concentration of 0.1% to NaCl before adding sargramostim to prevent adsorption; for a final concentration of 0.1% albumin, add 1 mg human albumin/1 ml 0.9% NaCl inj run over 2 hr; give within 6 hr after reconstitution

Y-site compatibilities: Amikacin, aminophylline, aztreonam, bleomycin, butorphanol, calcium gluconate, carboplatin, carmustine, cefazolin, cefepime, cefotaxime, cefotetan, ceftizoxime, ceftriaxone, cefuroxime, cimetidine, cisplatin, clindamycin, cyclophosphamide, cyclosporine, cytarabine, dacarbazine, dactinomycin, dexamethasone, diphenhydramine, dopamine, doxorubicin, doxycycline, droperidol, etoposide, famotidine, fentanyl, floxuridine, fluconazole, fluorouracil, furosemide, gentamicin, granisetron, heparin, idarubicin, ifosfamide, immune globulin, magnesium sulfate, mannitol, mechlorethamine, meperidine, mesna, methotrexate, metoclopramide, metronidazole, mezlocillin, miconazole, minocycline, mitoxantrone, netilmicin, pentostatin, piperacillin/tazobactam, potassium chloride, prochlorperazine, promethazine, ranitidine, teniposide, ticarcillin, ticarcillin/clavulanate, trimethoprimsulfamethoxazole, vinblastine, vincristine, zidovudine

Perform/provide:

• Storage in refrigerator; do not freeze

Evaluate:

• Therapeutic response: WBC and differential recovery

 = Nursing alert   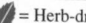 = Herb-drug interaction $\bigcirc$ = Do not crush

scopolamine (℞)

(skoe-pol′a-meen)

Func. class.: Cholinergic blocker
Chem. class.: Belladonna alkaloid

Action: Inhibits acetylcholine at receptor sites in autonomic nervous system, which controls secretions, free acids in stomach; blocks central muscarinic receptors, which decreases involuntary movements

Uses: Reduction of secretions before surgery, calm delirium, motion sickness, parkinsonian symptoms

Dosage and routes:

Parkinsonian symptoms
• *Adult:* IM/SC/IV 0.3-0.6 mg tid-qid using dilution provided

Preoperatively
• *Adult:* SC 0.4-0.6 mg

Nausea and vomiting
• *Child:* SC 0.006 mg/kg or 0.2 mg/m^2

Available forms: Inj 0.3, 0.4, 0.86, 1 mg/ml

Side effects/adverse reactions:

CNS: Confusion, anxiety, restlessness, irritability, delusions, hallucinations, headache, sedation, depression, incoherence, dizziness, excitement, delirium, flushing, weakness
INTEG: Urticaria
MISC: Suppression of lactation, nasal congestion, decreased sweating
EENT: Blurred vision, photophobia, dilated pupils, difficulty swallowing, mydriasis, cycloplegia
CV: Palpitations, tachycardia, postural hypotension, paradoxic bradycardia
GI: Dryness of mouth, constipation, nausea, vomiting, abdominal distress, ***paralytic ileus***
GU: Urinary hesitancy, retention

Contraindications: Hypersensitivity, narrow-angle glaucoma, myasthenia gravis, GI/GU obstruction, hypersensitivity to belladonna, barbiturates

Precautions: Pregnancy (C), elderly, lactation, prostatic hypertrophy, CHF, hypertension, dysrhythmia, children, gastric ulcer

Pharmacokinetics:
SC/IM: Peak 30-45 min, duration 7 hr
IV: Peak 10-15 min, duration 4 hr
Excreted in urine, bile, feces (unchanged)

Interactions:
• Increased anticholinergic effect: alcohol, narcotics, antihistamines, phenothiazines, tricyclics

NURSING CONSIDERATIONS

Assess:
• I&O ratio; retention commonly causes decreased urinary output
• Parkinsonism, EPS: shuffling gait, muscle rigidity, involuntary movements
• Urinary hesitancy, retention; palpate bladder if retention occurs
• Constipation; increase fluids, bulk, exercise if this occurs
• For tolerance over long-term therapy; dose may have to be increased or changed
• Mental status: affect, mood, CNS depression, worsening of mental symptoms during early therapy

Administer:
• Parenteral dose with patient recumbent to prevent postural hypotension
• Parenteral dose slowly; keep in bed for at least 1 hr after dose
• With or after meals for GI upset; may give with fluids other than H$_2$O
• At hs to avoid daytime drowsiness in patient with parkinsonism
• With analgesic to avoid behavioral changes when given as a preop

Additive compatibilities: Floxacillin, furosemide, meperidine, succinylcholine

S

Syringe compatibilities: Atropine, benzquinamide, butorphanol, chlorpromazine, cimetidine, diamorphine, dimenhydrinate, diphenhydramine, droperidol, fentanyl, glycopyrrolate, hydromorphone, hydroxyzine, meperidine, metoclopramide, midazolam, morphine, nalbuphine, pentazocine, pentobarbital, perphenazine, prochlorperazine, promazine, promethazine, ranitidine, sufentanil, thiopental

Y-site compatibilities: Heparin, hydrocortisone, potassium chloride, propofol, sufentanil, vit B/C

Perform/provide:
• Storage at room temp in light-resistant container
• Hard candy, frequent drinks, sugarless gum to relieve dry mouth

Evaluate:
• Therapeutic response: decreased secretions

Teach patient/family:
• Not to discontinue this drug abruptly; to taper off over 1 wk
• To avoid driving, other hazardous activities; drowsiness may occur
• To avoid OTC medication: cough, cold preparations with alcohol, antihistamines unless directed by prescriber

---

scopolamine (℞) (transdermal)

(skoe-pol′-a-meen)

Transderm-Scop

Func. class.: Antiemetic, anticholinergic

Chem. class.: Belladonna alkaloid

Action: Competitive antagonism of acetylcholine at receptor site in eye, smooth muscle, cardiac muscle, glandular cells; inhibition of vestibular input to the CNS, resulting in inhibition of vomiting reflex

Uses: Prevention of motion sickness

Dosage and routes:
• *Adult:* **PATCH** 1 placed behind ear 4-5 hr before travel, reapply q3 day, alternate ears
Not recommended for children

Available forms: Patch, 0.5 mg delivered in 72 hr

Side effects/adverse reactions:
INTEG: Rash, erythema
GU: Difficult urination
CNS: Dizziness, drowsiness, confusion, disorientation, memory disturbances, hallucinations
EENT: Blurred vision, altered depth perception, *dilated pupils,* photophobia, *dry mouth;* dry, itchy, red eyes; acute narrow-angle glaucoma

Contraindications: Hypersensitivity, glaucoma

Precautions: Children, elderly, pregnancy (C); pyloric, urinary, bladder neck, intestinal obstruction; liver, kidney disease

Pharmacokinetics:
Patch: Onset 4-5 hr, duration 72 hr

Interactions:
• Increased anticholinergic effects: antihistamines, antidepressants

NURSING CONSIDERATIONS
Teach patient/family:
• To avoid hazardous activities, activities requiring alertness; dizziness may occur
• To wash, dry hands before and after applying to surface behind ear
• To change patch q72h
• To apply at least 4 hr before traveling
• If blurred vision, severe dizziness, drowsiness occurs, to discontinue use, use another type of antiemetic
• To read label of all OTC medications; if any scopolamine is found in product, avoid use
• To keep out of children's reach

◆ = Nursing alert   ∥ = Herb-drug interaction   🚫 = Do not crush

secobarbital (℞)

(see-koe-bar'bi-tal)
Secogen Sodium*, Seconal
Sodium Pulvules, Seral*
Func. class.: Sedative/hypnotic-
barbiturate
Chem. class.: Barbitone (short
acting)

**Controlled Substance Schedule II
(USA), Schedule G (Canada)**
Action: Depresses activity in brain
cells primarily in reticular activating system in brain stem; selectively depresses neurons in posterior hypothalamus, limbic structures;
decreases seizure activity by inhibition of epileptic activity in CNS
Uses: Insomnia, sedation, preoper-
ative medication, status epilepticus,
acute tetanus convulsions
Dosage and routes:
Insomnia
• *Adult:* **PO/IM** 100-200 mg hs
• *Child:* **IM** 3-5 mg/kg, not to exceed 100 mg, not to inject >5 ml in
one site
Sedation/preoperatively
• *Adult:* **PO** 200-300 mg 1-2 hr preoperatively
• *Child:* **PO** 50-100 mg 1-2 hr preoperatively
Status epilepticus
• *Adult and child:* **IM/IV** 250-350
mg
Acute psychotic agitation
• *Adult and child:* **IM/IV** 5.5 mg/kg
q3-4h
Available forms: Caps 100 mg; inj
50 mg/ml
Side effects/adverse reactions:
*CNS: Lethargy, drowsiness, hang-
over,* dizziness, paradoxical stimulation in elderly and children, light-
headedness, dependency, CNS depression, mental depression, slurred
speech

GI: Nausea, vomiting, diarrhea, constipation
INTEG: Rash, urticaria, pain, abscesses at injection site, angioedema,
thrombophlebitis, ***Stevens-Johnson
syndrome***
CV: Hypotension, bradycardia
RESP: Depression, ***apnea, laryngospasm, bronchospasm***
*HEMA: Agranulocytosis, thrombo-
cytopenia, megaloblastic anemia*
(long-term treatment)
Contraindications: Hypersensitivity to barbiturates, pregnancy (D),
respiratory depression, addiction to
barbiturates, severe liver impairment, porphyria, uncontrolled severe pain
Precautions: Anemia, lactation, hepatic disease, renal disease, hypertension, elderly, acute/chronic pain
Pharmacokinetics:
IM: Onset 10-15 min, duration 4-
6 hr, metabolized by liver, excreted
by kidneys (metabolites); half-life
15-40 hr
Interactions:
• Do not mix with other drugs in sol
or syringe
• Increased CNS depression: alcohol, MAOIs, sedatives, narcotics
• Decreased effect of oral anticoagulants, corticosteroids, griseofulvin, quinidine
• Decreased half-life of doxycycline
⚠ Increased CNS depression: kava
Lab test interferences:
False increase: Sulfobromophtha-
lein
NURSING CONSIDERATIONS
Assess:
• VS q30min after parenteral route
for 2 hr
• Blood studies: Hct, Hgb, RBCs,
serum folate, vit D (if on long-term
therapy); pro-time in patients receiving anticoagulants

S

---

* = Canada only   Side effects: *italics* = common; ***bold italics*** = life-threatening

• Hepatic studies: AST, ALT, bilirubin; if increased, drug is usually discontinued

• Unresolved pain; drug may cause severe stimulation if pain is present

• Mental status: mood, sensorium, affect, memory (long, short)

• Physical dependency: frequent requests for medication, shakes, anxiety

◆ Barbiturate toxicity: hypotension; pulmonary constriction; cold, clammy skin; cyanosis of lips; insomnia; nausea; vomiting; hallucinations; delirium; weakness; mild symptoms may occur in 8-12 hr without drug

• Respiratory dysfunction: depression, character, rate, rhythm; hold drug if respirations <10/min or if pupils dilated

• Blood dyscrasias: fever, sore throat, bruising, rash, jaundice, epistaxis

• Perianal irritation if rectal forms used

Administer:
• After removal of cigarettes to prevent fires

• IM inj deep in large muscle mass to prevent tissue sloughing and abscesses

• After conservative measures for insomnia have been tried

• ½-1 hr before hs for sleeplessness

• On empty stomach for best absorption

• For <14 days, since drug is not effective after that; tolerance develops

• Crushed or whole

• Alone; do not mix with other drugs or inject if there is precipitate

• After cleansing enema is given rectally preoperatively in children

IV
• After diluting with sterile H_2O for inj; rotate; give 50 mg or less over 1 min; titrate to response

• Within 30 min of mixing with sterile water for inj; reconstitute after rotating ampule; do not shake; do not use cloudy sol; may be given directly or indirectly

• IV only with resuscitative equipment available; administer at <100 mg/min (only by qualified personnel)

Additive compatibilities: Amikacin, aminophylline

Perform/provide:
• Assistance with ambulation after receiving dose

• Safety measures: night-light, call bell within easy reach

• Checking to see if PO medication has been swallowed

• Storage of suppositories in refrigerator; do not use aqueous sol containing precipitate

Evaluate:
• Therapeutic response: ability to sleep at night, decreased early morning awakening if taking drug for insomnia, or decrease in number, severity of seizures if taking drug for seizure disorder

Teach patient/family:
• That morning hangover is common

• That drug is indicated only for short-term treatment of insomnia, probably ineffective after 2 wk

• That physical dependency may result when used for extended periods (45-90 days depending on dose)

• To avoid driving, other activities requiring alertness

• To avoid alcohol ingestion, CNS depressants; serious CNS depression may result

• Not to discontinue medication quickly after long-term use; drug should be tapered over 1-2 wk

• To tell all prescribers that barbiturate is being taken

• That withdrawal insomnia may occur after short-term use; not to start

---

◆ = Nursing alert   🥦 = Herb-drug interaction   🚫 = Do not crush

using drug again; insomnia will improve in 1-3 nights; may experience increased dreaming
• That effects may take 2 nights for benefits to be noticed
• Alternative measures to improve sleep (reading, exercise several hr before hs, warm bath, warm milk, TV, self-hypnosis, deep breathing)
Treatment of overdose: Lavage, activated charcoal, warming blanket, vital signs, hemodialysis, I&O ratio

selegiline (Ŗ)

(se-le′ji-leen)
Carbex, Eldepryl, Novo-Selegiline*, SD-Deprenyl
Func. class.: Antiparkinson agent
Chem. class.: Levorotatory acetylenic derivative of phenethylamine

Action: Increased dopaminergic activity by inhibition of MAO type B activity; not fully understood
Uses: Adjunct management of Parkinson's disease in patients being treated with levodopa/carbidopa who had poor response to therapy
Investigational uses: Alzheimer's disease
Dosage and routes:
• *Adult:* **PO** 10 mg/day given with levodopa/carbidopa in divided doses 5 mg at breakfast and lunch; after 2-3 days begin to reduce dose of levodopa/carbidopa 10%-30%
Available forms: Tabs 5 mg, caps 5 mg
Side effects/adverse reactions:
CNS: Increased tremors, chorea, restlessness, blepharospasm, increased bradykinesia, grimacing, tardive dyskinesia, dystonic symptoms, involuntary movements, increased apraxia, hallucinations, *dizziness,* mood changes, nightmares, delusions, lethargy, apathy, overstimulation, sleep disturbances, headache, migraine, numbness, muscle cramps, confusion, anxiety, tiredness, vertigo, personality change, back/leg pain
CV: Orthostatic hypotension, hypertension, dysrhythmia, palpitations, angina pectoris, hypotension, *tachycardia,* edema, *sinus bradycardia,* syncope
GI: Nausea, vomiting, constipation, weight loss, anorexia, diarrhea, heartburn, rectal bleeding, poor appetite, dysphagia
GU: Slow urination, nocturia, prostatic hypertrophy, urinary hesitation, retention, frequency, sexual dysfunction
INTEG: Increased sweating, alopecia, hematoma, rash, photosensitivity, facial hair
RESP: Asthma, shortness of breath
EENT: Diplopia, dry mouth, blurred vision, tinnitus
Contraindications: Hypersensitivity
Precautions: Pregnancy (C), lactation, children
Pharmacokinetics: Rapidly absorbed, peak ½-2 hr; rapidly metabolized (active metabolites: N-desmethyldeprenyl, amphetamine, methamphetamine), metabolites excreted in urine
Interactions:
◆ **Fatal interaction:** Opioids (especially meperidine); do not administer together
• Increased side effects of: levodopa/carbidopa
• **Serotonin syndrome** (confusion, seizures, fever, hypertension, agitation): fluoxetine, paroxitine, sertraline, fluvoxamine (discontinue 5 wk prior to selegiline); do not use together

S

• Do not use with tricyclics
• Drug/food: tyramine foods may increase hypertensive reactions

🍃 May decrease selegiline action: chaste tree fruit

Lab test interferences:

False positive: Urine ketones, urine glucose

False negative: Urine glucose (glucose oxidase)

False increase: Uric acid, urine protein

Decrease: VMA

NURSING CONSIDERATIONS
Assess:

• Decreased parkinsonian symptoms: rigidity, unsteady gait, weakness, tremors
• B/P, respiration throughout treatment
• Mental status: affect, mood behavioral changes, depression; perform suicide assessment

Administer:

• Drug until NPO before surgery
• Adjusting dosage to response
• With meals; limit protein taken with drug
• At doses <10 mg/day because of risks associated with nonselective inhibition of MAO

Perform/provide:

• Assistance with ambulation during beginning therapy

Evaluate:

• Therapeutic response: decrease in akathisia, improved mood

Teach patient/family:

• To change positions slowly to prevent orthostatic hypotension
• To report side effects: twitching, eye spasms; indicate overdose
• To use drug exactly as prescribed; if discontinued abruptly, parkinsonian crisis may occur
• To avoid foods high in tyramine: cheese, pickled products, wine, beer, large amounts of caffeine
• Not to exceed recommended dose

of 10 mg; might precipitate hypertensive crisis; report severe headache, other unusual symptoms

Treatment of overdose: IV fluids for hypertension, IV dilute pressure agent for B/P titration

---

senna (OTC)
(sen′na)
Black Draught, Dr. Caldwell Dosalax, Fletcher's Castoria, Gentlax, Senexon, Senna-Gen, Senokot, Senokotxtra

Func. class.: Laxative-stimulant
Chem. class.: Anthraquinone

Action: Stimulates peristalsis by action on Auerbach's plexus; softens feces by increasing water, electrolytes in large intestine

Uses: Acute constipation; bowel preparation for surgery or examination

Dosage and routes:

• *Adult:* **PO** 1-8 tabs (Senokot)/day or ½ to 4 tsp of granules (1 tsp-4 ml) added to water or juice; **RECT SUPP** 1-2 hs; **SYR** 1-4 tsp hs, 7.5-15 ml; (Black Draught) ¾ oz dissolved in 2.5 oz liquid given between 2-4 PM the day before procedure (X-Prep)
• *Child >27 kg:* **PO** ½ adult dose; do not use Black Draught for children
• *Child 1 mo-1 yr:* **SYR** 1.25-2.5 ml (Senokot) hs

Available forms: Supp 625 mg, 30 mg sennosides; powder 662 mg/g, 6, 15 mg sennosides/3g; tabs 8.6 mg sennosides, 180 mg; oral sol 3 mg sennosides/ml

Side effects/adverse reactions:

GI: Nausea, vomiting, anorexia, cramps, diarrhea, flatulence

META: Hypocalcemia, enteropathy, alkalosis, hypokalemia, **tetany**

GU: Pink, red or brown, black urine

◆ = Nursing alert   🍃 = Herb-drug interaction   🚫 = Do not crush

Contraindications: Hypersensitivity, GI bleeding, obstruction, CHF, lactation, abdominal pain, nausea/vomiting, appendicitis, acute surgical abdomen

Precautions: Pregnancy (C)

Pharmacokinetics:

PO: Onset 6-24 hr; metabolized by liver, excreted in feces

Interactions:

• Do not use with disulfiram (Antabuse)

NURSING CONSIDERATIONS
Assess:

• Stool: color, consistency, amount
• Blood, urine electrolytes if drug is used often
• I&O ratio to identify fluid loss
• Cause of constipation; fluids, bulk, exercise missing
• Cramping, rectal bleeding, nausea, vomiting; drug should be discontinued

Administer:

• In morning or evening (oral dose) with full glass of water
• Dissolve granules in water or juice before administration
• On empty stomach for more rapid results
• Shake oral sol before giving

Evaluate:

• Therapeutic response: decrease in constipation

Teach patient/family:

• That urine, feces may turn yellow-brown to red
• Not to use laxatives for long-term therapy; bowel tone will be lost
• That normal bowel movements do not always occur daily
• Not to use in presence of abdominal pain, nausea, vomiting
• To notify prescriber if constipation unrelieved or of symptoms of electrolyte imbalance: muscle cramps, pain, weakness, dizziness, excessive thirst

sertraline (R)

(ser′tra-leen)
Zoloft
Func. class.: Antidepressant
Chem. class.: SSRI

Action: Inhibits serotonin reuptake in CNS; increases action of serotonin; does not affect dopamine, norepinephrine

Uses: Major depression, obsessive-compulsive disorder (OCD)

Dosage and routes:

• *Adult:* **PO** 50 mg qd; may increase to max of 200 mg/day; do not change dose at intervals of <1 wk; administer qd in AM or PM
• *Geriatric:* **PO** 25 mg qd, increase by 25 mg q3 days to desired dose
• *Child 6-12 yr:* **PO** 25 mg qd
• *Child 13-17 yr:* **PO** 50 mg qd

Available forms: Tabs 25, 50, 100 mg

Side effects/adverse reactions:

CNS: Insomnia, agitation, somnolence, dizziness, headache, tremor, fatigue, paresthesia, twitching, confusion, ataxia, gait abnormality (elderly)

GU: Male sexual dysfunction, micturition disorder

GI: Diarrhea, nausea, constipation, anorexia, dry mouth, dyspepsia, *vomiting, flatulence*

CV: Palpitations, chest pain

EENT: Vision abnormalities

INTEG: Increased sweating, rash, hot flashes

ENDO: SIADH (elderly)

Contraindications: Hypersensitivity to this drug or SSRIs

Precautions: Pregnancy (B), lactation, elderly, hepatic, renal disease, epilepsy

Pharmacokinetics:

PO: Peak 4.5-8.4 hr; steady state 1 wk; plasma protein binding 99%,

S

elimination half-life 26-104 hr, extensively metabolized, metabolite excreted in urine, bile

Interactions:

• Increased effects of: antidepressants (tricyclics), diazepam, tolbutamide, warfarin, benzodiazepines

◆ **Fatal reactions:** MAOIs

• Increased sertraline levels: cimetidine, warfarin, other highly protein-bound drugs

• Altered lithium levels: lithium

🖊 Potentiation of SSRI: St. John's wort; do not use together

Lab test interferences:

Increase: AST, ALT

NURSING CONSIDERATIONS
Assess:

• Mental status: mood, sensorium, affect, suicidal tendencies, increase in psychiatric symptoms, depression, panic

• B/P (lying/standing), pulse q4h; if systolic B/P drops 20 mm Hg, hold drug, notify prescriber; take vital signs q4h in patients with cardiovascular disease

• Weight qwk; appetite may decrease with drug

• Urinary retention, constipation, especially in elderly

• Alcohol consumption; hold dose until morning

Administer:

• Increased fluids, bulk in diet for constipation, urinary retention

• With food, milk for GI symptoms

• Crushed if patient is unable to swallow medication whole

• Gum, hard candy, frequent sips of water for dry mouth

Perform/provide:

• Storage at room temp; do not freeze

• Assistance with ambulation during therapy, since drowsiness, dizziness occur

• Safety measures, including side rails, primarily for elderly

• Checking to see that PO medication is swallowed

Evaluate:

• Therapeutic response: significant improvement in depression, OCS

Teach patient/family:

• That therapeutic effect may take 1 wk

• To use caution in driving, other activities requiring alertness; drowsiness, dizziness, blurred vision may occur

• Not to discontinue medication quickly after long-term use; may cause nausea, headache, malaise

• To avoid alcohol, other CNS depressants

• To notify prescriber if pregnant or plan to become pregnant or breastfeed

---

sibutramine (℞)

(si-byoo′tra-meen)
Meridia
Func. class.: Appetite suppressant

Action: Inhibits reuptake of serotonin, norepinephrine, dopamine

Uses: Obesity in conjunction with other treatments

Dosage and routes:

• *Adult:* **PO** 10 mg qd; may be increased to 15 mg qd after 4 wk, or lowered to 5 mg qd depending on response

Available forms: Caps 5, 10, 15 mg

Side effects/adverse reactions:

CNS: Headache, insomnia, seizures, stimulation, drowsiness, dizziness, nervousness, emotional lability

CV: Hypotension, palpitations, vasodilation, *tachycardia*

GI: Anorexia, constipation, *dry mouth,* taste aberration, nausea, increased appetite

GU: Dysmenorrhea

◆ = Nursing alert   🖊 = Herb-drug interaction   🚫 = Do not crush

EENT: Laryngitis, pharyngitis, rhinitis, sinusitis

INTEG: Rash, sweating

Contraindications: Hypersensitivity, hypothyroidism, anorexia nervosa, severe hepatic/renal disease, uncontrolled hypertension, history of CAD, CHF, dysrhythmias, pregnancy, lactation, CVA

Precautions: History of seizures, elderly, children <16 yr, narrow-angle glaucoma

Interactions:

◆ Fatal serotonin syndrome: MAOIs, SSRIs, naratriptan, zolmitriptan, sumatriptan, dihydroergotamine, dextromethorphan, lithium, pentazocine, meperidine, fentanyl, tryptophan, or other centrally acting appetite suppressants; do not use together

• Hypertension: decongestants

• Increased levels of sibutramine: ketoconazole

Pharmacokinetics: Absorbed rapidly, peak 3-4 hr, extensively metabolized, widely distributed, half-life metabolites-14 hr, 16 hr

NURSING CONSIDERATIONS

Assess:

• B/P, pulse during treatment; if B/P or pulse rises or if palpitations, tachycardia occur, drug may need to be discontinued

• Patient's current dosage of antihypertensives, antidiabetics; these may need to be adjusted

• Need for medication and results when combined with other weight-loss strategies

Administer:

• PO with or without meals qd

Evaluate:

• Therapeutic response: decrease in weight over time

Teach patient/family:

• To discuss all other medications taken (including OTC) with health care provider; serious—even fatal—interactions can occur

• To take exactly as prescribed, and not to exceed recommended dose

---

sildenafil (R)

(sil-den'a-fill)

Viagra

Func. class: Erectile agent

Chem. class: Selective inhibitor of cGMP-PDE5

Action: Enhances the effect of nitric oxide (NO) by inhibiting phosphodiesterase type 5 (PDE5), which is necessary for degrading cGMP in the corpus cavernosum

Uses: Treatment of erectile dysfunction

Dosage and routes:

• *Adult:* **PO** 50 mg 1 hr before sexual activity, may be taken ½-4 hr before sexual activity; may be increased to 100 mg or decreased to 25 mg; max once/day

Available forms: Tabs 25, 50, 100 mg

Side effects/adverse reactions:

CNS: Headache, flushing, dizziness

MISC.: Dyspepsia, nasal congestion, UTI, abnormal vision, diarrhea, rash

Contraindication: Hypersensitivity

Precautions: Anatomical penile deformities, sickle cell anemia, leukemia, multiple myeloma, pregnancy (B)

Pharmacokinetics: Rapidly absorbed; bioavailability 40%; metabolized by liver (active metabolites); terminal half-life 4 hr, peak ½-1½ hr; reduced absorption with high-fat meal; excreted feces, urine

Interactions:

• Increased sildenafil levels: cimet-

S

idine, erythromycin, ketoconazole, itraconazole
• Decreased sildenafil levels: rifampin
• Decreased B/P: amlodipine
◆Do not use with nitrates; fatal fall in B/P

NURSING CONSIDERATIONS
Assess:
• Use of organic nitrates that should not be used with this drug
Administer:
PO
• Approximately 1 hr before sexual activity, do not use more than once a day
Teach patient/family:
• That drug does not protect against sexually transmitted diseases, including HIV
• That drug absorption is reduced with a high-fat meal
• That drug should not be used with nitrates in any form

---

silver nitrate (R)
Func. class.: Keratolytic

Action: Antiinfective, astringent, caustic
Uses: Cauterization of lesions, warts, burns (low concentrations)
Dosage and routes:
• *Adult and child:* **TOP** apply to area to be treated
Available forms: Sticks, sol 10%, 25%, 50%
Side effects/adverse reactions:
INTEG: Skin discoloration
Contraindications: Hypersensitivity
Interactions:
• Not to be used with alkalies, phosphates, thimerosal, benzalkonium chloride, halogenated acids
NURSING CONSIDERATIONS
Administer:
• After moistening stick with water

• To burns using a wet dressing (low concentrations 0.125%)
Perform/provide:
• Storage in cool area
Evaluate:
• Therapeutic response: absence of lesions, healing of burned areas
Teach patient/family:
• To avoid contact with clothing, unaffected areas; discoloration may occur

---

silver protein, mild (R, OTC)
Argyrol S.S. 10%, Argyrol S.S. 20%
Func. class.: Disinfectant
Chem. class.: Silver colloidal compound

Action: Destroys gram-positive, gram-negative organisms
Uses: Eye, nose, throat, swelling, infection
Dosage and routes:
• *Adult and child:* **TOP** sol use as needed
Available forms: Top sol 5%, 10%, 25%; eyedrops 20%
Side effects/adverse reactions:
INTEG: Irritation, discolored tissue
Contraindications: Hypersensitivity
Precautions: Pregnancy (C)
NURSING CONSIDERATIONS
Administer:
• To area to be treated only; do not apply to healthy skin
Perform/provide:
• Storage in tight container
Evaluate:
• Area of body involved: irritation, rash, breaks, dryness, scales

---

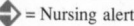

simethicone (OTC, ℞)

(si-meth'i-kone)
Extra Strength Gas-X,
Flatulex, Gas-X, Mylanta Gas,
Mylicon, Ovol*, Phazyme,
Phazyme 95, Phazyme 125
Func. class.: Antiflatulent

Action: Disperses, prevents gas pockets in GI system; does not decrease gas production
Uses: Flatulence
Dosage and routes:
• *Adult and child >12 yr:* PO 40-100 mg pc, hs
Available forms: Chew tabs 40, 80, 125 mg; tabs 60, 95 mg; drops 40 mg/0.6 ml; caps 125 mg; caps, soft gel 125 mg
Side effects/adverse reactions:
GI: Belching, rectal flatus
Contraindications: Hypersensitivity
Precautions: Pregnancy (C)
NURSING CONSIDERATIONS
Assess:
• Reason for excess gas production, decreased bowel sounds, recent surgery, other GI conditions
Administer:
• After meals; hs; shake susp well before giving; chew tabs should be chewed
Evaluate:
• Therapeutic response: absence of flatulence
Teach patient/family:
• That tablets must be chewed
• To shake suspension well before pouring

simvastatin (℞)

(sim-va-sta'tin)
Zocor
Func. class.: Antilipidemic
Chem. class.: HMG-CoA reductase inhibitor

Action: Inhibits HMG-CoA reductase enzyme, which reduces cholesterol synthesis
Uses: As an adjunct in primary hypercholesterolemia (types IIa, IIb), coronary artery disease
Dosage and routes:
• *Adult:* PO 5-10 mg qd in PM initially; usual range 5-40 mg/day qd in PM, not to exceed 40 mg/day; dosage adjustments may be made in 4-wk intervals or more
• *Elderly/renal disease:* PO 5 mg/day
Available forms: Tabs 5, 10, 20, 40, 80 mg
Side effects/adverse reactions:
INTEG: Rash, pruritus, alopecia
GI: Nausea, constipation, diarrhea, dyspepsia, flatus, abdominal pain, heartburn, *liver dysfunction,* pancreatitis
EENT: Lens opacities
MS: Muscle cramps, myalgia, *myositis, rhabdomyolysis*
CNS: Headache, tremor, vertigo, peripheral neuropathy
Contraindications: Hypersensitivity, pregnancy (X), lactation, active liver disease
Precautions: Past liver disease, alcoholism, severe acute infections, trauma, hypotension, uncontrolled seizure disorders, severe metabolic disorders, electrolyte imbalances
Pharmacokinetics: Peak 1-2½ hr, metabolized in liver (active metabolites), highly protein bound, excreted primarily in bile, feces

S

Interactions:
• Increased effects of warfarin
• Increased myalgia, myositis: cyclosporine, gemfibrozil, niacin, erythromycin
• Increased serum level of digoxin
Lab test interferences:
Increase: CPK, liver function tests
NURSING CONSIDERATIONS
Assess:
• 12 hr fasting lipid profile: LDL, ADL, TG, cholesterol at 6-8 wk, and q6mo
• Liver function studies q1-2mo during the first 1½ yr of treatment; AST, ALT, liver function tests may increase
• Renal studies in patients with compromised renal system: BUN, I&O ratio, creatinine
• Eyes with slit lamp before, 1 mo after treatment begins, annually; lens opacities may occur
Administer:
• Total daily dose in evening
Perform/provide:
• Storage in cool environment in tight container protected from light
Evaluate:
• Therapeutic response: decrease in cholesterol to desired level after 8 wk
Teach patient/family:
• That blood work and eye exam will be necessary during treatment
• To report blurred vision, severe GI symptoms, dizziness, headache
• That previously prescribed regimen will continue: low-cholesterol diet, exercise program

---

sirolimus
See appendix a—selected new drugs

---

sodium bicarbonate (℞, OTC)
Arm & Hammer Pure Baking Soda, Bellans, Citrocarbonate, Soda Mint, Neut
Func. class.: Alkalinizer
Chem. class.: $NaHCO_3$

Action: Orally neutralizes gastric acid, which forms water, $NaCl$, CO_2; increases plasma bicarbonate, which buffers H^+-ion concentration; reverses acidosis IV

Uses: Acidosis (metabolic), cardiac arrest, alkalinization (systemic/urinary) antacid
Dosage and routes:
Acidosis, metabolic
• *Adult and child:* **IV INF** 2-5 mEq/kg over 4-8 hr depending on CO_2, pH
Cardiac arrest
• *Adult and child:* **IV BOL** 1 mEq/kg of 7.5% or 8.4% sol, then 0.5 mEq/kg q10 min, then doses based on ABGs
• *Infant:* **IV INF** not to exceed 8 mEq/kg/day based on ABGs (4.2% sol)
Alkalinization of urine
• *Adult:* **PO** 325 mg-2 g qid or 48 mEq (4g), then 12-24 mEq q4h
• *Child:* **PO** 12-120 mg/kg/day (1-10 mEq/kg)
Antacid
• *Adult:* **PO** 300 mg-2 g chewed, taken with H_2O qd-qid
Available forms: Tabs 300, 325, 600, 650 mg; inj 4.2%, 5%, 7.5%, 8.4%
Side effects/adverse reactions:
CNS: Irritability, headache, confusion, stimulation, tremors, *twitching, hyperreflexia,* **tetany,** weakness, **convulsions** of alkalosis
CV: Irregular pulse, **cardiac arrest,** water retention, edema, weight gain
GI: Flatulence, *belching, distention,* **paralytic ileus,** acid rebound

---

◆ = Nursing alert   ∥ = Herb-drug interaction   ⊘ = Do not crush

META: Alkalosis
GU: Calculi
RESP: Shallow, slow respirations; cyanosis, ***apnea***

Contraindications: Hypertension, peptic ulcer, renal disease, hypocalcemia

Precautions: CHF, cirrhosis, toxemia, renal disease, pregnancy (C)

Pharmacokinetics:
PO: Onset 2 min, duration 10 min
IV: Onset 15 min, duration 1-2 hr, excreted in urine

Interactions:
• Increased effects: amphetamines, mecamylamine, quinine, quinidine, pseudoephedrine, flecainide, anorexiants
• Decreased effects: lithium, chlorpropamide, barbiturates, salicylates, benzodiazepines
• Increased Na and decreased K: corticosteroids

⬚ Decreased action of sodium bicarbonate: oak bark

Lab test interferences:
Increase: Urinary urobilinogen
False positive: Urinary protein, blood lactate

NURSING CONSIDERATIONS
Assess:
• Respiratory and pulse rate, rhythm, depth, lung sounds; notify prescriber of abnormalities
• Fluid balance (I&O, weight qd, edema); notify prescriber of fluid overload
• Electrolytes, blood pH, PO_2, HCO_3, during treatment; ABGs frequently during emergencies
• Urine pH, urinary output, during beginning treatment
• Extravasation with IV administration (tissue sloughing, ulceration, and necrosis)
• Weight qd with initial therapy
• Alkalosis: irritability, confusion, twitching, hyperreflexia stimulation, slow respirations, cyanosis, irregular pulse
• Milk-alkali syndrome: confusion, headache, nausea, vomiting, anorexia, urinary stones, hypercalcemia
• For GI perforation secondary to CO_2 in GI tract; may lead to perforation if ulcer is severe enough

Administer:
IV
• In prepared sol or diluted in an equal amount of compatible sol given 2-5 mEq/kg over 4-8 hr, not to exceed 50 mEq/hr; slower rate in children

Additive compatibilities: Amikacin, aminophylline, amobarbital, amphotericin B, atropine, bretylium, calcium chloride, calcium gluceptate, cefoxitin, ceftazidime, cephalothin, cephapirin, chloramphenicol, chlorothiazide, cimetidine, clindamycin, cytarabine, droperidol/fentanyl, ergonovine, erythromycin, esmolol, floxacillin, furosemide, heparin, hyaluronidase, hydrocortisone, kanamycin, lidocaine, mannitol, metaraminol, methotrexate, methyldopa, multivitamins, nafcillin, nalmefene, netilmicin, nizatidine, ofloxacin, oxacillin, oxytocin, phenobarbital, phenylephrine, phenytoin, phytonadione, potassium chloride, prochlorperazine, thiopental, verapamil

Syringe compatibilities: Milrinone, pentobarbital

Y-site compatibilities: Acyclovir, amifostine, asparaginase, aztreonam, cefepime, cefmetazole, ceftriaxone, cladribine, cyclophosphamide, cytarabine, daunorubicin, dexamethasone, dexchlorpheniramine, doxorubicin, etoposide, famotidine, filgrastim, fludarabine, gallium, granisetron, heparin, ifosfamide, indomethacin sodium trihydrate, insu-

lin, melphalan, mesna, methylprednisolone, morphine, paclitaxel,
piperacillin/tazobactam, potassium
chloride, propofol, remifentanil, tacrolimus, teniposide, thiotepa, tolazoline, vancomycin, vit B/C
Evaluate:
• Therapeutic response: ABGs, electrolytes, blood pH, HCO_3 WNL
Teach patient/family:
• To chew antacid tablets and drink
8 oz water
• Not to take antacid with milk, or
milk-alkali syndrome may result
• Not to use antacid for more than
2 wk
• To notify prescriber if indigestion
is accompanied by chest pain, dyspnea, diarrhea, dark, tarry stools
• About sodium-restricted diet; to
avoid use of baking soda for indigestion

---

sodium biphosphate/ sodium phosphate
(OTC)

Fleet Enema, Phospho-Soda
Func. class.: Laxative, saline

Action: Increases water absorption
in the small intestine by osmotic
action, laxative effect occurs by in-
creased peristalsis and water reten-
tion
Uses: Constipation, bowel or rectal
preparation for surgery, exam
Dosage and routes:
• *Adult:* **PO** 20-30 ml (Phospho-
Soda)
• *Child:* **PO** 5-15 ml (Phospho-
Soda)
• *Adult and child >12 yr:* **RECT** 1
enema (118 ml)
• *Child 2-12 yr:* **RECT** ½ enema
(59 ml)
Available forms: Enema 7 g
phosphate/19 g biphosphate/118 ml;

oral sol 18 g phosphate/48 g bi-
phosphate/100 ml
Side effects/adverse reactions:
GI: Nausea, cramps, diarrhea
META: Electrolyte, fluid imbalances
Contraindications: Hypersensitivity, rectal fissures, abdominal
pain, nausea/vomiting, appendicitis, acute surgical abdomen, ulcer-
ated hemorrhoids, Na-restricted
diets (Phospho-Soda)
Precautions: Pregnancy (C)
Pharmacokinetics: Excreted in
feces
NURSING CONSIDERATIONS
Assess:
• Stools: color, amount, consistency
• Bowel pattern, bowel sounds, flat-
ulence, distention, fever, dietary pat-
terns, exercise
• Blood, urine electrolytes if drug is
used often by patient
• Cramping, rectal bleeding, nausea, vomiting; if these symptoms
occur, drug should be discontinued
Administer:
• Alone for better absorption; do not
take within 1 hr of other drugs
Evaluate:
• Therapeutic response: decrease in
constipation
Teach patient/family:
• Not to use laxatives for long-term
therapy; bowel tone will be lost
• That normal bowel movements do
not always occur daily
• Not to use in presence of abdominal pain, nausea, vomiting
• To notify prescriber if constipation unrelieved or if symptoms of
electrolyte imbalance occur: mus-
cle cramps, pain, weakness, dizziness, excessive thirst
• To maintain fluid consumption

---

sodium polystyrene sulfonate (R)

(po-lee-stye'reen)
Kayexalate, SPS
Func. class.: Potassium-removing resin
Chem. class.: Cation exchange resin

Action: Removes potassium by exchanging sodium for potassium in body primarily in large intestine
Uses: Hyperkalemia in conjunction with other measures
Dosage and routes:
• *Adult:* **PO** 15 g qd-qid; **RECT** enema 30-50 g/100 ml of sorbitol warmed to body temp q6h
• *Child:* **PO/RECT** 1 mEq of K exchanged/g of resin, approximate dose 1g/kg q6h
Available forms: Susp 15 g polystyrene sulfonate, 21.5 ml sorbitol, 15 g (65 mEq) Na/60 ml; powder 15 g/4 level tsp
Side effects/adverse reactions:
GI: Constipation, anorexia, nausea, vomiting, diarrhea (sorbitol), fecal impaction, gastric irritation
META: Hypocalcemia, hypokalemia, hypomagnesemia, Na retention
Precautions: Pregnancy (C), renal failure, CHF, severe edema, severe hypertension
Interactions:
• Decreased effect of sodium polystyrene: antacids, laxatives
NURSING CONSIDERATIONS
Assess:
• Bowel function qd
• Hypotension: confusion, irritability, muscular pain, weakness
• Serum K, Ca, Mg, Na, acid-base balance
Administer:
• Oral dose as susp mixed with H_2O or syr (20-100 ml)

• Mild laxative as ordered to prevent constipation, fecal impaction
• Sorbitol as ordered to prevent constipation
• Retention enema after mixing with warm water; introduce by gravity, continue stirring, flush with 100 ml of fluid, clamp, and leave in place
Perform/provide:
• Retention of enema for at least ½-1 hr
• Irrigation of colon after enema with 1-2 qt nonsodium sol, drain
• Storage of freshly prepared sol 24 hr at room temp
Evaluate:
• Therapeutic response: K level WNL

somatropin (R)

(soe-ma-troe'pin)
Genotropin, Humatrope, Norditropin, Nutropin, Nutropin AQ, Serostim
Func. class.: Pituitary hormone
Chem. class.: Growth hormone

Action: Stimulates growth; somatropin similar to natural growth hormone; both preparations developed by recombinant DNA
Uses: Pituitary growth hormone deficiency (hypopituitary dwarfism), children with human growth hormone deficiency, AIDS wasting syndrome, cachexia, adults with somatropin deficiency syndrome (SDS)
Dosage and routes:
Genotropin
SC 0.16-0.24 mg/kg/wk divided into 6 or 7 inj, give in abd, thigh, buttocks
Humatrope
SC/IM 0.18 mg/kg divided into equal doses either on 3 alternate days or 6 ×/wk, max wk dose is 0.3 mg/kg

S

Nutropin/Nutropin AQ (growth hormone deficiency)
SC 0.3 mg/kg/wk
Serostim
SC at hs >55 kg, 6 mg; 45-55 kg, 5 mg; 35-45 kg, 4 mg
Norditropin
SC 0.024-0.034 mg/kg 6-7 ×/wk
Available forms: Powder for inj (lyophilized) 1.5 mg (4 IU/ml), 4 mg (12 IU/vial), 5 mg (13 IU/vial), 5 mg (15 IU/vial), 5 mg (15 IU/vial) rDNA origin, 5.8 mg (15 IU/ml), 6 mg (18 IU/ml), 8 mg (24 IU/vial), 10 mg (26 IU/vial); inj 10 mg (30 IU/vial)

Side effects/adverse reactions:
GU: Hypercalciuria
INTEG: Rash, urticaria, pain; inflammation at injection site
CNS: Headache, growth of intracranial tumor
ENDO: **Hyperglycemia, ketosis, hypothyroidism**
SYST: **Antibodies to growth hormone**
MS: Tissue swelling, joint and muscle pain

Contraindications: Hypersensitivity to benzyl alcohol, closed epiphyses, intracranial lesions
Precautions: Diabetes mellitus, hypothyroidism, pregnancy (C)
Pharmacokinetics: Half-life 15-60 min, duration 7 days; metabolized in liver
Interactions:
• Decreased growth: glucocorticosteroids
• Epiphyseal closure: androgens, thyroid hormones

NURSING CONSIDERATIONS
Assess:
• Growth hormone antibodies if patient fails to respond to therapy
• Thyroid function tests: T_3, T_4, T_7, TSH to identify hypothyroidism
• Allergic reaction: rash, itching, fever, nausea, wheezing

• Hypercalciuria: urinary stones; groin, flank pain; nausea, vomiting, urinary frequency, hematuria, chills
• Growth rate of child at intervals during treatment
Administer:
IM
• Rotate injection site
• Norditropin: after reconstituting 4 or 8 mg/2 ml diluent
• Humatrope: 5 mg/1.5-5 ml diluent, do not shake
• Nutropin/Nutropin AQ: reconstitute 5 mg/1-5 ml or 10 mg/1-10 ml bacteriostatic water for inj (benzyl alcohol preserved)
Perform/provide:
• Storage in refrigerator for <1 mo; if reconstituted <1 wk; do not use discolored or cloudy sol
Evaluate:
• Therapeutic response: growth in children
Teach patient/family:
• That treatment may continue for years; regular assessments are required

---

sotalol (℞)

(sot′ah-lahl)
Betapace, Sotacar*
Func. class.: Antidysrhythmic group II, III
Chem. class.: Nonselective β-blocker

Action: Blockade of β_1- and β_2-receptors leads to antidysrhythmic effect, prolongs action potential in myocardial fibers without affecting conduction, prolongs QT interval, no effect on QRS duration
Uses: Life-threatening ventricular dysrhythmias
Dosage and routes:
Renal dose
• CrCl 30-60 ml/min give q24h;

◆ = Nursing alert　　🌿 = Herb-drug interaction　　🚫 = Do not crush

CrCl 10-29 ml/min give q36-48h; CrCl <10 ml/min individualize dose
• *Adult:* **PO** initial 80 mg bid, may increase to 240-320 mg/day

Available forms: Tabs 80, 120, 160, 240 mg

Side effects/adverse reactions:

CV: Orthostatic hypotension, bradycardia, *CHF,* chest pain, ventricular dysrhythmias, AV block, peripheral vascular insufficiency, palpitations, prodysrhythmia, torsades de pointes

CNS: Dizziness, mental changes, drowsiness, fatigue, headache, catatonia, depression, anxiety, nightmares, paresthesia, lethargy, insomnia, decreased concentration

GI: Nausea, vomiting, diarrhea, dry mouth, flatulence, constipation, anorexia

INTEG: Rash, alopecia, urticaria, pruritus, fever

HEMA: Agranulocytosis, thrombocytopenic purpura (rare), *thrombocytopenia, leukopenia*

EENT: Tinnitus, visual changes, sore throat, double vision; dry, burning eyes

GU: Impotence, dysuria, ejaculatory failure, urinary retention

RESP: Bronchospasm, dyspnea, wheezing, nasal stuffiness, pharyngitis

MS: Joint pain, arthralgia, muscle cramps, pain

MISC.: Facial swelling, decreased exercise tolerance, weight change, Raynaud's disease

Contraindications: Hypersensitivity to β-blockers, cardiogenic shock, heart block (2nd or 3rd degree), sinus bradycardia, CHF, bronchial asthma, congenital or acquired long QT syndrome

Precautions: Major surgery, pregnancy (B), lactation, diabetes mellitus, renal disease, thyroid disease, COPD, well-compensated heart failure, CAD, nonallergic broncho-spasm, electrolyte disturbances, bradycardia, cardiac dysrhythmias, peripheral vascular disease

Pharmacokinetics:

PO: Onset 1-2 hr, peak 2-4 hr, duration 8-12 hr, half-life 12 hr; metabolized by liver (metabolites inactive), excreted unchanged in urine, crosses placenta, excreted in breast milk

Interactions:

• Increased hypotension: diuretics, other antihypertensives, nitroglycerin, prazosin

• Decreased β-blocker effects: sympathomimetics, nonsteroidal antiinflammatory agents, salicylates

• Increased hypoglycemia effect: insulin

• Increased effects of lidocaine

• Decreased bronchodilating effects of theophylline

• Decreased hypoglycemic effects of sulfonylureas

🌿 Potassium deficiency, increased antidysrhythmic effect: aloe, buckthorn, cascara sagrada, senna

Lab test interferences:

• *False increase:* Urinary catecholamines

• *Interference:* Glucose, insulin tolerance tests

NURSING CONSIDERATIONS
Assess:

• I&O, weight qd

• B/P, pulse q4h; note rate, rhythm, quality

• Apical/radial pulse before administration: notify prescriber of any significant changes

• Baselines in renal, liver function tests before therapy begins

• Edema in feet, legs qd

• Skin turgor, dryness of mucous membranes for hydration status

Administer:

• PO: ac, hs; tablet may be crushed or swallowed whole

• Reduced dosage in renal dysfunction

Perform/provide:
• Storage in dry area at room temp; do not freeze

Evaluate:
• Therapeutic response: absence of life-threatening dysrhythmias

Teach patient/family:
• Not to discontinue drug abruptly; taper over 2 wk or may precipitate angina
• Not to use OTC products containing α-adrenergic stimulants (nasal decongestants, OTC cold preparations) unless directed by prescriber
• To report bradycardia, dizziness, confusion, depression, fever
• To take pulse at home; advise when to notify prescriber
• To avoid alcohol, smoking, sodium intake
• To carry Medic Alert ID to identify drug being taken, allergies
• To avoid hazardous activities if dizziness is present
• To report symptoms of CHF including: difficulty in breathing, especially on exertion or when lying down; night cough, swelling of extremities
• To take medication to minimize orthostatic hypotension
• To wear support hose to minimize effects of orthostatic hypotension

Treatment of overdose: Lavage, IV atropine for bradycardia, IV theophylline for bronchospasm, digitalis, O_2, diuretic for cardiac failure; hemodialysis is useful for removal; administer vasopressor (norepinephrine) for hypotension, isoproterenol for heart block

---

sparfloxacin
(spar-floks'a-sin)
Zagam
Func. class.: Antiinfective
Chem. class.: Fluoroquinolone

Action: Interferes with conversion of intermediate DNA fragments into high-molecular-weight DNA in bacteria; DNA-gyrase inhibitor

Uses: Community-acquired pneumonia; chronic bronchitis caused by *Klebsiella pneumoniae, Haemophilus influenzae, H. parainfluenzae, Moraxella catarrhalis*

Dosage and routes:
Renal dose
• CrCl <50 ml/min day 400 mg on 1st day then 200 mg qod day 2-10
• *Adult:* **PO** 400 mg loading dose, then 200 mg q24h × 10 days
Available forms: Tabs 200 mg

Side effects/adverse reactions:
HEMA: **Leukopenia,** eosinophilia, anemia
CNS: Headache, dizziness, insomnia
GI: Nausea, flatulence, *vomiting,* diarrhea, *abdominal pain,* **pseudomembranous colitis**
CV: QT interval prolongation, vasodilation
INTEG: Rash, pruritus, photosensitivity

Contraindications: Hypersensitivity to quinolones, photosensitivity

Precautions: Pregnancy (C), lactation, children, renal disease, seizure disorders

Pharmacokinetics: Slow, erratic absorption, widely distributed; metabolized by liver, excreted in urine, feces; half-life 20 hr

Interactions:
• Decreased absorption of sparfloxacin: antacids with aluminum, mag-

---

 = Nursing alert   = Herb-drug interaction   ⊘ = Do not crush

nesium, iron products, zinc, sucralfate, give 4 hr apart
• Torsades de pointes: amiodarone, bepridil, disopyramide, erythromycin, pentamidine, phenothiazines, tricyclics, class Ia antidysrhythmics, class III antidysrhythmics

Lab test interferences:
Increase: AST, ALT

NURSING CONSIDERATIONS
Assess:
• For previous sensitivity reaction
• For signs and symptoms of infection: characteristics of sputum, WBC >10,000/mm^3, fever; obtain baseline information before and during treatment
• C&S before beginning drug therapy to identify if correct treatment has been initiated
• For allergic reactions: rash, urticaria, pruritus, chills, fever, joint pain; may occur a few days after therapy begins; epinephrine and resuscitation equipment should be available for anaphylactic reaction
• Blood studies: AST, ALT, alk phosphatase if patient is on long-term therapy
• Bowel pattern qd; if severe diarrhea occurs, drug should be discontinued
• For overgrowth of infection: perineal itching, fever, malaise, redness, pain, swelling, drainage, rash, diarrhea, change in cough, sputum

Administer:
• As directed only
• 4 hr before or 2 hr after antacids, zinc, calcium

Evaluate:
• Therapeutic response: absence of signs/symptoms of infection (WBC <10,000/mm^3, temp WNL)

Teach patient/family:
• To contact prescriber if vaginal itching, loose, foul-smelling stools, furry tongue occur (may indicate superinfection); report itching, rash, pruritus, urticaria
• To take all medication prescribed for the length of time ordered; drug must be taken as directed to maintain blood levels; do not give medication to others
• To notify prescriber of diarrhea with blood or pus
• To drink plenty of liquids
• To take 4 hr before or 2 hr after antacids, dairy products, zinc products
• To avoid direct sunlight

---

spectinomycin (R)
(spek-ti-noe-mye′sin)
Trobicin
Func. class.: Antiinfective
Chem. class.: Aminocyclitol

Action: Inhibits bacterial synthesis by binding to 30S subunit on ribosomes
Uses: Gonorrhea
Dosage and routes:
• *Adult:* **IM** 2-4 g as single dose
• *Child <45 kg:* **IM** 40 mg/kg single dose
Gonococcal infections in pregnancy
• *Adult:* **IM** 2 gm to treat those allergic to cephalosporins
Available forms: Powder for inj 400 mg/ml when reconstituted
Side effects/adverse reactions:
CNS: Dizziness, chills, fever, insomnia, headache, anxiety
HEMA: Anemia
GI: Nausea, vomiting, increased BUN
GU: Decreased urine output
INTEG: Pain at injection site, urticaria, rash, pruritus, fever
Contraindications: Hypersensitivity, syphilis

S

Precautions: Pregnancy (B), infants, children, lactation
Pharmacokinetics:
IM: Peak 1-2 hr, duration >8 hr, half-life 1-3 hr, excreted in urine (active form)

NURSING CONSIDERATIONS
Assess:
• Gonorrhea culture after treatment
• I&O ratio; report decreased output
• Liver studies: AST, ALT, serum alk phosphatase following multiple doses
• Blood studies: Hct, Hgb, BUN if multiple doses given
• Serologic test for gonorrhea 3 mo after treatment
• Allergies before treatment, reaction of each medication
Administer:
IM
• After shaking vial
• IM inj deep into large muscle mass (gluteus muscle only)
• With 20G needle; no more than 5 ml per site
Perform/provide:
• Storage at room temp; discard reconstituted sol after 24 hr
• Treatment of partner; report infection
Evaluate:
• Therapeutic response: negative gonorrhea culture after treatment

---

spironolactone (Ŗ)
(speer'on-oh-lak'tone)
Aldactone, Novo-Spiroton*
Func. class.: Potassium-sparing diuretic
Chem. class.: Aldosterone antagonist

Action: Competes with aldosterone at receptor sites in distal tubule, resulting in excretion of sodium chloride, water, retention of potassium, phosphate

Uses: Edema of CHF, hypertension, diuretic-induced hypokalemia, primary hyperaldosteronism (diagnosis, short-term treatment, long-term treatment), edema of nephrotic syndrome, cirrhosis of the liver with ascites

Edema/hypertension
• *Adult:* PO 25-200 mg/qd in single or divided doses
Edema
• *Child:* PO 3.3 mg/kg/day in single or divided doses
Hypertension
• *Child:* PO 1-2 mg/kg bid
Hypokalemia
• *Adult:* PO 25-100 mg/day; if **PO,** K supplements must not be used
Primary hyperaldosteronism diagnosis
• *Adult:* PO 400 mg/day × 4 days or 4 wk depending on test, then 100-400 mg/day maintenance
Available forms: Tabs 25, 50, 100 mg
Side effects/adverse reactions:
CNS: Headache, confusion, drowsiness, lethargy, ataxia
GI: Diarrhea, cramps, ***bleeding,*** gastritis, *vomiting,* anorexia, nausea
INTEG: Rash, pruritus, urticaria
ENDO: Impotence, gynecomastia, irregular menses, amenorrhea, postmenopausal bleeding, hirsutism, deepening voice
HEMA: ***Agranulocytosis***
ELECT: Hyperchloremic metabolic acidosis, ***hyperkalemia,*** hyponatremia
Contraindications: Hypersensitivity, anuria, severe renal disease, hyperkalemia, pregnancy (D)
Precautions: Dehydration, hepatic disease, lactation, renal impairment
Pharmacokinetics:
PO: Onset 24-48 hr, peak 48-72 hr;

◆ = Nursing alert   🍃 = Herb-drug interaction   🚫 = Do not crush

metabolized in liver, excreted in urine, crosses placenta

Interactions:

• Decreased effect of anticoagulants
• Increased action of antihypertensives, digitalis, lithium
• Increased hyperkalemia: K-sparing diuretics, K products, ACE inhibitors, salt substitutes
• Decreased effect of spironolactone: ASA

🍵 Hypokalemic alkalosis: licorice

Lab test interferences:

Interference: 17-OHCS, 17-KS, radioimmunoassay, digoxin assay

NURSING CONSIDERATIONS

Assess:

• Electrolytes: Na, Cl, K, BUN, serum creatinine, ABGs, CBC
• Weight, I&O qd to determine fluid loss; effect of drug may be decreased if used qd; ECG periodically (long-term therapy)
• Signs of metabolic acidosis: drowsiness, restlessness
• Rashes, temperature qd
• Confusion, especially in elderly; take safety precautions if needed
• Hydration: skin turgor, thirst, dry mucous membranes

Administer:

• In AM to avoid interference with sleep
• With food; if nausea occurs, absorption may be decreased slightly

Evaluate:

• Therapeutic response: improvement in edema of feet, legs, sacral area qd if medication is being used in CHF

Teach patient/family:

• To avoid foods with high K⁺ content: oranges, bananas, salt substitutes, dried apricots, dates
• That drowsiness, ataxia, mental confusion may occur; observe caution in driving
• To notify prescriber of cramps, diarrhea, lethargy, thirst, headache,

skin rash, menstrual abnormalities, deepening voice, breast enlargement

Treatment of overdose: Lavage if taken orally; monitor electrolytes, administer IV fluids, monitor hydration, renal, CV status

---

stavudine (℞)

(sta'vyoo-deen)
d4T, Zerit
Func. class.: Antiviral
Chem. class.: Thymidine nucleoside

Action: Prevents replication of HIV by the inhibition of the enzyme reverse transcriptase, causes DNA chain termination

Uses: Treatment of advanced HIV infection not responsive to other antivirals

Dosage and routes:

Renal dose

• *Wt >60 kg:* **PO** CrCl 26-50 ml/min 20 mg q12h; CrCl 10-25 ml/min 20 mg q24h
• *Wt <60 kg:* **PO** CrCl 26-50 ml/min 15 mg q12h; CrCl 10-25 ml/min 15 mg q24h
• *Adult >60 kg:* **PO** 40 mg q12h
• *Adult <60 kg:* **PO** 30 mg q12h
• *Child:* **PO** 2 mg/kg/day divided q12h

Available forms: Caps 15, 20, 30, 40 mg; PO powder for sol 1 mg/ml

Side effects/adverse reactions:

HEMA: **Bone marrow suppression**

CNS: Peripheral neuropathy, insomnia, anxiety, neuropathy, depression, dizziness, confusion, headache, chills/fever, malaise

GI: **Hepatotoxicity,** diarrhea, nausea, vomiting, anorexia, dyspepsia, constipation, stomatitis

MS: Myalgia, arthralgia

CV: Chest pain, vasodilation, hypertension

S

RESP: Dyspnea, pneumonia, asthma
INTEG: Rash, sweating, pruritus, benign neoplasms
EENT: Conjunctivitis, abnormal vision

Contraindications: Hypersensitivity to this drug or zidovudine, didanosine, zalcitabine; severe peripheral neuropathy

Precautions: Advanced HIV infection, pregnancy (C), lactation, bone marrow suppression; renal, liver disease, peripheral neuropathy

Interactions:

• Increased myelosuppression: other myelosuppressants

Pharmacokinetics: Excreted in urine, breast milk; peak 1 hr; half-life: elimination: 1-1.6 hr, intracellular: 3-3.5 hr

NURSING CONSIDERATIONS
Assess:

• Liver studies: AST, ALT
• Blood studies: WBC, differential, RBC, Hct, Hgb, platelets
• Renal studies: urinalysis, protein, blood
• C&S before drug therapy; drug may be given as soon as culture is taken
• Bowel pattern before, during treatment
• Weakness, tremors, confusion, dizziness; drug may have to be decreased or discontinued

Administer:

• With or without meals; absorption does not appear to be lowered when taken with food

Teach patient/family:

• The signs of peripheral neuropathy: burning, weakness, pain, prickling feeling in the extremities
• That drug should not be given with antineoplastics
• That drug is not a cure for AIDS, but will control symptoms

• To call prescriber if sore throat, swollen lymph nodes, malaise, fever occur; other drugs may be needed to prevent other infections
• That even with this drug, patient may pass AIDS virus to others
• That follow-up visits are necessary; serious toxicity may occur; blood counts must be done q2wk
• To take q12h around clock
• That serious drug interactions may occur if OTC products are ingested; see prescriber before taking aspirin, acetaminophen, indomethacin
• That drug may cause fainting or dizziness

Evaluate:

• Therapeutic response: decreased symptoms of HIV

---

streptokinase (℞)
(strep-toe-kye′nase)
Kabikinase, Streptase
Func. class.: Thrombolytic enzyme
Chem. class.: β-hemolytic streptococcus filtrate (purified)

Action: Activates conversion of plasminogen to plasmin (fibrinolysin): plasmin breaks down clots (fibrin), fibrinogen, factors V, VII; occlusion of venous access lines

Uses: Deep-vein thrombosis, pulmonary embolism, arterial thrombosis, arterial embolism, arteriovenous cannula occlusion, lysis of coronary artery thrombi after MI, acute evolving transmural MI

Dosage and routes:
Lysis of coronary artery thrombi
• *Adult:* IC 20,000 IU, then 2000 IU/min over 1 hr as **IV INF**
Arteriovenous cannula occlusion
• *Adult:* **IV INF** 250,000 IU/2 ml sol into occluded limb of cannula run over ½ hr; clamp for 2 hr; as-

◆ = Nursing alert   ∅ = Herb-drug interaction   ⊘ = Do not crush

pirate contents; flush with NaCl sol and reconnect

Thrombosis/embolism/DVT/ pulmonary embolism

• *Adult:* **IV INF** 250,000 IU over ½ hr, then 100,000 IU/hr for 72 hr for deep-vein thrombosis; 100,000 IU/hr over 24-72 hr for pulmonary embolism; 100,000 IU/hr × 24-72 hr for arterial thrombosis or embolism

Acute evolving transmural MI

• *Adult:* **IV INF** 1,500,000 IU diluted to a volume of 45 ml; give within 1 hr; intracoronary **INF** 20,000 IU by **BOL**, then 2,000 IU/min × 1 hr, total dose 140,000 IU

Available forms: Powder for inj, lyophilized, 250,000, 600,000, 750,000, 1,500,000 IU/vial

Side effects/adverse reactions:

CV: Dysrhythmias, hypotension, noncardiogenic pulmonary edema, *pulmonary embolism*

CNS: Headache, fever

EENT: Periorbital edema

GI: Nausea

HEMA: Decreased Hct, *bleeding*

INTEG: Rash, urticaria, phlebitis at IV inf site, itching, flushing

MS: Low back pain

RESP: Altered respirations, SOB, *bronchospasm*

SYST: **GI, GU, intracranial, retroperitoneal bleeding, surface bleeding, anaphylaxis**

Contraindications: Hypersensitivity, active bleeding, intraspinal surgery, CNS neoplasms, ulcerative colitis, enteritis, severe hypertension, severe renal disease, hepatic disease, hypocoagulation, COPD, subacute bacterial endocarditis, rheumatic valvular disease, cerebral embolism/thrombosis/hemorrhage, intraarterial diagnostic procedure or surgery (10 days), recent major surgery

Precautions: Arterial emboli from left side of heart, pregnancy (C)

Pharmacokinetics:

IV: Onset immediate, duration <12 hr; half-life <20 min; excreted in bile, urine

Interactions:

• Bleeding potential: aspirin, indomethacin, phenylbutazone, anticoagulants

Lab test interferences:

Increase: PT, aPTT, TT

Decrease: Plasminogen, fibrinogen

NURSING CONSIDERATIONS

Assess:

• Allergy: fever, rash, itching, chills; mild reaction may be treated with antihistamines

◆ For bleeding during 1st hr of treatment; hematuria, hematemesis, bleeding from mucous membranes, epistaxis, ecchymosis; may require tranfusion (rare), continue to assess for bleeding for 24 hr

• Blood studies (Hct, platelets, PTT, PT, TT, aPTT) before starting therapy; PT or aPTT must be less than 2× control before starting therapy; PTT or PT q3-4h during treatment

• For hypersensitive reactions: fever, rash, dyspnea; drug should be discontinued; for streptokinase reactions previously

• VS, B/P, pulse, respirations, neuro signs, temp at least q4h; temp >104° F (40° C) indicates internal bleeding; cardiac rhythm following intracoronary administration; systolic pressure increase >25 mm Hg should be reported to prescriber

◆ For neurologic changes that may indicate intracranial bleeding

◆ Retroperitoneal bleeding: back pain, leg weakness, diminished pulses

• For Guillain-Barré syndrome that may occur after treatment with this drug

• For respiratory depression

S

Administer:
IV

• As soon as thrombi identified; not useful for thrombi over 1 wk old

• Cryoprecipitate or fresh frozen plasma if bleeding occurs

• Loading dose at beginning of therapy; may require increased loading doses

• Heparin after fibrinogen level >100 mg/dl; heparin infusion to increase PTT to 1.5-2 × baseline for 3-7 days; IV heparin with loading dose is recommended after discontinuing streptokinase to prevent redevelopment of thrombi

• After reconstituting with 5 ml NS or D_5W; do not shake; further dilute to total volume of 45 ml; may be diluted to 500 ml in 45 ml increments; may dilute vial in 15 ml NS, further dilute 750,000 IU/50 ml NS or D_5W; further dilute 1,500,000 IU dose/100 ml or more

• About 10% patients have high streptococcal antibody titers requiring increased loading doses

• IV therapy using 0.8 μm filter

Y-site compatibilities: Dobutamine, dopamine, heparin, lidocaine, nitroglycerin

Perform/provide:

• Storage of reconstituted sol in refrigerator; discard after 24 hr

• Bed rest during entire course of treatment

• Avoidance of venous or arterial puncture, inj, rectal temp; any invasive treatment

• Treatment of fever with acetaminophen or aspirin

• Pressure for 30 sec to minor bleeding sites; inform prescriber if this does not attain hemostasis; apply pressure dressing

Evaluate:

• Therapeutic response: resolution of thrombosis, embolism

---

streptomycin (℞)
(strep-toe-mye′sin)

Func. class.: Antiinfective/antitubercular
Chem. class.: Aminoglycoside

Action: Interferes with protein synthesis in bacterial cell by binding to ribosomal subunit, causing inaccurate peptide sequence to form in protein chain, causing bacterial death

Uses: Sensitive strains of *Mycobacterium tuberculosis,* nontuberculous infections caused by sensitive strains of *Yersinia pestis, Brucella, Haemophilus influenzae, Klebsiella pneumoniae, Escherichia coli, E. aerogenes, Streptococcus viridans, Francisella tularensis, Proteus*

Dosage and routes:
Tuberculosis

• *Adult:* **IM** 15 mg/kg (max 1 g) qd × 2-3 mo, then 1 g 2-3 ×/week with other antitubercular drugs

• *Child:* **IM** 20-40 mg/kg/day in divided doses with other antitubercular drugs; max 15 mg/kg/day

Streptococcal endocarditis

• *Adult:* **IM** 1 g q12h × 1 wk with penicillin, then 500 mg bid × 1 wk

Enterococcal endocarditis

• *Adult:* **IM** 1 g q12h × 2 wk, then 500 mg q12h × 4 wk with penicillin, max 15 mg/kg/day

Available forms: Inj 400 mg/ml

Side effects/adverse reactions:

GU: **Oliguria, hematuria, renal damage, azotemia, renal failure, nephrotoxicity**

CNS: Confusion, depression, numbness, tremors, **convulsions,** muscle twitching, **neurotoxicity**

EENT: **Ototoxicity,** deafness, visual disturbances

HEMA: **Agranulocytosis, thrombo-**

◆ = Nursing alert   ∥ = Herb-drug interaction   ⊘ = Do not crush

cytopenia, leukopenia, eosinophilia, anemia

GI: Nausea, vomiting, anorexia, increased ALT, AST, bilirubin; hepatomegaly, ***hepatic necrosis,*** splenomegaly

CV: Hypotension, myocarditis, palpitations

INTEG: Rash, burning, urticaria, dermatitis, alopecia

Contraindications: Severe renal disease, hypersensitivity

Precautions: Neonates, mild renal disease, pregnancy (B), myasthenia gravis, lactation, hearing deficit, elderly, Parkinson's disease

Pharmacokinetics:

IM: Onset rapid, peak 1-2 hr; plasma half-life 2-2½ hr; not metabolized, excreted unchanged in urine, crosses placental barrier, poor penetration into CSF, small amounts enter breast milk

Interactions:

• Increased ototoxicity, neurotoxicity, nephrotoxicity: other aminoglycosides, amphotericin B, polymyxin, vancomycin, ethacrynic acid, furosemide, mannitol, methoxyflurane, cisplatin, cephalosporins, bacitracin

• Increased effects: nondepolarizing muscle relaxants, succinylcholine, warfarin

NURSING CONSIDERATIONS

Assess:

• Weight before treatment; calculation of dosage is usually based on ideal body weight, but may be calculated on actual body weight

• I&O ratio, urinalysis qd for proteinuria, cells, casts; report sudden change in urine output

• Serum peak 20-30 min after IM injection, trough level drawn 8 hr; acceptable levels—peak 5-25 µg/ml, trough should not be >5 µg/ml

• Urine pH if drug is used for UTI; urine should be kept alkaline

• Renal impairment by collecting urine for CrCl testing, BUN, serum creatinine; lower dosage should be given in renal impairment (CrCl <80 ml/min), monitor electrolytes: K, Na, Cl, Mg

• Deafness by audiometric testing, ringing, roaring in ears, vertigo; assess hearing before, during, after treatment

• Dehydration: high specific gravity, decrease in skin turgor, dry mucous membranes, dark urine

• Overgrowth of infection: fever, malaise, redness, pain, swelling, perineal itching, diarrhea, stomatitis, change in cough, sputum

• C&S before starting treatment to identify infecting organism

• Vestibular dysfunction: nausea, vomiting, dizziness, headache; drug should be discontinued if severe

• Inj sites for redness, swelling, abscesses; use warm compresses at site

Administer:

• IM inj in large muscle mass; rotate inj sites

• Drug in evenly spaced doses to maintain blood level

Additive compatibilities: Bleomycin

Syringe compatibilities: Penicillin G sodium

Y-site compatibilities: Esmolol

Perform/provide:

• Adequate fluids of 2-3 L/day unless contraindicated to prevent irritation of tubules

• Supervised ambulation, other safety measures with vestibular dysfunction

Evaluate:

• Therapeutic effect: absence of fever, draining wounds, negative C&S after treatment

Teach patient/family:

• To report headache, dizziness, symptoms of overgrowth of infection, renal impairment

S

Side effects: *italics* = common; ***bold italics*** = life-threatening

• To report loss of hearing, ringing, roaring in ears, fullness in head

Treatment of overdose: Hemodialysis; monitor serum levels of drug

---

succimer (℞)

(sux'i-mer)
Chemet
Func. class.: Heavy metal antagonist
Chem. class.: Chelating agent

Action: Binds with ions of lead to form a water-soluble complex excreted by kidneys

Uses: Lead poisoning in children with lead levels above 45 µg/dl; may be beneficial in mercury, arsenic poisoning

Dosage and routes:
• *Child:* **PO** 10 mg/kg or 350 mg/m^2 q8h × 5 days, then 10 mg/kg or 350 mg/m^2 q12h × 2 wk; another course may be required depending on lead levels; allow 2 wk between courses

Available forms: Caps 100 mg

Side effects/adverse reactions:
SYST: Back, stomach, head, rib, flank pain; abdominal cramps, chills, fever, flulike symptoms, head cold, headache
*HEMA: **Increased platelets, intermittent eosinophilia***
*GU: **Proteinuria,*** decreased urination, voiding difficulties
INTEG: Rash, urticaria, pruritus
META: Increased AST, ALT, alk phosphatase, cholesterol
GI: Nausea, vomiting, diarrhea, metallic taste, anorexia
CNS: Drowsiness, dizziness, paresthesia, sensorimotor neuropathy
EENT: Otitis media, watery eyes, film in eyes, plugged ears
RESP: Sore throat, rhinorrhea, nasal congestion, cough

Contraindications: Hypersensitivity

Precautions: Pregnancy (C), lactation, children <1 yr

Pharmacokinetics:
PO: Peak 1-2 hr, 49% excreted (39% in feces, 9% urine, 1% as CO_2 from lungs)

Interactions:
• Not recommended concurrently with other chelating agents

NURSING CONSIDERATIONS
Assess:
• Hepatic, renal studies: ALT, AST, alk phosphatase, BUN, creatinine, serum lead level
• I&O
• For lead sources in home, school
• Allergic reactions: rash, pruritus, urticaria; drug should be discontinued if antihistamines fail to help

Administer:
PO
• To children who cannot swallow capsule by separating the capsule and sprinkling content on food or in a spoon followed by a drink

Perform/provide:
• Adequate fluids; check hydration status qd

Evaluate:
• Therapeutic response: decrease in serum lead level

Teach patient/family:
• That therapeutic effect may take 1-3 mo
• To report urticaria, rash

---

succinylcholine (R)

(suk-sin-ill-koe'leen)
Anectine, Anectine Flo-Pack, Quelicin, succinylcholine chloride, Sucostrin, Suxamethonium

Func. class.: Neuromuscular blocker (depolarizing–ultra short)

Action: Inhibits transmission of nerve impulses by binding with cholinergic receptor sites, antagonizing action of acetylcholine; causes release of histamine

Uses: Facilitation of endotracheal intubation, skeletal muscle relaxation during orthopedic manipulations

Dosage and routes:
• *Adult:* **IV** 0.6 mg/kg, then 2.5 mg/min as needed; **IM** 2.5 mg/kg, not to exceed 150 mg
• *Child:* **IV/IM** 1-2 mg/kg, not to exceed 150 mg **IM**

Available forms: Inj 20, 50, 100 mg/ml; powder for inj 100, 500 mg/vial, 1 g/vial

Side effects/adverse reactions:
CV: Bradycardia, tachycardia; increased, decreased B/P; *sinus arrest, dysrhythmias*
RESP: Prolonged apnea, bronchospasm, cyanosis, respiratory depression
EENT: Increased secretions, increased intraocular pressure
MS: Weakness, muscle pain, fasciculations, prolonged relaxation
HEMA: Myoglobulinemia
INTEG: Rash, flushing, pruritus, urticaria

Contraindications: Hypersensitivity, malignant hyperthermia, decreased plasma pseudocholinesterase, penetrating eye injuries, acute narrow-angle glaucoma

Precautions: Pregnancy (C), cardiac disease, severe burns, fractures—fasciculations may increase damage—lactation, children <2 yr, electrolyte imbalances, dehydration, neuromuscular disease, respiratory disease, collagen diseases, glaucoma, eye surgery, elderly or debilitated patients

Pharmacokinetics:
IV: Onset 1 min, peak 2-3 min, duration 6-10 min
IM: Onset 2-3 min
Hydrolyzed in urine (active/inactive metabolites)

Interactions:
• Increased neuromuscular blockade: aminoglycosides, clindamycin, lincomycin, quinidine, local anesthetics, polymyxin antibiotics, lithium, narcotic analgesics, thiazides, enflurane, isoflurane, Mg salts, oxytocin
• Dysrhythmias: theophylline

NURSING CONSIDERATIONS
Assess:
• For electrolyte imbalances (K, Mg); may lead to increased action of this drug
• Vital signs (B/P, pulse, respirations, airway) until fully recovered; rate, depth, pattern of respirations, strength of hand grip
• I&O ratio; check for urinary retention, frequency, hesitancy
• Recovery: decreased paralysis of face, diaphragm, leg, arm, rest of body
• Allergic reactions: rash, fever, respiratory distress, pruritus; drug should be discontinued

Administer:
• Deep IM inj, preferably high in deltoid muscle
IV
• Using nerve stimulator by anesthesiologist to determine neuromuscular blockade
• Anticholinesterase to reverse neuromuscular blockade

S

• IV inf; dilute 1-2 mg/ml in D₅, isotonic saline sol, give 0.5-10 mg/min, titrate to response; may be given directly over 1 min

Additive compatibilities: Amikacin, cephapirin, isoproterenol, meperidine, methyldopate, morphine, norepinephrine, scopolamine

Syringe compatibilities: Heparin

Y-site compatibilities: Etomidate, heparin, potassium chloride, propofol, vit B/C

Perform/provide:
• Storage in refrigerator, powder at room temp; close tightly
• Reassurance if communication is difficult during recovery from neuromuscular blockade; postoperative stiffness is normal, soon subsides

Evaluate:
• Therapeutic response: paralysis of jaw, eyelid, head, neck, rest of body

Treatment of overdose: Edrophonium or neostigmine, atropine, monitor VS; may require mechanical ventilation

---

sucralfate (℞)
(soo-kral′fate)
Carafate, Sulcrate*
Func. class.: Protectant
Chem. class.: Aluminum hydroxide, sulfated sucrose

Action: Forms a complex that adheres to ulcer site, adsorbs pepsin

Uses: Duodenal ulcer, oral mucositis, stomatitis after radiation of head and neck

Investigational uses: Gastric ulcers, gastroesophageal reflux

Dosage and routes:
• *Adult:* **PO** 1 g qid 1 hr ac, hs
• *Child:* **PO** 40-80 mg/kg/day

Available forms: Tabs 1 g; oral susp 500 mg/5 ml

Side effects/adverse reactions:
CNS: Drowsiness, dizziness
GI: Dry mouth, constipation, nausea, gastric pain, vomiting
INTEG: Urticaria, rash, pruritus

Contraindications: Hypersensitivity

Precautions: Pregnancy (B), lactation, children, renal failure

Pharmacokinetics:
PO: Duration up to 5 hr

Interactions:
• Decreased action of tetracyclines, phenytoin, fat-soluble vitamins, cimetidine, digoxin, ketoconazole, ranitidine, theophylline
• Decreased absorption of fluoroquinolones
• Decreased absorption of sucralfate: antacids

NURSING CONSIDERATIONS
Assess:
• Gastric pH (>5 should be maintained)

Administer:
PO
• On an empty stomach, 1 hr before meals and hs

Perform/provide:
• Storage at room temp

Evaluate:
• Therapeutic response: absence of pain, GI complaints

Teach patient/family:
• To avoid black pepper, caffeine, alcohol, harsh spices, extremes in temp of food
• To take on empty stomach
• To take full course of therapy
• To avoid antacids within ½ hr of drug

◆ = Nursing alert   ∥ = Herb-drug interaction   ⃠ = Do not crush

sufentanil (R̵)

(soo-fen'ta-nil)

Sufenta

Func. class.: Opiate analgesic

Controlled Substance Schedule II

Action: Inhibits ascending pain pathways in CNS, increases pain threshold, alters pain perception

Uses: Primary anesthetic, adjunct to general anesthetic

Dosage and routes:

Primary anesthetic

• *Adult:* IV 8-30 µg/kg given with 100% O_2, a muscle relaxant

Adjunct

• *Adult:* IV 1-8 µg/kg given with nitrous oxide/O_2

Available forms: Inj 50 µg/ml

Side effects/adverse reactions:

CNS: Drowsiness, dizziness, confusion, headache, sedation, euphoria

GI: Nausea, vomiting, anorexia, constipation, cramps

GU: Increased urinary output, dysuria, urinary retention

INTEG: Rash, urticaria, bruising, flushing, diaphoresis, pruritus

EENT: Tinnitus, blurred vision, miosis, diplopia

CV: Palpitations, bradycardia, change in B/P

*RESP: **Respiratory depression***

Contraindications: Hypersensitivity, addiction (opiate)

Precautions: Addictive personality, pregnancy (C), lactation, increased intracranial pressure, MI (acute), severe heart disease, respiratory depression, hepatic disease, renal disease, child <18 yr

Pharmacokinetics: Onset 1½-3 hr, half-life 2½ hr

Interactions:

• Increased effects with other CNS depressants: alcohol, narcotics, sedative/hypnotics, antipsychotics, skeletal muscle relaxants, antihistamines

🖉 Increased CNS depression: kava

Lab test interferences:

Increase: Amylase

NURSING CONSIDERATIONS

Assess:

• I&O ratio; decreasing output may indicate urinary retention

• CNS changes: dizziness, drowsiness, hallucinations, euphoria, LOC, pupil reaction

• Allergic reactions: rash, urticaria

• Respiratory dysfunction: respiratory depression, character, rate, rhythm; notify prescriber if respirations are <10/min

• Need for pain medication, physical dependence

Administer:

• With antiemetic if nausea, vomiting occur

IV

• Undiluted over 1-2 min or give as inf

Y-site compatibilities: Amphotericin B cholesteryl, cisatracurium, remifentanil

Perform/provide:

• Storage in light-resistant area at room temp

• Safety measures: side rails, nightlight, call bell within easy reach

Evaluate:

• Therapeutic response: maintenance of anesthesia

Teach patient/family:

• To report any symptoms of CNS changes, allergic reactions

Treatment of overdose: Naloxone (Narcan) 0.2-0.8 mg IV, O_2, IV fluids, vasopressors

S

---

sulfadiazine (R)

(sul-fa-dye'a-zeen)
Sulfadiazine
Func. class.: Antiinfective
Chem. class.: Sulfonamide, intermediate acting

Action: Interferes with bacterial biosynthesis of proteins by competitive antagonism of PABA

Uses: UTIs, rheumatic fever prophylaxis, with pyrimethamine for *Toxoplasma gondii* encephalitis, chancroid, inclusion conjunctivitis, malaria, meningitis, *Haemophilus influenzae,* meningocococeal meningitis, nocardiosis, acute otitis media, trachoma

Dosage and routes:

UTIs

• *Adult:* **PO** 2-4 g, then 1-2 g q6h × 10 days

• *Child:* **PO** 75 mg/kg or 2 g/m², then 150 mg/kg/day or 4 g/m² in 4-6 divided doses, max 6 g/day

Rheumatic fever prophylaxis

• *Child >30 kg:* **PO** 1 g qd

• *Child <30 kg:* **PO** 500 mg qd

Available forms: Tabs 500 mg

Side effects/adverse reactions:

SYST: **Anaphylaxis**

GI: Nausea, vomiting, abdominal pain, stomatitis, *hepatitis,* glossitis, pancreatitis, diarrhea, *enterocolitis,* anorexia

CNS: Headache, insomnia, hallucinations, depression, vertigo, fatigue, anxiety, *convulsions,* drug fever, chills, drowsiness

HEMA: Leukopenia, thrombocytopenia, agranulocytosis, hemolytic anemia, aplastic anemia

INTEG: Rash, dermatitis, urticaria, *Stevens-Johnson syndrome,* erythema, photosensitivity, alopecia

GU: Renal failure, toxic nephrosis, increased BUN, creatinine, crystalluria, hematuria, proteinuria

CV: Allergic myocarditis

Contraindications: Hypersensitivity to sulfonamides, sulfonylureas, thiazide and loop diuretics, salicylates, sunscreens with PABA, lactation, infants <2 mo (except congenital toxoplasmosis), pregnancy at term, porphyria

Precautions: Pregnancy (B), impaired hepatic function, severe allergy, bronchial asthma, renal dysfunction

Pharmacokinetics:

PO: Rapidly absorbed, onset ½ hr; peak 3-6 hr, 30%-50% bound to plasma proteins, half-life 8-10 hr; excreted in urine, breast milk; crosses placenta, metabolized in liver

Interactions:

• Increased hypoglycemic response: sulfonylurea agents

• Increased anticoagulant effects: warfarin

• Decreased renal excretion of: methotrexate

• Decreased hepatic clearance of: phenytoin

• Increased effects of: barbiturates, tolbutamide, uricosurics

• Increased drug-free concentrations: indomethacin, probenecid, salicylates

• Increased thrombocytopenia: thiazide diuretics

• Increased nephrotoxicity; cyclosporine

Lab test interferences:

False positive: Urinary glucose test (Benedict's method)

NURSING CONSIDERATIONS

Assess:

• I&O ratio; note color, character, pH of urine if drug administered for UTIs; output should be 800 ml less than intake; if urine is highly acidic, alkalization may be needed

◆ = Nursing alert   🖋 = Herb-drug interaction   🚫 = Do not crush

• Kidney function studies: BUN, creatinine, urinalysis (long-term therapy)

• Blood dyscrasias: skin rash, fever, sore throat, bruising, bleeding, fatigue, joint pain, monitor CBC before and periodically

• Allergic reaction: rash, dermatitis, urticaria, pruritus, dyspnea, bronchospasm

Administer:

• On an empty stomach

• With full glass of H_2O to maintain adequate hydration; increase fluids to 2 L/day to decrease crystallization in kidneys

• Medication after C&S; repeat C&S after full course of medication

Perform/provide:

• Storage in tight, light-resistant container at room temp

Evaluate:

• Therapeutic response: absence of pain, fever, C&S negative

Teach patient/family:

• To take each oral dose with full glass of water to prevent crystalluria

• To complete full course of treatment to prevent superinfection

• To avoid sunlight or use sunscreen to prevent burns

• To avoid OTC medication (aspirin, vit C) unless directed by prescriber

• To notify prescriber of skin rash, sore throat, fever, mouth sores, unusual bruising, bleeding

sulfamethizole (℞)

(sul-fa-meth'i-zole)
Thiosulfil Forte
Func. class.: Antiinfective
Chem. class.: Sulfonamide, short acting

Action: Interferes with bacterial biosynthesis of proteins by competitive antagonism of PABA

Uses: UTIs

Dosage and routes:

• *Adult:* **PO** 0.5-1 g tid-qid

• *Child >2 mo:* **PO** 30-45 mg/kg/day in divided doses q6h

Available forms: Tabs 500 mg

Side effects/adverse reactions:

*SYST: **Anaphylaxis***

GI: Nausea, vomiting, abdominal pain, stomatitis, ***hepatitis,*** glossitis, pancreatitis, diarrhea, ***enterocolitis***

CNS: Headache, confusion, insomnia, hallucinations, depression, vertigo, fatigue, anxiety, ***convulsions,*** drug fever, chills

*HEMA: **Leukopenia, neutropenia, thrombocytopenia, agranulocytosis, hemolytic anemia***

INTEG: Rash, dermatitis, urticaria, ***Stevens-Johnson syndrome,*** erythema, photosensitivity

*GU: **Renal failure, toxic nephrosis,*** increased BUN, creatinine, crystalluria

*CV: **Allergic myocarditis***

Contraindications: Hypersensitivity to sulfonamides, sulfonylureas, thiazide/loop diuretics, salicylates, sunscreens with PABA, infants < 2 mo (except congenital toxoplasmosis), pregnancy at term

Precautions: Pregnancy (B), lactation, impaired hepatic function, severe allergy, bronchial asthma

Pharmacokinetics:

PO: Rapidly absorbed, peak 2 hr, 90% bound to plasma proteins; ex-

S

creted in urine, breast milk; crosses placenta

Interactions:

• Increased effects of: barbiturates, tolbutamide, uricosurics

• Increased drug-free concentrations: indomethacin, probenecid, salicylates

• Increased thrombocytopenia: thiazide diuretics

• Increased nephrotoxicity: cyclosporine

• Increased hypoglycemic response: sulfonylurea agents

• Increased anticoagulant effects: warfarin

• Decreased renal excretion of methotrexate

• Decreased hepatic clearance of phenytoin

Lab test interferences:

False positive: Urinary glucose test (Benedict's method)

NURSING CONSIDERATIONS
Assess:

• I&O ratio; note color, character, pH of urine if drug administered for UTIs; output should be 800 ml less than intake; if urine is highly acidic, alkalization may be needed

• Kidney function studies: BUN, creatinine, urinalysis if on long-term therapy

• Blood dyscrasias: skin rash, fever, sore throat, bruising, bleeding, fatigue, joint pain, monitor CBC before and periodically

• Allergic reaction: rash, dermatitis, urticaria, pruritus, dyspnea, bronchospasm

Administer:

• With full glass of H_2O to maintain adequate hydration; increase fluids to 2 L/day to decrease crystallization in kidneys

• Medication after C&S; repeat C&S after full course of medication

Perform/provide:

• Storage in tight, light-resistant container at room temp

Evaluate:

• Therapeutic response: absence of pain, fever, C&S negative

Teach patient/family:

• To take each oral dose with full glass of H_2O to prevent crystalluria

• To complete full course of treatment to prevent superinfection

• To avoid sunlight or use sunscreen to prevent burns

• To avoid OTC medication (aspirin, vit C) unless directed by prescriber

• To notify prescriber of skin rash, sore throat, fever, mouth sores, unusual bruising, bleeding

---

sulfamethoxazole (R)

(sul-fa-meth-ox'a-zole)
Apo-Sulfamethoxazole*,
Gantanol

Func. class.: Antiinfective
Chem. class.: Sulfonamide, intermediate acting

Action: Interferes with bacterial biosynthesis of proteins by competitive antagonism of PABA

Uses: UTIs, chancroid, inclusion conjunctivitis, malaria, meningococcal meningitis, nocardiosis, acute otitis media, toxoplasmosis, trachoma

Dosage and routes:
Renal dose

• CrCl <50 ml/min give 50% of dose

• *Adult:* PO 2 g, then 1 g bid or tid for 7-10 days

• *Child >2 mo:* PO 50-60 mg/kg × 1 dose then 25-30 mg/kg bid, not to exceed 75 mg/kg/day

Side effects/adverse reactions:
*SYST: **Anaphylaxis***

GI: Nausea, vomiting, abdominal pain, stomatitis, **hepatitis,** glossitis,

---

◆ = Nursing alert　　🌿 = Herb-drug interaction　　🚫 = Do not crush

pancreatitis, diarrhea, *enterocolitis*, anorexia

CNS: Headache, insomnia, hallucinations, depression, vertigo, fatigue, anxiety, *convulsions, drug fever,* chills, drowsiness

HEMA: Leukopenia, thrombocytopenia, agranulocytosis, hemolytic anemia, aplastic anemia

INTEG: Rash, dermatitis, urticaria, *Stevens-Johnson syndrome,* erythema, photosensitivity, alopecia

GU: Renal failure, toxic nephrosis, increased BUN, creatinine, crystalluria, hematuria, proteinuria

CV: Allergic myocarditis

Contraindications: Hypersensitivity to sulfonamides, sulfonylureas, thiazide and loop diuretics, salicylates, sunscreens with PABA, infants <2 mo (except congenital toxoplasmosis), pregnancy at term, porphyria

Precautions: Pregnancy (C), lactation, impaired hepatic/renal function, severe allergy, bronchial asthma

Pharmacokinetics:
PO: Poorly absorbed, peak 3-4 hr, 50%-70% bound to plasma proteins, half-life 7-12 hr; excreted in urine (unchanged 90%), breast milk; crosses placenta

Interactions:
• Increased effects of: barbiturates, uricosurics
• Increased drug-free concentrations: indomethacin, probenecid, salicylates
• Increased thrombocytopenia: thiazide diuretics
• Increased nephrotoxicity: cyclosporine
• Increased hypoglycemic response: sulfonylurea agents
• Increased anticoagulant effects: warfarin
• Decreased renal excretion of methotrexate
• Decreased hepatic clearance of phenytoin

Lab test interferences:
False positive: Urinary glucose test (Benedict's method)

NURSING CONSIDERATIONS
Assess:
• I&O ratio; note color, character, pH of urine if drug administered for UTIs; output should be 800 ml less than intake; if urine is highly acidic, alkalization may be needed
• Kidney function studies: BUN, creatinine, urinalysis (long-term therapy)
• Blood dyscrasias: skin rash, fever, sore throat, bruising, bleeding, fatigue, joint pain, monitor CBC before and periodically
• Allergic reaction: rash, dermatitis, urticaria, pruritus, dyspnea, bronchospasm

Administer:
PO
• On empty stomach
• With full glass of H_2O to maintain adequate hydration; increase fluids to 2 L/day to decrease crystallization in kidneys
• Medication after C&S; repeat C&S after full course of medication

Perform/provide:
• Storage in tight, light-resistant container at room temp

Evaluate:
• Therapeutic response: absence of pain, fever, C&S negative

Teach patient/family:
• To take each oral dose with full glass of H_2O to prevent crystalluria
• To complete full course of treatment to prevent superinfection
• To avoid sunlight or use sunscreen to prevent burns
• To avoid OTC medication (aspirin, vit C) unless directed by prescriber
• To notify prescriber of skin rash,

S

sore throat, fever, mouth sores, unusual bruising, bleeding

sulfasalazine (R)

(sul-fa-sal'a-zeen)

Azulfidine, Azulfidine EN-Tabs, PMS-Sulfasalazine*, S.A.S.*, Salazopyrin*, sulfasalazine

Func. class.: Antiinflammatory
Chem. class.: Sulfonamide

Action: Prodrug to deliver sulfapyridine and 5-aminosalicylic acid to colon; antiinflammatory in connective tissue also

Uses: Ulcerative colitis; rheumatoid arthritis in patients who inadequately respond to or are intolerant of analgesics/NSAIDs

Investigational uses: Ankylosing spondylitis, collagenous colitis, Crohn's disease, psoriasis

Dosage and routes:

Renal dose
• CrCl 10-30 ml/min give bid; CrCl <10 ml/min give qd
• *Adult:* **PO** 3-4 g/day in divided doses; maintenance 2 g/day in divided doses q6h
• *Child >2 yr:* **PO** 40-60 mg/kg/day in 4-6 divided doses, then 30 mg/kg/day in 4 doses, max 2 g/day

Rheumatoid arthritis
• *Adult:* **PO** 2g/day in evenly divided doses, initiate treatment with a lower dose of enteric-coated tab

Available forms: Tabs 500 mg

Side effects/adverse reactions:

*SYST: **Anaphylaxis***

GI: Nausea, vomiting, abdominal pain, stomatitis, *hepatitis,* glossitis, pancreatitis, diarrhea

CNS: Headache, confusion, insomnia, hallucinations, depression, vertigo, fatigue, anxiety, *convulsions,* drug fever, chills

*HEMA: **Leukopenia, neutropenia,*** *thrombocytopenia, agranulocytosis, hemolytic anemia*

INTEG: Rash, dermatitis, urticaria, ***Stevens-Johnson syndrome,*** erythema, photosensitivity

*GU: **Renal failure, toxic nephrosis,*** increased BUN, creatinine, crystalluria

*CV: **Allergic myocarditis***

Contraindications: Hypersensitivity to sulfonamides or salicylates, pregnancy at term, child <2 yr, intestinal, urinary obstruction

Precautions: Pregnancy (C), lactation, impaired hepatic function, severe allergy, bronchial asthma, impaired renal function

Pharmacokinetics:

PO: Partially absorbed, peak 1½-6 hr, duration 6-12 hr, half-life 6 hr, excreted in urine as sulfasalazine (15%), sulfapyridine (60%), 5-aminosalicylic acid and metabolites (20%-33%), in breast milk; crosses placenta

Interactions:
• Decreased absorption of digoxin
• Increased hypoglycemic response: oral hypoglycemics
• Increased anticoagulant effects: oral anticoagulants
• Decreased renal excretion of methotrexate
• Decreased hepatic clearance of phenytoin
• Drug/food: decreased iron/folic acid absorption

Lab test interferences:
False positive: Urinary glucose test

NURSING CONSIDERATIONS

Assess:
• Kidney function studies: BUN, creatinine, urinalysis (long-term therapy)
• Blood dyscrasias: skin rash, fever, sore throat, bruising, bleeding, fatigue, joint pain; monitor CBC before and q3mo

---

◆ = Nursing alert　　　📙 = Herb-drug interaction　　　🚫 = Do not crush

• Allergic reaction: rash, dermatitis, urticaria, pruritus, dyspnea, bronchospasm

Administer:

• With full glass of H_2O to maintain adequate hydration; increase fluids to 2 L/day to decrease crystallization in kidneys

• Total daily dose in evenly spaced doses and after meals to help minimize GI intolerance

Perform/provide:

• Storage in tight, light-resistant container at room temp

Evaluate:

• Therapeutic response: absence of fever, mucus in stools, pain in joints

Teach patient/family:

• To take each oral dose with full glass of H_2O to prevent crystalluria

• That contact lens, urine/skin may be yellow-orange

• To complete full course of treatment to prevent superinfection

• To avoid sunlight or use sunscreen to prevent burns

• To notify prescriber of skin rash, sore throat, fever, mouth sores, unusual bruising, bleeding

---

sulfinpyrazone (℞)

(sul-fin-peer'a-zone)
Anturane, sulfinpyrazone
Func. class.: Uricosuric
Chem. class.: Pyrazolone

Action: Inhibits tubular reabsorption of urates, with increased excretion of uric acid; inhibits prostaglandin synthesis, which decreases platelet aggregation

Uses: Inhibition of platelet aggregation, gout

Dosage and routes:

Inhibition of platelet aggregation

• *Adult:* PO 200 mg qid

Gout/gouty arthritis

• *Adult:* PO 100-200 mg bid × 1 wk, then 200-400 mg bid, not to exceed 800 mg/day

Available forms: Tabs 100 mg; caps 200 mg

Side effects/adverse reactions:

CNS: Dizziness, *convulsions, coma*

EENT: Tinnitus

GU: Renal calculi, hypoglycemia

GI: Gastric irritation, nausea, vomiting, anorexia, hepatic necrosis, GI bleeding

INTEG: Rash, dermatitis, pruritus, fever, photosensitivity

HEMA: Agranulocytosis (rare)

RESP: Apnea, irregular respirations

Contraindications: Hypersensitivity to pyrazolone derivatives, blood dyscrasias, CrCl <50 ml/min, active peptic ulcer, GI inflammation

Precautions: Pregnancy (C)

Pharmacokinetics:

PO: Peak 1-2 hr, duration 4-6 hr, half-life 4 hr; metabolized by liver, excreted in urine

Interactions:

• Increased toxicity: acetaminophen

• Increased effects of: warfarin, tolbutamide

• Decreased effects of: verapamil, theophylline

• Decreased effects of sulfinpyrazone: salicylates, niacin

Lab test interferences:

Increase: PSP, aminohippuric acid

False positive: Clinitest

NURSING CONSIDERATIONS

Assess:

• Uric acid levels (3-7 mg/dl); joint mobility, pain, swelling

• Respiratory rate, rhythm, depth; notify prescriber of abnormalities

• Renal function

• Bleeding tendencies, RBC, Hct

• I&O

• Electrolytes, CO_2 before, during treatment

• Urine pH, output, glucose during beginning treatment
Administer:
• With glass of milk
• With food for GI symptoms
• Increased fluids to prevent calculi; alkalinization of urine may be required
Evaluate:
• Therapeutic response: absence of pain, stiffness in joints
Teach patient/family:
• To avoid aspirin, alcohol, high-purine diet

---

sulfisoxazole (℞)

(sul-fi-sox′a-zole)
Gantrisin, Novosoxazole*, sulfisoxazole
Func. class.: Antiinfective
Chem. class.: Sulfonamide, short acting

Action: Interferes with bacterial biosynthesis of proteins by competitive antagonism of PABA
Uses: Urinary tract, systemic infections; chancroid; trachoma; toxoplasmosis; acute otitis media, malaria, *Haemophilus influenzae* meningitis, meningococcal meningitis, nocardiosis, eye infections
Dosage and routes:
Renal dose
• CrCl 10-50 ml/min give q8-12h; CrCl <10 ml/min give q12-24h
• *Adult:* **PO** 2-4 g loading dose, then 1-2 g qid × 7-10 days
• *Child >2 mo:* **PO** 75 mg/kg or 2 g/m^2 loading dose, then 120-150 mg/kg/day or 4 g/m^2/day in divided doses q6h, not to exceed 6 g/day
Available forms: Tabs 500 mg
Side effects/adverse reactions:
*SYST: **Anaphylaxis***
GI: Nausea, vomiting, abdominal pain, stomatitis, ***hepatitis,*** glossitis,

pancreatitis, diarrhea, ***enterocolitis,*** anorexia
CNS: Headache, insomnia, hallucinations, depression, vertigo, fatigue, anxiety, ***convulsions,*** drug fever, chills, drowsiness
*HEMA: **Leukopenia, thrombocytopenia, agranulocytosis, hemolytic anemia, aplastic anemia***
INTEG: Rash, dermatitis, urticaria, ***Stevens-Johnson syndrome,*** erythema, photosensitivity, alopecia
*GU: **Renal failure, toxic nephrosis,*** increased BUN, creatinine, crystalluria, hematuria, proteinuria
*CV: **Allergic myocarditis***
Contraindications: Hypersensitivity to sulfonamides and sulfonylureas, thiazide and loop diuretics, salicylates; sunscreen with PABA, lactation, infants < 2 mo (except congenital toxoplasmosis), pregnancy at term, porphyria
Precautions: Pregnancy (B), lactation, impaired hepatic/renal function, severe allergy, bronchial asthma
Pharmacokinetics:
PO: Rapidly absorbed, peak 2-4 hr, 85% protein bound; half-life 4-7 hr, excreted in urine, crosses placenta
Interactions:
• Increased effects of: barbiturates, tolbutamide, uricosurics
• Increased drug-free concentrations: indomethacin, probenecid, salicylates
• Increased thrombocytopenia: thiazides
• Increased nephrotoxicity: cyclosporine
• Increased hypoglycemic response: sulfonylurea agents
• Increased anticoagulant effect: warfarin
• Decreased renal excretion of methotrexate
• Decreased hepatic clearance of phenytoin

◆ = Nursing alert ∥ = Herb-drug interaction ⊘ = Do not crush

Lab test interferences:

False positive: Urinary glucose test

NURSING CONSIDERATIONS

Assess:

• I&O ratio; note color, character, pH of urine if drug administered for UTIs; output should be 800 ml less than intake; if urine is highly acidic, alkalization may be needed

• Kidney function studies: BUN, creatinine, urinalysis (long-term therapy)

• Blood dyscrasias: skin rash, fever, sore throat, bruising, bleeding, fatigue, joint pain, monitor CBC before and periodically

• Allergic reaction: rash, dermatitis, urticaria, pruritus, dyspnea, bronchospasm

Administer:

• On an empty stomach

• With full glass of H_2O to maintain adequate hydration; increase fluids to 2 L/day to decrease crystallization in kidneys

• Medication after C&S; repeat C&S after full course of medication

Perform/provide:

• Storage in tight, light-resistant container at room temp

Evaluate:

• Therapeutic response: absence of pain, fever, C&S negative

Teach patient/family:

• To take each oral dose with full glass of H_2O to prevent crystalluria

• To complete full course of treatment to prevent superinfection

• To avoid sunlight or use sunscreen to prevent burns; avoid hazardous activities if dizziness occurs

• To avoid OTC medication (aspirin, vit C) unless directed by prescriber

• To notify prescriber of skin rash, sore throat, fever, mouth sores, unusual bruising, bleeding

---

sulindac (℞)

(sul-in′dak)

Apo-Sulin*, Clinoril , NovoSundac*, sulindac

Func. class.: Nonsteroidal antiinflammatory

Chem. class.: Indeneacetic acid derivative

Action: Inhibits prostaglandin synthesis by decreasing an enzyme needed for biosynthesis; analgesic, antiinflammatory, antipyretic

Uses: Mild to moderate pain, osteoarthritis; rheumatoid, gouty arthritis; ankylosing spondylitis

Dosage and routes:

Arthritis

• *Adult:* **PO** 150 mg bid, may increase to 200 mg bid

Bursitis/acute arthritis

• *Adult:* **PO** 200 mg bid × 1-2 wk, then reduce dose

Available forms: Tabs 150, 200 mg

Side effects/adverse reactions:

GI: Nausea, anorexia, vomiting, diarrhea, jaundice, ***cholestatic hepatitis,*** constipation, flatulence, cramps, dry mouth, peptic ulcer, ***bleeding, ulceration, perforation***

CNS: Dizziness, drowsiness, fatigue, tremors, confusion, insomnia, anxiety, depression, headache

CV: Tachycardia, peripheral edema, palpitations, dysrhythmias

INTEG: Purpura, *rash, pruritus,* sweating, photosensitivity

*GU: **Nephrotoxicity: dysuria, hematuria, oliguria, azotemia***

*HEMA: **Blood dyscrasias*** with prolonged use

EENT: Tinnitus, hearing loss, blurred vision

Contraindications: Hypersensitivity, asthma, severe renal disease, severe hepatic disease, active ulcers

---

Side effects: *italics* = common; ***bold italics*** = life-threatening

Precautions: Pregnancy (C), lactation, children, bleeding disorders, GI disorders, cardiac disorders, hypersensitivity to other antiinflammatory agents, renal disease

Pharmacokinetics:

PO: Peak 2 hr, half-life 3-3½ hr; metabolized in liver; excreted in urine (metabolites), breast milk; 93% protein binding

Interactions:

• Increased risk of bleeding: anticoagulants

• Increased nephrotoxicity: cyclosporine

• Decreased sulindac effect: diflunisal, do not use together

• Increased toxicity: methotrexate, sulfonamides, sulfonylureas, probenecid

• GI side effects: aspirin

NURSING CONSIDERATIONS

Assess:

• Pain: frequency, intensity, characteristics, relief after med

• Asthma, aspirin hypersensitivity, nasal polyps; increased hypersensitivity

• Renal, liver, blood studies: BUN, creatinine, AST, ALT, Hgb, before treatment, periodically thereafter

• Have B/P checked qmo; drug causes Na retention

• Audiometric, ophthalmic exam before, during, after treatment

• For eye, ear problems: blurred vision, tinnitus may indicate toxicity

Administer:

• With food to decrease GI symptoms; best to take on empty stomach to facilitate absorption; tablet may be crushed

Perform/provide:

• Storage at room temp

Evaluate:

• Therapeutic response: decreased pain, stiffness, swelling in joints, ability to move more easily

Teach patient/family:

• To report blurred vision or ringing, roaring in ears (may indicate toxicity)

• To avoid driving, other hazardous activities if dizzy or drowsy

• To report change in urine pattern, weight increase, edema, pain increase in joints, fever, blood in urine (indicates nephrotoxicity)

• That therapeutic effects may take up to 1 mo

• To avoid alcohol and aspirin

• To take with full glass of water

• To use sunscreen

---

sumatriptan (℞)

(soo-ma-trip′tan)

Imitrex

Func. class.: Migraine agent

Chem. class.: 5-HT₁ receptor agonist

Action: Binds selectively to the vascular 5-HT₁ receptor subtype, exerts antimigraine effect; causes vasoconstriction in cranial arteries

Uses: Acute treatment of migraine with or without aura and cluster headache

Dosage and routes:

• *Adult:* **SC** 6 mg or less; may repeat in 1 hr; not to exceed 12 mg/24 hr; **PO** 25 mg with fluids, max 100 mg; **NASAL** one dose of 5, 10, or 20 mg in one nostril, may repeat in 2 hr, max 40 mg/24hr or >5 mo

Available forms: Inj 12 mg/ml; tabs 25, 50 mg, nasal spray 5 mg/100 mcl-U dose spray device, 20 mg/100 mcl-U

Side effects/adverse reactions:

NEURO: Tingling, hot sensation, burning, feeling of pressure, tightness, numbness, dizziness, sedation, headache, anxiety, fatigue, cold sensation

CV: Flushing

◆ = Nursing alert   ∅ = Herb-drug interaction   ⊘ = Do not crush

RESP: Chest tightness, pressure

EENT: Throat, mouth, nasal discomfort; vision changes

GI: Abdominal discomfort

MS: Weakness, neck stiffness, myalgia

INTEG: Injection site reaction, sweating

Contraindications: Angina pectoris, history of MI, documented silent ischemia, Prinzmetal's angina, ischemic heart disease, IV use, concurrent ergotamine-containing preparations, uncontrolled hypertension, hypersensitivity, basilar or hemiplegic migraine

Precautions: Postmenopausal women, men >40 yr, risk factors for CAD, hypercholesterolemia, obesity, diabetes, impaired hepatic or renal function, pregnancy (C), lactation, children, elderly

Pharmacokinetics: Onset of pain relief 10 min-2 hr, peak 10-20 min, 10%-20% plasma protein binding, metabolized in the liver (metabolite), excreted in urine, feces

Interactions:
• Extended vasospastic effects: ergot, ergot derivatives
• Increased sumatriptan effect: MAOIs

NURSING CONSIDERATIONS
Assess:
• B/P; signs/symptoms of coronary vasospasms
• Tingling, hot sensation, burning, feeling of pressure, numbness, flushing, injection site reaction
• For stress level, activity, recreation, coping mechanisms
• Neurologic status: LOC, blurring vision, nausea, vomiting, tingling in extremities preceding headache
• Ingestion of tyramine foods (pickled products, beer, wine, aged cheese), food additives, preservatives, colorings, artificial sweeteners, chocolate, caffeine, which may precipitate these types of headaches

Administer:
• SC only just below the skin; avoid IM or IV administration
🚫 PO, swallow whole

Perform/provide:
• Quiet, calm environment with decreased stimulation for noise, bright light, excessive talking

Evaluate:
• Therapeutic response: decrease in frequency, severity of migraine

Teach patient/family:
• The use of self-dosing system; not to exceed 12 mg/24 hr
• To report any side effects to prescriber
• To use contraception while taking drug
• To use nasal spray: one spray in one nostril, may repeat if headache returns, do not repeat if pain continues after 1st dose
• To have dark, quiet environment

---

tacrine (℞)

(tack'rin)

Cognex

Func. class.: Reversible cholinesterase

Action: Elevates acetylcholine concentrations (cerebral cortex) by slowing degradation of acetylcholine released in cholinergic neurons; does not alter underlying dementia

Uses: Treatment of mild to moderate dementia in Alzheimer's disease

Dosage and routes:
• *Adult:* PO 10 mg qid × 6 wk, then 20 mg qid × 6 wk, increase at 6-wk intervals if patient tolerating drug well and if transaminase is WNL

Available forms: Caps 10, 20, 30, 40 mg

Side effects/adverse reactions:
CNS: Dizziness, confusion, insom-

nia, tremor, *ataxia, somnolence, anxiety, agitation, depression, hallucinations, hostility, abnormal thinking,* chills, fever
CV: Hypotension or hypertension
GI: Nausea, vomiting, anorexia, abdominal pain, constipation, dyspepsia, flatulence, ***hepatotoxicity***
GU: Urinary frequency, UTI, incontinence
INTEG: Rash, flushing
RESP: Rhinitis, URI, cough, pharyngitis
Contraindications: Hypersensitivity to this drug or acridine derivatives, patients treated with this drug who developed jaundice with a total bilirubin of >3 mg/dl
Precautions: Sick sinus syndrome, history of ulcers, GI bleeding, hepatic disease, bladder obstruction, asthma, pregnancy (C), lactation, children, seizure disorders
Pharmacokinetics: Rapidly absorbed PO, 55% bound to plasma proteins, extensively metabolized to metabolites, elimination half-life 2-4 hr
Interactions:
• Decreased activity of anticholinergics
• Increased levels of tacrine: cimetidine
• Increased elimination half-life of theophylline
• Synergistic effect: succinylcholine, cholinesterase inhibitors, cholinergic agonists
NURSING CONSIDERATIONS
Assess:
• B/P: hypotension, hypertension
• Mental status: affect, mood, behavioral changes, depression; complete suicide assessment; hallucinations, confusion
• GI status: nausea, vomiting, anorexia, constipation, abdominal pain; add bulk, increase fluids for constipation

• GU status: urinary frequency, incontinence
• Serum ALT qo wk × 4-16 wk, then q3mo
Administer:
• Between meals; may be given with meals for GI symptoms
• Dosage adjusted to response no more than q6wk
Perform/provide:
• Assistance with ambulation during beginning therapy; dizziness, ataxia may occur
Evaluate:
• Therapeutic response: decrease in confusion, improved mood
Teach patient/family:
• To report side effects: twitching, eye spasms; indicate overdose
• To use drug exactly as prescribed: at regular intervals, preferably between meals; may be taken with meals for GI upset; drug is not a cure
• To notify prescriber of nausea, vomiting, diarrhea (dose increase or beginning treatment), or rash; very dark or very light stools, jaundice (delayed onset)
• Not to increase or abruptly decrease dose; serious consequences may result
Treatment of overdose: Withdraw drug, administer tertiary anticholinergics, provide supportive care

---

tacrolimus (℞)
(tak-roe-li′mus)
Prograf
Func. class.: Immunosuppressant
Chem. class.: Macrolide

Action: Produces immunosuppression by inhibiting T-lymphocytes
Uses: Organ transplants to prevent rejection

◆ = Nursing alert   ∅ = Herb-drug interaction   ⊘ = Do not crush

Dosage and routes:
• *Adult and child:* **IV** 0.03-0.05 mg/kg/day × 3 days then **PO** 0.15 mg/kg bid; adjust dose in renal impairment
Available forms: Inj 5 mg/ml; caps 1, 5 mg
Side effects/adverse reactions:
HEMA: **Anemia, leukocytosis, thrombocytopenia, purpura**
GI: Nausea, vomiting, diarrhea, constipation
CV: Hypertension
CNS: Tremors, headache, insomnia, paresthesia, chills, fever
GU: UTIs, **albuminuria, hematuria, proteinuria, renal failure**
META: Hirsutism, hyperglycemia, hyperkalemia, hyperuricemia, hypokalemia, hypomagnesemia
RESP: Pleural effusion, atelectasis, dyspnea
INTEG: Rash, flushing, itching, alopecia
EENT: Blurred vision, photophobia
Contraindications: Hypersensitivity to this drug or to some kinds of castor oil
Precautions: Severe renal, hepatic disease; pregnancy (C), diabetes mellitus, hyperkalemia, hyperuricemia, lymphomas, lactation, children <12, hypertension
Pharmacokinetics: Extensively metabolized, half-life 10 hr, 75% protein binding
Interactions:
• Increased toxicity: aminoglycosides, cisplatin, cyclosporine
• Increased blood levels: antifungals, calcium channel blockers, cimetidine, danazol, erythromycin
• Decreased blood levels: carbamazepine, phenobarbital, phenytoin, rifamycin
• Decreased effect of: vaccines
NURSING CONSIDERATIONS
Assess:
• Blood studies: Hgb, WBC, platelets during treatment qmo; if leukocytes <3000/mm^3 or platelets <100,000/mm^3, drug should be discontinued or reduced; decreased hemoglobulin level may indicate bone marrow suppression
• Liver function studies: alk phosphatase, AST, ALT, amylase, bilirubin, and for hepatotoxicity: dark urine, jaundice, itching, light-colored stools; drug should be discontinued
Administer:
• All medications PO if possible, avoiding IM injections; bleeding may occur
• With meals to reduce GI upset; nausea is common
• For several days before transplant surgery; patients should be placed in protective isolation
IV
• After diluting in 0.9% NaCl or D$_5$W to 0.004 to 0.02 mg/ml as a continuous infusion
Additive compatibilities: Cimetidine
Y-site compatibilities: Acyclovir, aminophylline, amphotericin B, ampicillin, ampicillin/sulbactam, benztropine, calcium gluconate, cefazolin, cefotetan, ceftazidime, ceftriaxone, cefuroxime, chloramphenicol, cimetidine, ciprofloxacin, clindamycin, dexamethasone, digoxin, diphenhydramine, dobutamine, dopamine, doxycycline, erythromycin, esmolol, fluconazole, furosemide, ganciclovir, gentamicin, haloperidol, heparin, hydrocortisone, imipenem/cilastatin, insulin (regular), isoproterenol, leucovorin, lorazepam, methylprednisolone, metoclopramide, metronidazole, mezlocillin, multivitamins, nitroglycerin, oxacillin, penicillin G potassium, perphenazine, phenytoin, piperacillin, potassium chloride, propranolol, ranitidine, sodium bicarbonate, sodium nitroprusside, trimethoprim-sulfamethoxazole, vancomycin

T

Evaluate:
• Therapeutic response: absence of graft rejection; immunosuppression in autoimmune disorders

Teach patient/family:
• To report fever, rash, severe diarrhea, chills, sore throat, fatigue; serious infections may occur; clay-colored stools, cramping (hepatotoxicity)
• To avoid crowds, persons with known infections to reduce risk of infection

---

tamoxifen (℞)

(ta-mox′i-fen)
Nolvadex, Nolvadex-D*, Novo-Tamoxifen*, Tamofen*, Tamone*

Func. class.: Antineoplastic
Chem. class.: Antiestrogen hormone

Action: Inhibits cell division by binding to cytoplasmic estrogen receptors; resembles normal cell complex but inhibits DNA synthesis and estrogen response of target tissue

Uses: Advanced breast carcinoma not responsive to other therapy in estrogen-receptor-positive patients (usually postmenopausal), prevention of breast cancer

Dosage and routes:
• *Adult:* **PO** 10-20 mg bid
Available forms: Tabs 10, 20 mg

Side effects/adverse reactions:
HEMA: **Thrombocytopenia, leukopenia,** DVT, PE
GI: Nausea, vomiting, altered taste (anorexia)
GU: Vaginal bleeding, pruritus vulvae
INTEG: Rash, alopecia
CV: Chest pain
CNS: Hot flashes, headache, light-headedness, depression
META: Hypercalcemia
EENT: Ocular lesions, retinopathy, corneal opacity, blurred vision (high doses)

Contraindications: Hypersensitivity, pregnancy (D)

Precautions: Leukopenia, thrombocytopenia, lactation, cataracts

Pharmacokinetics:
PO: Peak 4-7 hr, half-life 7 days (1 wk terminal), excreted primarily in feces

Interactions:
• Increased chance of bleeding: anticoagulants
• Increased tamoxifen levels: bromocriptine
• Increased thromboembolic events: cytotoxics

Lab test interferences:
Increase: Serum Ca

NURSING CONSIDERATIONS

Assess:
• CBC, differential, platelet count qwk; withhold drug if WBC is <3500 or platelet count is <100,000; notify prescriber
• Bleeding: hematuria, guaiac, bruising, petechiae, mucosa or orifices q8h
• Food preferences; list likes, dislikes
• Effects of alopecia on body image; discuss feelings about body changes
◆ Symptoms indicating severe allergic reactions: rash, pruritus, urticaria, purpuric skin lesions, itching, flushing

Administer:
• Antacid before oral agent; give drug after evening meal, before bedtime
• Antiemetic 30-60 min before giving drug to prevent vomiting

---

◆ = Nursing alert   ⑃ = Herb-drug interaction   ⃠ = Do not crush

Perform/provide:
• Liquid diet, if needed, including cola, Jell-O; dry toast or crackers may be added if patient is not nauseated or vomiting
• Increase fluid intake to 2-3 L/day to prevent dehydration
• Nutritious diet with iron, vitamin supplements as ordered
• Storage in light-resistant container at room temp

Evaluate:
• Therapeutic response: decreased tumor size, spread of malignancy

Teach patient/family:
• To report any complaints, side effects to prescriber
• That vaginal bleeding, pruritus, hot flashes are reversible after discontinuing treatment
• To report immediately decreased visual acuity, which may be irreversible; stress need for routine eye exams; care providers should be told about tamoxifen therapy
• To report vaginal bleeding immediately
• That tumor flare—increase in size of tumor, increased bone pain—may occur and will subside rapidly; may take analgesics for pain
• That premenopausal women must use mechanical birth control because ovulation may be induced
• That hair may be lost during treatment; a wig or hairpiece may make patient feel better; new hair may be different in color, texture

---

tamsulosin (℞)

(tam-sue-lo'sen)
Flomax
Func. class.: Selective α_1-adrenergic blocker
Chem. class.: Sulfamoylphenethylamine derivative

Action: Binds preferentially to α_{1A}-adrenoceptor subtype located mainly in the prostate

Uses: Symptoms of benign prostatic hyperplasia

Dosage and routes:
• *Adult:* **PO** 0.4 mg qd, increasing up to 0.8 mg qd if required

Available forms: Caps 0.4 mg

Side effects/adverse reactions:
CV: Chest pain
CNS: Dizziness, headache, asthenia
GI: Nausea, diarrhea
GU: Decreased libido, abnormal ejaculation
EENT: Amblyopia
MS: Back pain
RESP: Rhinitis, pharyngitis, cough

Contraindications: Hypersensitivity

Precautions: Pregnancy (C), children, lactation, hepatic disease, coronary artery disease, severe renal disease

Pharmacokinetics:
PO: Onset 2 hr, peak 2-6 hr, duration 6-12 hr; half-life 9-15 hr; metabolized in liver; excreted via urine; extensively protein bound (98%)

Interactions:
• Not to be taken with: prazosin, terazosin, doxazosin

NURSING CONSIDERATIONS

Assess:
• CBC with diff and liver function studies; B/P and heart rate
• BUN, uric acid, urodynamic studies (urinary flow rates, residual volume)

T

Administer:
PO

🚫 Whole; do not chew or crush tablets; may be given with food

Perform/provide:
• Storage in tight container in cool environment

Evaluate:
• Therapeutic response: decreased symptoms of benign prostatic hyperplasia

Teach patient/family:
• Not to drive or operate machinery for 4 hr after first dose or after dosage increase

---

telmisartan (Ɍ)
(tel-mih-sar′tan)
Micardis
Func. class.: Antihypertensive
Chem. class.: Angiotensin II receptor (Type AT_1)

Action: blocks the vasoconstrictor and aldosterone-secreting effects of angiotensin II; selectively blocks the binding of angiotensin II to the AT_1 receptor found in tissues

Uses: Hypertension, alone or in combination

Investigational uses: Heart failure

Dosage and routes:
• *Adult:* **PO** 40 mg qd; range 20-80 mg

Available forms: Tabs 40, 80 mg

Side effects/adverse reactions:
CNS: Dizziness, insomnia, *anxiety*
GI: Diarrhea, dyspepsia, *anorexia, vomiting*
MS: Myalgia, pain
RESP: Cough, *upper respiratory infection*

Contraindications: Hypersensitivity, pregnancy (D) 2nd and 3rd trimesters

Precautions: Hypersensitivity to ACE inhibitors: pregnancy (C) 1st trimester, lactation, children, elderly

Pharmacokinetics: Extensively metabolized, terminal half-life 24 hr, highly bound to plasma proteins, excreted in urine and feces

Interactions:
• Increased digoxin peak concentrations, and in trough concentrations: digoxin

NURSING CONSIDERATIONS
Assess:
• B/P, pulse q4h; note rate, rhythm, quality
• Electrolytes: K, Na, Cl
• Baselines in renal, liver function tests before therapy begins
• Edema in feet, legs qd
• Skin turgor, dryness of mucous membranes for hydration status

Administer:
• Without regard to meals
• Increased dose to black patients, B/P response may be reduced

Evaluate:
• Therapeutic response: decreased B/P

Teach patient/family:
• To comply with dosage schedule, even if feeling better
• To notify prescriber of mouth sores, fever, swelling of hands or feet, irregular heartbeat, chest pain
• That excessive perspiration, dehydration, vomiting, diarrhea may lead to fall in blood pressure; consult prescriber if these occur
• That drug may cause dizziness, fainting; light-headedness may occur

---

◆ = Nursing alert   𝕀 = Herb-drug interaction   🚫 = Do not crush

temazepam (℞)

(te-maz′e-pam)

Razepam, Restoril, temazepam

Func. class.: Sedative-hypnotic

Chem. class.: Benzodiazepine

Controlled Substance Schedule IV (USA), Schedule F (Canada)

Action: Produces CNS depression at limbic, thalamic, hypothalamic levels of the CNS; may be mediated by neurotransmitter γ-aminobutyric acid (GABA); results are sedation, hypnosis, skeletal muscle relaxation, anticonvulsant activity, anxiolytic action

Uses: Insomnia

Dosage and routes:

• *Adult:* **PO** 15-30 mg hs

Available forms: Caps 7.5, 15, 30 mg

Side effects/adverse reactions:

*HEMA: **Leukopenia, granulocytopenia** (rare)*

CNS: Lethargy, drowsiness, daytime sedation, dizziness, confusion, lightheadedness, headache, anxiety, irritability

GI: Nausea, vomiting, diarrhea, heartburn, abdominal pain, constipation, anorexia

CV: Chest pain, pulse changes

Contraindications: Hypersensitivity to benzodiazepines, pregnancy (X), lactation, intermittent porphyria

Precautions: Anemia, hepatic disease, renal disease, suicidal individuals, drug abuse, elderly, psychosis, children <15 yr, acute narrow-angle glaucoma, seizure disorders

Pharmacokinetics:

PO: Onset 30-45 min, duration 6-8 hr, half-life 10-20 hr; metabolized by liver, excreted by kidneys, crosses placenta, excreted in breast milk

Interactions:

• Increased effects of cimetidine, disulfiram, oral contraceptives

• Increased action of both drugs: alcohol, CNS depressants

• Decreased effect of antacids, theophylline, rifampin

🖋 Increased CNS depression: kava

Lab test interferences:

Increase: ALT, AST, serum bilirubin

Decrease: RAI uptake

False increase: Urinary 17-OHCS

NURSING CONSIDERATIONS

Assess:

• Blood studies: Hct, Hgb, RBCs (long-term therapy)

• Hepatic studies: AST, ALT, bilirubin (long-term therapy)

• Mental status: mood, sensorium, affect, memory (long, short)

• Blood dyscrasias: fever, sore throat, bruising, rash, jaundice, epistaxis (rare)

• Type of sleep problem: falling asleep, staying asleep

Administer:

• After removal of cigarettes to prevent fires

• After trying conservative measures for insomnia

• ½-1 hr before hs for sleeplessness

• On empty stomach for fast onset, but may be taken with food if GI symptoms occur

Perform/provide:

• Assistance with ambulation after receiving dose

• Safety measures: night-light, call bell within easy reach

• Checking to see if PO medication has been swallowed

• Storage in tight container in cool environment

Evaluate:

• Therapeutic response: ability to sleep at night, decreased early morning awakening if taking drug for insomnia

T

Teach patient/family:

• To avoid driving, other activities requiring alertness until stabilized

• To avoid alcohol ingestion, CNS depressants; serious CNS depression may result

• That effects may take 2 nights for benefits to be noticed

• Alternative measures to improve sleep: reading, exercise several hours before hs, warm bath, warm milk, TV, self-hypnosis, deep breathing

• That hangover, memory impairment are common in elderly but less common than with barbiturates

Treatment of overdose: Lavage, activated charcoal; monitor electrolytes, VS

---

temozolomide

See appendix a—selected new drugs

---

terazosin (℞)

(ter-ay'zoe-sin)
Hytrin

Func. class.: Antihypertensive
Chem. class.: Peripherally acting adrenergic blocker

Action: Decreases total vascular resistance, which is responsible for a decrease in B/P; this occurs by blockade of α_1-adrenoreceptors

Uses: Hypertension, as a single agent or in combination with diuretics or β-blockers, BPH

Dosage and routes:

• *Adult:* PO 1 mg hs, may increase dose slowly to desired response; not to exceed 20 mg/day

Available forms: Caps 1, 2, 5, 10 mg

Side effects/adverse reactions:

CV: Palpitations, orthostatic hypotension, tachycardia, edema, rebound hypertension

CNS: Dizziness, headache, drowsiness, anxiety, depression, vertigo, weakness, fatigue

GI: Nausea, vomiting, diarrhea, constipation, abdominal pain

GU: Urinary frequency, incontinence, impotence, priapism

EENT: Blurred vision, epistaxis, tinnitus, dry mouth, red sclera, nasal congestion, sinusitis

RESP: Dyspnea

Contraindications: Hypersensitivity

Precautions: Pregnancy (C), children, lactation

Pharmacokinetics: Peak 1 hr, half-life 9-12 hr, highly bound to plasma proteins; metabolized in liver, excreted in urine, feces

Interactions:

• Increased hypotensive effects: β-blockers, nitroglycerin, verapamil, nifedipine

NURSING CONSIDERATIONS

Assess:

• Urinary symptoms associated with BPH

• Orthostatic B/P, pulse, jugular venous distention q4h

• BUN, uric acid if on long-term therapy

• Weight qd, I&O

• Skin turgor, dryness of mucous membranes for hydration status

• Rales, dyspnea, orthopnea q30min

Perform/provide:

• Cool storage in tight container

Evaluate:

• Therapeutic response: decreased B/P, edema in feet, legs, decreased symptoms of BPH

Teach patient/family:

• That fainting occasionally occurs after first dose; not to drive or operate machinery for 4 hr after first dose or after an increase in dose; or take first dose hs

• To rise slowly from sitting/lying position

⬙ = Nursing alert 🖋 = Herb-drug interaction 🚫 = Do not crush

terbinafine (℞)

(ter-bin'a-feen)
Lamisil
Func. class.: Topical antifungal
Chem. class.: Synthetic allyl-amine derivative

Action: Interferes with cell membrane permeability in fungi such as *T. rubrum, T. mentagrophytes, T. tonsurans, E. floccosum, M. canis, M. audouinii, M. gypseum, Candida,* broad-spectrum antifungal
Uses: (TOP) Tinea cruris, tinea corporis, tinea pedis; (oral) onychomycosis of the toenail or fingernail due to dermatophytes
Investigational uses: Cutaneous candidiasis, tinea versicolor
Dosage and routes:

Topical
• Massage into affected area, surrounding area qd or bid, continue for 7-14 days, not to exceed 4 wk
Oral
• *Fingernail:* 250 mg/day × 6 wk
• *Toenail:* 250 mg/day × 12 wk
Available forms: Cream 1%, tabs 250 mg
Side effects/adverse reactions:

Topical
INTEG: Burning, stinging, dryness, itching, local irritation
Oral
HEME: **Neutropenia**
GI: Diarrhea, dyspepsia, abdominal pain, nausea
INTEG: Rash, pruritus, urticaria, **Stevens-Johnson syndrome**
MISC: Headache, liver enzyme changes, taste, visual disturbance
Contraindications: Hypersensitivity
Precautions: Pregnancy (B), lactation, children, liver/renal disease

Interactions:
• Decreased terbinafine clearance: cimetidine
• Increased terbinafine clearance: rifampin
• Increased clearance of: cyclosporine
NURSING CONSIDERATIONS
Assess:
• For continuing infection: increased size, number of lesions
Administer:
• To affected area, surrounding area; do not cover with occlusive dressings
Perform/provide:
• Storage below 30° C (86° F)
Evaluate:
• Therapeutic response: decrease in size, number of lesions
Teach patient/family:
• To wear cotton clothing
• To use clean towel, dry well
• To avoid contact with mucous membranes
• Not to cover areas unless directed by prescriber
• To report excessive itching, burning
• How to apply; massage cream into affected area and surrounding skin in AM, PM; effects observed within 1 wk, continue 1-2 wk after symptoms decrease

terbutaline (℞)

(ter-byoo'te-leen)
Brethaire, Brethine, Bricanyl
Func. class.: Selective β_2-agonist; bronchodilator
Chem. class.: Catecholamine

Action: Relaxes bronchial smooth muscle by direct action on β_2-adrenergic receptors through accumulation of cAMP at β-adrenergic receptor sites; bronchodilation, diuresis, CNS, cardiac stimulation occur; relaxes uterine smooth muscle

Uses: Bronchospasm, hyperkalemia

Investigational uses: Premature labor

Dosage and routes:

Bronchospasm

• *Adult and child >12 yr:* **INH** 2 puffs q1min, then q4-6h; **PO** 2.5-5 mg q8h; **SC** 0.25 mg q8h

Available forms: Tabs 2.5, 5 mg; aerosol 0.2 mg/actuation; inj 1 mg/ml

Side effects/adverse reactions:

CNS: Tremors, anxiety, insomnia, headache, dizziness, stimulation

CV: Palpitations, tachycardia, hypertension, dysrhythmias, *cardiac arrest*

GI: Nausea, vomiting

Contraindications: Hypersensitivity to sympathomimetics, narrow-angle glaucoma, tachydysrhythmias

Precautions: Pregnancy (B), cardiac disorders, hyperthyroidism, diabetes mellitus, prostatic hypertension, lactation, elderly, hypertension, glaucoma

Pharmacokinetics:

PO: Onset ½ hr, peak 1-2 hr, duration 4-8 hr

SC: Onset 6-15 min, peak ½-1 hr, duration 1½-4 hr

INH: Onset 5-30 min, peak 1-2 hr, duration 3-6 hr

Interactions:

• Increased effects of both drugs: other sympathomimetics

• Decreased action: β-blockers

• Hypertensive crisis: MAOIs

• Incompatible with bleomycin

NURSING CONSIDERATIONS

Assess:

• Respiratory function: vital capacity, forced expiratory volume, ABGs, B/P, pulse, respiratory pattern, lung sounds, sputum before and after treatment

• Tolerance over long-term therapy; dose may have to be changed; monitor for rebound bronchospasm

Administer:

• With food; may be crushed

• 2 hr before hs to avoid sleeplessness

IV

• IV after diluting each 5 mg/1 L D₅W for inf

• IV, run 5 μg/min; may increase 5 μg q10min, titrate to response; after ½-1 hr taper dose by 5 μg; switch to PO as soon as possible

Additive compatibilities: Aminophylline

Syringe compatibilities: Doxapram

Y-site compatibilities: Insulin (regular)

Perform/provide:

• Storage at room temp; do not use discolored sol

Evaluate:

• Therapeutic response: absence of dyspnea, wheezing

Teach patient/family:

• Not to use OTC medications; extra stimulation may occur

• The use of inhaler; review package insert with patient

• To avoid getting aerosol in eyes; burning, stinging will occur

• To wash inhaler in warm water and dry qd, rinse mouth after use

• All aspects of drug; avoid smoking, smoke-filled rooms, persons with respiratory infections

• To increase fluids >2 L/day; allow 15 min between inhalation of this drug and inhaler containing steroid

• To take on time; if missed, do not make up after 1 hr; wait until next dose

Treatment of overdose: Administer an α-blocker, then norepinephrine for severe hypotension

---

 = Nursing alert   = Herb-drug interaction   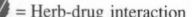 = Do not crush

testolactone (R)

(tess-toe-lak'tone)
Teslac
Func. class.: Antineoplastic
Chem. class.: Androgen hormone

Action: Acts on adrenal cortex to suppress activity; reduces estrone synthesis
Uses: Advanced breast carcinoma in postmenopausal women; prostatic cancer
Dosage and routes:
• *Adult:* **PO** 250 mg qid
Available forms: Tabs 50 mg
Side effects/adverse reactions:
GI: Nausea, vomiting, anorexia, glossitis
GU: Urinary retention, **renal failure**
INTEG: Rash, nail changes, facial hair growth
CV: Orthostatic hypertension, edema
CNS: Paresthesias, dizziness
EENT: Deepening voice
META: Hypercalcemia
Contraindications: Hypersensitivity, premenopausal women, carcinoma of male breast
Precautions: Renal disease, hypercalcemia, cardiac disease, pregnancy (C)
Pharmacokinetics: None known
Interactions:
• Enhanced effects of oral anticoagulants
Lab test interferences:
Increase: Urinary 17-OHCS
Decrease: Estradiol
NURSING CONSIDERATIONS
Assess:
• CA⁺ levels
• B/P q4h; tell patient to rise slowly from sitting or lying down
• Food preferences; list likes, dislikes

• Edema in feet; joint, stomach pain; shaking
◆ Symptoms indicating severe allergic reaction: rash, pruritus, urticaria, purpuric skin lesions, itching, flushing
• Anorexia, nausea, vomiting, constipation, weakness, loss of muscle tone (indicating hypercalcemia)
Administer:
PO
• For 1 mo or longer for desired response
Evaluate:
• Therapeutic response: decreased tumor size, spread of malignancy
Teach patient/family:
• To recognize and report signs of hepatotoxicity, hypercalcemia, virilization (in females), bleeding if on anticoagulants

testosterone (R)

Andro-Cyp 100, Andro-Cyp 200, Andro L.A. 200, Androderm, Andronate 100, Andronate 200, Delatest, Delatestryl, depAndro 100, depAndro 200, Depotest 100, Depotest 200, Depo-Testosterone, Duratest-100, Duratest-200, Durathate-200, Everone 100, Everone 200, Testex, Testoderm Transdermal, Testone LA 100, Testone LA 200, testosterone cypionate, testosterone enanthate, testosterone propionate, Testred Cypionate, Testrin PA

Func. class.: Androgenic anabolic steroid
Chem. class.: Halogenated testosterone derivative

Action: Increases weight by building body tissue, increases potassium, phosphorus, chloride, nitrogen levels, bone development

Uses: Female breast cancer, eunuchoidism, male climacteric, oligospermia, impotence, osteoporosis, weight loss in AIDS patients, vulvar dystrophies

Dosage and routes:

Replacement

• *Adult:* IM 25-50 mg 2-3 ×/wk (base or propionate) or 50-400 mg q2-4wk (enanthate or cypionate)

• *Adult:* **Trans Testoderm** 4-6 mg applied q24h; **Androderm** 5 mg applied q24h

Breast cancer

• *Adult:* **IM** 50-100 mg 3 ×/wk (propionate) or 200-400 mg q2-4wk (cypionate or enanthate)

Delayed male puberty

• *Child >12 yr:* **IM** up to 100 mg/mo for up to 6 mo

Available forms: Propionate inj 25, 50, 100 mg/ml, transdermal patches: Testoderm 4 mg/day (30 patches), 6 mg/day (30 patches), Androderm 2.5 mg/day (60 patches), 5 mg/day (60 patches); enanthate inj 100, 200 mg/ml; cypionate inj 50, 100, 200 mg/ml; 4, 6 mg/day

Side effects/adverse reactions:

INTEG: Rash, acneiform lesions, oily hair and skin, flushing, sweating, acne vulgaris, alopecia, hirsutism

CNS: Dizziness, headache, fatigue, tremors, paresthesias, flushing, sweating, anxiety, lability, insomnia, carpal tunnel syndrome

MS: Cramps, spasms

CV: Increased B/P

GU: Hematuria, amenorrhea, vaginitis, decreased libido, decreased breast size, clitoral hypertrophy, testicular atrophy

GI: Nausea, vomiting, constipation, weight gain, *cholestatic jaundice*

EENT: Conjunctival edema, nasal congestion

ENDO: Abnormal GTT

Contraindications: Severe renal, severe cardiac, severe hepatic disease, hypersensitivity, pregnancy (X), lactation, genital bleeding (rare)

Precautions: Diabetes mellitus, CV disease, MI

Pharmacokinetics:

PO: Metabolized in liver, excreted in urine, breast milk; crosses placenta

Interactions:

• Increased effects of oral antidiabetics, oxyphenbutazone

• Increased PT: anticoagulants

• Edema: ACTH, adrenal steroids

• Decreased effects of insulin

Lab test interferences:

Increase: Serum cholesterol, blood glucose, urine glucose

Decrease: Serum Ca, serum K, T_4, T_3, thyroid ^{131}I uptake test, urine 17-OHCS, 17-KS, PBI

NURSING CONSIDERATIONS

Assess:

• Weight qd; notify prescriber if weekly weight gain is >5 lb

• B/P q4h

• I&O ratio; be alert for decreasing urinary output, increasing edema

• Growth rate in children; growth rate may be uneven (linear/bone growth) with extended use

• Electrolytes: K, Na, Cl, Ca; cholesterol

• Liver function studies: ALT, AST, bilirubin

• Edema, hypertension, cardiac symptoms, jaundice

• Mental status: affect, mood, behavioral changes, aggression

• Signs of masculinization in female: increased libido, deepening of voice, decreased breast tissue, enlarged clitoris, menstrual irregularities; male: gynecomastia, impotence, testicular atrophy

• Hypercalcemia: lethargy, polyuria, polydipsia, nausea, vomiting, con-

⬥ = Nursing alert   **❱** = Herb-drug interaction   **⊘** = Do not crush stipation; drug may have to be decreased

• Hypoglycemia in diabetics; oral antidiabetic action is increased

Administer:

• Titrated dose; use lowest effective dose

• IM inj deep into upper outer quadrant of gluteal muscle

• Transdermal patches: Testoderm to skin of scrotum; Androderm to skin of back, upper arms, thighs, abdomen; area must be dry-shaved; may be reapplied after bathing, swimming

Perform/provide:

• Diet with increased calories, protein; decrease Na if edema occurs

Evaluate:

• Therapeutic response: 4-6 wk in osteoporosis

Teach patient/family:

• That drug must be combined with complete health plan: diet, rest, exercise

• To notify prescriber if therapeutic response decreases; if edema occurs

• Not to discontinue abruptly

• About changes in sex characteristics

• That women should report menstrual irregularities, voice changes, acne, facial hair growth

• That 1-3-mo course is necessary for response in breast cancer

• The proper application of patches

---

tetanus toxoid, adsorbed/tetanus toxoid (Rx)

Func. class.: Toxoid

Action: Produces specific antibodies to tetanus

Uses: Tetanus toxoid: used for prophylactic treatment of wounds

Dosage and routes:

• *Adult and child:* **IM** 0.5 ml q4-6 wk × 2 doses, then 0.5 ml 1 yr after dose 2 (adsorbed); **SC/IM** 0.5 ml q4-8wk × 3 doses, then 0.5 ml ½-1 yr after dose 3, booster dose 0.5 ml q10yr

Available forms: Inj adsorbed IM 5, 10 LfU/0.5 ml; inj IM, SC 4, 5 LfU/0.5 ml

Side effects/adverse reactions:

GI: Nausea, vomiting, anorexia

INTEG: Skin abscess, urticaria, itching, swelling, erythema, induration at injection site

CV: Tachycardia, hypotension

SYST: Lymphadenitis, ***anaphylaxis***

CNS: Crying, fretfulness, fever, drowsiness

Contraindications: Hypersensitivity, active infection, poliomyelitis outbreak, immunosuppression

Precautions: Pregnancy (C), elderly

NURSING CONSIDERATIONS

Assess:

• For skin reactions: swelling, rash, urticaria

• For history of allergies, skin conditions (eczema, psoriasis, dermatitis), reactions to vaccinations

• For anaphylaxis: inability to breathe, bronchospasm

Administer:

• At least 4 wk apart × 3 doses for children >6 wk old

• Only with epinephrine 1:1000 on unit to treat laryngospasm

Perform/provide:

• Written record of immunization

Teach patient/family:

• That doses are given at least 4 wk apart × 3 doses; booster needed at 10-yr intervals

T

tetracaine (℞)

(tet′ra-kane)
Pontocaine
Func. class.: Local anesthetic
Chem. class.: Ester

Action: Competes with calcium for sites in nerve membrane that control sodium transport across cell membrane; decreases rise of depolarization phase of action potential

Uses: Spinal anesthesia, epidural and peripheral nerve block, perineum, lower extremities

Dosage and routes:

Varies with route of anesthesia

Available forms: Inj 0.2%, 0.3%, 1%; powder

Side effects/adverse reactions:

CNS: Anxiety, restlessness, *convulsions, LOC,* drowsiness, disorientation, tremors, shivering

CV: Myocardial depression, cardiac arrest, dysrhythmias, bradycardia, hypotension, hypertension, fetal bradycardia

GI: Nausea, vomiting

EENT: Blurred vision, tinnitus, pupil constriction

INTEG: Rash, urticaria, allergic reactions, edema, burning, skin discoloration at injection site, tissue necrosis

RESP: Status asthmaticus, respiratory arrest, anaphylaxis

Contraindications: Hypersensitivity, severe liver disease, heart block

Precautions: Elderly, severe drug allergies, pregnancy (C), lactation, children

Pharmacokinetics: Onset 15 min, duration 3 hr; metabolized by liver, excreted in urine (metabolites)

Interactions:

• Dysrhythmias: epinephrine, halothane, enflurane

• Hypertension: MAOIs, tricyclic antidepressants, phenothiazines

• Decreased action of tetracaine: chloroprocaine

• Decreased action of sulfonamides

NURSING CONSIDERATIONS

Assess:

• B/P, pulse, respiration during treatment

• Fetal heart tones during labor

• Allergic reactions: rash, urticaria, itching

• Cardiac status: ECG for dysrhythmias, pulse, B/P, during anesthesia

Administer:

• Only if not cloudy, does not contain precipitate

• Only with crash cart, resuscitative equipment nearby

• Only without preservatives for epidural or caudal anesthesia

Perform/provide:

• Use of new sol, discard unused portions, store in refrigerator

Evaluate:

• Therapeutic response: anesthesia necessary for procedure

Treatment of overdose: Airway, O_2, vasopressor, IV fluids, anticonvulsants for seizures

tetracycline (℞)

(tet-ra-sye′kleen)
Achromycin V, Alatel, Apo-Tetra*, Novotetra*, Nu-Tetra*, Panmycin, Robitet, Sumycin, Teline, Tetracap, tetracycline HCl, Tetracyn, Tetralan, Tetram
Func. class.: Broad-spectrum antiinfective
Chem. class.: Tetracycline

Action: Inhibits protein synthesis and phosphorylation in microorganisms; bacteriostatic

Uses: Syphilis, *Chlamydia trachomatis,* gonorrhea, lymphogranuloma venereum; uncommon gram-positive, gram-negative organisms; rickettsial infections

Dosage and routes:
• *Adult:* PO 250-500 mg q6h
• *Child >8 yr:* PO 25-50 mg/kg/day in divided doses q6h

Gonorrhea
• *Adult:* PO 1.5 g, then 500 mg qid for a total of 9 g over 7 days

Chlamydia trachomatis
• *Adult:* PO 500 mg qid × 7 days

Syphilis
• *Adult:* PO 2-3 g in divided doses × 10-15 days; if syphilis duration >1 yr, must treat 30 days

Brucellosis
• *Adult:* PO 500 mg qid × 3 wk with 1 g streptomycin **IM** 2 × /day × 1 wk, and 1 × /day the second wk

Urethral syndrome in women
• *Adult:* PO 500 mg qid × 7 days

Acne
• *Adult:* 1 g/day in divided doses; maintenance 125-500 mg/day

Available forms: Oral susp 125 mg/5 ml; caps 200, 500 mg; tabs 250, 500 mg

Side effects/adverse reactions:
CNS: Fever, headache, paresthesia
HEMA: **Eosinophilia, neutropenia, thrombocytopenia, leukocytosis, hemolytic anemia**
EENT: Dysphagia, glossitis, decreased calcification, discoloration of deciduous teeth, oral candidiasis, oral ulcers
GI: Nausea, abdominal pain, *vomiting, diarrhea,* anorexia, enterocolitis, **hepatotoxicity,** flatulence, abdominal cramps, epigastric burning, stomatitis
CV: Pericarditis
GU: *Increased BUN*
INTEG: Rash, urticaria, photosensitivity, increased pigmentation, **exfoliative dermatitis,** pruritus, **angioedema**

Contraindications: Hypersensitivity to tetracyclines, children <8 yr, pregnancy (D), lactation

Precautions: Renal disease, hepatic disease

Pharmacokinetics:
PO: Peak 2-3 hr, duration 6 hr, half-life 6-10 hr; excreted in urine, breast milk; crosses placenta; 20%-60% protein bound

Interactions:
• Decreased effect of tetracycline: antacids, NaHCO₃, dairy products, alkali products, iron, kaolin/pectin, cimetidine
• Increased effect: warfarin, digoxin
• Decreased effect of penicillins, oral contraceptives
• Nephrotoxicity: methoxyflurane

Lab test interferences:
False negative: Urine glucose with Clinistix or Tes-Tape
False increase: Urinary catecholamines

NURSING CONSIDERATIONS
Assess:
• Signs of anemia: Hct, Hgb, fatigue
• I&O ratio
• Blood studies: PT, CBC, AST, ALT, BUN, creatinine
• Allergic reactions: rash, itching, pruritus, angioedema
• Nausea, vomiting, diarrhea; administer antiemetic, antacids as ordered
• Overgrowth of infection: fever, malaise, redness, pain, swelling, drainage, perineal itching, diarrhea, changes in cough or sputum

Administer:
• After C&S obtained
• 2 hr before or after iron products; 3 hr after antacid or kaolin/pectin products

Perform/provide:
• Storage in tight, light-resistant container at room temp

T

Side effects: *italics* = common; **bold italics** = life-threatening

Evaluate:

• Therapeutic response: decreased temp, absence of lesions, negative C&S

Teach patient/family:

• To avoid sun exposure; sunscreen does not seem to decrease photosensitivity

• That diabetic should avoid use of Clinistix, Diastix, or Tes-Tape for urine glucose testing

• That all prescribed medication must be taken to prevent superinfection

• To avoid milk products, antacids, or separate by 2 hr; take with a full glass of water

---

theophylline (R)

(thee-off'i-lin)

Accurbron, Aquaphyllin, Asmalix, Bronkodyl, Elixomin, Elixophyllin, Lanophyllin, Quibron-T Dividose, Quibron-T/SR Dividose, Respbid, Slo-bid Gyrocaps, Slo-Phyllin, Sustaire, Theo-24, Theobid Duracaps, Theochron, Theoclear-80, Theoclear L.A., Theo-Dur, Theolair-SR, Theo-Sav, Theospan-SR, Theostat 80, Theovent, Theo-X, T-Phyl, Uni-Dur, Uniphyl

Func. class.: Spasmolytic

Chem. class.: Xanthine, ethylenediamide

Action: Relaxes smooth muscle of respiratory system by blocking phosphodiesterase, which increases cAMP

Uses: Bronchial asthma, bronchospasm of COPD, chronic bronchitis

Dosage and routes:

Bronchospasm, bronchial asthma

• *Adult:* **PO** 100-200 mg q6h; dosage must be individualized; **RECT** 250-500 mg q8-12h

• *Child:* **PO** 50-100 mg q6h, not to exceed 12 mg/kg/24 hr

COPD, chronic bronchitis

• *Adult:* **PO** 330-660 mg q6-8h pc (sodium glycinate)

• *Child 1-9 yr:* **PO** 5 mg/kg loading dose, then 4 mg/kg q6h

• *Child 9-16 yr:* **PO** 5 mg/kg loading dose, then 3 mg/kg q6h

Apnea of prematurity

• *Neonate:* 2-10 mg/kg/day divided q8-12h (usual loading dose is 4 mg/kg **PO**)

Available forms: Caps 50, 100, 200, 250 mg; tabs 100, 125, 200, 225, 250, 300 mg; tabs, time rel 100, 200, 250, 300, 400, 500 mg; caps, time rel 50, 65, 100, 125, 130, 200, 250, 260, 300, 400, 500 mg; elix 80, 11.25 mg/15 ml; sol 80 mg/15 ml; liq 80, 150, 160 mg/15 ml; susp 300 mg/15 ml

Side effects/adverse reactions:

CNS: Anxiety, restlessness, insomnia, dizziness, **convulsions,** headache, light-headedness, muscle twitching, tremors

CV: Palpitations, sinus tachycardia, hypotension, other dysrhythmias, fluid retention with tachycardia

ENDO: Hyperglycemia

GI: Nausea, vomiting, anorexia, diarrhea, bitter taste, dyspepsia, gastric distress

RESP: Increased rate

INTEG: Flushing, urticaria

Contraindications: Hypersensitivity to xanthines, tachydysrhythmias

Precautions: Elderly, CHF, cor pulmonale, hepatic disease, active peptic ulcer disease, diabetes mellitus, hyperthyroidism, hypertension, children, pregnancy (C)

Pharmacokinetics:

PO: Peak 2 hr

SOL: Peak 1 hr

Metabolized in liver, excreted in urine and breast milk, crosses placenta

---

⬥ = Nursing alert   🖋 = Herb-drug interaction   🚫 = Do not crush

Interactions:

• Decreased theophylline level: phenytoin, phenobarbital, carbamazepine, rifampin, smoking

• Increased action of theophylline: cimetidine, propranolol, erythromycin, troleandomycin, ciprofloxacin, oral contraceptives

• May increase effects of anticoagulants

• Cardiotoxicity: β-blockers

• Decreased effect of lithium

🌿 Toxicity: ephedra (ma huang)

NURSING CONSIDERATIONS

Assess:

◆ Theophylline blood levels (therapeutic level is 5-15 µg/ml); toxicity may occur with small increase above 20 µg/ml

• Monitor I&O; diuresis occurs; elderly or child may be dehydrated

• Signs of toxicity: irritability, insomnia, restlessness, tremors, nausea, vomiting

• Respiratory rate, rhythm, depth; auscultate lung fields bilaterally; notify prescriber of abnormalities

• Allergic reactions: rash, urticaria; drug should be discontinued

Administer:

• PO after meals for GI symptoms; absorption may be affected

IV

Additive compatibilities: Cefepime, chlorpromazine, fluconazole, furosemide, hydrocortisone, lidocaine, methylprednisolone, verapamil

Y-site compatibilities: Acyclovir, ampicillin, ampicillin/sulbactam, aztreonam, cefazolin, cefotetan, ceftazidime, ceftriaxone, cimetidine, cisatracurium, clindamycin, dexamethasone, diltiazem, dobutamine, dopamine, doxycycline, erythromycin, famotidine, fluconazole, gentamicin, haloperidol, heparin, hydrocortisone, lidocaine, methyldopa, methylprednisolone, metronidazole, midazolam, nafcillin, nitroglycerin, penicillin G potassium, piperacillin, potassium chloride, ranitidine, remifentanil, sodium nitroprusside, ticarcillin, ticarcillin/clavulanate, tobramycin, vancomycin

Evaluate:

• Therapeutic response: ability to breathe more easily

Teach patient/family:

• To check OTC medications, current prescription medications for ephedrine, which will increase stimulation; to avoid alcohol, caffeine

• To avoid hazardous activities; dizziness may occur

• That if GI upset occurs, to take drug with 8 oz H_2O; avoid food; absorption may be decreased

🚫 Not to break, crush, chew, or dissolve slow-release products

• That contents of bead-filled capsule may be sprinkled over food for children's use

• To notify prescriber of toxicity: nausea, vomiting, anxiety, insomnia, convulsions

• To notify prescriber of change in smoking habit; dosage may have to be changed

---

thiabendazole (℞)

(thye-a-ben′da-zole)

Mintezol

Func. class.: Anthelmintic

Chem. class.: Benzimidazole derivative

Action: Inhibits anaerobic metabolism, disrupts microtubules

Uses: Pinworm, roundworm, threadworm, whipworm, trichinosis, hookworm, cutaneous larva migrans (creeping eruption)

Dosage and routes:

• *Adult and child:* **PO** 25 mg/kg in

---

2 doses qd × 2-5 days, not to exceed 3 g/day

Available forms: Tabs, chew 500 mg; oral susp 500 mg/5 ml

Side effects/adverse reactions:

SYST: **Anaphylaxis**

GU: **Hematuria, nephrotoxicity,** enuresis, abnormal smell of urine

INTEG: Rash, pruritus, erythema, **Stevens-Johnson syndrome**

CNS: Dizziness, headache, drowsiness, fever, flushing, **convulsions,** behavioral changes

EENT: Tinnitus, blurred vision, xanthopsia

GI: Nausea, vomiting, anorexia, diarrhea, jaundice, **liver damage,** epigastric distress

CV: Hypotension, bradycardia

Contraindications: Hypersensitivity

Precautions: Severe malnutrition, hepatic disease, renal disease, anemia, severe dehydration, child <14 kg, pregnancy (C)

Pharmacokinetics:

PO: Peak 1-2 hr, metabolized completely by liver, excreted in feces and urine

NURSING CONSIDERATIONS

Assess:

• Stools periodically during entire treatment

Administer:

• Susp after shaking

• PO after meals to avoid GI symptoms

Perform/provide:

• Storage in tight container

Evaluate:

• Therapeutic response: stools negative for helminths

Teach patient/family:

• Proper hygiene after BM, including hand-washing technique; tell patient not to put fingers in mouth

• That infected person should sleep alone; not to shake bed linen; to change bed linen qd

• To clean toilet qd with disinfectant (green soap solution)

• The need for compliance with dosage schedule, duration of treatment

• To drink fruit juice to remove mucus that intestinal tapeworms burrow in; aids in expulsion of worms

• To avoid hazardous activities if drowsiness occurs

Treatment of overdose: Induce emesis or gastric lavage

---

thiamine (vit B₁)
(PO-OTC, IM-℞)
Betaxin*, Betalin S, Biamine, Revitonus, Thiamilate, thiamine HCl

Func. class.: Vit B₁

Chem. class.: Water soluble

Action: Needed for pyruvate metabolism, carbohydrate metabolism

Uses: Vit B₁ deficiency or polyneuritis, cheilosis adjunct with thiamine beriberi, Wernicke-Korsakoff syndrome, pellagra, metabolic disorders

Dosage and routes:

RDA

• *Adult:* male 1.2-1.5 mg, females 1.1 mg; pregnancy 1.5 mg; lactation 1.6 mg

• *Child 7-10 yr:* 1.3 mg

• *Child 4-6 yr:* 0.9 mg

• *Child 1-3 yr:* 0.7 mg

• *Infants 6 mo-1 yr:* 0.4 mg

• *Neonates and infants <6 mo:* 0.3 mg

Beriberi

• *Adult:* **IM** 10-20 mg tid × 2 wk, then 5-10 mg qd × 1 mo

Beriberi with cardiac failure

• *Adult and child:* **IV** 10-30 mg tid

Available forms: Tabs 50, 100, 250, 500 mg; inj 100 mg/ml; enteric coated tabs 20 mg

---

◆ = Nursing alert   ⏐⏐ = Herb-drug interaction   ⃠ = Do not crush

Side effects/adverse reactions:
CNS: Weakness, restlessness
GI: Hemorrhage, *nausea, diarrhea*
CV: ***Collapse, pulmonary edema,*** hypotension
INTEG: ***Angioneurotic edema,*** cyanosis, sweating, warmth
SYST: ***Anaphylaxis***
EENT: Tightness of throat
Contraindications: Hypersensitivity
Precautions: Pregnancy (A)
Pharmacokinetics:
PO/INJ: Unused amounts excreted in urine (unchanged)

NURSING CONSIDERATIONS
Assess:
• Thiamine levels throughout treatment
• Nutritional status: yeast, beef, liver, whole or enriched grains, legumes
Administer:
• By IM injection; rotate sites if pain and inflammation occur; do not mix with alkaline sols; Z-track to minimize pain
IV
• Undiluted over 5 min or diluted with IV sol and given as an inf at 100 mg or less/5 min or more
Syringe compatibilities: Doxapram
Y-site compatibilities: Famotidine
Perform/provide:
• Storage in tight, light-resistant container
• Application of cold to help decrease pain
Evaluate:
• Therapeutic response: absence of nausea, vomiting, anorexia, insomnia, tachycardia, paresthesias, depression, muscle weakness
Teach patient/family:
• The necessary foods to be included in diet: yeast, beef, liver, legumes, whole grain

thiethylperazine (℞)
(thye-eth-il-per′a-zeen)
Norzine, Torecan
Func. class.: Antiemetic
Chem. class.: Phenothiazine, piperazine derivative

Action: Acts centrally by blocking chemoreceptor trigger zone, which in turn acts on vomiting center
Uses: Nausea, vomiting
Dosage and routes:
• *Adult:* **PO/IM** 10 mg/qd-tid
Available forms: Tabs 10 mg; inj 5 mg/ml
Side effects/adverse reactions:
GU: Urinary retention, dark urine
CNS: *Euphoria, depression,* restlessness, tremor, EPS, ***convulsions,*** drowsiness
GI: Nausea, vomiting, anorexia, dry mouth, diarrhea, constipation, weight loss, metallic taste, cramps
CV: ***Circulatory failure, tachycardia,*** postural hypotension, ECG changes
RESP: ***Respiratory depression***
Contraindications: Hypersensitivity to phenothiazines, coma, seizure, encephalopathy, bone marrow depression, pregnancy (X)
Precautions: Children <2 yr, elderly, lactation
Pharmacokinetics:
PO: Onset 45-60 min
RECT: Onset 45-60 min, metabolized by liver, crosses placenta, excreted in urine, breast milk
Interactions:
• Decreased effect of thiethylperazine: barbiturates, antacids
• Increased anticholinergic action: anticholinergics, antiparkinson drugs, antidepressants

NURSING CONSIDERATIONS
Assess:
• VS, B/P; check patients with cardiac disease more often

T

• Respiratory status before, during, after administration of emetic; check rate, rhythm, character; respiratory depression can occur rapidly with elderly or debilitated patients

Administer:
• IM inj in large muscle mass; aspirate to avoid IV administration; patient should remain recumbent 1 hr after inj

Syringe compatibilities: Butorphanol, hydromorphone, midazolam, ranitidine

Y-site compatibilities: Aldesleukin

Evaluate:
• Therapeutic response: absence of nausea, vomiting

Teach patient/family:
• To avoid hazardous activities, activities requiring alertness; dizziness may occur

---

thioguanine (6-TG) (℞)

(thye-oh-gwah'neen)
thioguanine, Lanvis*
Func. class.: Antineoplastic-antimetabolite
Chem. class.: Purine analog

Action: Interferes with synthesis, utilization of purine nucleotides; S phase of cell cycle specific

Uses: Acute leukemias, chronic granulocytic leukemia, lymphomas, multiple myeloma, solid tumors

Dosage and routes:
• *Adult and child:* **PO** 2 mg/kg/day, then increase slowly to 3 mg/kg/day after 4 wk
Available forms: Tabs 40 mg

Side effects/adverse reactions:
*HEMA: **Thrombocytopenia, leukopenia, myelosuppression, anemia***
*GI: Nausea, vomiting, anorexia, di-*arrhea, stomatitis, **hepatotoxicity,** gastritis, jaundice
*GU: **Renal failure,** hyperuricemia, oliguria*
INTEG: Rash, dermatitis, dry skin

Contraindications: Prior drug resistance, leukopenia (<2500/mm^3), thrombocytopenia (<100,000/mm^3), anemia, pregnancy (D)

Precautions: Liver disease

Pharmacokinetics: Oral form absorbed only 30%, metabolized in liver, only small amounts excreted in urine (unchanged)

Interactions:
• Increased toxicity: radiation, other antineoplastics

Lab test interferences:
Increase: Uric acid (blood, urine)

NURSING CONSIDERATIONS
Assess:
• CBC, differential, platelet count qwk; withhold drug if WBC is <3500/mm^3 or platelet count is <100,000/mm^3; notify prescriber; drug should be discontinued
• Renal function studies: BUN, serum uric acid, urine CrCl, electrolytes before, during therapy
• I&O ratio; report fall in urine output to <30 ml/hr
• Monitor temp q4h; fever may indicate beginning infection
• Liver function tests before, during therapy: bilirubin, alk phosphatase, AST, ALT
• Bleeding time, coagulation time during treatment
• Bleeding: hematuria, guaiac, bruising, petechiae, mucosa or orifices q8h
• Hepatotoxicity: jaundiced skin, sclera; dark urine, clay-colored stools, pruritus, abdominal pain, fever, diarrhea
• Buccal cavity q8h for dryness, sores, ulceration, white patches, oral pain, bleeding, dysphagia

---

◆ = Nursing alert   🌿 = Herb-drug interaction   ⊘ = Do not crush

◆ Symptoms indicating severe allergic reaction: rash, urticaria, itching, flushing

Administer:

• Antacid before oral agent; give drug after evening meal before bedtime

• Antiemetic 30-60 min before giving drug to prevent vomiting

• Allopurinol or sodium bicarbonate to maintain uric acid levels, alkalinization of urine

• Transfusion for anemia

Perform/provide:

• Strict medical asepsis, protective isolation if WBC levels are low

• Liquid diet: carbonated beverage, Jell-O; dry toast, crackers may be added when patient is not nauseated or vomiting

• Increase fluid intake to 2-3 L/day to prevent urate deposits, calculi formation, unless contraindicated

• Diet low in purines: no organ meats (kidney, liver), dried beans, peas to maintain alkaline urine

• Rinsing of mouth tid-qid with water, club soda, brushing of teeth bid-tid with soft brush or cotton-tipped applicators for stomatitis; use unwaxed dental floss

• Nutritious diet with iron, vitamin supplements as ordered

• Storage in tightly closed container in cool environment

Evaluate:

• Therapeutic response: decreased tumor size, spread of malignancy

Teach patient/family:

• Why protective isolation precautions are needed

• To report any complaints, side effects to prescriber: black tarry stools, chills, fever, sore throat, bleeding, bruising, cough, shortness of breath, dark, bloody urine

• To avoid foods with citric acid, hot or rough texture if stomatitis is present

• To report stomatitis: any bleeding, white spots, ulcerations in mouth; to examine mouth qd, report symptoms

• That contraceptive measures are recommended during therapy

• To drink 10-12 (8 oz) glasses of fluid/day

---

thiopental (℞)
(thye-oh-pen′tal)
Pentothal, thiopental sodium
Func. class.: General anesthetic
Chem. class.: Barbiturate

Controlled Substance Schedule III

Action: Acts in reticular-activating system to produce anesthesia, raises seizure threshold

Uses: Short, general anesthesia; narcoanalysis, induction anesthesia before other anesthetics

Investigational uses: Increased intracranial pressure

Dosage and routes:
Induction
• *Adult:* **IV** 210-280 mg or 3-5 ml/kg
General anesthetic
• *Child:* **IV** 3-8 mg/kg then 1 mg/kg as needed
• *Adult:* **IV** 50-75 mg given at 20-40 sec intervals
Narcoanalysis
• *Adult:* **IV** 100 mg/min, not to exceed 50 ml/min
Sedation or narcosis
• *Adult:* **RECT** 12-20 mg/lb
Available forms: Powder for inj 2%, 2.5%

Side effects/adverse reactions:
RESP: ***Respiratory depression, bronchospasm***
CNS: Retrograde amnesia, prolonged somnolence

T

CV: Tachycardia, hypotension, *myocardial depression, dysrhythmias*
EENT: Sneezing, coughing
INTEG: Chills, *shivering*, necrosis, pain at injection site
MS: Muscle irritability
Contraindications: Hypersensitivity, status asthmaticus, hepatic/intermittent porphyrias
Precautions: Severe cardiovascular disease, renal disease, hypotension, liver disease, myxedema, myasthenia gravis, asthma, increased intracranial pressure, pregnancy (C)
Pharmacokinetics:
IV: Onset 30-40 sec; half-life 11½ hr; crosses placenta
Interactions:
• Increased action: CNS depressants
⚫ Increased CNS depression: kava
NURSING CONSIDERATIONS
Assess:
• VS q3-5min during IV administration, after dose, q4h postoperatively
• Extravasation; if it occurs, use nitroprusside or chloroprocaine to decrease pain, increase circulation
• Dysrhythmias or myocardial depression
Administer:
• Only with crash cart, resuscitative equipment nearby
IV
• After diluting 500 mg/20 ml sterile H₂O for inj; give each 25 mg or less/min, titrate to response
Additive compatibilities: Chloramphenicol, hydrocortisone sodium succinate, oxytocin, pentobarbital, phenobarbital, potassium chloride, sodium bicarbonate
Solution compatibilities: D₅/0.45% NaCl, D₅W, multiple electrolyte sol, 0.45% NaCl, 0.9% NaCl, 1/6 M sodium lactate
Syringe compatibilities: Aminophylline, hyaluronidase, hydro-

cortisone sodium succinate, neostigmine, pentobarbital, propofol, scopolamine, tubocurarine
Y-site compatibilities: Doxacurium, fentanyl, heparin, milrinone, mivacurium, nitroglycerin, ranitidine, remifentanil
Evaluate:
• Therapeutic response: maintenance of anesthesia

---

thioridazine (℞)

(thye-or-rid′a-zeen)
Apo-Thioridazine*, Mellaril, Mellaril Concentrate, Mellaril-5, Novo-Ridazine*, PMS-Thioridazine*, thioridazine HCl
Func. class.: Antipsychotic, neuroleptic
Chem. class.: Phenothiazine piperidine

Action: Depresses cerebral cortex, hypothalamus, limbic system, which control activity, aggression; blocks neurotransmission produced by dopamine at synapse; exhibits strong α-adrenergic, anticholinergic blocking action; mechanism for antipsychotic effects is unclear
Uses: Psychotic disorders, schizophrenia, behavioral problems in children, anxiety, major depressive disorders, organic brain syndrome
Dosage and routes:
Psychosis
• *Adult:* PO 25-100 mg tid, max dose 800 mg/day; dose is gradually increased to desired response, then reduced to minimum maintenance
Depression/behavioral problems/ organic brain syndrome
• *Adult:* PO 25 mg tid, range from 10 mg bid-qid to 50 mg tid-qid; decreased dose in elderly
• *Geriatric:* PO 10-25 mg qd-bid,

◆ = Nursing alert   ⚫ = Herb-drug interaction   🚫 = Do not crush

increase 4-7 days by 10-25 mg to desired dose
• *Child 2-12 yr:* PO 0.5-3 mg/kg/day in divided doses
Available forms: Tabs 10, 15, 25, 50, 100, 150, 200 mg; conc 30, 100 mg/ml; susp 25, 100 mg/5 ml; syr 10 mg/15 ml
Side effects/adverse reactions:
RESP: **Laryngospasm,** dyspnea, *respiratory depression*
CNS: EPS (rare): pseudoparkinsonism, akathisia, dystonia, tardive dyskinesia, **seizures,** *headache,* confusion, **neuroleptic malignant syndrome**
HEMA: Anemia, **leukopenia, leukocytosis, agranulocytosis**
INTEG: Rash, photosensitivity, dermatitis
EENT: Blurred vision, glaucoma, dry eyes
GI: Dry mouth, nausea, vomiting, anorexia, constipation, diarrhea, jaundice, weight gain
GU: Urinary retention, urinary frequency, enuresis, impotence, amenorrhea, gynecomastia
CV: Orthostatic hypotension, **cardiac arrest,** ECG changes, **tachycardia**
Contraindications: Hypersensitivity, blood dyscrasias, coma, children <2 yr, brain damage, bone marrow depression
Precautions: Pregnancy (C), lactation, seizure disorders, hypertension, hepatic disease, cardiac disease
Pharmacokinetics:
PO: Onset erratic, peak 2-4 hr; metabolized by liver, excreted in urine, breast milk; crosses placenta, half-life 26-36 hr
Interactions:
• Oversedation: other CNS depressants, alcohol, barbiturate anesthetics

• Decreased thioridazine effect: lithium, barbiturates
• Decreased antihypertensive effect: centrally acting antihypertensives
• Decreased absorption: aluminum hydroxide, magnesium hydroxide antacids
• Increased anticholinergic effects: anticholinergics
⚕ Increased CNS depression: kava
Lab test interferences:
Increase: Liver function tests, cardiac enzymes, cholesterol, blood glucose, prolactin, bilirubin, PBI, cholinesterase, ^{131}I
Decrease: Hormones (blood, urine)
False positive: Pregnancy test, PKU
False negative: Urinary steroid, pregnancy test
NURSING CONSIDERATIONS
Assess:
• Mental status before first dose
• Swallowing of PO medication; check for hoarding or giving of medication to other patients
• I&O ratio; palpate bladder if low urinary output occurs
• Bilirubin, CBC, liver function studies qmo
• Urinalysis is recommended before and during prolonged therapy
• Affect, orientation, LOC, reflexes, gait, coordination, sleep pattern disturbances
• B/P standing and lying; also include pulse and respirations q4h during initial treatment; establish baseline before starting treatment; report drops of 30 mm Hg
• Dizziness, faintness, palpitations, tachycardia on rising
• EPS including akathisia (inability to sit still, no pattern to movements), tardive dyskinesia (bizarre movements of jaw, mouth, tongue, extremities), pseudoparkinsonism (rigidity, tremors, pill rolling, shuffling gait)
◆ For neuroleptic malignant syn-

drome: altered mental status, muscle rigidity, increased CPK, hyperthermia

• Skin turgor qd

• Constipation, urinary retention qd; increase bulk, water in diet

Administer:

• Antiparkinsonian agent on order from prescriber for EPS

• Concentrate mixed in citrus juices or distilled or acidified tap water

• Decreased dose in elderly

Perform/provide:

• Decreased sensory input by dimming lights, avoiding loud noises

• Supervised ambulation until stabilized on medication if needed; do not involve in strenuous exercise program because fainting is possible; patient should not stand still for long periods

• Increased fluids to prevent constipation

• Sips of water, candy, gum for dry mouth

• Storage in tight, light-resistant container; avoid contact with skin

Evaluate:

• Therapeutic response: decrease in emotional excitement, hallucinations, delusions, paranoia, reorganization of patterns of thought, speech

Teach patient/family:

• That orthostatic hypotension occurs frequently, to rise from sitting or lying position gradually; to avoid hazardous activities until stabilized on medication

• To remain lying down after IM injection for at least 30 min

• To avoid hot tubs, hot showers, tub baths; hypotension may occur

• To avoid abrupt withdrawal of thioridazine, or EPS may result; drug should be withdrawn slowly

• To avoid OTC preparations (cough, hay fever, cold) unless approved by prescriber; serious drug interactions may occur; avoid use with alcohol, CNS depressants; increased drowsiness may occur

• To use a sunscreen

• About compliance with drug regimen

• About the necessity for meticulous oral hygiene, since oral candidiasis may occur

• To report sore throat, malaise, fever, bleeding, mouth sores; if these occur, CBC should be drawn and drug discontinued

• That in hot weather, heat stroke may occur; take extra precautions to stay cool

Treatment of overdose: Lavage if orally ingested, provide an airway; do not induce vomiting

---

thiotepa (R)

(thye-oh-tep'a)
Thioplex
Func. class.: Antineoplastic
Chem. class.: Alkylating agent

Action: Responsible for crosslinking DNA strands leading to cell death; activity is not cell cycle phase specific

Uses: Hodgkin's disease, lymphomas; breast, ovarian, lung, bladder cancer; neoplastic effusions

Dosage and routes:

• *Adult:* IV 0.3-0.4 mg/kg at 1-4 wk intervals

Neoplastic effusions

• *Adult:* **INTRACAVITY** 0.6-0.8 mg/kg

Bladder cancer

• *Adult:* **INSTILL** 60 mg/30-60 ml water for inj instilled in bladder for 2 hr once weekly × 4 wk

Available forms: Powder for inj 15 mg

Side effects/adverse reactions:
CNS: Dizziness, headache

◆ = Nursing alert   ⫽ = Herb-drug interaction   ⊘ = Do not crush

HEMA: **Thrombocytopenia, leukopenia, pancytopenia**
GI: Nausea, vomiting, anorexia
GU: Hyperuricemia, **hematuria,** amenorrhea, azoospermia
INTEG: Rash, pruritus

Contraindications: Hypersensitivity, pregnancy (D)

Precautions: Radiation therapy, bone marrow suppression, impaired renal or hepatic function

Pharmacokinetics: Onset slow, metabolized in liver, excreted in urine

Interactions:
• Increased apnea: neuromuscular blockers

NURSING CONSIDERATIONS
Assess:
• CBC, differential, platelet count qwk; withhold drug if WBC is <4000/mm^3 or platelet count is <75,000/mm^3; notify prescriber
• Renal function studies: BUN, serum uric acid, urine CrCl before, during therapy
• I&O ratio, report fall in urine output of 30 ml/hr
• Monitor temp q4h (may indicate beginning infection)
• Liver function tests before, during therapy (bilirubin, AST, ALT, LDH) as needed or monthly
• Bleeding: hematuria, guaiac, bruising or petechiae, mucosa or orifices q8h
• Jaundiced skin, sclera; dark urine, clay-colored stools, itchy skin, abdominal pain, fever, diarrhea
• Buccal cavity q8h for dryness, sores, ulceration, white patches, oral pain, bleeding, dysphagia
◆ Symptoms indicating severe allergic reaction: rash, pruritus, urticaria, itching, flushing

Administer:
• Antiemetic 30-60 min before giving drug to prevent vomiting

IV
• After diluting 15 mg/1.5 ml of sterile H$_2$O for inj; give over 1-3 min; may be further diluted in 50-100 ml compatible sol, use a 0.22 μ filter

Y-site compatibilities: Acyclovir, allopurinol, amifostine, amikacin, aminophylline, amphotericin B, ampicillin, ampicillin/sulbactam, aztreonam, bleomycin, bumetanide, buprenorphine, butorphanol, calcium gluconate, carboplatin, carmustine, cefazolin, cefepime, cefoperazone, cefonicid, cefotaxime, cefotetan, cefoxitin, ceftazidime, ceftizoxime, ceftriaxone, cefuroxime, chlorpromazine, cimetidine, ciprofloxacin, clindamycin, cyclophosphamide, cytarabine, dacarbazine, dactinomycin, daunorubicin, diphenhydramine, dobutamine, dopamine, doxorubicin, doxycycline, droperidol, enalaprilat, etoposide, famotidine, floxuridine, fluconazole, fludarabine, fluorouracil, furosemide, gallium, ganciclovir, gentamicin, granisetron, haloperidol, heparin, hydrocortisone, hydromorphone, hydroxyzine, idarubicin, ifosfamide, imipenem-cilastatin, leucovorin, lorazepam, magnesium sulfate, mannitol, melphalan, meperidine, mesna, methotrexate, methylprednisolone, metoclopramide, metronidazole, mezlocillin, miconazole, mitomycin, mitoxantrone, morphine, nalbuphine, netilmicin, ofloxacin, ondansetron, paclitaxel, piperacillin, piperacillin/tazobactam, plicamycin, potassium chloride, prochlorperazine, promethazine, ranitidine, sodium bicarbonate, streptozocin, teniposide, ticarcillin, ticarcillin/clavulanate, tobramycin, trimethoprim - sulfamethoxazole, vancomycin, vinblastine, vincristine, zidovudine

---

Side effects: *italics* = common; **bold italics** = life-threatening

Perform/provide:

• Storage in light-resistant container; refrigerate

• Strict medical asepsis, protective isolation if WBC levels are low

• Increase fluid intake to 2-3 L/day to prevent urate deposits, calculi formation

• Warm compresses at injection site for inflammation

Evaluate:

• Therapeutic response: decreased tumor size, spread of malignancy

Teach patient/family:

• About protective isolation

• That azoospermia or amenorrhea can occur; reversible after discontinuing treatment; to use effective contraception during treatment

• To report any bleeding, white spots or ulcerations in mouth to prescriber; to examine mouth qd

• To report signs of infection: fever, sore throat, flulike symptoms

• To report signs of anemia: fatigue, headache, faintness, shortness of breath, irritability

• To avoid use of razors, commercial mouthwash

• To avoid use of aspirin products, ibuprofen

---

thiothixene (R)

(thye-oh-thix′een)

Navane, thiothixene

Func. class.: Antipsychotic, neuroleptic

Chem. class.: Thioxanthene

Action: Depresses cerebral cortex, hypothalamus, limbic system, which control activity, aggression; blocks neurotransmission produced by dopamine at synapse; exhibits strong α-adrenergic blocking action; mechanism for antipsychotic effects is unclear

Uses: Psychotic disorders, schizophrenia, acute agitation

Dosage and routes:

• *Adult:* **PO** 2-5 mg bid-qid depending on severity of condition; dose gradually increased to 15-30 mg if needed; **IM** 4 mg bid-qid; max dose 30 mg qd; administer **PO** dose as soon as possible

• *Geriatric:* **PO** 1-2 mg qd-bid, increase by 1-2 mg q4-7 days to desired dose

Available forms: Caps 1, 2, 5, 10, 20 mg; conc 5 mg/ml; inj 2 mg/ml; powder for inj 5 mg/ml

Side effects/adverse reactions:

RESP: **Laryngospasm,** dyspnea, **respiratory depression**

CNS: EPS: pseudoparkinsonism, akathisia, dystonia, tardive dyskinesia; **seizures,** headache, **neuroleptic malignant syndrome**

HEMA: Anemia, **leukopenia, leukocytosis, agranulocytosis**

INTEG: Rash, photosensitivity, dermatitis

EENT: Blurred vision, glaucoma

GI: Dry mouth, nausea, vomiting, anorexia, constipation, diarrhea, jaundice, weight gain

GU: Urinary retention, urinary frequency, enuresis, impotence, amenorrhea, gynecomastia

CV: Orthostatic hypotension, hypertension, **cardiac arrest,** ECG changes, **tachycardia**

Contraindications: Hypersensitivity, blood dyscrasias, child <12 yr, bone marrow depression, circulatory collapse, CNS depression, coma, alcoholism, CV disease, hepatic disease, Reye's syndrome, narrow-angle glaucoma

Precautions: Pregnancy (C), lactation, seizure disorders, hypertension, hepatic disease, elderly

Pharmacokinetics:

PO: Onset slow, peak 2-8 hr, duration up to 12 hr

◆ = Nursing alert　　🍃 = Herb-drug interaction　　🚫 = Do not crush

IM: Onset 15-30 min, peak 1-6 hr, duration up to 12 hr

Metabolized by liver, excreted in urine, breast milk; crosses placenta, half-life 34 hr

Interactions:

• Oversedation: other CNS depressants, alcohol, barbiturate anesthetics

⚕ Increased CNS depression: kava

Lab test interferences:

Increase: Liver function tests, cardiac enzymes, cholesterol, blood glucose, prolactin, bilirubin, PBI, cholinesterase, ^{131}I

Decrease: Uric acid

NURSING CONSIDERATIONS

Assess:

• For oculogyric crisis

• Mental status before initial administration

• Swallowing of PO medication; check for hoarding or giving of medication to other patients

• I&O ratio, palpate bladder if low urinary output occurs

• Bilirubin, CBC, liver function studies qmo

• Urinalysis is recommended before and during prolonged therapy

• Affect, orientation, LOC, reflexes, gait, coordination, sleep pattern disturbances

• B/P standing and lying; pulse and respirations q4h during initial treatment; establish baseline before starting treatment; report drops of 30 mm Hg

• Dizziness, faintness, palpitations, tachycardia on rising

• EPS including akathisia (inability to sit still, no pattern to movements), tardive dyskinesia (bizarre movements of jaw, mouth, tongue, extremities), pseudoparkinsonism (rigidity, tremors, pill rolling, shuffling gait)

◆ For neuroleptic malignant syndrome: muscle rigidity, altered mental status, increased CPK, hyperthermia

• Constipation, urinary retention daily; increase bulk, water in diet

Administer:

• Antiparkinsonian agent on order from prescriber for EPS

• Concentrate mixed in citrus juices or distilled or acidified tap water

• IM injection into large muscle mass

Syringe compatibilities: Benztropine, diphenhydramine, hydroxyzine

Perform/provide:

• Decreased sensory input by dimming lights, avoiding loud noises

• Supervised ambulation until stabilized on medication; do not involve in strenuous exercise program because fainting is possible; patient should not stand still for long periods

• Increased fluids to prevent constipation

• Sips of water, candy, gum for dry mouth

• Storage in tight, light-resistant container; keep reconstituted sol at room temp for up to 48 hr; avoid contact with skin

Evaluate:

• Therapeutic response: decrease in emotional excitement, hallucinations, delusions, paranoia, reorganization of patterns of thought, speech

Teach patient/family:

• That orthostatic hypotension occurs frequently, and to rise from sitting or lying position gradually; to avoid hazardous activities until stabilized on medication

• To remain lying down after IM inj for at least 30 min

• To avoid hot tubs, hot showers, tub baths; hypotension may occur

• To avoid abrupt withdrawal of this

T

---

drug, or EPS may result; drug should be withdrawn slowly

• To avoid OTC preparations (cough, hay fever, cold) unless approved by prescriber; serious drug interactions may occur; avoid use with alcohol, CNS depressants; increased drowsiness may occur

• To use a sunscreen

• About compliance with drug regimen

• About EPS

• The necessity for meticulous oral hygiene, since oral candidiasis may occur

• To report sore throat, malaise, fever, bleeding, mouth sores; if these occur, CBC should be drawn and drug discontinued

• That in hot weather, heat stroke may occur; take extra precautions to stay cool

Treatment of overdose: Lavage if orally ingested; provide an airway; do not induce vomiting

---

thyroid USP (desiccated) (℞)

(thye′roid)

Armour Thyroid, Cholaxin*, S-P-T, Thyrar, Thyroid Strong, Thyroid USP

Func. class.: Thyroid hormone
Chem. class.: Active thyroid hormone in natural state and ratio

Action: Increases metabolic rates, increases cardiac output, O_2 consumption, body temp, blood volume, growth, development at cellular level

Uses: Hypothyroidism, cretinism (juvenile hypothyroidism), myxedema

Dosage and routes:
Hypothyroidism

• *Adult:* **PO** 65 mg qd, increased by 65 mg q30d until desired response; maintenance dose 65-195 mg qd

• *Elderly:* **PO** 7.5-15 mg qd, double dose q6-8wk until desired response

Cretinism/juvenile hypothyroidism

• *Child over 1 yr:* **PO** up to 180 mg qd titrated to response

• *Child 4-12 mo:* **PO** 30-60 mg qd

• *Child 1-4 mo:* **PO** 15-30 mg qd; may increase q2wk; titrated to response; maintenance dose 30-45 mg qd

Myxedema

• *Adult:* **PO** 16 mg qd, double dose q2wk, maintenance 65-195 mg/day

Available forms: Tabs 16, 32, 65, 98, 130, 195, 260, 325 mg; tabs enteric coated 32, 65, 130 mg; sugar-coated tabs 32, 65, 130, 195 mg; caps 65, 130, 195, 325 mg

Side effects/adverse reactions:
CNS: Insomnia, tremors, headache, *thyroid storm*

CV: Tachycardia, palpitations, angina, dysrhythmias, hypertension, *cardiac arrest*

GI: Nausea, diarrhea, increased or decreased appetite, cramps

MISC: Menstrual irregularities, weight loss, sweating, heat intolerance, fever

Contraindications: Adrenal insufficiency, MI, thyrotoxicosis

Precautions: Elderly, angina pectoris, hypertension, ischemia, cardiac disease, pregnancy (A), lactation

Pharmacokinetics:
PO: Peak 12-48 hr, half-life 6-7 days

Interactions:

• Decreased absorption of thyroid: cholestyramine

• Increased effects of anticoagulants, sympathomimetics, tricyclic antidepressants, catecholamines

• Decreased effects of digitalis drugs, insulin, hypoglycemics

• Decreased effects of thyroid: estrogens

⬥ = Nursing alert   🌿 = Herb-drug interaction   🚫 = Do not crush

⚠ Do not use with: bugleweed

Lab test interferences:

Increase: CPK, LDH, AST, PBI, blood glucose

Decrease: TSH, ^{131}I uptake test, uric acid, triglycerides

NURSING CONSIDERATIONS

Assess:

• B/P, pulse before each dose
• I&O ratio
• Weight qd in same clothing, using same scale, at same time of day
• Height, growth rate of child
• T_3, T_4, which are decreased; radioimmunoassay of TSH, which is increased; radio uptake, which is decreased if dosage is too low
• Pro-time may require decreased anticoagulant; check for bleeding, bruising
• Increased nervousness, excitability, irritability; may indicate too high dose of medication, usually after 1-3 wk of treatment
• Cardiac status: angina, palpitation, chest pain, change in VS

Administer:

• In AM if possible as a single dose to decrease sleeplessness
• At same time each day to maintain drug level
• Only for hormone imbalances; not to be used for obesity, male infertility, menstrual disorders, lethargy
• Lowest dose that relieves symptoms

Perform/provide:

• Removal of medication 4 wk before RAIU test

Evaluate:

• Therapeutic response: absence of depression; increased weight loss, diuresis, pulse, appetite; absence of constipation, peripheral edema, cold intolerance; pale, cool, dry skin; brittle nails, alopecia, coarse hair, menorrhagia, night blindness, paresthesias, syncope, stupor, coma, rosy cheeks

Teach patient/family:

• That hair loss will occur in child, is temporary
• To report excitability, irritability, anxiety; indicates overdose
• Not to switch brands unless directed by prescriber
• That hypothyroid child will show almost immediate behavior/personality change
• That treatment drug is not to be taken to reduce weight
• To avoid OTC preparations with iodine; read labels
• To avoid iodine food, iodized salt, soybeans, tofu, turnips, some seafood, some bread

---

tiagabine (℞)

(tie-ah-ga′been)

Gabatril

Func. class.: Anticonvulsant

Action: Mechanism unknown; may increase seizure threshold; structurally similar to GABA; tiagabine binding sites in neocortex, hippocampus

Uses: Adjunct treatment of partial seizures

Dosage and routes:

• *Adult:* **PO** 4 mg qd, may increase by 4-8 mg qwk until desired response, max 32 mg/day
• *Child 12-18 yr:* **PO** 4 mg qd, may increase by 4 mg at beginning of wk 2; may increase by 4-8 mg qwk until desired response; max 32 mg/day

Available forms: Tabs 4, 12, 16, 20 mg

Side effects/adverse reactions:

CNS: Dizziness, anxiety, somnolence, ataxia, amnesia, unsteady gait, depression

CV: Vasodilation

GI: Nausea, vomiting, diarrhea

INTEG: Pruritus, rash

RESP: Pharyngitis, coughing

T

Contraindications: Hypersensitivity to this drug

Precautions: Hepatic disease, renal disease, pregnancy (C), lactation, children <12 yr, elderly

Pharmacokinetics: Absorption >95%, half-life 7-9 hrs

Interactions:
Unknown

NURSING CONSIDERATIONS
Assess:
• Renal studies: urinalysis, BUN, urine creatinine q3mo
• Hepatic studies: ALT, AST, bilirubin
• Description of seizures
• Mental status: mood, sensorium, affect, behavioral changes; if mental status changes, notify prescriber
• Eye problems, need for ophthalmic examinations before, during, after treatment (slit lamp, funduscopy, tonometry)
• Allergic reaction: purpura, red raised rash; if these occur, drug should be discontinued

Perform/provide:
• Storage at room temp away from heat and light
• Hard candy, frequent rinsing of mouth, gum for dry mouth
• Assistance with ambulation during early part of treatment; dizziness occurs
• Seizure precautions: padded side rails; move objects that may harm patient
• Increased fluids, bulk in diet for constipation

Evaluate:
• Therapeutic response: decreased seizure activity; document on patient's chart

Teach patient/family:
• To carry Medic Alert ID stating patient's name, drugs taken, condition, prescriber's name and phone number

• To avoid driving, other activities that require alertness
• Not to discontinue medication quickly after long-term use

Treatment of overdose: Lavage, VS

---

ticarcillin (R)
(tye-kar-sill′in)
Ticar
Func. class.: Broad-spectrum antiinfective
Chem. class.: Extended-spectrum penicillin

Action: Interferes with cell wall replication of susceptible organisms; osmotically unstable cell wall swells, bursts from osmotic pressure.

Uses: Respiratory, soft tissue, urinary tract infections, bacterial septicemia; effective for gram-positive cocci *(Staphylococcus aureus, Streptococcus faecalis, S. pneumoniae),* gram-negative cocci *(Neisseria gonorrhoeae),* gram-positive bacilli *(Clostridium perfringens, C. tetani),* gram-negative bacilli *(Bacteroides, Fusobacterium nucleatum, Escherichia coli, Proteus mirabilis, Salmonella, Morganella morganii, Proteus rettgeri, Enterobacter, Pseudomonas aeruginosa, Serratia, Peptococcus, Peptostreptococcus, Eubacterium)*

Dosage and routes:
• Dosage reduction needed for renal impairment CrCl <30 ml/min
• *Adult:* **IV/IM** 4-24 g/day in divided doses q4-6h; infuse over ½-2 hr
• *Child:* **IV/IM** 50-300 mg/kg/day in divided doses q4-8h
• *Neonate:* **IV INF** 75-100 mg/kg/ 8-12 hr

Available forms: Inj 1, 3, 6, 20, 30 g

Side effects/adverse reactions:
HEMA: Anemia, increased bleeding

◆ = Nursing alert   ∮ = Herb-drug interaction   ⊘ = Do not crush time, ***bone marrow depression, granulocytopenia***

GI: Nausea, vomiting, diarrhea; increased AST, ALT; abdominal pain, glossitis, colitis

GU: Oliguria, proteinuria, hematuria, *vaginitis, moniliasis, **glomerulonephritis***

CNS: Lethargy, hallucinations, anxiety, depression, twitching, ***coma, convulsions***

INTEG: Rash

META: Hypokalemia

Contraindications: Hypersensitivity to penicillins

Precautions: Hypersensitivity to cephalosporins, pregnancy (B), lactation, renal disease

Pharmacokinetics:

IM: Peak 1 hr, duration 4-6 hr

IV: Peak 30-45 min, duration 4 hr, half-life 70 min; small amount metabolized in liver; excreted in urine, breast milk

Interactions:

• Decreased antimicrobial effect of ticarcillin: tetracyclines, aminoglycosides IV

• Increased effect of: neuromuscular blockers, heparin

• Increased ticarcillin concentrations: aspirin, probenecid

🚩 Delayed/reduced absorption: khat, separate by ≥2 hr

Lab test interferences:

False positive: Urine glucose, urine protein

NURSING CONSIDERATIONS

Assess:

• I&O ratio; report hematuria, oliguria, since penicillin in high doses is nephrotoxic

🔻 Any patient with compromised renal system, since drug is excreted slowly in poor renal system function; toxicity may occur rapidly

• Liver studies: AST, ALT

• Blood studies: WBC, RBC, Hgb, Hct, bleeding time

• Renal studies: urinalysis, protein, blood, BUN, creatinine

• C&S before drug therapy; drug may be given as soon as culture is taken

• Bowel pattern before, during treatment

• Skin eruptions after administration of penicillin to 1 wk after discontinuing drug

• Respiratory status: rate, character, wheezing, tightness in chest

• Allergies before initiation of treatment, reaction of each medication; highlight allergies on chart

Administer:

• Drug after C&S has been completed

IV

• After diluting 1 g or less/4 ml sterile H$_2$O for inj; dilute further with 10-20 ml or more D$_5$W, NS, or sterile H$_2$O for inj sol; give 1 g or less/5 min or more or by intermittent inf over ½-2 hr or by continuous inf at prescribed rate

Additive compatibilities: Ranitidine, verapamil

Y-site compatibilities: Acyclovir, allopurinol, amifostine, aztreonam, cisatracurium, cyclophosphamide, diltiazem, doxorubicin, famotidine, filgrastim, fludarabine, granisetron, heparin, hydromorphone, IL-2, insulin (regular), magnesium sulfate, melphalan, meperidine, morphine, ondansetron, perphenazine, propofol, remifentanil, sargramostim, teniposide, theophylline, thiotepa, verapamil, vinorelbine

Perform/provide:

• Adrenalin, suction, tracheostomy set, endotracheal intubation equipment

• Adequate fluid intake (2 L) during diarrhea episodes

• Scratch test to assess allergy on

order from prescriber; usually done when penicillin is only drug of choice

• Storage at room temp, reconstituted sol 72 hr at room temp

Evaluate:

• Therapeutic response: absence of fever, purulent drainage, redness, inflammation

Teach patient/family:

• That culture may be taken after completed course of medication

• To report sore throat, fever, fatigue (may indicate superinfection)

• To wear or carry Medic Alert ID if allergic to penicillins

• To notify nurse of diarrhea

Treatment of overdose: Withdraw drug, maintain airway, administer epinephrine, aminophylline, O_2, IV corticosteroids for anaphylaxis

---

ticarcillin/ clavulanate (℞)

Timentin

Func. class.: Broad-spectrum antiinfective

Chem. class.: Extended-spectrum penicillin

Action: Interferes with cell wall replication of susceptible organisms; osmotically unstable cell wall swells, bursts from osmotic pressure

Uses: Respiratory, soft tissue, and urinary tract infections, bacterial septicemia; effective for gram-positive cocci *(Staphylococcus aureus, Streptococcus faecalis, S. pneumoniae),* gram-negative cocci *(Neisseria gonorrhoeae),* gram-positive bacilli *(Clostridium perfringens, C. tetani),* gram-negative bacilli *(Bacteroides, Fusobacterium nucleatum, Escherichia coli, Proteus mirabilis, Salmonella, Morganella morganii, Proteus rettgeri, Enterobacter, Pseu-* *domonas aeruginosa, Serratia, Peptococcus, Peptostreptococcus, Eubacterium)*

Dosage and routes:

• Dosage reduction indicated in renal impairment (CrCl <30 ml/min)

• *Adult:* **IV INF** 1 vial containing ticarcillin 3 g, clavulanate 0.1 g q4-6h, infuse over 30 min

• *Child <60 kg:* **IV INF** 200-300 mg ticarcillin/kg/day in divided doses q4-6h

Available forms: Inj 3 g ticarcillin, 0.1 g clavulanate; IV inf 3 g ticarcillin, 0.1 g clavulanate; discs 75 µg ticarcillin, 10 µg clavulanate; powder for inj 3 g ticarcillin, 0.1 g clavulanate; 30 g ticarcillin, 1 g clavulanate

Side effects/adverse reactions:

HEMA: Anemia, increased bleeding time, *bone marrow depression, granulocytopenia*

GI: Nausea, vomiting, diarrhea; increased AST, ALT; abdominal pain, glossitis, colitis

GU: Oliguria, proteinuria, hematuria, *vaginitis, moniliasis, glomerulonephritis*

CNS: Lethargy, hallucinations, anxiety, depression, twitching, *coma, convulsions*

META: Hyperkalemia, hypokalemia, alkalosis, hypernatremia

Contraindications: Hypersensitivity to penicillins; neonates

Precautions: Hypersensitivity to cephalosporins, pregnancy (B), renal disease

Pharmacokinetics:

IV: Peak 30-45 min, duration 4 hr, half-life 64-68 min; excreted in urine

Interactions:

• Decreased antimicrobial effect of ticarcillin: tetracyclines, aminoglycosides IV

• Increased effect of: neuromuscular blockers, heparin

◆ = Nursing alert   🖉 = Herb-drug interaction   🚫 = Do not crush

• Increased ticarcillin concentrations: aspirin, probenecid

🖉 Delayed/reduced absorption: khat, separate by ≥2 hr

Lab test interferences:

False positive: Urine glucose, urine protein, Coombs' test

NURSING CONSIDERATIONS

Assess:

• I&O ratio; report hematuria, oliguria, since penicillin in high doses is nephrotoxic

◆ Any patient with compromised renal system, since drug is excreted slowly in poor renal system function; toxicity may occur rapidly

• Liver studies: AST, ALT

• Blood studies: WBC, RBC, Hct, Hgb, bleeding time

• Renal studies: urinalysis, protein, blood, BUN, creatinine

• C&S before drug therapy; drug may be given as soon as culture is taken

• Bowel pattern before, during treatment

• Skin eruptions after administration of penicillin to 1 wk after discontinuing drug

• Respiratory status: rate, character, wheezing, and tightness in chest

• Allergies before initiation of treatment, reaction of each medication; highlight allergies on chart

Administer:

• Drug after C&S

IV

• After diluting 3.1 g or less/13 ml of sterile H_2O or NaCl (200 mg/ml), shake; may further dilute in 50-100 ml or more NS, D_5W, or LR sol and run over ½ hr

Y-site compatibilities: Allopurinol, amifostine, aztreonam, cefepime, cyclophosphamide, diltiazem, doxorubicin liposome, famotidine, filgrastim, fluconazole, fludarabine, foscarnet, gallium, granisetron, heparin, insulin (regular) melphalan, meperidine, morphine, ondansetron, perphenazine, propofol, remifentanil, sargramostim, teniposide, theophylline, thiotepa, vinorelbine

Perform/provide:

• Adrenaline, suction, tracheostomy set, endotracheal intubation equipment

• Adequate fluid intake (2 L) during diarrhea episodes

• Scratch test to assess allergy on order from prescriber; usually done when penicillin is only drug of choice

• Storage of reconstituted sol 12-24 hr at room temp, or 3-7 days refrigerated

Evaluate:

• Therapeutic response: absence of fever, purulent drainage, redness, inflammation

Teach patient/family:

• To report persistent diarrhea

• That culture may be taken after completed course of medication

• To report sore throat, fever, fatigue (may indicate superinfection)

• To wear or carry Medic Alert ID if allergic to penicillins

Treatment of overdose: Withdraw drug, maintain airway, administer epinephrine, O_2, IV corticosteroids for anaphylaxis

---

ticlopidine (℞)

(tye-cloe'pi-deen)

Ticlid

Func. class.: Platelet aggregation inhibitor

Action: Inhibits first and second phases of ADP-induced effects in platelet aggregation

Uses: Reducing the risk of stroke in high-risk patients

Investigational uses: Intermittent claudication, chronic arterial occlusion, subarachnoid hemorrhage, ure-

---

Side effects: *italics* = common; ***bold italics*** = life-threatening

mic patients with AV shunts/fistulas, open heart surgery, coronary artery bypass grafts, primary glomerulonephritis, sickle cell disease

Dosage and routes:
• *Adult:* **PO** 250 mg bid with food
Available forms: Tabs 250 mg

Side effects/adverse reactions:
INTEG: Rash, pruritus
GI: Nausea, vomiting, *diarrhea,* GI discomfort, *cholestatic jaundice, hepatitis,* increased cholesterol, LDL, VLDL, TG
HEMA: Bleeding (epistaxis, hematuria, conjunctival hemorrhage, GI bleeding), agranulocytosis, neutropenia, thrombocytopenia, thrombotic thombocytopenic purpura
CNS: Dizziness

Contraindications: Hypersensitivity, active liver disease, blood dyscrasias, active bleeding

Precautions: Past liver disease, renal disease, elderly, pregnancy (B), lactation, children, increased bleeding risk

Pharmacokinetics: Peak 1-3 hr, metabolized by liver, excreted in urine, feces; half-life increases with repeated dosing

Interactions:
• Increased bleeding tendencies: anticoagulants, aspirin
• Decreased plasma levels of ticlopidine: antacids
• Decreased plasma levels of digoxin
• Increased effects of ticlopidine: cimetidine
• Increased effects of theophylline

NURSING CONSIDERATIONS
Assess:
• Liver function studies: AST, ALT, bilirubin, creatinine (long-term therapy)
• Blood studies: CBC; CBC q2 wk × 3 mo, Hct, Hgb, pro-time (long-term therapy)

Administer:
• With food to decrease gastric symptoms

Evaluate:
• Therapeutic response: absence of stroke

Teach patient/family:
• That blood work will be necessary during treatment
• To report any unusual bleeding to prescriber
• To take with food or just after eating to minimize GI discomfort
• To report side effects such as diarrhea, skin rashes, subcutaneous bleeding, signs of cholestasis (jaundiced skin and sclera, dark urine, light-colored stools)

---

tiludronate (℞)
(till-oo'droe-nate)
Skelid
Func. class.: Parathyroid agent (calcium regulator)
Chem. class.: Bisphosphonate

Action: Decreases bone resorption and new bone development
Uses: Paget's disease
Dosage and routes:
• *Adult:* **PO** 400 mg qd, with 8 oz water × 3 mo
Available forms: Tabs 240 mg (equal to 200/mg tiludronic acid)

Side effects/adverse reactions:
GI: Nausea, diarrhea, dry mouth, gastritis, vomiting, flatulence, gastric ulcers
RESP: Rhinitis, rales, sinusitis, URI
CNS: Headache, somnolence, dizziness, anxiety, vertigo, nervousness, involuntary movements
ENDO: Hyperparathyroidism
INTEG: Rash, epidermal necrosis, pruritus, sweating
GU: Nephrotoxicity, UTI
MS: Bone pain, decreased mineral-

⬦ = Nursing alert   ⫸ = Herb-drug interaction   ⊘ = Do not crush ization of nonaffected bones, pathological fractures

Contraindications: Hypersensitivity to bisphosphonates, pathologic fractures, children, colitis, severe renal disease with creatinine >5 mg/dl

Precautions: Pregnancy (C), renal disease, lactation, restricted vit D/Ca, GI disease

Pharmacokinetics:

Half-life 150 hr; duration 6 mo

Interactions:

• Decreased absorption of tiludronate: antacids, mineral supplements with magnesium, calcium, aluminum, aspirin

• Increased effect of tiludronate: indomethacin

NURSING CONSIDERATIONS
Assess:

• GI symptoms, polyuria, flushing, head swelling, tingling, headache—may indicate hypercalcemia; nervousness, irritability, twitching, seizures, spasm, paresthesia indicates hypocalcemia at start of treatment

• Nutritional status; evaluate diet for sources of vitamin D (milk, some seafood), calcium (dairy products, dark green vegetables), phosphates

• BUN, creatinine, uric acid, chloride, electrolytes, urine pH, urinary calcium, magnesium, phosphate, urinalysis (calcium should be kept at 9-10 mg/dl), albumin, alk phosphatase baseline and q3-6 mo; check urine sediment for casts throughout treatment

• For increased drug level—toxic reactions occur rapidly; have calcium chloride or gluconate on hand if calcium level drops too low; check for tetany

Administer:

• On empty stomach to improve absorption (2 hr ac), with 6-8 oz water

Evaluate:

• Therapeutic response: calcium levels 9-10 mg/dl; decreasing symptoms of Paget's disease

Teach patient/family:

• To notify prescriber of hypercalcemic relapse: renal calculi, nausea, vomiting, thirst, lethargy, deep bone or flank pain

• To follow a low-calcium diet as prescribed (Paget's disease, hypercalcemia)

• To notify prescriber of diarrhea, nausea; dose may be divided to lessen these symptoms

---

timolol (℞)

(tye′moe-lole)

Blocadren, timolol maleate

Func. class.: Antihypertensive

Chem. class.: Nonselective β-blocker

Action: Competitively blocks stimulation of β-adrenergic receptor within vascular smooth muscle (decreases rate of SA node discharge, increases recovery time), slows conduction of AV node, decreases heart rate, which decreases O_2 consumption in myocardium; also decreases renin-aldosterone-angiotensin system, at high doses inhibits $β_2$-receptors in bronchial system

Uses: Mild to moderate hypertension, sinus tachycardia, persistent atrial extrasystoles, tachydysrhythmias, prophylaxis of angina pectoris, reduction of mortality after MI, migraine prevention

Investigational uses: Mitral valve prolapse, hypertrophic cardiomyopathy, thyrotoxicosis, tremors, anxiety, pheochromocytoma, tachydysrhythmias, angina pectoris

Dosage and routes:

Hypertension

• *Adult:* **PO** 10 mg bid, or 20 mg qd,

T

Side effects: *italics* = common; ***bold italics*** = life-threatening

may increase by 10 mg q2-3d, not to exceed 60 mg/day

Myocardial infarction

• *Adult:* **PO** 10 mg bid beginning 1-4 wks after MI

Migraine headache prevention

• *Adult:* **PO** 10 mg bid or 20 mg qd; may increase to 30 mg/day, 20 mg in AM, 10 mg in PM

Available forms: Tabs 5, 10, 20 mg

Side effects/adverse reactions:

CV: Hypotension, bradycardia, *CHF,* edema, chest pain, claudication

CNS: Insomnia, dizziness, hallucinations, anxiety

GI: Nausea, vomiting, *ischemic colitis,* diarrhea, *abdominal pain, mesenteric arterial thrombosis*

INTEG: Rash, alopecia, pruritus, fever

HEMA: Agranulocytosis, thrombocytopenia, purpura

EENT: Visual changes, sore throat, *double vision,* dry burning eyes

GU: Impotence, urinary frequency

RESP: Bronchospasm, dyspnea, cough, rales

META: Hypoglycemia

MUSC: Joint pain, muscle pain

Contraindications: Hypersensitivity to β-blockers, cardiogenic shock, heart block (2nd or 3rd degree), sinus bradycardia, CHF, cardiac failure

Precautions: Major surgery, pregnancy (C), lactation, diabetes mellitus, renal disease, thyroid disease, COPD, well-compensated heart failure, CAD, nonallergic bronchospasm

Pharmacokinetics:

PO: Peak 2-4 hr; half-life 3-4 hr; excreted 30%-45% unchanged; 60%-65% metabolized by liver; excreted in urine, breast milk

Interactions:

• Increased hypotension, bradycardia: reserpine, hydralazine, methyldopa, prazosin, anticholinergics, alcohol, reserpine, nitrates

• Decreased antihypertensive effects: indomethacin, thyroid

• Increased hypoglycemic effects: insulin, sulfonylureas

• Decreased bronchodilation: theophyllines

Lab test interferences:

Increase: Liver function tests, renal function tests, K, uric acid

Decrease: Hct, Hgb, HDL

NURSING CONSIDERATIONS

Assess:

• I&O, weight qd

• B/P during initial treatment, periodically thereafter, pulse q4h; note rate, rhythm, quality

• Apical/radial pulse before administration; notify prescriber of any significant changes

• Baselines in renal, liver function tests before therapy begins

• Edema in feet, legs qd

• Skin turgor, dryness of mucous membranes for hydration status

Administer:

• PO ac, hs, tablet may be crushed or swallowed whole

• Reduced dosage in renal dysfunction

Perform/provide:

• Dry storage at room temp; do not freeze

Evaluate:

• Therapeutic response: decreased B/P after 1-2 wk

Teach patient/family:

• To take with or immediately after meals

• Not to discontinue drug abruptly; taper over 2 wk; may cause precipitate angina

• Not to use OTC products containing α-adrenergic stimulants (nasal decongestants, cold preparations) unless directed by prescriber

• To report bradycardia, dizziness, confusion, depression, fever, sore throat, shortness of breath to prescriber

◆ = Nursing alert   ⫸ = Herb-drug interaction   ⊘ = Do not crush

• To take pulse at home; advise when to notify prescriber
• To avoid alcohol, smoking, sodium intake
• To comply with weight control, dietary adjustments, modified exercise program
• To carry Medic Alert ID to identify drug, allergies
• To avoid hazardous activities if dizziness is present
• To report symptoms of CHF: difficult breathing, especially on exertion or when lying down; night cough; swelling of extremities
• To take medication hs to minimize effect of orthostatic hypotension
• To wear support hose to minimize effects of orthostatic hypotension

Treatment of overdose: Lavage, IV atropine for bradycardia, IV theophylline for bronchospasm, digitalis, O_2, diuretic for cardiac failure, hemodialysis; administer vasopressor (norepinephrine)

---

tioronin (℞)

(tye-o-pro'nen)
Thiola
Func. class.: Cystine-depleting agent
Chem. class.: Active reducing, complexing thiol compound

Action: Prevents cystine (kidney) stone formation by increasing amount of water-soluble cystine
Uses: Prevention of kidney stone formation in patients with severe homozygous cystinuria with urinary cystine greater than 500 mg/day, who are resistant to conservative treatment

Dosage and routes:
• *Adult:* PO 800-1000 mg/day, given

in divided doses tid at least 1 hr before or 2 hr after meals
• *Child:* PO 15 mg/kg/day, given in divided doses tid at least 1 hr before or 2 hr after meals
Available forms: Tabs 100 mg
Side effects/adverse reactions:
MISC: Blunting of taste
INTEG: Erythema, maculopapular rash, wrinkling skin, lupuslike syndrome (fever, arthralgia, lymphadenopathy), pruritus
CNS: Drug fever
META: Vit B_6 deficiency
Contraindications: History of agranulocytosis, thrombocytopenia, aplastic anemia
Precautions: Pregnancy (C), lactation, myasthenia gravis, Goodpasture's syndrome, children <9 yr
Pharmacokinetics: Reduction of urinary cystine of 250-500 mg on 1-2 g/day may be expected; excreted in urine 78% in 3 days
NURSING CONSIDERATIONS
Assess:
• I&O during treatment; check urine for stones; strain all urine, keep output at 2 L/day
• Diet for alkaline foods: dairy products; prevent overindulgence of Na, alkali foods, since hypercalcinuria results
• Urine pH; notify prescriber of pH over 7
• Urinary cystine 1 mo after treatment, q3mo thereafter
Administer:
PO
• After adequate hydration, conservative treatment: 3 L/day fluid, 16 oz fluid at meals and hs
Perform/provide:
• Storage at room temp
Evaluate:
• Therapeutic response: decrease in urinary cystine to <250 mg/L, absence of pain, hematuria

T

Teach patient/family:
• To watch for lupuslike syndrome: fever, joint pain, swollen lymph glands; drug may have to be discontinued

---

tirofiban (℞)

(tie-roh-fee′ban)
Aggrastat
Func. class.: Antiplatelet
Chem. class.: Nonpeptide antagonist

Action: Activation of platelet glycoprotein (GP) IIb/IIIa receptor that leads to binding of fibrinogen and von Willebrand's factor, which causes platelet aggregation

Uses: Acute coronary syndrome

Dosage and routes:
• *Adult:* **IV** 0.4 µg/kg/min×30 min, then 0.1 µg/kg/min; give ½ dose in renal disease

Available forms: Inj for sol 250 µg/ml, inj 50 µg/ml

Side effects/adverse reactions:
CV: Bradycardia
CNS: Dizziness
INTEG: Rash
*HEMA: **Bleeding***
OTHER: Dissection, coronary artery edema, pain in legs/pelvis, sweating

Contraindications: Hypersensitivity, active internal bleeding, stroke, major surgery, severe trauma, intracranial neoplasm, aneurysm, hemorrhage

Precautions: Pregnancy (B), lactation, elderly, renal disease, bleeding tendencies

Pharmocokinetics: Half-life 2 hr, excretion via urine/feces; plasma clearance 20%-25% lower in elderly; renal insufficiency decreases plasma clearance

Interactions:
• Increased bleeding: aspirin, heparin

• Increased clearance of tirofiban: levothyroxine, omeprazole

NURSING CONSIDERATIONS
Assess:
• B/P pulse during treatment until stable; take B/P lying, standing; orthostatic hypotension is common
• Platelet counts, Hct, Hgb, prior to treatment, within 6 hr of loading dose and at least qd thereafter

Administer:
• IV: Give ½ dose in renal disease
• Dilute inj: withdraw and discard 100 ml from a 500 ml bag of sterile 0.9% NaCl or D₅W and replace this vol with 50 ml of tirofiban inj from one vial
• Tirofiban inj for sol is premixed in containers of 500 ml 0.9% NaCl (50 mg/ml)
• Minimize other arterial/venous punctures; IM inj, catheter use, intubation, to reduce bleeding risks

Evaluate:
• Therapeutic response: decreased platelet count

Teach patient/family:
• That it is necessary to quit smoking to prevent excessive vasoconstriction
• To avoid hazardous activities; dizziness may occur

---

tizanidine

(ti-za′nih-deen)
Zanaflex
Func. class.: Skeletal muscle relaxant, α₂-adrenergic agonist
Chem. class.: Imidazoline

Action: Increases presynaptic inhibition of motor neurons and reduces spasticity by α₂-adrenergic agonism

Uses: Acute/intermittent management of increased muscle tone associated with spasticity

---

 = Nursing alert   = Herb-drug interaction   ⊘ = Do not crush

Dosage and routes:
• *Adult:* **PO** 8 mg, increase gradually by 2-4 mg increments, may repeat dose q6-8h, not to exceed 36 mg/24 hr
Available forms: Tabs 4 mg
Side effects/adverse reactions:
GI: Dry mouth, vomiting, increased ALT, abnormal liver function studies, constipation
CNS: Somnolence, dizziness, speech disorder, dyskinesia, nervousness, hallucination, psychosis
OTHER: UTI, infection, blurred vision, urinary frequency, flulike syndrome, pharyngitis, rhinitis
Contraindications: Hypersensitivity
Precautions: Hypotension, liver disease, pregnancy (C), lactation, elderly, children, renal disease
Pharmacokinetics: Completely absorbed, widely distributed; half-life 2.5 hr, peak 1½ hr; protein binding 30%; metabolized by liver, excreted in urine, feces
Interactions:
• Increased CNS depression: alcohol
• Decreased clearance of tizanidine: oral contraceptives
NURSING CONSIDERATIONS
Assess:
• For hypotension, gradual dosage increase should lessen hypotensive effects; have patient rise slowly from supine to upright; watch those patients receiving antihypertensives for increased effects
• For increased sedation, dizziness, hallucinations, psychosis; drug may need to be discontinued
• Vision by ophthalmic exam, corneal opacities may occur
• Liver function studies: 1, 3, 6 mo during treatment and periodically thereafter

Teach patient/family:
• To rise slowly from lying or sitting to upright position
• To ask for assistance if dizziness, sedation occur; to avoid drinking alcohol, to avoid operating machinery or driving until effects are known

---

tobramycin (℞)
(toe-bra-mye′sin)
Nebcin, TOBI, tobramycin sulfate, Tobrax
Func. class.: Antiinfective
Chem. class.: Aminoglycoside

Action: Interferes with protein synthesis in bacterial cell by binding to ribosomal subunit, causing inaccurate peptide sequence to form in protein chain, causing bacterial death
Uses: Severe systemic infections of CNS, respiratory, GI, urinary tract, bone, skin, soft tissues caused by *Pseudomonas aeruginosa, Escherichia coli, Enterobacter, Providencia, Citrobacter, Staphylococcus, Proteus, Klebsiella, Serratia;* cystic fibrosis (nebulizer) for *Pseudomonas aeruginosa*
Dosage and routes:
• *Adult:* **IM/IV** 3 mg/kg/day in divided doses q8h; may give up to 5 mg/kg/day in divided doses q6-8h; once qd dosing is an option
• *Child:* **IM/IV** 6-7.5 mg/kg/day in 3-4 equal divided doses
• *Child ≥6 yr:* **NEB** 300 mg bid in repeating cycles of 28 days on/28 days off of drug; give **INH** over 10-15 min using a hand-held PARI LC PLUS reusable nebulizer with a DeVilbiss Pulmo-Aid compressor
• *Neonate <1 wk:* **IM** up to 4 mg/kg/day in divided doses q12h; **IV** up to 4 mg/kg/day in divided doses q12h diluted in 50-100 mg NS or D_5W; give over 30-60 min

T

Available forms: Inj 10, 40 mg/ml; powder for inj 1.2 g; inj 20 mg/2 ml; neb sol 300 mg/5 ml

Side effects/adverse reactions:

*GU: **Oliguria, hematuria, renal damage, azotemia, renal failure, nephrotoxicity***

CNS: Confusion, depression, numbness, tremors, ***convulsions,*** muscle twitching, ***neurotoxicity,*** dizziness, vertigo

*EENT: **Ototoxicity,** deafness, visual disturbances, tinnitus*

*HEMA: **Agranulocytosis, thrombocytopenia, leukopenia, eosinophilia,** anemia*

GI: Nausea, vomiting, anorexia; increased ALT, AST, bilirubin, hepatomegaly, ***hepatic necrosis,*** splenomegaly

CV: Hypotension, hypertension, palpitation

INTEG: Rash, burning, urticaria, dermatitis, alopecia

Contraindications: Severe renal disease, hypersensitivity to aminoglycosides

Precautions: Neonates, mild renal disease, pregnancy (C), myasthenia gravis, lactation, hearing deficits, Parkinson's disease, elderly

Pharmacokinetics:

IM: Onset rapid, peak 1 hr

IV: Onset immediate, peak 1 hr
Plasma half-life 2-3 hr prolonged in neonates; not metabolized, excreted unchanged in urine, crosses placental barrier, poor penetration into CSF

Interactions:

• Increased ototoxicity, neurotoxicity, nephrotoxicity: other aminoglycosides, amphotericin B, polymyxin, vancomycin, ethacrynic acid, furosemide, mannitol, methoxyflurane, cisplatin, cephalosporins, bacitracin, acyclovir, penicillins

NURSING CONSIDERATIONS

Assess:

• Weight before treatment; dosage is usually based on ideal body weight, but may be calculated on actual body weight

• I&O ratio, urinalysis qd for proteinuria, cells, casts; report sudden change in urine output

• VS during infusion; watch for hypotension, change in pulse

• IV site for thrombophlebitis, including pain, redness, swelling q30min; change site if needed; apply warm compresses to discontinued site

• Serum peak, drawn at 30-60 min after IV infusion or 60 min after IM injection, trough drawn just before next dose, peak 4-12 µg/ml, trough 1-2 µg/ml

• Urine pH if drug is used for UTI; urine should be kept alkaline

• Renal impairment by securing urine for CrCl testing, BUN, serum creatinine; lower dosage should be given in renal impairment (CrCl <80 ml/min); monitor electrolytes: potassium, sodium, chloride, magnesium monthly, if patient is on long-term therapy

• Deafness by audiometric testing; ringing, roaring in ears; vertigo; assess hearing before, during, after treatment

• Dehydration: high specific gravity, decrease in skin turgor, dry mucous membranes, dark urine

• Overgrowth of infection: fever, malaise, redness, pain, swelling, perineal itching, diarrhea, stomatitis, change in cough, sputum

• C&S before starting treatment to identify infecting organism

• Vestibular dysfunction: nausea, vomiting, dizziness, headache; drug should be discontinued if severe

• Inj sites for redness, swelling, abscesses; use warm compresses at site

Administer:

• IM inj in large muscle mass; rotate inj sites

◆ = Nursing alert   ∥ = Herb-drug interaction   ⊘ = Do not crush

• Drug in evenly spaced doses to maintain blood level; separate aminoglycosides and penicillins by ≥1 hr

• Bicarbonate to alkalinize urine if ordered in treating UTI, as drug is most active in an alkaline environment

IV

• Diluted in 50-100 ml 0.9% NaCl or D_5W (adult), infuse over 20-60 min

Additive compatibilities: Aztreonam, bleomycin, calcium gluconate, cefoxitin, ciprofloxacin, clindamycin, furosemide, metronidazole, ofloxacin, ranitidine, verapamil

Syringe compatibilities: Doxapram

Y-site compatibilities: Acyclovir, amifostine, amiodarone, amsacrine, aztreonam, ciprofloxacin, cisatracurium, cyclophosphamide, diltiazem, doxorubicin liposome, enalaprilat, esmolol, filgrastim, fluconazole, fludarabine, foscarnet, furosemide, granisetron, hydromorphone, IL-2, insulin (regular), labetalol, magnesium sulfate, melphalan, meperidine, midazolam, morphine, perphenazine, remifentanil, tacrolimus, teniposide, theophylline, thiotepa, tolazoline, vinorelbine, zidovudine

Nebulizer

• Give as close to q12hr apart as possible; do not use <6hr apart

• Do not mix with dornase alfa in the nebulizer

Perform/provide:

• Adequate fluids of 2-3 L/day unless contraindicated to prevent irritation of tubules

• Flush of IV line with NS or D_5W after infusion

• Supervised ambulation, other safety measures with vestibular dysfunction

Evaluate:

• Therapeutic response: absence of fever, draining wounds, negative C&S after treatment

Teach patient/family:

• To report headache, dizziness, symptoms of overgrowth of infection, renal impairment

• To report loss of hearing; ringing, roaring in ears; feeling of fullness in head

Nebulizer

• Have patient inhale sitting or standing, breathe normally through the mouthpiece, may use noseclips

• To use multiple therapies first, then tobramycin

Treatment of overdose: Hemodialysis; monitor serum levels of drug

---

tocainide (℞)

(toe-kay'nide)

Tonocard

Func. class.: Antidysrhythmic (Class Ib)

Chem. class.: Lidocaine analog

Action: Suppresses automaticity of tissue conduction and spontaneous depolarization of ventricles during diastole; does not affect heart rate

Uses: Life-threatening ventricular dysrhythmias (multifocal/unifocal PVCs), ventricular tachycardia

Dosage and routes:

• *Adult:* **PO** 400 mg q8h

Available forms: Tabs 400, 600 mg

Side effects/adverse reactions:

CNS: Headache, dizziness, involuntary movement, confusion, psychosis, restlessness, irritability, paresthesias, tremors, *seizures*

EENT: Tinnitus, blurred vision, hearing loss

GI: Nausea, vomiting, anorexia, diarrhea, hepatitis

CV: Hypotension, bradycardia, angina, PVCs, *heart block, cardio-*

---

vascular collapse, arrest, CHF, chest pain, tachycardia, prodysrhythmia

RESP: Dyspnea, *respiratory depression, pulmonary fibrosis*

INTEG: Rash, urticaria, edema, swelling

HEMA: Blood dyscrasias: leukopenia, agranulocytosis, hypoplastic anemia, thrombocytopenia

Contraindications: Hypersensitivity to amides, severe heart block

Precautions: Pregnancy (C), lactation, children, renal disease, liver disease, CHF, respiratory depression, myasthenia gravis, blood dyscrasias

Pharmacokinetics:

PO: Peak 0.5-3 hr; half-life 10-17 hr; metabolized by liver, excreted in urine

Interactions:

• Increased effects: propranolol, quinidine, all other antidysrhythmics

• Decreased tocainide effects: cimetidine, rifampin

 Potassium deficiency, antidysrhythmic action: aloe, buckthorn, cascara sagrada, senna

Lab test interferences:

Increase: CPK

False positive: ANA titer

NURSING CONSIDERATIONS

Assess:

• Chest x-ray film, pulmonary function tests, liver enzymes during treatment

• CBC during beginning treatment

• I&O ratio; check for decreasing output

• Blood levels (therapeutic level 4-10 µg/ml)

• B/P continuously for fluctuations

• Lung fields; bilateral rales may occur in CHF patient

• Increased respiration, increased pulse; drug should be discontinued

• Toxicity: fine tremors, dizziness

• Blood dyscrasias: fatigue, sore throat, fever, bruising

• Cardiac status, respiration: rate, rhythm, character

Evaluate:

• Therapeutic response: decreased dysrhythmia

Treatment of overdose: O₂, artificial ventilation, ECG; administer dopamine for circulatory depression, diazepam or thiopental for convulsions

---

tolazoline (℞)

(toe-laz′a-leen)

Priscoline

Func. class.: Peripheral vasodilator

Chem. class.: Imidazoline derivative

Action: Peripheral vasodilation occurs by direct relaxation on vascular smooth muscle; also has weak α- and β-adrenergic properties

Uses: Persistent pulmonary hypertension and hypoxic pulmonary hypertension of newborn

Dosage and routes:

• *Neonate:* **IV** 1-2 mg/kg via scalp vein; **IV INF** 1-2 mg/kg/hr

Available forms: Inj 25 mg/ml

Side effects/adverse reactions:

CV: Hypotension, tachycardia, dysrhythmias, hypertension, *cardiovascular collapse*

RESP: Pulmonary hemorrhage

GU: Edema, oliguria, hematuria

GI: Vomiting, diarrhea, peptic ulcer, *GI hemorrhage, hepatitis*

INTEG: Flushing, tingling, rash, chills, sweating, increased pilomotor activity

HEMA: Thrombocytopenia, leukopenia

Contraindications: Hypersensitivity, CVA, CAD

Precautions: Pregnancy (C), mitral stenosis
Pharmacokinetics:
IM/SC: Peak 30-60 min, duration 3-4 hr, excreted in urine, half-life 3-10 hr
Interactions:
• Increased effects with β-blockers, antihypertensives
• Decreased B/P, rebound hypertension: epinephrine
NURSING CONSIDERATIONS
Assess:
• ABGs, electrolytes, VS in newborn
• B/P, pulse during treatment until stable; take B/P lying; orthostatic hypotension is common
• Hepatic tests: AST, ALT, bilirubin; liver enzymes may increase
• Blood studies: CBC, platelets; watch for thrombocytopenia, agranulocytosis
• Hepatic involvement: vomiting, jaundice; drug should be discontinued
• For bleeding from GI tract: coffee grounds vomitus, increased pulse, pain in upper gastric area
• Affected areas for changes in temp, color
Administer:
IV
• Undiluted; give 10 mg or less over 1 min; in scalp vein may be diluted in D_5, D_5NS, LR, NS, ½NS, Ringer's sol; run over 1 hr
• Decreased dose for patients with low urine output (<1 ml/kg/h)
Additive compatibilities: Verapamil
Y-site compatibilities: Aminophylline, ampicillin, calcium gluconate, cefotaxime, cimetidine, dobutamine, dopamine, furosemide, gentamicin, phytonadione, sodium bicarbonate, tobramycin, vancomycin

Perform/provide:
• Dark storage at room temp
Evaluate:
• Therapeutic response: decrease in pulmonary hypertension or pulse volume, increased temp in extremities
Teach patient/family:
• To report jaundice, dark urine, joint pain, fatigue, malaise, bruising, easy bleeding; may indicate blood dyscrasias
Treatment of overdose: Administer IV fluids, head-low position

---

tolcapone (℞)
(toll'cah'pone)
Tasmar
Func. class.: Antiparkinson agent
Chem. class.: Catecholamine inhibitor

Action: Selective, reversible inhibitor of catecholamine; used as adjunct to levodopa/carbidopa therapy
Uses: Parkinsonism
Dosage and routes:
• *Adult:* **PO** 100-200 mg tid, with levodopa/carbidopa therapy; max 600 mg/day
Available forms: Tabs 100, 200 mg
Side effects/adverse reactions:
CNS: Dystonia, dyskinesia, dreaming, *fatigue, headache, confusion,* psychosis, hallucination, dizziness
CV: Orthostatic hypotension, chest pain, hypotension
EENT: Cataract, eye inflammation
GI: Nausea, vomiting, anorexia, abdominal distress, diarrhea, constipation, **fatal liver failure**
GU: UTI, urine discoloration, uterine tumor, micturition disorder
HEMA: **Hemolytic anemia, leukopenia, agranulocytosis**
INTEG: Sweating, alopecia

Contraindications: Hypersensitivity

Precautions: Renal disease, cardiac disease, hepatic disease, hypertension, pregnancy (C), asthma, lactation

Pharmacokinetics: Rapidly absorbed, peak 2 hr, protein binding 99%, extensively metabolized, half-life 2-3 hr, excreted in urine (60%), feces (40%)

Interactions:

• Inhibition of normal catecholamine metabolism: MAOIs, MAO-B inhibitor may be used

• May influence pharmacokinetics of: α-methyldopa, dobutamine, apomorphine, isoproterenol

NURSING CONSIDERATIONS
Assess:

• Liver function enzymes: AST, ALT, alk phosphatase, LDH, bilirubin, CBC, monitor ALT, AST q2wk × 1 yr, then q4wk × 6 mo, and q8wk thereafter; if LFTs are elevated, this drug should not be used

• Involuntary movements in parkinsonism: akinesia, tremors, staggering gait, muscle rigidity, drooling

• B/P, respiration during initial treatment; hypo/hypertension should be reported

• Mental status: affect, mood, behavioral changes

Administer:

• PO tid with levodopa/carbidopa therapy, only to be used if levodopa/carbidopa does not provide satisfactory result

Perform/provide:

• Assistance with ambulation during beginning therapy

Evaluate:

• Therapeutic response: decrease in akathisia, increased mood

Teach patient/family:

• To change positions slowly to prevent orthostatic hypotension

• That urine, sweat may change color

• That food taken within 1 hr ac or 2 hr pc decreases action of drug by 20%

• To report signs of liver injury: clay-colored stools, jaundice, fatigue, appetite loss, lethargy

• To report nausea, vomiting, anorexia

---

tolmetin (℞)

(tole′met-in)
Tolectin DS, Tolectin 200, Tolectin 600, tolmetin sodium
Func. class.: Nonsteroidal antiinflammatory
Chem. class.: Pyrrole acetic acid derivative

Action: Inhibits prostaglandin synthesis by decreasing an enzyme needed for biosynthesis; analgesic, antiinflammatory, antipyretic

Uses: Mild to moderate pain, osteoarthritis, rheumatoid arthritis

Dosage and routes:

• *Adult:* **PO** 400 mg tid-qid, not to exceed 2 g/day

• *Child >2 yr:* **PO** 15-30 mg/kg/day in 3 or 4 divided doses

Available forms: Caps 400 mg; tabs 200, 600 mg

Side effects/adverse reactions:

GI: Nausea, anorexia, vomiting, diarrhea, jaundice, *cholestatic hepatitis,* constipation, flatulence, cramps, dry mouth, peptic ulcer, ulceration, bleeding, perforation

CNS: Dizziness, drowsiness, fatigue, tremors, confusion, insomnia, anxiety, depression, headache

CV: Tachycardia, peripheral edema, palpitations, dysrhythmias, hypertension

INTEG: Purpura, rash, pruritus, sweating

GU: **Nephrotoxicity: dysuria, he-**

---

maturia, oliguria, azotemia, pseudoproteinuria
HEMA: **Blood dyscrasias**
EENT: Tinnitus, hearing loss, blurred vision
Contraindications: Hypersensitivity, asthma, severe renal disease, severe hepatic disease, ulcer disease
Precautions: Pregnancy (B), lactation, children, bleeding disorders, GI disorders, cardiac disorders, hypersensitivity to other antiinflammatory agents, peptic ulcer disease
Pharmacokinetics:
PO: Peak 2 hr, half-life 3-3½ hr; metabolized in liver, excreted in urine (metabolites), excreted in breast milk, 99% protein binding
Interactions:

• Increased action of warfarin, phenytoin, sulfonamides
NURSING CONSIDERATIONS
Assess:

• Renal, liver, blood studies: BUN, creatinine, AST, ALT, Hgb before treatment, periodically thereafter
• I&O ratio
• Audiometric, ophthalmic exam before, during, after treatment
• For eye, ear problems: blurred vision, tinnitus (may indicate toxicity)
Administer:

• With food to decrease GI symptoms; best to take on empty stomach to facilitate absorption; tab may be crushed
Perform/provide:

• Storage at room temp
Evaluate:

• Therapeutic response: decreased pain, stiffness, swelling in joints, ability to move more easily
Teach patient/family:

• To report blurred vision, ringing, roaring in ears (may indicate toxicity)
• To avoid driving, other hazardous activities if dizzy or drowsy

• To report change in urine pattern, weight increase, edema, pain increase in joints, fever, blood in urine (indicates nephrotoxicity)
• That therapeutic effects may take up to 1 mo
• To drink 8 glasses water daily
• About drug interactions

---

tolterodine (℞)
(toll-tehr′oh-deen)
Detrol
Func. class.: Overactive bladder product
Chem. class.: Muscarinic receptor antagonist

Action: Relaxes smooth muscles in urinary tract by inhibiting acetylcholine at postganglionic sites
Uses: Overactive bladder (urinary frequency, urgency)
Dosage and routes:
• *Adult:* **PO** 2 mg bid, hepatic disease 1 mg bid
Available forms: Tabs 1, 2 mg
Side effects/adverse reactions:
CNS: Anxiety, paresthesia, fatigue, *dizziness,* headache
CV: Chest pain, hypertension
EENT: Vision abnormalities, xerophthalmia
GI: Nausea, vomiting, anorexia, abdominal pain, constipation, dry mouth, dyspepsia
GU: Dysuria, urinary retention, frequency, UTI
INTEG: Rash, pruritus
RESP: Bronchitis, cough, pharyngitis, URI
Contraindications: hypersensitivity, uncontrolled narrow-angle glaucoma, urinary retention, gastric retention
Precautions: Pregnancy (C), lactation, children, renal/hepatic disease, controlled narrow-angle glaucoma

Pharmacokinetics: Rapidly absorbed, highly protein bound, extensively metabolized, excreted in urine/feces

Interactions:

• Increased action of tolterodine: macrolide antibiotics, antifungals
Food increases the bioavailability of tolterodine

NURSING CONSIDERATIONS
Assess:

• Urinary patterns: distention, nocturia, frequency, urgency, incontinence

• Allergic reactions: rash; if this occurs, drug should be discontinued

Evaluate:

• Urinary status: dysuria, frequency, nocturia, incontinence

Teach patient/family:

• To avoid hazardous activities; dizziness may occur

---

topiramate (R)

(toh-pire'ah-mate)

Topamax

Func. class.: Anticonvulsant, miscellaneous

Chem. class.: Carbamate derivative

Action: Mechanism of action unknown; may prevent seizure spread as opposed to an elevation of seizure threshold

Uses: Partial seizures, with or without generalization in adults

Dosage and routes:

Renal dose

• CrCl <70 ml/min give ½ dose

Adjunctive therapy

• *Adult:* **PO** add 400 mg in 2 divided doses

Available forms: Tabs 25, 100, 200 mg; sprinkle cap 15, 25, 50 mg

Side effects/adverse reactions:

RESP: URI, pharyngitis, sinusitis

EENT: Diplopia, vision abnormality

INTEG: Rash

MISC: Weight loss, leukopenia

CNS: Dizziness, fatigue, cognitive disorder, insomnia, anxiety, depression, paresthesia

ENDO: Weight loss

GI: Diarrhea, anorexia, nausea, dyspepsia, abdominal pain, constipation, dry mouth

GU: Breast pain, dysmenorrhea, menstrual disorder

Contraindications: Hypersensitivity

Precautions: Hepatic, renal, cardiac disease, elderly, lactation, children, pregnancy (C)

Pharmacokinetics: Well absorbed, terminal half-life 21 hr; excreted in urine (55%-97% unchanged), crosses placenta, excreted in breast milk, protein binding (9%-17%); steady state 4 days

Interactions:

• Decreased levels of: oral contraceptives, digoxin

• Increased levels of: alcohol, CNS depressants, carbonic anhydrase inhibitors

• Decreased levels of topiramate: food, phenytoin, carbamazepine, valproic acid

NURSING CONSIDERATIONS
Assess:

• Renal studies: urinalysis, BUN, urine creatinine q3mo

• Hepatic studies: ALT, AST, bilirubin

• CBC during long-term therapy

• Description of seizures

• Mental status: mood, sensorium, affect, behavioral changes; if mental status changes, notify prescriber

• Body weight, evidence of cognitive disorder

Administer:

🚫 Whole; do not break, crush, or chew tabs, very bitter

• May take with food

Perform/provide:
• Storage at room temp away from heat and light
• Assistance with ambulation during early part of treatment; dizziness occurs
• Seizure precautions: padded side rails, move objects that may harm patient

Evaluate:
• Therapeutic response: decreased seizure activity

Teach patient/family:
• To carry Medic Alert ID stating patient's name, drugs taken, condition, prescriber's name, phone number
• To avoid driving, other activities that require alertness
• Not to discontinue medication quickly after long-term use

Treatment of overdose: Lavage, VS

---

topotecan

(toh-poh-tee'kan)
Hycamtin
Func. class.: Antineoplastic hormone
Chem. class.: Semi-synthetic derivative of camptothecin (topoisomerase inhibitor)

Action: Antitumor drug with topoisomerase I–inhibitory activity topoisomerase I relieves torsional strain in DNA by causing single-strand breaks; causes double-strand DNA damage

Uses: Metastatic carcinoma of the ovary after failure of traditional chemotherapy

Dosage and routes:
• *Adult:* **IV INF** 1.5 mg/m^2 over 30 min qd × 5 days starting on day 1 of a 21-day course × 4 courses; may be reduced to 0.25 mg/m^2 for subsequent courses if severe neutropenia occurs

Available forms: Lyophilized powder for inj 4 mg (free base)

Side effects/adverse reactions:
HEMA: **Neutropenia, leukopenia, thrombocytopenia, anemia, sepsis**
GI: Abdominal pain, constipation, diarrhea, obstruction, nausea, stomatitis, vomiting; increased ALT, AST; anorexia
CNS: Arthralgia, asthenia, headache, myalgia, pain
RESP: Dyspnea
INTEG: Total alopecia

Contraindications: Hypersensitivity, lactation, severe bone marrow depression

Precautions: Children, pregnancy (C)

Interactions:
• Increased duration of neutropenia when used with: G-CSF
• Increased myelosuppression when used with: cisplatin

Pharmacokinetics: Rapidly and completely absorbed; excreted in urine and feces as metabolites; half-life 6 hr, geriatric half-life 8 hr; 94% bound to plasma proteins

NURSING CONSIDERATIONS

Assess:
• Liver function studies: AST, ALT, alk phosphatase, which may be elevated
• For CNS symptoms: drowsiness, confusion, depression, anxiety
• CBC, differential, platelet count weekly; withhold drug if WBC is <3500/mm^3 or platelet count is <100,000/mm^3; notify prescriber of these results; drug should be discontinued
• Buccal cavity q8h for dryness, sores or ulceration, white patches, oral pain, bleeding, dysphagia
• GI symptoms: frequency of stools, cramping
• Signs of dehydration: rapid respi-

T

ration, poor skin turgor, decreased urine output, dry skin, restlessness, weakness

Perform/provide:

• Increased fluid intake to 2-3 L/day to prevent dehydration, unless contraindicated

• Changing of IV site q48h

• Rinsing of mouth tid-qid with water, club soda; brushing of teeth bid-tid with soft brush or cotton-tipped applicator for stomatitis; use unwaxed dental floss

• Nutritious diet with iron, vit K supplements, low fiber, few dairy products

Evaluate:

• Therapeutic response: decreased tumor size, spread of malignancy

Teach patient/family:

• To avoid foods with citric acid or hot or rough texture if stomatitis is present; to drink adequate fluids

• To report stomatitis; any bleeding, white spots, ulcerations in mouth; tell patient to examine mouth qd; report symptoms

• To report signs of anemia: fatigue, headache, faintness, shortness of breath, irritability

• To use contraception during therapy

---

toremifene (℞)

(tor-em'ih-feen)
Fareston
Func. class.: Antineoplastic
Chem. class.: Antiestrogen hormone

Action: Inhibits cell division by binding to cytoplasmic estrogen receptors; resembles normal cell complex but inhibits DNA synthesis and estrogen response of target tissue
Uses: Advanced breast carcinoma not responsive to other therapy in estrogen-receptor-positive patients (usually postmenopausal)

Dosage and routes:
• *Adult:* **PO** 60 mg qd
Available forms: Tabs 60 mg

Side effects/adverse reactions:
HEMA: **Thrombocytopenia, leukopenia**
GI: Nausea, *vomiting,* altered taste (anorexia)
GU: Vaginal bleeding, pruritus vulvae
INTEG: Rash, alopecia
CV: Chest pain
CNS: Hot flashes, headache, lightheadedness, depression
META: Hypercalcemia
EENT: Ocular lesions, retinopathy, corneal opacity, blurred vision (high doses)

Contraindications: Hypersensitivity, pregnancy (D)
Precautions: Leukopenia, thrombocytopenia, lactation, cataracts
Pharmacokinetics:
PO: Peak 3 hr, excreted primarily in feces

Lab test interferences:
Increase: Serum Ca

NURSING CONSIDERATIONS
Assess:
• CBC, differential, platelet count qwk; withhold drug if WBC is <3500/mm³ or platelet count is <100,000/mm³; notify prescriber
• Bleeding: hematuria, guaiac, bruising, petechiae, mucosa or orifices q8h
• Effects of alopecia on body image; discuss feelings about body changes
◆ Symptoms indicating severe allergic reactions: rash, pruritus, urticaria, purpuric skin lesions, itching, flushing
Administer:
• Antacid before oral agent; give drug after evening meal, before bedtime

---

◆ = Nursing alert   🖋 = Herb-drug interaction   ⊘ = Do not crush

• Antiemetic 30-60 min before giving drug to prevent vomiting

Perform/provide:
• Liquid diet, if needed, including cola, Jell-O; dry toast or crackers may be added if patient is not nauseated or vomiting
• Increase fluid intake to 2-3 L/day to prevent dehydration
• Nutritious diet with iron, vitamin supplements as ordered
• Storage in light-resistant container at room temp

Evaluate:
• Therapeutic response: decreased tumor size, spread of malignancy

Teach patient/family:
• To report any complaints, side effects to prescriber
• That vaginal bleeding, pruritus, hot flashes are reversible after discontinuing treatment
• To report immediately decreased visual acuity, which may be irreversible; stress need for routine eye exams; care providers should be told about tamoxifen therapy
• To report vaginal bleeding immediately
• That tumor flare—increase in size of tumor, increased bone pain—may occur and will subside rapidly; may take analgesics for pain
• That premenopausal women must use mechanical birth control because ovulation may be induced
• That hair may be lost during treatment; a wig or hairpiece may make patient feel better; new hair may be different in color, texture.

torsemide (℞)
(tor'suh-mide)
Demadex
Func. class.: Loop diuretic
Chem. class.: Sulfonamide derivative

Action: Acts on loop of Henle, proximal, distal tubule by inhibiting absorption of chloride, sodium, water
Uses: Treatment of hypertension and edema in CHF, hepatic disease, renal disease

Dosage and routes:
CHF
• *Adult:* **PO/IV** 10-20 mg/day, may increase as needed up to 200 mg/day
Chronic renal failure
• *Adult:* **PO/IV** 20 mg/day, may increase up to 200 mg/day
Hepatic cirrhosis
• *Adult:* **PO/IV** 5-10 mg/day may increase as needed up to 40 mg/day
Hypertension
• *Adult:* **PO** 5 mg/day may increase to 10 mg/day
Available forms: Tabs 5, 10, 20, 100 mg; inj 10 mg/ml vials of 2, 5 ml

Side effects/adverse reactions:
CNS: Headache, dizziness, asthenia, insomnia, nervousness
CV: Orthostatic hypotension, chest pain, ECG changes, *circulatory collapse,* ventricular tachycardia
EENT: Loss of hearing, ear pain, tinnitus, blurred vision
ENDO: Hyperglycemia, hyperuricemia
ELECT: Hypokalemia, hypochloremic alkalosis, hypomagnesemia, hypocalcemia, hyponatremia, metabolic alkalosis
GI: Nausea, diarrhea, dyspepsia, GI hemorrhage, rectal bleeding, cramps

T

*GU: Polyuria, **renal failure,** gly-cosuria*

INTEG: Rash, photosensitivity

MS: Cramps, stiffness

RESP: Rhinitis, cough increase

Contraindications: Hypersensitivity to sulfonamides, anuria, hypovolemia, infants, lactation, electrolyte depletion

Precautions: Diabetes mellitus, dehydration, severe renal disease, pregnancy (C)

Pharmacokinetics:

PO: Rapidly absorbed; duration 6 hr; excreted in urine, feces, breast milk; crosses placenta; half-life 2-4 hr, plasma protein binding 97%-99%

Interactions:

• Increased toxicity: lithium, nondepolarizing skeletal muscle relaxants, digitalis

• Increased action of antihypertensives, oral anticoagulants, nitrates

• Increased ototoxicity: aminoglycosides, cisplatin, vancomycin

• Decreased antihypertensive effect of torsemide: indomethacin, metolazone

• Incompatible with acidic sol, vit C, corticosteroids, diphenhydramine, dobutamine, esmolol, epinephrine, gentamicin, meperidine, milrinone, netilmicin, norepinephrine, reserpine, spironolactone, tetracyclines in sol

• Incompatible with any drug in syringe

Lab test interferences:

Interference: GTT

NURSING CONSIDERATIONS

Assess:

• Hearing when giving high doses

• Weight, I&O daily to determine fluid loss; effect of drug may be decreased if used qd

• Rate, depth, rhythm of respiration, effect of exertion

• B/P lying, standing; postural hypotension may occur

• Electrolytes: K, Na, Cl; include BUN, blood sugar, CBC, serum creatinine, blood pH, ABGs, uric acid, Ca, Mg

• Glucose in urine of diabetic

• Signs and symptoms of metabolic alkalosis: drowsiness, restlessness

• Signs and symptoms of hypokalemia: postural hypotension, malaise, fatigue, tachycardia, leg cramps, weakness

• Rashes, temp elevation qd

• Confusion, especially in elderly; take safety precautions if needed

Administer:

• In AM to avoid interference with sleep if using drug as a diuretic

• K replacement if K <3 mg/dl

• With food if nausea occurs; absorption may be decreased slightly

Evaluate:

• Therapeutic response: improvement in edema of feet, legs, sacral area qd if medication is being used in CHF

Teach patient/family:

• To rise slowly from lying, sitting position

• To recognize adverse reactions: muscle cramps, weakness, nausea, dizziness

• To take with food or milk for GI symptoms

• To take early in day to prevent nocturia

Treatment of overdose: Lavage if taken orally; monitor electrolytes, administer dextrose in saline; monitor hydration, CV, renal status

---

◆ = Nursing alert   ▦ = Herb-drug interaction   ⊘ = Do not crush

trace elements (R)

Concentrated Multiple Trace Elements, ConTE-PAK-4, M.T.E.-4, M.T.E.-4 Concentrated, M.T.E.-5, M.T.E.-5 Concentrated, M.T.E.-6, M.T.E.-6 Concentrated, M.T.E.-7, MulTE-PAK-4, MulTE-PAK-5, Multiple Trace Element, Multiple Trace Element Neonatal, Multiple Trace Element Pediatric, Neotrace 4, PedTE-PAK-4, Pedtrace-4, P.T.E.-4, P.T.E.-5

Func. class.: Mineral supplements

Action: Needed for adequate absorption and synthesis of amino acids

Uses: Prevention of trace element deficiency

Dosage and routes:
Usual dosage may be given in TPN sol

Chromium
• *Adult:* IV 10-15 µg qd
• *Child:* IV 0.14-0.20 µg/kg/day

Copper
• *Adult:* IV 0.5-1.5 mg/day
• *Child:* IV .05-0.2 mg/kg/day

Iodine
• *Adult:* IV 1 µg/kg/day

Manganese
• *Adult:* IV 1-3 mg/day

Selenium
• *Adult:* IV 40-120 µg/day
• *Child:* IV 3 µg/kg/day

Zinc
• *Adult:* IV 2-4 mg/day
• *Child:* IV 0.05 mg/kg/day

Available forms: Many forms available—see particular elements

Side effects/adverse reactions: Depends on element

Precautions: Liver, biliary disease, pregnancy (C), lactation, vomiting, diarrhea

NURSING CONSIDERATIONS
Assess:
• Trace element levels; notify prescriber if low; copper 0.07-0.15 mg/ml, zinc 0.05-0.15 mg/100 ml, manganese 4-20 µg/100 ml, selenium 0.1-0.19 µg/ml
• Trace element deficiency of patient receiving TPN for extended period

Administer:
• By IV infusion, often mixed with TPN solution

Evaluate:
• Therapeutic response: absence of element deficiency

tramadol (R)

(tram′a-dole)
Ultram
Func. class.: Central analgesic

Action: Not completely understood, binds to opioid receptors, inhibits reuptake of norepinephrine, serotonin; does not cause histamine release or affect heart rate

Uses: Management of moderate to severe pain

Dosage and routes:
Renal dose
• CrCl <30 ml/min give q12h, max 200 mg/day
• *Adult:* PO 50-100 mg prn q4-6h; not to exceed 400 mg/day
• *Elderly (>75 years):* PO <300 mg/day in divided doses

Hepatic impairment
• PO 50 mg q12h

Available forms: Tabs 50 mg

Side effects/adverse reactions:
CNS: Dizziness, CNS stimulation, somnolence, headache, anxiety, confusion, euphoria, *seizures,* hallucinations
GI: Nausea, constipation, vomiting, dry mouth, diarrhea, abdominal pain, anorexia, flatulence, *GI bleeding*

CV: Vasodilation, orthostatic hypotension, tachycardia, hypertension, abnormal ECG

INTEG: Pruritus, rash, urticaria, vesicles

GU: Urinary retention/frequency, menopausal symptoms, dysuria, menstrual disorder

Interactions:
• Decreased levels of tramadol: carbamazepine
• Inhibition of norepinephrine and serotonin reuptake: MAO inhibitors, use together with caution
• Increased CNS depression: alcohol, sedatives, hypnotics, opiates
🌿 Increased CNS depression: kava

Lab test interferences:
Increase: Creatinine, liver enzymes
Decrease: Hgb

Contraindications: Hypersensitivity, acute intoxication with any CNS depressant

Precautions: Seizure disorder, pregnancy (C), lactation, children, elderly, renal or hepatic disease, respiratory depression, head trauma, increased intracranial pressure, acute abdominal condition, drug abuse

Pharmacokinetics: Rapidly and almost completely absorbed, steady state 2 days, may cross blood-brain barrier, extensively metabolized, 30% excreted in the urine as unchanged drug

NURSING CONSIDERATIONS
Assess:
• Pain: location, type, character, give before pain becomes extreme
• I&O ratio: check for decreasing output; may indicate urinary retention
• Need for drug
• For constipation: increase fluids, bulk in diet
• CNS changes: dizziness, drowsiness, hallucinations, euphoria, LOC, pupil reaction
• Allergic reactions: rash, urticaria

Administer:
PO
• With antiemetic for nausea, vomiting
• When pain is beginning to return; determine dosage interval by patient response

Perform/provide:
• Storage in cool environment, protected from sunlight
• Assistance with ambulation
• Safety measures: side rails, nightlight, call bell within easy reach

Evaluate:
• Therapeutic response: decrease in pain

Teach patient/family:
• To report any symptoms of CNS changes, allergic reactions
• That drowsiness, dizziness, and confusion may occur, to call for assistance
• To make position changes slowly, orthostatic hypotension may occur
• To avoid OTC medications and alcohol unless approved by prescriber

---

trandolapril (℞)
(tran-doe'la-prill)
Mavik
Func. class.: Antihypertensive
Chem. class.: Angiotension-converting enzyme inhibitor

Action: Selectively suppresses renin-angiotensin-aldosterone system; inhibits ACE; prevents conversion of angiotensin I to angiotensin II, dilates arterial and venous vessels, lowers B/P

Uses: Hypertension, heart failure, post-MI/left ventricular dysfunction post MI

Dosage and routes:
Hypertension
• *Adult:* **PO** 1 mg/day, 2 mg/day in

◆ = Nursing alert   🌿 = Herb-drug interaction   🚫 = Do not crush

African-Americans, make dosage adjustment ≥wk; up to 8 mg/day

Heart failure post MI/left ventricular dysfunction post MI
• *Adult:* **PO** 1 mg/day, titrate upward to 4 mg/day if tolerated

Renal dose
• CrCl <30 ml/min give 0.5 mg/day, may increase gradually

Available forms: Tabs 1, 2, 4 mg

Side effects/adverse reactions:
*CV: Hypotension, **MI**,* palpitations, angina, TIAs, *stroke,* bradycardia, dysrhythmias
CNS: Dizziness, paresthesias, headache, fatigue, drowsiness, depression, sleep disturbances
GI: Nausea, vomiting, cramps, diarrhea, constipation, ileus, pancreatitis, hepatitis, *dyspepsia*
INTEG: Rash, purpura
*HEMA: **Agranulocytosis, neutropenia, leukopenia, anemia***
*GU: **Proteinuria, renal failure***
RESP: Dyspnea, *cough*
MISC: Hyperkalemia, hyponatremia, impotence, *myalgia*

Contraindications: Hypersensitivity, history of angioedema, pregnancy (D) (2nd/3rd trimester)

Precautions: Renal disease, hyperkalemia, hepatic disease, bilateral renal stenosis, post kidney transplant, aorta/mitral valve stenosis, cirrhosis, severe renal disease, untreated CHF, autoimmune disease, severe hypertension

Pharmacokinetics:
PO: Peak 4-10 hr; half-life 0.6-1.1 hr, 16-24 hr; metabolized by liver, excreted in urine

Interactions:
• Hypersensitivity: allopurinol
• Severe hypotension: diuretics, other antihypertensives
• Decreased effects of trandolapril: aspirin, antacids
• Increased K levels: salt substitutes, K-sparing diuretics, K supplements
• May increase effects of ergots, neuromuscular blocking agents, antihypertensives, hypoglycemics, barbiturates, reserpine, levodopa
• Effects may be increased by phenothiazines, diuretics, phenytoin, quinidine, nifedipine

NURSING CONSIDERATIONS
Assess:
• B/P, pulse q4h; note rate, rhythm, quality
• Electrolytes: K, Na, Cl
• Baselines in renal, liver function tests before therapy begins
• Edema in feet, legs daily
• Skin turgor, dryness of mucous membranes for hydration status
• Symptoms of CHF: edema, dyspnea, wet rales

Evaluate:
• Therapeutic response: decreased B/P

Teach patient/family:
• Not to use OTC (cough, cold, orallergy) products unless directed by prescriber
• To avoid sunlight or wear sunscreen for photosensitivity
• To comply with dosage schedule, even if feeling better
• To notify prescriber of mouth sores, sore throat, fever, swelling of hands or feet, irregular heartbeat, chest pain, signs of angioedema
• That excessive perspiration, dehydration, vomiting, diarrhea may lead to fall in blood pressure; consult prescriber if these occur
• That drug may cause dizziness, fainting; light-headedness may occur during 1st few days of therapy
• That drug may cause skin rash or impaired perspiration
• Not to discontinue drug abruptly
• Not to use OTC products unless directed by prescriber

• To rise slowly to sitting or standing position to minimize orthostatic hypotension

---

tranylcypromine (Ŗ)
(tran-ill-sip´roe-meen)
Parnate
Func. class.: Antidepressant-MAOI
Chem. class.: Nonhydrazine

Action: Increases concentrations of endogenous epinephrine, norepinephrine, serotonin, dopamine in storage sites in CNS by inhibition of MAO; increased concentration reduces depression

Uses: Depression, when uncontrolled by other means

Investigational uses: Bulimia, cocaine addiction, migraines, seasonal affective disorder, panic disorder

Dosage and routes:
• *Adult:* PO 10 mg bid; may increase to 30 mg/day after 2 wk; up to 60 mg/day

Available forms: Tabs 10 mg

Side effects/adverse reactions:
HEMA: Anemia
CNS: Dizziness, drowsiness, confusion, headache, anxiety, tremors, stimulation, weakness, hyperreflexia, mania, insomnia, fatigue
GI: Constipation, dry mouth, nausea, vomiting, *anorexia,* diarrhea, weight gain
GU: Change in libido, urinary frequency
INTEG: Rash, flushing, increased perspiration
CV: Orthostatic hypotension, hypertension, dysrhythmias, **hypertensive crisis**
EENT: Blurred vision
ENDO: **SIADH-like syndrome**
Contraindications: Hypersensitivity to MAOIs, elderly, hypertension, CHF, severe hepatic disease, pheochromocytoma, severe renal disease, severe cardiac disease

Precautions: Suicidal patients, convulsive disorders, severe depression, schizophrenia, hyperactivity, diabetes mellitus, pregnancy (C), lactation

Pharmacokinetics: Metabolized by liver, excreted by kidneys, crosses placenta, excreted in breast milk

Interactions:
• Increased pressor effects: guanethidine, clonidine, indirect-acting sympathomimetics (ephedrine), buspirone
• Increased effects of: direct-acting sympathomimetics (epinephrine), alcohol, barbiturates, benzodiazepines, CNS depressants, levodopa, β-blockers, antidiabetics, sulfonamide, rauwolfia alkaloids, methyldopa, L-tryptophan, thiazide diuretics, sumatriptan
• *Serotonin-syndrome:* fluoxetine, fluvoxamine, sertraline, paroxetine
• *Hypertensive crisis:* tricyclic antidepressants, meperidine, dibenzazepine agents, methylphenidate, dextromethorphan

🖋 Increased sympathomimetic action: ephedra

🖋 Increased B/P: brewer's yeast

NURSING CONSIDERATIONS
Assess:
• B/P (lying, standing), pulse; if systolic B/P drops 20 mm Hg, stop drug, notify prescriber
• Blood studies: CBC, leukocytes, cardiac enzymes (long-term therapy)
• Hepatic studies: ALT, AST, bilirubin; hepatotoxicity may occur

◆ Toxicity: increased headache, palpitation; discontinue drug immediately; prodromal signs of hypertensive crisis

---

◆ = Nursing alert   🖋 = Herb-drug interaction   🚫 = Do not crush

• Mental status changes: mood, sensorium, affect, memory (long, short), increase in psychiatric symptoms
• Urinary retention, constipation, edema: take weight weekly
• Withdrawal symptoms: headache, nausea, vomiting, muscle pain, weakness

Administer:
• Increased fluids, bulk in diet if constipation occurs
• With food or milk for GI symptoms
• Crushed if patient is unable to swallow medication whole
• Dosage hs if oversedation occurs during day
• Gum, hard candy, frequent sips of water for dry mouth
• Phentolamine for severe hypertension

Perform/provide:
• Cool storage in tight container
• Assistance with ambulation during beginning therapy for drowsiness/dizziness
• Safety measures including side rails
• Checking to see if PO medication swallowed

Evaluate:
• Therapeutic response: decreased depression

Teach patient/family:
• That therapeutic effects may take 48 hr-3 wks
• To avoid driving, other activities requiring alertness
• To avoid alcohol ingestion, CNS depressants, OTC medications: cold, weight loss, hay fever, cough syrup
• Not to discontinue medication quickly after long-term use
• To avoid high-tyramine foods: cheese (aged), sour cream, yogurt, beer, wine, pickled products, liver, raisins, bananas, figs, avocados, meat tenderizers, chocolate, increased caffeine, ginseng

• To report headache, palpitation, neck stiffness

Treatment of overdose: Lavage, activated charcoal; monitor electrolytes, vital signs; diazepam IV, NaHCO$_3$

---

trastuzumab (℞)

(tras-tuz'uh-mab)
Herceptin
Func. class.: Miscellaneous antineoplastic
Chem. class.: Humanized monoclonal antibody

Action: DNA-derived monoclonal antibody selectively binds to extracellular portion of human epidermal growth factor receptor 2; it inhibits proliferation of cancer cells

Uses: Breast cancer; metastatic with overexpression of HER2

Dosage and routes:
• *Adult:* IV 4 mg/kg given over 90 min, then maintenance 2 mg/kg given over 30 min; do not give as IV push or BOL

Available forms: Lyophilized powder 440 mg

Side effects/adverse reactions:
CNS: Dizziness, numbness, paresthesias, depression, insomnia, neuropathy, peripheral neuritis
*CV: **Tachycardia, CHF***
INTEG: Rash, acne, herpes simplex
GI: Nausea, vomiting, anorexia, diarrhea
MISC: Flulike syndrome; fever, headache, chills
HEMA: Anemia, ***leukopenia***
MS: Arthralgia, bone pain
META: Edema, peripheral edema
RESP: Cough, dyspnea, pharyngitis, rhinitis, sinusitis

Contraindications: Hypersensitivity to this drug, Chinese hamster ovary cell protein

T

Precautions: Pregnancy (B), lactation, children, elderly, cardiac disease, anemia, leukopenia

Pharmacokinetics: Half-life 1.7-12 days

NURSING CONSIDERATIONS

Assess:
• For symptoms of infection; may be masked by drug
• CNS reaction: LOC, mental status, dizziness, confusion

Administer:
• Acetaminophen as ordered to alleviate fever and headache

IV
• After reconstituting vial with 20 ml bacteriostatic water for inj, 1.1% benzyl alcohol preserved (supplied) to yield 21 mg/ml, mark date on vial 28 days from reconstitution date, if patient is allergic to benzyl alcohol, reconstitute with sterile water for inj—use immediately
• Do not mix or dilute with other drugs or dextrose sol

Perform/provide:
• Increased fluid intake to 2-3 L/day

Evaluate:
• Therapeutic response: decrease in size of tumors

Teach patient/family:
• To take acetaminophen for fever
• To avoid hazardous tasks, since confusion, dizziness may occur
• To report signs of infection: sore throat, fever, diarrhea, vomiting
• Emotional lability is common; notify presriber if severe or incapacitating

---

trazodone (R)

(tray´zoe-done)

Desyrel, Desyrel Dividose, trazodone HCl

Func. class.: Antidepressant, miscellaneous

Chem. class.: Triazolopyridine

Action: Selectively inhibits serotonin uptake by brain, potentiates behavioral changes

Uses: Depression

Investigational uses: Chronic pain

Dosage and routes:
• *Adult:* PO 150 mg/day in divided doses; may increase by 50 mg/day q3-4d, not to exceed 600 mg/day
• *Geriatric:* PO 25-50 mg hs, increase by 25-50 mg q3-7days to desired dose

Available forms: Tabs 50, 100, 150, 300 mg

Side effects/adverse reactions:

*HEMA: **Agranulocytosis, thrombocytopenia, eosinophilia, leukopenia***

CNS: Dizziness, drowsiness, confusion, headache, anxiety, tremors, stimulation, weakness, insomnia, nightmares, EPS (elderly), increase in psychiatric symptoms

GI: Diarrhea, dry mouth, nausea, vomiting, **paralytic ileus,** increased appetite, cramps, epigastric distress, jaundice, **hepatitis,** stomatitis

*GU: Urinary retention, **acute renal failure,** priapism*

INTEG: Rash, urticaria, sweating, pruritus, photosensitivity

*CV: Orthostatic hypotension, ECG changes, tachycardia, **hypertension,*** palpitations

EENT: Blurred vision, tinnitus, mydriasis

Contraindications: Hypersensitivity to tricyclic antidepressants, re-

---

◆ = Nursing alert   ∥ = Herb-drug interaction   ⊘ = Do not crush

covery phase of MI, convulsive disorders, prostatic hypertrophy

Precautions: Suicidal patients, severe depression, increased intraocular pressure, narrow-angle glaucoma, urinary retention, cardiac disease, hepatic disease, hyperthyroidism, electroshock therapy, elective surgery, pregnancy (C)

Pharmacokinetics: Metabolized by liver, excreted by kidneys, feces; half-life 4.4-7.5 hr

Interactions:

• Decreased effects of guanethidine, clonidine, indirect-acting sympathomimetics (ephedrine)

• Increased effects of direct-acting sympathomimetics (epinephrine), alcohol, barbiturates, benzodiazepines, CNS depressants

➤ Hyperpyretic crisis, convulsions, hypertensive episode: MAOI (pargyline [Eutonyl])

🖊 Increased CNS depression: kava

Lab test interferences:

Increase: Serum bilirubin, blood glucose, alk phosphatase

False increase: Urinary catecholamines

Decrease: VMA, 5-HIAA

NURSING CONSIDERATIONS
Assess:

• B/P (lying, standing), pulse q4h; if systolic B/P drops 20 mm Hg, hold drug, notify prescriber; take vital signs q4h in patients with cardiovascular disease

• Blood studies: CBC, leukocytes, differential, cardiac enzymes if patient is receiving long-term therapy

• Hepatic studies: AST, ALT, bilirubin

• Weight qwk; appetite may increase with drug

• ECG for flattening of T wave, bundle branch block, AV block, dysrhythmias in cardiac patients

• EPS, primarily in elderly: rigidity, dystonia, akathisia

• Mental status changes: mood, sensorium, affect, suicidal tendencies, increase in psychiatric symptoms, depression, panic

• Urinary retention, constipation; constipation most likely in children

• Withdrawal symptoms: headache, nausea, vomiting, muscle pain, weakness; not usual unless drug discontinued abruptly

• Alcohol consumption; hold dose until morning

Administer:

• Increased fluids, bulk in diet if constipation occurs, especially in elderly

• With food, milk for GI symptoms

• Dosage hs for oversedation during day; may take entire dose hs; elderly may not tolerate qd dosing

• Gum, hard candy, frequent sips of water for dry mouth

Perform/provide:

• Storage in tight, light-resistant container at room temp

• Assistance with ambulation during beginning therapy for drowsiness/dizziness

• Safety measures, including side rails, primarily for elderly

• Checking to see if PO medication swallowed

Evaluate:

• Therapeutic response: decreased depression

Teach patient/family:

• That therapeutic effects may take 2-3 wk

• To use caution in driving, other activities requiring alertness because of drowsiness, dizziness, blurred vision

• To avoid alcohol ingestion, other CNS depressants

• Not to discontinue medication quickly after long-term use; may cause nausea, headache, malaise

T

• To wear sunscreen or large hat, since photosensitivity occurs

Treatment of overdose: ECG monitoring; induce emesis; lavage, activated charcoal; administer anticonvulsant

---

tretinoin (vit A acid, retinoic acid) (Ŗ)
(tret′i-noyn)
Retin-A, Stievaa*, Tretinoin LF, IV, Vesanoid
Func. class.: Vit A acid, acne product; antineoplastic (misc.)
Chem. class.: Tretinoin derivative

Action: Decreases cohesiveness of follicular epithelium, decreases microcomedone formation (TOP); induces maturation of acute promyelocytic leukemia, exact action is unknown (PO)

Uses: Acne vulgaris (grades 1-3) (top); (PO) acute promyelocytic leukemia

Investigational uses: Skin cancer
Dosage and routes:
• *Adult and child:* **TOP** cleanse area, apply hs; cover lightly
Promyelocytic leukemia
• *Adult:* **PO** 45 mg/m²/day given as 2 evenly divided doses until remission, discontinue treatment 30 days after remission or 90 days of treatment, whichever is first

Available forms: Cream 0.01%, 0.05%; gel 0.01%, 0.025%; liq 0.05%; caps 10 mg

Side effects/adverse reactions:
INTEG: (top) Rash, stinging, warmth, redness, erythema, blistering, crusting, peeling, contact dermatitis, hypopigmentation, hyperpigmentation
Oral
CNS: Headache, fever, sweating

GI: Nausea, vomiting, **hemorrhage**, abdominal pain, diarrhea, constipation, dyspepsia, distention, hepatitis

Contraindications: Hypersensitivity to retinoids or sensitivity to parabens, pregnancy (D) (PO)

Precautions: Lactation, eczema, sunburn, pregnancy (C) (top)

Pharmacokinetics:
TOP: Poor systemic absorption

Interactions:
• Increase peeling: medication containing agents such as sulfur, benzoyl peroxide, resorcinol, salicylic acid (top)
• Use with caution: medicated, abrasive soaps, cleansers that have drying effect, products with high concentrations of alcohol astringents (top)
• Increased plasma concentrations of tretinoin: ketoconazole (oral)

NURSING CONSIDERATIONS
Assess:
Topical
• Area of body involved, what helps or aggravates condition; cysts, dryness, itching; lesions may worsen at beginning of treatment
Oral
• Liver function, coagulation, hematologic parameters, also cholesterol, triglyceride

Administer:
Topical
• Once daily before hs; cover area lightly using gauze; use gloves to apply

Perform/provide:
Topical
• Storage at room temp
• Hand washing after application

Evaluate:
• Therapeutic response: decrease in size and number of lesions

Teach patient/family:
Topical
• To avoid application on normal

◆ = Nursing alert   🌿 = Herb-drug interaction   ⊘ = Do not crush

skin, getting cream in eyes, nose, other mucous membranes
• To avoid sunlight, sunlamps, or use protective clothing, sunscreen
• That treatment may cause warmth, stinging, dryness, peeling will occur
• That cosmetics may be used over drug; not to use shaving lotions
• That rash may occur during first 1-3 wk of therapy
• That drug does not cure condition; only relieves symptoms
• That therapeutic results may be seen in 2-3 wk but may not be optimal until after 6 wk

triamcinolone (R_x)

(trye-am-sin'oh-lone)
Amcort, Aristocort, Aristocort Forte, Aristocort Intralesional, Aristospan Intra-Articular, Aristospan Intralesional, Articulose L.A., Atolone, Azmacort, Cenocort A-40, Cenocort Forte, Kenacort, Kenaject-40, Kenalog, Kenalog-10, Kenalog-40, Tac-40, Tac-40, Triam-A, triamcinolone, triamcinolone acetonide, Triam Forte, Triamolone 40, Triamonide 40, Tri-Kort, Trilog, Trilone, Trisoject
Func. class.: Corticosteroid
Chem. class.: Glucocorticoid, intermediate-acting

Action: Decreases inflammation by suppression of migration of polymorphonuclear leukocytes, fibroblasts, reversal to increase capillary permeability and lysosomal stabilization
Uses: Severe inflammation, immunosuppression, neoplasms, asthma (steroid dependent), collagen, respiratory, dermatologic disorders

Dosage and routes:
• *Adult:* **PO** 4-12 mg/day in divided doses qd-qid; **IM** 40 mg qwk (acetonide, or diacetate), 5-48 mg into neoplasms (diacetate, acetonide), 2-40 mg into joint or soft tissue (diacetate, acetonide), 0.5 mg/in^2 of affected intralesional skin (hexacetonide), 2-20 mg into joint or soft tissue (hexacetonide)
• *Child:* **PO** 117 µg/kg/day as a single or divided dose
Asthma
• *Adult:* **INH** 2 tid-qid, not to exceed 16 **INH**/day
• *Child 6-12 yr:* **INH** 1-2 tid-qid, not to exceed 12 **INH**/day
Available forms: Tabs 1, 2, 4, 8 mg; syr 2 mg/5 ml, 4.85 mg/5 ml; inj 25, 40 mg/ml diacetate; inj 3, 10, 40 mg/ml acetonide; inj 20, 5 mg/ml hexacetonide; aerosol actuation/100 µg (acetonide)
Side effects/adverse reactions:
INTEG: Acne, poor wound healing, ecchymosis, petechiae
CNS: Depression, flushing, sweating, headache, mood changes
CV: Hypertension, ***circulatory collapse, thrombophlebitis, embolism,*** tachycardia, edema
*HEMA: **Thrombocytopenia***
MS: Fractures, osteoporosis, weakness
*GI: Diarrhea, nausea, abdominal distention, **GI hemorrhage,*** *increased appetite, **pancreatitis***
EENT: Fungal infections, increased intraocular pressure, blurred vision
Contraindications: Psychosis, hypersensitivity, idiopathic thrombocytopenia, acute glomerulonephritis, amebiasis, fungal infections, nonasthmatic bronchial disease, child <2 yr, AIDS, TB
Precautions: Pregnancy (C), diabetes mellitus, glaucoma, osteoporosis, seizure disorders, ulcerative colitis, CHF, myasthenia gravis, re-

nal disease, esophagitis, peptic ulcer

Pharmacokinetics:
PO/IM: Peak 1-2 hr, half-life 2-5 hr
Interactions:
• Decreased action of triamcinolone: cholestyramine, colestipol, barbiturates, rifampin, ephedrine, phenytoin, theophylline
• Decreased effects of anticoagulants, anticonvulsants, antidiabetics, ambenonium, neostigmine, isoniazid, toxoids, vaccines, anticholinesterases, salicylates, somatrem
• Increased side effects: alcohol, salicylates, indomethacin, amphotericin B, digitalis, cyclosporine, diuretics
• Increased action of triamcinolone: salicylates, estrogens, indomethacin, oral contraceptives, ketoconazole, macrolide antibiotics

⧸ Increased potassium loss: aloe, buckthorn, rhubarb, senna

Lab test interferences:
Increase: Cholesterol, Na, blood glucose, uric acid, Ca, urine glucose
Decrease: Ca, K, T$_4$, T$_3$, thyroid ^{131}I uptake test, urine 17-OHCS, 17-KS, PBI
False negative: Skin allergy tests

NURSING CONSIDERATIONS
Assess:
• K, blood sugar, urine glucose while on long-term therapy; hypokalemia and hyperglycemia
• Weight qd; notify prescriber if weekly gain >5 lb
• B/P q4h, pulse; notify prescriber if chest pain occurs
• I&O ratio; be alert for decreasing urinary output, increasing edema
• Plasma cortisol levels during long-term therapy (normal level: 138-635 nmol/L SI units when drawn at 8 AM)
• Infection: increased temp, WBC, even after withdrawal of medication; drug masks infection

• K depletion: paresthesias, fatigue, nausea, vomiting, depression, polyuria, dysrhythmias, weakness
• Edema, hypertension, cardiac symptoms
• Mental status: affect, mood, behavioral changes, aggression

Administer:
• After shaking susp (parenteral)
• Titrated dose; use lowest effective dose
• IM injection deep in large muscle mass; rotate sites; avoid deltoid; use 21G needle
• In one dose in AM to prevent adrenal suppression; avoid SC administration; may damage tissue
• With food or milk to decrease GI symptoms

Perform/provide:
• Assistance with ambulation for patient with bone tissue disease to prevent fractures
• Use of spacer device for elderly patients with inhaler

Evaluate:
• Therapeutic response: ease of respirations, decreased inflammation

Teach patient/family:
• That ID as steroid user should be carried
• To notify prescriber if therapeutic response decreases; dosage adjustment may be needed
• Not to discontinue abruptly; adrenal crisis can result
• To avoid OTC products: salicylates, alcohol in cough products, cold preparations unless directed by prescriber
• About cushingoid symptoms
• The symptoms of adrenal insufficiency: nausea, anorexia, fatigue, dizziness, dyspnea, weakness, joint pain

---

⬥ = Nursing alert   *⧸* = Herb-drug interaction   ⊘ = Do not crush

triamcinolone (topical-oral) (OTC)
(trye-am-sin'oh-lone)
Kenalog in Orabase, Oralone Dental
Func. class.: Topical anesthetic
Chem. class.: Synthetic fluorinated adrenal corticosteroid

Action: Inhibits nerve impulses from sensory nerves
Uses: Oral pain
Dosage and routes:
• *Adult and child:* **TOP** press ¼ inch into affected area until film appears, repeat bid-tid
Available forms: Paste 0.1%
Side effects/adverse reactions:
INTEG: Rash, irritation, sensitization

Contraindications: Hypersensitivity, infants <1 yr, application to large areas, presence of fungal, viral, or bacterial infections of mouth or throat
Precautions: Child <6 yr, sepsis, pregnancy (C), denuded skin
NURSING CONSIDERATIONS
Assess:
• Allergy: rash, irritation, reddening, swelling
• Infection: if affected area is infected, do not apply
Administer:
• After cleansing oral cavity
Evaluate:
• Therapeutic response: absence of pain in affected area
Teach patient/family:
• To report rash, irritation, redness, swelling
• How to apply paste

triamterene (Rx)
(trye-am'ter-een)
Dyrenium
Func. class.: Potassium-sparing diuretic
Chem. class.: Pteridine derivative

Action: Acts on distal tubule to inhibit reabsorption of sodium, chloride; increase potassium retention
Uses: Edema, may be used with other diuretics; hypertension
Dosage and routes:
• *Adult:* **PO** 100 mg bid pc, not to exceed 300 mg/day
• *Geriatric:* **PO** 50 mg qd, max 100 mg/day
Available forms: Caps 50, 100 mg
Side effects/adverse reactions:
GI: Nausea, diarrhea, vomiting, dry mouth, jaundice, *liver disease*
ELECT: Hyperkalemia, hyponatremia, hypochloremia
CNS: Weakness, headache, dizziness, fatigue
INTEG: Photosensitivity, rash
HEMA: Thrombocytopenia, megaloblastic anemia, low folic acid levels
GU: Azotemia, interstitial nephritis, increased BUN, creatinine, renal stones, bluish discoloration of urine
Contraindications: Hypersensitivity, anuria, severe renal disease, severe hepatic disease, hyperkalemia, lactation
Precautions: Dehydration, hepatic disease, CHF, renal disease, pregnancy (B), cirrhosis
Pharmacokinetics:
PO: Onset 2 hr, peak 6-8 hr, duration 12-16 hr; half-life 3 hr; metabolized in liver, excreted in bile and urine
Interactions:
• Nephrotoxicity: indomethacin

T

• Enhanced action of antihypertensives, amantadine

• Increased hyperkalemia: other K-sparing diuretics, K products, ACE inhibitors, salt substitutes

• Decreased renal clearance of triamterene: cimetidine

Lab test interferences:

Interference: Quinidine serum levels, LDH

NURSING CONSIDERATIONS
Assess:

• Weight, I&O qd to determine fluid loss; effect of drug may be decreased if used qd

• Electrolytes: K, Na, Cl; include BUN, blood sugar, CBC, serum creatinine, blood pH, ABGs, liver function tests

• Improvement in CVP q8h

• Signs of metabolic acidosis: drowsiness, restlessness

• Rashes, temp qd

• Confusion, especially in elderly; take safety precautions if needed

• Hydration: skin turgor, thirst, dry mucous membranes

Administer:

• In AM to avoid interference with sleep

• With food if nausea occurs; absorption may be decreased slightly

Evaluate:

• Therapeutic response: improvement in edema of feet, legs, sacral area qd if medication is being used in CHF

Teach patient/family:

• To take medication after meals for GI upset

• To avoid prolonged exposure to sunlight; photosensitivity may occur; may turn urine blue

• To avoid foods high in K: oranges, bananas, salt substitutes, dried apricots, dates

• To notify prescriber of weakness, headache, nausea, vomiting, dry mouth, fever, sore throat, mouth sores, unusual bleeding or bruising

Treatment of overdose: Lavage if taken orally; monitor electrolytes; administer IV fluids, dialysis; monitor hydration, CV, renal status

---

triazolam (Ŗ)
(trye-ay′zoe-lam)
Apo-Triazo*, Halcion, Novotriolam*, Nu-Triazol*
Func. class.: Sedative-hypnotic
Chem. class.: Benzodiazepine

Controlled Substance Schedule IV (USA), Schedule F (Canada)
Action: Produces CNS depression at limbic, thalamic, hypothalamic levels of CNS; may be mediated by neurotransmitter γ-aminobutyric acid (GABA); results are sedation, hypnosis, skeletal muscle relaxation, anticonvulsant activity, anxiolytic action

Uses: Insomnia, sedative, hypnotic
Dosage and routes:
• *Adult:* **PO** 0.125-0.5 mg hs
• *Elderly:* **PO** 0.625-0.125 mg hs
Available forms: Tabs 0.125, 0.25 mg

Side effects/adverse reactions:
*HEMA: **Leukopenia, granulocytopenia*** (rare)
CNS: Headache, lethargy, drowsiness, daytime sedation, dizziness, confusion, light-headedness, anxiety, irritability, amnesia, poor coordination
GI: Nausea, vomiting, diarrhea, heartburn, abdominal pain, constipation
CV: Chest pain, pulse changes

Contraindications: Hypersensitivity to benzodiazepines, pregnancy (X), lactation, intermittent porphyria

Precautions: Anemia, hepatic di-

---

sease, renal disease, suicidal individuals, drug abuse, elderly, psychosis, child <15 yr, acute narrow-angle glaucoma, seizure disorders

Pharmacokinetics:

PO: Onset 30-45 min, duration 6-8 hr; metabolized by liver, excreted by kidneys (inactive metabolites), crosses placenta, excreted in breast milk; half-life 2-3 hr

Interactions:

• Increased effects of cimetidine, disulfiram, erythromycin, macrolides, probenecid, isoniazid, oral contraceptives

• Increased action of both drugs: alcohol, CNS depressants

• Decreased effect of antacids, theophylline, rifampin, smoking

🍃 Increased CNS depression: kava

Lab test interferences:

Increase: ALT, AST, serum bilirubin

Decrease: RAI uptake

False increase: Urinary 17-OHCS

NURSING CONSIDERATIONS

Assess:

• Blood studies: Hct, Hgb, RBC if blood dyscrasias suspected (rare)

• Hepatic studies: AST, ALT, bilirubin if liver damage has occurred

• Mental status: mood, sensorium, affect, memory (long, short)

• Blood dyscrasias: fever, sore throat, bruising, rash, jaundice, epistaxis (rare)

• Type of sleep problem: falling asleep, staying asleep

Administer:

• After removal of cigarettes to prevent fires

• After trying conservative measures for insomnia

• ½ hr before hs for sleeplessness

• On empty stomach for fast onset, but may be taken with food if GI symptoms occur

Perform/provide:

• Assistance with ambulation after receiving dose

• Safety measures: side rails, night-light, call bell within easy reach

• Checking to see if PO medication has been swallowed

• Cool storage in tight container

Evaluate:

• Therapeutic response: ability to sleep at night, decreased amount of early morning awakening if taking drug for insomnia

Teach patient/family:

• That dependence is possible after long-term use

• To avoid driving, other activities requiring alertness until drug is stabilized

• To avoid alcohol ingestion, CNS depressants; serious CNS depression may result

• That effects may take 2 nights for benefits to be noticed; for short-term use only

• Alternative measures to improve sleep: reading, exercise several hours before hs, warm bath, warm milk, TV, self-hypnosis, deep breathing

• That hangover is common in elderly but less common than with barbiturates; rebound insomnia may occur for 1-2 nights after discontinuing drug

Treatment of overdose: Lavage, activated charcoal; monitor electrolytes, VS

T

trifluoperazine (℞)

(trye-floo-oh-per'a-zeen)
Novoflurazine*, Solazine*,
Stelazine, Suprazine,
Terfluzine, trifluoperazine
HCl, Triflurin

Func. class.: Antipsychotic, neuroleptic

Chem. class.: Phenothiazine, piperazine

Action: Depresses cerebral cortex, hypothalamus, limbic system, which control activity, aggression; blocks neurotransmission produced by dopamine at synapse; exhibits strong α-adrenergic, anticholinergic blocking action; mechanism for antipsychotic effects is unclear

Uses: Psychotic disorders, nonpsychotic anxiety, schizophrenia

Dosage and routes:

Psychotic disorders

• *Adult:* **PO** 2-5 mg bid, usual range 15-20 mg/day, may require 40 mg/day or more; **IM** 1-2 mg q4-6h

• *Geriatric:* **PO** 0.5-1 mg qd-bid, increase q4-7 days by 0.5-1 mg/day to desired dose

• *Child >6 yr:* **PO** 1 mg qd or bid; **IM** not recommended for children, but 1 mg may be given qd or bid

Nonpsychotic anxiety

• *Adult:* **PO** 1-2 mg bid, not to exceed 5 mg/day; do not give longer than 12 wk

Available forms: Tabs 1, 2, 5, 10 mg; conc 10 mg/ml; inj 2 mg/ml

Side effects/adverse reactions:

RESP: **Laryngospasm,** dyspnea, ***respiratory depression***

CNS: EPS: *pseudoparkinsonism, akathisia, dystonia, tardive dyskinesia,* **seizures,** *headache*

HEMA: Anemia, **leukopenia, leukocytosis, agranulocytosis**

INTEG: *Rash,* photosensitivity, dermatitis

EENT: Blurred vision, glaucoma, dry eyes

GI: Dry mouth, nausea, vomiting, anorexia, constipation, diarrhea, jaundice, weight gain

GU: Urinary retention, urinary frequency, enuresis, impotence, amenorrhea, gynecomastia

CV: Orthostatic hypotension, hypertension, ***cardiac arrest,*** ECG changes, ***tachycardia***

Contraindications: Hypersensitivity, cardiovascular disease, coma, blood dyscrasias, severe hepatic disease, child <6 yr, glaucoma

Precautions: Breast cancer, seizure disorders, pregnancy (C), lactation, diabetes mellitus, respiratory conditions, prostatic hypertrophy, elderly

Pharmacokinetics:

PO: Onset rapid, peak 2-3 hr, duration 12 hr

IM: Onset immediate, peak 1 hr, duration 12 hr

Metabolized by liver, excreted in urine, breast milk; crosses placenta

Interactions:

• Oversedation: other CNS depressants, alcohol, barbiturate anesthetics

• Toxicity: epinephrine

• Decreased absorption: aluminum hydroxide, magnesium hydroxide antacids

• Decreased effects of lithium, levodopa

• Increased effects of both drugs: β-adrenergic blockers, alcohol

• Increased anticholinergic effects: anticholinergics

🌿 Increased CNS depression: kava

Lab test interferences:

Increase: Liver function tests, cardiac enzymes, cholesterol, blood glucose, prolactin, bilirubin, PBI, cholinesterase, ^{131}I

Decrease: Hormones (blood, urine)

⬥ = Nursing alert   🌿 = Herb-drug interaction   🚫 = Do not crush

False positive: Pregnancy tests, PKU
False negative: Urinary steroids, 17-OHCS, pregnancy tests

NURSING CONSIDERATIONS

Assess:

• Mental status before initial administration

• Swallowing of PO medication; check for hoarding or giving of medication to other patients

• I&O ratio; palpate bladder if low urinary output occurs

• Bilirubin, CBC, liver function studies qmo

• Urinalysis is recommended before and during prolonged therapy

• Affect, orientation, LOC, reflexes, gait, coordination, sleep pattern disturbances

• For hypo-/hyperglycemia; appetite patterns

• B/P standing and lying; also include pulse, respirations q4h during initial treatment; establish baseline before starting treatment; report drops of 30 mm Hg

• Dizziness, faintness, palpitations, tachycardia on rising

• EPS including akathisia (inability to sit still, no pattern to movements), tardive dyskinesia (bizarre movements of jaw, mouth, tongue, extremities), pseudoparkinsonism (rigidity, tremors, pill rolling, shuffling gait)

• Skin turgor qd

• Constipation, urinary retention qd; if these occur increase bulk, water in diet

Administer:

• Reduced dose in elderly

• Antiparkinsonian agent on order from prescriber for EPS

PO

• Conc in 120 ml of tomato or fruit juice, milk, orange, carbonated beverage, coffee, tea, water, or semisolid foods (soup, pudding)

Perform/provide:

• Decreased stimulus by dimming lights, avoiding loud noises

• Supervised ambulation until stabilized on medication if needed; do not involve in strenuous exercise program because fainting is possible; patient should not stand still for long periods

• Increased fluids and bulk in diet to prevent constipation

• Sips of water, candy, gum for dry mouth

• Storage in tight, light-resistant container, oral sol in amber bottles; slight yellowing of inj or conc is common, does not affect potency

Evaluate:

• Therapeutic response: decrease in emotional excitement, hallucinations, delusions, paranoia, reorganization of patterns of thought, speech

Teach patient/family:

• That orthostatic hypotension occurs frequently, and to rise from sitting or lying position gradually; avoid hazardous activities until stabilized on medication

• To remain lying down after IM injection for at least 30 min

• To avoid hot tubs, hot showers, tub baths; hypotension may occur

• To avoid abrupt withdrawal of this drug, or EPS may result; drug should be withdrawn slowly

• To avoid OTC preparations (cough, hay fever, cold) unless approved by prescriber, since serious drug interactions may occur; avoid use with alcohol, CNS depressants; increased drowsiness may occur

• To use a sunscreen

• About compliance with drug regimen

• About the necessity for meticulous oral hygiene; oral candidiasis may occur

- To report sore throat, malaise, fever, bleeding, mouth sores; CBC should be drawn and drug discontinued
- That in hot weather, heat stroke may occur; take extra precautions to stay cool

Treatment of overdose: Lavage if orally ingested; provide an airway; do not induce vomiting

---

triflupromazine (℞)

(trye-floo-proe′ma-zeen)

Vesprin

Func. class.: Antipsychotic, neuroleptic

Chem. class.: Phenothiazine, aliphatic

Action: Depresses cerebral cortex, hypothalamus, limbic system, which control activity, aggression; blocks neurotransmission produced by dopamine at synapse; exhibits strong α-adrenergic, anticholinergic blocking action; mechanism for antipsychotic effects is unclear

Uses: Psychotic disorders, schizophrenia, acute agitation, nausea, vomiting

Dosage and routes:

Psychosis

- *Adult:* **PO** 10-50 mg bid-tid depending on severity of condition; dose is gradually increased to desired dose; **IM** 60 mg; not to exceed 150 mg/day
- *Child >2 yr:* **PO** 0.5-2 mg/kg/day in 3 divided doses; may increase to 10 mg if needed; **IM** 0.2 to 0.25 mg/kg to a maximum total dose of 10 mg/day

Nausea/vomiting

- *Adult:* **PO** 20-30 mg qd; **IV** 1-3 mg; **IM** 5-15 mg, q4h, max 60 mg qd

- *Child >2 yr:* **PO/IM** 0.2 mg/kg, max 10 mg qd

Acute agitation

- *Adult:* **IM** 60-150 mg/day in 3 divided doses
- *Child >2 yr:* **IM** 0.2-0.25 mg/kg/day in divided doses, max 10 mg qd

Available forms: Tabs 10, 25, 50 mg*; inj 10, 20 mg/ml

Side effects/adverse reactions:

*RESP: **Laryngospasm,** dyspnea, **respiratory depression***

*CNS: EPS: pseudoparkinsonism, akathisia, dystonia, tardive dyskinesia; drowsiness, headache, **seizures***

HEMA: Anemia, **leukopenia, leukocytosis, agranulocytosis**

INTEG: Rash, photosensitivity, dermatitis

EENT: Blurred vision, glaucoma

GI: Dry mouth, nausea, vomiting, anorexia, constipation, diarrhea, jaundice, weight gain

GU: Urinary retention, urinary frequency, enuresis, impotence, amenorrhea, gynecomastia

CV: Orthostatic hypotension, hypertension, **cardiac arrest,** ECG changes, **tachycardia**

Contraindications: Hypersensitivity, blood dyscrasias, coma, child <2½ yr, brain damage, bone marrow depression

Precautions: Pregnancy (C), lactation, seizure disorders, hepatic disease, cardiac disease

Pharmacokinetics:

PO: Onset erratic, peak 2-4 hr, duration 4-6 hr

IM: Onset 15-30 min, peak 1 hr, duration 4-6 hr

Metabolized by liver, excreted in urine, breast milk; feces, crosses placenta

Interactions:

- Oversedation: other CNS depressants, alcohol, barbiturate anesthetics

---

⬥ = Nursing alert   🌿 = Herb-drug interaction   Ⓢ = Do not crush

• Toxicity: epinephrine

• Decreased absorption: aluminum hydroxide, magnesium hydroxide antacids

• Decreased effects of lithium, levodopa

• Increased effects of both drugs: β-adrenergic blockers, alcohol

• Increased anticholinergic effects: anticholinergics

🖉 Increased CNS depression: kava

Lab test interferences:

Increase: Liver function tests, cardiac enzymes, cholesterol, blood glucose, prolactin, bilirubin, PBI, cholinesterase, ^{131}I

Decrease: Hormones (blood, urine)

False positive: Pregnancy tests, PKU

False negative: Urinary steroids, pregnancy tests

NURSING CONSIDERATIONS

Assess:

• Swallowing of PO medication; check for hoarding or giving of medication to other patients

• I&O ratio; palpate bladder if low urinary output occurs

• Bilirubin, CBC, liver function studies qmo

• Urinalysis is recommended before and during prolonged therapy

• Affect, orientation, LOC, reflexes, gait, coordination, sleep pattern disturbances

• B/P standing and lying; pulse, respirations q4h during initial treatment; establish baseline before starting treatment; report drops of 30 mm Hg

◆ For neuroleptic malignant syndrome: altered mental status, muscle rigidity, increased CPK, hyperthermia

• Dizziness, faintness, palpitations, tachycardia on rising

• EPS, including akathisia (inability to sit still, no pattern to movements), tardive dyskinesia (bizarre movements of jaw, mouth, tongue, extremities), pseudoparkinsonism (rigidity, tremors, pill rolling, shuffling gait)

• Assess for hypo-/hyperglycemia; appetite patterns

• Constipation, urinary retention qd; if these occur, increase bulk, water in the diet

Administer:

• Reduced dose to elderly

• Antiparkinsonian agent on order from prescriber for EPS

• IM inj into large muscle mass; avoid contact with skin

IV

• IV after diluting 10 mg/9 ml of NS; give 1 mg or less/2 min

Additive compatibilities: Meperidine, netilmicin

Syringe compatibilities: Glycopyrrolate

Perform/provide:

• Decreased stimulus by dimming lights, avoiding loud noises

• Supervised ambulation until stabilized on medication; do not involve in strenuous exercise program because fainting is possible; patient should not stand still for long periods

• Increased fluids to prevent constipation

• Sips of water, candy, gum for dry mouth

• Storage in tight, light-resistant container

Evaluate:

• Therapeutic response: decrease in emotional excitement, hallucinations, delusions, paranoia, reorganization of patterns of thought, speech

Teach patient/family:

• That orthostatic hypotension occurs frequently, and to rise from sitting or lying position gradually; to avoid hazardous activities until stabilized on medication

• To remain lying down for at least 30 min after IM inj

• To avoid hot tubs, hot showers, tub baths; hypotension may occur

• To avoid abrupt withdrawal; or EPS may result; drug should be withdrawn slowly

• To avoid OTC preparations (cough, hay fever, cold) unless approved by prescriber; serious drug interactions may occur; avoid use with alcohol, CNS depressants; increased drowsiness may occur

• To use sunscreen

• About compliance with drug regimen

• About the necessity for meticulous oral hygiene, since oral candidiasis may occur

• To report sore throat, malaise, fever, bleeding, mouth sores; if these occur, CBC should be drawn and drug discontinued

• That in hot weather, heat stroke may occur; take extra precautions to stay cool

Treatment of overdose: Lavage if orally ingested; provide an airway; *do not induce vomiting*

---

trihexyphenidyl (R)

(trye-hex-ee-fen'i-dill)
Artane, Artane Sequels, Novohexidyl*, Trihexane, Trihexy-2, Trihexy-5, trihexyphenidyl HCl
Func. class.: Cholinergic blocker
Chem. class.: Synthetic tertiary amine

Action: Blocks central muscarinic receptors, which decreases involuntary movements, sweating, salivation

Uses: Parkinson symptoms, drug-induced EPS

Dosage and routes:
Parkinson symptoms
• *Adult:* PO 1 mg, increased by 2 mg q3-5d to a total of 6-10 mg/day
Drug-induced EPS
• *Adult:* PO 1 mg/day; usual dose 5-15 mg/day
Available forms: Tabs 2, 5 mg; caps sus rel 5 mg; elix 2 mg/5 ml

Side effects/adverse reactions:
CNS: Confusion, anxiety, restlessness, irritability, delusions, hallucinations, headache, sedation, depression, incoherence, dizziness, flushing, weakness
EENT: Blurred vision, photophobia, dilated pupils, difficulty swallowing, dry eyes, increased intraocular tension, angle-closure glaucoma
CV: Palpitations, tachycardia, postural hypotension
INTEG: Urticaria, rash
MISC: Suppression of lactation, nasal congestion, decreased sweating, increased temp, hyperthermia, heat stroke, numbness of fingers
MS: Weakness, cramping
GI: Dryness of mouth, constipation, nausea, vomiting, abdominal distress, ***paralytic ileus***
GU: Urinary hesitancy, retention, dysuria

Contraindications: Hypersensitivity, narrow-angle glaucoma, myasthenia gravis, GI/GU obstruction, myocardial ischemia, unstable CV disease, prostatic hypertrophy

Precautions: Pregnancy (C), elderly, lactation, tachycardia, abdominal obstruction, infection, children, gastric ulcer

Pharmacokinetics:
PO: Onset 1 hr, peak 2-3 hr, duration 6-12 hr, excreted in urine, half-life 5-10 hr

Interactions:
• Increased anticholinergic effects: antihistamines, phenothiazines, amantadine

---

⬥ = Nursing alert   🌿 = Herb-drug interaction   🚫 = Do not crush

• Decreased action of haloperidol
• Increased CNS depression: analgesics, alcohol, sedatives/hypnotics
• Increased levels of: digoxin

NURSING CONSIDERATIONS
Assess:
• I&O ratio; retention commonly causes decreased urinary output
• B/P, pulse frequently while dose is being determined
• Urinary hesitancy, retention; palpate bladder if retention occurs
• Constipation; increase fluids, bulk, exercise
• For tolerance over long-term therapy; dosage may have to be increased or medication changed
• Mental status: affect, mood, CNS depression, worsening of mental symptoms during early therapy

Administer:
• With or after meals for GI upset; may give with fluids other than water
• At hs to avoid daytime drowsiness in patient with parkinsonism

Perform/provide:
• Storage at room temp in light-resistant container
• Hard candy, frequent drinks, sugarless gum to relieve dry mouth

Evaluate:
• Therapeutic response: parkinsonism: shuffling gait, muscle rigidity, involuntary movements

Teach patient/family:
• Not to discontinue this drug abruptly; to taper off over 1 wk
• To avoid driving, other hazardous activities; drowsiness may occur
• To avoid OTC medications: cough, cold preparations with alcohol, antihistamines unless directed by prescriber
• To avoid sudden position changes
• To avoid hot climates; overheating may occur

---

trimethobenzamide (℞)
(trye-meth-oh-ben'za-mide)
Arrestin, Benzacot, Brogan, Stemetic, T-Gen, Tebamide, Ticon, Tigan, Tiject-20, Triban, Trimazide, Trimethobenzamide, trimethobenzamide HCl
Func. class.: Antiemetic, anticholinergic
Chem. class.: Ethanolamine derivative

Action: Acts centrally by blocking chemoreceptor trigger zone, which in turn acts on vomiting center
Uses: Nausea, vomiting, prevention of postoperative vomiting
Dosage and routes:

Postoperative vomiting
• *Adult:* **IM/RECT** 200 mg before or during surgery; may repeat 3 hr after

Discontinuing anesthesia
• *Child 13-40 kg:* **PO/RECT** 100-200 mg tid-qid
• *Child <13 kg:* **PO/RECT** 100 mg tid-qid

Nausea/vomiting
• *Adult:* **PO** 250 mg tid-qid; **IM/RECT** 200 mg tid-qid

Available forms: Caps 100, 250 mg; supp 100, 200 mg; inj 100 mg/ml
Side effects/adverse reactions:

CNS: Drowsiness, restlessness, headache, dizziness, insomnia, confusion, nervousness, tingling, *vertigo,* EPS
GI: Nausea, anorexia, diarrhea, vomiting, constipation
CV: Hypertension, hypotension, palpitation
INTEG: Rash, urticaria, fever, chills, flushing
EENT: Dry mouth, blurred vision, diplopia, nasal congestion, photosensitivity

T

Contraindications: Hypersensitivity to narcotics, shock, children (parenterally)

Precautions: Children, cardiac dysrhythmias, elderly, asthma, pregnancy (C), prostatic hypertrophy, bladder-neck obstruction, narrow-angle glaucoma, stenosing peptic ulcer, pyloroduodenal obstruction

Pharmacokinetics:

PO: Onset 20-40 min, duration 3-4 hr

IM: Onset 15 min, duration 2-3 hr Metabolized by liver, excreted by kidneys

Interactions:

• Increased effect: CNS depressants

• May mask ototoxic symptoms associated with antibiotics

NURSING CONSIDERATIONS

Assess:

• For nausea, vomiting before, after treatment

• VS, B/P; check patients with cardiac disease more often

• Signs of toxicity of other drugs or masking of symptoms of disease: brain tumor, intestinal obstruction

• Observe for drowsiness, dizziness

Administer:

• IM inj in large muscle mass; aspirate to avoid IV administration

• Tablets may be swallowed whole, chewed, allowed to dissolve

Syringe compatibilities: Glycopyrrolate, hydromorphone, midazolam, nalbuphine

Y-site compatibilities: Heparin, hydrocortisone, potassium chloride, vit B/C

Evaluate:

• Therapeutic response: decreased nausea, vomiting

Teach patient/family:

• To avoid hazardous activities, activities requiring alertness; dizziness may occur; to request assistance with ambulation

• To avoid alcohol, other depressants

• To keep out of children's reach

---

trimethoprim (Ŗ)

(trye-meth'oh-prim)

Proloprim, Trimethoprim, Trimpex

Func. class.: Urinary antiinfective

Chem. class.: Folate antagonist

Action: Prevents bacterial synthesis by blocking enzyme reduction of dihydrofolic acid

Uses: *Escherichia coli, Proteus mirabilis, Klebsiella, Enterobacter* UTIs

Dosage and routes:

Renal dose

• CrCl 15-30 ml/min 50 mg q12h; CrCl <15 ml/min avoid use

• *Adult:* **PO** 100 mg q12h × 10 days

• *Child:* 4 mg/kg/day divided q12h

Available forms: Tabs 100, 200 mg

Side effects/adverse reactions:

INTEG: **Exfoliative dermatitis,** pruritus, rash

HEMA: **Thrombocytopenia, leukopenia, neutropenia, megaloblastic anemia** (rare)

GI: Nausea, vomiting, abdominal pain, abnormal taste, increased AST, ALT, bilirubin, creatinine

CNS: Fever

Contraindications: Hypersensitivity, CrCl <15 ml/min, megaloblastic anemia

Precautions: Folate deficiency, pregnancy (C), lactation, fragile X chromosome, child <12 yr old, renal disease, hepatic disease

Pharmacokinetics:

PO: Peak 1-4 hr, half-life 8-11 hr; metabolized in liver, excreted in urine (unchanged 60%), breast milk; crosses placenta

---

◆ = Nursing alert   🖋 = Herb-drug interaction   🚫 = Do not crush

Interactions:
• Increased action of phenytoin
NURSING CONSIDERATIONS
Assess:
• Nocturia; may indicate drug resistance
• Signs of infection, anemia
• AST, ALT, BUN, bilirubin, creatinine, urine cultures
• C&S; drug may be given as soon as culture is obtained
• Skin eruptions
Administer:
• With full glass of water
Perform/provide:
• Storage in tight, light-resistant container
• Adequate intake of fluids (2 L) to decrease bacteria in bladder
Evaluate:
• Therapeutic response: absence of pain in bladder area, negative C&S
Teach patient/family:
• All aspects of drug therapy: need to complete entire course of medication to ensure organism death (10-14 days); culture may be taken after completed course of medication
• That drug must be taken in equal intervals around clock to maintain blood levels
• To notify nurse of nausea, vomiting, rash, severe fatigue, sore throat

trimethoprim-sulfamethoxazole (Ŗ)

(trye-meth'oh-prim–sul-fa-meth-ox'a-zole)
Apo-Sulfatrim*, Bactrim, Bactrim IV, Bethaprim, Comoxol, Cotrim, Septra, Sulfatrim
Func. class.: Antiinfective
Chem. class.: Miscellaneous sulfonamide

Action: Sulfamethoxazole (SMZ) interferes with bacterial biosynthesis of proteins by competitive antagonism of PABA when adequate levels are maintained; trimethoprim (TMP) blocks synthesis of tetrahydrofolic acid; combination blocks 2 consecutive steps in bacterial synthesis of essential nucleic acids, protein

Uses: UTI, otitis media, acute and chronic prostatitis, shigellosis, *Pneumocystis carinii* pneumonitis, chronic bronchitis, chancroid, traveler's diarrhea

Dosage and routes: Based on TMP content
UTI
• *Adult:* **PO** 160 mg TMP q12h × 10-14 days
• *Child:* **PO** 8 mg/kg TMP qd in 2 divided doses q12h
Otitis media
• *Child:* **PO** 8 mg/kg TMP qd in 2 divided doses q12h × 10 days
Chronic bronchitis
• *Adult:* **PO** 160 mg TMP q12h × 14 days
Pneumocystis carinii *pneumonitis*
• *Adult and child:* **PO** 20 mg/kg TMP qd in 4 divided doses q6h × 14 days; **IV** 15-20 mg/kg/day (based on TMP) in 3-4 divided doses for up to 14 days
• Dosage reduction necessary in

T

moderate to severe renal impairment (CrCl <30 ml/min)

Available forms: Tabs 80 mg trimethoprim/400 mg sulfamethoxazole, 160 mg trimethoprim/800 mg sulfamethoxazole; susp 40 mg/200 mg/5 ml; IV 16 mg/80 mg/ml

Side effects/adverse reactions:

CNS: Headache, insomnia, hallucinations, depression, vertigo, fatigue, anxiety, *convulsions, drug fever,* chills, *aseptic meningitis*

CV: Allergic myocarditis

GI: Nausea, vomiting, abdominal pain, stomatitis, *hepatitis,* glossitis, pancreatitis, diarrhea, *enterocolitis,* anorexia

GU: Renal failure, toxic nephrosis; increased BUN, creatinine; crystalluria

HEMA: Leukopenia, neutropenia, thrombocytopenia, agranulocytosis, hemolytic anemia, hypoprothrombinemia, Henoch-Schönlein purpura, methemoglobinemia, eosinophilia I

INTEG: Rash, dermatitis, urticaria, *Stevens-Johnson syndrome,* erythema, photosensitivity, pain, inflammation at injection site

RESP: Cough, shortness of breath

SYST: Anaphylaxis, SLE

Contraindications: Hypersensitivity to trimethoprim or sulfonamides, pregnancy at term, megaloblastic anemia, infants <2 mo, CrCl <15 ml/min, lactation, porphyria

Precautions: Pregnancy (C), renal disease, elderly, G6PD deficiency, impaired hepatic/renal function, possible folate deficiency, severe allergy, bronchial asthma

Pharmacokinetics:

PO: Rapidly absorbed, peak 1-4 hr; half-life 8-13 hr, excreted in urine (metabolites and unchanged), breast milk; crosses placenta; 68% bound to plasma proteins; TMP achieves high levels in prostatic tissue and fluid

Interactions:

• Increased hypoglycemic response: sulfonylurea agents

• Increased anticoagulant effects: oral anticoagulants

• Decreased hepatic clearance of phenytoin

• Decreased response: cyclosporine

• Increased bone marrow depressant effects: methotrexate

• Thrombocytopenia: thiazide diuretics

Lab test interferences:

Increase: Alk phosphatase, creatinine, bilirubin

False positive: Urinary glucose test

NURSING CONSIDERATIONS

Assess:

• Allergic reactions: rash, fever (AIDS patients more susceptible)

• I&O ratio; note color, character, pH of urine if drug administered for UTI; output should be 800 ml less than intake; if urine is highly acidic, alkalization may be needed

• Kidney function studies: BUN, creatinine, urinalysis (long-term therapy)

• Type of infection; obtain C&S before starting therapy

• Blood dyscrasias, skin rash, fever, sore throat, bruising, bleeding, fatigue, joint pain

• Allergic reaction: rash, dermatitis, urticaria, pruritus, dyspnea, bronchospasm

Administer:

PO

• Medication after C&S; repeat C&S after full course of medication

• With resuscitative equipment, epinephrine available; severe allergic reactions may occur

• With full glass of water to maintain adequate hydration; increase flu-

---

 = Nursing alert   = Herb-drug interaction $\bigcirc$ = Do not crush ids to 2 L/day to decrease crystallization in kidneys

IV

• After diluting 5 ml of drug/125 ml D_5W, run over 1-1½ hr

Syringe compatibilities: Heparin

Y-site compatibilities: Acyclovir, aldesleukin, allopurinol, amifostine, amphotericin B cholesteryl, atracurium, aztreonam, cefepime, cyclophosphamide, diltiazem, doxorubicin liposome, enalaprilat, esmolol, filgrastim, fludarabine, gallium, granisetron, hydromorphone, labetalol, lorazepam, magnesium sulfate, melphalan, meperidine, morphine, pancuronium, perphenazine, piperacillin/tazobactam, remifentanil, sargramostim, tacrolimus, teniposide, thiotepa, vecuronium, zidovudine

Perform/provide:

• Storage in tight, light-resistant container at room temp

Evaluate:

• Therapeutic response: absence of pain, fever, C&S negative

Teach patient/family:

• To take each oral dose with full glass of water to prevent crystalluria; drink 8-10 glasses of water/day; to take on an empty stomach 1 hr ac, 2 hr pc

• To complete full course of treatment to prevent superinfection

• To avoid sunlight or use sunscreen to prevent burns

• To avoid OTC medications (aspirin, vit C) unless directed by prescriber

• If diabetic, to use Clinistix or Tes-Tape

• To use alternative contraceptive measures; decreased effectiveness of oral contraceptives may result

• To notify prescriber if skin rash, sore throat, fever, mouth sores, unusual bruising, bleeding occur

trimetrexate (R)
(tri-me-trex′ate)
Neutrexin
Func. class.: Antiinfective-misc.
Chem. class.: Nonclassical folic acid antagonist

Action: Inhibits an enzyme that reduces folic acid, which is needed for purine biosynthesis in all cells; result is disruption of RNA, DNA, cell death; leucovorin usually transported into cells by active, carrier-mediated process; however, *Pneumocystis carinii* organisms lack carrier system; trimetrexate must be given with leucovorin to protect normal cells

Uses: Moderate to severe *Pneumocystis carinii* pneumonia as an alternative to TMP/SMZ; may be useful in treating non–small cell lung, prostate, colorectal cancer

Dosage and routes:

Leucovorin must be given concurrently and for 72 hr past last trimetrexate dose

• *Adult:* **IV** 45 mg/m² qd over 60-90 min; with leucovorin **IV** 20 mg/m² over 5-10 min q6h for a daily dose of 80 mg/m² or **PO** qid 20 mg/m² evenly spaced during the day; **PO** dose should be rounded to the next higher 25 mg; course is trimetrexate 21 days, leucovorin 24 days; modifications in dose must be based on hematologic toxicity

Available forms: Powder for inj lyophilized 25 mg

Side effects/adverse reactions:

CNS: Confusion, fatigue, fever

GI: Nausea, vomiting, **hepatotoxicity,** ulcer, stomatitis

GU: Increased serum creatinine

HEMA: **Thrombocytopenia, anemia**

INTEG: Rash, pruritus

META: Hyponatremia, hypocalcemia

Contraindications: Hypersensitivity to trimetrexate, leucovorin, methotrexate, thrombocytopenia ($<25,000/mm^3$), severe anemia, neutropenia ($<500/mm^3$), pregnancy (D)

Precautions: Renal disease, hepatic disease, lactation, children, seizures

Pharmacokinetics:

Terminal half-life 7-15 hr; may be 95%-98% protein bound

Interactions:

Specific interactions not known; these interactions may occur:

• Increased toxicity: aspirin, sulfa drugs, other antineoplastics, radiation

• Decreased effect of trimetrexate: erythromycin, ketoconazole, fluconazole, rifampin, rifabutin, cimetidine

NURSING CONSIDERATIONS
Assess:

• CBC, differential, platelet count qwk; withhold drug if neutrophils $<500/mm^3$ or platelet count $<25,000/mm^3$; notify prescriber; drug should be discontinued; hematologic toxicity should be graded 1-4, 4 most severe

• Renal function studies: BUN, serum uric acid, urine CrCl, electrolytes before, during therapy; treatment should be interrupted when creatinine >2.5 mg/dl

• I&O ratio; report urine output <30 ml/hr

• Monitor temp q4h; fever may indicate beginning infection; no rectal temps

• Liver function tests before, during therapy: bilirubin, alk phosphatase, AST, ALT; treatment should be interrupted when alk phosphatase or transaminase $>5 \times$ upper normal limit

• Bleeding time, coagulation time during treatment

Administer:

• Antiemetic 30-60 min before giving drug to prevent vomiting

• Transfusion for anemia

IV

• Reconstitute with 2 ml D_5 or sterile H_2O (12.5 mg/ml) filter 0.22 μ prior to dilution; dilute reconstituted sol with D_5 for concentration of 0.25-2 mg/ml; give over 60 min; flush IV line thoroughly with 10 ml D_5 before, after dose

• Trimetrexate and leucovorin sol separately; leucovorin may be given before or after trimetrexate; IV line must be flushed between infusions

• If trimetrexate comes in contact with skin, wash with soap, water immediately

Y-site compatibilities: Amifostine, zidovudine

Perform/provide:

• Strict medical asepsis and protective isolation if WBC levels low

• Liquid diet: carbonated beverage, Jell-O; dry toast, crackers may be added when patient is not nauseated or vomiting

• Rinsing of mouth tid-qid with water, club soda; brushing of teeth bid-tid with soft brush or cotton-tipped applicators for stomatitis; use unwaxed dental floss

• Nutritious diet with iron, vitamin supplements

• Storage after reconstitution up to 24 hr refrigerated; do not freeze reconstituted sol; discard after 24 hr

Evaluate:

• Therapeutic response: decreased symptoms of pneumocystis

• Bleeding: hematuria, guaiac, bruising or petechiae, mucosa or orifices q8h

• Food preferences; list likes, dislikes

◆Hepatotoxicity: jaundiced skin,

sclera; dark urine, clay-colored stools, pruritus, abdominal pain, fever, diarrhea
• Buccal cavity q8h for dryness, sores, ulceration, white patches, oral pain, bleeding, dysphagia
• Symptoms of severe allergic reaction: rash, urticaria, itching, flushing

Teach patient/family:

• About protective isolation
• To report any complaints, side effects to nurse or prescriber: black, tarry stools; chills, fever, sore throat, bleeding, bruising, cough, shortness of breath, dark or bloody urine
• To avoid foods with citric acid, hot or rough texture if stomatitis is present
• To report to prescriber stomatitis: any bleeding, white spots, ulcerations in mouth; to examine mouth qd, report symptoms to nurse
• To drink 10-12 glasses of fluid/day
• To avoid alcohol, salicylates
• To avoid use of razors, commercial mouthwash

---

trimipramine (℞)

(tri-mip´ra-meen)
Surmontil, Trimipramine Maleate, Trisoralen
Func. class.: Antidepressant—tricyclic
Chem. class.: Tertiary amine

Action: Selectively inhibits serotonin uptake by brain; potentiates behavioral changes

Uses: Depression, enuresis in children

Dosage and routes:
• *Adult:* **PO** 75 mg/day in divided doses, may be increased to 200 mg/day
• *Geriatric:* **PO** 25 mg hs, increase by 25 mg q3-7 days, max 100 mg/day
• *Child >6 yr:* 25 mg hs, may increase to 50 mg in child <12 yr or 75 mg in child >12 yr

Available forms: Caps 25, 50, 100 mg

Side effects/adverse reactions:

HEMA: **Agranulocytosis, thrombocytopenia, eosinophilia, leukopenia**
CNS: Dizziness, drowsiness, confusion, headache, anxiety, tremors, stimulation, weakness, insomnia, nightmares, EPS (elderly), increase in psychiatric symptoms
GI: Diarrhea, *dry mouth,* nausea, vomiting, *paralytic ileus,* increased appetite, cramps, epigastric distress, jaundice, *hepatitis,* stomatitis, *constipation*
GU: Urinary retention, **acute renal failure**
INTEG: Rash, urticaria, sweating, pruritus, photosensitivity
CV: Orthostatic hypotension, ECG changes, tachycardia, **hypertension,** palpitations
EENT: Blurred vision, tinnitus, mydriasis

Contraindications: Hypersensitivity to tricyclic antidepressants, recovery phase of MI, convulsive disorders, prostatic hypertrophy

Precautions: Suicidal patients, severe depression, increased intraocular pressure, narrow-angle glaucoma, urinary retention, cardiac disease, hepatic disease, hyperthyroidism, electroshock therapy, elective surgery, pregnancy (C), elderly

Pharmacokinetics: Metabolized by liver, excreted by kidneys, steady state 2-6 days; half-life 7-30 hr

Interactions:
• Decreased effects of: guanethidine, clonidine, indirect-acting sympathomimetics (ephedrine)

T

- Increased effects of direct-acting sympathomimetics (epinephrine), alcohol, barbiturates, benzodiazepines, CNS depressants
- Hyperpyretic crisis, convulsions, hypertensive episode: MAOI (pargyline [Eutonyl])

/// Increased anticholinergic effect: belladonna, henbane

/// Increased antidepressant action: scopola

Lab test interferences:

Increase: Serum bilirubin, blood glucose, alk phosphatase

False increase: Urinary catecholamines

Decrease: VMA, 5-HIAA

NURSING CONSIDERATIONS
Assess:

- B/P (lying, standing), pulse q4h; if systolic B/P drops 20 mm Hg, hold drug, notify prescriber; take vital signs q4h in patients with cardiovascular disease
- Blood studies: CBC, leukocytes, differential, cardiac enzymes if patient is receiving long-term therapy
- Hepatic studies: AST, ALT, bilirubin, creatinine
- Weight qwk; appetite may increase with drug
- ECG for flattening of T wave, bundle branch block, AV block, dysrhythmias in cardiac patients
- EPS primarily in elderly: rigidity, dystonia, akathisia
- Mental status changes: mood, sensorium, affect, suicidal tendencies, increase in psychiatric symptoms, depression, panic
- Urinary retention, constipation; constipation is more likely to occur in children, elderly
- Withdrawal symptoms: headache, nausea, vomiting, muscle pain, weakness; not usual unless drug is discontinued abruptly
- Alcohol consumption; hold dose until morning

Administer:

- Increased fluids, bulk in diet for constipation, urinary retention
- With food, milk for GI symptoms
- Dosage hs for oversedation during day; may take entire dose hs; elderly may not tolerate once/day dosing
- Gum, hard candy, or frequent sips of water for dry mouth

Perform/provide:

- Storage in tight, light-resistant container at room temp
- Assistance with ambulation during beginning therapy for drowsiness/dizziness
- Safety measures, including side rails, primarily for elderly
- Checking to see if PO medication swallowed

Evaluate:

- Therapeutic response: decreased depression or enuresis

Teach patient/family:

- That therapeutic effects may take 2-3 wk
- To use caution in driving, other activities requiring alertness because of drowsiness, dizziness, blurred vision
- To avoid alcohol ingestion, other CNS depressants
- Not to discontinue medication quickly after long-term use; may cause nausea, headache, malaise
- To wear sunscreen or large hat, since photosensitivity occurs

Treatment of overdose: ECG monitoring; induce emesis; lavage, activated charcoal; administer anticonvulsant

◆ = Nursing alert   /// = Herb-drug interaction   ⊘ = Do not crush

triprolidine (OTC, ℞)

(trye-proe'li-deen)
Actidil, Alleract, Myidil,
triprolidine HCl
Func. class.: Antihistamine
Chem. class.: Alkylamine, H$_1$-receptor antagonist

Action: Acts on blood vessels, GI, respiratory system by competing with histamine for H$_1$-receptor site; decreases allergic response by blocking histamine

Uses: Rhinitis, allergy symptoms

Dosage and routes:
• *Adult:* PO 2.5 mg tid-qid
• *Child >6 yr:* PO 1.25 mg tid-qid
• *Child 4-6 yr:* PO 0.9 mg tid-qid
• *Child 2-4 yr:* PO 0.6 mg tid-qid
• *Child 4 mo-2 yr:* 0.3 mg tid-qid

Available forms: Tabs 2.5 mg; syr 1.25 mg/5 ml

Side effects/adverse reactions:
CNS: Dizziness, drowsiness, poor coordination, fatigue, anxiety, euphoria, confusion, paresthesia, neuritis
CV: Hypotension, palpitations, tachycardia
RESP: Increased thick secretions, wheezing, chest tightness
HEMA: **Thrombocytopenia, agranulocytosis, hemolytic anemia**
GI: Constipation, dry mouth, nausea, vomiting, anorexia, diarrhea
INTEG: Rash, urticaria, photosensitivity
GU: Urinary retention, dysuria, frequency
EENT: Blurred vision, dilated pupils, tinnitus, nasal stuffiness, dry nose, throat, mouth

Contraindications: Hypersensitivity to H$_1$-receptor antagonist, acute asthma attack, lower respiratory tract disease

Precautions: Increased intraocular pressure, renal disease, cardiac disease, hypertension, bronchial asthma, seizure disorder, stenosed peptic ulcers, hyperthyroidism, prostatic hypertrophy, bladder neck obstruction, pregnancy (C)

Pharmacokinetics:
PO: Onset 20-60 min, duration 8-12 hr; detoxified in liver, excreted by kidneys (metabolites/free drug), half-life 20-24 hr

Interactions:
• Increased CNS depressants: barbiturates, narcotics, hypnotics, tricyclic antidepressants, alcohol
• Decreased effect of oral anticoagulants, heparin
• Increased effect of triprolidine: MAOIs
⚠ Increased anticholinergic effect: henbane

Lab test interferences:
False negative: Skin allergy tests

NURSING CONSIDERATIONS
Assess:
• I&O ratio; be alert for urinary retention, frequency, dysuria; drug should be discontinued
• CBC during long-term therapy; blood dyscrasias
• Respiratory status: rate, rhythm, increase in bronchial secretions, wheezing, chest tightness
• Cardiac status: palpitations, increased pulse, hypotension
Administer:
• With meals for GI symptoms; absorption may slightly decrease
Perform/provide:
• Hard candy, gum, frequent rinsing of mouth for dryness
• Storage in tight container at room temp
Evaluate:
• Therapeutic response: decreased itching associated with pruritus
Teach patient/family:
• All aspects of drug use; to notify

T

prescriber of confusion, sedation, hypotension
• To avoid driving, other hazardous activity if drowsiness occurs
• To avoid concurrent use of alcohol, other CNS depressants
Treatment of overdose: Administer ipecac syrup or lavage, diazepam, vasopressors, barbiturates (short-acting)

---

tromethamine (℞)
(troe-meth′a-meen)
Tham, Tham-E
Func. class.: Alkalinizer
Chem. class.: Amine

Action: Proton acceptor that corrects acidosis by combining with hydrogen ions to form bicarbonate and buffer; acts as diuretic (osmotic)
Uses: Acidosis (metabolic) associated with cardiac disease, COPD
Dosage and routes:
• *Adult:* IV 0.3 M required = kg of weight × HCO_3 deficit (mEq/L)
• *Child:* IV same as above given over 3-6 hr, not to exceed 40 ml/kg
Available forms: Inj 36 mg/ml, powder for inj 36 g
Side effects/adverse reactions:
CV: Irregular pulse, ***cardiac arrest***
META: Alkalosis, hypoglycemia
RESP: Shallow, slow respirations, cyanosis, ***apnea***
GI: ***Hepatic necrosis***
INTEG: Infection at injection site, extravasation, phlebitis
Contraindications: Hypersensitivity, anuria, uremia
Precautions: Severe respiratory disease/respiratory depression, pregnancy (C), cardiac edema, renal disease, infants
Pharmacokinetics:
IV: Excreted in urine

Interactions:
⊘ Decreased alkaline effect: oak bark
NURSING CONSIDERATIONS
Assess:
• Respiratory rate, rhythm, depth; notify prescriber of abnormalities that may indicate acidosis
• Electrolytes, blood glucose, chloride; CO_2 before, during treatment
• Urine pH, urinary output, urine glucose during beginning treatment
• I&O ratio, report large increase or decrease
• IV site for extravasation, phlebitis, thrombosis
• For signs of K^+ depletion
Administer:
• IV slowly to avoid pain at infusion site and toxicity
• IV undiluted as inf or added to priming fluid or ACD blood; give 5 ml or less/min
Evaluate:
• Therapeutic response: decreased metabolic acidosis
Teach patient/family:
• To increase K^+ in diet: bananas, oranges, cantaloupe, honeydew, spinach, potatoes, dried fruit

---

tubocurarine (℞)
(too-boe-kyoor-ar′een)
Tubarine*, Tubocuraine
Func. class.: Neuromuscular blocker
Chem. class.: Curare alkaloid

Action: Inhibits transmission of nerve impulses by binding with cholinergic receptor sites, antagonizing action of acetylcholine
Uses: Facilitation of endotracheal intubation, skeletal muscle relaxation during mechanical ventilation, surgery, or general anesthesia

---

◆ = Nursing alert   ⊘ = Herb-drug interaction   ⊘ = Do not crush

Dosage and routes:
• *Adult:* **IV BOL** 0.4-0.5 mg/kg, then 0.08-0.10 mg/kg 20-45 min after 1st dose if needed for long procedures
Available forms: Inj 3 mg/ml, 20 U/ml
Side effects/adverse reactions:
CV: Bradycardia, tachycardia, increased, decreased B/P
RESP: ***Prolonged apnea, bronchospasm, cyanosis, respiratory depression***
EENT: Increased secretions
INTEG: Rash, flushing, pruritus, urticaria
Contraindications: Hypersensitivity
Precautions: Pregnancy (C), cardiac disease, lactation, children <2 yr, electrolyte imbalances, dehydration, neuromuscular disease, respiratory disease
Pharmacokinetics:
IV: Onset 15 sec, peak 2-3 min, duration ½-1½ hr; half-life 1-3 hr; degraded in liver, kidney (minimally); excreted in urine (unchanged) crosses placenta
Interactions:
• Increased neuromuscular blockade: aminoglycosides, clindamycin, lincomycin, quinidine, local anesthetics, polymyxin antibiotics, lithium, narcotic analgesics, thiazides, enflurane, isoflurane, trimethaphan, magnesium salts
• Dysrhythmias: theophylline
NURSING CONSIDERATIONS
Assess:
• For electrolyte imbalances (K, Mg); may lead to increased action of this drug
• Vital signs (B/P, pulse, respirations, airway) q15min until fully recovered; rate, depth, pattern of respirations, strength of hand grip
• I&O ratio; check for urinary retention, frequency, hesitancy

• Recovery: decreased paralysis of face, diaphragm, leg, arm, rest of body; allow to recover fully before completing neurologic assessment
• Allergic reactions: rash, fever, respiratory distress, pruritus; drug should be discontinued
Administer:
• With diazepam or morphine when used for therapeutic paralysis; provides no sedation alone
• Using nerve stimulator by anesthesiologist to determine neuromuscular blockade
• Anticholinesterase to reverse neuromuscular blockade
• IV undiluted 3 mg/ml; give single dose over 1-1½ sec by qualified person; diluted to 4 ml in NS given 0.5 ml/2 min for myasthenia testing
Solution compatibilities: D_5, $D_{10}W$, 0.9% NaCl, 0.45% NaCl, Ringer's, LR, dextrose/Ringer's or dextrose/LR combinations
Syringe compatibilities: Pentobarbital, thiopental
Perform/provide:
• Storage in light-resistant area; use only fresh sol
• Reassurance if communication is difficult during recovery from neuromuscular blockade
Evaluate:
• Therapeutic response: paralysis of jaw, eyelid, head, neck, rest of body
Treatment of overdose: Edrophonium or neostigmine, atropine, monitor VS; may require mechanical ventilation

T

urea (Ŗ)

(yoor-ee'a)

Ureaphil, Carbamex*

Func. class.: Diuretic, osmotic

Chem. class.: Carbonic acid diamide salt

Action: Elevates plasma osmolality, increasing flow of water into plasma from ocular and cranial fluids

Uses: To decrease intracranial pressure, intraocular pressure

Dosage and routes:

• *Adult:* IV 1-1.5 g/kg of 30% sol over 1-3 hr, not to exceed 4 ml/min; do not exceed 120 g/day

• *Child >2 yr:* IV 0.5-1.5 g/kg, not to exceed 4 ml/min

• *Child <2 yr:* IV 0.1 g/kg, not to exceed 4 ml/min

Available forms: Inj 40 g/150 ml

Side effects/adverse reactions:

CNS: Dizziness, disorientation, fever, syncope, *headache*

GI: Nausea, vomiting

INTEG: Venous thrombosis, phlebitis, extravasation

Contraindications: Severe renal disease, active intracranial bleeding, marked dehydration, liver failure

Precautions: Hepatic disease, renal disease, pregnancy (C), electrolyte imbalances, lactation

Pharmacokinetics:

IV: Onset ½-1 hr, peak 1 hr, duration 3-10 hr (diuresis), 5-6 hr (intraocular pressure); half-life 1 hr; excreted in urine, breast milk; crosses placenta

Interactions:

• Incompatible with whole blood, alkalies in sol or syringe

• Increased renal excretion of lithium

NURSING CONSIDERATIONS

Assess:

• Weight, I&O qd to determine fluid loss; effect of drug may be decreased if used qd; for hourly urinary output

• Rate, depth, rhythm of respiration, effect of exertion

• B/P lying, standing, postural hypotension may occur

• Electrolytes: K, Na, Cl; include BUN, blood sugar, CBC, serum creatinine, blood pH, ABGs, liver function tests

• Fever, signs of extravasation

• Confusion, especially in elderly; take safety precautions if needed

• Hydration: skin turgor, thirst, dry mucous membranes

Administer:

• IV after diluting 30 g/100 ml diluent with D_5, D_{10}; run 30% sol over 1-2 hr; check for extravasation; do not exceed 4 ml/min; may cause bleeding; use IV filter

• Within minutes of reconstitution; sol becomes ammonia on standing

Evaluate:

• Therapeutic response: improvement in edema of feet, legs, sacral area daily in CHF

Teach patient/family:

• That drug will cause diuresis in ½ hr

Treatment of overdose: Lavage if taken orally; monitor electrolytes, administer IV fluids, monitor BUN, hydration, CV status

⬦ = Nursing alert   🔌 = Herb-drug interaction   🚫 = Do not crush

urokinase (R)

(yoor-oh-kin'ase)
Abbokinase, Abbokinase
Open-Cath
Func. class.: Thrombolytic enzyme
Chem. class.: β-Hemolytic streptococcus filtrate (purified)

Action: Promotes thrombolysis by directly converting plasminogen to plasmin

Uses: Venous thrombosis, pulmonary embolism, arterial thrombosis, arterial embolism, arteriovenous cannula occlusion, lysis of coronary artery thrombi after MI

Dosage and routes:

Lysis of pulmonary emboli

• *Adult and child:* IV 4400 IU/kg/hr × 12-24 hr, not to exceed 200 ml; then **IV** heparin, then anticoagulants

Coronary artery thrombosis

• *Adult:* **INSTILL** 6000 IU/min into occluded artery for 1-2 hr after giving **IV BOL** of heparin 2500-10,000 U

• May also give as **IV INF** 2 million-3 million U over 45-90 min

Venous catheter occlusion

• *Adult and child:* **INSTILL** 5000 IU into line, wait 5 min, then aspirate, repeat aspiration attempts q5min × ½ hr; if occlusion has not been removed, cap line and wait ½-1 hr, then aspirate; may need 2nd dose if still occluded

Available forms: Powder for inj, lyophilized: 250,000 IU/vial; powder for catheter clearance

Side effects/adverse reactions:

HEMA: Decreased Hct, **bleeding**
INTEG: Rash, *urticaria*, phlebitis at IV infusion site, itching, flushing
CNS: Headache, fever
GI: Nausea, vomiting

RESP: Altered respirations, SOB, **bronchospasm,** cyanosis
MS: Low back pain
CV: Hypertension, dysrhythmias
EENT: Periorbital edema
SYST: **GI, GU, intracranial, retroperitoneal bleeding,** surface bleeding, **anaphylaxis** (rare)

Contraindications: Hypersensitivity, active bleeding, intraspinal surgery, neoplasms of CNS, ulcerative colitis/enteritis, severe hypertension, renal disease, hepatic disease, hypocoagulation, COPD, subacute bacterial endocarditis, rheumatic valvular disease, cerebral embolism/thrombosis/hemorrhage, intraarterial diagnostic procedure or surgery (10 days), recent major surgery

Precautions: Arterial emboli from left side of heart, pregnancy (B)

Pharmacokinetics:

IV: Half-life 10-20 min; small amounts excreted in urine

Interactions:

• Bleeding potential: aspirin, indomethacin, phenylbutazone, anticoagulants

Lab test interferences:

Increase: PT, APTT, TT

NURSING CONSIDERATIONS

Assess:

• VS, B/P, pulse, resp, neurologic signs, temp at least q4h; temp >104° F (40° C) is an indicator of internal bleeding; cardiac rhythm following intracoronary administration

• For neurologic changes that may indicate intracranial bleeding

• Retroperitoneal bleeding: back pain, leg weakness, diminished pulses

• Peripheral pulses, lung sounds, respiratory function

• Allergy: fever, rash, itching, chills; mild reaction may be treated with antihistamines

• Bleeding during 1st hr of treatment (hematuria, hematemesis, bleeding from mucous membranes, epistaxis, ecchymosis)

• Blood studies (Hct, platelets, PTT, PT, TT, APTT) before starting therapy; PT or APTT must be less than 2 × control before starting therapy TT; or PT q3-4h during treatment

Administer:
IV

• Using infusion pump, terminal filter (0.45 μm or smaller)

• Reconstituting only with 5.2 ml sterile water for inj (not bacteriostatic water), and roll (not shake) to enhance reconstitution; further dilute with 190 ml; give as intermittent inf or give to clear cannula by using 1 ml of diluted drug; inject into cannula slowly, clamp 5 min, aspirate clot; avoid excessive pressure when urokinase is injected into catheter; force could rupture catheter or expel clot into circulation

• As soon as thrombi identified; not useful for thrombi over 1 wk old

• Cryoprecipitate or fresh frozen plasma if bleeding occurs

• Loading dose at beginning of therapy; may require increased loading doses

• Heparin therapy after thrombolytic therapy is discontinued, TT or APTT less than 2 × control (about 3-4 hr)

Y-site compatibilities: TPN 55, 56
Perform/provide:

• Storage in refrigerator; use immediately after reconstitution

• Bed rest during entire course of treatment; use caution in handling patients

• Avoidance of venous, arterial puncture procedures, inj, rectal temp

• Treatment of fever with acetaminophen or aspirin

• Placement of sign above patient's bed stating urokinase therapy

• Pressure for 30 sec to minor bleeding sites; 30 min to sites of arterial puncture followed by pressure dressing; inform prescriber if hemostasis not attained, apply pressure dressing

Evaluate:

• Therapeutic response: decreased clotting, thrombosis, embolism

---

ursodiol (R)
(ur-soh-die'-ohl)
Actigall
Func. class.: Gallstone solubilizing agent
Chem. class.: Ursodeoxycholic acid

Action: Suppresses hepatic synthesis, secretion of cholesterol; inhibits intestinal absorption of cholesterol

Uses: Dissolution of radiolucent, noncalcified gallbladder stones (less than 20 mm in diameter) in which surgery is not indicated

Dosage and routes:

• *Adult:* **PO** 8-10 mg/kg/day in 2-3 divided doses using gallbladder ultrasound q6mo; determine if stones have dissolved; if so, continue therapy, repeat ultrasound within 1-3 mo

Available forms: Caps 300 mg

Side effects/adverse reactions:

GI: Diarrhea, nausea, vomiting, abdominal pain, constipation, stomatitis, flatulence, dyspepsia, biliary pain

INTEG: Pruritus, rash, urticaria, dry skin, sweating, alopecia

CNS: Headache, anxiety, depression, insomnia, fatigue

MS: Arthralgia, myalgia, back pain

OTHER: Cough, rhinitis

Contraindications: Calcified cholesterol stones, radiopaque stones, radiolucent bile pigment stones,

---

◆ = Nursing alert   ∥ = Herb-drug interaction   ⊘ = Do not crush

chronic liver disease, hypersensitivity

Precautions: Pregnancy (B), lactation, children

Pharmacokinetics: 80% excreted in feces, 20% metabolized, excreted into bile, lost in feces

Interactions:

• Reduced action of ursodiol: cholestyramine, colestipol, aluminum-based antacids

• Increased risk of stone formation: clofibrate, gemfibrozil, estrogens, oral contraceptives

NURSING CONSIDERATIONS
Assess:

• GI status: diarrhea, abdominal pain, nausea, vomiting; drug may have to be discontinued if side effects are severe

• Skin for pruritus, rash, urticaria, dry skin; provide soothing lotion to lesions

• Musculoskeletal status: aches or stiffness in joints

Administer:

• For up to 9-12 mo; if no improvement is seen, discontinue drug

Evaluate:

• Therapeutic response: decreasing size of stones on ultrasound

Teach patient/family:

• That anxiety, depression, insomnia are side effects and are reversible after discontinuing drug

---

valacyclovir (℞)

(val-a-sye'kloh-vir)

Valtrex

Func. class.: Antiviral

Chem. class.: Acyclic purine nucleoside analog

Action: Interferes with DNA synthesis by conversion to acyclovir, causing decreased viral replication, time of lesional healing

Uses: Herpes zoster (not immunosuppressed), recurrent genital herpes (not immunosuppressed)

Dosage and routes:

Genital herpes

• *Adult:* **PO** 1 g bid × 10 days initially; 1 g qd or 500 mg bid in those with <10 recurrences/yr

Herpes zoster

• *Adult:* **PO** 1 g tid × 1 wk

Available forms: Tabs 500 mg

Side effects/adverse reactions:

CNS: Tremors, lethargy, *dizziness, headache,* weakness

GI: Nausea, vomiting, diarrhea, abdominal pain, constipation

INTEG: Rash

Contraindications: Hypersensitivity to this drug or acyclovir

Precautions: Lactation, hepatic disease, renal diseae, electrolyte imbalance, dehydration, pregnancy (B)

Pharmacokinetics:

PO: Onset unknown, terminal half-life 2½-3½ hr; converted to acyclovir that crosses placenta and enters breast milk

Interactions:

• Increased blood levels of valacyclovir: cimetidine, probenecid

NURSING CONSIDERATIONS
Assess:

• Signs of infection; characteristics of lesions

• C&S before drug therapy; drug may be taken as soon as culture is taken; repeat C&S after treatement; determine the presence of other sexually transmitted diseases

• Bowel pattern before, during treatment

• Skin eruptions: rash

• Allergies before treatment, reaction of each medication; place allergies on chart in bright red letters

Evaluate:

• Therapeutic response: absence of itching, painful lesions; crusting and healed lesions

---

Teach patient/family:
• To take as prescribed; if dose is missed, take as soon as remembered up to 1 hr before next dose; do not double dose
• That drug may be taken orally before infection occurs; drug should be taken when itching or pain occurs, usually before eruptions
• That partners need to be told that patient has herpes; they can become infected; condoms must be worn to prevent reinfections
• That drug does not cure infection. just controls symptoms and does not prevent infection of others

Treatment of overdose: Discontinue drug, hemodialysis, resuscitate if needed

---

valproate
(val'proh-ate)
Depacon
valproic acid
(val'proh-ik)
Depakene, Myproic acid
divalproex sodium
(dye-val'proh-ex)
Depakote, Epival*
Func. class: Anticonvulsant
Chem. class: Carboxylic acid derivative

Action: Increases levels of γ-aminobutyric acid (GABA) in brain, which decreases seizure activity

Uses: Simple (petit mal), complex (petit mal) absence, mixed, manic episodes associated with bipolar disorder, migraine

Investigational uses: Tonic-clonic (grand mal), myoclonic seizures, migraines

Dosage and routes:
Epilepsy
• *Adult and child:* **PO** 15 mg/kg/ day divided in 2-3 doses, may increase by 5-10 mg/kg/day qwk, not to exceed 60 mg/kg/day in 2-3 divided doses; **IV** ≤20 mg/min over 1 hr

Mania (divalproex sodium)
• *Adult:* **PO** 750 mg qd in divided doses, max 60 mg/kg/day
Migraine
• *Adult:* **PO** 250 mg bid, may increase to 1000 mg/day if needed

Available forms: Valproic acid: caps 250 mg; divalproex: tabs delayed rel 125, 250, 500 mg; 125 mg sprinkle cap; valproate: syr 250 mg/5 ml; inj: 5 ml

Side effects/adverse reactions:
*HEMA: **Thrombocytopenia, leukopenia, lymphocytosis,** increased protime
CNS: Sedation, drowsiness, dizziness, headache, incoordination, paresthesia, depression, hallucinations, behavioral changes, tremors, aggression, weakness
GI: Nausea, vomiting, constipation, diarrhea, heartburn, anorexia, cramps, **hepatic failure, pancreatitis, toxic hepatitis,** stomatitis
INTEG: Rash, alopecia, bruising
GU: Enuresis, irregular menses
EENT: Visual disturbances

Contraindications: Hypersensitivity, pregnancy (D), hepatic disease
Precautions: Lactation, child <2 yr
Pharmacokinetics:
PO: Onset 15-30 min, peak 1-4 hr, duration 4-6 hr
Metabolized by liver; excreted by kidneys, breast milk; crosses placenta; half-life 9-16 hr
Interactions:
• Increased effects: CNS depressants
• Increased toxicity of valproic acid: salicylates
• Increased toxicity of: warfarin
• Increased action of: phenytoin

◆ = Nursing alert   ⫻ = Herb-drug interaction   ⊘ = Do not crush

• Increased CNS effects of: phenobarbital, primadone
• Increased sedation: benzodiazepines
• Decreased metabolism of valproic acid: cimetidine

Lab test interferences:
False positive: Ketones
Interference: Thyroid function tests

NURSING CONSIDERATIONS
Assess:
• Blood studies: Hct, Hgb, RBC, serum folate, pro-time, platelets, vit D if on long-term therapy
• Hepatic studies: AST, ALT, bilirubin, hepatic failure
• Blood levels: therapeutic level 50-100 μg/ml
• Mental status: mood, sensorium, affect, memory (long, short)
• Respiratory dysfunction: respiratory depression, character, rate, rhythm; hold drug if respirations are <12/min or if pupils are dilated

Administer:
PO
🚫 Tablets or capsules whole; do not break, crush, or chew
• Elixir alone; do not dilute with carbonated beverage; do not give syrup to patients on sodium restriction
• Give with food or milk to decrease GI symptoms

Evaluate:
• Therapeutic response: decreased seizures

Teach patient/family:
• That physical dependency may result from extended use
• To avoid driving, other activities that require alertness
• Not to discontinue medication quickly after long-term use; convulsions may result
• To report visual disturbances, rash, diarrhea, light-colored stools, jaundice, protracted vomiting to prescriber

valrubicin (℞)
(val-roo'bih-sin)
Valstar
Func. class.: Antineoplastic, antibiotic
Chem. class.: Anthracycline glycoside

Action: A semisynthetic analog of doxorubicin that inhibits DNA synthesis primarily; replication is decreased by binding to DNA, which causes strand splitting; active throughout entire cell cycle; a vesicant

Uses: Bladder cancer

Dosage and routes:
• *Adult:* Intravesically 800 mg qwk ×6 wk, delay administration ≥2 wks after transurethral resection of fulguration

Available forms: Sol for intravesical instillation: 40 mg/ml

Side effects/adverse reactions:
*HEMA: **Thrombocytopenia, leukopenia,** anemia*
GI: Nausea, vomiting, anorexia, diarrhea
GU: UTI, urinary retention, hematuria
INTEG: Rash
CV: Chest pain

Contraindications: Hypersensitivity to anthracyclines or *Cremophor El*, urinary tract infection, small bladder

Precautions: Pregnancy (C), lactation, children

Pharmacokinetics: Penetrates into bladder wall, not metabolized

NURSING CONSIDERATIONS
Assess:
• I&O ratio; report fall in urine output to <30 ml/hr
• Monitor temperature q4h; fever may indicate beginning infection

• Local irritation, pain, burning at injection site

Administer:

• After urinary catheter is inserted under aseptic conditions, drain bladder and instill the diluted 75 ml valrubicin by gravity for several min, withdraw catheter, drug should be retained for 2 hr, then void

• Use procedure for handling and disposal of cytotoxic agents

• Do not use polyvinyl chloride (PVC) or IV tubing

• Prepare/store valrubicin sol in glass, polypropylene, or polyolefin tubing/containers

• For instillation, 5 ml vials (200 mg valrubicin/5 ml/vial) should be warmed to room temp, withdraw 20 ml for the 4 vials and dilute with 55 ml 0.9% NaCl inj to 75 ml of diluted valrubicin sol

• Valrubicin sol is clear red, at lower temps a waxy precipitate may form, warm in hand until sol is clear

Perform/provide:

• Strict hand-washing technique, gloves, protective clothing

• Increased fluid intake to 2-3 L/day to prevent urate, calculi formation

• Storage at room temperature for 12 hr after reconstituting

Evaluate:

• Therapeutic response: decreased tumor size, spread of malignancy

Teach patient/family:

• To report any complaints, side effects to nurse or prescriber

• That urine and other body fluids may be red-orange for 48 hr

• That contraceptive measures are recommended during therapy

---

valsartan (℞)
(val'sahr-tan)
Diovan
Func. class.: Antihypertensive
Chem. class.: Angiotensin II receptor (Type AT_1)

Action: Blocks the vasoconstrictor and aldosterone-secreting effects of angiotensin II; selectively blocks the binding of angiotensin II to the AT_1 receptor found in tissues

Uses: Hypertension, alone or in combination

Dosage and routes:

• *Adult:* **PO** 80-160 mg qd alone or in combination with other antihypertensives

Available forms: Tabs 80, 160 mg

Side effects/adverse reactions:

CNS: Dizziness, insomnia, depression, drowsiness, vertigo

CV: Angina pectoris, 2nd degree AV block, *cerebrovascular accident,* hypotension, *myocardial infarction, dysrhythmias*

EENT: Conjunctivitis

GI: Diarrhea, abdominal pain, nausea, *hepatotoxicity*

GU: Impotence, *nephrotoxicity*

HEMA: Anemia, neutropenia

MS: Cramps, myalgia, pain, stiffness

RESP: Cough

Contraindications: Hypersensitivity, pregnancy, severe hepatic disease, bilateral renal artery stenosis

Precautions: Hypersensitivity to ACE inhibitors: congestive heart failure, hypertrophic cardiomyopathy aortic/mitral valve stenosis, CAD; lactation, children, elderly

Pharmacokinetics:

Peak 2 hr, duration >24 hr, extensively metabolized, half-life 9 hr; excreted in feces, urine, breast milk

---

NURSING CONSIDERATIONS
Assess:
- B/P, pulse q4h; note rate, rhythm, quality
- Blood studies: BUN, creatinine, LFTs before treatment
- Electrolytes: K, Na, Cl, total CO_2
- Baselines in renal, liver function tests before therapy begins
- Edema in feet, legs qd
- Skin turgor, dryness of mucous membranes for hydration status

Administer:
PO
- Without regard to meals

Evaluate:
- Therapeutic response: decreased B/P

Teach patient/family:
- To comply with dosage schedule, even if feeling better
- To notify prescriber of fever, swelling of hands or feet, irregular heartbeat, chest pain
- That excessive perspiration, dehydration, diarrhea may lead to fall in blood pressure; consult prescriber if these occur
- That drug may cause dizziness, fainting; light-headedness may occur
- To rise slowly to sitting or standing position to minimize orthostatic hypotension
- Not to take this medication if pregnant or breastfeeding, or have had an allergic reaction to this drug
- That if a dose is missed, to take it as soon as possible, unless it is within an hour before next dose

---

vancomycin (℞)

(van-koe-mye'sin)
Vancocin, Vancoled, vancomycin HCl
Func. class.: Antiinfective-misc.
Chem. class.: Tricyclic glycopeptide

Action: Inhibits bacterial cell wall synthesis

Uses: Resistant staphylococcal infections, pseudomembranous colitis, staphylococcal enterocolitis, endocarditis prophylaxis for dental procedures, diphtheroid endocarditis

Dosage and routes:
Serious staphylococcal infections
- *Adult:* **IV** 500 mg q6h or 1 g q12h
- *Child:* **IV** 40 mg/kg/day divided q6-8h
- *Neonate:* **IV** 15 mg/kg initially followed by 10 mg/kg q8-24h

Pseudomembranous/staphylococcal enterocolitis
- *Adult:* **PO** 500 mg/day in divided doses for 7-10 days
- *Child:* **PO** 40 mg/kg/day divided q6h, not to exceed 2 g/day

Endocarditis prophylaxis
- *Adult:* **IV** 1 g over 1 hr, 1 hr before dental procedure

Available forms: Pulvules 125, 250 mg; powder for oral sol 1, 10 g; powder for inj 500 mg, 1, 5, 10 g

Side effects/adverse reactions:
*CV: **Cardiac arrest, vascular collapse** (rare)*
*EENT: **Ototoxicity, permanent deafness,** tinnitus*
*HEMA: **Leukopenia, eosinophilia, neutropenia***
*GI: **Nausea,** pseudomembranous colitis*
RESP: Wheezing, dyspnea
*SYST: **Anaphylaxis***
*GU: **Nephrotoxicity,** increased BUN, creatinine, albumin, **fatal uremia***

INTEG: Chills, fever, rash, thrombophlebitis at injection site, urticaria, pruritus, necrosis (Red Man's syndrome)

Contraindications: Hypersensitivity, previous hearing loss

Precautions: Renal disease, pregnancy (C), lactation, elderly, neonates

Pharmacokinetics:

IV: Peak 5 min; half-life 4-8 hr; excreted in urine (active form); IV; feces PO crosses placenta

PO: Absorption: poor

Interactions:

• Ototoxicity or nephrotoxicity: aminoglycosides, cephalosporins, colistin, polymyxin, bacitracin, cisplatin, amphotericin B, nondepolarizing muscle relaxants

NURSING CONSIDERATIONS
Assess:

• I&O ratio; report hematuria, oliguria; nephrotoxicity may occur

◆ Any patient with compromised renal system; drug is excreted slowly in poor renal system function; toxicity may occur rapidly; BUN, creatinine

• Blood studies: WBC

• Serum levels: peak 1 hr after 1 hr inf 25-40 mg/ml, trough prior to next dose 5-10 mg/ml

• C&S; drug may be given as soon as culture is taken

• Auditory function during, after treatment

• B/P during administration; sudden drop may indicate Red Man's syndrome

• Signs of infection

• Hearing loss, ringing, roaring in ears; drug should be discontinued

• Skin eruptions

• Respiratory status: rate, character, wheezing, tightness in chest

• Allergies before treatment, reaction of each medication; place allergies on chart in bright red letters; notify all people giving drugs

Administer:

• Antihistamine if Red Man's syndrome occurs: decreased B/P, flushing of neck, face

• Dose based on serum concentration

IV

• After reconstitution with 10 ml sterile water for injection (500 mg/10 ml); further dilution is needed for IV, 500 mg/100 ml 0.9%NaCl, D_5W given as int inf over 1 hr; decrease rate of infusion if Red Man's syndrome occurs

Additive compatibilities: Amikacin, atracurium, calcium gluconate, cefepime, cimetidine, corticotropin, dimenhydrinate, famotidine, hydrocortisone, meropenem, ofloxacin, potassium chloride, ranitidine, verapamil, vit B/C

Y-site compatibilities: Acyclovir, allopurinol, amifostine, amiodarone, amsacrine, atracurium, cisatracurium, cyclophosphamide, diltiazem, doxorubicin liposome, enalaprilat, esmolol, filgrastim, fluconazole, fludarabine, gallium, granisetron, hydromorphone, insulin (regular), labetalol, lorazepam, magnesium sulfate, melphalan, meperidine, meropenem, midazolam, morphine, ondansetron, paclitaxel, pancuronium, perphenazine, propofol, remifentanil, sodium bicarbonate, tacrolimus, teniposide, theophylline, thiotepa, tolazoline, vecuronium, vinorelbine, warfarin, zidovudine

Perform/provide:

• Storage at room temp for up to 2 wk after reconstitution

• Adrenaline, suction, tracheostomy set, endotracheal intubation equipment on unit; anaphylaxis may occur

---

◆ = Nursing alert   ✐ = Herb-drug interaction   ⊘ = Do not crush

• Adequate intake of fluids (2 L/day) to prevent nephrotoxicity

Evaluate:

• Therapeutic response: absence of fever, sore throat; neg culture

Teach patient/family:

• All aspects of drug therapy: need to complete entire course of medication to ensure organism death (7-10 days); culture may be taken after completed course of medication

• To report sore throat, fever, fatigue; could indicate superinfection

• That drug must be taken in equal intervals around clock to maintain blood levels

---

vecuronium (R̷)

(vek-yoo-roe'nee-um)
Norcuron

Func. class.: Neuromuscular blocker

Chem. class.: Monoquaternary analog of pancuronium

Action: Inhibits transmission of nerve impulses by binding with cholinergic receptor sites, antagonizing action of acetylcholine

Uses: Facilitation of endotracheal intubation, skeletal muscle relaxation during mechanical ventilation, surgery, general anesthesia

Dosage and routes:

• *Adult and child >9 yr:* **IV BOL** 0.08-0.10 mg/kg, then 0.01-0.015 mg/kg for prolonged procedures

Available forms: 10 mg/5 ml vial

Side effects/adverse reactions:

CNS: Skeletal muscle weakness or paralysis (rare)

*RESP: **Prolonged apnea, possible respiratory paralysis***

Contraindications: Hypersensitivity

Precautions: Pregnancy (C), cardiac disease, lactation, children <2 yr, electrolyte imbalances, dehydration, neuromuscular disease, respiratory disease, hepatic disease

Pharmacokinetics:

IV: Onset 15 min, peak 3-5 min, duration 45-60 min; half-life 65-75 min; not metabolized; excreted in feces; crosses placenta

Interactions:

• Increased neuromuscular blockade: aminoglycosides, clindamycin, lincomycin, quinidine, local anesthetics, polymyxin antibiotics, lithium, opioid analgesics, thiazides, enflurane, isoflurane, succinylcholine

• Dysrhythmias: theophylline

NURSING CONSIDERATIONS

Assess:

• For electrolyte imbalances (K, Mg); may lead to increased action of this drug

• Vital signs (B/P, pulse, respirations, airway) q15min until fully recovered; rate, depth, pattern of respirations, strength of hand grip

• I&O ratio; check for urinary retention, frequency, hesitancy

• Recovery: decreased paralysis of face, diaphragm, leg, arm, rest of body; allow to recover fully before completing neurologic assessment

• Allergic reactions: rash, fever, respiratory distress, pruritus; drug should be discontinued

Administer:

• With diazepam or morphine when used for therapeutic paralysis; provides no sedation alone

• Using nerve stimulator by anesthesiologist to determine neuromuscular blockade

• Anticholinesterase to reverse neuromuscular blockade

• IV after diluting with diluent provided; give by direct IV over 1 min; may give as continuous inf 10-20

V

mg/100 ml; titrate to patient response (only by qualified person)

Y-site compatibilities: Aminophylline, cefazolin, cefuroxime, cimetidine, diltiazem, dobutamine, dopamine, epinephrine, esmolol, fentanyl, fluconazole, gentamicin, heparin, hydrocortisone, hydromorphone, isoproterenol, labetalol, lorazepam, midazolam, milrinone, morphine, nicardipine, nitroglycerin, norepinephrine, propofol, ranitidine, sodium nitroprusside, trimethoprim-sulfamethoxazole, vancomycin

Perform/provide:

• Storage in refrigerator; discard in 24 hr

• Reassurance if communication is difficult during recovery from neuromuscular blockade

Evaluate:

• Therapeutic response: paralysis of jaw, eyelid, head, neck, rest of body

Treatment of overdose: Edrophonium or neostigmine, atropine, monitor VS; may require mechanical ventilation

---

venlafaxine (℞)

(ven-la-fax′een)

Effexor

Func. class.: Antidepressant (misc)

Action: Potent inhibitor of neuronal serotonin and norepinephrine uptake, weak inhibitor of dopamine; no muscarinic, histaminergic, or α-adrenergic receptors in vitro

Uses: Depression

Dosage and routes:

Renal dose

• Mild-moderate impairment, 75% of dose

Hepatic dose

• Moderate impairment, 50% of dose

Depression

• *Adult:* **PO** 75 mg/day in 2 or 3 divided doses; taken with food, may be increased to 150 mg/day; if needed, may be further increased to 225 mg/day; increments of 75 mg/day at intervals of no less than 4 days; some hospitalized patients may require up to 375 mg/day in 3 divided doses; ext rel 37.5-75 mg PO qd, max 225 mg/day

Available forms: Tabs scored 25, 37.5, 50, 75, 100 mg; cap ext rel 37.5, 75, 150 mg

Side effects/adverse reactions:

CNS: Emotional lability, vertigo, apathy, ataxia, CNS stimulation, euphoria, hallucinations, hostility, increased libido, hypertonia, hypotonia, psychosis

CV: Migraine, angina pectoris, hypertension, extrasystoles, postural hypotension, syncope, thrombophlebitis

EENT: Abnormal vision, ear pain, cataract, conjunctivitis, corneal lesions, dry eyes, otitis media, photophobia

GI: Dysphagia, eructation, colitis, gastritis, gingivitis, ***rectal hemorrhage,*** stomatitis, stomach and mouth ulceration

GU: Anorgasmia, dysuria, hematuria, metrorrhagia, vaginitis, impaired urination, albuminuria, amenorrhea, kidney calculus, cystitis, nocturia, breast and bladder pain, polyuria, ***uterine hemorrhage, vaginal hemorrhage,*** moniliasis

INTEG: Ecchymosis, acne, alopecia, brittle nails, dry skin, photosensitivity

META: Peripheral edema, weight loss or gain, diabetes mellitus, edema, glycosuria, hyperlipemia, hypokalemia

MS: Arthritis, bone pain, bursitis, myasthenia tenosynovitis

RESP: Bronchitis, dyspnea, asthma, chest congestion, epistaxis, hyperventilation, laryngitis

---

SYST: Accidental injury, malaise, neck pain, enlarged abdomen, cyst, facial edema, hangover, hernia

Contraindications: Hypersensitivity

Precautions: Mania, pregnancy (C), lactation, children, elderly, hypertension, seizure disorder

Pharmacokinetics: Well absorbed, extensively metabolized in the liver to an active metabolite; 87% of drug recovered in urine; 27% protein binding; half-life 5-7, 11-13 hr (active metabolite) respectively

Interactions:

◆ Hyperthermia, rigidity, rapid fluctuations of vital signs, mental status changes, neuroleptic malignant syndrome: MAOIs

NURSING CONSIDERATIONS

Assess:

• B/P lying, standing; pulse q/4 h; if systolic B/P drops 20 mm Hg, hold drug, notify prescriber; take VS q4h in patients with cardiovascular disease

• Blood studies: CBC, leukocytes, differential cardiac enzymes if patient is receiving long-term therapy

• Hepatic studies: AST, ALT, bilirubin

• Weight qwk; weight loss or gain; appetite may increase

• With food, milk for GI symptoms

• Gum, hard candy, frequent sips of water for dry mouth

• Mental status: mood, sensorium, affect, suicidal tendencies, increase in psychiatric symptoms; depression, panic

• Withdrawal symptoms: headache, nausea, vomiting, muscle pain, weakness; not usual unless drug is discontinued abruptly

Perform/provide:

• Storage in tight container at room temp; do not freeze

• Assistance with ambulation during beginning therapy, since drowsiness, dizziness occur

• Checking to see if PO medication swallowed

Evaluate:

• Therapeutic response; decreased depression

Teach patient/family:

• To dispense in small amounts because of suicide potential, especially in the beginning of therapy

• To use with caution when driving or other activities requiring alertness because of drowsiness, dizziness, blurred vision

• To avoid alcohol ingestion, other CNS depressants

• Not to discontinue medication quickly after long-term use; may cause nausea, headache, malaise

• To wear sunscreen or large hat, since photosensitivity occurs

Treatment of overdose: ECG monitoring; induce emesis; lavage, activated charcoal; administer anticonvulsant

---

verapamil (℞)

(ver-ap′a-mill)
Calan, Calan SR, Isoptin, Isoptin SR , verapamil HCl, verapamil HCl SR, Verelan

Func. class.: Calcium channel blocker; antihypertensive; antianginal

Chem. class.: Phenylalkylamine

Action: Inhibits calcium ion influx across cell membrane during cardiac depolarization; produces relaxation of coronary vascular smooth muscle; dilates coronary arteries; decreases SA/AV node conduction; dilates peripheral arteries

Uses: Chronic stable angina pectoris, vasospastic angina, dysrhythmias, hypertension

Investigational uses: Prevention of migraine headaches, ventricular outflow obstruction in hypertrophic cardiomyopathy

Dosage and routes:
• *Adult:* **PO** 80 mg tid or qid, increase qwk; **IV BOL** 5-10 mg >2 min, repeat if necessary in 30 min
• *Child 1-15 yr:* **IV BOL** 0.1-0.3 mg/kg >2 min, repeat in 30 min, not to exceed 10 mg in a single dose
Available forms: Tabs 40, 80, 120 mg; sus rel tabs 120, 180, 240 mg; inj 5 mg/ml; sus rel caps 120, 180, 240, 360 mg

Side effects/adverse reactions:
*CV: Edema, **CHF**,* bradycardia, hypotension, palpitations, AV block
GI: Nausea, diarrhea, gastric upset, *constipation,* increased liver function studies
GU: Nocturia, polyuria
CNS: Headache, drowsiness, dizziness, anxiety, depression, weakness, insomnia, confusion, light-headedness

Contraindications: Sick sinus syndrome, 2nd- or 3rd-degree heart block, hypotension less than 90 mm Hg systolic, cardiogenic shock, severe CHF

Precautions: CHF, hypotension, hepatic injury, pregnancy (C), lactation, children, renal disease, concomitant β-blocker therapy

Pharmacokinetics:
IV: Onset 3 min, peak 3-5 min, duration 10-20 min
PO: Onset variable, peak 3-4 hr, duration 17-24 hr, half-life (biphasic) 4 min, 3-7 hr (terminal)
Metabolized by liver, excreted in urine (96% as metabolites)

Interactions:
• Increased hypotension: prazosin, quinidine
• Increased effects: β-blockers, antihypertensives, cimetidine, digoxin
• Decreased effects of lithium

• Increased levels of digoxin, theophylline, cyclosporine, carbamazepine, nondepolarizing muscle relaxants
• Food/drug: increased hypotensive effects: grapefruit

Lab test interferences:
Increase: Liver function tests

NURSING CONSIDERATIONS
Assess:
• Cardiac status: B/P, pulse, respiration, ECG intervals (PR, QRS, QT)
Administer:
• Before meals, hs; sus rel give with food
IV
• Undiluted through Y-tube or 3-way stopcock of compatible sol; give over 2 min, or 3 min elderly

Additive compatibilities: Amikacin, amiodarone, ascorbic acid, atropine, bretylium, calcium chloride, calcium gluconate, cefamandole, cefazolin, cefotaxime, cefoxitin, cephapirin, chloramphenicol, cimetidine, clindamycin, dexamethasone, diazepam, digoxin, dopamine, epinephrine, erythromycin, gentamicin, heparin, hydrocortisone sodium phosphate, hydrocortisone, hydromorphone, insulin (regular), isoproterenol, lidocaine, magnesium sulfate, mannitol, meperidine, metaraminol, methicillin, methyldopa, methylprednisolone, metoclopramide, mezlocillin, morphine, moxalactam, multivitamins, naloxone, nitroglycerin, norepinephrine, oxytocin, pancuronium, penicillin G potassium, penicillin G sodium, pentobarbital, phenobarbital, phentolamine, phenytoin, piperacillin, potassium chloride, potassium phosphates, procainamide, propranolol, protamine, quinidine, sodium bicarbonate, sodium nitroprusside, theophylline, ticarcillin, tobramycin,

◆ = Nursing alert   🖋 = Herb-drug interaction   🚫 = Do not crush

tolazoline, vancomycin, vasopressin, vit B/C

Syringe compatibilities: Amrinone, heparin, milrinone

Y-site compatibilities: Amrinone, ciprofloxacin, dobutamine, dopamine, famotidine, hydralazine, meperidine, methicillin, milrinone, penicillin G potassium, piperacillin, propofol, ticarcillin

Evaluate:

• Therapeutic response: decreased anginal pain, decreased B/P, dysrhythmias

Teach patient/family:

• To increase fluids/fiber to counteract constipation

• How to take pulse before taking drug; to keep record or graph

• To avoid hazardous activities until stabilized on drug, dizziness no longer a problem

• To limit caffeine consumption; no alcohol products

• To avoid OTC drugs unless directed by prescriber

• To comply with all areas of medical regimen: diet, exercise, stress reduction, drug therapy

• To change positions slowly to prevent syncope

Treatment of overdose: Defibrillation, atropine for AV block, vasopressor for hypotension

---

vidarabine (℞)

(vih-dar′ah-been)

Vira-A

Func. class.: Antibacterial, antiviral

Chem. class.: Purine nucleoside

Action: Inhibits bacterial/viral replication by preventing DNA synthesis

Uses: Herpes simplex virus encephalitis, varicella-zoster encephalomyelitis, herpes zoster in immunosuppressed

Dosage and routes:

Herpes simplex encephalitis

• *Adult and child:* **IV INF** 15 mg/kg/day × 10 days; infuse over 12-24 hr

Herpes zoster in immunocompromised patients

• *Adult and child:* **IV** 10 mg/kg/day × 5 day

Herpes simplex

• *Neonate:* **IV** 15 mg/kg/day × 10 days

Available forms: Susp for inj 200 mg/ml

Side effects/adverse reactions:

CNS: Psychosis, hallucinations, dizziness, weakness, tremors, *fatal metabolic encephalopathy,* confusion, malaise, headache

META: SIADH

HEMA: **Anemia, thrombocytopenia, neutropenia**

GI: Nausea, vomiting, anorexia, diarrhea, weight loss

INTEG: Pain, thrombophlebitis at injection site

Contraindications: Hypersensitivity

Precautions: Renal disease, liver disease, lactation, pregnancy (C)

Pharmacokinetics: Crosses blood-brain barrier, excreted by kidneys (metabolites), crosses placenta, half-life 1½-3 hr

Interactions:

• Increased neurologic side effects: allopurinol

• Incompatible with blood, protein products

NURSING CONSIDERATIONS

Assess:

• Liver studies: AST, ALT

• Blood studies: WBC, differential, RBC, Hct, Hgb, platelets

• Renal studies: urinalysis, protein, blood

Side effects: *italics* = common; **bold italics** = life-threatening

• C&S; drug may be given as soon as culture is taken; C&S may be taken after therapy
• Bowel pattern before, during treatment
• Fluid overload; drug requires large volume to stay in sol
• Weakness, tremors, confusion, dizziness, psychosis; drug may have to be decreased or discontinued

Administer:
• Shake sol; dilute to 450 mg/L IV; give fluid at constant rate over 12-24 hr, using in-line filter with mean pore diameter of 0.45 mm or less

Evaluate:
• Therapeutic response: decreased infection

---

vinblastine (VLB) (℞)
(vin-blast'een)
Velban, Velbe*, vinblastine sulfate
Func. class.: Antineoplastic
Chem. class.: Vinca rosea alkaloid

Action: Inhibits mitotic activity, arrests cell cycle at metaphase; inhibits RNA synthesis, blocks cellular use of glutamic acid needed for purine synthesis; a vesicant

Uses: Breast, testicular cancer, lymphomas, neuroblastoma; Hodgkin's, non-Hodgkin's lymphomas; mycosis fungoides, histiocytosis, Kaposi's sarcoma

Dosage and routes:
• *Adult:* **IV** 0.1 mg/kg or 3.7 mg/m^2 qwk or q2wk, not to exceed 0.5 mg/kg or 18.5 mg/m^2 qwk
• *Child:* 2.5 mg/m^2 then 3.75, 5, 6.25, 7.5 at 7-day intervals

Available forms: Inj, powder 10 mg for 10 ml IV

Side effects/adverse reactions:
HEMA: **Thrombocytopenia, leukopenia, myelosuppression**

GI: *Nausea, vomiting,* ileus, *anorexia, stomatitis,* constipation, abdominal pain, **GI, rectal bleeding, hepatotoxicity,** pharyngitis
GU: Urinary retention, **renal failure**
INTEG: *Rash,* alopecia, photosensitivity
RESP: **Fibrosis, pulmonary infiltrate**
CV: Tachycardia, orthostatic hypotension
CNS: Paresthesias, peripheral neuropathy, depression, headache, **convulsions**
META: SIADH

Contraindications: Hypersensitivity, infants, pregnancy (D)

Precautions: Renal disease, hepatic disease

Pharmacokinetics: Half-life (triphasic) 35 min, 53 min, 19 hr; metabolized in liver, excreted in urine, feces; crosses blood-brain barrier

Interactions:
• Increased action of methotrexate
• Do not use with radiation
• Synergism: bleomycin
• Decreased phenytoin level: phenytoin
• Bronchospasm: mitomycin

NURSING CONSIDERATIONS
Assess:
• CBC, differential, platelet count qwk; withhold drug if WBC is <4000/mm^3 or platelet count is <75,000/mm^3; notify prescriber
• Pulmonary function tests, chest x-ray studies before, during therapy; chest x-ray film should be obtained q2wk during treatment
• Neurologic status: sensory-vibratory evaluation if side effects occur
• Renal function studies: BUN, serum uric acid, urine CrCl, electrolytes before, during therapy
• I&O ratio; report fall in urine output of 30 ml/hr

◆ = Nursing alert　　🖋 = Herb-drug interaction　　🚫 = Do not crush

• Monitor temp q4h; may indicate beginning infection
• Liver function tests before, during therapy (bilirubin, AST, ALT, LDH) as needed or qmo
• RBC, Hct, Hgb, since these may be decreased
• Bleeding: hematuria, guaiac, bruising or petechiae, mucosa of orifices q8h
• Dyspnea, rales, unproductive cough, chest pain, tachypnea, fatigue, increased pulse, pallor, lethargy
• Effects of alopecia on body image; discuss feelings about body changes
• Sensitivity of feet/hands, which precedes neuropathy
• Jaundiced skin, sclera; dark urine, clay-colored stools, itchy skin, abdominal pain, fever, diarrhea
• Buccal cavity q8h for dryness, sores or ulceration, white patches, oral pain, bleeding, dysphagia
• Local irritation, pain, burning, discoloration at injection site
• Symptoms indicating severe allergic reaction: rash, pruritus, urticaria, purpuric skin lesions, itching, flushing
• Frequency of stools and characteristics: cramping; acidosis; signs of dehydration: rapid respirations, poor skin turgor, decreased urine output, dry skin, restlessness, weakness

Administer:
• Antiemetic 30-60 min before giving drug and prn to prevent vomiting
• Transfusion for anemia

IV
• After diluting 10 mg/10 ml NaCl; give through Y-tube or 3-way stopcock or directly over 1 min
• Hyaluronidase 150 U/ml in 1 ml NaCl, warm compress for extravasation for vesicant activity treatment

Additive compatibilities: Bleomycin

Syringe compatibilities: Bleomycin, cisplatin, cyclophosphamide, droperidol, fluorouracil, leucovorin, methotrexate, metoclopramide, mitomycin, vincristine

Y-site compatibilities: Allopurinol, amifostine, amphotericin B cholesteryl, aztreonam, bleomycin, cisplatin, cyclophosphamide, doxorubicin, doxorubicin liposome, droperidol, filgrastim, fludarabine, fluorouracil, granisetron, heparin, leucovorin, melphalan, methotrexate, metoclopramide, mitomycin, ondansetron, paclitaxel, piperacillin/tazobactam, sargramostim, teniposide, thiotepa, vincristine, vinorelbine

Perform/provide:
• Deep-breathing exercises with patient 3-4 ×/day; place in semi-Fowler's position
• Liquid diet: cola, Jell-O; dry toast or crackers may be added if patient is not nauseated or vomiting
• Increase fluid intake to 2-3 L/day to prevent urate deposits, calculi formation
• Rinsing of mouth tid-qid with water
• Brushing of teeth bid-tid with soft brush or cotton-tipped applicators for stomatitis; use unwaxed dental floss
• Nutritious diet with iron, vitamin supplements
• HOB raised to facilitate breathing

Evaluate:
• Therapeutic response: decreased tumor size, spread of malignancy

Teach patient/family:
• To report any complaints or side effects to nurse or prescriber

---

- To report any changes in breathing or coughing
- That hair may be lost during treatment, a wig or hairpiece may make patient feel better; tell patient that new hair may be different in color, texture
- To report change in gait or numbness in extremities; may indicate neuropathy
- To avoid foods with citric acid, hot or rough texture
- To report any bleeding, white spots or ulcerations in mouth to prescriber; to examine mouth qd

---

vincristine (VCR) (℞)

(vin-kris′teen)

Oncovin, Vincasar PFS, vincristine sulfate

Func. class.: Antineoplastic-misc

Chem. class.: Vinca alkaloid

Action: Inhibits mitotic activity, arrests cell cycle at metaphase; inhibits RNA synthesis, blocks cellular use of glutamic acid needed for purine synthesis; a vesicant

Uses: Breast, lung cancer, lymphomas, neuroblastoma, Hodgkin's disease, acute lymphoblastic and other leukemias, rhabdomyosarcoma, Wilms' tumor, osteogenic and other sarcomas

Dosage and routes:
- *Adult:* IV 1-2 mg/m²/wk, not to exceed 2 mg
- *Child:* IV 1.5-2 mg/m²/wk, not to exceed 2 mg

Available forms: Inj 1 mg/ml

Side effects/adverse reactions:

INTEG: Alopecia

HEMA: **Thrombocytopenia, leukopenia, myelosuppression, anemia**

GI: Nausea, vomiting, anorexia, stomatitis, constipation, **paralytic ileus,** abdominal pain, **hepatotoxicity**

CV: Orthostatic hypotension

CNS: Decreased reflexes, numbness, weakness, motor difficulties, CNS depression, cranial nerve paralysis, *seizures*

Contraindications: Hypersensitivity, infants, pregnancy (D)

Precautions: Renal disease, hepatic disease, hypertension, neuromuscular disease

Pharmacokinetics: Half-life (triphasic) 0.85 min, 7.4 min, 164 min; metabolized in liver; excreted in bile, feces; crosses placental barrier, blood-brain barrier

Interactions:
- Increased action of methotrexate, anticoagulants
- Do not use with radiation
- Neurotoxicity: peripheral nervous system drugs
- Decreased digoxin level: digoxin
- Decreased action of vincristine: L-asparaginase
- Acute pulmonary reactions: mitomycin-c

NURSING CONSIDERATIONS

Assess:
- CBC, differential, platelet count qwk; withhold drug if WBC is <4000/mm³ or platelet count is <75,000/mm³; notify prescriber
- Renal function studies: BUN, serum uric acid, urine CrCl, electrolytes before, during therapy
- I&O ratio, report fall in urine output of 30 ml/hr
- Monitor temp q4h; may indicate beginning infection
- Liver function tests before, during therapy (bilirubin, AST, ALT, LDH) as needed or monthly
- RBC, Hct, Hgb; may be decreased
- Deep tendon reflexes; drug is neurotoxic
- Sensitivity of feet/hands, which precedes neuropathy

⬥ = Nursing alert   🖋 = Herb-drug interaction   🚫 = Do not crush

• Bleeding: hematuria, guaiac, bruising or petechiae, mucosa of orifices q8h
• Effects of alopecia on body image, discuss feelings about body changes
• Jaundiced skin, sclera; dark urine, clay-colored stools, itchy skin, abdominal pain, fever, diarrhea
• Buccal cavity q8h for dryness, sores or ulceration, white patches, oral pain, bleeding, dysphagia
• Symptoms indicating severe allergic reaction: rash, pruritus, urticaria, purpuric skin lesions, itching, flushing
• Frequency of stools, characteristics: cramping, acidosis; signs of dehydration: rapid respirations, poor skin turgor, decreased urine output, dry skin, restlessness, weakness

Administer:
• Agents to prevent constipation
• Antiemetic 30-60 min before giving drug and prn
• Transfusion for anemia
• Antispasmodic for GI symptoms
IV
• After diluting with diluent provided or 1 mg/10 ml of sterile H_2O or NaCl; give through Y-tube or 3-way stopcock or directly over 1 min
• Hyaluronidase 150 U/ml in 1 ml NaCl; apply warm compress for extravasation

Additive compatibilities: Bleomycin, cytarabine, fluorouracil, methotrexate

Syringe compatibilities: Bleomycin, cisplatin, cyclophosphamide, doxapram, doxorubicin, droperidol, fluorouracil, heparin, leucovorin, methotrexate, metoclopramide, mitomycin, vinblastine

Y-site compatibilities: Allopurinol, amifostine, amphotericin B cholesteryl, aztreonam, bleomycin, cisplatin, cladribine, cyclophosphamide, doxorubicin, doxorubicin liposome, droperidol, filgrastim, fludarabine, fluorouracil, granisetron, heparin, leucovorin, melphalan, methotrexate, metoclopramide, mitomycin, ondansetron, paclitaxel, piperacillin/tazobactam, sargramostim, teniposide, thiotepa, vinblastine, vinorelbine

Perform/provide:
• Liquid diet: cola, Jell-O; dry toast or crackers may be added if patient is not nauseated or vomiting
• Rinsing of mouth tid-qid with water
• Brushing of teeth bid-tid with soft brush or cotton-tipped applicators for stomatitis; use unwaxed dental floss
• Nutritious diet with iron, vitamin supplements

Evaluate:
• Therapeutic response: decreased tumor size, spread of malignancy

Teach patient/family:
• To report change in gait or numbness in extremities; may indicate neuropathy
• To report any complaints or side effects to nurse or prescriber
• To report any bleeding, white spots or ulcerations in mouth to prescriber; to examine mouth qd

---

vinorelbine (℞)
(vi-nor′el-bine)
Navelbine
Func. class.: Antineoplastic-misc
Chem. class.: Semisynthetic vinca alkaloid

Action: Inhibits mitotic activity, arrests cell cycle at metaphase; inhibits RNA synthesis, blocks cellular use of glutamic acid needed for purine synthesis; a vesicant

Uses: Unresectable advanced non-small cell lung cancer (NSCLC) stage IV; may be used alone or in combination with cisplatin for stage III or IV NSCLC breast cancer

Dosage and routes:
• *Adult:* IV 30 mg/m^2 qwk

Available forms: Powder 10 mg for 10 ml inj

Side effects/adverse reactions:
CV: Chest pain
RESP: Shortness of breath
HEMA: **Neutropenia, anemia, thrombocytopenia, granulocytopenia**
GI: Nausea, vomiting, ileus, anorexia, stomatitis, constipation, abdominal pain, diarrhea, **hepatotoxicity**
INTEG: Rash, alopecia, photosensitivity
CNS: Paresthesias, peripheral neuropathy, depression, headache, **convulsions,** weakness, jaw pain
META: SIADH
MS: Myalgia

Contraindications: Hypersensitivity, infants, pregnancy (D), granulocyte count <1000 cells/mm^3 pretreatment

Precautions: Renal, hepatic disease, elderly, lactation, children

Pharmacokinetics: Half-life 27-43 hr, peak 1-2 hr

Interactions:
• Possible increased toxicity: fluorouracil

NURSING CONSIDERATIONS
Assess:
• B/P (baseline and q15min) during administration
• CBC, differential, platelet count weekly; withhold drug if WBC is <4000/mm^3 or platelet count is <75,000/mm^3; notify prescriber of results, recovery will take 3 wk
• For dyspnea, rales, unproductive cough, chest pain, tachypnea
• Renal function studies: BUN, serum uric acid, urine CrCl before, during therapy; I&O ratio; report fall in urine output to <30 ml/hr; for decreased hyperuricemia
• For cold, fever, sore throat (may indicate beginning infection); notify prescriber if these occur
• For bleeding: hematuria, guaiac, bruising or petechiae, mucosa or orifices q8h, no rectal temps; avoid IM injections; use pressure to venipuncture sites
• Nutritional status: an antiemetic may be needed
◆For symptoms of severe allergic reactions: rash, pruritus, urticaria, itching, flushing, bronchospasm, hypotension, epinephrine and crash cart should be nearby

Administer:
• Antiemetic 30-60 min before giving drug and prn to prevent vomiting

IV
• Hyaluronidase 150 U/ml in 1 ml NaCl, warm compress for extravasation for vesicant activity treatment
• By cont inf: 40 mg/m^2 q3wk after an IV bol of 8 mg/m^2; may be given in combination with doxorubicin, fluorouracil, cisplatin

Y-site compatibilities: Amikacin, aztreonam, bleomycin, bumetanide, buprenorphine, butorphanol, calcium gluconate, carboplatin, carmustine, cefotaxime, ceftazidime, ceftizoxime, chlorpromazine, cimetidine, cisplatin, clindamycin, cyclophosphamide, cytarabine, dacarbazine, dactinomycin, daunorubicin, dexamethasone, diphenhydramine, doxorubicin, doxorubicin liposome, doxycycline, droperidol, enalaprilat, etoposide, famotidine, filgrastim, floxuridine, fluconazole, fludarabine, gallium, gentamicin, granisetron, haloperidol, heparin, hydrocortisone, hydromorphone, hydroxyzine, idarubicin, ifosfamide, imipenem-cilastatin, lorazepam, mannitol, mechlorethamine, melphalan, meperidine, mesna, methotrexate, metoclopramide, metronidazole, minocycline, mitoxantrone, morphine, nalbuphine, netilmicin, ondansetron, plicamycin, streptozocin, teniposide, ticarcillin, ticarcillin/clavulanate, tobramycin, vancomycin, vinblastine, vincristine, zidovudine

Perform/provide:

• Liquid diet: cola, Jell-O; dry toast or crackers if patient not nauseated or vomiting

• Brushing of teeth bid-tid with soft brush or cotton-tipped applicators for stomatitis; unwaxed dental floss

• Nutritious diet with iron, vitamin supplements

Evaluate:

• Therapeutic response: decreased tumor size, spread of malignancy

Teach patient/family:

• To report change in gait or numbness in extremities; may indicate neuropathy

• To report any complaints or side effects to nurse or prescriber

• To examine mouth qd for bleeding, white spots, ulcerations; notify prescriber

---

vitamin A (℞, OTC)
Aquasol A, Del-Vi-A, Vitamin A
Func. class.: Vitamin, fat soluble
Chem. class.: Retinol

Action: Needed for normal bone, tooth development, visual dark adaptation, skin disease, mucosa tissue repair, assists in production of adrenal steroids, cholesterol, RNA
Uses: Vit A deficiency

Dosage and routes:

• *Adult and child >8 yr:* **PO** 100,000-500,000 IU qd × 3 days, then 50,000 qd × 2 wk; dose based on severity of deficiency; maintenance 10,000-20,000 IU for 2 mo

• *Child 1-8 yr:* **IM** 5000-15,000 IU qd × 10 days

• *Infant <1 yr:* **IM** 5000-15,000 IU × 10 days

Maintenance

• *Child 4-8 yr:* **IM** 15,000 IU qd × 2 mo

• *Child <4 yr:* **IM** 10,000 IU qd × 2 mo

Available forms: Caps 10,000, 25,000, 50,000 IU; drops 5000 IU; inj 50,000 IU/ml; tabs 10,000, 25,000, 50,000 IU

Side effects/adverse reactions:

GI: Nausea, vomiting, anorexia, abdominal pain, ***jaundice***

CNS: Headache, ***increased intracranial pressure, intracranial hypertension,*** lethargy, malaise

EENT: Gingivitis, papilledema, exophthalmos, inflammation of tongue and lips

INTEG: Drying of skin, pruritus, increased pigmentation, night sweats, alopecia

MS: Arthralgia, retarded growth, hard areas on bone

META: Hypomenorrhea, hypercalcemia

Contraindications: Hypersensitivity to vit A, malabsorption syndrome (PO)

Precautions: Lactation, impaired renal function, pregnancy (C)

Pharmacokinetics: Stored in liver, kidneys, fat; excreted (metabolites) in urine, feces

Interactions:

• Decreased absorption of vit A: mineral oil, cholestyramine, colestipol

• Increased levels of vit A: corticosteroids, oral contraceptives

V

• Do not administer IV because of risk of anaphylactic shock

Lab test interferences:

False increase: Bilirubin, serum cholesterol

NURSING CONSIDERATIONS

Assess:

• Nutritional status: yellow and dark green vegetables, yellow/orange fruits, vit A-fortified foods, liver, egg yolks

• Vit A deficiency: decreased growth, night blindness, dry, brittle nails; hair loss; urinary stones; increased infection, hyperkeratosis of skin; drying of cornea

Administer:

PO

• With food (PO) for better absorption

Perform/provide:

• Storage in tight, light-resistant container

Evaluate:

• Therapeutic response: increased growth rate, weight; absence of dry skin and mucous membranes, night blindness

Teach patient/family:

• That if dose is missed, it should be omitted

• That ophthalmic exams may be required periodically throughout therapy

• Not to use mineral oil while taking this drug

• To notify prescriber of nausea, vomiting, lip cracking, loss of hair, headache

• Not to take more than the prescribed amount

Treatment of overdose: Discontinue drug

---

vitamin D (cholecalciferol, vitamin D₃ or ergocalciferol, vitamin D₂) (Ŗ, OTC)
Calciferol, Delta-D, Drisdol, Radiostol*, Radiostol Forte*, Vitamin D, Vitamin D₃
Func. class.: Vit D
Chem. class.: Fat soluble

Action: Needed for regulation of calcium, phosphate levels, normal bone development, parathyroid activity, neuromuscular functioning

Uses: Vit D deficiency, rickets, renal osteodystrophy, hypoparathyroidism, hypophosphatemia, psoriasis, rheumatoid arthritis

Dosage and routes:

Deficiency

• *Adult:* **PO/IM** 12,000 IU qd, then increased to 500,000 IU/day

• *Child:* **PO/IM** 1500-5000 IU qd × 2-4 wk, may repeat after 2 wk or 600,000 IU as single dose

Hypoparathyroidism

• *Adult and child:* **PO/IM** 200,000 IU given with 4 g Ca tab

Available forms: Tabs 400, 1000, 50,000 IU; caps 25,000, 50,000 IU; liq 8000 IU/ml; inj 500,000 IU/ml, 500,000 IU/5 ml

Side effects/adverse reactions:

GI: Nausea, vomiting, anorexia, cramps, diarrhea, constipation, metallic taste, dry mouth

CNS: Fatigue, weakness, drowsiness, *convulsions,* headache, psychosis

GU: Polyuria, nocturia, *hematuria, albuminuria, renal failure,* decreased libido

CV: Hypertension, dysrhythmias

MS: Decreased bone growth, early joint pain, early muscle pain

INTEG: Pruritus, photophobia

◆ = Nursing alert ∮ = Herb-drug interaction ⊘ = Do not crush

Contraindications: Hypersensitivity, hypercalcemia, renal dysfunction, hyperphosphatemia

Precautions: Cardiovascular disease, renal calculi, pregnancy (C)

Pharmacokinetics: Half-life 7-12 hr; stored in liver, duration 2 mo; excreted in bile (metabolites) and urine

Interactions:

• Decreased effects of vit D: cholestyramine, colestipol, phenobarbital, phenytoin

• Increased toxicity: diuretics (thiazides), antacids, verapamil

NURSING CONSIDERATIONS
Assess:

• Vit D levels q2wk during treatment

• Ca, PO_4, Mg, BUN, alk phosphatase, urine Ca, creatinine

• In children, monitor height and weight

• Nutritional status: egg yolk, fortified dairy products, cod, halibut, salmon, sardines

Administer:

• IM inj deep in large muscle mass; administer slowly; aspirate carefully; rotate inj sites; avoid IV administration

Evaluate:

• Therapeutic response: absence of rickets/osteomalacia, adequate Ca/phosphate levels, decrease in bone pain

Teach patient/family:

• That if dose is missed, to omit

• The necessary foods in diet

• To avoid vitamin supplements unless directed by prescriber

• To keep appointments with health care providers; line between therapeutic and toxic doses is narrow

• To report weakness, lethargy, headache, anorexia, loss of weight

• To report nausea, vomiting, abdominal cramps, diarrhea, constipation, excessive thirst, polyuria, muscle and bone pain

• To decrease intake of antacids and laxatives containing Mg

---

vitamin E (OTC)

Amino-Opti-E, Aquasol E, Daltose*, E-Complex-600, E-Ferol, E-Vitamin Succinate, E-200 I.U. Softgels, Gordo-Vite E, Tocopherol, Vitamin E, Vita-Plus E Softgells, Vitec

Func. class.: Vit E
Chem. class.: Fat soluble

Action: Needed for digestion and metabolism of polyunsaturated fats, decreases platelet aggregation, decreases blood clot formation, promotes normal growth and development of muscle tissue, prostaglandin synthesis

Uses: Vit E deficiency, impaired fat absorption, hemolytic anemia in premature neonates, prevention of retrolental fibroplasia, sickle cell anemia, supplement in malabsorption syndrome

Dosage and routes:

Deficiency

• *Adult:* **PO** 60-75 IU qd

• *Child:* **PO** 1 mg/0.6 g of dietary fat

Prevention of deficiency

• *Adult:* **PO** 30 IU/day; **TOP** apply to affected areas

• *Infants:* **PO** 5 IU/day

Available forms: Caps 100, 200, 400, 500, 600, 1000 IU; tabs 100, 200, 400 IU; drops 50 mg/ml; chew tabs 400 U; ointment, cream, lotion, oil

Side effects/adverse reactions:

META: Altered metabolism of hormones: thyroid, pituitary, adrenal; altered immunity

MS: Weakness

CNS: Headache, fatigue

GI: Nausea, cramps, diarrhea

GU: Gonadal dysfunction

CV: Increased risk of thrombophlebitis

EENT: Blurred vision

INTEG: Sterile abscess, contact dermatitis

Contraindications: None significant

Precautions: Pregnancy (A)

Pharmacokinetics:

PO: Metabolized in liver, excreted in bile

Interactions:

• Increased action of oral anticoagulants

• Decreased absorption: cholestyramine, colestipol, mineral oil, sucralfate

NURSING CONSIDERATIONS
Assess:

• Vit E levels during treatment

• Nutritional status: wheat germ, dark green leafy vegetables, nuts, eggs, liver, vegetable oils, dairy products, cereals

Administer:

PO

• Administer with or after meals

• *Chewable tabs:* Chew well

• *Sol:* May be dropped in mouth or mixed with food

TOP

• To moisturize dry skin

Perform/provide:

• Storage in tight, light-resistant container

Evaluate:

• Therapeutic response: absence of hemolytic anemia, adequate vit E levels, improvement in skin lesions, decreased edema

Teach patient/family:

• The necessary foods in diet

• To omit if dose is missed

• To avoid vitamin supplements unless directed by prescriber

---

warfarin (℞)

(war′far-in)

Coumadin, Sofarin, warfarin sodium, Warfilone Sodium*

Func. class.: Anticoagulant

Action: Interferes with blood clotting by indirect means; depresses hepatic synthesis of vit K-dependent coagulation factors (II, VII, IX, X)

Uses: Pulmonary emboli, deep-vein thrombosis, MI, atrial dysrhythmias, postcardiac valve replacement

Dosage and routes:

• *Adult:* **PO/IV** 10-15 mg/day × 3 days, then titrated to prothrombin time qd

• *Child:* 0.1 mg/kg/day titrated to INR

Available forms: Tabs 1, 2, 2.5, 5, 7.5, 10 mg; inj 50 mg/2 ml

Side effects/adverse reactions:

GI: Diarrhea, nausea, vomiting, anorexia, stomatitis, cramps, *hepatitis*

GU: Hematuria

INTEG: Rash, dermatitis, urticaria, alopecia, pruritus

CNS: Fever

HEMA: Hemorrhage, agranulocytosis, leukopenia, eosinophilia

Contraindications: Hypersensitivity, hemophilia, leukemia with bleeding, peptic ulcer disease, thrombocytopenic purpura, hepatic disease (severe), severe hypertension, subacute bacterial endocarditis, acute nephritis, blood dyscrasias, pregnancy (D), eclampsia, preeclampsia, lactation

Precautions: Alcoholism, elderly

Pharmacokinetics:

PO: Onset 12-24 hr, peak 1½-3 days, duration 3-5 days, half-life 1½-2½ days; metabolized in liver, excreted in urine/feces (active/inactive metabolites), crosses pla-

---

◆ = Nursing alert   ▮ = Herb-drug interaction   ⊘ = Do not crush

centa, 99% bound to plasma proteins

Interactions:

• Increased action of warfarin: allopurinol, chloramphenicol, amiodarone, diflunisal, heparin, steroids, cimetidine, disulfiram, thyroid, glucagon, metronidazole, quinidine, sulindac, sulfinpyrazone, sulfonamides, clofibrate, salicylates, ethacrynic acids, indomethacin, mefenamic acid, oxyphenbutazones, phenylbutazone, cefamandole, chloral hydrate, cotrimoxazole, erythromycin, quinolone antibiotics, isoniazid, thrombolytic agents, tricyclic antidepressants

• Decreased action of warfarin: barbiturates, griseofulvin, ethchlorvynol, carbamazepine, rifampin, oral contraceptives, phenytoin, estrogens, vit K, cholestyramine, corticosteroids, mercaptopurine, sucralfate, vit K foods, vit supplements

• Increased toxicity: oral sulfonylureas, phenytoin

🖉 Increased risk of bleeding: bromelain, cinchona, cayenne, feverfew, garlic, danshen, ginkgo biloba, quinine, ginger

🖉 Decreased anticoagulation: ginseng, alfalfa

Lab test interferences:

Increase: T$_3$ uptake

Decrease: Uric acid

NURSING CONSIDERATIONS

Assess:

• Blood studies (Hct, platelets, occult blood in stools) q3mo

• Prothrombin time, which should be 1½-2 × control; PT often done qd initially or INR (international normalized ratio)

• Bleeding gums, petechiae, ecchymosis, black tarry stools, hematuria

• Fever, skin rash, urticaria

• Needed dosage change q1-2wk; when stable, PT q3wk

Administer:

• At same time each day to maintain steady blood levels

• Tabs whole or crushed

• Avoiding all IM injections that may cause bleeding

IV

• After diluting with diluent provided (50 mg/2 ml); rotate vial, give through Y-tube or 3-way stopcock at [dH]25 mg/min

Y-site compatibilities: Amikacin, ascorbic acid, cefazolin, ceftriaxone, cephapirin, dopamine, epinephrine, heparin, lidocaine, metaraminol, morphine, nitroglycerin, oxytocin, potassium chloride, ranitidine

Perform/provide:

• Storage in tight container

Evaluate:

• Therapeutic response: decrease of deep-vein thrombosis

Teach patient/family:

• To avoid OTC preparations that may cause serious drug interactions unless directed by prescriber

• To use soft-bristle toothbrush to avoid bleeding gums, and to use electric razor

• To carry a Medic Alert ID identifying drug taken

• The importance of compliance

• To report any signs of bleeding: gums, under skin, urine, stools

• To avoid hazardous activities (football, hockey, skiing), dangerous work

• The importance of avoiding unusual changes in vitamin intake, diet or lifestyle

• To inform dentists and other physicians of anticoagulant intake

• That smoking increases dose requirements

• To limit foods high in vit K

Treatment of overdose: Administer vit K

zafirlukast (Ŗ)

(za-feer'loo-cast)
Accolate
Func. class.: Bronchodilator
Chem class: Leukotriene receptor antagonist

Action: Antagonizes the contractile action of leukotrienes (LTC_4, LTD_4, LTE_4) in airway smooth muscle; inhibits bronchoconstriction caused by antigens

Uses: Prophylaxis and chronic treatment of asthma in adults/children >12 yr

Dosage and routes:
• *Adult:* **PO** 20 mg bid, take 1 hr ac or 2 hr pc
Available forms: Tabs 20 mg

Contraindications: Hypersensitivity

Precautions: Pregnancy (B), elderly, lactation, children, hepatic disease

Interactions:
• Increased plasma levels of zafirlukast: aspirin
• Decreased plasma levels of zafirlukast: erythromycin, terfenadine, theophylline
• Increased pro-time: warfarin
• Drug/food: decreased bioavailability

Side effects/adverse reactions:
CNS: Headache, dizziness
GI: Nausea, diarrhea, abdominal pain, vomiting
OTHER: Infections, pain, asthenia, myalgia, fever, dyspepsia, increased ALT

Pharmacokinetics: Unknown

NURSING CONSIDERATIONS
Assess:

◈ Adult patients carefully for symptoms of Churg-Strauss syndrome (rare), including eosinophilia, vasculitic rash, worsening pulmonary symptoms, cardiac complications, and/or neuropathy
• Respiratory rate, rhythm, depth; auscultate lung fields bilaterally; notify prescriber of abnormalities

Administer:
• PO after meals for GI symptoms; absorption may be affected

Evaluate:
• Therapeutic response: ability to breathe more easily

Teach patient/family:
• To check OTC medications, current prescription medications, which will increase stimulation
• To avoid hazardous activities; dizziness may occur
• That if GI upset occurs, to take drug with 8 oz water; avoid food if possible, absorption may be decreased
• To notify prescriber of nausea, vomiting, diarrhea, abdominal pain

---

zalcitabine (Ŗ)

(zal-sit'a-bin)
ddC, dideoxycytidine HIVID
Func. class.: Antiviral
Chem. class.: Synthetic pyrimidine nucleoside analog of 2'-deoxycytidine

Action: Inhibits HIV replication by the conversion of this drug by cellular enzymes to an active antiviral metabolite

Uses: Advanced HIV infections in adults, children >13 yr who cannot use zidovudine or who do not respond to treatment

Dosage and routes:
• *Adult:* **PO** combined with zidovudine in advanced HIV infection: 0.75 mg concomitantly with 200 mg zidovudine q8h; dosage reduction not necessary for patients weighing >30 kg; in presence of peripheral

---

◈ = Nursing alert   ⁄⁄ = Herb-drug interaction   ⊘ = Do not crush

neuropathy initiate dose at 0.375 mg q8h of zalcitabine
Renal dose
• CrCl <40 ml/min, reduce dose
Available forms: Tabs 0.375, 0.75 mg
Side effects/adverse reactions:
GI: Pancreatitis, *diarrhea, nausea, vomiting,* abdominal pain, constipation, stomatitis, dysplasia, liver abnormalities, *oral ulcers,* flatulence, taste perversion, dry mouth, oral thrush, melena, *increased ALT, AST, alk phosphatase, amylase*
GU: Uric acid, **toxic nephropathy,** polyuria
CNS: Headache, peripheral neuropathy, **seizures,** confusion, anxiety, hypertonia, abnormal thinking, asthenia, insomnia, CNS depression, pain, *dizziness,* chills, *fever*
RESP: Cough, pneumonia, dyspnea, asthma, hypoventilation
ENDO: Hypoglycemia, hyponatremia, hyperbilirubinemia, hyperglycemia
INTEG: Rash, pruritus, alopecia, sweating, acne
MS: Myalgia, arthritis, myopathy, muscular atrophy
CV: Hypertension, vasodilation, dysrhythmia, syncope, palpitation, tachycardia
EENT: Ear pain, otitis, photophobia, visual impairment
HEMA: **Leukopenia, granulocytopenia, thrombocytopenia,** anemia
Contraindications: Hypersensitivity
Precautions: Renal, hepatic disease, pregnancy (C), lactation, child <13 yr, peripheral neuropathy, heart failure
Pharmacokinetics:
PO: Elimination half-life 1.62 hr; administration within 5 min of food will decrease absorption; elimination via kidneys

Interactions:
• Increased risk of pancreatitis with agents that can cause pancreatitis
• Increased risk of peripheral neuropathy with other agents that can cause peripheral neuropathy: aminoglycosides, amphotericin B, chloramphenicol, cimetidine, cisplatin, dapsone, disulfiram, ethionamide, foscarnet, glutethimide, gold, hydralazine, iodoquinol, isoniazid, metronidazole, nitrofurantoin, phenytoin, probenecid, ribavirin, vincristine; use with didanosine is not recommended
• Decreased absorption: ketoconazole, dapsone, food, antacids, metoclopramide
• Do not administer with tetracyclines
• Decreased concentrations of fluoroquinolone antibiotics
NURSING CONSIDERATIONS
Assess:
• Neuropathy: tingling or pain in hands and feet, distal numbness
• Pancreatitis: abdominal pain, nausea, vomiting, elevated liver enzymes; drug should be discontinued, since condition can be fatal
• Children by dilated retinal examination q6mo to rule out retinal depigmentation
• CBC, differential, platelet count qwk; withhold drug if WBC is <4000/mm^3 or platelet count is <75,000/mm^3; notify prescriber
• Renal function studies: BUN, serum uric acid, urine CrCl before, during therapy
• Temp q4h; may indicate beginning infection
• Liver function tests before, during therapy (bilirubin, AST, ALT), triglycerides, amylase prn or qmo
Administer:
• Antibiotics: for prophylaxis of infection

Perform/provide:

• Strict medical asepsis, protective isolation if WBC levels are low

Evaluate:

• Therapeutic response: absence of infection; symptoms of HIV

Teach patient/family:

• To report signs of infection: fever, sore throat, flu symptoms

• To report signs of anemia: fatigue, headache, faintness, shortness of breath, irritability

• To report bleeding; avoid use of razors, commercial mouthwash

• That hair may be lost during therapy; a wig or hairpiece may make patient feel better

---

zaleplon
See appendix a—selected new drugs

---

zanamivir
See appendix a—selected new drugs

---

zidovudine (R)
(zye-doe'-vue-deen)
Apo-Zidovudine*,   Azidothymidine, AZT, Novo-AZT*, Retrovir
Func. class.: Antiviral
Chem. class.: Thymidine analog

Action: Inhibits replication of HIV virus by incorporating into cellular DNA by viral reverse transcriptase, thereby terminating the cellular DNA chain

Uses: Symptomatic/asymptomatic HIV infections (AIDS, ARC), confirmed *Pneumocystis carinii* pneumonia, absolute CD4 lymphocytes of <200/mm^3, prevention of maternal-fetal HIV transmission

Dosage and routes:

• *Adult:* PO 200 mg q4h; may have to stop treatment if severe bone marrow depression occurs, and restart after bone marrow recovery; IV 1-2 mg/kg q4h, initiate PO as soon as possible

• *Child:* PO 90-180 mg/m^2/dose q6h; IV same as adult

• *Neonates:* PO 2-3 mg/kg/dose q6h; IV same as adult

Prevention of maternal-fetal HIV transmission

• *Neonatal:* PO 2 mg/kg/dose q6h × 6 wk beginning 8-12 hr after birth; IV 1.5 mg/kg/dose over 30 min q6h until able to take PO

• *Maternal (>14 wk gestation):* PO 100 mg 5×/day until start of labor, then IV 2 mg/kg over 1 hr followed by IV INF 1 mg/kg/hr until umbilical cord clamped

Asymptomatic HIV infection

• *Child 3 mo to 12 yr:* PO 90-180 mg/m^2 q6h (max 200 mg q6h); IV 1-2 mg/kg over 1 hr q4h

• *Adult:* PO 100 mg q4h while awake (5×/day)

Symptomatic HIV infection

• *Child 3 mo to 12 yr:* PO 90-180 mg/m^2 q6h (max 200 mg q6h); IV 1-2 mg/kg over 1 hr q4h

• *Adult:* PO 100 mg q4h; IV 1-2 mg/kg over 1 hr q4h

Prevention of HIV following needlestick

• *Adult:* PO 200 mg tid plus lamivudine 150 mg bid, plus a protease inhibitor for high-risk exposure; begin within 2 hr of exposure

Available forms: Caps 100 mg; inj 200 mg/20 ml; oral syr 50 mg/5 ml

Side effects/adverse reactions:

*HEMA: **Granulocytopenia, anemia***

CNS: Fever, headache, malaise, diaphoresis, *dizziness, insomnia,* paresthesia, somnolence, chills, tremor, twitching, anxiety, confusion, de-

---

⬦ = Nursing alert   🖉 = Herb-drug interaction   🚫 = Do not crush pression, lability, vertigo, loss of mental acuity

GI: Nausea, vomiting, diarrhea, anorexia, cramps, *dyspepsia,* constipation, dysphagia, *flatulence,* rectal bleeding, mouth ulcer

RESP: Dyspnea

EENT: Taste change, hearing loss, photophobia

INTEG: Rash, acne, pruritus, urticaria

MS: Myalgia, arthralgia, muscle spasm

GU: Dysuria, polyuria, urinary frequency, hesitancy

Contraindications: Hypersensitivity

Precautions: Granulocyte count $<1000/mm^3$ or Hgb <9.5 g/dl, pregnancy (C), lactation, child, severe renal disease, impaired hepatic disease

Pharmacokinetics:

PO: Rapidly absorbed from GI tract, peak ½-1½ hr, metabolized in liver (inactive metabolites), excreted by kidneys

Interactions:

• Toxicity: amphotericin B, dapsone, flucytosine, adriamycin, interferon, vincristine, vinblastine, pentamidine, probenecid, experimental nucleoside analogs, benzodiazepines, cimetidine, morphine, sulfonamides, acyclovir, ganciclovir, doxorubicin, acetaminophen, indomethacin, fluconazole, phenytoin, trimethoprim

• Granulocytopenia: acetaminophen, aspirin, indomethacin

NURSING CONSIDERATIONS

Assess:

• Blood counts q2wk; watch for decreasing granulocytes, Hgb; if low, therapy may have to be discontinued and restarted after hematologic recovery; blood transfusions may be required

Administer:

• By mouth; capsules should be swallowed whole

• Trimethoprim-sulfamethoxazole, pyrimethamine, or acyclovir as ordered to prevent opportunistic infections; if these drugs are given, watch for neurotoxicity

IV

• After diluting each 1 mg/0.25 ml or more D_5W to 4 mg/ml or less; give over 1 hr

Y-site compatibilities: Acyclovir, allopurinol, amifostine, amikacin, amphotericin B, amphotericin B cholesteryl, aztreonam, cefepime, ceftazidime, ceftriaxone, cimetidine, cisatracurium, clindamycin, dexamethasone, dobutamine, dopamine, doxorubicin liposome, erythromycin, filgrastim, fluconazole, fludarabine, gentamicin, granisetron, heparin, imipenem/cilastatin, lorazepam, melphalan, metoclopramide, morphine, nafcillin, ondansetron, oxacillin, paclitaxel, pentamidine, phenylephrine, piperacillin, piperacillin/tazobactam, potassium chloride, ranitidine, remifentanil, sargramostim, teniposide, thiotepa, tobramycin, trimethoprim-sulfamethoxazole, trimetrexate, vancomycin, vinorelbine

Perform/provide;

• Storage in cool environment; protect from light

Evaluate:

• Blood dyscrasias (anemia, granulocytopenia): bruising, fatigue, bleeding, poor healing

Teach patient/family:

• That GI complaints and insomnia resolve after 3-4 wk of treatment

• That drug is not cure for AIDS but will control symptoms

• To notify prescriber of sore throat, swollen lymph nodes, malaise, fever; other infections may occur

z

• That patient is still infective, may pass AIDS virus on to others

• That follow-up visits must be continued since serious toxicity may occur; blood counts must be done q2wk

• That drug must be taken q4h around clock, even during night; to take 30 min ac or in pc

• That serious drug interactions may occur if OTC products are ingested; check with prescriber before taking aspirin, acetaminophen, indomethacin

• That other drugs may be necessary to prevent other infections

• That drug may cause fainting or dizziness

---

zileuton (R)
(zye'loo-tahn)
Zyflo
Func. class.: Bronchodilator, leukotriene pathway inhibitor
Chem. class.: 5-lipoxygenase inhibitor

Action: Inhibits leukotriene (LT) formation; leukotrienes exert their effects by increasing neutrophil, eosinophil migration; aggregation of neutrophils, monocytes; smooth muscle contraction, capillary permeability; these actions further lead to bronchoconstriction, inflammation, edema

Uses: Allergic rhinitis, asthma
Investigational uses: Ulcerative colitis, rheumatoid arthritis
Dosage and routes:

Asthma
• *Adult and child:* 12 yr: **PO** 600 mg qid, may be given with meal and hs

Ulcerative colitis
• *Adult:* **PO** 600 mg bid
Available forms: Tabs 600 mg

Side effects/adverse reactions:
CNS: Dizziness, insomnia, fatigue, paresthesias, headache
GI: Nausea, abdominal pain, dyspepsia, diarrhea, LFT abnormalities
INTEG: Hives
MS: Myalgia, asthenia
Contraindications: Hepatic disease, elevations in LFTs 3× upper limits, hypersensitivity
Precautions: Acute attacks of asthma, alcohol consumption, pregnancy (C)
Pharmacokinetics:
PO: Rapidly absorbed, peak 1-3 hr, half-life 2.1-2.5 hr, protein binding 93% (albumin); metabolized by liver, excretion in urine
Interactions:
• Increased action of zileuton: theophylline, propranolol
• May increase effects of anticoagulants
NURSING CONSIDERATIONS
Assess:
• CBC, blood chemistry during treatment
• LFTs before and qmo × 3 mo, then q2-3mo during treatment
• Respiratory rate, rhythm, depth; auscultate lung fields bilaterally; notify prescriber of abnormalities
• Allergic reactions: rash, urticaria; drug should be discontinued
Administer:
PO
• After meals for GI symptoms; absorption may be affected
Evaluate:
• Therapeutic response: ability to breathe more easily
Teach patient/family:
• To check OTC medications, current prescription medications for ephedrine, which will increase stimulation; to avoid alcohol
• To avoid hazardous activities; dizziness may occur

◆ = Nursing alert   ⫸ = Herb-drug interaction   Ⓢ = Do not crush

• That if GI upset occurs to take drug with 8 oz water or food; absorption may be decreased slightly
• To notify prescriber of nausea, vomiting, anxiety, insomnia

---

zinc (R, OTC)
Orazinc, PMS Egozine*, Verazinc, Zinca-Pak, Zincate, Zinc 15, Zinc-220, zinc sulfate
Func. class.: Trace element; nutritional supplement

Action: Needed for adequate healing, bone and joint development (23% zinc)
Uses: Prevention of zinc deficiency, adjunct to vit A therapy
Investigational uses: Wound healing
Dosage and routes:
Dietary supplement
• *Adult:* PO 25-50 mg/day
Nutritional supplement (IV)
• *Adult:* IV 2.5-4 mg/day; may increase by 2 mg/day if needed
• *Child 1-5 yr:* IV 100 µg/kg/day
• *Infant <1.5-3 kg:* IV 300 µg/kg/day
Available forms: Tabs 66, 110 mg; caps 220 mg; inj 1 mg, 5 mg/ml
Side effects/adverse reactions:
GI: Nausea, vomiting, cramps, heartburn, ulcer formation
Overdose: Diarrhea, rash, dehydration, restlessness
Precautions: Pregnancy (A)
Interactions:
• Decreased absorption of other covalent cations
NURSING CONSIDERATIONS
Assess:
• Zinc levels during treatment
Administer:
• With meals to decrease gastric upset; avoid dairy products

Evaluate:
• Therapeutic response: absence of zinc deficiency
Teach patient/family:
• That element must be taken for 2 mo to be effective
• To report immediately nausea, diarrhea, rash, severe vomiting, restlessness, abdominal pain, tarry stools

---

zolmitriptan (R)
(zole-mih-trip′tan)
Zomig
Func. class.: Migraine agent
Chem. class.: 5-HT$_1$ receptor agonist

Action: Binds selectively to the vascular 5-HT$_1$ receptor subtype, exerts antimigraine effect; causes vasoconstriction in cranial arteries
Uses: Acute treatment of migraine with or without aura
Dosage and routes:
• *Adult:* PO ≥2.5 mg (tab may be broken), may repeat after 2 hr, max 10 mg/24 hr
Available forms: Tabs 2.5, 5 mg
Side effects/adverse reactions:
CV: Palpitations
GI: Abdominal discomfort
MS: Weakness, neck stiffness, myalgia
NEURO: Tingling, hot sensation, burning, feeling of pressure, tightness, numbness, dizziness, sedation
RESP: Chest tightness, pressure
Contraindictions: Angina pectoris, history of MI, documented silent ischemia, ischemic heart disease, concurrent ergotamine-containing preparations, uncontrolled hypertension, hypersensitivity, basilar or hemiplegic migraine
Precautions: Postmenopausal women, men >40 yr, risk factors for CAD, hypercholesterolemia, obesity, diabetes, impaired hepatic or

Z

---

renal function, pregnancy (C), lactation, children, elderly

Pharmacokinetics: Duration 2-3½ hr, 25% plasma protein binding, half-life 3-3½ hr, metabolized in the liver (metabolite), excreted in urine, feces

Interactions:

• Extended vasospastic effects: ergot, ergot derivatives

• Do not use within 2 wk of MAOIs

• Increased half-life of zolmitriptan: cimetidine

• Weakness, hyperreflexia, incoordination: SSRIs (fluoxetine, fluvoxamine, paroxetine, sertraline)

NURSING CONSIDERATIONS
Assess:

• Tingling, hot sensation, burning, feeling of pressure, numbness, flushing

• For stress level, activity, recreation, coping mechanisms

• Neurologic status: LOC, blurring vision, nausea, vomiting, tingling in extremities preceding headache

• Ingestion of tyramine foods (pickled products, beer, wine, aged cheese), food additives, preservatives, colorings, artifical sweeteners, chocolate, caffeine, which may precipitate these types of headaches

• For serotonin syndrome, if also taking an SSRI

Administer:

• Take with fluids as soon as symptoms of migraine occur

Perform/provide:

• Quiet, calm environment with decreased stimulation for noise, bright light, excessive talking

Evaluate:

• Therapeutic response: decrease in frequency, severity of headache

Teach patient/family:

• To report any side effects to prescriber

• To use contraception while taking drug

zolpidem (℞)

(zole′pih-dem)

Ambien

Func. class.: Sedative-hypnotic

Chem. class.: Nonbenzodiazepine of imidazopyridine class

Controlled Substance Schedule IV

Action: Produces CNS depression at limbic, thalamic, hypothalamic levels of CNS; may be mediated by neurotransmitter γ-aminobutyric acid (GABA); results are sedation, hypnosis, skeletal muscle relaxation, anticonvulsant activity, anxiolytic action

Uses: Insomnia, short-term treatment

Dosage and routes:

• *Adult:* **PO** 10 mg hs × 7-10 days only; total dose should not exceed 10 mg

• *Geriatric:* **PO** 5 mg hs

Available forms: Tabs 5, 10 mg

Side effects/adverse reactions:

HEMA: ***Leukopenia, granulocytopenia*** (rare)

CNS: Headache, lethargy, drowsiness, daytime sedation, dizziness, confusion, light-headedness, anxiety, irritability, amnesia, poor coordination

GI: Nausea, vomiting, diarrhea, heartburn, abdominal pain, constipation

CV: Chest pain, palpitation

Contraindications: Hypersensitivity to benzodiazepines

Precautions: Anemia, hepatic disease, renal disease, suicidal individuals, drug abuse, elderly, psychosis, child <18 yr, seizure disorders, pregnancy (B), lactation

Pharmacokinetics:

PO: Onset 1.5 hr, metabolized by liver, excreted by kidneys (inactive metabolites), crosses placenta, excreted in breast milk; half-life 2-3 hr

Interactions:

• Increased action of both drugs: alcohol, CNS depressants

🔻 Increased CNS depression: kava

Lab test interferences:

Increase: ALT, AST, serum bilirubin

Decrease: RAI uptake

False increase: Urinary 17-OHCS

NURSING CONSIDERATIONS

Assess:

• Blood studies: Hct, Hgb, RBC, if blood dyscrasias are suspected (rare)

• Hepatic studies: AST, ALT, bilirubin if liver damage has occurred

• Mental status: mood, sensorium, affect, memory (long, short)

• Blood dyscrasias: fever, sore throat, bruising, rash, jaundice, epistaxis (rare)

• Type of sleep problem: falling asleep, staying asleep

Administer:

• After removal of cigarettes to prevent fires

• After trying conservative measures for insomnia

• ½-1 hr before hs for sleeplessness

• On empty stomach for fast onset but may be taken with food if GI symptoms occur

Perform/provide:

• Assistance with ambulation after receiving dose

• Safety measures: side rails, nightlight, call bell within easy reach

• Checking to see if PO medication has been swallowed

• Storage in tight container in cool environment

Evaluate:

• Therapeutic response: ability to sleep at night, decreased amount of early morning awakening if taking drug for insomnia

Teach patient/family:

• That dependence is possible after long-term use

• To avoid driving or other activities requiring alertness until drug is stabilized

• To avoid alcohol ingestion, CNS depressants; serious CNS depression may result

• That effects may take 2 nights for benefits to be noticed

• Alternative measures to improve sleep: reading, exercise several hours before hs, warm bath, warm milk, TV, self-hypnosis, deep breathing

• That hangover is common in elderly but less common than with barbiturates; rebound insomnia may occur for 1-2 nights after discontinuing drug

Treatment of overdose: Lavage, activated charcoal; monitor electrolytes, vital signs

Z

Appendix a

Selected new drugs

abacavir (R)
(ah-bak'ah-veer)
Ziagen
Func. class.: Antiviral
Chem. class.: Nucleoside analog

Action: A synthetic nucleoside analog with inhibitory action against HIV. Inhibits replication of the virus by incorporating into cellular DNA by viral reverse transcriptase, thereby terminating the cellular DNA chain
Uses: In combination with other antiretroviral agents for HIV-1 infection

Dosage and routes:
• *Adult:* PO 300 mg bid with other antiretrovirals
• *Adolescents and child ≥3 mo:* 8 mg/kg bid, max 300 mg bid with other antiretrovirals
Available forms: Tabs 300 mg; oral sol 20 mg/ml
Side effects/adverse reactions:
*HEMA: **Granulocytopenia, anemia***
CNS: Fever, headache, malaise, insomnia, paresthesia
GI: Nausea, vomiting, diarrhea, anorexia, cramps, abdominal pain
RESP: Dyspnea
*INTEG: Rash, **fatal hypersensitivity reactions,** urticaria*
*META: **Lactic acidosis***
Contraindications: Hypersensitivity
Precautions: Granulocyte count <1000/mm^3 or Hgb <9.5 g/dl, pregnancy (C), lactation, children, severe renal disease, impaired hepatic function
Pharmacokinetics: 50% plasma protein binding, metabolized to inactive metabolites, half-life 1½-2 hr
Interactions:
• Increased abacavir levels: alcohol
NURSING CONSIDERATIONS
Assess:
◆ For lactic acidosis and severe hepatomegaly with steatosis
◆ For fatal hypersensitivity reactions: fever, rash, nausea, vomiting, diarrhea, abdominal discomfort; treatment should be discontinued and not restarted
• For blood dyscrasias (anemia, granulocytopenia): bruising, fatigue, bleeding, poor healing
• For increased temp, may indicate beginning infection
• Renal function studies: BUN, serum uric acid, CrCl before, during therapy; these may be elevated throughout treatment
• Liver function tests before and during therapy: bilirubin, AST, ALT, amylase, alkaline phosphatase q mo
• Blood counts q2wk; watch for decreasing granulocytes, Hgb; if low, therapy may have to be discontinued and restarted after hematologic recovery; blood transfusions may be required
Administer:
• Give in combination with other antiretrovirals with food

Perform/provide:

• Storage in cool environment; protect from light

Teach patient/family:

• That drug is not cure for AIDS but will control symptoms

• To notify prescriber of sore throat, swollen lymph nodes, malaise, fever; other infections may occur

• That patient is still infective, may pass AIDS virus on to others

• That follow-up visits must be continued since serious toxicity may occur; blood counts must be done

• To use contraception during treatment

• Give patient Medication Guide and Warning Card, discuss points on guide

• That other drugs may be necessary to prevent other infections

---

alitretinoin (R)

Panretin

Func. class.: Retinoid, 2nd generation

Action: Controls cellular differentiation and proliferation of neoplastic and healthy cells

Uses: Kaposi's sarcoma cutaneous lesions

Dosage and routes:

• *Adult:* **TOP** Apply enough gel to cover lesions with a generous coating, allow to dry for 3-5 min, before covering with clothing, do not apply near mucosal areas, apply as long as benefit occurs

Available forms: Gel 0.1%

Side effects/adverse reactions:

INTEG: Rash, stinging, warmth, redness, erythema, blistering, crusting, peeling, contact dermatitis, pain

Contraindications: Hypersensitivity to retinoids, pregnancy (D)

Precautions: Lactation, eczema,

sunburn, elderly, cutaneous T-cell lymphoma

Pharmacokinetics:

TOP: Poor systemic absorption

Interactions:

• Do not use around DEET (an insect repellant agent)

NURSING CONSIDERATIONS

Assess:

• Area of body involved, what helps or aggravates condition; cysts, dryness, itching; lesions may worsen at beginning of treatment

Administer:

• Bid initially to lesions, can be increased to tid-qid according to tolerance, discontinue for a few days if severe reactions occur

Perform/provide:

• Storage at room temp

• Hand washing after application

Evaluate:

• Therapeutic response: decrease in size and number of lesions

Teach patient/family:

• To avoid application on normal skin, getting cream in eyes, nose, other mucous membranes

• To avoid sunlight, sunlamps, or use protective clothing, sunscreen

• That treatment may cause warmth, stinging, dryness, peeling will occur

• That drug does not cure condition; only relieves symptoms

• That therapeutic results may be seen in 2-3 wk but may not be optimal until after 6 wk

---

aminolevulinic acid (R)

Levulan Kerastick

Func. class.: Photochemotherapy

Action: ALA is the 1st step resulting in heme synthesis; a protopor-

---

◆ = Nursing alert   ⫸ = Herb-drug interaction   Ⓝ = Do not crush phyrin IX precursor that is a photosensitizer

Uses: Face/scalp nonhyperkeratotic actinic keratoses

Dosage and routes:

• *Adult:* **TOP** 1 application of solution and 1 dose of illumination/treatment site × 8wk

Available forms: Sol 20% (354 mg)

Side effects/adverse reactions:

INTEG: Crusting, hypopigmentation, hyperpigmentation, ulceration, pain, itching, bleeding, pustules

Contraindications: Hypersensitivity to porphyrins

Precautions: Lactation, sunburn, pregnancy (C), inherited or acquired coagulation defects

Pharmacokinetics: Unknown

Interactions:

• May increase photosensitivity: phenothiazines, sulfonylureas, thiazides, tetracyclines

NURSING CONSIDERATIONS

Assess:

• Area of body involved, what helps or aggravates condition

Administer:

• Preparing ALA top sol by holding applicator cap pointing up. Crush the bottom ampule containing sol vehicle by applying pressure to position A on cardboard sleeve; crush top ampule containing ALA powder by applying pressure to position B on sleeve; hold applicator between thumb and forefinger, point away from the face, shake gently for about 3 min to dissolve powder; sol is applied to lesions after cleaning and drying

Evaluate:

• Therapeutic response: decrease in size and number of lesions

Teach patient/family:

• To avoid sunlight, sunlamps, or use protective clothing, sunscreen

• That treatment may cause pain, crusting

• After application of ALA, to return the next day for treatment

---

amprenavir (℞)

(am-pren'ah-veer)

Agenerase

Func. class.: Antiviral

Chem. class.: Synthetic peptide-like substrate analog

Action: Inhibits human immunodeficiency virus (HIV) protease, which prevents maturation of the infectious virus

Uses: HIV in combination with other antiretroviral agents

Dosage and routes:

• *Adult:* **PO** (cap) 1200 mg bid

• *Child 13-16 yr:* **PO** (cap) 1200 mg bid

• *Child 4-12 yr or wt <50 kg:* **PO** Caps: 20 mg/kg qd or 15 mg/kg tid, max 2400 mg; sol: 22.5 mg/kg bid or 17 mg/kg tid qd, max 2800 mg

Available forms: Caps 50, 150 mg; oral sol 15 mg/ml

Side effects/adverse reactions:

GI: Diarrhea, abdominal pain, nausea

CNS: Paresthesia, headache

INTEG: Rash, **Stevens-Johnson syndrome**

*HEMA: **Acute hemolytic anemia***

ENDO: New onset diabetes, hyperglycemia, exacerbation of preexisting diabetes mellitus

Contraindications: Hypersensitivity

Precautions: Liver disease, pregnancy (C), lactation, children, hemophilia, sulfonamide sensitivity, elderly

Pharmacokinetics: Rapidly absorbed, peak 1-2 hr, 90% protein bound, metabolized in liver, excreted unchanged in urine/feces (minimal)

Interactions:
• Do not use with: loratadine, midazolam, triazolam, ergots

◆ Serious life-threatening interactions: amiodarone, lidocaine, quinidine, tricyclics

• Increased amprenavir levels: ketoconazole, ritonavir, cimetidine, itraconazole, indinavir, clarithromycin, erythromycin

• Decreased amprenavir levels: rifamycins, antacids, carbamazepine, phenobarbital, phenytoin

• Drug/food: decreased bioavailability after high-fat meal

Lab test interferences: CPK, glucose (low)

NURSING CONSIDERATIONS
Assess:
• Signs of infection, anemia
• Liver function studies: ALT, AST
• C&S before drug therapy; drug may be taken as soon as culture is taken; repeat C&S after treatment; determine the presence of other sexually transmitted diseases

• Bowel pattern before, during treatment; if severe abdominal pain with bleeding occurs, drug should be discontinued; monitor hydration

• Skin eruptions, rash, urticaria, itching

• Allergies before treatment, reaction of each medication; place allergies on chart

Teach patient/family:
• To take as prescribed with or without food; if dose is missed, take as soon as remembered up to 1 hr before next dose; do not double dose

• That drug must be taken in equal intervals around the clock to maintain blood levels for duration of therapy

• That caps and sol are not interchangeable on a mg/mg basis

---

bexarotene (R)
Targretin
Func. class.: Retinoid, 2nd generation

Action: Selectively binds and activates retinoid X receptors (RXRs) that are partially responsible for cellular proliferation and differentiation. Inhibits some tumor cells

Uses: Cutaneous T-cell lymphoma

Investigational uses: Breast cancer

Dosage and routes:
• *Adult:* **PO** 300 mg/day/m², may increase to 400 mg/day with proper monitoring

Available forms: Cap 75 mg

Side effects/adverse reactions:
CNS: Headache, fatigue, lethargy
*GI: Nausea, abdominal pain, diarrhea, **acute pancreatitis***
INTEG: Rash, asthenia, dry skin
*HEMA: **Leukopenia, neutropenia,*** anemia
SYST: Infection, hypothyroidism

Contraindications: Hypersensitivity to retinoids, pregnancy (X)

Precautions: Lactation, sunburn, hepatic, renal disease

Pharmacokinetics: Unknown

Interactions:
• Increased bexarotene levels: azole antiinfectives, grapefruit juice
• Decreased bexarotene levels: barbiturates, rifampins
• Limit intake of vit A ≤15,000 IU/day

NURSING CONSIDERATIONS
Assess:
• Area of body involved, what helps or aggravates condition; cysts, dryness, itching
• Cholesterol, HDL, triglycerides may be elevated
• CBC for leukopenia, neutropenia, anemia

◆ = Nursing alert   ∥ = Herb-drug interaction   ⊘ = Do not crush

Administer:
• With food
Perform/provide:
• Storage at room temp
Evaluate:
• Therapeutic response: decrease in size and number of lesions
Teach patient/family:
• To avoid sunlight, sunlamps, or use protective clothing, sunscreen

---

cilostazol (℞)

(sih-los'tah-zol)
Pletal
Func. class.: Platelet aggregation inhibitor
Chem. class.: Quinolone derivative

Action: Inhibits cellular phosphodiesterase; reversibly inhibits thrombin, ADP, collagen

Uses: Intermittent claudication

Dosage and routes:
• *Adult:* **PO** 100 mg bid taken ≥30 min ac or 2 hr pc breakfast and dinner or 50 mg bid if using drugs that inhibit CYP3A4; 12 wk of treatment may be needed for beneficial effect

Available forms: Tabs 50, 100 mg

Side effects/adverse reactions:
CNS: Dizziness, vertigo, anxiety, insomnia, neuralgia
CV: Palpitations, tachycardia, *atrial fibrillation/flutter, cerebral infarct, cerebral ischemia, CHF, cardiac arrest, MI, nodal dysrhythmia*
GI: Nausea, vomiting, *diarrhea,* GI discomfort, colitis, cholelithiasis, ulcer, esophagitis, gastritis
HEMA: Bleeding (epistaxis, hematuria, conjunctival hemorrhage, GI bleeding), agranulocytosis, neutropenia, thrombocytopenia
INTEG: Rash

MISC: Back pain, headache, infection, myalgia, peripheral edema, chills, fever, malaise, diabetes mellitus
RESP: Cough, pharyngitis, rhinitis

Contraindications: Hypersensitivity, CHF, active liver disease, blood dyscrasias, active bleeding

Precautions: Past liver disease, renal disease, elderly, pregnancy (C), lactation, children, increased bleeding risk

Pharmacokinetics: 95%-98% protein binding, metabolism-hepatic extensively by cytochrome P450 enzymes, excreted urine (74%), feces (20%), half-life 11-13 hr

Interactions:
• Increased bleeding tendencies: anticoagulants, aspirin
• Increased cilostazol levels: diltiazem, erythromycin, fluvoxamine, fluoxetine, nefazodone, omeprazole, ketoconazole, itraconazole, fluconazole, macrolides
• Drug/food: do not use with grapefruit juice

NURSING CONSIDERATIONS
Assess:
• For underlying CV disease since CV risk is great
• For CV lesions with repeated oral administration
• Liver function studies: AST, ALT, bilirubin, creatinine
• Blood studies: CBC; CBC q2 wk, Hct, Hgb, pro-time
Administer:
• Give bid ≥30 min ac or 2 hr pc
Evaluate:
• Therapeutic response: absence of stroke
Teach patient/family:
• That blood work will be necessary during treatment
• To report any unusual bleeding to prescriber

---

* = Canada only   Side effects: *italics* = common; ***bold italics*** = life-threatening

• To report side effects such as diarrhea, skin rashes, subcutaneous bleeding

• That effects may take 2-4 wk, treatment of up to 12 wk may be required for necessary effect

• About potential CV risks in patients with cardiac disease

• To take ≥30 min ac or 2 hr pc

• That reading the patient package insert is necessary

---

coagulation factor VIIa, recombinant (℞)

NovoSeven

Func. class.: Antihemophilic

Action: Promotes hemostasis by activating the intrinsic pathway of coagulation

Uses: Bleeding in hemophilia A or B, with inhibitors to Factor VIII or IX

Dosage and routes:

• *Adult:* **IV BOL** 90 µg/kg q2h until hemostasis occurs, or until therapy is deemed to be inadequate; posthemostatic doses q3-6h may be required

Available forms: Lyophilized powder, 1.2 mg/vial (1200 µg/vial), 4.8 mg/vial (4800 µg/vial) recombinant human coagulation factor VIIa (rFVIIa)

Side effects/adverse reactions:

CNS: Fever, headache

SYST: **Hemorrhage NOS, hemarthrosis, fibrinogen plasma decreased,** hypertension, bradycardia, **DIC, coagulation disorder, thrombosis**

INTEG: Pain, redness at inj site, pruritus, purpura, rash

Contraindications: Hypersensitivity to this product or mouse, hamster, or bovine products

Precautions: Pregnancy (B), lactation, children

Pharmacokinetics: Half-life 2.3 hr

Interactions:

• Do not use with activated prothrombin complex concentrates or prothrombin complex concentrate

NURSING CONSIDERATIONS

Assess:

• VS, B/P, pulse, respirations, neurologic signs, temperature at least q4h, temperature 104° F (40° C) or indicators of internal bleeding, cardiac rhythm

• Pro-time, aPTT, plasma FVII clotting

• For thrombosis, dose should be reduced or stopped

Administer:

IV

• Bring to room temp; for 1.2 mg vial/2.2 ml sterile water for inj; 4.8 mg vial/8.5 ml sterile water for inj

• Remove caps from stop, cleanse stopper with alcohol, allow to dry, draw back plunger of sterile syringe and allow air into syringe, insert needle of syringe into sterile water for inj, inject the air and withdraw amount required, insert syringe needle with diluent into drug vial, aim to side so liquid runs down vial wall, gently swirl until dissolved, use within 3 hr, give by bol over 3-5 min

• Do not admix, keep refrigerated until ready to use, avoid sunlight

Evaluate:

• Therapeutic response: hemostasis

---

denileukin diftitox (℞)
(den-ih-loo'kin dif'tih-tox)
Ontak
Func. class.: Antineoplastic—misc.

Action: A recombinant DNA-derived cytotoxic protein; inhibits cellular protein synthesis

Uses: Cutaneous T-cell lymphoma that expresses CD25 component of the IL-2 receptor

Dosage and routes:
• *Adult:* IV 9-18 µg/kg/day given for 5 days q21 days, given over ≥15 min

Available forms: Sol for inj, frozen 150 µg/ml

Side effects/adverse reactions:
CNS: Dizziness, paresthesia, nervousness, confusion, insomnia
CV: Hypotension, vasodilation, tachycardia, thrombosis, hypertension, dysrhythmias
GI: Nausea, anorexia, vomiting, diarrhea, constipation, dyspepsia, dysphagia
GU: Hematuria, albuminuria, pyuria, creatinine increase
HEMA: **Thrombocytopenia, leukopenia,** anemia
INTEG: Rash, pruritus, sweating
META: Hypoalbuminemia, edema, hypocalcemia, weight decrease, dehydration, hypokalemia
MISC: Fever, chills, asthenia, infection, pain, headache, chest pain, flu-like symptoms
MS: Myalgia, arthralgia
RESP: Dyspnea, cough, pharyngitis, rhinitis

Contraindications: Hypersensitivity to denileukin, diphtheria toxin, interleukin-2

Precautions: Radiation therapy, pregnancy (C), lactation, elderly, children

Pharmacokinetics: Concentrates in liver/kidneys; metabolized by proteolytic degradation

Interactions:
• Increased bone marrow depression: radiation, other antineoplastics
• Decreased antibody reaction: live vaccines

NURSING CONSIDERATIONS
Assess:
• CBC, differential, platelet count weekly; withhold drug if WBC <4000/mm³ or platelet count <75,000/mm³; notify prescriber of results
• Monitor temp q4h (may indicate beginning infection)
• Liver function tests before, during therapy (bilirubin, AST, ALT, LDH) as needed or monthly
• Bleeding: hematuria, guaiac, bruising or petechiae, mucosa or orifices q8h
• Jaundice of skin, sclera; dark urine; clay-colored stools; itchy skin; abdominal pain; fever; diarrhea
• For vascular leak syndrome after 2wk of treatment, hypotension, edema, hypoalbuminemia; monitor weight, B/P, serum albumin, edema
• Obtain CD25 expression on skin biopsy samples

Administer:
• Antiemetic 30-60 min before giving drug to prevent vomiting
• Antibiotics for prophylaxis of infection

IV
• Prepare and hold sol in plastic syringes or soft plastic IV bags only
• Draw calculated dose from vial, inject into empty IV infusion bag, for each 1 ml of drug removed from vial, no more than 9 ml of sterile saline without preservative should be added to IV bag; infuse over ≥ 15 min; do not give by bolus; do not

Side effects: *italics* = common; ***bold italics*** = life-threatening

admix with other drugs; do not use a filter
• Use within 6 hr, discard unused portions
Perform/provide:
• Storage in light-resistant container, dry area
• Warm compresses at infusion site for inflammation
Evaluate:
• Therapeutic response: decreased tumor size, spread of malignancy
Teach patient/family:
• To report signs of infection: fever, sore throat, flu symptoms
• To report signs of anemia: fatigue, headache, faintness, shortness of breath, irritability
• To report bleeding; avoid use of razors, commercial mouthwash
• To avoid use of aspirin products or ibuprofen

---

dexmedetomidine
Precedex
Func. class.: Sedative, alpha$_2$ adrenoceptor agonist

Action: Produces alpha$_2$ activity seen at low and moderate doses, also alpha$_1$ at high doses
Uses: Sedation in mechanically ventilated, intubated patients ICU
Dosage and routes:
• *Adult:* **IV** loading dose of 1 µg/kg over 10 min then 0.2-0.7 µg/kg/hr, do not use for more than 24 hr
Available forms: Inj 100 µg/ml
Side effects/adverse reactions:
GI: Nausea, thirst
GU: Oliguria
CV: Bradycardia, hypotension, hypertension, ***atrial fibrillation, infarction***
RESP: Pulmonary edema, pleural effusion, hypoxia
HEMA: Leukocytosis, anemia

Contraindications: Hypersensitivity
Precautions: Elderly, respiratory depression, severe respiratory disorders, cardiac dysrhythmias, pregnancy (C), lactation, children, renal disease
Pharmacokinetics: Rapid distribution, excreted in urine; metabolized in liver
Interactions:
• Increased CNS depression: alcohol, opioids, sedative/hypnotics, antipsychotics, skeletal muscle relaxants, inhalational anesthetics
NURSING CONSIDERATIONS
Assess:
• Injection site: phlebitis, burning, stinging
• ECG for changes: atrial fibrillation
• CNS changes: movement, jerking, tremors, dizziness, LOC, pupil reaction
• Respiratory dysfunction: respiratory depression, character, rate, rhythm; notify prescriber if respirations are <10/min
Administer:
IV
• After diluting with D$_5$W 0.9% NaCl, withdraw 2 ml of drug and add to 48 ml of 0.9% NaCl to a total of 50 ml, shake to mix well
• Only with resuscitative equipment available
• Only by qualified persons trained in ICU sedation
Solution compatibilities: LR, D$_5$W, 0.9% NaCl, 20% mannitol
Additive compatibilities: Thiopental, etomidate, vecuronium, pancuronium, succinylcholine, atracurium, mivacurium, glycopyrrolate, phenylephrine, atropine, midazolam, morphine, fentanyl
Perform/provide:
• Safety measures: side rails, nightlight, call bell within easy reach

---

⬥ = Nursing alert   ⫽ = Herb-drug interaction   ⊘ = Do not crush

Evaluate:
• Therapeutic response: induction of anesthesia

---

dofetilide (R)
Tikosyn
Func. class.: Antidysrhythmic (Class III)

Action: Blocks cardiac ion channel carrying the rapid component of delayed potassium current, no effect on sodium channels

Uses: Atrial fibrillation, flutter

Dosage and routes:
• *Adult:* PO 125-500 µg bid depending on CrCl
Renal dose
• CrCl <20 ml/min do not use

Available forms: Caps 125, 250, 500 µg

Side effects/adverse reactions:
CNS: Syncope, dizziness
GI: Nausea, vomiting, severe diarrhea, anorexia
CV: Hypotension, postural hypotension, bradycardia, angina, PVCs, substernal pressure, transient hypertension, precipitation of angina

Contraindications: Hypersensitivity, digitalis toxicity, aortic stenosis, pulmonary hypertension, children, QT syndromes, severe renal disease

Precautions: Renal disease, pregnancy (C), lactation

Pharmacokinetics: Well absorbed

Interactions:
• Increased hypokalemia: potassium-depleting diuretics
• Do not use with cimetidine, ketoconazole, verapamil, prochlorperazine, trimethoprim, sulfamethizole, amiloride, metformin, megestrol, prochlorperazine, triamterene

NURSING CONSIDERATIONS
Assess:
• ECG continuously to determine drug effectiveness, PVCs, other dysrhythmias; renal function, QTc q3mo
• B/P continuously for hypotension, hypertension; orthostatic hypotension; keep supine until hypotension subsides
• Cardiac status: rate, rhythm, character, continuously

Administer:
PO
• For 3 days hospitalized

Perform/provide:
• Place patient in supine position unless otherwise ordered; assist with ambulation

Evaluate:
• Therapeutic response: atrial fibrillation

Teach patient/family:
• To make position changes slowly; orthostatic hypotension may occur
• Notify prescriber if fast heartbeats with fainting or dizziness occur
• Notify all prescribers of all medications and supplements taken

---

doxercalciferol (R)
Hectorol
Func. class.: Parathyroid agent (calcium regulator)
Chem. class.: Vit D hormone

Action: Synthetic vit D analog, reduces parathyroid hormone

Uses: To lower high parathyroid hormone levels in patients undergoing chronic kidney dialysis

Dosage and routes:
• *Adult:* PO 10 µg 3×/wk at dialysis

Available forms: Caps 2.5 µg

Side effects/adverse reactions:
CNS: Drowsiness, headache, lethargy
GI: Nausea, diarrhea, vomiting, anorexia, dry mouth, constipation, cramps, metallic taste

---

* = Canada only   Side effects: *italics* = common; ***bold italics*** = life-threatening

MS: Myalgia, arthralgia, decreased bone development

GU: Polyuria, hypercalciuria, hyperphosphatemia, hematuria

RESP: SOB

Contraindications: Hypersensitivity, hyperphosphatemia, hypercalcemia, vit D toxicity

Precautions: Pregnancy (C), renal calculi, lactation, CV disease

Pharmacokinetics: Unknown

Interactions:

• Decreased absorption of doxercalciferol: cholestyramine, magnesium antacids, mineral oil, do not use together

NURSING CONSIDERATIONS

Assess:

• BUN, urinary calcium, AST, ALT, cholesterol, creatinine, albumin, uric acid, chloride, magnesium, electrolytes, urine pH, phosphate; may increase calcium, should be kept at 9-10 mg/dl, vit D 50-135 IU/dl, phosphate 70 mg/dl

• Alk phosphatase; may be decreased

• For increased drug level, since toxic reactions may occur rapidly

• For dry mouth, metallic taste, polyuria, bone pain, muscle weakness, headache, fatigue, change in LOC, dysrhythmias, increased respirations, anorexia, nausea, vomiting, cramps, diarrhea, constipation; may indicate hypercalcemia

• Renal status: decreased urinary output (oliguria, anuria), edema in extremities, weight gain 5-7 lb, periorbital edema

• Nutritional status, diet for sources of vit D (milk, some seafood); calcium (dairy products, dark green vegetables), phosphates (dairy products) must be avoided

Perform/provide:

• Storage protected from light, heat, moisture

• Restriction of sodium, potassium if required

• Restriction of fluids if required for chronic renal failure

Evaluate:

• Therapeutic response: calcium 9-10 mg/dl, decreasing symptoms of hypocalcemia, hypoparathyroidism

Teach patient/family:

• The symptoms of hypercalcemia

• About foods rich in calcium

• To avoid products with sodium: cured meats, dairy products, cold cuts, olives, beets, pickles, soups, meat tenderizers in chronic renal failure

• To avoid products with potassium: oranges, bananas, dried fruit, peas, dark green leafy vegetables, milk, melons, beans in chronic renal failure

• To avoid OTC products containing calcium, potassium, or sodium in chronic renal failure

• To avoid all preparations containing vit D

• To monitor weight weekly

🚫 Not to break, crush, or chew caps

---

entacapone (℞)

(en'ta-kah-pone)

Comtan

Func. class.: Antiparkinson agent

Chem. class.: COMT inhibitor

Action: Inhibits COMT (catechol-O-methyltransferase) and alters the plasma pharmacokinetics of levodopa. Given with levodopa/carbidopa

Uses: Parkinsonism in those experiencing end of dose, decreased effect

Dosage and routes:

• *Adult:* **PO** 200 mg given with

◆ = Nursing alert   🌿 = Herb-drug interaction   🚫 = Do not crush

carbidopa/levodopa, max 1600 mg/
day
Available forms: Tabs 200 mg film
coated
Side effects/adverse reactions:
*CNS: Involuntary choreiform move-
ments, hand tremors, fatigue, headache, anxiety, twitching, numbness,
dyskinesia, hypokinesia, hyperkine-
sia, weakness, confusion, agitation,
nightmares,* psychosis, hallucination, hypomania, severe depression,
dizziness
*GI: Nausea, vomiting, anorexia, ab-
dominal distress, dry mouth, flatulence, bitter taste, diarrhea, constipation, dyspepsia,* gastritis, GI disorder
INTEG: Rash, sweating, alopecia
CV: Orthostatic hypotension
MISC: Dark urine, back pain, dyspnea, purpura, fatigue, asthenia,
infection-bacterial
Contraindications: Hypersensitivity
Precautions: Renal disease, hepatic
disease, pregnancy (C), affective
disorders, psychosis, lactation,
children
Pharmacokinetics: Excreted in
urine, feces; well absorbed, protein
binding 98%, metabolized liver extensively, enters breast milk, half-
life of levodopa is extended
Interactions:
• Increased CV reactions, avoid use:
bitolterol, apomorphine, dopamine,
dobutamine, epinephrine, methyldopa, isoetharine, norepinephrine
• Decreased excretion: ampicillin,
chloramphenicol, probenecid, erythromycin, rifampin
• Prevents catecholamine metabolism, do not use together: MAOIs
NURSING CONSIDERATIONS
Assess:
• Liver function enzymes: AST,
ALT, alk phosphatase, LDH, bilirubin, CBC

• Involuntary movements in parkinsonism: akinesia, tremors, staggering gait, muscle rigidity, drooling
when given with levodopa/carbidopa
• B/P, respiration during initial treatment
• Mental status: affect, mood, behavioral changes, depression; complete suicide assessment
Administer:
• Only after MAOIs have been discontinued for 2 wk
Perform/provide:
• Assistance with ambulation during beginning therapy
Evaluate:
• Therapeutic response: decrease in
akathisia, increased mood when
given with levodopa/carbidopa
Teach patient/family:
• That hallucinations, mental
changes, nausea, dyskinesia can
occur
• To change positions slowly to prevent orthostatic hypotension; not to
drive or operate machinery until stabilized on medication and mental
performance is not affected
• To use drug exactly as prescribed
• That urine, sweat may darken
• To notify prescriber if pregnancy
is suspected; or if lactating, drug is
excreted in breast milk

---

epirubicin (℞)

(ep-ih-roo'bi-sin)
Ellence
Func. class.: Antineoplastic, an-
tibiotic
Chem. class.: Anthracycline

Action: Inhibits DNA synthesis primarily; replication is decreased by
binding to DNA, which causes strand
splitting; maximum cytotoxic effects at Sand G_2 phases, a vesicant
Uses: Breast cancer as an adjuvant

therapy, with axillary node involvement following resection

Dosage and routes:
• *Adult:* **IV Inf** 100-120 mg/m^2 initially, given with other antineoplastics; given in repeated cycles; 3-4 wk cycles

Available forms: Inj 2 mg/ml

Side effects/adverse reactions:
*HEMA: **Thrombocytopenia, leukopenia, anemia, neutropenia, secondary AML***

GI: Nausea, vomiting, anorexia, mucositis, diarrhea

GU: Amenorrhea, hot flashes, hyperuricemia

INTEG: Rash, necrosis at injection site, reversible alopecia

MISC: Infection, febrile neutropenia, lethargy, fever, conjunctivitis

*CV: Increased B/P, **sinus tachycardia, PVCs,** chest pain, **bradycardia, extrasystoles***

Contraindications: Hypersensitivity to this drug, anthracyclines, anthracenediones, severe hepatic disease, baseline neutrophil count <1500 cell/mm^3, severe myocardial insufficiency, recent MI, pregnancy (D), lactation, systemic infections

Precautions: Renal, hepatic, cardiac disease; gout, bone marrow depression (severe), elderly, children

Pharmacokinetics: Triphasic pattern of elimination; half-life 3 min, 2.5 hr, 33 hr; metabolized by liver; crosses placenta; excreted in urine, bile, breast milk

Interactions:
• Increased toxicity: other antineoplastics or radiation, cimetidine
• Decreased antibody response: live virus vaccine

NURSING CONSIDERATIONS
Assess:
• CBC, differentials, platelet count weekly; withhold drug if WBC is <4000/mm^3 or platelet count is <75,000/mm^3; notify prescriber of these results

• Blood, urine uric acid levels; swelling, joint pain primarily in extremities, patient should be well hydrated to prevent urate deposits

• Renal function studies: BUN, serum uric acid, urine CrCl, electrolytes before, during therapy

• I&O ratio; report fall in urine output to <30 ml/hr; dosage adjustment is needed if serum creatinine >5 mg/dl

• Monitor temp q4h; fever may indicate beginning infection

• Liver function tests before, during therapy: bilirubin, AST, ALT, alk phosphatase as needed or monthly

• ECG, LVEF, MUCA scan, or ECHO; watch for ST-T wave changes, low QRS and T, possible dysrhythmias (sinus tachycardia, heart block, PVCs)

• Bleeding: hematuria, guaiac, bruising, or petechiae, mucosa or orifices q8h

• Effects of alopecia on body image; discuss feelings about body changes

• Alkalosis if severe vomiting is present

• Local irritation, pain, burning at injection site

• GI symptoms: frequency of stools, cramping

• Acidosis, signs of dehydration: rapid respirations, poor skin turgor, decreased urine output, dry skin, restlessness, weakness

• Cardiac status: B/P, pulse, character, rhythm, rate, ABGs, ECG

Administer:
• Antiemetic 30-60 min before giving drug to prevent vomiting

• Allopurinol or sodium bicarbonate to maintain uric acid levels, alkalinization of urine

• Transfusion for anemia

◆ = Nursing alert   ✎ = Herb-drug interaction   ⊘ = Do not crush

IV

• Hydrocortisone, dexamethasone, or sodium bicarbonate (1 mEq/1 ml) for extravasation; apply ice compresses

• Given into tubing of free-flowing IV infusion (0.9% NaCl or D_5) give over 3-5 min

Perform/provide:

• Strict hand-washing technique, gloves, protective clothing

• Liquid diet: carbonated beverages, gelatin may be added if patient is not nauseated or vomiting

• Increased fluid intake to 2-3 L/day to prevent urate, calculi formation

Evaluate:

• Therapeutic response: decreased tumor size, spread of malignancy

Teach patient/family:

• To report any complaints, side effects to nurse or prescriber

• That hair may be lost during treatment and wig or hairpiece may make patient feel better; tell patient that new hair may be different in color, texture

• To avoid crowds and persons with infections when granulocyte count is low

• That contraceptive measures are recommended during therapy

• To avoid vaccinations; reactions may occur

---

exemestane (℞)

(ex-em′eh-stane)

Aromasin

Func. class.: Antineoplastic

Chem. class.: Aromatase inhibitor

Action: Lowers serum estradiol concentrations; many breast cancers have strong estrogen receptors

Uses: Advanced breast carcinoma not responsive to other therapy in estrogen-receptor-positive patients (postmenopausal)

Dosage and routes:

• *Adult:* **PO** 25 mg qd pc

Available forms: Tabs 25 mg

Side effects/adverse reactions:

GI: Nausea, vomiting, fatigue, diarrhea, constipation, abdominal pain, increased appetite

CV: Hypertension

CNS: Hot flashes, headache, depression, insomnia, anxiety

RESP: Cough, dyspnea

Contraindications: Hypersensitivity, pregnancy (D), premenopausal women

Precautions: Lactation, children, elderly, liver disease, renal disease

Pharmacokinetics: Half-life 24 hr, excreted in feces, urine

NURSING CONSIDERATIONS

Assess:

• B/P, hypertension may occur

Perform/provide:

• Liquid diet, if needed including cola, gelatin; dry toast or crackers may be added if patient is not nauseated or vomiting

• Increase fluid intake to 2-3 L/day to prevent dehydration

• Nutritious diet with iron, vitamin supplements as ordered

• Storage in light-resistant container at room temp

Evaluate:

• Therapeutic response: decreased tumor size, spread of malignancy

Teach patient/family:

• To report any complaints, side effects to prescriber

• That hot flashes are reversible after discontinuing treatment

---

ganirelix (℞)
Antagon
Func. class.: Gonadotropin-releasing hormone antagonist
Chem. class.: Synthetic deca-peptide

Action: Inhibitor of pituitary gonadotropin secretion; initially increases LH and FSH, induces a rapid suppression of gonadotropin secretion

Uses: For inhibition of premature LH surges in women undergoing controlled ovarian hyperstimulation

Dosage and routes:
• *Adult:* SC 250 μg qd during early to mid follicular phase, continue until the day of hCG administration

Available forms: Inj 250 μg/0.5 ml

Side effects/adverse reactions:
CNS: Headache
ENDO: Ovarian hyperstimulation syndrome, abdominal pain (gyn)
GI: Nausea
GU: Spotting, breakthrough bleeding
INTEG: Pain on injection
SYST: Fetal death

Contraindications: Hypersensitivity, pregnancy (X), latex allergy, lactation

Pharmacokinetics: Excreted in feces/urine, half-life 13-16 hr, metabolized to metabolites, protein binding 82%

NURSING CONSIDERATIONS
Assess:
• For suspected pregnancy, drug should not be used
• For latex allergy, drug should not be used

Administer:
• SC using abdomen, around navel or upper thigh, swab inj area with disinfectant, clean a 2 in circle and allow to dry, pinch up area between thumb and finger, insert needle at 45-90° to surface, if positioned correctly, no blood will be drawn back into syringe, if blood is drawn into syringe, reposition needle without removing it

Perform/provide:
• Protection from light

Evaluate:
• Therapeutic response: pregnancy

Teach patient/family:
• To report abdominal pain, vaginal bleeding

gatifloxacin (℞)
(gat-ih-floks'ah-sin)
Tequin
Func. class.: Broad-spectrum antiinfective
Chem. class.: Fluoroquinolone antibacterial

Action: Interferes with conversion of intermediate DNA fragments into high–molecular weight DNA in bacteria; DNA gyrase inhibitor

Uses: Infection caused by susceptible *Escherichia coli, Staphylococcus aureus, Haemophilus influenzae, H. parainfluenzae, Klebsiella pneumoniae, Moraxella catarrhalis, Neisseria gonorrhoeae, Proteus mirabilis,* and other microorganisms: *Chlamydia pneumoniae, Legionella pneumophila, Mycoplasma pneumoniae,* acute bacterial exacerbation of chronic bronchitis, acute sinusitis, community-acquired pneumonia, gonorrhea

Dosage and routes:
Renal dose
• CrCl ≥40 ml/min 400 mg qd; <40 ml/min 200 mg qd after 400 mg initially; hemodialysis 200 mg qd after 400 mg initially

◆ = Nursing alert   🌿 = Herb-drug interaction   🚫 = Do not crush

Uncomplicated urinary tract infections
• *Adult:* **PO/IV** 400 mg single dose
Complicated/severe urinary tract infections
• *Adult:* **PO/IV** 400 mg × 7-10 days
Chronic bronchitis
• *Adult:* **PO/IV** 400 mg × 7-10 days
Acute sinusitis
• *Adult:* **PO/IV** 400 mg × 10 days
Community-acquired pneumonia
• *Adult:* **PO/IV** 400 mg × 7-14 days
Gonorrhea
• *Adult:* **PO/IV** 400 mg single dose
Available forms: Tabs 200, 400 mg; inj 20 ml (200 mg), 40 ml (400 mg)
Side effects/adverse reactions:
CNS: Headache, dizziness, insomnia, paresthesia, tremor, vasodilation
GI: Nausea, diarrhea, increased ALT, AST, ***pseudomembranous colitis***
INTEG: Rash, pruritus, urticaria, photosensitivity, flushing, fever, chills
RESP: Dyspnea, pharyngitis
Contraindications: Hypersensitivity to quinolones
Precautions: Pregnancy (C), lactation, children, renal disease
Pharmacokinetics: Half-life 6½-14 hr; excreted in urine unchanged
Interactions:
• Decreased absorption of gatifloxacin: magnesium antacids, aluminum hydroxide, sucralfate, calcium
• Increased serum levels of gatifloxacin: probenecid
NURSING CONSIDERATIONS
Assess:
• CNS symptoms: headache, dizziness, insomnia
• Kidney, liver function studies: BUN, creatinine, AST, ALT
• I&O ratio, urine pH <5.5 is ideal
• Allergic reactions: fever, flushing, rash, urticaria, pruritus

Administer:
PO
• 2 hr before or 2 hr after antacids, zinc, iron, calcium
IV
• Do not use flexible containers in series connections, air embolism may occur
• Do not use if particulate matter is present
• Do not admix with other drugs
• Dilute with compatible sol to 2 mg/ml before administration
Solution compatibilities: D_5, 0.9% NaCl, D_5/0.9% NaCl, LR/D_5, water for inj
Perform/provide:
• Limited intake of alkaline foods, drugs: milk, dairy products, alkaline antacids, sodium bicarbonate
Evaluate:
• Therapeutic response: decreased pain, frequency, urgency, C&S; absence of infection
Teach patient/family:
• Not to take any products containing magnesium or calcium (such as antacids), iron, or aluminum with this drug or within 2 hr of drug
• That photosensitivity may occur; patient should avoid sunlight or use sunscreen to prevent burns
• If dizziness occurs, to ambulate, perform activities with assistance
• To complete full course of drug therapy
• To contact prescriber if adverse reaction occurs or if inflammation or pain in tendon occurs

---

**interferon alfa-n1
lymphoblastoid** (℞)
(in-ter-feer′on al′fa n one lim-
foh-blast′oid)
Wellferon
Func. class.: Recombinant type
1 interferon

Action: Induces biologic responses
and has antiviral, antiproliferative
and immunomodulatory effects;
mixture of alpha interferons isolated from human cells after induction with parainfluenza virus
Uses: Chronic hepatitis C infections
Dosage and routes:
• *Adult:* **SC/IM** 3 MU × 3×/wk ×
48 wk
Available forms: Solution 3 MU/ml
Side effects/adverse reactions:
*CNS: Headache, fever, insomnia, diz-
ziness, anxiety, hostility, lability, nervousness, depression, confusion, abnormal thinking, amnesia*
*GI: Abdominal pain, nausea, diar-
rhea, anorexia, vomiting*
MS: Back pain
*INTEG: Alopecia, pruritus, rash, er-
ythema, dry skin*
*HEMA: **Granulocytopenia, thrombocytopenia, leukopenia,** ecchymosis*
*RESP: Pharyngitis, upper respira-
tory infection, cough, epistaxis, dyspnea, bronchitis*
Contraindications: Hypersensitivity to alpha interferons, history of
anaphylaxis to bovine or ovine immunoglobulins, egg protein, polymyxin B, neomycin sulfate
Precautions: Thyroid disorders, myelosuppression, hepatic, cardiac disease, lactation, children <18 yr,
depression/suicide
Pharmacokinetics: Peak 24-36 hr

Interactions:
• Use caution when giving with theophylline, myelosuppressive agents
NURSING CONSIDERATIONS
Assess:
• ALT, HCV viral load; patients that
show no reduction in ALT, HCV are
unlikely to show benefit of treat-
ment after 16 wk
• Platelet counts, heme concentration, ANC, serum creatinine
concentration, albumin, bilirubin,
TSH, T4
• For myelosuppression, hold dose
if neutrophil count is <500 × 10⁶/L
or if platelets are <50 × 10⁹/L
• For hypersensitivity: discontinue
immediately if hypersensitivity occurs
Administer:
• Same brand of product during
course of treatment
Evaluate:
• Therapeutic response: decreased
chronic hepatitis C signs/symptoms
Teach patient/family:
• Provide patient or family member
with written, detailed information
about drug
• Instructions for home use if ap-
propriate

levalbuterol (℞)
(lev-al-byoo′ter-ole)
Xopenex
Func. class.: Adrenergic β₂-
agonist

Action: Causes bronchodilation by
action on β₂ (pulmonary) receptors
by increasing levels of cAMP, which
relaxes smooth muscle; produces
bronchodilation, CNS, cardiac stimulation, as well as increased diuresis and gastric acid secretion; longer
acting than isoproterenol
Uses: Treatment or prevention of

⬥ = Nursing alert   🌿 = Herb-drug interaction   🚫 = Do not crush

bronchospasm (reversible obstructive airway disease)
Dosage and routes:
• *Adult and child ≥12 yr:* **INH** 0.63 mg tid, q6-8h by nebulization
Available forms: Sol, inh 0.63 mg, 1.25 mg/3 ml
Side effects/adverse reactions:
CNS: Tremors, anxiety, insomnia, headache, dizziness, stimulation, *restlessness,* hallucinations, flushing, irritability
EENT: Dry nose, irritation of nose and throat
CV: Palpitations, tachycardia, hypertension, angina, hypotension, dysrhythmias
GI: Heartburn, nausea, vomiting
MS: Muscle cramps
Contraindications: Hypersensitivity to sympathomimetics, tachydysrhythmias, severe cardiac disease
Precautions: Lactation, pregnancy (C), cardiac disorders, hyperthyroidism, diabetes mellitus, hypertension, prostatic hypertrophy, narrow-angle glaucoma, seizures
Pharmacokinetics: Metabolized in the liver and tissues, crosses placenta, breast milk, blood-brain barrier
INH: Onset 5-15 min, peak 1-1½ hr, duration 6-8 hr
Interactions:
• Increased action of aerosol bronchodilators
• Increased action of levalbuterol: tricyclic antidepressants, MAOIs, other adrenergics
• May inhibit action of levalbuterol: other β-blockers
NURSING CONSIDERATIONS
Assess:
• Respiratory function: vital capacity, forced expiratory volume, ABGs, lung sounds, heart rate and rhythm (baseline)

• That patient has not received theophylline therapy before giving dose
• For evidence of allergic reactions
Administer:
• By nebulization q6-8h
Evaluate:
• Therapeutic response: absence of dyspnea, wheezing after 1 hr, improved airway exchange, improved ABGs
Teach patient/family:
• Not to use OTC medications; excess stimulation may occur
• To avoid getting aerosol in eyes; blurring may result
• To wash inhaler in warm water qd and dry
• To avoid smoking, smoke-filled rooms, persons with respiratory infections
◆ That paradoxic bronchospasm may occur and to stop drug immediately
• To limit caffeine products such as chocolate, coffee, tea, and colas
Treatment of overdose: Administer a β_1-adrenergic blocker

---

levetiracetam (℞)
(lev-eh-teer-ass'eh-tam)
Keppra
Func. class.: Anticonvulsant

Action: Inhibits nerve impulses by limiting influx of sodium ions across cell membrane in motor cortex
Uses: Partial onset seizures
Dosage and routes:
• *Adult:* **PO** 500 mg bid
Available forms: Tabs 250, 500, 750 mg
Side effects/adverse reactions:
HEMA: Lowered Hct, Hgb, infection
CNS: Dizziness, somnolence, asthenia
Contraindications: Hypersensitivity

Precautions: Hepatic disease, renal disease, cardiac disease, psychosis, pregnancy (C), lactation, children

Pharmacokinetics: Rapidly absorbed, not protein bound, excreted via kidneys 66% unchanged; half-life 6-8 hr, longer in elderly

NURSING CONSIDERATIONS

Assess:

• Renal studies: urinalysis, BUN, urine creatinine q3mo

• Blood studies: RBC, Hct, Hgb

• Hepatic studies: ALT, AST, bilirubin

• Description of seizures

• Mental status: mood, sensorium, affect, behavioral changes; if mental status changes, notify prescriber

Administer:

• With food, milk to decrease GI symptoms

Perform/provide:

• Storage at room temperature

• Assistance with ambulation during early part of treatment; dizziness occurs

Evaluate:

• Therapeutic response: decreased seizure activity, document on patient's chart

Teach patient/family:

• To carry Medic Alert ID stating patient's name, drugs taken, condition, prescriber's name, phone number

• To avoid driving, other activities that require alertness

• Not to discontinue medication quickly after long-term use

---

levobupivacaine (R)

(lee-voh-bu-piv′ah-kane)
Chirocaine
Func. class.: Local anesthetic
Chem. class.: Amide

Action: Competes with calcium for sites in nerve membrane that control sodium transport across cell membrane; decreases rise of depolarization phase of action potential

Uses: Local, regional anesthesia, surgical anesthesia, pain management, continuous epidural analgesia

Dosage and routes:

• Varies with route of anesthesia

Available forms: Inj 2.5, 5, 7.5 mg/ml

Side effects/adverse reactions:

CNS: Anxiety, restlessness, *convulsions, loss of consciousness,* drowsiness, disorientation, tremors, shivering

CV: Myocardial depression, cardiac arrest, dysrhythmias, bradycardia, hypotension, hypertension, *fetal bradycardia*

GI: Nausea, vomiting

EENT: Blurred vision, tinnitus, pupil constriction

INTEG: Rash, urticaria, allergic reactions, edema, burning, skin discoloration at injection site, tissue necrosis

RESP: Status asthmaticus, respiratory arrest, anaphylaxis

Contraindications: Hypersensitivity, children <12 yr, elderly, severe liver disease

Precautions: Severe drug allergies, pregnancy (B)

Pharmacokinetics: Onset 2-8 min, duration 3-6 hr; metabolized by liver, excreted in urine (metabolites)

Interactions:

• Dysrhythmias: epinephrine, halothane, enflurane

• Hypertension: MAOIs, tricyclic antidepressants, phenothiazines

• Decreased action of levobupivacaine: chloroprocaine

NURSING CONSIDERATIONS

Assess:

• B/P, pulse, respiration during treatment

• Fetal heart tones during labor

◆ = Nursing alert   ∥ = Herb-drug interaction   ⊘ = Do not crush

• Allergic reactions: rash, urticaria, itching
• Cardiac status: ECG for dysrhythmias, pulse, B/P during anesthesia
Administer:
• Only with crash cart, resuscitative equipment nearby
• Only drugs without preservatives for epidural or caudal anesthesia
Perform/provide:
• Use of new sol; discard unused portions
Evaluate:
• Therapeutic response: anesthesia necessary for procedure
Treatment of overdose: Airway, O_2, vasopressor, IV fluids, anticonvulsants for seizures

---

lymphocyte immune globulin (anti-thymocyte) (R)
Atgam
Func. class.: Immune globulins—immunosuppressant

Action: Produces immunosuppression by inhibiting the function of lymphocytes (T)
Uses: Organ transplants to prevent rejection, aplastic anemia
Dosage and routes:
Renal allograft
• *Adult:* IV 10-30 mg/kg/day
• *Child:* IV 5-25 mg/kg/day
Available forms: Inj 50 mg/ml
Side effects/adverse reactions:
Renal transplant
CNS: Fever, chills, headache, dizziness, weakness, faintness, *seizures*
INTEG: Rash, pruritus, urticaria, wheal
GI: Diarrhea, nausea, vomiting, epigastric pain
CV: Chest pain, hypertension, tachycardia

SYST: **Anaphylaxis**
Aplastic anemia
CNS: Fever, chills, headache, *seizures,* lightheadedness, encephalitis, postviral encephalopathy
CV: Bradycardia, myocarditis, irregularity
GI: Nausea, LFTs abnormality
Contraindications: Hypersensitivity
Precautions: Severe renal disease, severe hepatic disease, pregnancy (C), lactation, children
Pharmacokinetics: Onset rapid, half-life 5.7 days
Interactions: None known
NURSING CONSIDERATIONS
Assess:
• For infection; if infection occurs evaluation will be needed to continue therapy
• Renal studies: BUN, creatinine at least monthly during treatment, 3 mo after treatment
• Liver function studies: alk phosphatase, AST, ALT, bilirubin
Administer:
• Do not infuse <4 hr
Delaying the onset of allograft rejection
• For 14 doses qod over 28 days. Start 1st dose within 24 hr of transplant
Treatment of rejection
• For 14 days, alternate day therapy up to 21 days
Aplastic anemia
• For 8-14 days, or alternate day treatment up to 21 days
• Skin testing must be completed prior to treatment; use intradermal inj of 0.1 ml of a 1:1000 dilution (5 µg horse IgG) in 0.9% NaCl, if a wheal or rash >10 mm or both, use caution during inf
• Dilute in saline sol before inf, invert IV bag, so undiluted drug does not contact the air inside, concentration should not be >1 mg/ml

---

• Keep emergency equip nearby for severe allergic reaction
Evaluate:
• Therapeutic response: absence of rejection; hematologic recovery (aplastic anemia)
Teach patient/family:
• To report fever, chills, sore throat, fatigue, since serious infections may occur
• To use contraceptive measures during treatment, for 12 wk after ending therapy

---

modafinil (℞)
(moh-daf'ih-nil)
Provigil
Func. class.: Cerebral stimulant

Action: Promotes wakefulness, exact mechanism is unknown
Uses: Narcolepsy
Dosage and routes:
Narcolepsy
• *Adult:* **PO** 200 mg qd in the AM, may increase to 400 mg qd if needed
Hepatic dose
• Reduce dose by 50%
Available forms: Tabs 100, 200 mg
Side effects/adverse reactions:
META: Hyperglycemia, albuminuria
RESP: Rhinitis, pharyngitis, lung disorder, dyspnea, asthma, epistaxis
EENT: Abnormal vision, amblyopia
CNS: Hyperactivity, insomnia, restlessness, dizziness, headache, chills, stimulation
GI: Anorexia, dry mouth, diarrhea, nausea, vomiting, mouth ulcer, gingivitis, thirst
GU: Urinary retention, abnormal ejaculation
CV: Palpitations, tachycardia, hypertension, *dysrhythmias*
INTEG: Herpes simplex, dry skin
Contraindications: Hypersensitivity, hyperthyroidism, hypertension, glaucoma, severe arteriosclerosis,

drug abuse, cardiovascular disease, anxiety
Precautions: Gilles de la Tourette's disorder, pregnancy (C), elderly, lactation, children <16 yr
Pharmacokinetics: Absorbed rapidly, well distributed, protein binding 60%, metabolized extensively, half-life 15 hr with multiple dosing, peak 2-4 hr
Interactions:
• Increased levels of: clomipramine, phenytoin, warfarin, tricyclics
• Decreased levels of: cyclosporine, oral contraceptives
• Decreased modafinil absorption: methylphenidate
• Use cautiously with MAOIs
NURSING CONSIDERATIONS
Assess:
• For improvement in narcolepsy
Administer:
• Gum, hard candy, frequent sips of water for dry mouth
Evaluate:
• Therapeutic response: increased CNS stimulation, decreased drowsiness
Teach patient/family:
• To decrease caffeine consumption (coffee, tea, cola, chocolate); may increase irritability, stimulation
• To avoid OTC preparations unless approved by prescriber
• To notify prescriber if rash or other symptoms of allergy occur
• To notify prescriber if pregnancy is suspected, or if breast-feeding; another form of contraception is needed if using hormonal contraception while on this drug and for a month afterwards
• To avoid hazardous activities until stabilized on medication

---

◆ = Nursing alert   ∅ = Herb-drug interaction   ⊘ = Do not crush

moxifloxacin

Avelox

Func. class.: Antiinfective
Chem. class.: Fluoroquinolone

Action: Interferes with conversion of intermediate DNA fragments into high-molecular-weight DNA in bacteria; DNA gyrase inhibitor

Uses: Acute bacterial sinusitis: *Streptococcus pneumoniae, Haemophilus influenzae, Moraxella catarrhalis;* acute bacterial exacerbation of chronic bronchitis: *S. pneumoniae, H. influenzae, Haemophilus parainfluenzae, Klebsiella pneumoniae, Staphylococcus aureus, M. catarrhalis;* community-acquired pneumonia: *S. pneumoniae, H. influenzae, Mycoplasma pneumoniae, Chlamydia pneumoniae, M. catarrhalis*

Dosage and routes:

• *Adult:* 400 mg qd × 5-10 days depending on condition

Available forms: Tabs 400 mg

Side effects/adverse reactions:

CV: Prolonged QT interval

CNS: Headache, dizziness, fatigue, insomnia, depression, *restlessness, seizures,* confusion

GI: Nausea, diarrhea, increased ALT, AST, flatulence, heartburn, *vomiting,* oral candidiasis, dysphagia

INTEG: Rash, pruritus, urticaria, photosensitivity, flushing, fever, chills

MS: Tremor, arthralgia, tendon rupture

Contraindications: Hypersensitivity to quinolones

Precautions: Pregnancy (C), lactation, children, renal disease, epilepsy, uncorrected hypokalemia, prolonged QT interval, patients receiving class IA, III antidysrhythmics

Pharmacokinetics: Excreted in urine as active drug, metabolites

Interactions:

• Decreased absorption of moxifloxacin: magnesium antacids, aluminum hydroxide, zinc, iron, sucralfate, calcium, enteral feeding, didanosine

• Increased serum levels of moxifloxacin: probenecid

• Increased toxicity: caffeine, theophylline, cyclosporine

• Increased warfarin, cyclosporine effect

• Prolonged QT: antidysrythmics class IA, III

NURSING CONSIDERATIONS

Assess:

• CNS symptoms: headache, dizziness, fatigue, insomnia, depression

• Kidney, liver function studies: BUN, creatinine, AST, ALT

• I&O ratio, urine pH <5.5 is ideal

• Allergic reactions: fever, flushing, rash, urticaria, pruritus

Administer:

• 2 hr before or 2 hr after antacids, zinc, iron, calcium

Perform/provide:

• Limited intake of alkaline foods, drugs: milk, dairy products, alkaline antacids, sodium bicarbonate

Evaluate:

• Therapeutic response: decreased pain, C&S; absence of infection

Teach patient/family:

• Not to take any products containing magnesium or calcium (such as antacids), iron, or aluminum with this drug or within 2 hr of drug

• That photosensitivity may occur; patient should avoid sunlight or use sunscreen to prevent burns

• That fluids must be increased to

3 L/day to avoid crystallization in kidneys

• If dizziness occurs, to ambulate, perform activities with assistance

• To complete full course of drug therapy

• To contact prescriber if adverse reaction occurs or if inflammation or pain in tendon occurs

---

nitric oxide (℞)

(nye'trik ok'side)

INOmax

Func. class.: Respiratory inhalant

Action: Increases partial pressure of arterial oxygen (Pao$_2$) by dilating pulmonary vessels

Uses: Treatment of term and near-term (>34 wk) neonates with hypoxic respiratory failure associated with pulmonary hypertension; used with other agents and ventilatory support

Dosage and routes:

• *Neonate:* **INH** 20 ppm × up to 2 wk until O$_2$ desaturation has been resolved and neonate is ready to be weaned from therapy

Available forms: Gas 100, 800 ppm

Side effects/adverse reactions:

RESP: ***Pulmonary hemorrhage,*** atelectasis

SYST: ***Intracranial hemorrhage,*** hematuria, hyperglycemia, ***sepsis,*** cellulitis, ***stridor,*** withdrawal syndrome, ***methemoglobinemia, seizures, cerebral infarction, posttreatment infection,*** hypotension

Contraindications: Dependence on right to left shunting of blood, hypersensitivity

Precautions: Bradycardia, rales, infections, pregnancy (C)

Pharmacokinetics: Unknown

NURSING CONSIDERATIONS

Assess:

• Respiratory rate, rhythm, character, chest expansion, color, transcutaneous saturation, ABGs, methemoglobinemia

Administer:

• Only by persons trained in neonatal ventilation, inhalation

• Only in neonates; not indicated for other populations

Perform/provide:

• Weaning off therapy; do not discontinue abruptly

Evaluate:

• Therapeutic response: significant improvement in respiratory status and pulmonary hypertension

---

octreotide (℞)

(ok-tree'oh-tide)

Sandostatin, Sandostatin LAR Depot

Func. class.: Hormone, antidiarrheal

Chem. class.: Octapeptide

Action: A potent growth hormone similar to somatostatin

Uses: Sandostatin: acromegaly, carcinoid tumors, vasoactive intestinal peptide tumors (VIPomas); LAR Depot: long-term maintenance of acromegaly, carcinoid tumors, VIPomas

Investigational uses: GI fistula, variceal bleeding, diarrheal conditions, pancreatic fistula, irritable bowel syndrome, dumping syndrome

Dosage and routes:

Initial dose

• *Adult:* **IV/SC** 50 μg bid-tid CSI (continuous SC inf) has been used but is not approved

Acromegaly

• *Adult:* **SC** 50 μg tid, adjust q2wk based on somatomedin C

◆ = Nursing alert   ▌ = Herb-drug interaction   ⊘ = Do not crush

VIPomas
• *Adult:* **SC** 0.2-0.3 mg qd in 2-4 doses for 2 wk, not to exceed 0.45 mg qd

Carcinoid tumors
• *Adult:* **SC** 0.1-0.6 mg qd in 2-4 doses for 2 wk, titrated to patient response

GI fistula
• *Adult:* **SC** 50-200 µg q8h

Irritable bowel syndrome
• *Adult:* **SC** 100 µg single dose to 125 µg bid

Dumping syndrome
• *Adult:* **SC** 50-150 µg/day

Variceal bleeding
• *Adult:* **IV** 25-50 µg/hr cont **IV** inf for 18 hr-5 days

Available forms: Sandostatin: inj 0.05, 0.1, 0.2 0.5, 1 mg/ml; LAR Depot: inj 10, 20, 30 mg/5 ml

Side effects/adverse reactions:

CNS: Headache, dizziness, fatigue, weakness, depression, anxiety, tremors, **seizure,** paranoia

*CV: Sinus bradycardia, conduction abnormalities, **dysrhythmias,** chest pain, SOB, thrombophlebitis, ischemia, **CHF,** hypertension, palpitations*

ENDO: Hyperglycemia, ketosis, hypothyroidism, hypoglycemia, galactorrhea, diabetes insipidus

*GI: Diarrhea, nausea, abdominal pain, vomiting, flatulence, distention, constipation, **hepatitis,** increased LFTs, **GI bleeding, pancreatitis***

GU: UTI, pollakiuria

HEMA: Hematoma of inj site, bruise

INTEG: Rash, urticaria, pain; inflammation at injection site

MS: Joint and muscle pain

Contraindications: Hypersensitivity

Precautions: Diabetes mellitus, hypothyroidism, pregnancy (B), elderly, lactation, children, renal disease

Pharmacokinetics: Absorbed rapidly, completely, peak ½ hr, half-life 1.7 hr, duration 12 hr, excreted unchanged in urine

Interactions:
• Cyclosporine: Possible ↑ rejection
• Drug/food: ↓ absorption of dietary fat, ↓ vit B_{12} levels

NURSING CONSIDERATIONS

Assess:
• Growth hormone antibodies, IGF-1, 1-4 hr intervals for 8-12 hr post dose in acromegaly; 5-HIAA, plasma serotonin, plasma substance P in carcinoid; VIP in VIPomas
• Thyroid function tests: T_3, T_4, T_7, TSH to identify hypothyroidism
• Fecal fat, serum carotene
• Allergic reaction: rash, itching, fever, nausea, wheezing
• For cardiac status: bradycardia, conduction abnormalities, dysrhythmias; monitor ECG for QT prolongation, low voltage, axis shifts, early repolarization, R/S transition, early wave progression

Administer:

SC
• Rotate injection site

Perform/provide:
• Storage in refrigerator for unopened amps, vials; or room temp for 2 wk, protect from light; do not use discolored or cloudy sol

Evaluate:
• Therapeutic response: growth in children

Teach patient/family:
• Regular assessments are required
• Regarding SC injection if patient or other persons will be giving injection

---

orlistat (℞)

(or'lih-stat)
Xenical
Func. class.: Lipase inhibitor

Action: Inhibits the absorption of dietary fats
Uses: Obesity management
Dosage and routes:
• *Adult:* **PO** 120 mg tid with each main meal containing fat
Available forms: Caps 120 mg
Side effects/adverse reactions:
MS: Back pain, arthritis, myalgia, tendinitis
CNS: Insomnia, depression, anxiety, dizziness, headache, fatigue
GI: Oily spotting, flatus with discharge, fecal urgency, fatty/oily stool, oily evacuation, fecal incontinence, nausea, vomiting, abdominal pain, infectious diarrhea, rectal pain, tooth disorder
GU: UTI, vaginitis, menstrual irregularity
RESP: Influenza, URI, LRI, EENT symptoms
INTEG: Dry skin, rash
Contraindications: Hypersensitivity, malabsorption syndrome, cholestasis
Precautions: Hypothyroidism, other organic causes of obesity, lactation, children, pregnancy (B)
Pharmacokinetics: Minimal absorption, peak 8 hr, 99% protein binding, excretion in feces, half-life 1-2 hr
Interactions:
• Decreased absorption: fat-soluable vitamins, cyclosporine
• Increased lipid-lowering effect: pravastatin
NURSING CONSIDERATIONS
Assess:
• Weight weekly, diabetic patients may need reduction in oral hypoglycemics
• For misuse in certain population (anorexia nervosa, bulimia)
Administer:
• For obesity only if patient is on weight-reduction program that includes dietary changes, exercise; patient should be on a diet with 30% of calories from fat, omit dose of orlistat if a meal contains no fat
Evaluate:
• Therapeutic response: decrease in weight
Teach patient/family:
• Safety and effectiveness beyond 2 yr have not been determined
• By instructing patient to read patient's information sheet
• To take a multivitamin containing fat-soluble vitamins 2 hr before or after orlistat
• To avoid hazardous activities until pt is stabilized on medication

oseltamivir (℞)

(oss-el-tam'ih-veer)
Tamiflu
Func. class.: Antiviral
Chem. class.: Ethyl ester prodrug

Action: Inhibits influenza virus neuraminidase with possible alteration of virus particle aggregation and release
Uses: Treatment of influenza type A
Dosage and routes:
• *Adult:* **PO** 75 mg × 5 days, begin treatment within 2 days of onset of symptoms
Available forms: Caps 75 mg
Side effects/adverse reactions:
CNS: Headache, dizziness, fatigue, *insomnia*
GI: Nausea, vomiting, diarrhea, abdominal pain
RESP: Cough

Contraindications: Hypersensitivity

Precautions: Hepatic disease, renal disease, elderly, pregnancy (C)

Pharmacokinetics: Rapidly absorbed, protein binding low, converted to oseltamivir carboxylate, half-life 1-3 hr

NURSING CONSIDERATIONS
Assess:
• Bowel pattern before, during treatment
• Signs of infection
Administer:
• Within 2 days of symptoms of influenza; continue for 5 days
• At least 4 hr before hs to prevent insomnia
Perform/provide:
• Storage in tight, dry container
Evaluate:
• Therapeutic response: absence of fever, malaise, cough, dyspnea in infection
Teach patient/family:
• About aspects of drug therapy
• To avoid hazardous activities if dizziness occurs

---

perindopril (R̥)
(per-in'doe-pril)
Aceon
Func. class.: Antihypertensive
Chem. class.: Angiotensin-converting enzyme inhibitor

Action: Selectively suppresses renin-angiotensin-aldosterone system; inhibits ACE; prevents conversion of angiotensin I to angiotensin II, dilation of arterial, venous vessels
Uses: Hypertension
Dosage and routes:
Hypertension
• *Adult:* **PO** 4 mg/day, may increase or decrease to desired response range 4-8 mg/day; may give in 2 divided doses or as a single dose
Patients on diuretics
• Discontinue diuretic 2-3 days prior to perindopril then resume diuretic if needed
Renal impairment
• CrCl <30 ml/min 2 mg/day, max 8 mg/day
Available forms: Tabs scored 2, 4, 8 mg
Side effects/adverse reactions:
CV: Hypotension, chest pain, tachycardia, dysrhythmias, syncope
CNS: Insomnia, dizziness, paresthesias, headache, fatigue, anxiety
GI: Nausea, vomiting, colitis, cramps, diarrhea, constipation, flatulence, dry mouth, loss of taste
INTEG: Rash, purpura, alopecia, hyperhidrosis
*HEMA: **Agranulocytosis, neutropenia***
EENT: Tinnitus, visual changes, sore throat, double vision, dry burning eyes
*GU: **Proteinuria, renal failure,*** increased frequency of polyuria or oliguria
RESP: Dyspnea, dry cough, rales, angioedema
META: Hyperkalemia
Contraindications: Hypersensitivity, history of angioedema
Precautions: Renal disease, hyperkalemia, pregnancy (C), lactation, hepatic failure, dehydration, bilateral renal artery stenosis
Pharmacokinetics: Metabolized by liver, excreted in urine
Interactions:
• Hypersensitivity: allopurinol
• Severe hypotension: diuretics, other antihypertensives
• Increased K levels: salt substitutes, K-sparing diuretics, K supplements

---

• May increase effects of neuromuscular blocking agents, antihypertensives, lithium
• Effects may be increased by diuretics

Lab test interferences:
Interference: Glucose/insulin tolerance tests

NURSING CONSIDERATIONS
Assess:
• B/P, pulse q4h; note rate, rhythm, quality
• Electrolytes: K, Na, Cl during 1st 2 wk of therapy
• Baselines in renal, liver function tests before therapy begins and 1 wk into therapy
• Edema in feet, legs daily
• Skin turgor, dryness of mucous membranes for hydration status
• Symptoms of CHF: edema, dyspnea, wet rales

Administer:
• **PO** as a single dose or in 2 divided doses

Evaluate:
• Therapeutic response: decreased B/P

Teach patient/family:
• Not to use OTC (cough, cold, or allergy) products unless directed by prescriber; to avoid salt substitutes
• To avoid sunlight or wear sunscreen for photosensitivity
• To comply with dosage schedule, even if feeling better
• To notify prescriber of mouth sores, sore throat, fever, swelling of hands or feet, irregular heartbeat, chest pains, signs of angioedema
• That excessive perspiration, dehydration, vomiting, diarrhea may lead to fall in blood pressure; consult prescriber if these occur
• That drug may cause dizziness, fainting; light-headedness may occur during 1st few days of therapy

• That drug may cause skin rash or impaired perspiration; angioedema may occur and to D/C if it occurs
• Not to discontinue drug abruptly
• That CV adverse reactions may reoccur
• To rise slowly to sitting or standing position to minimize orthostatic hypotension

Treatment of overdose: Lavage, IV atropine for bradycardia, IV theophylline for bronchospasm, digitalis, O_2, diuretic for cardiac failure

---

pioglitazone (R)
(pie-oh-glye′ta-zone)
Actos
Func. class.: Antidiabetic, oral
Chem. class.: Thiazolidinedione

Action: Improves insulin resistance by hepatic glucose metabolism, insulin receptor kinase activity, insulin receptor phosphorylation
Uses: Stable adult-onset diabetes mellitus (type II) NIDDM
Dosage and routes:
Monotherapy
• *Adult:* **PO** 15-30 qd, may increase to 45 mg/day
Combination therapy
• *Adult:* **PO** 15-30 mg qd with a sulfonylurea, metformin, or insulin. Decrease sulfonylurea dose if hypoglycemia occurs. Decrease insulin dose by 10-25% if hypoglycemia occurs or if plasma glucose is <100 mg/dl, max 45 mg/day
Hepatic dose
• Do not use in active liver disease or if ALT >2.5 times ULN
Available forms: Tabs 15, 30, 45 mg
Side effects/adverse reactions:
MISC: Myalgia, sinusitis, URI, pharyngitis

◆ = Nursing alert   ⫽ = Herb-drug interaction   ⊘ = Do not crush

CNS: Headache
ENDO: Aggravated diabetes mellitus

Contraindications: Hypersensitivity to thiazolidinedione, lactation, children, diabetic ketoacidosis

Precautions: Pregnancy (C), elderly, thyroid disease, hepatic, renal disease

Pharmacokinetics: Maximal reduction in FBS after 12 wk; half-life 3-7 hr, total 16-24 hr

Interactions:

• Decreased effect of: oral contraceptives, use an alternate contraceptive method

NURSING CONSIDERATIONS
Assess:

• For hypoglycemic reactions (sweating, weakness, dizziness, anxiety, tremors, hunger), hyperglycemic reactions soon after meals

• CBC (baseline, q3mo) during treatment; check liver function tests periodically AST, LDH, renal studies: BUN, creatinine, urinary glucose

• FBS, glycosylated Hgb, fasting plasma insulin, plasma lipids/lipoproteins, B/P, body weight during treatment

Administer:

• Once a day; give with meals to decrease GI upset and provide best absorption

• Tabs crushed and mixed with food or fluids for patients with difficulty swallowing

Perform/provide:

• Conversion from other oral hypoglycemic agents; change may be made without gradual dosage change; monitor serum or urine glucose and ketones tid during conversion

• Storage in tight container in cool environment

Teach patient/family:

• To use capillary blood glucose test or Chemstrip tid; that periodic liver function testing is mandatory

• The symptoms of hypo/hyperglycemia, what to do about each

• That the drug must be continued on daily basis; explain consequence of discontinuing drug abruptly

• To avoid OTC medications or herbal preparations unless approved by prescriber

• That diabetes is lifelong illness; that this drug is not a cure; only controls symptoms

• That all food included in diet plan must be eaten to prevent hypoglycemia

• To carry Medic Alert ID and glucagon emergency kit for emergencies

• To notify prescriber if oral contraceptives are used

• Not to use if breast-feeding

Evaluate:

• Therapeutic response: Decrease in polyuria, polydipsia, polyphagia; clear sensorium; absence of dizziness; stable gait, blood glucose at normal level

---

poractant alfa (℞)
Curosurf
Func. class.: Lung surfactant extract

Action: Replenishes surfactant and restores surface activity to the lungs in premature infants

Uses: Treatment (rescue) of respiratory distress syndrome in premature infants

Investigational uses: Prophylaxis of RDS, adult RDS due to viral pneumonia, HIV-infected infants with *Pneumocystis carinii* pneumonia, treatment of adult RDS in near drowning

---

Dosage and routes:

• INTRATRACHEAL INSTILL

Available forms: Susp 120 mg (1.5 ml); 240 mg (3 ml), phospholipids

Side effects/adverse reactions:

(Concurrent illnesses that have occurred during treatment are in bold)

*RESP: **Pulmonary air leaks, pulmonary interstitial emphysema, apnea, pulmonary hemorrhage***

*SYST: **Patent ductus arteriosus, intracranial hemorrhage, severe intracranial hemorrhage, necrotizing enterocolitis, posttreatment sepsis, posttreatment infection,*** bradycardia, oxygen desaturation, pallor, vasoconstriction, hypotension, hypertension

Precautions: Bradycardia, rales, infections

Pharmacokinetics: Becomes lung associated within hours of administration

NURSING CONSIDERATIONS

Assess:

• Respiratory rate, rhythm, character, chest expansion, color, transcutaneous saturation, ABGs

• Endotracheal tube placement before dosing; for apnea after endotracheal administration

• Reflux of drug into the endotracheal tube during administration; stop drug if this occurs, and if needed, increase peak inspiratory pressure on the ventilator by 4-5 cm H_2O until tube is cleared

• Infant for repeat dosing using radiographic confirmation of RDS; repeat doses should be given as above; ventilator settings for repeat doses FIo_2 were decreased by 0.2 or amount to prevent cyanosis; ventilator rate of 30/min; inspiratory time <1 sec; if infant's pretreatment rate was >30, it was left unchanged during dosing; resume usual ventilator management after dosing

Administer:

• After suctioning

• By endotracheal administration only by persons trained in neonatal intubation and ventilation

• After using a No. 5 Fr end-hole catheter inserted into the endotracheal tube with the tip at distal end of endotracheal tube just beyond the end of the endotracheal tube; shorten the catheter before insertion; insert the drug into the main bronchi by positioning infant with either right or left side dependent

• Divide doses and administer with infant in different positions

• Determine dosing by weight of infant; slowly withdraw contents into plastic syringe through 20G needle; do not filter or shake; attach premeasured No. 5 Fr catheter to syringe; fill with drug and discard excess through catheter so only dose to be given remains in syringe

• For prevention dosing, stabilize, weigh, and intubate infant; give drug within 15 min of birth if possible; position infant and inject first dose through catheter over 2-3 sec; remove catheter and manually ventilate with O_2 to prevent cyanosis (60 bpm) and sufficient positive pressure to promote adequate air exchange and chest wall excursion

• For rescue dosing, give dosing as soon as infant is placed on ventilator after birth; immediately before administering dose, change ventilator settings to 60/min, inspiratory time 0.5 sec, FIo_2 1; position infant and inject first dose through catheter over 2-3 sec; remove catheter; return to mechanical ventilator

• Ventilate infant for >30 sec or until stable after prevention or rescue strategy; reposition for next dose; same procedure for subsequent dosing; do not suction for at least 1 hr

---

◆= Nursing alert   ∥= Herb-drug interaction   ⊘= Do not crush

after dosing unless airway obstruction is evident; resume ventilator therapy after dosing
Perform/provide:

• Reduction in peak ventilator inspiratory pressures immediately if chest expansion improves substantially after dose

• Reduction in FIo$_2$ in small, repeated steps when infant becomes pink and transcutaneous oxygen saturation is in excess of 95%; oxygen saturation should remain between 90% and 95%

• Suctioning of all infants before administration to prevent mucus plugging; if endotracheal tube obstruction is suspected, remove obstruction and replace tube immediately

• Storage in refrigeration; protect from light; warm to room temperature for >20 min or warm in hand >8 min before giving; do not use artificial warming methods; enter a vial only once; unopened, unused vials that have been warmed to room temperature may be rerefrigerated within 8 hr of warming; do not warm and return to refrigerator more than once
Evaluate:

• Therapeutic response: significant improvement in respiratory status

---

rabeprazole (℞)
(rah-bep′rah-zole)
Aciphex
Func. class.: Proton pump inhibitor
Chem. class.: Benzimidazole

Action: Suppresses gastric secretion by inhibiting hydrogen/potassium ATPase enzyme system in gastric parietal cell; characterized as gastric acid pump inhibitor, since it blocks final step of acid production

Uses: Gastroesophageal reflux disease (GERD), severe erosive esophagitis, poorly responsive systemic GERD, pathologic hypersecretory conditions (Zollinger-Ellison syndrome, systemic mastocytosis, multiple endocrine adenomas); treatment of active duodenal ulcers with or without antiinfectives for *H. pylori*

Dosage and routes:
Healing of duodenal ulcers
• *Adult:* **PO** 20 mg qd × ≤4 wk to be taken after breakfast
Healing of erosive esophagitis or ulcerative GERD
• *Adult:* **PO** 20 mg qd × 4-8 wk
Pathologic hypersecretory conditions
• *Adult:* **PO** 60 mg/day; may increase to 120 mg in 2 divided doses
Available forms: Tabs, delayed rel 20 mg
Side effects/adverse reactions:
CNS: Headache, dizziness, asthenia
GI: Diarrhea, abdominal pain, vomiting, nausea, constipation, flatulence, acid regurgitation, abdominal swelling, anorexia, irritable colon, esophageal candidiasis, dry mouth
RESP: Upper respiratory infections, cough, epistaxis
INTEG: Rash, dry skin, urticaria, pruritus, alopecia
META: Hypoglycemia, increased hepatic enzymes, weight gain
EENT: Tinnitus, taste perversion
CV: Chest pain, angina, tachycardia, bradycardia, palpitations, peripheral edema
GU: UTI, urinary frequency, increased creatinine, ***proteinuria, hematuria,*** testicular pain, glycosuria
*HEMA: **Pancytopenia, thrombocytopenia, neutropenia, leukocytosis,*** anemia

---

MISC: Back pain, fever, fatigue, malaise

Contraindications: Hypersensitivity

Precautions: Pregnancy (C), lactation, children

Pharmacokinetics: Eliminated in urine as metabolites and in feces

Interactions:
• Increased serum levels of rabeprazole: benzodiazepines, phenytoin, clarithromycin
• Decreased levels of rabeprazole: sucralfate

NURSING CONSIDERATIONS
Assess:
• GI system: bowel sounds q8h, abdomen for pain, swelling, anorexia
• Hepatic enzymes: AST, ALT, alk phosphatase during treatment
Administer:
🚫 After breakfast qd; do not crush, break, chew delayed rel tab
Evaluate:
• Therapeutic response: absence of epigastric pain, swelling, fullness
Teach patient/family:
• To report severe diarrhea; drug may have to be discontinued
• That diabetic patient should know hypoglycemia may occur
• To avoid hazardous activities; dizziness may occur
• To avoid alcohol, salicylates, ibuprofen; may cause GI irritation

---

rapacuronium (℞)
(rap-ah-cure-oh'nee-um)
Raplon
Func. class.: Neuromuscular blocker (nondepolarizing)
Chem. class.: Synthetic curariform

Action: Inhibits transmission of nerve impulses by competing for cholinergic receptor sites
Uses: Facilitation of endotracheal intubation, skeletal muscle relaxation during mechanical ventilation, surgery, or general anesthesia

Dosage and routes:
Tracheal intubation
• *Adult:* **IV** 1.5 mg/kg for short procedures, max block 90 sec, lasting about 15 min
Repeat dosing in adults
• *Adult:* **IV** after intubating dose, may give up to 3 maintenance doses of 0.5 mg/kg
• *Children 1 mo-12 yr:* **IV** 2 mg/kg under halothane anesthesia
Available forms: Inj 100, 200 mg
Side effects/adverse reactions:
CV: Bradycardia; tachycardia; increased, decreased B/P; extrasystoles
RESP: **Prolonged apnea, bronchospasm, cyanosis, respiratory depression**
MS: Weakness
INTEG: Rash, flushing, pruritus, urticaria, sweating, salivation
Contraindications: Hypersensitivity
Precautions: Pregnancy (C), renal disease, cardiac disease, lactation, electrolyte imbalances, dehydration, neuromuscular disease, respiratory disease, ICP, malignant hyperthermia
Pharmacokinetics:
IV: Metabolized (small amounts), excreted in urine (unchanged), crosses placenta, elimination half-life 22 days; protein binding 50-88%
Interactions:
• Increased neuromuscular blockade: antibiotics, inhalation anesthetics, magnesium salts, lithium, local anesthetics, procainamide, quinidine
• Decreased neuromuscular blockade: anticonvulsants
Lab test interferences:
Decrease: Cholinesterase

◆ = Nursing alert   🖉 = Herb-drug interaction   🚫 = Do not crush

NURSING CONSIDERATIONS
Assess:
• For electrolyte imbalances (K, Mg); may lead to increased action of this drug
• Vital signs (B/P, pulse, respirations, airway) until fully recovered; rate, depth, pattern of respirations, strength of hand grip
• I&O ratio; check for urinary retention, frequency, hesitancy
• Recovery: decreased paralysis of face, diaphragm, leg, arm, rest of body; allow to recover fully before neuro assessment
• Allergic reactions: rash, fever, respiratory distress, pruritus; drug should be discontinued
Administer:
IV, direct
• With diazepam or morphine when used for therapeutic paralysis; this drug provides no sedation
• Using nerve stimulator by anesthesiologist to determine neuromuscular blockade
• Atropine to counteract muscarinic effects
• After succinylcholine effects subside
• Anticholinesterase to reverse neuromuscular blockade
Additive compatibilities: Alfentanil, atropine, droperidol, epinephrine, fentanyl, gentamicin, glycopyrrolate, heparin, ketamine, labetalol, lidocaine, methohexital, metoclopramide, midazolam, morphine, potassium chloride, propranolol, ranitidine, remifentanil, sufentanil, verapamil
Solution compatibilities: 0.9% NaCl, D_5W, D_5 NaCl, sterile water for inj, LR, bacteriostatic water for inj
Perform/provide:
• Storage in refrigerator; do not store in plastic; use only fresh sol

• Reassurance if communication is difficult during recovery from neuromuscular blockade
• Frequent (q2h) instillation of artificial tears and covering eyes to prevent drying of cornea
Evaluate:
• Therapeutic response: paralysis of jaw, eyelid, head, neck, rest of body
Treatment of overdose: Edrophonium or neostigmine, atropine, monitor VS; may require mechanical ventilation

---

rofecoxib (℞)
(roh-fih-kox′ib)
Vioxx
Func. class.: Nonsteroidal antiinflammatory

Action: May inhibit prostaglandin synthesis by decreasing enzyme needed for biosynthesis; analgesic, antiinflammatory, antipyretic properties
Uses: Acute, chronic osteoarthritis pain, primary dysmenorrhea
Dosage and routes:
Osteoarthritis
• *Adult:* **PO** 12.5 mg/day as a single dose may increase to 25 mg if needed
Primary dysmenorrhea
• *Adult:* **PO** 50 mg qd, use for <5 days
Available forms: Tabs 12.5, 25 mg; susp 12.5, 25 mg/5 ml
Side effects/adverse reactions:
CNS: Fatigue, anxiety, depression, nervousness, paresthesia
CV: ***Tachycardia,*** *angina,* ***MI,*** *palpitations,* ***dysrhythmias,*** *hypertension, fluid retention*
EENT: Tinnitus, hearing loss, blurred vision, glaucoma, cataract, conjunctivitis, eye pain
GI: Nausea, anorexia, vomiting, constipation, dry mouth, diverticulitis, gastritis, gastroenteritis, hemor-

rhoids, hiatal hernia, stomatitis, GI bleeding

GU: Nephrotoxicity: dysuria, hematuria, oliguria, azotemia, cystitis, UTI

HEMA: Blood dyscrasias, epistaxis, bruising, anemia

INTEG: Purpura, *rash, pruritus, sweating, erythema, petechiae, photosensitivity, alopecia*

RESP: Pharyngitis, shortness of breath, pneumonia, coughing

Contraindications: Hypersensitivity to aspirin, iodides, other NSAIDs, asthma

Precautions: Pregnancy (C), lactation, children, bleeding disorders, GI disorders, cardiac disorders, hypersensitivity to other antiinflammatory agents

Pharmacokinetics: Well absorbed, crosses placenta, bound to plasma proteins

Interactions:

• Decreased effect, increased adverse reactions: aspirin, ACE inhibitors

• Increased bleeding: aspirin, other NSAIDs, anticoagulants

• Decreased effect of: diuretics

• Increased toxicity: lithium, antineoplastics

• Increased adverse reaction: glucocorticosteroids

NURSING CONSIDERATIONS
Assess:

• For pain of rheumatoid arthritis, osteoarthritis; check ROM, inflammation of joints, characteristics of pain

• Blood counts during therapy; watch for decreasing platelets; if low, therapy may need to be discontinued, restarted after hematologic recovery; and for blood dyscrasias (thrombocytopenia): bruising, fatigue, bleeding, poor healing

Administer:
PO

• With food or milk to decrease gastric symptoms

🚫 Do not crush, dissolve, or chew

Evaluate:

• Therapeutic response: decreased pain in arthritic conditions; decreased inflammation in arthritic conditions

Teach patient/family:

• That drug must be continued for prescribed time to be effective; to avoid other NSAIDs

• To report bleeding, bruising, fatigue, malaise, since blood dyscrasia do occur

• To take with a full glass of water to enhance absorption

---

rosiglitazone (℞)
(ros-ih-glit′ah-zone)
Avandia
Func. class.: Antidiabetic, oral
Chem. class.: Thiazolidinedione

Action: Improves insulin resistance by hepatic glucose metabolism, insulin receptor kinase activity, insulin receptor phosphorylation

Uses: Stable adult-onset diabetes mellitus (type II) NIDDM

Dosage and routes:
Monotherapy

• *Adult:* **PO** 4 mg qd or in 2 divided doses, may increase to 8 mg qd or in 2 divided doses after 12 wk

Combination therapy

• *Adult:* **PO** This drug should be added to metformin at the adult dose

Available forms: Tabs 2, 4, 8 mg

Side effects/adverse reactions:

MISC: Accidental injury, URI, sinusitis, anemia, back pain, diarrhea, edema

CNS: Fatigue, headache

ENDO: Hyper/hypoglycemia

Contraindications: Hypersensitivity to thiazolidinediones, children, lactation, diabetic ketoacidosis

Precautions: Pregnancy (C), elderly, thyroid disease, hepatic, renal disease

Pharmacokinetics: Maximal reductions in FBS after 6-12 wk, protein binding 99.8%, excreted in urine, feces, elimination half-life 3-4 hr

Interactions:

• May decrease effect of: oral contraceptives, alternate method advised

NURSING CONSIDERATIONS
Assess:

• For hypoglycemic reactions (sweating, weakness, dizziness, anxiety, tremors, hunger), hyperglycemic reactions soon after meals

• CBC (baseline, q3mo) during treatment; check liver function tests periodically AST, LDH, renal studies: BUN, creatinine, urinary glucose

• FBS, glycosylated Hgb, fasting plasma insulin, plasma lipids/lipoproteins, B/P, body weight during treatment

Administer:

• Once or in 2 divided doses

• Tabs crushed and mixed with food or fluids for patients with difficulty swallowing

Perform/provide:

• Conversion from other oral hypoglycemic agents if needed; change may be made without gradual dosage change; monitor serum or urine glucose and ketones tid during conversion

• Storage in tight container in cool environment

Teach patient/family:

• To use capillary blood glucose test or Chemstrip tid; that periodic liver function testing is mandatory

• The symptoms of hypo/hyperglycemia, what to do about each

• That the drug must be continued on daily basis: explain consequence of discontinuing drug abruptly

• To avoid OTC medications or herbal preparations unless approved by prescriber

• That diabetes is lifelong illness; that this drug is not a cure; only controls symptoms

• That all food included in diet plan must be eaten to prevent hypoglycemia

• To carry Medic Alert ID and glucagon emergency kit for emergencies

• To notify prescriber if oral contraceptives are used

• Not to use if breast-feeding

Evaluate:

• Therapeutic response: Decrease in polyuria, polydipsia, polyphagia; clear sensorium; absence of dizziness; stable gait, blood glucose at normal level

---

sirolimus (℞)

(seer-oh-lie′mus)

Rapamune

Func. class.: Immunosuppressant

Chem. class.: Macrolide

Action: Produces immunosuppression by inhibiting T-lymphocyte activation and proliferation

Uses: Organ transplants to prevent rejection, recommended use is with cyclosporine and corticosteroids

Investigational uses: Psoriasis

Dosage and routes:

• *Adult:* **PO** 2 mg qd with a 6 mg loading dose, may use 5 mg qd with a 15 mg loading dose

• *Child >13 yr weighing <40 kg (88 lb):* to 1 mg/m^2/day, 3 mg/m^2 loading dose

---

Hepatic dose
• Reduce by 33% in maintenance dose

Available forms: Oral sol 1 mg/ml

Side effects/adverse reactions:

HEMA: **Anemia, leukopenia, thrombocytopenia, purpura**

GI: Nausea, vomiting, diarrhea, constipation

CV: Hypertension, *atrial fibrillation, CHF, hypotension, palpitation, tachycardia*

CNS: Tremors, headache, insomnia, *paresthesia,* chills, fever

GU: UTIs, **albuminuria, hematuria, proteinuria, renal failure**

META: Hyperglycemia, increased creatinine, edema, hypercholesterolemia, hyperlipemia, hypophosphatemia, weight gain, hyperkalemia, hyperuricemia, hypokalemia, hypomagnesemia

RESP: **Pleural effusion, atelectasis,** dyspnea

INTEG: Rash, acne

EENT: Blurred vision, photophobia

SYST: **Lymphoma**

Contraindications: Hypersensitivity to this drug or to components of the drug

Precautions: Severe renal, hepatic disease; pregnancy (C), diabetes mellitus, hyperkalemia, hyperuricemia, lymphomas, lactation, children <13 yr, hypertension

Pharmacokinetics: Rapidly absorbed, peak 1 hr single dose, 2 hr multiple dosing, protein binding 92%

Interactions:
• Increased blood levels: antifungals, calcium channel blockers, cimetidine, danazol, erythromycin, cyclosporine, metoclopramide, bromocriptine, HIV-protease inhibitors
• Decreased blood levels: carbamazepine, phenobarbital, phenytoin, rifamycin, rifapentine
• Decreased effect of: vaccines

• Drug/food: alters bioavailability; use consistently with or without food; do not use with grapefruit juice

NURSING CONSIDERATIONS

Assess:
• Blood levels in those that may have altered metabolism, trough level ≥15 ng/ml are associated with increased adverse reactions
• Lipid profile: cholesterol, triglycerides, a lipid-lowering agent may be needed
• For infection and development of lymphoma
• Blood studies: Hgb, WBC, platelets during treatment qmo; if leukocytes <3000/mm^3 or platelets <100,000/mm^3, drug should be discontinued or reduced; decreased hemoglobulin level may indicate bone marrow suppression
• Liver function studies: alk phosphatase, AST, ALT, amylase, bilirubin, and for hepatotoxicity: dark urine, jaundice, itching, light-colored stools; drug should be discontinued

Administer:
• Prophylaxis for *Pneumocystis carinii* pneumonia for 1 yr after transplantation; prophylaxis for cytomegalovirus (CMV) is recommended for 90 days after transplantation in those at increased risk for CMV
• All medications PO if possible, avoiding IM injections; bleeding may occur
• For 3 days before transplant surgery; patients should be placed in protective isolation
• Use amber oral dose syringe and withdraw amount needed oral sol from the bottle, empty correct dose into plastic/glass container holding 60 ml of water/orange juice, stir vigorously and have patient drink at once, refill container with additional 120 ml water/orange juice, stir vigorously and drink at once, if using

⬥ = Nursing alert   🌿 = Herb-drug interaction   🚫 = Do not crush

a pouch squeeze entire contents into container and follow above directions
• Store protected from light, refrigerate, stable for 24 mo

Evaluate:
• Therapeutic response: absence of graft rejection; immunosuppression in autoimmune disorders

Teach patient/family:
• To report fever, rash, severe diarrhea, chills, sore throat, fatigue; serious infections may occur; clay-colored stools, cramping (hepatotoxicity)
• To avoid crowds, persons with known infections to reduce risk of infection
• To use contraception before, during and 12 wk after drug has been discontinued

---

temozolomide (R)
(tem-oh-zole′oh-mide)
Temodar
Func. class.: Antineoplastic-misc agent
Chem. class.: Imidazotetrazine derivative

Action: A prodrug that undergoes conversion to MTIC. MTIC action prevents DNA transcription

Uses: Anaplastic astrocytoma with relapse

Dosage and routes:
• *Adult:* **PO** Adjust dose based on nadir neutrophil and platelet counts 150 mg/m²/day × 5 days during a 28-day cycle

Available forms: Caps 5, 20, 100, 250 mg

Side effects/adverse reactions:
HEMA: ***Thrombocytopenia, leukopenia,*** anemia
GI: *Nausea, anorexia, vomiting*
CNS: ***Seizures,*** hemiparesis, dizzi-

ness, *poor coordination, amnesia, insomnia, paresthesia, somnolence, paresis, ataxia, anxiety, dysphagia, depression, confusion*
INTEG: *Rash, pruritus*
GU: Urinary incontinence, UTI, frequency
RESP: URI, pharyngitis, sinusitis, coughing
MISC: Headache, fatigue, asthenia, fever, edema, back pain, weight increase, diplopia

Contraindications: Hypersensitivity to this drug or carbazine, pregnancy (D), lactation

Precautions: Radiation therapy, renal, hepatic disease

Pharmacokinetics: Absorption complete, rapid; crosses blood-brain barrier, excreted urine/feces, half-life 1.8 hr, peak 1 hr

Interactions:
• Increased myelosuppression: radiation, other antineoplastics
• Decreased antibody reaction: live virus vaccines

NURSING CONSIDERATIONS
Assess:
• CBC on day 22 (21 days after 1st dose), CBC weekly until recovery if ANC is <1.5 × 10⁹/L and platelets <100 × 10⁹/L, do not administer to patients that do not tolerate 100 mg/m², myelosuppression usually occurs late in the treatment cycle
• Monitor temp q4h (may indicate beginning infection)
• Liver function tests before, during therapy (bilirubin, AST, ALT, LDH), as needed or monthly
• Bleeding: hematuria, guaiac, bruising or petechiae, mucosa or orifices q8h

Administer:
• Antiemetic 30-60 min before giving drug to prevent vomiting
• Antibiotics for prophylaxis of infection

• Fluids IV or PO before chemotherapy to hydrate patient

• Caps should not be opened; if accidentally damaged, do not allow contact with skin, or inhale

• Give on empty stomach to prevent nausea/vomiting

Perform/provide:

• Storage in light-resistant container, dry area

Evaluate:

• Therapeutic response: decreased tumor size, spread of malignancy

Teach patient/family:

• To report signs of infection: fever, sore throat, flu symptoms

• To report signs of anemia: fatigue, headache, faintness, shortness of breath, irritability

• To report bleeding; avoid use of razors, commercial mouthwash

• To avoid use of aspirin products or ibuprofen

---

zaleplon (℞)

(zal´eh-plon)

Sonata

Func. class.: Sedative/hypnotic

Chem. class.: Pyrazolopyrimidine

Action: Binds selectively to omega-1 receptor of the $GABA_A$ receptor complex; results are sedation, hypnosis, skeletal muscle relaxation, anticonvulsant activity, anxiolytic action

Uses: Insomnia

Dosage and routes:

• *Adult:* **PO** 10 mg hs; may increase dose to 20 mg hs if needed; 5 mg may be used in low weight persons

Available forms: Caps 5, 10 mg

Side effects/adverse reactions:

CNS: Lethargy, drowsiness, daytime sedation, dizziness, confusion, anxiety, amnesia, depersonalization, hal-lucinations, hypesthesia, paresthesia, somnolence, tremor, vertigo

GI: Nausea, abdominal pain, constipation, anorexia, colitis, dyspepsia, dry mouth

EENT: Vision change, ear/eye pain, hyperacusis, parosmia

MISC: Asthenia, fever, headache, myalgia, dysmenorrhea

Contraindications: Hypersensitivity

Precautions: Hepatic disease, renal disease, elderly, psychosis, child <15 yr, pregnancy (C), lactation

Pharmacokinetics:

PO: Rapid onset, metabolized by liver extensively; excreted by kidneys (inactive metabolites); half-life 1 hr

Interactions:

• Increased effects of zaleplon: cimetidine

• Decreased effect of zaleplon: rifampin

• Food: prolonged absorption, sleep onset reduced: high-fat/heavy meal

NURSING CONSIDERATIONS

Assess:

• Mental status: mood, sensorium, affect, memory (long, short)

• Type of sleep problem: falling asleep, staying asleep

Administer:

• After removal of cigarettes to prevent fires

• After trying conservative measures for insomnia

• Immediately before hs for sleeplessness

• On empty stomach for fast onset

Perform/provide:

• Assistance with ambulation after receiving dose

• Safety measure: nightlight, call bell within easy reach

• Checking to see if PO medication has been swallowed

• Storage in tight container in cool environment

◆ = Nursing alert   🖋 = Herb-drug interaction   ⊘ = Do not crush

Evaluate:
• Therapeutic response: ability to sleep at night, decreased amount of early morning awakening

Teach patient/family:
• To avoid driving or other activities requiring alertness until drug is stabilized
• To avoid alcohol ingestion or CNS depressants
• Alternative measures to improve sleep: reading, exercise several hr before hs, warm bath, warm milk, TV, self-hypnosis, deep breathing
• That drug may cause memory problems, dependence (if used for longer periods of time), changes in behavior/thinking
• That drug is for short-term use only
• To take immediately before going to bed
• Not to ingest a high-fat/heavy meal before taking

---

zanamivir (℞)
(zan′ah-mih-veer)
Relenza
Func. class.: Antiviral

Action: Inhibits the enzyme needed for influenza virus replication
Uses: Treatment of influenza type A for those that have been symptomatic for no more than 2 days
Dosage and routes:
• *Adult and child >12 yr:* **INH** 2 inhalations (two 5 mg blisters) q12h × 5 days, on the 1st day 2 doses should be taken at least 2 hr between doses
Available forms: Blisters of powder for inhalation: 5 mg
Side effects/adverse reactions:
CNS: Headache, dizziness, fatigue
EENT: Ear, nose, throat infections
GI: Nausea, vomiting, diarrhea

RESP: Nasal symptoms, cough, sinusitis, bronchitis
Contraindications: Hypersensitivity
Precautions: Lactation, children <12 yr, respiratory disease, elderly, pregnancy (B)
Pharmacokinetics: Half-life 2½-5 hr, not metabolized, excreted in urine unchanged
Interactions:
• None known
NURSING CONSIDERATIONS
Assess:
• Bowel pattern before, during treatment
• Skin eruptions, photosensitivity after administration of drug
• Respiratory status: rate, character, wheezing, tightness in chest
• Allergies before initiation of treatment, reaction of each medication
• Signs of infection
Administer:
• Within 2 days of symptoms of influenza; continue for 5 days
• Give patient "Patient's Instruction for Use" and review all points before using delivery system
Perform/provide:
• Storage in tight, dry container
Evaluate:
• Therapeutic response: absence of fever, malaise, cough, dyspnea in infection
Teach patient/family:
• That this drug does not reduce transmission risk of influenza to others
• Patients with asthma or COPD to carry a fast-acting inhaled bronchodilator since bronchospasm may occur; to use scheduled inhaled bronchodilators before using this drug
• To avoid hazardous activities if dizziness occurs
• To take drug exactly as prescribed

Appendix b

Recent FDA drug approvals

Generic name	Trade name	Use
alosetron	Lotronex	Irritable bowel syndrome
cevimeline	Evoxac	Dry mouth in Sjögren's syndrome
linezolid	Zyvox	Antibiotic-resistant infections
oxcarbazepine	Trileptal	Partial seizures
pemirolast	Alamast	Allergic conjunctivitis
pneumococcal 7-valent conjugate vaccine	Prevnar	Immunization against *Streptococcus pneumoniae*
progestogen emergency contraceptive	Plan B	Prevention of pregnancy

Appendix c

Ophthalmic, otic, nasal, and topical products

OPHTHALMIC PRODUCTS

α-ADRENERGIC BLOCKER
dapiprazole (R)
(da-pip'ra-zole)
Rev-Eyes

ANESTHETICS
proparacaine (R)
(proe-par'a-kane)
AK-Taine, Alcaine, Diocane*,
Ocu-Caine, Ophthaine,
Ophthestic, Spectro-Caine
tetracaine (R)
(tet'ra-kane)
Minims Tetracaine,
Pontocaine Eye, Pontocaine
HCl, tetracaine

ANTIHISTAMINES
emedastine (R)
(ee-med'ah-steen)
Emadine
levocabastine (R)
(lee-voh-cab'ah-steen)
Livostin
olopatadine (R)
(oh-loh-pat'ah-deen)
Patanol

ANTIINFECTIVES
bacitracin (R)
(bass-i-tray'sin)
AK-Tracin, Bacitracin
Ophthalmic

brimonidine (R)
(bri-moe'ni-deen)
Alphagan
chloramphenicol (R)
(klor-am-fen'i-kole)
AK-Chlor, Chloramphenicol,
Chloramphenicol
Ophthalmic, Chloromycetin
Ophthalmic, Chloroptic,
Chloroptic S.O.P., Fenicol*,
Isopto Fenical*, Pentamycin*
ciprofloxacin (R)
(sip-ro-floks'a-sin)
Ciloxan
erythromycin (R)
(er-ith-roe-mye'sin)
AK-Mycin, Erythromycin,
Ilotycin
gentamicin (R)
(jen-ta-mye'sin)
Garamycin Ophthalmic,
Genoptic Ophthalmic,
Genoptic S.O.P., Gentacidin,
Gent-AK, gentamicin,
Gentamicin Ophthalmic
Liquifilm, Gentak
idoxuridine-IDU (R)
(eye-dox-yoor'i-deen)
Herplex, Stoxil
natamycin (R)
(nat-a-mye'sin)
Natacyn
norfloxacin (R)
(nor-floks'a-sin)
Chibroxin, Ofloxacin, Ocuflox

---

* = Canada only   Side effects: *italics* = common; ***bold italics*** = life-threatening

ofloxacin (R)
(oh-flox'a-sin)
Ocuflox

polymyxin B (R)
(pol-ee-mix'in)
Aerosporin, polymyxin B
sulfate

silver nitrate 1% (R)
sulfacetamide
sodium (R)
(sul-fa-seet'a-mide)
AK-Sulf, Bleph-10 Liquifilm,
Bleph-10 S.O.P., Isopto
Cetamide, Ophthacet,
Sodium Sulamyd, sodium
sulfacetamide 10%, sodium
sulfacetamide 15%, sodium
sulfacetamide 30%, SOSS-10,
Sulfair 15

tetracycline (R)
(tet-ra-sye'kleen)
Achromycin Ophthalmic

tobramycin (R)
(toe-bra-mye'sin)
Tobrex

trifluridine (R)
(trye-floor'i-deen)
Viroptic

vidarabine (R)
(vye-dare'a-been)
Vira-A

β-ADRENERGIC BLOCKERS
betaxolol (R)
(beh-tax'oh-lole)
Betoptic, Betoptic 5

carteolol (R)
(kar-tee'oh-lole)
Ocupress

levobunolol (R)
(lee-voe-byoo'no-lole)
Betagen

metipranolol (R)
(met-ee-pran'oh-lole)
Optipranolol

timolol (R)
(tye'moe-lole)
Apo-Timop*, Betimol,
Timoptic

CHOLINERGICS
(Direct-acting)
carbachol (R)
(kar'ba-kole)
Iosopto Carbachol, Miostat

pilocarpine (R)
(pye-loe-kar'peen)
Adsorbocarpine, Akarpine,
Isopto Carpine, Ocu-Carpine,
Ocusert-Pilo, Pilagan, Pilocar,
pilocarpine, Pilopine HS,
Piloptic-1, Piloptic-2, Pilostat,
Pilopto-Carpine

CHOLINESTERASE
INHIBITORS
demecarium (R)
(dem-e-kare'ee-um)
Humorsol

ecothiophate (R)
(ek-oh-thye'eh-fate)
Ecostigmine Iodide,
Phospholine Iodide

isoflurophate (R)
(eye-soe-floor'oh-fate)
Floropryl

physostigmine (R)
(fi-zoe-stig'meen)
Eserine Salicylate, Isopto
Eserin

CYCLOPLEGIC
MYDRIATICS
atropine (R)
(a'troe-peen)
Atropine-1, Atropine Care
Ophthalmic, Atropine Sulfate

⬦ = Nursing alert　　🮥 = Herb-drug interaction　　🚫 = Do not crush

Ophthalmic, Atropine Sulfate
S.O.P., Atropisol, Isopto
Atropine

cyclopentolate (℞)
(sye-kloe-pen'toe-late)
AK-Pentolate, Cyclogly,
I-Pentolate

homatropine (℞)
(home-a'troe-peen)
AK-Homatropine,
I-Homatrine, Isopto
Homatropine, Minims
Homatropine*, Spectro-
Homatropine

physostigmine (℞)
(fi-zoe-stig'meen)
Fisostin, Isopto Eserine Solu-
tion/Eserine Sulfate Ointment

scopolamine (℞)
(skoe-pol'a-meen)
Isopto-Hyoscine

tropicamide (℞)
(troe-pik'a-mide)
Mydriacyl, Tropicacyl, I-Pir-
amide

GLUCOCORTICOIDS
dexamethasone (℞)
(dex-a-meth'a-sone)
AK-Dex, Decadron
Phosphate, Dexamethasone
Ophthalmic Suspension,
Maxidex

fluorometholone (℞)
(flure-oh-meth'oh-lone)
Flarex, Fluor-Op, FML, FML
Forte, FML Liquifilm

medrysone (℞)
(me'dri-sone)
HMS

prednisolone (℞)
(pred-niss'oh-lone)
Econopred, Econopred Plus,
AK-Pred, Inflamase Forte,
Inflamase Mild Ophthalmic,

Metreton Ophthalmic, Pred-
Forte, Pred-Mild

rimexolone (℞)
(ri-mex'a-lone)
Vexol

NONSTEROIDAL
ANTIINFLAMMATORIES
diclofenac (℞)
(dye-kloe'fen-ak)
Voltaren

flurbiprofen (℞)
(flure-bih-proh'fen)
Ocufen

ketorolac (℞)
(kee-toe'role-ak)
Acular

suprofen (℞)
(soo-proe'fen)
Profenal

SYMPATHOMIMETICS
apraclonidine (℞)
(a-pra-klon'i-deen)
Lopidine

brimonidine (℞)
(brih-moh'nih-deen)
Alphagan

dipivefrin (℞)
(dye-pi'vef-rin)
Propine

**epinephrine
bitartrate/epinephrine
HCl/epinephryl
borate** (℞)
(ep-i-nef'rin)
Epitrate, Mytrate/Epifrin,
Glaucon/Epinal, Eppy*

---

* = Canada only   Side effects: *italics* = common; ***bold italics*** = life-threatening

OPHTHALMIC DECONGESTANTS/ VASOCONSTRICTORS

naphazoline (OTC, ℞)
(naf-az'oh-leen)
AK-Con Ophthalmic, Albalon Liquifilm Ophthalmic, Allerest Eye Drops, Clear Eyes, Comfort Eye Drops, Degest 2, Nafazair, naphazoline HCl, Naphcon, Naphcon Forte, Opcon, Vasoclear, Vasocon Regular, Estivin II

oxymetazoline (℞)
(ox-i-meth'oh-lone)
OcuClear, Visine, LR

phenylephrine (OTC)
(fen-ill-ef'rin)
AK-Dilate Ophthalmic, AK-Nefrin Ophthalmic, Isopto Frin, Neo-Synephrine 2.5%, Neo-Synephrine 10% Plain, Neo-Synephrine Viscous, phenylephrine HCl, 2.5% Mydfrin Ophthalmic, Phenoptic Relief, Prefrin

tetrahydrozoline (OTC)
(tet-ra-hye-dro'zoe-leen)
Collyrium Fresh Eye Drops, Eyesine, Murine Plus Eye Drops, Optigene 3 Eye Drops, Soothe Eye Drops, tetrahydrozoline HCl, Tyzine HCl, Tyzine Pediatric, Visine Eye Drops

MISCELLANEOUS OPHTHALMICS

brinzolamide (℞)
(brin-zoh'la-mide)
Azopt

latanoprost
(la-tan'oh-proest)
Xalatan

dorzolamide (℞)
(dor-zol'a-mide)
Trusopt

ketotifen (℞)
(kee-toh-tif'en)
Zaditor

lodoxamide
(loe-dox'a-mide)
Alomide

Pregnancy categories: Demecarium, isoflurophate (X); apraclonidine, cyclopentolate, ecothiophate, glucocorticoids, levobunalol, metipranolol, pilocarpine, proparacaine, suprofen, tetracaine (C); dapiprazole, dipivefrin (B)

β-*Adrenergic blockers*
Action: Reduces production of aqueous humor by unknown mechanism
Uses: Ocular hypertension, chronic open-angle glaucoma

Anesthetics
Action: Decreases ion permeability by stabilizing neuronal membrane
Uses: Cataract extraction, tonometry, gonioscopy, removal of foreign objects, corneal suture removal, glaucoma surgery (ophth); pruritus, sunburn, toothache, sore throat, cold sores, oral pain, rectal pain and irritation, control of gagging (top)

Antiinfectives
Action: Inhibits folic acid synthesis by preventing PABA use, which is necessary for bacterial growth
Uses: Conjunctivitis, superficial eye infections, corneal ulcers, prophylaxis against infection after removal of foreign matter from the eye

Antiinflammatories
Action: Decreases inflammation, resulting in decreased pain, photophobia, hyperemia, cellular infiltration

---

◆ = Nursing alert   ⫸ = Herb-drug interaction   ⊘ = Do not crush

Uses: Inflammation of eye, eyelids, conjunctiva, cornea; uveitis, iridocyclitis, allergic conditions, burns, foreign bodies, postoperatively in cataract

Carbonic anhydrase inhibitor

Action: Converted to epinephrine, which decreases aqueous production and increases outflow

Uses: Open-angle glaucoma, ocular hypertension

Direct-acting miotic

Action: Acts directly on cholinergic receptor sites; induces miosis, spasm of accommodation, fall in intraocular pressure, caused by stimulation of ciliary, pupillary sphincter muscles, which leads to pulling away of iris from filtration angle, resulting in increased outflow of aqueous humor

Uses: Primary glaucoma, early stages of wide-angle glaucoma (less useful in advanced stages), chronic open-angle glaucoma, acute narrow-angle glaucoma before emergency surgery; also neutralizes mydriatics used during eye exam; may be used alternately with mydriatics to break adhesions between iris and lens

Side effects/adverse reactions:

CNS: Headache

CV: Hypertension, tachycardia, dysrhythmias

EENT: Burning, stinging

GI: Bitter taste

Contraindications: Hypersensitivity

Precautions: Pregnancy, lactation, children, aphakia, hypersensitivity to carbonic anhydrase inhibitors, sulfonamides, thiazide diuretics, ocular inhibitors, hepatic and renal insufficiency

NURSING CONSIDERATIONS

Assess:

• Ophth exams and intraocular pressure readings

• Blood counts; liver, renal function tests and serum electrolytes during long-term treatment

Perform/provide:

• Storage at room temp away from light

Evaluate:

• Positive therapeutic response

• Absence of increased intraocular pressure

Teach patient/family:

• How to instill drops

• That drug may cause burning, itching, blurring, dryness of eye area

NASAL AGENTS

NASAL DECONGESTANTS

azelastine (R)

(ay-zell′ah-steen)

Astelin

desoxyephedrine (OTC)

(des-oxy-e-fed′rin)

Vicks Inhaler

ephedrine (OTC)

(e-fed′rin)

Kondon's Nasal Jelly, Pretz-D, Vicks Vatronol

epinephrine (OTC)

(ep-i-neff′rin)

Adrenalin

naphazoline (OTC)

(naff-a-zoe′leen)

Privine

oxymetazoline (OTC)

(ox-i-met-az′oh-leen)

Afrin, Afrin Children's Nose Drops, Allerest 12-Hour Nasal, Chlorphed-LA, Coricidin Nasal Mist, Dristan Long Lasting, Duramist Plus, Duration, Genasal, NTZ

Long-Acting Nasal, Nafrine*, Neo-Synephrine 12 Hour, Nostrilla, oxymetazoline HCl, Sinarest 12-Hour, Sinex Long-Acting, Twice-A-Day Nasal, 4-Way Long Acting Nasal

phenylephrine (OTC)
(fen-ill-eff'rin)
Alconefrin 12, Children's Nostril, Neo-Synephrine, Sinex

propylhexadrine (OTC)
(proe-pil-hex'a-dreen)
Benzedrex Inhaler

tetrahydrozoline (OTC)
(tet-ra-hye-dro'zoe-leen)
Tyzine

xylometazoline (OTC)
(zye-loh-meh-tazz'oh-leen)
Otrivin, Otrivin Pediatric Nasal Drops, xylometazoline HCl

NASAL STEROIDS
beclomethasone (℞)
(be-kloe-meth'a-sone)
Beconase AQ Nasal, Beconase Inhalation, Vancenase AQ Nasal, Vancenase Nasal

dexamethasone (℞)
(dex-a-meth'a-sone)
Decadron Phosphate Turbinaire

Pregnancy category: C
Action: Produces vasoconstriction (rapid, long acting) of arterioles, thereby decreasing fluid exudation, mucosal engorgement by stimulation of α-adrenergic receptors in vascular smooth muscle
Uses: Nasal congestion
Dosage and routes:
Desoxyephedrine
• *Adult and child >6 yr:* 1-2 **INH** in each nostril q2h or less

Ephedrine
• *Adult:* Fill dropper to the level marked, then use in each nostril q4h or less
Epinephrine
• *Adult and child >6 yr:* Apply with swab, drops, spray prn
Naphazoline
• *Adult and child >6 yr:* 1-2 drops/spray q6h or less
Oxymetazoline
• *Adult and child >6 yr:* **INSTILL** 2-3 gtt or sprays to each nostril bid
• *Child 2-6 yr:* **INSTILL** 2-3 gtt or sprays 0.025 sol bid, not to exceed 3 days
Phenylephrine
• *Adult and child >12 yr:* 2-3 drops/spray (0.25-0.5) in each nostril q3-4h or less; or 2-3 drops/spray (1%) in each nostril q4h or less
• *Child 6-12 yr:* 2-3 drops/spray (0.25%) in each nostril q3-4h
• *Infant >6 mo:* 1-2 drops (0.16%) in each nostril q3h
Propylhexadrine
• *Adult and child >6 yr:* 1-2 **INH** in each nostril q2h or less
Tetrahydrozoline
• *Adult and child >6 yr:* 2-4 drops (0.1%) q3-4h prn or 3-4 sprays in each nostril q4h prn
• *Child 2-6 yr:* 2-3 drops (0.05%) in each nostril q4-6h prn
Xylometazoline
• *Adult and child >12 yr:* 2-3 drops/spray (0.1%) in each nostril q8-10h
• *Child 2-12 yr:* 2-3 drops (0.05%) in each nostril q8-10h
Available forms: Nasal sol 0.025%, 0.05%
Side effects/adverse reactions:
CNS: Anxiety, restlessness, tremors, weakness, insomnia, dizziness, fever, headache
EENT: Irritation, burning, sneezing, stinging, dryness, rebound congestion
GI: Nausea, vomiting, anorexia

◆ = Nursing alert   🌿 = Herb-drug interaction   🚫 = Do not crush

INTEG: Contact dermatitis

Contraindications: Hypersensitivity to sympathomimetic amines

Precautions: Children <6 yr, elderly, diabetes, cardiovascular disease, hypertension, hyperthyroidism, increased intracranial pressure, prostatic hypertrophy, pregnancy (C), glaucoma

NURSING CONSIDERATIONS
Assess:
• For redness, swelling, pain in nasal passages before and during treatment
• For syst absorption; hypertension, tachycardia; notify prescriber; syst absorption occurs at high doses or after prolonged use

Administer:
• Having patient tilt head back, squeeze bulb to create a vacuum, and draw correct amount of sol into dropper; insert 2 gtt of sol into nostril; repeat in other nostril
• Store in light-resistant container; do not expose to high temp or let sol come into contact with aluminum
• For <4 consecutive days
• Environmental humidification to decrease nasal congestion, dryness

Evaluate:
• Therapeutic response: decreased nasal congestion

Teach patient/family:
• That stinging may occur for several applications; drying of mucosa may be decreased by environmental humidification
• To notify prescriber if irregular pulse, insomnia, dizziness, or tremors occur
• Proper administration to avoid syst absorption
• To rinse dropper with very hot water to prevent contamination

TOPICAL GLUCOCORTICOIDS

alclometasone (℞)
(al-kloe-met′a-sone)
Adovate

amcinonide (℞)
(am-sin′oh-nide)
Cyclocort

betamethasone (℞)
(bay-ta-meth′a-sone)
Alphatrex, Beben*, Betacort*, Betaderm, Betatrex, Beta-Val, Bethovate*, Betmethacort, Celestoderm*, Dermabet, Diprolene, Diprosone, Ectosonel*, Maxivate, Metaderm*, Novobetamet, Psorion, Uticort, Valisone, Valnac

clobetasol (℞)
(kloe-bay′ta-sol)
Dermovate*, Temovate

clocortolone (℞)
(kloe-kore′toe-lone)
Cloderm

desonide (℞)
(dess′oh-nide)
Des Owen, Tridesilon

desoximetasone (℞)
(dess-ox-i-met′a-sone)
Topicort

dexamethasone (℞)
(dex-a-meth′a-sone)
Aeroseb-Dex, Decaderm, Decaspray

diflorasone (℞)
(dye-flor′a-sone)
Florone, Maxiflor, Psorcon

fluocinolone (℞)
(floo-oh-sin′oh-lone)
Fluocin, Licon, Lidemol*, Lidex, Lyderm*, Topsyn*, Vasoderm

---

flurandrenolide (℞)

(flure-an-dren'oh-lide)
Cordran, Cordran SP,
Cordran Tape, Drenison
1/4*, Drenison Tape*

fluticasone (℞)

(floo-tik'a-sone)
Cutivate

halcinonide (℞)

(hal-sin'oh-nide)
Halog, Halog-E

halobetasol (℞)

(hal-oh-bay'ta-sol)
Ultravate

hydrocortisone (℞)

(hye-droe-kor'ti-sone)
Actiocort, Aeroseb-HC, Ala-
Cort, Allercort, Alphaderm,
Anusol HC, Bactine, Barriere-
HC*, Calde-CORT Anti-Itch,
Carmol HC, Cetacort, Corta-
cet*, Cortaid, Cortate*, Cort-
Dome, Cortef*, Corticaine,
Corticreme*, Cortifair, Corti-
zone, Cortoderm*, Cortril,
Delcort, Dermacort,
DemiCort, Dermtex HC,
Emo-Cort, Epifoam,
FoilleCort, Gly-Cort, Gyne-
cort, Hi-Cor, Hycort, Hy-
derm*, Hydro-Tex, Hytone,
Lacti-Care-HC, Lanacort,
Lemoderm, Locoid, My Cort,
Novoehydrocort*, Nutracort
Pharm, Pharmacort, Penta-
cort, Rederm, Rhulicort S-T
Cort, Synacort, Sarna HC*,
Texa-Cort, Unicort*, Westcort

methylprednisolone
(℞)

(meth-ill-pred-niss'oh-lone)
Depo-Medrol

mometasone (℞)

(moe-met'a-sone)
Elocon

prednicarbate (℞)

(pred-ni-kar'bate)
Dermatop

triamcinolone (℞)

(trye-am-sin'oh-lone)
Aristocort, Flutex, Kenac,
Kenalog, Kenonel,
Triaderm*, Trianide*,
Triderm, Trymex

Pregnancy category: C
Action: Antipruritic, antiinflamma-
tory
Uses: Psoriasis, eczema, contact der-
matitis, pruritus; usually reserved
for severe dermatoses that have not
responded to less potent formula-
tion
Dosage and routes:
• *Adult and child:* Apply to affected
area
Side effects/adverse reactions:
*INTEG: Acne, atrophy, epidermal
thinning, purpura, striae*
Contraindications: Hypersensitivity, viral infections, fungal infections
Precautions: Pregnancy (C)
NURSING CONSIDERATIONS
Assess:
• Temp; if fever develops, drug
should be discontinued
• For systemic absorption, increased
temp, inflammation, irritation
Administer:
• Only to affected areas; do not get
in eyes
• Leaving site uncovered or lightly
covered; occlusive dressing is not
recommended—systemic absorption
may occur
• Use only on dermatoses; do not
use on weeping, denuded, or infected area
• Cleansing before application of
drug
• Continuing treatment for a few
days after area has cleared

◆ = Nursing alert   ✎ = Herb-drug interaction   ⊘ = Do not crush

- Store at room temp
Evaluate:
- Therapeutic response: absence of severe itching, patches on skin, flaking
Teach patient/family:
- To avoid sunlight on affected area, burns may occur
- To limit treatment to 14 days

TOPICAL ANTIFUNGALS

amphotericin B (OTC)
(am-foe-ter'i-sin)
Fungizone

butenafine (℞)
(byoo-tin'a-feen)
Mentex

ciclopirox (OTC)
(sye-kloe-peer'ox)
Loprox

clioquinol (OTC)
(klye-oh-kwin'ole)
Vioforim

clotrimazole (OTC)
(kloe-trye'ma-zole)
Canestew*, Clotrimaderm*, Lotrimin, Lotrimin AF, Mycelex, Mycelex OTC, Myclo*, Neozol*

econazole (OTC)
(ee-kon'a-zole)
Spectazole

haloprogin (OTC)
(hal-oh-proe'jin)
Halotex

ketoconazole (OTC)
(kee-toe-kon'a-zole)
Nizoral

miconazole (OTC)
(mye-kon'a-zole)
Micatin, Monistat-Derm

naftifine (OTC)
(naff'ti-feen)
Naftin

nystatin (OTC)
(nye-stat'in)
Mycostatin, Nodostine*, Nilstat, Nyoderm*, Nystex

oxiconazole (OTC)
(ox-i-kon'a-zole)
Oxistat

selenium (OTC)
(see-leen'ee-um)
Exsel, Head and Shoulders Intensive Treatment, Selenium Sulfide, Selsun, Selsun Blue

terbinafine (OTC)
(ter-bin'a-feen)
Lamisil

tolnaftate (OTC)
(tole-naf'tate)
Absorbine Antifungal, Absorbine Jock Itch, Absorbine Jr. Antifungal, Aftate For Athlete's Foot, Aftate for Jock Itch, Desenex Spray, Genaspor, NP-27, Quinsana Plus, Tinactin, Ting, tolnaftate, Zeasorb-AF

undecylenic acid (OTC)
(un-deh-sih-len'ik)
Caldesene, Cruex, Decylenes, Desenex, Desenex Maximum Strength, Protectol

Pregnancy category: B
Action: Interferes with fungal cell membrane permeability
Uses: Tinea cruris, tinea pedis, diaper rash, minor skin irritations; amphotericin B is used for *Candida* infections
Dosage and routes:
- Massage into affected area, surrounding area qd or bid, con-

tinue for 7-14 days, not to exceed 4 wk

Side effects/adverse reactions:
INTEG: Burning, stinging, dryness, itching, local irritation

Contraindications: Hypersensitivity

Precautions: Pregnancy (B), lactation, children

Interactions: None

NURSING CONSIDERATIONS
Assess:

• Skin for fungal infections; peeling, dryness, itching before and throughout treatment

• For continuing infection; increased size, number of lesions

Administer:
Topical route

• To affected area, surrounding area; do not cover with occlusive dressings

• Store below 30° C (86° F)

Evaluate:

• Therapeutic response: decrease in size, number of lesions

Teach patient/family:

• To apply with glove to prevent further infection; not to cover with occlusive dressings

• That long-term therapy may be needed to clear infection (2 wk-6 mo depending on organism); compliance is needed even after feeling better

• Proper hygiene; hand-washing technique, nail care, use of concomitant top agents if prescribed

• To avoid use of OTC creams, ointments, lotions unless directed by prescriber

• To use medical asepsis (hand washing) before, after each application; to change socks and shoes once a day during treatment of tinea pedis

• To report to health care prescriber if infection persists or recurs; if blis-

ters, burning, oozing, swelling occur

• To avoid alcohol because nausea, vomiting, hypertension may occur

• To use sunscreen or avoid direct sunlight to prevent photosensitivity

• To notify health-care prescriber of sore throat, fever, skin rash, which may indicate overgrowth of organisms

---

TOPICAL ANTIINFECTIVES

bacitracin (OTC)
(bass-i-tray'sin)
Baciguent, Bacitin*,
Bacitracin

chloramphenicol (Ŗ)
(klor-am-fen'i-kole)
Chloromycetin

erythromycin (OTC)
(er-ith-roe-mye'sin)
A/T/S, Akne-Mycin, C-Solve 2,
Erycette, Eryderm, Erygel,
Erymax, Erythromycin,
E-Solve 2, ETS-2%, Staticin,
Theramycin Z, T-Statd

gentamicin (Ŗ)
(jen-ta-mye'sin)
G-Myticin, Garamycin,
gentamicin

mafenide (Ŗ)
(ma'fe-nide)
Sulfamylon

mupirocin (Ŗ)
(myoo-peer'oh-sin)
Bactroban, Pseudomonic
Acid A

neomycin (OTC)
(nee-oh-mye'sin)
Myciguent, Neomycin Sulfate

nitrofurazone (Ŗ)
(nye-troe-fyoor'a-zone)
Furacin, Nitrofurazone

◆ = Nursing alert   ⫽ = Herb-drug interaction   ⊘ = Do not crush

silver sulfadiazine (Ŗ)
(sul-fa-dye'a-zeen)
Flamazine*, Silvadene, SSD,
SSD AF, Thermazene
sodium sulfacetamide lotion 10% (Ŗ)
(sul-fa-see'ta-mide)

Klaron
tetracycline (Ŗ)
(tet-ra-sye'kleen)
Achromycin, Topicycline

Pregnancy category: C
Action: Interferes with bacterial protein synthesis
Uses: Skin infections, minor burns, wounds, skin grafts, primary pyodermas, otitis externa
Side effects/adverse reactions:
INTEG: Rash, urticaria, scaling, redness
Contraindications: Hypersensitivity, large areas, burns, ulcerations
Precautions: Pregnancy (C), lactation, impaired renal function, external ear or perforated eardrum
NURSING CONSIDERATIONS
Assess:
• Allergic reaction: burning, stinging, swelling, redness
• For signs of nephrotoxicity or ototoxicity
Administer:
• Enough medication to cover lesions completely
• After cleansing with soap, water before each application; dry well
• To less than 20% of body surface area when patient has impaired renal function
Perform/provide:
• Storage at room temp in dry place
Evaluate:
• Therapeutic response: decrease in size, number of lesions

TOPICAL ANTIVIRALS

acyclovir (Ŗ)
(ay-sye'kloe-ver)
Zovirax
penciclovir (Ŗ)
(pen-sye'kloe-ver)
Denavir

Pregnancy category: C
Action: Interferes with viral DNA replication
Uses: Simple mucocutaneous herpes simplex, in immunocompromised clients with initial herpes genitalis
Side effects/adverse reactions:
INTEG: Rash, urticaria, stinging, burning, pruritus, vulvitis
Contraindications: Hypersensitivity
Precautions: Pregnancy (C), lactation
NURSING CONSIDERATIONS
Assess:
• Allergic reaction: burning, stinging, swelling, redness, rash, vulvitis, pruritus
Administer:
• Using finger cot or rubber glove to prevent further infection
• Enough medication to cover lesions completely
• After cleansing with soap, water before each application; dry well
Perform/provide:
• Storage at room temp in dry place
Evaluate:
• Therapeutic response: decrease in size, number of lesions
Teach patient/family:
• Not to use in eyes or when there is no evidence of infection
• To apply with glove to prevent further infection
• To avoid use of OTC creams, ointments, lotions unless directed by prescriber

---

• To use medical asepsis (hand washing) before, after each application and avoid contact with eyes

• To adhere strictly to prescribed regimen to maximize successful treatment outcome

• To begin taking drug when symptoms arise

TOPICAL ANESTHETICS

benzocaine (OTC)
(ben'zoe-kane)
Anbesol Maximum Strength, Baby Anbesol, Children's Chloraseptic, Medamint, Orabase Baby, Oracin, Ora-Jel, Oratect, Spec-T Anesthetic, T-Caine, Tyrobenz

dibucaine (OTC)
(dye'byoo-kane)
dibucaine, Nupercainal

lidocaine (OTC, ℞)
(lye'doe-kane)
Aloe Extra, Anestacon, Burn Relief, Derma Flex, lidocaine HCl topical, lidocaine viscous, Solarcaine, Xylocaine, Xylocaine Viscous, Zilactin-L

pramoxine (OTC)
(pra-mox'een)
Fleet Relief, Prax, ProctoFoam, Tronolane, Tronothane

tetracaine (OTC)
(tet'ra-cane)
Pontocaine

Pregnancy category: C
Action: Inhibits conduction of nerve impulses from sensory nerves
Uses: Oral irritation, sore throat, toothache, cold sore, canker sore, sunburn, minor cuts, insect bites, pain, itching

Dosage and routes:
• *Adult and child:* **TOP** apply qid as needed; **RECT** insert tid and after each BM
Side effects/adverse reactions:
INTEG: Rash, irritation, sensitization

Contraindications: Hypersensitivity, infants <1 yr, application to large areas
Precautions: Child <6 yr, sepsis, pregnancy (C), denuded skin
NURSING CONSIDERATIONS
Assess:
• Pain: location, duration, characteristics before and after administration

• For infection: redness, drainage, inflammation; this drug should not be used until infection is treated
Perform/provide:
• Storage in tight, light-resistant container; do not freeze, puncture, or incinerate aerosol container
Evaluate:
• Therapeutic response: decreased redness, swelling, pain
Teach patient/family:
• To avoid contact with eyes

• Not to use for prolonged periods: use for <1 wk; if condition remains, prescriber should be contacted

VAGINAL ANTIFUNGALS

butoconazole (OTC)
(byoo-toh-kone'ah-zole)
Femstat

clotrimazole (OTC)
(kloe-trye'ma-zole)
Canesten*, Gyne-Lotrimin, Mycelex G, Mycelex Twin Pak, Myclo*

miconazole (OTC)
(mye-kon'a-zole)
Monistat, Monistat 3, Monistat 7, Monistat Dual Pak

nystatin (OTC)
(nye-stat'in)
mycostatin, Nadostine*, Nilstat, Nyoderm*, O-V Statin

terconazole (OTC)
(ter-kone'ah-zole)
Terazol

tioconazole (OTC)
(tye-oh-kone'ah-zole)
Gyne-Trosyd*, Vagistat

Pregnancy category: Nystatin (A); clotrimazole (B); butoconazole, terconazole, tioconazole (C)
Action: Interferes with fungal DNA replication; binds sterols in fungal cell membranes, which increases permeability, leaking of nutrients
Uses: Vaginal, vulval, vulvovaginal candidiasis (moniliasis)
Dosage and routes:
Butoconazole
• *Adult:* VAG 5 g (1 applicator) hs × 3-6 days
Clotrimazole
• *Adult:* 100 mg (1 vag tab, 100 mg) hs × 1 wk, or 200 mg (2 vag tab, 100 mg) hs × 3 nights, or 500 mg (1 vag tab, 500 mg); or 5 g (1 applicator) hs × 1-2 wks

Miconazole
• *Adult:* 200 mg supp hs × 3 days or 100 mg supp × 1 wk
Nystatin
• *Adult:* 100,000 U qd × 2 wk
Terconazole
• *Adult:* VAG 5 g (1 applicator) hs × 7 days
Tioconazole
• *Adult:* 1 applicator hs × 1 wk
Side effects/adverse reactions:
GU: Vulvovaginal burning, itching, pelvic cramps
INTEG: Rash, urticaria, stinging, burning
MISC: **Headache**, body pain
Contraindications: Hypersensitivity
Precautions: Children <2 yr, pregnancy, lactation
Interactions: None
NURSING CONSIDERATIONS
Assess:
• For allergic reaction: burning, stinging, itching, discharge, soreness
Administer:
Topical route
• One full applicator every night high into the vagina
• Store at room temp in dry place
Evaluate:
• Therapeutic outcome: decrease in itching or white discharge (vaginal)
Teach patient/family:
• About asepsis (hand washing) before, after each application
• To apply with applicator only; to avoid use of any other vaginal product unless directed by prescriber; sanitary napkin may prevent soiling of undergarments
• To abstain from sexual intercourse until treatment is completed; reinfection and irritation may occur
• To notify prescriber if symptoms persist

OTIC STEROIDS

OTIC ANTIINFECTIVES

hydrocortisone
(hye-droe-kor′ti-sone)
Cortamed*, Otall (R)

Pregnancy category: C
Action: Antiinflammatory, antipruritic
Uses: Ear canal inflammation
Side effects/adverse reactions:
EENT: Itching, irritation in ear
INTEG: Rash, urticaria
Contraindications: Hypersensitivity, perforated eardrum
Precautions: Pregnancy (C)
NURSING CONSIDERATIONS
Assess:
• For redness, swelling, fever, pain in ear, which indicates infection
Administer:
• After removing impacted cerumen by irrigation
• After cleaning stopper with alcohol
• After restraining child if necessary
• After warming sol to body temp
Evaluate:
• Therapeutic response: decreased ear pain, inflammation
Teach patient/family:
• The correct method of instillation using aseptic technique, including not touching dropper to ear
• That dizziness may occur after instillation

chloramphenicol (R)
(klor-am-fen′i-kole)
Chloromycetin Otic,
Sopamycetin*
neomycin (R)
(nee-oh-mye′sin)
Drotic, Otocort

Pregnancy category: C
Action: Inhibits protein synthesis in susceptible microorganisms
Uses: Ear infection (external), short-term use
Side effects/adverse reactions:
EENT: Itching, irritation in ear
INTEG: Rash, urticaria
Contraindications: Hypersensitivity, perforated eardrum
Precautions: Pregnancy (C)
NURSING CONSIDERATIONS
Assess:
• For redness, swelling, fever, pain in ear, which indicates superinfection
Administer:
• After removing impacted cerumen by irrigation
• After cleaning stopper with alcohol
• After restraining child if necessary
• After warming sol to body temp
Evaluate:
• Therapeutic response: decreased ear pain
Teach patient/family:
• The correct method of instillation using aseptic technique, including not touching dropper to ear
• That dizziness may occur after instillation

Appendix d

Commonly used antiinfectives in adults and children

amoxicillin
  Adult: **PO** 750 mg-1.5 g qd in divided doses q8h
  Child: **PO** 20-40 mg/kg/day in divided doses q8h
ampicillin
  Adult: **PO** 1-2 g qd in divided doses q6h
      IM/IV 2-8 g qd in divided doses q4-6h
  Child: **PO** 50-100 mg/kg/day in divided doses q6h
      IM/IV 100-200 mg/kg/day in divided doses q6h
cefaclor
  Adult: **PO** 250-500 mg q8h
  Child: **PO** 24-40 mg/kg/day in divided doses q8h
cephalexin
  Adult: **PO** 250-500 mg q6h
  Child: **PO** 25-50 mg/kg/day in 4 equal doses
chloramphenicol
  Adult and child >3 mo: 50-100 mg/kg/day in divided doses q6h
clindamycin
  Adult: **PO** 150-450 mg q6h
      IM/IV 300 mg q6-12h
  Child >1 mo: **PO** 8-25 mg/kg/day in divided doses q6-8h
          IM/IV 15-40 mg/kg/day in divided doses q6-8h
erythromycin
  Adult: 250-500 mg q6h
  Child: 30-50 mg/kg/day in divided doses q6h
gentamicin
  Adult: **IV INF** 3-5 mg/kg/day in divided doses q8h
  Child: **IV/IM** 2-2.5 mg/kg q8h
  Neonate and infant: **IV/IM** 2.5 mg/kg q8h
kanamycin
  Adult and child: **IV INF/IM** 15 mg/kg/day in divided doses
            q8-12h
methicillin
  Adult: **IM/IV** 4-12 g/day in divided doses q4-6h
  Child: **IM/IV** 50-300 mg/kg/day in divided doses q4-12h
      PO 25-50 mg/kg/day in divided doses q6h
  Neonate: **IM** 10 mg/kg q12h

* = Canada only   Side effects: *italics* = common; ***bold italics*** = life-threatening

nafcillin

Adult: **PO/IM/IV** 2-6 g/day in divided doses q4-6h
Child: **IM** 25 mg/kg q12h

nitrofurantoin

Adult and child >12 yr: **PO** 50-100 mg qid pc

oxacillin

Adult: **PO** 2-6 g/day in divided doses q4-6h
   IM/IV 2-12 g/day in divided doses q4-6h
Child: **PO/IM/IV** 50-100 mg/kg/day in divided doses q6h

penicillin G benzathine

Adult: **IM** 1.2 million U

penicillin G potassium

Adult: **PO** 400,000-500,000 U q6-8h
Child <12 yr: **PO** 25,000-90,000 U/kg/day in 3-6 divided doses

penicillin G procaine

Adult and child: **IM** 600,000-1.2 million U in 1-2 doses/day
Neonate: **IM** 50,000 U/kg qd

sulfisoxazole

Adult: **PO** 2-4 g loading dose, then 1-2 g qid
Child >2 mo: **PO** 75 mg/kg or 2 g/m^2 loading dose, then 150
   mg/kg/day or 4 g/m^2/day in divided doses q6h

ticarcillin

Adult: **IV/IM** 12-24 g/day in divided doses q3-6h
Child: **IV/IM** 50-300 mg/kg/day in divided doses q4-8h
Neonate: **IV INF** 75-100 mg/kg q8-12h

⬥ = Nursing alert   🌿 = Herb-drug interaction   🚫 = Do not crush

Appendix e

Combination products

A-200 Shampoo:
0.33% pyrethrins
4% piperonyl butoxide
Uses: Scabicide, pediculicide

Acid-X:
acetaminophen 500 mg
calcium carbonate 250 mg
Uses: Analgesic, antacid

Actifed:
pseudoephedrine 60 mg
triprolidine 2.5 mg
Uses: Decongestant

Actifed, Allergy, Nighttime:
pseudoephedrine 30 mg
diphenhydramine 25 mg
Uses: Decongestant, antihistamine

Actifed Plus:
pseudoephedrine 30 mg
triprolidine 1.25 mg
acetaminophen 500 mg
Uses: Decongestant, antihistamine

Actifed Sinus Daytime:
pseudoephedrine 30 mg
acetaminophen 500 mg
Uses: Decongestant

Actifed Sinus Nighttime:
pseudoephedrine 30 mg
diphenhydramine 25 mg
acetaminophen 500 mg
Uses: Decongestant, antihistamine

Adderall 10 mg:
dextroamphetamine sulfate 5 mg
dextroamphetamine saccharate 2.5 mg
amphetamine sulfate 2.5 mg
amphetamine aspartate 2.5 mg
Uses: CNS stimulant

Adderall 20 mg:
dextroamphetamine sulfate 5 mg
dextroamphetamine saccharate 5 mg
amphetamine sulfate 5 mg
amphetamine aspartate 5 mg
Uses: CNS stimulant

Advil Cold & Sinus Caplets:
pseudoephedrine 30 mg
ibuprofen 200 mg
Uses: Decongestant

AK-Cide Ophthalmic Suspension/ Ointment:
10% sulfacetamide sodium
0.5% prednisolone acetate
Uses: Ophth antiinfective, antiinflammatory

Aldactazide 25/25:
spironolactone 25 mg
hydrochlorothiazide 25 mg
Uses: Diuretic

Aldactazide 50/50:
spironolactone 50 mg
hydrochlorothiazide 50 mg
Uses: Diuretic

Aldoclor-150:
methyldopa 250 mg
chlorothiazide 150 mg
Uses: Antihypertensive

Aldoclor-250:
methyldopa 250 mg
chlorothiazide 250 mg
Uses: Antihypertensive

Aldoril-15:
methyldopa 250 mg
hydrochlorothiazide 15 mg
Uses: Antihypertensive

Aldoril-25:
methyldopa 250 mg
hydrochlorothiazide 25 mg
Uses: Antihypertensive

Alka-Seltzer Effervescent, Original:
sodium bicarbonate 1916 mg

---

* = Canada only   Side effects: *italics* = common; ***bold italics*** = life-threatening

citric acid 1000 mg
aspirin 325 mg
Uses: Antacid, adsorbent, antiflatulent

Alka-Seltzer Plus Allergy Liqui-Gels:
pseudoephedrine 30 mg
chlorpheniramine 2 mg
acetaminophen 325 mg
Uses: Decongestant, antihistamine

Alka-Seltzer Plus Night-Time Cold Liqui-Gels:
doxylamine 6.25 mg
dextromethorphan 10 mg
pseudoephedrine 30 mg
acetaminophen 250 mg
Uses: Antitussive, decongestant

Alka-Seltzer Plus Cold & Cough Liqui-Gels:
dextromethorphan 10 mg
pseudoephedrine 30 mg
chlorpheniramine 2 mg
acetaminophen 250 mg
Uses: Antitussive, decongestant

Alka-Seltzer Plus Cold & Cough:
phenylpropanolamine 20 mg
chlorpheniramine 2 mg
dextromethorphan 10 mg
aspirin 325 mg
Uses: Antitussive, decongestant

Alka-Seltzer Plus Cold Liqui-Gels:
pseudoephedrine 30 mg
chlorpheniramine 2 mg
acetaminophen 250 mg
Uses: Decongestant, antihistamine

Alka-Seltzer Plus Cold Medicine:
chlorpheniramine 2 mg
phenylpropanolamine 20 mg
aspirin 325 mg
Uses: Antihistamine, analgesic

Alka-Seltzer Plus Flu & Body Aches Non-Drowsy Liqui-Gels:
pseudoephedrine 30 mg
dextromethorphan 10 mg
acetaminophen 250 mg
Uses: Decongestant, antitussive, analgesic

Alka-Seltzer Plus Night-Time Cold:
phenylpropanolamine 20 mg
doxylamine 6.25 mg
dextromethorphan 15 mg
aspirin 500 mg
Uses: Antitussive, analgesic

Alka-Seltzer Plus Sinus:
phenylpropanolamine 20 mg
aspirin 325 mg
Uses: Analgesic

Allerest Headache Strength Advanced Formula:
pseudoephedrine 30 mg
chlorpheniramine 2 mg
acetaminophen 325 mg
Uses: Decongestant, antihistamine

Allerest Maximum Strength Caplets:
pseudoephedrine 30 mg
chlorpheniramine 2 mg
Uses: Decongestant, antihistamine

Allerest Maximum Strength 12 Hour Caplets:
phenylpropanolamine 75 mg
chlorpheniramine 12 mg
Uses: Antihistamine

Allerest No-Drowsiness:
pseudoephedrine 30 mg
acetaminophen 325 mg
Uses: Decongestant, analgesic

Allerest Sinus Pain Formula:
pseudoephedrine 30 mg
chlorpheniramine 2 mg
acetaminophen 500 mg
Uses: Decongestant, antihistamine, analgesic

All-Nite Cold Formula Liquid:
Per 5 ml:
pseudoephedrine 10 mg
doxylamine 1.25 mg
dextromethorphan 5 mg
acetaminophen 167 mg
Uses: Decongestant, antihistamine, analgesic

◆ = Nursing alert   🔯 = Herb-drug interaction   🚫 = Do not crush

Alor 5/500:
hydrocodone 5 mg
aspirin 500 mg
Uses: Analgesic

Amaphen:
acetaminophen 325 mg
butalbital 50 mg
caffeine 40 mg
Uses: Analgesic, barbiturates

Ambenyl Cough Syrup:
Per 5 ml:
bromodiphenhydramine 12.5 mg
codeine 10 mg
5% alcohol
Uses: Antihistamine, opioid analgesic

Anacin:
aspirin 400 mg
caffeine 32 mg
Uses: Analgesic

Anacin Maximum Strength:
aspirin 500 mg
caffeine 32 mg
Uses: Analgesic

Anacin PM (Aspirin Free):
diphenhydramine 25 mg
acetaminophen 500 mg
Uses: Analgesic

Anaplex HD Syrup:
Per 5 ml:
hydrocodone 1.7 mg
phenylephrine 5 mg
chlorpheniramine 2 mg
Uses: Analgesic, adrenergic, antihistamine

Anaplex Liquid:
Per 5 ml:
chlorpheniramine 2 mg
pseudoephedrine 30 mg
Uses: Antihistamine, decongestant

Anatuss:
guaifenesin 100 mg
dextromethorphan 15 mg
phenylpropanolamine 25 mg
acetaminophen 325 mg
Uses: Antitussive, expectorant, analgesic

Anatuss DM:
guaifenesin 400 mg
pseudoephedrine 60 mg
dextromethorphan 20 mg
Uses: Expectorant, adrenergic, antitussive

Anatuss DM Syrup:
Per 5 ml:
guaifenesin 100 mg
pseudoephedrine 30 mg
dextromethorphan 10 mg
Uses: Expectorant, adrenergic, antitussive

Anatuss LA:
pseudoephedrine 120 mg
guaifenesin 400 mg
Uses: Adrenergic, expectorant

Anatuss Syrup:
Per 5 ml:
guaifenesin 100 mg
dextromethorphan 15 mg
phenylpropanolamine 25 mg
Uses: Expectorant, antitussive

Anexsia 5/500:
hydrocodone 5 mg
acetaminophen 500 mg
Uses: Analgesic

Anexsia 7.5/650:
hydrocodone 7.5 mg
acetaminophen 650 mg
Uses: Analgesic

Anexsia 10/660:
hydrocodone 10 mg
acetaminophen 660 mg
Uses: Analgesic

Antihist-D:
clemastine 1.34 mg
phenylpropanolamine 75 mg
Uses: Antihistamine

Antrocol Elixir:
Per 5 ml:
atropine 0.195 mg
phenobarbital 16 mg
alcohol 20%
Uses: Anticholinergic, barbiturate

---

* = Canada only   Side effects: *italics* = common; ***bold italics*** = life-threatening

Apresazide 25/25:
hydralazine 25 mg
hydrochlorothiazide 25 mg
Uses: Antihypertensive

Aprodine w/Codeine Syrup:
Per 5 ml:
pseudoephedrine 30 mg
triprolidine 1.25 mg
codeine 10 mg
Uses: Adrenergic, analgesic

Aprodine Syrup:
Per 5 ml:
pseudoephedrine 30 mg
triprolidine 1.25 mg
Uses: Adrenergic, analgesic

A.R.M.:
phenylpropanolamine 25 mg
chlorpheniramine 4 mg
Uses: Antihistamine

Arthritis Pain Formula:
aspirin 500 mg
aluminum hydroxide 27 mg
magnesium hydroxide 100 mg
Uses: Analgesic, antacid

Arthrotec:
diclofenac 50 or 75 mg
misoprostol 200 µg
Uses: NSAID, gastric protectant

Asbron G Elixir:
theophylline 150 mg
guaifenesin 100 mg
alcohol 15%
Uses: Bronchodilator, expectorant

Asbron G Inlay:
theophylline 150 mg
guaifenesin 100 mg
sucrose
Uses: Bronchodilator, expectorant

Ascriptin A/D:
aspirin 325 mg
aluminum hydroxide 75 mg
magnesium hydroxide 75 mg
calcium carbonate 75 mg
Uses: Analgesic

Aspirin-Free Bayer Select Allergy Sinus:
pseudoephedrine 30 mg
chlorpheniramine 2 mg
acetaminophen 500 mg
Uses: Adrenergic, antihistamine, analgesic

Aspirin-Free Bayer Select Head & Chest Cold:
pseudoephedrine 30 mg
guaifenesin 100 mg
dextromethorphan 10 mg
acetaminophen 325 mg
Uses: Adrenergic, antitussive, expectorant, analgesic

Aspirin Free Excedrin:
acetaminophen 500 mg
caffeine 65 mg
Uses: Analgesic

Aspirin Free Excedrin Dual:
acetaminophen 500 mg
calcium carbonate 111 mg
magnesium carbonate 64 mg
magnesium oxide 30 mg
Uses: Analgesic, antacid

Augmentin 250:
amoxicillin 250 mg
clavulanic acid 125 mg
Uses: Antiinfective

Augmentin 500:
amoxicillin 500 mg
clavulanic acid 125 mg
Uses: Antiinfective

Augmentin 875:
amoxicillin 875 mg
clavulanic acid 125 mg
Uses: Antiinfective

Augmentin 125 Chewable:
amoxicillin 125 mg
clavulanic acid 31.25 mg
Uses: Antiinfective

Augmentin 250 Chewable:
amoxicillin 250 mg
clavulanic acid 62.5 mg
Uses: Antiinfective

◆ = Nursing alert   🖉 = Herb-drug interaction   ⊘ = Do not crush

Augmentin 125 mg/5 ml Suspension:
Per 5 ml:
amoxicillin 125 mg
clavulanic acid 31.25 mg
Uses: Antiinfective

Augmentin 250 mg/5 ml Suspension:
Per 5 ml:
amoxicillin 250 mg
clavulanic acid 62.5 mg
Uses: Antiinfective

Auralgan Otic Solution:
5.4% antipyrine
1.4% benzocaine
Uses: Otic analgesic

B&O Supprettes No. 15A Supps:
belladonna extract 15 mg
opium 30 mg
Uses: Anticholinergic, narcotic analgesic

B&O Supprettes No. 16A Supps:
belladonna extract 16.2 mg
opium 60 mg
Uses: Anticholinergic, narcotic analgesic

Bactrim:
trimethoprim 80 mg
sulfamethoxazole 400 mg
Uses: Antiinfective

Bactrim DS:
trimethoprim 160 mg
sulfamethoxazole 800 mg
Uses: Antiinfective

Bactrim I.V.:
trimethoprim 80 mg
sulfamethoxazole 400 mg
Uses: Antiinfective

Bancap HC:
acetaminophen 500 mg
hydrocodone 5 mg
Uses: Analgesic

Bayer Plus, Extra Strength:
aspirin 500 mg
calcium carbonate
magnesium carbonate
magnesium oxide
Uses: Analgesic, antacid

Bayer Select Chest Cold:
dextromethorphan 15 mg
acetaminophen 500 mg
Uses: Antitussive, analgesic

Bayer Select Flu Relief:
acetaminophen 500 mg
pseudoephedrine 30 mg
dextromethorphan 15 mg
chlorpheniramine 2 mg
Uses: Analgesic, adrenergic, antitussive, antihistamine

Bayer Select Head & Chest Cold, Aspirin Free Caplets:
pseudoephedrine 30 mg
dextromethorphan 10 mg
guaifenesin 100 mg
acetaminophen 325 mg
Uses: Adrenergic, antitussive, expectorant, analgesic

Bayer Select Head Cold:
pseudoephedrine 30 mg
acetaminophen 500 mg
Uses: Adrenergic, analgesic

Bayer Select Maximum Strength Headache:
acetaminophen 500 mg
caffeine 65 mg
Uses: Nonnarcotic analgesic

Bayer Select Maximum Strength Menstrual:
acetaminophen 500 mg
pamabrom 25 mg
Uses: Nonnarcotic analgesic

Bayer Select Maximum Strength Night-Time Pain Relief:
acetaminophen 500 mg
diphenhydramine 25 mg
Uses: Analgesic, antihistamine

Bayer Select Maximum Strength Sinus Pain Relief:
acetaminophen 500 mg
pseudoephedrine 30 mg
Uses: Analgesic, adrenergic

Bayer Select Night Time Cold:
acetaminophen 500 mg
pseudoephedrine 30 mg
dextromethorphan 15 mg
triprolidine 1.25 mg
Uses: Analgesic, adrenergic, antitussive, antihistamine

Bellatal:
phenobarbital 16.2 mg
hyoscyamine sulfate 0.1037 mg
atropine sulfate 0.0194 mg
scopolamine hydrobromide 0.0065 mg
Uses: Barbiturate, anticholinergic

Bellergal-S:
ergotamine 0.6 mg
belladonna alkaloids 0.2 mg
phenobarbital 40 mg
Uses: α-Adrenergic blocker, anticholinergic, barbiturate

Bel-Phen-Ergot-SR:
phenobarbital 40 mg
ergotamine tartrate 0.6 mg
belladonna alkaloids 0.2 mg
Uses: α-Adrenergic blocker, anticholinergic, barbiturate

Benadryl Allergy Decongestant Liquid:
Per 5 ml:
diphenhydramine 12.5 mg
pseudoephedrine 30 mg
Uses: Antihistamine, adrenergic

Benadryl Allergy/Sinus Headache Caplets:
diphenhydramine 12.5 mg
pseudoephedrine 30 mg
acetaminophen 500 mg
Uses: Antihistamine, adrenergic, analgesic

Benadryl Decongestant Allergy:
pseudoephedrine 60 mg
diphenhydramine 25 mg
Uses: Adrenergic, antihistamine

Benylin Expectorant Liquid:
Per 5 ml:
dextromethorphan 5 mg
guaifenesin 100 mg
5% alcohol
Uses: Expectorant, antitussive

Benylin Multi-Symptom Liquid:
Per 5 ml:
dextromethorphan 5 mg
pseudoephedrine 15 mg
guaifenesin 100 mg
Uses: Antitussive, adrenergic, expectorant

Betoptic-Pilo:
0.25% betaxolol
1.75% pilocarpine
Uses: Ophthalmic

Biohist-LA Tablets:
pseudoephedrine 120 mg
carbinoxamine 8 mg
Uses: Adrenergic

Blephamide Ophthalmic Suspension/Ointment:
0.2% prednisolone
10% sodium sulfacetamide
Uses: Ophthalmic antiinfective, antiinflammatory

Bromatapp Tablets:
phenylpropanolamine 75 mg
brompheniramine 12 mg
Uses: Decongestant, antihistamine

Bromfed Capsules:
pseudoephedrine 120 mg
brompheniramine 12 mg
Uses: Antihistamine, adrenergic

Bromfed-PD Capsules:
pseudoephedrine 60 mg
brompheniramine 6 mg
Uses: Adrenergic, antihistamine

Bromfed Tablets:
pseudoephedrine 60 mg
brompheniramine 4 mg
Uses: Antihistamine, adrenergic

Bromfenex:
brompheniramine 12 mg
pseudoephedrine 120 mg
Uses: Antihistamine, adrenergic

Bromfenex PD:
brompheniramine 6 mg
pseudoephedrine 60 mg
Uses: Antihistamine, adrenergic

Bromo-Seltzer:
sodium bicarb 2781 mg
acetaminophen 325 mg
citric acid 2224 mg
Uses: Antacid, analgesic

Bromophen T.D.:
phenylephrine 15 mg
phenylpropanolamine 15 mg
brompheniramine 12 mg
Uses: Antihistamine, decongestant

Brondelate Elixir:
theophylline 192 mg
guaifenesin 150 mg
Uses: Bronchodilator, expectorant

Brontex:
codeine 10 mg
guaifenesin 300 mg
Uses: Analgesic, expectorant

Bufferin:
aspirin 325 mg
calcium carbonate 158 mg
magnesium oxide 63 mg
magnesium carbonate 34 mg
Uses: Analgesic, antacid

Bufferin AF Nite-Time:
acetaminophen 500 mg
diphenhydramine 38 mg
Uses: Analgesic, antihistamine

Butibel:
belladonna extract 15 mg
butabarbital 15 mg
Uses: Anticholinergic, barbiturate

Cafatine PB:
ergotamine 1 mg
caffeine 100 mg
belladonna alkaloids 0.125 mg
pentobarbital 30 mg
Uses: Migraine agent

Cafergot:
ergotamine 1 mg
caffeine 100 mg
Uses: Adrenergic blocker

Cafergot Suppositories:
ergotamine 2 mg
caffeine 100 mg
Uses: Adrenergic blocker

Caladryl:
8% calamine, camphor
2.2% alcohol
1% pramoxine
Uses: Top antihistamine

Caladryl Clear:
1% pramoxine
0.1% zinc acetate
2% alcohol
camphor
Uses: Top antihistamine

Calcet:
calcium 152.8 mg
vitamin D 100 IU
Uses: Supplement

Calcidrine Syrup:
Per 5 ml:
codeine 8.4 mg
calcium iodide 152 mg
Uses: Analgesic

Caltrate 600+D:
vitamin D 200 IU
calcium 600 mg
Uses: Supplement

Cama Arthritis Pain Reliever:
aspirin 500 mg
magnesium oxide 150 mg
aluminum hydroxide 125 mg
Uses: Nonnarcotic analgesic, antacid

Capozide 25/15:
captopril 25 mg
hydrochlorothiazide 15 mg
Uses: Antihypertensive

Capozide 25/25:
captopril 25 mg
hydrochorothiazide 25 mg
Uses: Antihypertensive

Capozide 50/15:
captopril 50 mg
hydrochlorothiazide 15 mg
Uses: Antihypertensive

Capozide 50/25:
captopril 50 mg
hydrochlorothiazide 25 mg
Uses: Antihypertensive

Cardec DM Syrup:
Per 5 ml:
pseudoephedrine 60 mg
carbinoxamine 4 mg
dextromethorphan 15 mg
Uses: Adrenergic, antitussive

Cetacaine Topical:
14% benzocaine
2% tetracaine
0.5% benzalkonium chloride
0.005% cetyl dimethyl ethyl ammonium bromide
Uses: Local analgesic

Ceta Plus:
hydrocodone 5 mg
acetaminophen 500 mg
Uses: Analgesic

Cetapred Ophthalmic Ointment:
0.25% prednisolone
10% sodium sulfacetamide
Uses: Ophthalmic antiinfective, antiinflammatory

Cheracol Syrup:
Per 5 ml:
codeine 10 mg
guaifenesin 100 mg
Uses: Analgesic, expectorant

Cheracol Plus Liquid:
Per 5 ml:
phenylpropanolamine 8.3 mg
chlorpheniramine 1.3 mg
dextromethorphan 6.7 mg
8% alcohol
Uses: Antihistamine, antitussive

Children's Cepacol Liquid:
Per 5 ml:
acetaminophen 160 mg
pseudoephedrine 15 mg
Uses: Analgesic, adrenergic

Chlor-Trimeton Allergy-Sinus Caplets:
phenylpropanolamine 12.5 mg
chlorpheniramine 2 mg
acetaminophen 500 mg
Uses: Antihistamine, analgesic

Chlor-Trimeton 4 Hour Relief:
pseudoephedrine 60 mg
chlorpheniramine 4 mg
Uses: Antihistamine, adrenergic

Chlor-Trimeton 12 Hour Relief:
pseudoephedrine 120 mg
chlorpheniramine 8 mg
Uses: Antihistamine, adrenergic

Chromagen:
ferrous fumarate 66 mg
vitamin B_{12} 10 µg
vitamin C 250 mg
intrinsic factor 100 mg
Uses: Supplement

Claritin-D:
loratidine 5 mg
pseudoephedrine 120 mg
Uses: Antihistamine, adrenergic

Claritin-D 24-Hour:
loratidine 10 mg
pseudoephedrine 240 mg
Uses: Antihistamine, adrenergic

Clindex:
chlordiazepoxide 5 mg
clidinium 2.5 mg
Uses: Antianxiety, anticholinergic

Clomycin Ointment:
bacitracin 500 U
neomycin sulfate 3.5 g
polymyxin B sulfate 500 U
lidocaine 40 mg
Uses: Antiinfective, local anesthetic

Co-Apap:
pseudoephedrine 30 mg
chlorpheniramine 2 mg
dextromethorphan 15 mg
acetaminophen 325 mg
Uses: Adrenergic, antihistamine, antitussive, analgesic

Co-Gesic:
acetaminophen 500 mg
hydrocodone 5 mg
Uses: Analgesic

◆ = Nursing alert   ∅ = Herb-drug interaction   ⊘ = Do not crush

Codamine Syrup:
Per 5 ml:
hydrocodone 5 mg
phenylpropanolamine 25 mg
Uses: Analgesic

Codehist DH Elixir:
Per 5 ml:
pseudoephedrine 30 mg
chlorpheniramine 2 mg
codeine 10 mg
Uses: Adrenergic, antihistamine, analgesic

Codiclear DH Syrup:
Per 5 ml:
hydrocodone 5 mg
guaifenesin 100 mg
Uses: Analgesic, expectorant

Codimal:
pseudoephedrine 30 mg
chlorpheniramine 2 mg
acetaminophen 500 mg
Uses: Adrenergic, antihistamine, analgesic

Codimal DH Syrup:
Per 5 ml:
hydrocodone 1.66 mg
phenylephrine 5 mg
pyrilamine 8.33 mg
Uses: Analgesic, adrenergic

Codimal DM Syrup:
Per 5 ml:
phenylephrine 5 mg
pyrilamine 8.33 mg
dextromethorphan 10 mg
Uses: Adrenergic, antitussive

Codimal LA:
chlorpheniramine 8 mg
pseudoephedrine 120 mg
Uses: Antihistamine, adrenergic

Codimal PH Syrup:
Per 5 ml:
codeine 10 mg
phenylephrine 5 mg
pyrilamine 8.33 mg
Uses: Analgesic, adrenergic

Col-Probenecid:
probenecid 500 mg
colchicine 0.5 mg
Uses: Antigout agent

ColBenemid:
probenecid 500 mg
colchicine 0.5 mg
Uses: Antigout agent

Coldrine:
pseudoephedrine 30 mg
acetaminophen 500 mg
Uses: Decongestant, nonnarcotic analgesic

Coly-Mycin S Otic Suspension:
1% hydrocortisone
neomycin base 3.3 mg/ml
colistin 3 mg/ml
0.05% thonzonium bromide
Uses: Otic antiinfective

Combipres 0.1:
chlorthalidone 15 mg
clonidine 0.1 mg
Uses: Antihypertensive

Combipres 0.2:
chlorthalidone 15 mg
clonidine 0.2 mg
Uses: Antihypertensive

Combipres 0.3:
chlorthalidone 15 mg
clonidine 0.3 mg
Uses: Antihypertensive

Combivent:
ipratropium bromide 18 µg
albuterol 103 µg/actuation
Uses: Bronchodilator

Combivir:
lamivudine 150 mg
zidovudine 300 mg
Uses: Antiviral

Comhist Tablets:
phenylephrine 10 mg
chlorpheniramine 2 mg
phenyltoloxamine 25 mg
Uses: Adrenergic, antihistamine

Comhist LA:
phenylephrine 20 mg

---

* = Canada only   Side effects: *italics* = common; ***bold italics*** = life-threatening

chlorpheniramine 4 mg
phenyltoloxamine 50 mg
Uses: Adrenergic, antihistamine

Comtrex Liquid:
Per 5 ml:
chlorpheniramine 0.67 mg
acetaminophen 108.3 mg
dextromethorphan 3.3 mg
pseudoephedrine 10 mg
Uses: Antihistamine, analgesic, antitussive, decongestant

Comtrex Allergy-Sinus:
chlorpheniramine 2 mg
acetaminophen 500 mg
pseudoephedrine 30 mg
Uses: Antihistamine, analgesic, decongestant

Comtrex Liqui-Gels:
acetaminophen 325 mg
phenylpropanolamine 12.5 mg
chlorpheniramine 2 mg
dextromethorphan 10 mg
Uses: Analgesic, decongestant, antihistamine, antitussive

Comtrex Maximum Strength Caplets:
acetaminophen 500 mg
pseudoephedrine 30 mg
chlorpheniramine 2 mg
dextromethorphan 15 mg
Uses: Analgesic, decongestant, antihistamine, antitussive

Comtrex Maximum Strength Liqui-Gels:
acetaminophen 500 mg
phenylpropanolamine 12.5 mg
chlorpheniramine 2 mg
dextromethorphan 15 mg
Uses: Analgesic, decongestant, antihistamine, antitussive

Comtrex Maximum Strength Multi-Symptoms Cold, Flu Relief:
pseudoephedrine 30 mg
dextromethorphan 15 mg
chlorpheniramine 2 mg
acetaminophen 500 mg
Uses: Analgesic, decongestant, antihistamine, antitussive

Comtrex Maximum Strength Multi-Symptom Cold & Flu Relief Liqui-Gels:
acetaminophen 500 mg
phenylpropanolamine 12.5 mg
chlorpheniramine 2 mg
dextromethorphan 15 mg
Uses: Analgesic, decongestant, antihistamine, antitussive

Comtrex Maximum Strength Non-Drowsy Caplets:
acetaminophen 500 mg
pseudoephedrine 30 mg
dextromethorphan 15 mg
Uses: Analagesic, decongestant, antitussive

Congess SR:
guaifenesin 250 mg
pseudoephedrine 120 mg
Uses: Expectorant, decongestant

Congestac:
guaifenesin 400 mg
pseudoephedrine 60 mg
Uses: Expectorant, decongestant

Contac Cough & Chest Cold Liquid:
Per 5 ml:
pseudoephedrine 15 mg
dextromethorphan 5 mg
guaifenesin 50 mg
acetaminophen 125 mg
Uses: Decongestant, antitussive, expectorant, analgesic

Contac Cough & Sore Throat Liquid:
Per 5 ml:
dextromethorphan 5 mg
acetaminophen 125 mg
Uses: Antitussive, analgesic

Contac Day Allergy/Sinus:
pseudoephedrine 60 mg
acetaminophen 650 mg
Uses: Decongestant, analgesic

◆ = Nursing alert ／ = Herb-drug interaction ◯ = Do not crush

Contac Day Cold and Flu:
pseudoephedrine 60 mg
dextromethorphan 30 mg
acetaminophen 650 mg
Uses: Decongestant, antitussive, analgesic
Contac 12 Hour Capsules:
phenylpropanolamine 75 mg
chlorpheniramine 8 mg
Uses: Antihistamine
Contac Maximum Strength 12 Hour:
phenylpropanolamine 75 mg
chlorpheniramine 12 mg
Uses: Antihistamine
Contac Night Allergy Sinus:
pseudoephedrine 60 mg
diphenhydramine 50 mg
acetaminophen 650 mg
Uses: Decongestant, antihistamine, analgesic
Contac Night Cold and Flu Caplets:
pseudoephedrine 60 mg
diphenhydramine 50 mg
acetaminophen 650 mg
Uses: Decongestant, antihistamine, antitussive, analgesic
Contac Severe Cold & Flu Nighttime Liquid:
Per 5 ml:
pseudoephedrine 10 mg
chlorpheniramine 0.67 mg
dextromethorphan 5 mg
acetaminophen 167 mg
18.5% alcohol
Uses: Decongestant, antihistamine, antitussive, analgesic
Contuss Liquid:
Per 5 ml:
phenylpropanolamine 20 mg
phenylephrine 5 mg
guaifenesin 100 mg
Uses: Adrenergic, expectorant
Coricidin:
chlorpheniramine 2 mg
acetaminophen 325 mg
Uses: Antihistamine, analgesic
Coricidin 'D':
phenylpropanolamine 12.5 mg
chlorpheniramine 2 mg
acetaminophen 325 mg
Uses: Antihistamine, analgesic
Coricidin Maximum Strength Sinus Headache Caplets:
phenylpropanolamine 12.5 mg
chlorpheniramine 2 mg
acetaminophen 500 mg
Uses: Antihistamine, analgesic
Cortisporin Ophthalmic/Otic Suspension:
0.35% neomycin polymyxin B 10,000 U/ml
1% hydrocortisone
Uses: Ophthalmic antiinfective, antiinflammatory
Cortisporin Ophthalmic Ointment:
0.35% neomycin base
bacitracin 400 U
polymyxin B 10,000 U
hydrocortisone 1%
Uses: Ophthalmic antiinfective
Cortisporin Topical Cream:
0.5% neomycin sulfate
polymyxin B 10,000 U
0.5% hydrocortisone
Uses: Topical antiinfective
Cortisporin Topical Ointment:
0.5% neomycin sulfate
bacitracin 400 U
polymyxin B 5,000 U
1% hydrocortisone
Uses: Topical antiinfective
Corzide 40/5:
nadolol 40 mg
bendroflumethiazide 5 mg
Uses: Antihypertensive
Cough-X:
dextromethorphan 5 mg
benzocaine 2 mg
Uses: Antitussive, local anesthetic

---

* = Canada only   Side effects: *italics* = common; ***bold italics*** = life-threatening

Creon:
lipase 8,000 U
amylase 30,000 U
protease 13,000 U
pancreatin 300 mg
Uses: Digestive enzyme

Cyclomydril Ophthalmic Solution:
0.2% cyclopentolate
1% phenylephrine
Uses: Mydriatic

Dallergy Caplets:
chlorpheniramine 8 mg
phenylephrine 20 mg
methscopolamine 2.5 mg
Uses: Antihistamine, adrenergic

Dallergy Syrup:
Per 5 ml:
chlorpheniramine 2 mg
phenylephrine 10 mg
methscopolamine 0.625 mg
Uses: Antihistamine, adrenergic

Dallergy Tablets:
chlorpheniramine 4 mg
phenylephrine 10 mg
methscopolamine 1.25 mg
Uses: Antihistamine, adrenergic

Dallergy-D Syrup:
Per 5 ml:
phenylephrine 5 mg
chlorpheniramine 2 mg
Uses: Antihistamine, adrenergic

Damason-P:
hydrocodone 5 mg
aspirin 500 mg
Uses: Analgesic

Darvocet-N 100:
propoxyphene-N 100 mg
acetaminophen 650 mg
Uses: Analgesic

Darvon Compound-65:
propoxyphene 65 mg
aspirin 389 mg
caffeine 32.4 mg
Uses: Analgesic

Deconamine:
pseudoephedrine 60 mg

chlorpheniramine 4 mg
Uses: Antihistamine, decongestant

Deconamine CX:
hydrocodone 5 mg
pseudoephedrine 30 mg
guaifenesin 300 mg
Uses: Analgesic, decongestant, expectorant

Deconamine SR:
pseudoephedrine 120 mg
chlorpheniramine 8 mg
Uses: Antihistamine, decongestant

Deconamine Syrup:
Per 5 ml:
pseudoephedrine 30 mg
chlorpheniramine 2 mg
Uses: Antihistamine, decongestant

Defen-LA:
pseudoephedrine 60 mg
guaifenesin 600 mg
Uses: Decongestant, expectorant

Demazin:
phenylpropanolamine 25 mg
chlorpheniramine 4 mg
Uses: Antihistamine

Demi-Regroton:
chlorthalidone 25 mg
reserpine 0.125 mg
Uses: Antihypertensive

Demulen 1/50:
ethinyl estradiol 50 µg
ethynodiol diacetate 1 mg
Uses: Oral contraceptive

Dexacidin Ophthalmic Ointment/ Suspension:
Per ml:
0.1% dexamethasone
0.35% neomycin
polymyxin B 10,000 U/g
Uses: Ophth, antiinfective/antiinflammatory

Dexasporin Ophthalmic Ointment:
Per gram:
0.1% dexamethasone
0.35% neomycin
polymyxin B 10,000 U

Uses: Ophth, antiinfective/antiinflammatory

DHC Plus:
dihydrocodeine 16 mg
acetaminophen 356.4 mg
caffeine 30 mg
Uses: Analgesic

Dialose Plus:
docusate sodium 100 mg
yellow phenolphthalein 65 mg
Uses: Laxative

Dieutrim T.D.:
benzocaine 9 mg
phenylpropanolamine 75 mg
carboxymethylcellulose 75 mg
Uses: Top anesthetic

Di-Gel Advanced Formula:
magnesium hydroxide 128 mg
calcium carbonate 280 mg
simethicone 20 mg
Uses: Antacid, adsorbent, antiflatulent

Di-Gel Liquid:
Per 5 ml:
aluminum hydroxide 200 mg
magnesium hydroxide 200 mg
simethicone 20 mg
Uses: Antacid, adsorbent, antiflatulent

Dihistine DH Liquid:
Per 5 ml:
pseudoephedrine 30 mg
chlorpheniramine 2 mg
codeine 10 mg
Uses: Decongestant, antihistamine, analgesic

Dilaudid Cough Syrup:
Per 5 ml:
guaifenesin 100 mg
hydromorphone 1 mg
5% alcohol
Uses: Expectorant, analgesic

Dilor-G Liquid:
dyphylline 300 mg
guaifenesin 300 mg
Uses: Bronchodilator, expectorant

Dilor-G Tablets:
dyphylline 200 mg
guaifenesin 200 mg
Uses: Bronchodilator, expectorant

Dimetane Decongestant:
brompheniramine 4 mg
phenylephrine 10 mg
Uses: Antihistamine, adrenergic

Dimetane-DC Cough Syrup:
Per 5 ml:
brompheniramine 2 mg
phenylpropanolamine 12.5 mg
codeine 10 mg
Uses: Antihistamine, analgesic

Dimetane-DX Cough Syrup:
Per 5 ml:
brompheniramine 2 mg
pseudoephedrine 30 mg
dextromethorphan 10 mg
Uses: Antihistamine, decongestant, antitussive

Dimetapp:
brompheniramine 4 mg
phenylpropanolamine 25 mg
Uses: Antihistamine

Dimetapp Cold & Allergy Chewable:
phenylpropanolamine 6.25 mg
brompheniramine 1 mg
Uses: Antihistamine

Dimetapp Cold & Flu:
phenylpropanolamine 12.5 mg
brompheniramine 2 mg
acetaminophen 500 mg
Uses: Antihistamine, analgesic

Dimetapp DM Elixir:
Per 5 ml:
phenylpropanolamine 12.5 mg
brompheniramine 2 mg
dextromethorphan 10 mg
Uses: Antihistamine, antitussive

Dimetapp Elixir:
Per 5 ml:
phenylpropanolamine 12.5 mg
brompheniramine 2 mg
Uses: Antihistamine

---

* = Canada only   Side effects: *italics* = common; ***bold italics*** = life-threatening

Dimetapp Extentabs:
phenylpropanolamine 75 mg
brompheniramine 12 mg
Uses: Antihistamine

Dimetapp Sinus:
pseudoephedrine 30 mg
ibuprofen 200 mg
Uses: Decongestant, analgesic

Diutensin-R:
methylclothiazide 2.5 mg
reserpine 0.1 mg
Uses: Antihypertensive

Doan's PM Extra Strength:
magnesium salicylate 500 mg
diphenhydramine 25 mg
Uses: Analgesic, antihistamine

Dolacet:
hydrocodone 5 mg
acetaminophen 500 mg
Uses: Analgesic

Donnatal:
phenobarbital 16.2 mg
hyoscyamine 0.1037 mg
atropine 0.0194 mg
scopolamine 0.0065 mg
Uses: Anticholinergic, barbiturate

Donnatal Elixir:
Per 5 ml:
phenobarbital 16.2 mg
hyoscyamine 0.1037 mg
atropine 0.0194 mg
scopolamine 0.0065 mg
23% alcohol
Uses: Anticholinergic, barbiturate

Donnatal Extentabs:
phenobarbital 48.6 mg
hyoscyamine 0.3111 mg
atropine 0.0582 mg
scopolamine 0.0195 mg
Uses: Anticholinergic, barbiturate

Donnazyme:
pancreatin 500 mg
lipase 1000 U
protease 12,500 U
amylase 12,500 U
Uses: Pancreatic enzymes

Dorcol Children's Cold Formula Liquid:
Per 5 ml:
pseudoephedrine 15 mg
chlorpheniramine 1 mg
Uses: Decongestant, antihistamine

Doxidan:
docusate calcium 60 mg
phenolphthalein 65 mg
Uses: Stool softener

Dristan Cold:
pseudoephedrine 30 mg
acetaminophen 500 mg
Uses: Decongestant, analgesic

Dristan Cold Maximum Strength Caplets:
pseudoephedrine 30 mg
brompheniramine 2 mg
acetaminophen 500 mg
Uses: Decongestant, antihistamine, analgesic

Dristan Cold Multi-Symptom Formula:
acetaminophen 325 mg
phenylephrine 5 mg
chlorpheniramine 2 mg
Uses: Analgesic, adrenergic, antihistamine

Dristan Sinus:
pseudoephedrine 30 mg
ibuprofen 200 mg
Uses: Decongestant, analgesic

Drixoral Allergy Sinus:
pseudoephedrine 60 mg
dexbrompheniramine 3 mg
acetaminophen 500 mg
Uses: Decongestant, antihistamine, analgesic

Drixoral Cold & Allergy:
pseudoephedrine 120 mg
dexbrompheniramine 6 mg
Uses: Decongestant, antihistamine

Drixoral Cold & Flu:
pseudoephedrine 60 mg
dexbrompheniramine 3 mg
acetaminophen 500 mg

⬥ = Nursing alert   🖉 = Herb-drug interaction   🚫 = Do not crush

Uses: Decongestant, antihistamine, analgesic

Drixoral Cough & Congestion Liquid Caps:

pseudoephedrine 60 mg
dextromethorphan 30 mg
Uses: Decongestant, antitussive

Drixoral Cough & Sore Throat Liquid Caps:

dextromethorphan 15 mg
acetaminophen 325 mg
Uses: Antitussive, analgesic

Drixoral Plus:

pseudoephedrine 60 mg
dexbrompheniramine 3 mg
acetaminophen 500 mg
Uses: Decongestant, antihistamine, analgesic

DT:

Per 5 ml dose:
diphtheria toxoid 2LfU
tetanus toxoid 5LfU
Uses: Vaccine

DTP:

Per 0.5 ml dose:
diphtheria toxoid 6.5LfU
tetanus toxoid 5LfU
pertussis 4LfU
Uses: Vaccine

Dura-Vent:

phenylpropanolamine 75 mg
guaifenesin 600 mg
Uses: Expectorant

Dura-Vent/A:

phenylpropanolamine 75 mg
chlorpheniramine 10 mg
Uses: Antihistamine

Dura-Vent/DA:

phenylephrine 20 mg
chlorpheniramine 8 mg
methscopolamine 2.5 mg
Uses: Adrenergic, antihistamine

Dyazide:

hydrochlorothiazide 25 mg
triamterene 37.5 mg
Uses: Diuretic

Dylline-GG Liquid:

dyphylline 300 mg
guaifenesin 300 mg
Uses: Bronchodilator, expectorant

Dynafed Asthma Relief:

ephedrine 25 mg
guaifenesin 200 mg
Uses: Adrenergic, expectorant

Dynafed Plus Maximum Strength:

pseudoephedrine 30 mg
acetaminophen 500 mg
Uses: Decongestant, analgesic

Dyphylline-GG Elixir:

Per 5 ml:
dyphylline 100 mg
guaifenesin 100 mg
Uses: Bronchodilator, expectorant

E-Pilo-1 Ophthalmic Solution:

1% epinephrine bitartrate
1% pilocarpine
Uses: Miotic

E-Pilo-2 Ophthalmic Solution:

1% epinephrine bitartrate
2% pilocarpine
Uses: Miotic

E-Pilo-4 Ophthalmic Solution:

1% epinephrine bitartrate
4% pilocarpine
Uses: Miotic

Elase-Chloromycetin Ointment:

Per gram:
fibrinolysin 1 U
desoxyribonuclease 666.6 U
chloramphenicol 10 mg
Uses: Enzyme, antiinfective

Elase Ointment:

Per gram:
fibrinolysin 1 U
desoxyribonuclease 666.6 U
Uses: Enzyme

Elixophyllin GG Liquid:

Per 5 ml:
theophylline 100 mg
guaifenesin 100 mg
Uses: Expectorant, bronchodilator

EMLA Cream:
lidocaine 2.5 mg
prilocaine 2.5 mg
Uses: Local anesthetic
Empirin w/Codeine #3:
aspirin 325 mg
codeine phosphate 30 mg
Uses: Analgesic
Empirin w/Codeine #4:
aspirin 325 mg
codeine phosphate 60 mg
Uses: Analgesic
Enduronyl:
methyclothiazide 5 mg
deserpidine 0.25 mg
Uses: Diuretic
Entex:
phenylephrine 5 mg
phenylpropanolamine 45 mg
guaifenesin 200 mg
Uses: Adrenergic, expectorant
Entex LA:
phenylpropanolamine 75 mg
guaifenesin 400 mg
Uses: Adrenergic, expectorant
Entex PSE:
pseudoephedrine 120 mg
guaifenesin 600 mg
Uses: Adrenergic, expectorant
Epifoam Aerosol Foam:
1% hydrocortisone
1% pramoxine
Uses: Topical corticosteroid
Esgic-Plus:
butalbital 50 mg
acetaminophen 500 mg
caffeine 40 mg
Uses: Barbiturate, analgesic
Esimil:
guanethidine 10 mg
hydrochlorothiazide 25 mg
Uses: Antihypertensive
Estratest:
esterified estrogens 1.25 mg
methyltestosterone 2.5 mg
Uses: Androgen, estrogen

Etrafon:
perphenazine 2 mg
amitriptyline 25 mg
Uses: Antipsychotic, antidepressant
Etrafon Forte:
perphenazine 4 mg
amitriptyline 25 mg
Uses: Antipsychotic, antidepressant
Excedrin Migraine:
aspirin 250 mg
acetaminophen 250 mg
caffeine 65 mg
Uses: Migraine agent
Excedrin P.M.:
acetaminophen 500 mg
diphenhydramine citrate 38 mg
Uses: Analgesic, antihistamine
Excedrin P.M. Liquid:
Per 30 ml:
acetaminophen 1000 mg
diphenhydramine 50 mg
Uses: Analgesic, antihistamine
Excedrin P.M. Liquigels:
acetaminophen 500 mg
diphenhydramine 25 mg
Uses: Analgesic, antihistamine
Excedrin Sinus Extra Strength:
pseudoephedrine 30 mg
acetaminophen 500 mg
Uses: Decongestant, analgesic
Fansidar:
sulfidoxine 500 mg
pyrimethamine 25 mg
Uses: Antimalarial
Fedahist:
pseudoephedrine 60 mg
chlorpheniramine 4 mg
Uses: Decongestant, antihistamine
Fedahist Expectorant Syrup:
Per 5 ml:
guaifenesin 200 mg
pseudoephedrine 20 mg
Uses: Expectorant, decongestant
Fedahist Gyrocaps:
pseudoephedrine 65 mg

◆ = Nursing alert   ⫽ = Herb-drug interaction   🚫 = Do not crush

chlorpheniramine 10 mg
Uses: Decongestant, antihistamine
Fedahist Timecaps:
pseudoephedrine 120 mg
chlorpheniramine 8 mg
Uses: Decongestant, antihistamine
Feen-A-Mint Pills:
docusate sodium 100 mg
phenolphthalein 65 mg
Uses: Laxative
Fem-1:
acetaminophen 500 mg
pamabrom 25 mg
Uses: Nonnarcotic analgesic
Ferro-Sequels:
docusate sodium 100 mg
ferrous fumarate 150 mg
Uses: Laxative, hematinic
Fioricet:
acetaminophen 325 mg
caffeine 40 mg
butalbital 50 mg
Uses: Analgesic, barbiturate
Fioricet w/Codeine:
acetaminophen 325 mg
caffeine 40 mg
butalbital 50 mg
codeine 30 mg
Uses: Analgesic, barbiturate
Fiorinal:
aspirin 325 mg
caffeine 40 mg
butalbital 50 mg
Uses: Analgesic, barbiturate
Fiorinal with Codeine:
aspirin 325 mg
caffeine 40 mg
butalbital 50 mg
codeine 30 mg
Uses: Analgesic, barbiturate
FML-S Ophthalmic Suspension:
0.1% flurometholone
10% sulfacetamide
Uses: Ophth, antiinfective/antiinflammatory

Gas-Ban:
calcium carbonate 500 mg
simethicone 40 mg
Uses: Antiflatulent, antacid
Gas-Ban DS Liquid:
Per 5 ml:
aluminum hydroxide 400 mg
magnesium hydroxide 400 mg
simethicone 40 mg
Uses: Antiflatulent, antacid
Gaviscon:
magnesium trisilicate 20 mg
aluminum hydroxide 80 mg
Uses: Antacid, adsorbent, antiflatulent
Gaviscon Liquid:
Per 5 ml:
aluminum hydroxide 31.7 mg
magnesium carbonate 119.3 mg
Uses: Antacid, adsorbent, antiflatulent
Gelprin:
acetaminophen 125 mg
aspirin 240 mg
caffeine 32 mg
Uses: Analgesic
Gelusil:
aluminum hydroxide 200 mg
magnesium hydroxide 200 mg
simethicone 25 mg
Uses: Antacid, adsorbent, antiflatulent
Genatuss DM Syrup:
Per 5 ml:
guaifenesin 100 mg
dextromethorphan 10 mg
Uses: Expectorant, antitussive
Granulex Aerosol:
Per 0.82 ml:
trypsin 0.1 mg
balsam peru 72.5 mg
castor oil 650 mg
Uses: Top enzyme
Guaifenex PPA 75:
guaifenesin 600 mg

---

phenylpropanolamine 75 mg
Uses: Expectorant, decongestant
Guaifenex PSE 60:
pseudoephedrine 60 mg
guaifenesin 600 mg
Uses: Decongestant, expectorant
Guaifenex PSE 120:
pseudoephedrine 120 mg
guaifenesin 600 mg
Uses: Decongestant, expectorant
Haley's M-O Liquid:
Per 15 ml:
magnesium hydroxide 900 mg
mineral oil 3.75 ml
Uses: Laxative
Halotussin-DM Sugar Free Liquid:
Per 5 ml:
guaifenesin 100 mg
dextromethorphan 10 mg
Uses: Expectorant, antitussive
Helidac:
In a compliance package:
bismuth subsalicylate 262.4 mg tabs
metronidazole 250 mg tabs
tetracycline 500 mg caps
Uses: Antiinfective
Humibid DM Sprinkle Caps:
dextromethorphan 15 mg
guaifenesin 300 mg
Uses: Expectorant, antitussive
Humibid DM Tablets:
dextromethorphan 30 mg
guaifenesin 600 mg
Uses: Expectorant, antitussive
Hycodan:
hydrocodone 5 mg
homatropine 1.5 mg
Uses: Analgesic, mydriatic
Hycodan Syrup:
Per 5 ml:
hydrocodone 5 mg
homatropine 1.5 mg
Uses: Analgesic, mydriatic
Hycomine Compound:
chlorpheniramine 2 mg

acetaminophen 250 mg
phenylephrine 10 mg
hydrocodone 5 mg
caffeine 30 mg
Uses: Antihistamine, analgesic, adrenergic
Hycomine Syrup:
Per 5 ml:
hydrocodone 5 mg
phenylpropanolamine 25 mg
Uses: Analgesic, decongestant
Hycotuss Expectorant:
Per 5 ml:
guaifenesin 100 mg
hydrocodone 5 mg
10% alcohol
Uses: Expectorant
Hydro-Serp:
hydrochlorothiazide 50 mg
reserpine 0.125 mg
Uses: Antihypertensive
Hydrocet:
hydrocodone 5 mg
acetaminophen 500 mg
Uses: Narcotic, opioid analgesic
Hydrogesic:
hydrocodone 5 mg
acetaminophen 500 mg
Uses: Narcotic, opioid analgesic
Hydropres-50:
hydrochlorothiazide 50 mg
reserpine 0.125 mg
Uses: Antihypertensive
Hydroserpin #1:
hydrochlorothiazide 25 mg
reserpine 0.125 mg
Uses: Antihypertensive
Hyzaar:
losartan potassium 50 mg
hydrochlorothiazide 12.5 mg
potassium 4.24 mg
Uses: Antihypertensive
Iberet Filmtab:
ferrous sulfate 105 mg
ascorbic acid 150 mg

◆ = Nursing alert   ∅ = Herb-drug interaction   ⊘ = Do not crush

B-complex vitamins
Uses: Supplement
Iberet Liquid:
Per 5 ml:
ferrous sulfate 78.75 mg
ascorbic acid 112.5 mg
B-complex vitamins
Uses: Supplement
Imodium Advanced:
loperamide 2 mg
simethicone 125 mg
Uses: Antidiarrheal, antiflatulent
Inderide 40/25:
propranolol 40 mg
hydrochlorothiazide 25 mg
Uses: Antihypertensive
Innovar:
Per ml:
droperidol 2.5 mg
fentanyl 0.05 mg
Uses: Narcotic analgesic, general anesthetic
Iofed:
brompheniramine 12 mg
pseudoephedrine 120 mg
Uses: Antihistamine, adrenergic
Iofed PD:
brompheniramine 6 mg
pseudoephedrine 60 mg
Uses: Antihistamine, adrenergic
Iophen-C Liquid:
Per 5 ml:
iodinated glycerol 30 mg
codeine 10 mg
Uses: Expectorant, analgesic
Iophen-DM Liquid:
Per 5 ml:
iodinated glycerol 30 mg
dextromethorphan 10 mg
Uses: Expectorant, antitussive
Kondremul with Phenolphthalein:
Per 15 ml:
phenolphthalein 150 mg
55% mineral oil
Irish moss
Uses: Laxative

Lactinex:
Mixed culture of:
Lactobacillus acidophilus and
Lactobacillus bulgaricus
Uses: Supplement
Levsin PB Drops:
Per ml:
hyoscyamine 0.125 mg
phenobarbital 15 mg
5% alcohol
Uses: Anticholinergic, barbiturate
Levsin with Phenobarbital:
hyoscyamine 0.125 mg
phenobarbital 15 mg
Uses: Anticholinergic, barbiturate
Lexxel:
enalapril 5 mg
felodipine 5 mg
Uses: Antihypertensive
Librax:
chlordiazepoxide 5 mg
clidinium 2.5 mg
Uses: Antianxiety, anticholinergic
Lida-Mantel-HC-Cream:
0.5% hydrocortisone
3% lidocaine
Uses: Antiinflammatory, analgesic
Limbitrol DS 10-25:
chlordiazepoxide 10 mg
amitriptyline 25 mg
Uses: Antidepressant, antianxiety
Lobac:
salicylamide 200 mg
phenyltoloxamine 20 mg
acetaminophen 300 mg
Uses: Skeletal muscle relaxant, analgesic
Loestrin Fe 1.5/30:
norethindrone acetate 1.5 mg
ethinyl estradiol 30 μg
Uses: Oral contraceptive
Lomotil:
diphenoxylate 2.5 mg
atropine 0.025 mg
Uses: Antidiarrheal, anticholinergic

---

* = Canada only   Side effects: *italics* = common; ***bold italics*** = life-threatening

Lomotil Liquid:
Per 5 ml:
diphenoxylate 2.5 mg
atropine 0.025 mg
Uses: Antidiarrheal, anticholinergic

Lo Ovral:
ethinyl estradiol 30 μg
norgestrel 0.3 mg
Uses: Oral contraceptive

Lopressor HCT 50/25:
metoprolol 50 mg
hydrochlorothiazide 25 mg
Uses: Antihypertensive

Lopressor HCT 100/25:
metoprolol 100 mg
hydrochlorothiazide 25 mg
Uses: Antihypertensive

Lopressor HCT 100/50:
metoprolol 100 mg
hydrochlorothiazide 50 mg
Uses: Antihypertensive

Lorcet 10/650:
acetaminophen 650 mg
hydrocodone 10 mg
Uses: Analgesic

Lortab 2.5/500:
hydrocodone 2.5 mg
acetaminophen 500 mg
Uses: Analgesic

Lortab 5/500:
hydrocodone 5 mg
acetaminophen 500 mg
Uses: Analgesic

Lortab 7.5/500:
hydrocodone 7.5 mg
acetaminophen 500 mg
Uses: Analgesic

Lortab 10/500:
hydrocodone 10 mg
acetaminophen 500 mg
Uses: Analgesic

Lortab ASA:
aspirin 500 mg
hydrocodone 5 mg
Uses: Analgesic

Lortab Elixir:
Per 5 ml:
hydrocodone 2.5 mg
acetaminophen 167 mg
Uses: Analgesic

Lotensin HCT 5/6.25:
benazepril 5 mg
hydrochlorothiazide 6.25 mg
Uses: Antihypertensive

Lotensin HCT 10/12.5:
benazepril 10 mg
hydrochlorothiazide 12.5 mg
Uses: Antihypertensive

Lotensin HCT 20/12.5:
benazepril 20 mg
hydrochlorothiazide 12.5 mg
Uses: Antihypertensive

Lotensin HCT 20/25:
benazepril 20 mg
hydrochlorothiazide 25 mg
Uses: Antihypertensive

Lotrel 2.5/10:
amlopidine 2.5 mg
benazepril 10 mg
Uses: Antihypertensive

Lotrel 5/10:
amlodipine 5 mg
benazepril 10 mg
Uses: Antihypertensive

Lotrel 5/20:
amlodipine 5 mg
benazepril 20 mg
Uses: Antihypertensive

Lotrisone Topical:
0.05% betamethasone
1% clotrimazole
Uses: Local antiinfective, antiinflammatory

Lufyllin-EPG Elixir:
Per 5 ml:
dyphylline 150 mg
ephedrine 24 mg
guaifenesin 300 mg
phenobarbital 24 mg
Uses: Bronchodilator, expectorant

◆ = Nursing alert   ∥ = Herb-drug interaction   ⊘ = Do not crush

Lufyllin-EPG Tablets:
dyphylline 100 mg
ephedrine 16 mg
guaifenesin 200 mg
phenobarbital 16 mg
Uses: Bronchodilator, adrenergic, expectorant, barbiturate

Lufyllin-GG:
dyphylline 200 mg
guaifenesin 200 mg
Uses: Bronchodilator, expectorant

Lufyllin-GG Elixir:
dyphylline 100 mg
guaifenesin 100 mg
alcohol 17%
Uses: Bronchodilator, expectorant

M-M-R-II:
measles
mumps
rubella
Uses: Vaccine, toxoid

M-R Vax II:
measles
rubella
Uses: Vaccine, toxoid

Maalox:
aluminum hydroxide 200 mg
magnesium hydroxide 200 mg
Uses: Antacid, adsorbent, antiflatulent

Maalox Plus:
aluminum hydroxide 200 mg
magnesium hydroxide 200 mg
simethicone 25 mg
Uses: Antacid, adsorbent, antiflatulent

Maalox Plus Extra Strength Suspension:
Per 5 ml:
aluminum hydroxide 500 mg
magnesium hydroxide 450 mg
simethicone 40 mg
Uses: Antacid, adsorbent, antiflatulent

Maalox Suspension:
Per 5 ml:
aluminum hydroxide 225 mg
magnesium hydroxide 200 mg
Uses: Antacid, adsorbent, antiflatulent

Mapap Cold Formula:
acetaminophen 325 mg
chlorpheniramine 2 mg
pseudoephedrine 30 mg
dextromethorphan 15 mg
Uses: Bronchodilator, expectorant

Marax:
ephedrine 25 mg
theophylline 130 mg
hydroxyzine 10 mg
Uses: Bronchodilator, sedative/hypnotic

Maxitrol Ophthalmic Suspension/Ointment:
Per ml:
0.35% neomycin
0.1% dexamethasone
polymyxin B 10,000 U
Uses: Ophthalmic antiinfective, antiinflammatory

Maxzide:
hydrochlorothiazide 50 mg
triamterene 75 mg
Uses: Antihypertensive, diuretic

Maxzide-25 MG:
hydrochlorothiazide 25 mg
triamterene 37.5 mg
Uses: Diuretic

Medi-Flu Liquid:
Per 5 ml:
pseudoephedrine 10 mg
chlorpheniramine 0.67 mg
dextromethorphan 5 mg
acetaminophen 167 mg
18.5% alcohol
Uses: Decongestant, antihistamine, antitussive, analgesic

Mepergan Fortis:
meperidine 50 mg
promethazine 25 mg
Uses: Analgesic, antihistamine

Mepergan Injection:
meperidine 25 mg

promethazine 25 mg
Uses: Analgesic

Metimyd Ophthalmic Suspension/ Ointment:
0.5% prednisolone
10% sodium sulfacetamide
Uses: Ophthalmic antiinfective, anti-inflammatory

Midol Maximum Strength Multi-Symptom Menstrual Gelcaps:
acetaminophen 500 mg
pyrilamine 15 mg
caffeine 60 mg
Uses: Analgesic

Midol PM:
acetaminophen 500 mg
diphenhydramine 25 mg
Uses: Analgesic, antihistamine

Midol PMS Maximum Strength Caplets:
acetaminophen 500 mg
pyrilamine 15 mg
pamabrom 25 mg
Uses: Analgesic

Midol, Teen:
acetaminophen 400 mg
pamabrom 25 mg
Uses: Analgesic

Midrin:
isometheptene 65 mg
acetaminophen 325 mg
dichloralphenazone 100 mg
Uses: Analgesic

Minizide 1:
prazosin 1 mg
polythiazide 0.5 mg
Uses: Antihypertensive

Minizide 2:
prazosin 2 mg
polythiazide 0.5 mg
Uses: Antihypertensive

Minizide 5:
prazosin 5 mg
polythiazide 0.5 mg
Uses: Antihypertensive

Modane Plus:
docusate sodium 100 mg
phenolphthalein 65 mg
Uses: Laxative

Moduretic:
hydrochlorothiazide 50 mg
amiloride 5 mg
Uses: Diuretic

Motrin IB Sinus:
pseudoephedrine 30 mg
ibuprofen 200 mg
Uses: Adrenergic, analgesic

Murocoll-2 Ophthalmic Drops:
0.3% scopolamine
10% phenylephrine
Uses: Ophth anticholinergic, mydriatic

Mycolog II Topical:
Per gram:
0.1% triamcinolone acetonide
nystatin 100,000 U
Uses: Local antiinfective, antiinflammatory

Mylanta:
aluminum hydroxide 200 mg
magnesium hydroxide 200 mg
simethicone 20 mg
Uses: Antacid, adsorbent, antiflatulent

Mylanta Double Strength Liquid:
Per 5 ml:
aluminum hydroxide 400 mg
magnesium hydroxide 400 mg
simethicone 40 mg
Uses: Antacid, adsorbent, antiflatulent

Mylanta Gelcaps:
calcium carbonate 311 mg
magnesium carbonate 232 mg
Uses: Antacid, adsorbent, antiflatulent

Naldecon Tablets:
phenylpropanolamine 40 mg
phenylephrine 10 mg
phenyltoloxamine 15 mg

chlorpheniramine 5 mg
Uses: Antihistamine, decongestant
Naldecon CX Adult Liquid:
Per 5 ml:
guaifenesin 200 mg
phenylpropanolamine 12.5 mg
codeine 10 mg
Uses: Antihistamine
Naldecon DX Adult Liquid:
Per 5 ml:
dextromethorphan 10 mg
guaifenesin 200 mg
phenylpropanolamine 12.5 mg
Uses: Expectorant, decongestant
Naldecon DX Children's Syrup:
Per 5 ml:
dextromethorphan 5 mg
guaifenesin 100 mg
phenylpropanolamine 6.25 mg
Uses: Antihistamine, decongestant
Naldecon DX Pediatric Drops:
Per ml:
phenylpropanolamine 6.25 mg
dextromethorphan 5 mg
guaifenesin 50 mg
Uses: Antihistamine, decongestant
Naldecon EX Children's Syrup:
Per 5 ml:
guaifenesin 100 mg
phenylpropanolamine 6.25 mg
Uses: Antihistamine, decongestant
Naldecon EX Pediatric Drops:
Per ml:
phenylpropanolamine 6.25 mg
guaifenesin 50 mg
Uses: Antihistamine, decongestant
Naldecon Pediatric Drops:
Per ml:
phenylpropanolamine 5 mg
phenylephrine 1.25 mg
chlorpheniramine 0.5 mg
phenyltoloxamine 2 mg
Uses: Antihistamine, decongestant
Naldecon Pediatric Syrup:
Per 5 ml:
phenylpropanolamine 5 mg

phenylephrine 1.25 mg
chlorpheniramine 0.5 mg
phenyltoloxamine 2 mg
Uses: Antihistamine, decongestant
Naldecon Senior DX Liquid:
Per 5 ml:
dextromethorphan 10 mg
guaifenesin 200 mg
Uses: Expectorant, antitussive
Naldecon Syrup:
Per 5 ml:
chlorpheniramine 2.5 mg
phenylephrine 5 mg
phenylpropanolamine 20 mg
phenyltoloxamine 7.5 mg
Uses: Antihistamine, decongestant
Naphcon-A Ophthalmic Solution:
0.25% naphazoline
0.3% pheniramine
Uses: Ophth vasoconstrictor
Nasatab LA:
guaifenesin 500 mg
pseudoephedrine 120 mg
Uses: Expectorant, decongestant
NeoDecadron Ophthalmic Ointment:
0.35% neomycin
0.05% dexamethasone
Uses: Ophth antiinfective, antiinflammatory
NeoDecadron Ophthalmic Solution:
0.35% neomycin
0.1% dexamethasone
Uses: Ophth antiinfective, antiinflammatory
NeoDecadron Topical:
neomycin 0.5%
dexamethasone 0.1%
Uses: Top antiinfective, antiinflammatory
Neosporin Cream:
Per gram:
polymyxin B 10,000 U

neomycin 3.5 mg
Uses: Top antiinfective
Neosporin G.U. Irrigant:
Per ml:
neomycin 40 mg
polymyxin B 200,000 U
Uses: Antiinfective
Neosporin Ointment:
Per gram:
polymyxin B 5000 U
bacitracin zinc 400 U
neomycin 3.5 mg
Uses: Top antiinfective
Neosporin Ophthalmic Solution:
Per ml:
neomycin 1.75 mg
polymyxin B 10,000 U
gramicidin 0.025 mg
Uses: Ophthalmic antiinfective
Neosporin Ophthalmic Ointment:
Per gram:
neomycin 3.5 mg
polymyxin B 10,000 U
bacitracin zinc 400 U
Uses: Ophthalmic antiinfective
Neosporin Plus Cream:
polymyxin B 10,000 U
neomycin 3.5 mg
lidocaine 40 mg
Uses: Top antiinfective
Niferex-150 Forte:
ferrous sulfate 150 mg
vitamin B_{12} 25 μg
folic acid 1 mg
Uses: Supplement
Norgesic:
orphenadrine 25 mg
aspirin 385 mg
caffeine 30 mg
Uses: Skeletal muscle relaxant, analgesic
Norgesic Forte:
orphenadrine 50 mg
aspirin 770 mg
caffeine 60 mg

Uses: Skeletal muscle relaxant, analgesic
Novacet Lotion:
sodium sulfacetamine 10%
sulfur 5%
Uses: Acne agent
Novafed A:
pseudoephedrine 120 mg
chlorpheniramine 8 mg
Uses: Adrenergic, antihistamine
NuLytely:
PEG 3350/420 g
sodium bicarbonate 5.72 g
sodium chloride 11.2 g
potassium chloride 1.48 g
Uses: Laxative
NyQuil Hot Therapy:
Per packet:
acetaminophen 1000 mg
pseudoephedrine 60 mg
dextromethorphan 30 mg
doxylamine 12.5 mg
Uses: Analgesic, adrenergic, antitussive
NyQuil Nightime Cold/Flu Medicine Liquid:
Per 5 ml:
pseudoephedrine 10 mg
doxylamine 1.25 mg
dextromethorphan 5 mg
acetaminophen 167 mg
25% alcohol
Uses: Adrenergic, antitussive, analgesic
Octicair Otic Suspension:
hydrocortisone 1%
neomycin 5 mg/ml
polymyxin B 10,000 U/ml
Uses: Otic antiinflammatory, antiinfective
Opcon-A Ophthalmic Solution:
0.027% naphazoline
0.315% pheniramine
Uses: Ophth vasoconstrictor
Ornade:
phenylpropanolamine 75 mg

◆ = Nursing alert   ∥ = Herb-drug interaction   ⊘ = Do not crush

chlorpheniramine 12 mg
Uses: Antihistamine, decongestant
Ornex:
pseudoephedrine 30 mg
acetaminophen 500 mg
Uses: Adrenergic, analgesic
Ornex No Drowsiness Caplets:
acetaminophen 325 mg
pseudoephedrine 30 mg
Uses: Adrenergic, analgesic
Ortho-cept:
ethinyl estradiol 30 μg
desogestrel 0.15 mg
Uses: Oral contraceptive
Ortho-Novum 7/7/7:
Phase I:
0.5 mg norethindrone
35 μg ethinyl estradiol
Phase II:
0.75 mg norethindrone
35 μg ethinyl estradiol
Phase III:
1 mg norethinidrone
35 μg estradiol
Uses: Oral contraceptive
Otocort Otic Suspension:
hydrocortisone 1%
neomycin 5 mg/ml
polymyxin B 10,000 U
Uses: Otic antiinflammatory, antiinfective
Pain-X Topical:
0.05% capsaicin
5% menthol
4% camphor
Uses: Top analgesic
Pamprin Maximum Pain Relief:
acetaminophen 250 mg
pamabrom 25 mg
magnesium salicylate 250 mg
Uses: Analgesic
Pamprin Multi-Symptom:
acetaminophen 500 mg
pamabrom 25 mg
pyrilamine 15 mg
Uses: Analgesic

Panacet 5/500:
hydrocodone 5 mg
acetaminophen 500 mg
Uses: Analgesic
Panasal 5/500:
hydrocodone 5 mg
aspirin 500 mg
Uses: Analgesic
Pancrease Capsules:
amylase 20,000 U
protease 25,000 U
lipase 4500 U (microspheres)
Uses: Digestive enzyme
Pedia Care Cold-Allergy Chewable:
pseudoephedrine 15 mg
chlorpheniramine 1 mg
Uses: Adrenergic, antihistamine
Pedia Care Cough-Cold Liquid:
Per 5 ml:
pseudoephedrine 15 mg
chlorpheniramine 1 mg
dextromethorphan 5 mg
Uses: Adrenergic, antihistamine, antitussive
Pedia Care NightRest Cough-Cold Liquid:
Per 5 ml:
pseudoephedrine 15 mg
chlorpheniramine 1 mg
dextromethorphan 7.5 mg
Uses: Adrenergic, antihistamine, antitussive
Pediacof Syrup:
Per 5 ml:
codeine 5 mg
phenylephrine 2.5 mg
chlorpheniramine 0.75 mg
potassium iodide 75 mg
5% alcohol
Uses: Opioid, narcotic analgesic, antihistamine
Pediacon DX Children's Syrup:
Per 5 ml:
phenylpropanolamine 6.25 mg
guaifenesin 100 mg

dextromethorphan 5 mg
Uses: Expectorant, antitussive
Pediacon DX Pediatric Drops:
Per ml:
phenylpropanolamine 6.25 mg
guaifenesin 50 mg
dextromethorphan 5 mg
Uses: Expectorant, antitussive
Pediacon EX Drops:
phenylpropanolamine 6.25 mg
guaifenesin 50 mg
Uses: Antitussive, decongestant
Pediazole Suspension:
Per 5 ml:
erythromycin 200 mg
sulfisoxazole 600 mg
Uses: Antiinfective
Percocet:
oxycodone 5 mg
acetaminophen 325 mg
Uses: Analgesic
Percodan:
oxycodone 4.88 mg
aspirin 325 mg
Uses: Analgesic
Percogesic:
phenyltoloxamine 30 mg
acetaminophen 325 mg
Uses: Analgesic
Perdiem Granules:
Per teaspoon:
senna 0.74 g
psyllium 3.25 g
sodium 1.8 mg
potassium 35.5 mg
Uses: Laxative
Peri-Colace Capsules:
docusate sodium 100 mg
casanthranol 30 mg
Uses: Laxative
Peri-Colace Syrup:
Per 15 ml:
docusate sodium 60 mg
casanthranol 30 mg
Uses: Laxative

Phenerbel-S:
ergotamine tartrate 0.6 mg
belladonna alkaloids 0.2 mg
phenobarbital 40 mg
Uses: α-Adrenergic blocker, anticholinergic
Phenergan VC Syrup:
Per 5 ml:
phenylephrine 5 mg
promethazine 6.25 mg
Uses: Adrenergic, antihistamine
Phenergan VC w/Codeine Syrup:
Per 5 ml:
phenylephrine 5 mg
promethazine 6.25 mg
codeine 10 mg
Uses: Adrenergic, antihistamine, opioid analgesic
Phenergan w/Codeine Syrup:
Per 5 ml:
promethazine 6.25 mg
codeine 10 mg
Uses: Antihistamine, analgesic
Phenylfenesin LA:
phenylpropanolamine 75 mg
guaifenesin 400 mg
Uses: Decongestant, expectorant
Pherazine DM Syrup:
Per 5 ml:
dextromethorphan 15 mg
promethazine 6.25 mg
7% alcohol
Uses: Antitussive, antihistamine
Phillips' Laxative Gelcaps:
docusate sodium 83 mg
phenolphthalein 90 mg
Uses: Laxative
PMB-400:
conjugated estrogens 0.45 mg
meprobamate 400 mg
Uses: Oral contraceptive
Polaramine Expectorant Liquid:
Per 5 ml:
guaifenesin 100 mg
dexchlorpheniramine 2 mg

◆ = Nursing alert   ⫽ = Herb-drug interaction   ⃠ = Do not crush

pseudoephedrine 20 mg
7.5% alcohol
Uses: Expectorant
Polycillin-PRB Oral Suspension:
Per single dose:
ampicillin 3.5 g
probenecid 1 g
Uses: Antiinfective
Polycitra Syrup:
Per 5 ml:
potassium citrate 550 mg
sodium citrate 500 mg
citric acid 334 mg
Uses: Laxative
Poly-Histine Elixir:
Per 5 ml:
pheniramine 4 mg
pyrilamine 4 mg
phenyltoloxamine 4 mg
4% alcohol
Uses: Antihistamine
Poly-Histine DM Syrup:
Per 5 ml:
brompheniramine 2 mg
phenylpropanolamine 12.5 mg
dextromethorphan 10 mg
Uses: Antihistamine, antitussive
Poly-Histine CS Syrup:
Per 5 ml:
phenylpropanolamine 12.5 mg
brompheniramine 2 mg
codeine 10 mg
Uses: Antihistamine, analgesic
Poly-Pred Ophthalmic Suspension:
Per ml:
0.5% prednisolone acetate
0.35% neomycin
polymyxin B 10,000 U
Uses: Ophth antiinflammatory, anti-
    infective
Polysporin Ointment:
Per gram:
polymyxin B 10,000 U
bacitracin zinc 500 U
Uses: Top antiinfective

Polysporin Ophthalmic Ointment:
Per gram:
polymyxin B 10,000 U
bacitracin zinc 500 U
Uses: Ophthalmic antiinfective
Polytrim Ophthalmic:
Per ml:
trimethoprim 1 mg
polymyxin B 10,000 U
Uses: Ophthalmic antiinfective
Premphase:
In a compliance package:
conjugated estrogens 0.625 mg
medroxyprogesterone 5 mg
Uses: Oral contraceptive
Prempro:
In a compliance package:
conjugated estrogens 0.625 mg
medroxyprogesterone 2.5 mg
Uses: Oral contraceptive
Premsyn PMS:
acetaminophen 500 mg
pamabrom 25 mg
pyrilamine 15 mg
Uses: Analgesic
Prevpac:
In a compliance package:
amoxicillin 500 mg caps
clarithromycin 500 mg tabs
lansoprazole 30 mg caps
Uses: Antiinfective
Primatene:
theophylline 130 mg
ephedrine 24 mg
phenobarbital 7.5 mg
Uses: Bronchodilator, barbiturate
Primatene Dual Action:
theophylline 60 mg
ephedrine 12.5 mg
guaifenesin 100 mg
Uses: Bronchodilator, expectorant, ad-
    renergic
Primaxin 250 mg
I.V. for Injection:
imipenem 250 mg

---

* = Canada only   Side effects: *italics* = common; ***bold italics*** = life-threatening

cilastatin sodium 250 mg
Uses: Antiinfective
Primaxin 500 mg
I.V. for Injection:
imipenem 500 mg
cilastatin sodium 500 mg
Uses: Antiinfective
Prinzide 10-12.5:
lisinopril 10 mg
hydrochlorothiazide 12.5 mg
Uses: Antihypertensive
Prinzide 20-12.5:
lisinopril 20 mg
hydrochlorothiazide 12.5 mg
Uses: Antihypertensive
Prinzide 20-25:
lisinopril 20 mg
hydrochlorothiazide 25 mg
Uses: Antihypertensive
Probampacin Oral Suspension:
Per single dose:
ampicillin 3.5 g
probenecid 1 g
Uses: Antiinfective
Proben-C:
colchicine 0.5 mg
probenecid 500 mg
Uses: Antigout agent
Proctofoam-HC Aerosol Foam:
1% hydrocortisone
1% pramoxine
Uses: Topical corticosteroid
Propacet 100:
propoxyphene-N 100 mg
acetaminophen 650 mg
Uses: Analgesic
Pseudo-Chlor:
pseudoephedrine 120 mg
chlorpheniramine 8 mg
Uses: Antihistamine
Pseudo-Gest Plus:
pseudoephedrine 60 mg
chlorpheniramine 4 mg
Uses: Antihistamine
P-V-Tussin:
phenindamine 25 mg

guaifenesin 200 mg
hydrocodone 5 mg
Uses: Antihistamine, analgesic
Quadrinal:
ephedrine 24 mg
theophylline 65 mg
potassium iodide 320 mg
phenobarbital 24 mg
Uses: Adrenergic, bronchodilator, barbiturate
Quelidrine Cough Syrup:
Per 5 ml:
dextromethorphan 10 mg
phenylephrine 5 mg
ephedrine 5 mg
chlorpheniramine 2 mg
ammonium chloride 40 mg
ipecac 0.005 ml
Uses: Expectorant, adrenergic, antihistamine
Quibron-300:
theophylline 300 mg
guaifenesin 180 mg
Uses: Bronchodilator, expectorant
Quibron:
theophylline, 150 mg
guaifenesin 90 mg
Uses: Bronchodilator, expectorant
R&C Shampoo:
0.3% pyrethrins
3% piperonyl butoxide
Uses: Scabicide, pediculicide
Rauzide:
bendroflumethiazide 4 mg
powdered rauwolfia serpentina 50 mg
Uses: Diuretic, antihypertensive
Regroton:
chlorthalidone 50 mg
reserpine 0.25 mg
Uses: Diuretic, antihypertensive
Regulace:
docusate sodium 100 mg
casanthranol 30 mg
Uses: Laxative
Renese-R:
polythiazide 2 mg

◆ = Nursing alert   ∥ = Herb-drug interaction   ⊘ = Do not crush

reserpine 0.25 mg
Uses: Diuretic, antihypertensive
Respahist:
pseudoephedrine 60 mg
brompheniramine 6 mg
Uses: Adrenergic, antihistamine
Respaire-60:
guaifenesin 200 mg
pseudoephedrine 60 mg
Uses: Expectorant, adrenergic
RID Shampoo:
0.3% pyrethrins
3% piperonyl butoxide
Uses: Scabicide, pediculicide
Rifamate:
isoniazid 150 mg
rifampin 300 mg
Uses: Antitubercular, antileprotic
Rifater:
rifampin 120 mg
isoniazid 50 mg
pyrazinamide 300 mg
Uses: Antitubercular
Riopan Plus Suspension:
Per 5 ml:
magaldrate 540 mg
simethicone 40 mg
Uses: Antacid, adsorbent, antiflatulent
Robaxisal:
methocarbamol 400 mg
aspirin 325 mg
Uses: Skeletal muscle relaxant, analgesic
Robitussin A-C Syrup:
Per 5 ml:
codeine 10 mg
guaifenesin 100 mg
3.5% alcohol
Uses: Analgesic, expectorant
Robitussin-CF Liquid:
Per 5 ml:
guaifenesin 100 mg
dextromethorphan 10 mg
phenylpropanolamine 12.5 mg
4.75% alcohol

Uses: Antitussive, expectorant
Robitussin Cold & Cough Liqui-Gels:
pseudoephedrine 30 mg
guaifenesin 200 mg
dextromethorphan 10 mg
Uses: Antitussive, expectorant
Robitussin-DAC Syrup:
Per 5 ml:
codeine 10 mg
guaifenesin 100 mg
pseudoephedrine 30 mg
1.4% alcohol
Uses: Analgesic, expectorant, adrenergic
Robitussin-DM Liquid:
Per 5 ml:
guaifenesin 100 mg
dextromethorphan 10 mg
Uses: Expectorant, antitussive
Robitussin Maximum Strength Cough and Cold Liquid:
dextromethorphan 15 mg
pseudoephedrine 30 mg
Uses: Antitussive, adrenergic
Robitussin Night Relief Liquid:
dextromethorphan 5 mg
pyrilamine 8.3 mg
pseudoephedrine 10 mg
acetaminophen 108.3 mg
Uses: Antitussive, adrenergic
Robitussin Pediatric Cough & Cold Liquid:
Per 5 ml:
pseudoephedrine 15 mg
dextromethorphan 7.5 mg
Uses: Antitussive, adrenergic
Robitussin-PE Syrup:
guaifenesin 100 mg
pseudoephedrine 30 mg
1.4% alcohol
Uses: Expectorant, adrenergic
Robitussin Severe Congestion Liqui-Gels:
guaifenesin 200 mg
pseudoephedrine 30 mg

---

* = Canada only   Side effects: *italics* = common; ***bold italics*** = life-threatening

Uses: Expectorant, adrenergic
Rolaids Calcium Rich:
magnesium hydroxide 80 mg
calcium carbonate 412 mg
Uses: Antacid, adsorbent, antiflatulent
Rondec:
pseudoephedrine 60 mg
carbinoxamine 4 mg
Uses: Adrenergic
Rondec DM Drops:
Per ml:
pseudoephedrine 25 mg
carbinoxamine 2 mg
dextromethorphan 4 mg
Uses: Adrenergic, antitussive
Rondec DM Syrup:
Per 5 ml:
pseudoephedrine 60 mg
carbinoxamine 4 mg
dextromethorphan 15 mg
Uses: Adrenergic, antitussive
Rondec Oral Drops:
Per 5 ml:
pseudoephedrine 25 mg
carbinoxamine 2 mg
Uses: Adrenergic
Roxicet:
Per 5 ml:
acetaminophen 325 mg
oxycodone 5 mg
Uses: Opioid analgesic
Roxicet 5/500:
oxycodone 5 mg
acetaminophen 500 mg
Uses: Opioid analgesic
Ru-Tuss:
phenylephrine 25 mg
phenylpropanolamine 50 mg
chlorpheniramine 8 mg
hyoscyamine 0.19 mg
atropine 0.04 mg
scopolamine 0.01 mg
Uses: Antihistamine, anticholinergic
Ru-Tuss DE:
pseudoephedrine 120 mg

guaifenesin 600 mg
Uses: Adrenergic, expectorant
Ru-Tuss Expectorant Liquid:
Per 5 ml:
guaifenesin 100 mg
pseudoephedrine 30 mg
dextromethorphan 10 mg
10% alcohol
Uses: Adrenergic, expectorant, antitussive
Ru-Tuss w/Hydrocodone Liquid:
Per 5 ml:
hydrocodone 1.7 mg
phenylephrine 5 mg
pyrilamine 3.3 mg
pheniramine 3.3 mg
phenylpropanolamine 3.3 mg
5% alcohol
Uses: Analgesic, adrenergic, decongestant
Ryna-C Liquid:
Per 5 ml:
pseudoephedrine 30 mg
chlorpheniramine 2 mg
codeine 10 mg
Uses: Adrenergic, antihistamine, analgesic
Ryna Liquid:
Per 5 ml:
pseudoephedrine 30 mg
chlorpheniramine 2 mg
Uses: Adrenergic, antihistamine
Rynatan:
phenylephrine 25 mg
chlorpheniramine 8 mg
pyrilamine 25 mg
Uses: Adrenergic, antihistamine
Rynatan Pediatric Suspension:
Per 5 ml:
phenylephrine 5 mg
chlorpheniramine 2 mg
pyrilamine 12.5 mg
Uses: Adrenergic, antihistamine
Rynatuss:
ephedrine 10 mg
carbetapentane 60 mg

◆ = Nursing alert   ∥ = Herb-drug interaction   🚫 = Do not crush

chlorpheniramine 5 mg
phenylephrine 10 mg
Uses: Adrenergic, antihistamine
Salutensin:
hydroflumethiazide 50 mg
reserpine 0.125 mg
Uses: Antihypertensive
Salutensin Demi:
hydroflumethiazide 25 mg
reserpine 0.125 mg
Uses: Antihypertensive
Scot-Tussin DM Liquid:
Per 5 ml:
chlorpheniramine 2 mg
dextromethorphan 15 mg
Uses: Antihistamine, antitussive
**Scot-Tussin Original 5-Action
  Liquid:**
phenylephrine 4.2 mg
pheniramine 13.3 mg
sodium citrate 83.3 mg
sodium salicylate 83.3 mg
caffeine citrate 25 mg
Uses: Adrenergic, analgesic
Scot-Tussin Senior Clear Liquid:
Per 5 ml:
guaifenesin 200 mg
dextromethorphan 15 mg
Uses: Antitussive, expectorant
Sedapap-10:
acetaminophen 650 mg
butalbital 50 mg
Uses: Analgesic, barbiturate
Semprex-D:
acrivastine 8 mg
pseudoephedrine 60 mg
Uses: Adrenergic, bronchodilator
Senokot-S:
docusate 50 mg
senna concentrate 187 mg
Uses: Laxative
Septra:
sulfamethoxazole 400 mg
trimethroprim 80 mg
Uses: Antiinfective

Septra DS:
sulfamethoxazole 800 mg
trimethroprim 160 mg
Uses: Antiinfective
Septra I.V. for Injection:
Per 5 ml:
trimethoprim 80 mg
sulfamethoxazole 400 mg
Uses: Antiinfective
Septra Suspension:
Per 5 ml:
trimethoprim 40 mg
sulfamethoxazole 200 mg
Uses: Antiinfective
Ser-Ap-Es:
hydrochlorothiazide 15 mg
reserpine 0.1 mg
hydralazine 25 mg
Uses: Diuretic, antihypertensive
Silafed Syrup:
Per 5 ml:
pseudoephedrine 30 mg
triprolidine 1.25 mg
Uses: Adrenergic, antihistamine
Silaminic Cold Syrup:
Per 5 ml:
phenylpropanolamine 12.5 mg
chlorpheniramine 2 mg
Uses: Antihistamine
Silaminic Expectorant Liquid:
Per 5 ml:
phenylpropanolamine 12.5 mg
guaifenesin 100 mg
Uses: Expectorant
Sinarest Extra Strength:
pseudoephedrine 30 mg
chlorpheniramine 2 mg
acetaminophen 500 mg
Uses: Adrenergic, antihistamine, an-
  algesic
Sinarest No Drowsiness:
pseudoephedrine 30 mg
acetaminophen 500 mg
Uses: Adrenergic, analgesic
Sinarest Sinus:
pseudoephedrine 30 mg
chlorpheniramine 2 mg

acetaminophen 325 mg
Uses: Adrenergic, antihistamine, analgesic
Sine-Aid IB:
pseudoephedrine 30 mg
ibuprofen 200 mg
Uses: Adrenergic, analgesic
Sine-Aid Maximum Strength:
pseudoephedrine 30 mg
acetaminophen 500 mg
Uses: Adrenergic, analgesic
Sinemet 10/100:
carbidopa 10 mg
levodopa 100 mg
Uses: Antiparkinsonian
Sinemet 25/100:
carbidopa 25 mg
levodopa 100 mg
Uses: Antiparkinsonian
Sinemet 25/250:
carbidopa 25 mg
levodopa 250 mg
Uses: Antiparkinsonian
Sinemet CR 25-100:
carbidopa 25 mg
levodopa 100 mg
Uses: Antiparkinsonian
Sinemet CR 50-200:
carbidopa 50 mg
levodopa 200 mg
Uses: Antiparkinsonian
Sine-Off Maximum Strength No Drowsiness Formula Caplets:
pseudoephedrine 30 mg
acetaminophen 500 mg
Uses: Adrenergic, analgesic
Sine-Off Sinus Medicine:
pseudoephedrine 30 mg
chlorpheniramine 2 mg
acetaminophen 500 mg
Uses: Adrenergic, antihistamine, analgesic
Sinutab Maximum Strength Sinus Allergy:
acetaminophen 500 mg
pseudoephedrine 30 mg
chlorpheniramine 2 mg
Uses: Analgesic, adrenergic, antihistamine
Sinutab Maximum Strength Without Drowsiness:
acetaminophen 500 mg
pseudoephedrine 30 mg
Uses: Analgesic, adrenergic
Sinutab Non-Drying:
pseudoepedrine 30 mg
guaifenesin 200 mg
Uses: Adrenergic, expectorant
Slo-Phyllin GG Syrup:
theophylline 150 mg
guaifenesin 90 mg
Uses: Bronchodilator, expectorant
Synophylate-GG Syrup:
theophylline 150 mg
guaifenesin 100 mg
alcohol 15%
Uses: Bronchodilator, expectorant
Soma Compound:
carisoprodol 200 mg
aspirin 325 mg
Uses: Skeletal muscle relaxant, analgesic
Spec-T Lozenge:
dextromethorphan 10 mg
benzocaine 10 mg
Uses: Antitussive, topical anesthetic
St. Joseph Cold Tablets for Children:
phenylpropanolamine 3.125 mg
acetaminophen 80 mg
Uses: Decongestant, analgesic
Sudafed Cold & Cough Liquicaps:
pseudoephedrine 30 mg
dextromethorphan 10 mg
guaifenesin 100 mg
acetaminophen 250 mg
Uses: Adrenergic, antitussive, expectorant, analgesic
Sudafed Plus:
pseudoephedrine 60 mg
chlorpheniramine 4 mg
Uses: Adrenergic, antihistamine

⬥ = Nursing alert   🌿 = Herb-drug interaction   🚫 = Do not crush

Sudafed Severe Cold:
pseudoephedrine 30 mg
dextromethorphan 15 mg
Uses: Adrenergic, antitussive
Sudafed Sinus Maximum Strength:
pseudoephedrine 30 mg
acetaminophen 500 mg
Uses: Adrenergic, analgesic
Sudal 60/500:
pseudoephedrine 60 mg
guaifenesin 500 mg
Uses: Adrenergic, expectorant
Sudal 120/600:
pseudoephedrine 120 mg
guaifenesin 600 mg
Uses: Adrenergic, expectorant
Sultrin Triple Sulfa Vaginal Cream:
3.42% sulfathiazole
2.86% sulfacetamine
3.7% sulfabenzamide
Uses: Antiinfective
Sultrin Triple Sulfa Vaginal Tablets:
sulfathiazole 172.5 mg
sulfacetamide 143.75
sulfabenzamide 184 mg
Uses: Antiinfective
Synalgos-DC:
aspirin 356.4 mg
caffeine 30 mg
dihydrocodeine 16 mg
Uses: Analgesic
Synercid:
quinupristin 150 mg
dalfopristin 350 mg
Uses: Antiinfective
Talacen:
acetaminophen 650 mg
pentazocine 25 mg
Uses: Analgesic
Talwin Compound:
aspirin 325 mg
pentazocine 12.5 mg
Uses: Analgesic
Talwin NX:
pentazocine 50 mg

naloxone 0.5 mg
Uses: Analgesic, opioid antagonist
Tarka 182:
trandolapril 2 mg (immed rel)
verapamil 180 mg (sus rel)
Uses: Antihypertensive, calcium channel blocker
Tarka 241:
trandolapril 1 mg (immed rel)
verapamil 240 mg (sus rel)
Uses: Antihypertensive, calcium channel blocker
Tarka 242:
trandolapril 2 mg (immed rel)
verapamil 240 mg (sus rel)
Uses: Antihypertensive, calcium channel blocker
Tarka 244:
trandolapril 4 mg (immed rel)
verapamil 240 mg (sus rel)
Uses: Antihypertensive, calcium channel blocker
Tavist-D:
clemastine 1.34 mg
phenylpropanolamine 75 mg
Uses: Antihistamine, decongestant
Tavist Sinus:
acetaminophen 500 mg
pseudoephedrine 30 mg
Uses: Analgesic, adrenergic
Teczem:
enalapril 5 mg (extended release)
diltiazem 180 mg (extended release)
Uses: Antihypertensive, calcium channel blocker
Tedrigen:
ephedrine 22.5 mg
theophylline 120 mg
phenobarbital 7.5 mg
Uses: Adrenergic, bronchodilator, barbiturate
Tegrin-LT Shampoo:
0.33% pyrethrins
3.15% piperonyl butoxide
Uses: Scabicide, pediculicide

---

* = Canada only   Side effects: *italics* = common; ***bold italics*** = life-threatening

Tenoretic 50:
atenolol 50 mg
chlorthalidone 25 mg
Uses: Antihypertensive

Tenoretic 100:
atenolol 100 mg
chlorthalidone 25 mg
Uses: Antihypertensive

Terra-Cortril Ophthalmic Suspension:
1.5% hydrocortisone acetate
0.5% oxytetracycline
Uses: Ophth antiinflammatory, antiinfective

Terramycin with Polymycin B Sulfate Ophthalmic Ointment:
Per gram:
polymyxin B 10,000 units
oxytetracycline 5 mg
Uses: Ophth antiinfective

T-Gesic:
hydrocodone 5 mg
acetaminophen 500 mg
Uses: Analgesic

Theodrine:
ephedrine 22.5 mg
theophylline 120 mg
Uses: Adrenergic, bronchodilator

Theolate Liquid:
theophylline 150 mg
guaifenesin 90 mg
Uses: Bronchodilator, expectorant

Theophylline Kl Elixir:
theophylline 80 mg
potassium iodide 130 mg
Uses: Bronchodilator, expectorant

Thera-Flu, Flu & Cold Medicine Powder:
Per packet:
pseudoephedrine 60 mg
chlorpheniramine 4 mg
acetaminophen 650 mg
Uses: Adrenergic, antihistamine, analgesic

Thera-Flu, Flu, Cold & Cough Powder:
Per packet:
pseudoephedrine 60 mg
chlorpheniramine 4 mg
dextromethorphan 20 mg
acetaminophen 650 mg
Uses: Adrenergic, antihistamine, antitussive, analgesic

Thera-Flu NightTime Powder:
Per packet:
pseudoephedrine 60 mg
chlorpheniramine 4 mg
dextromethorphan 30 mg
acetaminophen 1000 mg
Uses: Adrenergic, antihistamine, antitussive, analgesic

Thera-Flu Non-Drowsy Flu, Cold & Cough Maximum Strength Powder
Per packet:
pseudoephedrine 60 mg
dextromethorphan 30 mg
acetaminophen 1000 mg
Uses: Adrenergic, antitussive, analgesic

Thera-Flu Non-Drowsy Formula Maximum Strength Caplets:
pseudoephedrine 30 mg
dextromethorphan 15 mg
acetaminophen 500 mg
Uses: Adrenergic, antitussive, analgesic

Timentin for Injection:
Per 3.1-g vial:
ticarcillin 3 g
clavulanic acid 0.1 g
Uses: Antiinfective

Timolide 10/25:
timolol 10 mg
hydrochlorothiazide 25 mg
Uses: Antihypertensive

Titralac Plus:
calcium carbonate 420 mg
simethicone 21 mg
Uses: Antacid, adsorbent, antiflatulent

◆ = Nursing alert   ∥ = Herb-drug interaction   ⊘ = Do not crush

Tobra Dex Ophthalmic Suspension/ Ointment:
tobramycin 0.3%
dexamethasone 0.1%
Uses: Ophth antiinfective, antiinflammatory

Triacin-C Cough Syrup:
Per 5 ml:
codeine 10 mg
pseudoephedrine 30 mg
triprolidine 1.25 mg
Uses: Analgesic, adrenergic, antihistamine

Tri-Hydroserpine:
hydralazine 25 mg
hydrochlorothiazide 15 mg
reserpine 0.1 mg
Uses: Antihypertensive

Tri-Levlen:
Phase I:
levonorgestrel 0.05 mg
ethinyl estradiol 30 µg
Phase II:
levonorgestrel 0.075 mg
ethinyl estradiol 40 µg;
Phase III:
levonorgestrel 0.125 mg
ethinyl estradiol 30 µg
Uses: Oral contraceptive

Triaminic Allergy:
phenylpropanolamine 25 mg
chlorpheniramine 4 mg
Uses: Antihistamine

Triaminic AM Cough & Decongestant Formula Liquid:
Per 5 ml:
pseudoephedrine 15 mg
dextromethorphan 7.5 mg
Uses: Adrenergic, antitussive

Triaminic Cold:
phenylpropanolamine 12.5 mg
chlorpheniramine 2 mg
Uses: Decongestant, antihistamine

Triaminic-DM Syrup:
Per 5 ml:
dextromethorphan 5 mg
phenylpropanolamine 6.25 mg
Uses: Antitussive, decongestant

Triaminic Expectorant Liquid:
Per 5 ml:
guaifenesin 50 mg
phenylpropanolamine 6.25 mg
Uses: Expectorant, decongestant

Triaminic Expectorant DH Liquid:
Per 5 ml:
guaifenesin 100 mg
hydrocodone 1.67 mg
phenylpropanolamine 12.5 mg
pheniramine 6.25 mg
pyrilamine 6.25 mg
5% alcohol
Uses: Analgesic, expectorant, decongestant

Triaminic Expectorant w/Codeine Liquid:
Per 5 ml:
phenylpropanolamine 12.5 mg
codeine 10 mg
guaifenesin 100 mg
Uses: Expectorant, decongestant, analgesic

Triaminic Nite Light Liquid:
Per 5 ml:
pseudoephedrine 15 mg
chlorpheniramine 1 mg
dextromethorphan 7.5 mg
Uses: Adrenergic, antihistamine, antitussive

Triaminic Oral Infant Drops:
Per ml:
phenylpropanolamine 20 mg
pyrilamine 10 mg
pheniramine 10 mg
Uses: Decongestant, antihistamine

Triaminic Sore Throat Formula Liquid:
Per 5 ml:
pseudoephedrine 15 mg
dextromethorphan 7.5 mg
acetaminophen 160 mg
Uses: Adrenergic, antitussive

Triaminic Syrup:
Per 5 ml:
phenylpropanolamine 6.25 mg
chlorpheniramine 1 mg
Uses: Decongestant, antihistamine

Triaminicin Cold, Allergy, Sinus:
phenylpropanolamine 25 mg
chlorpheniramine 4 mg
acetaminophen 650 mg
Uses: Decongestant, antihistamine analgesic

Triaminicol Multi-Symptom Cough, Cold:
phenylpropanolamine 12.5 mg
chlorpheniramine 2 mg
dextromethorphan 10 mg
Uses: Decongestant, antihistamine, antitussive

Triaminicol Multi-Symptom Relief Liquid:
Per 5 ml:
phenylpropanolamine 12.5 mg
chlorpheniramine 2 mg
dextromethorphan 10 mg
Uses: Decongestant, antihistamine, antitussive

Triavil 2-10:
perphenazine 2 mg
amitriptyline 10 mg
Uses: Antidepressant, antipsychotic

Triavil 4-10:
perphenazine 4 mg
amitriptyline 10 mg
Uses: Antidepressant, antipsychotic

Triavil 2-25:
perphenazine 2 mg
amitriptyline 25 mg
Uses: Antidepressant, antipsychotic

Triminol Cough Syrup:
Per 5 ml:
dextromethorphan 10 mg
chlorpheniramine 2 mg
phenylpropanolamine 12.5 mg
Uses: Antitussive, antihistamine, decongestant

Trinalin Repetabs:
azatadine maleate 1 mg
pseudoephedrine 120 mg
Uses: Antihistamine

Triphasil:
Phase I:
levonorgestrel 0.05 mg
ethinyl estradiol 30 µg
Phase II:
levonorgestrel 0.075 mg
ethinyl estradiol 40 µg
Phase III:
levonorgestrel 0.125 mg
ethinyl estradiol 30 µg
Uses: Oral contraceptive

Triple Antibiotic Ophthalmic Ointment:
Per gram:
polymyxin B 10,000 U
neomycin 3.5 mg
bacitracin 400 U
Uses: Antiinfective

Tuinal 100 mg:
amobarbital 50 mg
secobarbital 50 mg
Uses: Sedative-hypnotic

Tuinal 200 mg:
amobarbital 100 mg
secobarbital 100 mg
Uses: Sedative-hypnotic

Tusibron-DM Syrup:
Per 5 ml:
guaifenesin 100 mg
dextromethorphan 15 mg
Uses: Expectorant, antitussive

Tussionex Pennkinetic Suspension:
Per 5 ml:
chlorpheniramine 8 mg
hydrocodone 10 mg
Uses: Antihistamine, analgesic

Tussi-Organidin NR Liquid:
Per 5 ml:
codeine 10 mg
guaifenesin 100 mg
Uses: Analgesic, expectorant

◆ = Nursing alert   🖋 = Herb-drug interaction   ⊘ = Do not crush

Tussi-Organidin DM NR Liquid:
Per 5 ml:
guaifenesin 100 mg
dextromethorphan 10 mg
Uses: Expectorant, antitussive

Tylenol Allergy Sinus, Maximum Strength Gelcaps:
acetaminophen 500 mg
chlorpheniramine 2 mg
pseudoephedrine 30 mg
Uses: Antihistamine, adrenergic, analgesic

Tylenol Children's Cold:
acetaminophen 80 mg
chlorpheniramine 0.5 mg
pseudoephedrine 7.5 mg
Uses: Antihistamine, adrenergic, analgesic

Tylenol Children's Cold Liquid:
Per 5 ml:
acetaminophen 160 mg
chlorpheniramine 1 mg
pseudoephedrine 15 mg
Uses: Antihistamine, adrenergic, analgesic

Tylenol Children's Cold Multi-Symptom Plus Cough Liquid:
Per 5 ml:
acetaminophen 160 mg
dextromethorphan 5 mg
chlorpheniramine 1 mg
pseudoephedrine 15 mg
Uses: Antihistamine, adrenergic, analgesic

Tylenol Children's Cold Plus Cough Chewable:
acetaminophen 80 mg
pseudoephedrine 7.5 mg
dextromethorphan 2.5 mg
chlorpheniramine 0.5 mg
Uses: Antihistamine, adrenergic, analgesic

Tylenol Cold Multi-Symptom:
acetaminophen 325 mg
chlorpheniramine 2 mg
pseudoephedrine 30 mg

dextromethorphan 15 mg
Uses: Antihistamine, adrenergic, analgesic

Tylenol Cold No Drowsiness:
acetaminophen 325 mg
pseudoephedrine 30 mg
dextromethorphan 15 mg
Uses: Analgesic, adrenergic, antitussive

Tylenol Flu Maximum Strength Gelcaps:
dextromethorphan 15 mg
pseudoephedrine 30 mg
acetaminophen 500 mg
Uses: Analgesic, adrenergic, antitussive

Tylenol Flu NightTime Maximum Strength Gelcaps:
pseudoephedrine 30 mg
chlorpheniramine 2 mg
acetaminophen 500 mg
Uses: Adrenergic, antihistamine, analgesic

Tylenol Flu NightTime Maximum Strength Powder:
pseudoephedrine 60 mg
diphenhydramine 50 mg
acetaminophen 1000 mg
Uses: Adrenergic, antihistamine, analgesic

Tylenol Headache Plus, Extra Strength:
acetaminophen 500 mg
calcium carbonate 250 mg
Uses: Analgesic, antacid

Tylenol Multi-Symptom Cough Liquid:
Per 5 ml:
dextromethorphan 10 mg
acetaminophen 216.7 mg
5% alcohol
Uses: Antitussive, analgesic

Tylenol Multi-Symptom Cough w/Decongestant Liquid:
Per 5 ml:
dextromethorphan 10 mg

acetaminophen 200 mg
pseudoephedrine 20 mg
Uses: Antitussive, analgesic, adrenergic

Tylenol Multi-Symptom Hot Medication:
Per packet:
acetaminophen 650 mg
chlorpheniramine 4 mg
pseudoephedrine 60 mg
dextromethorphan 30 mg
Uses: Analgesic, antihistamine, adrenergic, antitussive

Tylenol PM, Extra Strength:
acetaminophen 500 mg
diphenhydramine 25 mg
Uses: Analgesic, antihistamine

Tylenol Severe Allergy:
diphenhydramine 12.5 mg
acetaminophen 500 mg
Uses: Analgesic, antihistamine

Tylenol Sinus Maximum Strength:
pseudoephedrine 30 mg
acetaminophen 500 mg
Uses: Adrenergic, analgesic

Tylenol with Codeine Elixir:
Per 5 ml:
acetaminophen 120 mg
codeine 12 mg
Uses: Analgesic

Tylenol with Codeine No. 2:
acetaminophen 300 mg
codeine 15 mg
Uses: Analgesic

Tylenol with Codeine No. 3:
acetaminophen 300 mg
codeine 30 mg
Uses: Analgesic

Tylenol with Codeine No. 4:
acetaminophen 300 mg
codeine 60 mg
Uses: Analgesic

Tylox:
oxycodone 5 mg
acetaminophen 500 mg
Uses: Analgesic

Tyrodone Liquid:
Per 5 ml:
hydrocodone 5 mg
pseudoephedrine 60 mg
5% alcohol
Uses: Analgesic, adrenergic

Unasyn for Injection 1.5 g:
ampicillin 1 g
sulbactam 0.5 g
Uses: Antiinfective

Unasyn for Injection 3 g:
ampicillin 2 g
sulbactam 1 g
Uses: Antiinfective

Uniretic:
moexipril 7.5 mg
hydrochlorothiazide 12.5 mg
or moexipril 15 mg
hydrochlorothiazide 25 mg
Uses: Antihypertensive, diuretic

Unituss HC Syrup:
hydrocodone 2.5 mg
phenylephrine 5 mg
chlorpheniramine 2 mg
Uses: Analgesic, adrenergic, antihistamine

Urised:
methenamine 40.8 mg
phenylsalicylate 18.1 mg
atropine 0.03 mg
hyoscyamine 0.03 mg
benzoic acid 4.5 mg
methylene blue 5.4 mg
Uses: Antiinfective

Ursinus Inlay:
pseudoephedrine 30 mg
aspirin 325 mg
Uses: Adrenergic, analgesic

Vanquish:
aspirin 227 mg
acetaminophen 194 mg
caffeine 33 mg
Uses: Nonnarcotic analgesic

Vaseretic 10-25:
enalapril 10 mg

hydrochlorothiazide 25 mg
Uses: Antihypertensive, diuretic
Vasocidin Ophthalmic Ointment:
sulfacetamide 10%
prednisolone 0.5%
Uses: Ophthalmic antiinfective, anti-inflammatory
Vasocidin Ophthalmic Solution:
sulfacetamide 10%
prednisolone 0.25%
Uses: Ophthalmic antiinfective, anti-inflammatory
Vasocon-A Ophthalmic Solution:
naphazoline 0.05%
antazoline 0.5%
Uses: Ophthalmic vasoconstrictor
Vicks 44D Cough & Head Congestion Liquid:
Per 5 ml:
dextromethorphan 10 mg
pseudoephedrine 20 mg
Uses: Antitussive, adrenergic
Vicks 44E Liquid:
Per 5 ml:
dextromethorphan 6.7 mg
guaifenesin 66.7 mg
Uses: Antitussive, expectorant
Vicks 44M Cold, Flu, & Cough LiquiCaps:
dextromethorphan 10 mg
pseudoephedrine 30 mg
chlorpheniramine 2 mg
acetaminophen 250 mg
Uses: Antitussive, adrenergic, antihistamine, analgesic
Vicks 44 Non-Drowsy Cold & Cough LiquiCaps:
dextromethorphan 30 mg
pseudoephedrine 60 mg
Uses: Antitussive, adrenergic
Vicks Children's NyQuil Nighttime Cough/Cold Liquid:
Per 5 ml:
pseudoephedrine 10 mg
chlorpheniramine 0.67 mg

dextromethorphan 5 mg
Uses: Adrenergic, antihistamine, antitussive
Vicks Cough Silencers:
dextromethorphan 2.5 mg
benzocaine 1 mg
Uses: Antitussive, top anesthetic
Vicks DayQuil Allergy Relief 4 Hour:
phenylpropanolamine 25 mg
brompheniramine 4 mg
Uses: Decongestant, antihistamine
Vicks DayQuil Allergy Relief 12 Hour ER:
phenylpropanolamine 75 mg
brompheniramine 12 mg
Uses: Decongestant, antihistamine
Vicks DayQuil Liquid:
Per 5 ml:
dextromethorphan 3.3 mg
pseudoephedrine 10 mg
acetaminophen 108.3 mg
guaifenesin 33.3 mg
Uses: Antitussive, adrenergic, analgesic, expectorant
Vicks DayQuil Sinus Pressure & Pain Relief:
pseudoephedrine 30 mg
acetaminophen 500 mg
Uses: Adrenergic, analgesic
Vicks NyQuil Liquicaps:
pseudoephedrine 30 mg
doxylamine 6.25 mg
dextromethorphan 10 mg
acetaminophen 250 mg
Uses: Adrenergic, antihistamine, antitussive, analgesic
Vicks NyQuil Multi-Symptom Cold Flu Relief Liquid:
pseudoephedrine 10 mg
doxylamine 2.1 mg
dextromethorphan 5 mg
acetaminophen 167 mg
Uses: Adrenergic, antihistamine, antitussive, analgesic

Vicks Pediatric Formula 44e Liquid:
Per 5 ml:
dextromethorphan 3.3 mg
guaifenesin 33.3 mg
Uses: Expectorant, antitussive

Vicks Pediatric Formula 44 m Multi-Symptom Cough & Cold Liquid
pseudoephedrine 10 mg
chlorpheniramine 0.67 mg
dextromethorphan 5 mg
Uses: Adrenergic, antihistamine, antitussive

Vicodin:
acetaminophen 500 mg
hydrocodone 5 mg
Uses: Analgesic

Vicodin ES:
acetaminophen 750 mg
hydrocodone 7.5 mg
Uses: Analgesic

Vicodin HP:
hydrocodone 10 mg
acetaminophen 660 mg
Uses: Analgesic

VicodinTuss:
Per 5 ml:
hydrocodone 5 mg
guaifenesin 100 mg
Uses: Analgesic, expectorant

Vicoprofen:
hydrocodone 7.5 mg
ibuprofen 200 mg
Uses: Analgesic

Wigraine Suppositories:
ergotamine 2 mg
caffeine 100 mg
Uses: α-adrenergic blocker

Zestoretic 10/12.5:
lisinopril 10 mg
hydrochlorothiazide 12.5 mg
Uses: Antihypertensive

Zestoretic 20/12.5:
lisinopril 20 mg
hydrochlorothiazide 12.5 mg
Uses: Antihypertensive

Zestoretic 20/25:
lisinopril 20 mg
hydrochlorothiazide 25 mg
Uses: Antihypertensive

Ziac 2.5:
bisoprolol 2.5 mg
hydrochlorothiazide 6.25 mg
Uses: Antihypertensive

Ziac 5:
bisoprolol 5 mg
hydrochlorothiazide 6.25 mg
Uses: Antihypertensive

Ziac 10:
bisoprolol 10 mg
hydrochlorothiazide 6.25 mg
Uses: Antihypertensive

Zydone:
hydrocodone 5 mg
acetaminophen 500 mg
Uses: Analgesic

◆ = Nursing alert   ✦ = Herb-drug interaction   🚫 = Do not crush

Appendix f

Rarely used drugs

abciximab (℞)
(ab-six′i-mab)
ReoPro
Functional class.: Platelet aggregation inhibitor

Dosage and routes: *Adult:* **IV** 250 µg (0.25 mg)/kg bolus 10-60 min prior to PTCA, followed by 10 µg/min **CONT INF** for 12 hr
Uses: Used with heparin and aspirin to prevent acute cardiac ischemia following percutaneous transluminal angioplasty (PTCA) in patients at high risk for reclosure of affected arteries
Contraindications: Hypersensitivity to this drug or murine protein; GI, GU bleeding; CVA within 2 yr, bleeding disorders, intracranial neoplasm, intracranial arteriovenous malformations, intracranial aneurysm, platelet count >100,000/mm^3, recent surgery, aneurysm, uncontrolled severe hypertension, vasculitis

aminocaproic acid (℞)
(a-mee-noe-ka-proe′ik)
Amicar, aminocaproic acid, EACA
Functional class.: Hemostatic

Dosage and routes: *Adult:* **PO/IV** 5 g loading dose, then 1-1.25 g q1h if needed, not to exceed 30 g/day
Uses: Hemorrhage from hyperfibrinolysis, adjunctive therapy in hemophilia

Contraindications: Hypersensitivity, abnormal bleeding, postpartum bleeding, DIC, upper urinary tract bleeding, new burns

ammonium chloride (PO-OTC, IV-℞)
(ah-mohn′ee-um klor′ide)
ammonium chloride
Functional class.: Acidifier

Dosage and routes:
Alkalosis: Adult and child: **IV INF** 0.9-1.3 ml/min of a 2.14% sol, not to exceed 5 ml/min
Acidifier: Adult: **PO** 4-12 g/day in divided doses; *Child:* **PO** 75 mg/kg/day in divided doses
Expectorant: Adult: **PO** 250-500 mg q2-4h as needed
Uses: Alkalosis (metabolic), systemic and urinary acidifier, expectorant, diuretic
Contraindications: Hypersensitivity, severe hepatic disease, severe renal disease

amyl nitrite (℞)
(am′il nye′trite)
amyl nitrite, Amyl Nitrite Aspirols, Amyl Nitrite Vaporole
Functional class.: Coronary vasodilator

Dosage and routes:
Angina: Adult: **INH** 0.18-0.3 ml as needed, 1-6 inhalations from 1 cap, may repeat in 3-5 min

Cyanide poisoning: Adult: **INH** 0.3 ml ampule inhaled 15 sec until preparation of sodium nitrite infusion is ready

Uses: Acute angina pectoris, cyanide poisoning

Investigational uses: Cardiac murmur diagnosis

Contraindications: Hypersensitivity to nitrites, severe anemia, increased intracranial pressure, hypertension, pregnancy (X)

benzonatate (℞)
(ben-zoe'na-tate)
Tessalon Perles

Functional class.: Antitussive, nonnarcotic

Dosage and routes: *Adult and child:* **PO** 100 mg tid, not to exceed 600 mg/day; *Child <10 yr:* **PO** 8 mg/kg in 3-6 divided doses

Uses: Nonproductive cough
Contraindications: Hypersensitivity

benzoyl peroxide (OTC)
(ben'zoe-ill per-ox'ide)

Functional class.: Antiacne medication

Dosage and routes: *Adult and child:* **TOP** apply to affected area qd or bid

Uses: Mild to moderate acne
Contraindications: Hypersensitivity to benzoic acid derivatives

benzquinamide (℞)
(benz-kwin'a-mide)
Emete-Con

Functional class.: Antiemetic

Dosage and routes: *Adult:* **IM** 50 mg or 0.5-1 mg/kg, may be repeated in 1 hr, then q3-4h prn; **IV** 25 mg or 0.2-0.4 mg/kg as a one-time dose

Uses: To inhibit nausea, vomiting associated with anesthetic, surgery
Contraindications: Hypersensitivity, hypertension

beractant (℞)
(ber-ak'tant)
Survanta

Functional class.: Natural lung surfactant

Dosage and routes: **INTRATRACHEAL INSTILL:** 4 doses can be administered in the 1st 48 hrs of life; give doses no more frequently than q6h; each dose is 100 mg of phospholipids/kg birth weight (4 ml/kg)

Uses: Prevention and treatment (rescue) of respiratory distress syndrome in premature infants

cabergoline (℞)
(ka-bear'joe-leen)
Dostinex

Functional class.: Dopamine receptor/agonist

Dosage and routes:

Hyperprolactinemic indications:
Adult: **PO** 0.25 mg 2×/wk, may increase by 0.25 mg 2×/wk at 4 wk intervals, max 1 mg 2×/wk; maintenance therapy may be needed for 6 mo

Uses: Reduced prolactin/secretion in postpartum lactation
Contraindications: Hypersensitivity, uncontrolled hypertension

◆ = Nursing alert   🖋 = Herb-drug interaction   🚫 = Do not crush

chlorpropamide (℞)

(klor-proe'pa-mide)

Chloronase*, Chlorpropamide, Diabinese, Novopropamide*

Functional class.: Antidiabetic

Dosage and routes: *Adult:* **PO** 100-250 mg qd, initially, then 100-500 mg maintenance according to response; not to exceed 750 mg/day

Uses: Stable adult-onset diabetes mellitus (type II) NIDDM

Contraindications: Hypersensitivity to sulfonylureas, juvenile or brittle diabetes, pregnancy (D), lactation, renal failure

colfosceril (℞)

(kole-foss'er-ill)

Exosurf Neonatal

Functional class.: Synthetic lung surfactant

Dosage and routes:
Prophylactic treatment: Endotracheally: 5 ml/kg as soon as possible after birth and repeat doses 12 and 24 hr later to infants remaining on mechanical ventilation

Rescue treatment: Endotracheally: Administer in two 2.5 ml/kg doses; give initial dose after treatment of RDS, then second dose in 12 hr

Uses: Treatment of respiratory distress syndrome (RDS) in premature infants

cosyntropin (℞)

(koe-sin-troe'pin)

Cortrosyn, Synacthen*, Tetracosactrin

Functional class.: Pituitary hormone

Dosage and routes: *Adult and child >2 yr:* **IM/IV** 0.25-1 mg between blood sampling; *Child <2 yr:* **IM/IV** 0.125 mg

Uses: Testing adrenocortical function

Contraindications: Hypersensitivity

crotamiton (℞)

(kroe-tam'i-ton)

Functional class.: Scabicide

Dosage and routes:
Scabies: Adult and child: **CREAM** wash area with soap, water; remove visible crusts, apply cream, apply another coat in 24 hr, remove with soap, water in 48 hr

Pruritus: Massage into affected area, repeat as necessary

Uses: Scabies, pruritus

Contraindications: Hypersensitivity, skin inflammation, abrasions, breaks in skin, mucous membranes

deferoxamine (℞)

(de-fer-ox'a-meen)

Desferal

Functional class.: Heavy metal antagonist

Dosage and routes:
Acute iron toxicity: Adult and child: **IM/IV** 1 g, then 500 mg q4h × 2 doses, then 500 mg q4-12h × 2 doses, not to exceed 15 mg/kg/hr or 6 g/24 hr

Chronic iron toxicity: Adult and child: **IM** 500 mg-1 g/day plus **IV INF** 2 g given by separate line with each blood transfusion, not to exceed 15 mg/kg/hr or 6 g/24 hr; **SC** 1-2 g over 8-24 hr by SC infusion pump

Uses: Acute, chronic iron intoxication, hemochromatosis, hemosiderosis

---

Contraindications: Hypersensitivity, anuria, severe renal disease, child <3 yr

---

delavirdine (R)
(de-la-veer'din)
Rescriptor
Functional class.: Non-nucleoside reverse transcriptase inhibitor (NNRTI)

Dosage and routes: *Adult and child ≥16 yr:* 400 mg tid in combination with zidovudine or didanosine
Uses: HIV-1 in combination with zidovudine or didanosine
Contraindications: Hypersensitivity to this drug or atevirdine

---

desipramine (R)
(dess-ip'ra-meen)
desipramine HCl, Norpramin, Pertofrane
Functional class.: Antidepressant tricyclic

Dosage and routes: *Adult:* PO 75-150 mg/day in divided doses; may increase to 300 mg/day or may give daily dose hs; *Adolescent and elderly:* PO 25-50 mg/day, may increase to 100 mg/day
Uses: Depression
Contraindications: Hypersensitivity to tricyclic antidepressants, recovery phase of myocardial infarction, narrow-angle glaucoma, convulsive disorders, prostatic hypertrophy, child <12 yr

---

dienestrol (R)
(dye-en-ess'trole)
DV, Ortho Dienestrol
Functional class.: Estrogen

Dosage and routes: *Adult:* **VAG CREAM** 1-2 applications qd × 2 wk, then ½ dose × 2 wk, then 1 application
Uses: Atrophic vaginitis, kraurosis vulvae
Contraindications: Breast cancer, thromboembolic disorders, reproductive cancer, genital bleeding (abnormal, undiagnosed), pregnancy (X), lactation

---

dimercaprol (R)
(dye-mer-cap'role)
BAL in Oil, British Anti-Lewisite*, dimercaptopropanol
Functional class.: Heavy metal antagonist

Dosage and routes:
Severe gold/arsenic poisoning: *Adult:* **IM** 3 mg/kg q4h × 2 days then qid × 1 day, then bid × 10 days
Mild gold/arsenic poisoning: *Adult:* **IM** 2.5 mg/kg qid × 2 days, then bid × 1 day, then qd × 10 days
Acute lead poisoning: *Adult:* **IM** 4 mg/kg, then q4h with edetate calcium disodium 12.5 mg/kg **IM,** not to exceed 5 mg/kg/dose
Mercury poisoning: *Adult:* **IM** 5 mg/kg, then 2.5 mg/kg/day or bid × 10 days
Uses: Arsenic, gold, mercury, lead poisoning
Contraindications: Hypersensitivity, anuria, hepatic insufficiency, poisoning of other metals, severe renal disease, child <3 yr, pregnancy (D)

◆ = Nursing alert   ▦ = Herb-drug interaction   ⊘ = Do not crush

disulfiram (℞)

(dye-sul'fi-ram)
Antabuse, disulfiram
Functional class.: Alcohol deterrent

Dosage and routes: *Adult:* **PO** 250-500 mg qd × 1-2 wk, then 125-500 mg qd until fully socially recovered
Uses: Chronic alcoholism (as adjunct)
Contraindications: Hypersensitivity, alcohol intoxication, psychoses, CV disease, pregnancy (X), lactation

ᴅ-penicillamine (℞)

(pen-i-sill'a-meen)
Cuprimine, Depen
Functional class.: Heavy metal antagonist

Dosage and routes:
Cystinuria: Adult: **PO** 250 mg qid ac, not to exceed 5 g/day; *Child:* **PO** 30 mg/kg/day in divided doses qid ac
Wilson's disease: Adult: **PO** 250 mg qid ac; *Child:* **PO** 20 mg/kg/day in divided doses ac
Rheumatoid arthritis: Adult: **PO** 125-250 mg/day, then increased 250 mg q2-3mo if needed, not to exceed 1 g/day; *Child:* **PO** 3 mg/kg/day, increase to max 10 mg/kg/day
Uses: Wilson's disease, rheumatoid arthritis, cystinuria, lead poisoning
Contraindications: Hypersensitivity to penicillins, anuria, agranulocytosis, severe renal disease, pregnancy (D), lactation

edetate calcium disodium (℞)

(ee'de-tate)
calcium disodium versenate, calcium EDTA, edathamil calcium disodium, sodium calcium edetate
Functional class.: Heavy metal antagonist (antidote)

Dosage and routes:
Acute lead encephalopathy: Adult and child: 1.5 g/m²/day × 3-5 days, with dimercaprol; may be given again after 4 days off drug
Lead poisoning: Adult: **IV** 1 g/250-500 ml D₅W or 0.9% NaCl over 1-2 hr or q12h × 3-5 days; may repeat after 2 days; not to exceed 50 mg/kg/day; may be given as **CONT INF** over 8-24 hr
• *Adult:* **IM** 35 mg/kg bid
• *Child:* **IM** 35 mg/kg/day in divided doses q8-12h, not to exceed 50 mg/kg/day; may give for 3-5 days, off 4 days before next course
Uses: Lead poisoning, acute lead encephalopathy
Contraindications: Hypersensitivity, anuria, poisoning of other metals, severe renal disease, child <3 yr

edetate disodium (℞)

(ee'de-tate)
Chealamide, Disodium EDTA, Disotate, Endrate
Functional class.: Metal antagonist

Dosage and routes: *Adult and child:* **IV INF** 15-50 mg/kg/day in 2 divided doses, diluted in 500 ml D₅W or 0.9% NaCl, given over 3-4 hr, not to exceed 3 g/day (adult) or 70 mg/kg/day (child); allow 5 days between courses (child), 2 days (adult)
Uses: Hypercalcemic crisis, control

of ventricular dysrhythmias associated with digitalis toxicity

Contraindications: Hypersensitivity, anuria, hepatic insufficiency, poisoning of other metals, severe renal disease, child <3 yr, seizure disorders, active/inactive TB

estramustine (℞)

(ess-tra-muss'teen)

Emcyt

Functional class.: Antineoplastic

Dosage and routes: *Adult:* **PO** 10-16 mg/kg in 3-4 divided doses/day; treatment may continue for ≥3 mo or 600 mg/m²/day in 3 divided doses

Uses: Metastatic prostate cancer

Contraindications: Hypersensitivity to estradiol, thromboembolic disorders, pregnancy (D)

etomidate (℞)

(e-tom'i-date)

Amidate

Functional class.: General anesthetic

Dosage and routes: *Adult and child >10 yr:* **IV** 0.2-0.6 mg/kg over ½-1 min

Uses: Induction of general anesthesia

Contraindications: Hypersensitivity, labor/delivery

felbamate (℞)

(fell'ba-mate)

Felbatol

Functional class.: Anticonvulsant

Dosage and routes:

Adjunctive therapy: *Adult:* **PO** add 1.2 g/day in 3-4 divided doses; reduce other anticonvulsants (valp-

roic acid, phenytoin, carbamazepine and derivatives) by 20% to control plasma concentrations; may increase felbamate 1.2 g/day increments qwk, up to 3.6 g/day

Monotherapy: *Adult:* **PO** 1.2 g/day in 3-4 divided doses; titrate with close supervision; increase dose by 600-mg increments q2wk to 3.6 g/day if needed

Lennox-Gastaut syndrome adjunctive therapy: *Child 2-14 yr:* **PO** add 15 mg/kg/day in 3-4 divided doses; reduce other anticonvulsants (valproic acid, phenytoin, carbamazepine and derivatives) by 20% to control plasma concentrations; may increase felbamate 15 mg/kg/day qwk up to 45 mg/day

Uses: Partial seizures, with or without generalization in adults; partial and generalized seizures in children with Lennox-Gastaut syndrome

Contraindications: Hypersensitivity to this drug, other carbamates, blood dyscrasia, hepatic disease

floxuridine (℞)

(flox-yoor'i-deen)

Floxuridine, FUDR

Functional class.: Antineoplastic, antimetabolite

Dosage and routes: *Adult:* **INTRAARTERIAL** by continuous inf 0.1-0.6 mg/kg/day × 1-6 wk; **HEPATIC ARTERY INJ** 0.4-0.6 mg/kg/day × 1-6 wk

Uses: GI adenocarcinoma metastatic to liver; cancer of breast, head, neck, liver, brain, gallbladder, bile duct

Contraindications: Hypersensitivity, myelosuppression, pregnancy (D), poor nutritional status, serious infections

◆ = Nursing alert　　　🖉 = Herb-drug interaction　　　🚫 = Do not crush

fludarabine (℞)
(floo-dar'a-been)
Fludara
Functional class.: Antineoplastic, antimetabolite

Dosage and routes: *Adult:* **IV** 25 mg/m^2 over 30 min qd × 5 days, may repeat q28d; reconstitute with 2 ml of sterile water for inj; dissolution should occur in <15 sec
Uses: Chronic lymphocytic leukemia, non-Hodgkin's lymphoma
Contraindications: Hypersensitivity, pregnancy (D), lactation

glycerin, anhydrous (℞)
(gli'ser-in, an-hye'drus)
Functional class.: Ophthalmic

Dosage and routes: *Adult:* **IN-STILL** 1-2 gtt after local anesthetic
Uses: Reduce corneal edema
Contraindications: Hypersensitivity

halcinonide (℞)
(hal-sin'oh-nide)
Functional class.: Corticosteroid, synthetic

Dosage and routes: *Adult:* **TOP** apply to affected area bid-tid
Uses: Inflammation of corticosteroid-responsive dermatoses
Contraindications: Hypersensitivity, viral infections, fungal infections

hydroquinone (℞)
(hye-droh'quin-ohn)
Functional class.: Depigmenting agent

Dosage and routes: *Adult and child:* **TOP** apply to affected area qd-bid
Uses: Bleaching skin, including age spots, freckles, lentigo, chloasma
Contraindications: Hypersensitivity, inflamed skin, prickly heat, sunburn

hydroxyprogesterone (℞)
(hye-drox-ee-pro-jess'te-rone)
Functional class.: Progestin, hormone

Dosage and routes:
Menstrual disorders: Adult: **IM** 125-375 mg q4wk; discontinue after 4 cycles
Uterine cancer: Adult: **IM** 1-5 g/wk
Uses: Uterine carcinoma, menstrual disorders (abnormal uterine bleeding, amenorrhea)
Contraindications: Breast cancer, hypersensitivity, thromboembolic disorders, genital bleeding (abnormal, undiagnosed), pregnancy (X)

idoxuridine-IDU (℞)
(eye-dox-yoor'i-deen)
Herplex, Stoxil
Functional class.: Antiviral

Dosage and routes: *Adult and child:* **INSTILL** 1 gtt q1h during day and 2 hr during night
Uses: Herpes simplex keratitis, CMV, varicella zoster alone or with corticosteroids
Contraindications: Hypersensitivity

indecainide (℞)
(in-de-kane'ide)

Functional class.: Antidysrhythmic (Class IC)

Dosage and routes: *Adult:* **PO** 100-200 mg/day in divided dose q12h; 50 mg q12h initially, then increase dose by 25 mg increments q4d, max 400 mg/day
Uses: Life-threatening dysrhythmias, sustained ventricular tachycardia
Contraindications: 2nd- or 3rd-degree AV block, right bundle branch block, cardiogenic shock, hypersensitivity

iodoquinol (℞)
(eye-oh-doh-kwin'ole)

Functional class.: Amebicide

Dosage and routes: *Adult:* **PO** 630-650 mg tid × 20 days, not to exceed 2 g/day; *Child:* **PO** 30-40 mg/kg/day in 2-3 divided doses × 20 days, not to exceed 1.95 g/24 hr × 20 days; do not repeat treatment before 2-3 wk
Uses: Intestinal amebiasis
Contraindications: Hypersensitivity to this drug or iodine, renal disease, hepatic disease, severe thyroid disease, preexisting optic neuropathy

isotretinoin (℞)
(eye-soe-tret'i-noyn)

Functional class.: Antiacne agent

Dosage and routes: *Adult:* **PO** 0.5-2 mg/kg/day in 2 divided doses × 15-20 wk; if relapse occurs, repeat after 2 mo off drug
Uses: Severe recalcitrant cystic acne

Contraindications: Hypersensitivity, inflamed skin, pregnancy (X)

isoxsuprine (℞)
(eye-sox'syoo-preen)

Functional class.: Peripheral vasodilator

Dosage and routes: *Adult:* **PO** 10-20 mg tid or qid
Uses: Symptoms of cerebrovascular insufficiency, peripheral vascular disease including arteriosclerosis obliterans, thromboangiitis obliterans, Raynaud's disease
Contraindications: Hypersensitivity, postpartum, arterial bleeding

ketamine (℞)
(keet'a-meen)
Ketalar

Functional class.: General anesthetic

Dosage and routes: *Adult and child:* **IV** 1-4.5 mg/kg over 1 min; **IM** 6.5-13 mg/kg; *Maintenance:* ½ to full induction dose may be repeated
Uses: Short anesthesia for diagnostic/surgical procedures
Contraindications: Hypersensitivity, CVA, increased intracranial pressure, severe hypertension, cardiac decompensation, child <2 yr

lincomycin (℞)
(lin-koe-mye'sin)

Functional class.: Antibacterial

Dosage and routes: *Adult:* **PO** 500 mg q6-8h, not to exceed 8 g/d; **IM** 600 mg/d or q12h; **IV** 600 mg-1 g q8-12h; dilute in 100 ml **IV sol;** infuse over 1 hr, not to exceed 8 g/day; *Child > 1 mo:* **PO** 30-60 mg/kg/d in divided doses q6-8h; **IM** 10

◆ = Nursing alert   ▰ = Herb-drug interaction   ⊘ = Do not crush

mg/kg/d q12h; **IV** 10-20 mg/kg/d in divided doses q8-12h; dilute to 100 ml **IV sol**; infuse over 1 hr
Uses: Infections caused by group A β-hemolytic streptococci, pneumococci, staphylococci (respiratory tract, skin, soft tissue, urinary tract infections, osteomyelitis, septicemia)
Contraindications: Hypersensitivity, ulcerative colitis/enteritis, infants <1 mo

masoprocol (℞)

(mas-o-proe′cole)

Functional class.: Miscellaneous topical product

Dosage and routes: *Adult:* **TOP** apply to lesion bid × 2-4 wk
Uses: Actinic keratoses
Contraindications: Hypersensitivity, children

mazindol (℞)

(may′zin-dole)

Functional class.: Anorexiant

Dosage and routes: *Adult:* **PO** 1 mg ac, or 2 mg 1 hr ac lunch
Uses: Exogenous obesity
Contraindications: Hypersensitivity to sympathomimetic amine, glaucoma, drug abuse, cardiovascular disease, children <12 yr, hypertension, severe arteriosclerosis, agitated states, hyperthyroidism

mefenamic acid (℞)

(me-fe-nam′ik)

Functional class.: Nonsteroidal antiinflammatory

Dosage and routes: *Adult and child >14 yr:* **PO** 500 mg, then 250 mg q6h, use not to exceed 1 wk

Uses: Mild to moderate pain, dysmenorrhea, inflammatory disease
Contraindications: Hypersensitivity, asthma, severe renal disease, severe hepatic disease, ulcer disease

mefloquine (℞)

(meh′floh-quin)

Functional class.: Antimalarial

Dosage and routes: *Adult:* **PO** 1250 mg as a single dose (treatment); 250 mg qwk × 4 wk, then 250 mg q2wk (prevention)
Uses: Treatment and prevention of *Plasmodium falciparum* malaria, *P. vivax*
Contraindications: Hypersensitivity

mepenzolate (℞)

(me-pen′zoe-late)

Functional class.: GI anticholinergic

Dosage and routes: *Adult:* **PO** 25-50 mg qid with meals, hs; titrate to patient response
Uses: Treatment of peptic ulcer disease, irritable bowel syndrome in combination with other drugs; for other GI disorders
Contraindications: Hypersensitivity to anticholinergics, narrow-angle glaucoma, GI obstruction, myasthenia gravis, paralytic ileus, GI atony, toxic megacolon

methohexital (℞)

(meth-oh-hex′i-tal)
Brevital Sodium, Brietal Sodium*
Functional class.: General anesthetic

Dosage and routes: *Adult and child:* **IV** 50-120 mg given 1 ml/5 sec

Maintenance: Adult and child: **IV** 20-40 mg q4-7min 0.1% sol; **CONT IV** 3 ml/min (6 mg/min) 0.2% sol
Uses: General anesthesia for electroshock therapy, reduction of fractures, adjunct with other anesthetics, balanced anesthesia
Contraindications: Hypersensitivity, status asthmaticus, hepatic/intermittent porphyrias, pregnancy (D)

methoxsalen (℞)

(meth-ox'a-len)

Functional class.: Pigmenting agent

Dosage and routes:
Vitiligo: Adult and child >12 yr: **PO** 20 mg qd 2-4 hr before exposure to therapeutic ultraviolet rays; administer on alternate days; **TOP** apply 1-2 hr before exposure to UVA light; treatment intervals regulated by erythema response
Psoriasis: Adult: **PO** dosage individualized to weight; taken 2 hr before exposure to therapeutic ultraviolet rays
Uses: Vitiligo, psoriasis
Contraindications: Hypersensitivity, melanoma, LE, albinism, sunburn, cataracts, squamous cell cancer, child ≤12 yr, diseases associated with photosensitivity

methscopolamine (℞)

(meth-skoe-pol'a-meen)

Functional class.: GI anticholinergic

Dosage and routes: *Adult:* **PO** 2.5-5 mg 1/2 hr ac, hs
Uses: Peptic ulcer disease
Contraindications: Hypersensitivity to anticholinergics, narrow-angle glaucoma, GI obstruction, myasthenia gravis, paralytic ileus, GI atony, toxic megacolon

methsuximide (℞)

(meth-sux'i-mide)

Functional class.: Anticonvulsant

Dosage and routes: *Adult and child:* **PO** 300 mg/day; may increase by 300 mg/wk, not to exceed 1.2 g/day in divided doses
Uses: Refractory absence seizures (petit mal)
Contraindications: Hypersensitivity to succinimide derivatives

mitotane (℞)

(mye'toe-tane)
Lysodren, p'-DDD
Functional class.: Antineoplastic

Dosage and routes: *Adult:* **PO** 9-10 g/day in divided doses tid or qid; may have to decrease dose for severe reaction
Uses: Adrenocortical carcinoma
Contraindications: Hypersensitivity

molindone (℞)

(moe-lin'done)

Functional class.: Antipsychotic/neuroleptic

Dosage and routes: *Adult:* **PO** 50-75 mg/day increasing to 225 mg/day if needed
Uses: Psychotic disorders
Contraindications: Hypersensitivity, coma, child

◆ = Nursing alert   / = Herb-drug interaction   ⊘ = Do not crush

papaverine (℞)
(pa-pav′er-een)

Functional class.: Peripheral vaso-dilator

Dosage and routes: *Adult:* **PO** 100-300 mg 3-5×/day; **SUS REL** 150-300 mg q8-12h; **IM/IV** 30-120 mg q3h prn

Uses: Arterial spasm resulting in cerebral and peripheral ischemia; myocardial ischemia associated with vascular spasm or dysrhythmias; angina pectoris; peripheral pulmonary embolism; visceral spasm as in ureteral, biliary, GI colic, peripheral vascular disease

Contraindications: Hypersensitivity, complete AV heart block

paraldehyde (℞)
(par-al′de-hyde)

Functional class.: Anticonvulsant

Dosage and routes:
Seizures: Adult: **IM** 5-10 ml; divide 10 ml into 2 inj; **IV** 0.2-0.4 ml/kg in **NS** inj; *Child:* **IM** 0.15 ml/kg; **RECT** 0.3 ml/kg q4-6h or 1 ml/yr of age, not to exceed 5 ml; may repeat in 1 hr prn; **IV** 5 ml/90 ml **NS** inj; begin infusion at 5 ml/hr; titrate to patient response
Alcohol withdrawal: Adult: **PO/RECT** 5-10 ml, not to exceed 60 ml; **IM** 5 ml q4-6h × 24 hr, then q6h on following days, not to exceed 30 ml
Sedation: Adult: **PO/REC** 4-10 ml; **IM** 5 ml; **IV** 3-5 ml in emergency only; *Child:* **PO/REC/IM** 0.15 ml/kg
Tetanus: Adult: **IV** 4-5 ml or 12 ml by gastric tube q4h diluted with water; **IM** 5-10 ml prn
Uses: Refractory seizures, status epilepticus, sedation, insomnia, alcohol withdrawal, tetanus, eclampsia
Contraindications: Hypersensitivity, gastroenteritis with ulceration

paramethadione (℞)
(par-a-meth-a-dye′one)

Functional class.: Anticonvulsant

Dosage and routes: *Adult:* **PO** 300 mg tid; may increase by 300 mg/wk, not to exceed 600 mg qid; *Child >6 yr:* **PO** 0.9 g/day in divided doses tid or qid; *Child 2-6 yr:* **PO** 0.6 g/day in divided doses tid or qid; *Child <2 yr:* **PO** 0.3 g/day in divided doses tid or qid
Uses: Refractory absence (petit mal) seizures
Contraindications: Hypersensitivity, blood dyscrasias, pregnancy (D), lactation

paromomycin (℞)
(par-oh-moe-mye′sin)

Functional class.: Amebicide

Dosage and routes:
Intestinal amebiasis: Adult and child: **PO** 25-35 mg/kg/day in 3 divided doses × 5-10 day pc
Hepatic coma: Adult: 4 g qd in divided doses × 5-6 day
Uses: Intestinal amebiasis, adjunct in hepatic coma
Contraindications: Hypersensitivity, renal disease, GI obstruction

permethrin (otc, ℞)
(per-meth′ren)

Functional class.: Pediculicide

Dosage and routes:
Lice (head): Adult and child: Wash hair, towel dry; apply liberally to hair, leave on 10 min, rinse with water

Scabies: Adult and child: **TOP** 5% cream applied and massaged into all skin surfaces; leave cream on 8-14 hr, then wash
Uses: Lice, nits, ticks, flea nits
Contraindications: Hypersensitivity

phenacemide (℞)
(fe-nass'e-mide)
Functional class.: Anticonvulsant

Dosage and routes: *Adult:* **PO** 500 mg tid, may increase by 500 mg/wk, not to exceed 5 g/day; *Child 5-10 yr:* **PO** 250 mg tid, may increase by 250 mg/wk, not to exceed 1.5 g/day prn
Uses: Refractory, generalized tonic-clonic (grand mal), complex-partial (psychomotor), absence (petit mal), atypical seizures
Contraindications: Hypersensitivity, psychiatric condition, pregnancy (D), lactation

phendimetrazine (℞)
(fen-dye-me'tra-zeen)
Functional class.: Anorexiant

Dosage and routes: *Adult:* **PO** 35 mg bid-tid 1 hr ac, not to exceed 70 mg tid; **SUS REL** 105 mg qd ac AM
Uses: Exogenous obesity
Contraindications: Hypersensitivity, hyperthyroidism, hypertension, glaucoma, severe arteriosclerosis, severe cardiovascular disease, children <12 yr, agitated states, drug abuse

phenoxybenzamine (℞)
(fen-ox-ee-ben'za-meen)
Functional class.: Antihypertensive

Dosage and routes: *Adult:* **PO** 10 mg qd, increase by 10 mg qod, usual range: 20-40 mg bid-tid; *Child:* **PO** 0.2 mg/kg or 6 mg/m^2/day, max 10 mg; may increase q4d; maintenance dose 0.4-1.2 mg/kg/day or 12-36 mg/m^2/day divided doses tid or qid
Uses: Pheochromocytoma
Contraindications: Hypersensitivity, CHF, angina, cerebral vascular insufficiency, coronary arteriosclerosis

phentermine (℞)
(fen'ter-meen)
Functional class.: Cerebral stimulant

Dosage and routes: *Adult:* **PO** 8 mg tid 30 min before meals or 15-37.5 mg qd before breakfast
Uses: Exogenous obesity
Contraindications: Hypersensitivity, hyperthyroidism, hypertension, glaucoma, severe arteriosclerosis, angina pectoris, cardiovascular disease, pregnancy (C), child <12 yr

physostigmine (℞)
(fi-zoe-stig'meen)
Antilirium
Functional class.: Antidote, reversible anticholinesterase

Dosage and routes:
Overdose of anticholinergics: *Adult:* **IM/IV** 2 mg; give no more than 1 mg/min; may repeat; *Child:* **IM/IV** inj 0.02 mg/kg, not more than 0.5 mg/min; may repeat at 5-10 min intervals until max dose of 2 mg

Postanesthesia: Adult: **IM/IV** 0.5-1 mg; give no more than 1 mg/min **(IV)**; can repeat at 10 to 30 min intervals

Uses: To reverse CNS effects of diazepam; anticholinergic, tricyclic antidepressant, Alzheimer's disease, hereditary ataxia

Contraindications: Hypotension, obstruction of intestine or renal system , asthma, gangrene, CV disease, choline esters, depolarizing neuromuscular blocking agents, diabetes

pinacidil (℞)
(pye-na'si-dill)
Functional class.: Antihypertensive

Dosage and routes: *Adult:* **PO** 12.5-25 mg bid
Uses: Severe hypertension not responsive to other therapy
Contraindications: Acute MI, dissecting aortic aneurysm, hypersensitivity, pheochromocytoma

pralidoxime (℞)
(pra-li-dox'eem)
Protopam Chloride
Functional class.: Cholinesterase reactivator

Dosage and routes:
Anticholinesterase overdose: Adult: **IV** 1-2 g, then 250 mg q5min until desired response
Organophosphate poisoning: Adult: **IV INF** 1-2 g/100 ml 0.9% NaCl over 15-30 min; may repeat in 1 hr; **PO** 1-3 g q5h; *Child:* **IV INF** 20-40 mg/kg/dose diluted in 100 ml 0.9% NaCl over 15-30 min
Uses: Cholinergic crisis in myasthenia gravis, organophosphate poisoning antidote (early), relief of paralysis of respiratory muscles; used

as an adjunct to systemic atropine administration
Contraindications: Hypersensitivity, carbamate insecticide poisoning

streptozocin (℞)
(strep-toe-zoe'sin)
Zanosar
Functional class.: Antineoplastic alkylating agent

Dosage and routes: *Adult:* **IV** 500 mg/m^2 × 5 days q6wk until desired response; or 1 g/m^2 qwk × 2 wk, not to exceed 1.5 g/m^2 in 1 dose
Uses: Metastatic islet cell carcinoma of pancreas
Investigational uses: Prevention of spread of Hodgkin's disease, metastatic carcinoid tumor, pancreatic adenocarcinoma, colon malignancies
Contraindications: Hypersensitivity

teniposide (℞)
(ten-i-poe'side)
Vumon, VM 26
Functional class.: Antineoplastic

Dosage and routes: *Child:* **IV INF** combo teniposide 165 mg/m^2 and cytarabine 300 mg/m^2 2×/wk × 8-9 doses or combo teniposide 250 mg/m^2 and vincristine 1.5 mg/m^2 qwk × 4-8 wk and prednisone 40 mg/m^2 **PO** × 28 days
Uses: Childhood acute lymphoblastic leukemia (ALL), refractory childhood acute lymphocytic leukemia
Contraindications: Hypersensitivity, bone marrow depression, severe hepatic disease, severe renal disease, bacterial infection, pregnancy (D)

tolazamide (R)

(tole-az'a-mide)
Tolamide, tolazimide, Tolinase
Functional class.: Antidiabetic

Dosage and routes: *Adult:* **PO** 100 mg/day for FBS <200 mg/dl or 250 mg/day for FBS >200 mg/dl; dose should be titrated to response (1 g or less/day)

Uses: Type II (NIDDM) diabetes mellitus

Contraindications: Hypersensitivity to sulfonylureas, juvenile or brittle diabetes

tolbutamide (R)

(tole-byoo'ta-mide)
Mobenol*, Novobutamide*, Orinase, tolbutamide, Tolbutone*
Functional class.: Antidiabetic

Dosage and routes: *Adult:* **PO** 1-2 g/day in divided doses, titrated to patient response; **IV** 1 g (Fajans test)
Uses: Type II (NIDDM) diabetes mellitus
Contraindications: Hypersensitivity to sulfonylureas, juvenile or brittle diabetes

trientine (R)

(tri'en-teen)
Syprine
Functional class.: Heavy-metal antagonist

Dosage and routes: *Adult:* **PO** 750-2000 mg in divided doses bid-qid; *Child:* **PO** 500-1500 mg in divided doses bid-qid
Uses: Wilson's disease
Contraindications: Hypersensitivity, cystinuria, rheumatoid arthritis, biliary cirrhosis

vasopressin (R)

(vay-soe-press'in)
Pitressin Synthetic
Functional class.: Pituitary hormone

Dosage and routes:
Diabetes insipidus: *Adult:* **IM/SC** 5-10 units bid-qid as needed; **IM/SC** 2.5-5 units q2-3 days (Pitressin Tannate) for chronic therapy; *Child:* **IM/SC** 2.5-10 units bid-qid as needed; **IM/SC** 1.25-2.5 units q2-3 days (Pitressin Tannate) for chronic therapy

Abdominal distention: *Adult:* **IM** 5 units, then q3-4h, increasing to 10 units if needed (aqueous)

Uses: Diabetes insipidus (nonnephrogenic/nonpsychogenic), abdominal distention postoperatively, bleeding esophageal varices

Contraindications: Hypersensitivity, chronic nephritis

◆ = Nursing alert   ∥ = Herb-drug interaction   ⊘ = Do not crush

Appendix g Less frequently used antihistamines

GENERIC NAME	TRADE NAME(S)	USES	DOSAGES AND ROUTES	AVAILABLE FORMS	INTERACTIONS	CONTRAINDICATIONS
acrivastine/ pseudoephedrine (R)	Semprex-D	• Rhinitis • Allergy symptoms • Chronic idiopathic urticaria	• Adult, child >12 yr: PO 8 mg q4-6h	• Caps 8 mg/60 mg	• Increased CNS depression: alcohol, narcotics, sedatives, hypnotics • Hypertensive crisis: MAOIs ♣ May increase CNS depression: kava ♣ May increase anticholinergic effect: henbane leaf	• Hypersensitivity to this drug or triprolidine • Severe hypertension • Cardiac disease
azatadine (R)	Optimine	• Allergy symptoms • Rhinitis • Chronic urticaria	• Adult: PO 1-2 mg bid, not to exceed 4 mg/day • Geriatric: PO 1 mg qd-bid	• Tabs 1 mg	• Increased CNS depression: barbiturates, narcotics, hypnotics, tricyclic antidepressants, alcohol • Decreased effect of: oral anticoagulants • Increased effect of: azatadine: MAOIs ♣ Increased CNS depression: kava ♣ Increased anticholinergic effect: henbane leaf	• Hypersensitivity to H$_1$-receptor antagonists • Acute asthma attack • Lower respiratory tract disease • Child <12 yr
buclizine (R)	Bucladin-S, Softabs	• Motion sickness • Dizziness • Nausea • Vomiting • Antihistamine	• Adult: PO 25-50 mg, prn ½ hr before travel; may be repeated q4-6h prn	• Tabs 50 mg	• Increased anticholinergic effect: henbane leaf ♣ Increased CNS depression: kava	• Hypersensitivity to cyclizines • Shock

KEY: ✦ = Canada only; ♣ = herb/drug interaction

Continued

Appendix g Less frequently used antihistamines—cont'd

GENERIC NAME	TRADE NAME(S)	USES	DOSAGES AND ROUTES	AVAILABLE FORMS	INTERACTIONS	CONTRAINDICATIONS
cyclizine (otc, **B**)	Marezine	• Motion sickness • Prevention of postoperative vomiting • Antihistamine	*Vomiting* • Adult: IM 25-50 mg ½ hr before termination of surgery; then q4-6h prn (lactate) • Child: IM 3 mg/kg divided in 3 equal doses *Motion sickness* • Adult: PO 50 mg then q4-6h prn, not to exceed 200 mg/day (HCl) • Child: PO 25 mg q4-6h prn	• Tabs 50 mg • Inj 50 mg/ml	• May increase CNS effect: alcohol, tranquilizers, narcotics ♣ Increased CNS depression: kava	• Hypersensitivity to cyclizines • Shock
dexchlorpheniramine (**B**)	Dexchlor, dexchlorpheniramine maleate, Poladex, Polaramine	• Allergy symptoms • Rhinitis • Pruritus • Contact dermatitis	• Adult: PO 1-2 mg tid-qid; repeat action 4-6 mg bid-tid • Child 6-11 yr: PO 1 mg q4-6h, or time rel 4 mg hs • Child 2-5 yr: PO 0.5 mg q4-6h; do not use repeat action form	• Tabs 2 mg • Repeat action tabs 4, 6 mg • Syr 2 mg/5 ml	• Increased CNS depression: barbiturates, narcotics, hypnotics, tricyclic antidepressants, alcohol • Decreased effect: oral anticoagulants, heparin • Increased effect of dexchlorpheniramine: MAOIs ♣ Increased anticholinergic effect: henbane leaf	• Hypersensitivity to H_1-receptor antagonists • Acute asthma attack • Lower respiratory tract disease

trimeprazine (R)	Panectyl*, Temaril	• Pruritus	• Adult: PO 2.5 mg qid; time-rel 5 mg bid • Geriatric: PO 2.5 mg bid • Child 3-12 yr: PO 2.5 mg tid or hs • Child 6 mo-1 yr: PO 1.25 mg tid or hs	• Tabs 2.5 mg • Time-rel spanules 5 mg • Syr 2.5 mg/5 ml	• Increased CNS depression: barbiturates, narcotics, hypnotics, tricyclic antidepressants, alcohol • Decreased effect of oral anticoagulants, heparin • Increased effect of trimeprazine: MAOIs ♣ Increased anticholinergic effect: henbane leaf	• Hypersensitivity to H_1-receptor antagonists • Acute asthma attack • Lower respiratory tract disease
tripelennamine (R)	PBZ, PBZ-SR, Pelamine, tripelennamine HCl	• Rhinitis • Allergy symptoms	• Adults: PO 25-50 mg q4-6h, not to exceed 600 mg/day; time-rel 100 mg bid-tid, not to exceed 600 mg/day • Child >5 yr: PO timerel 50 mg q8-12h, not to exceed 300 mg/day • Child <5 yr: PO 5 mg/kg/day in 4-6 divided doses, not to exceed 300 mg/day	• Tabs 25, 50 mg • Time-rel tabs 100 mg • Elix 37.5 mg/5 ml	• Increased CNS depression: barbiturates, narcotics, hypnotics, tricyclic antidepressants, alcohol • Decreased effect of oral anticoagulants, heparin • Increased effect of tripelennamine: MAOIs ♣ Increased anticholinergic effect: henbane leaf	• Hypersensitivity to H_1-receptor antagonists • Acute asthma attack • Lower respiratory tract disease

KEY: * = Canada only;   ♣ = herb/drug interaction

Appendix h

Look-alike/sound-alike drug names

acetohexamide	acetazolamide	clomipramine	clomiphene
Adriamycin	Aredia	clomipramine	Norpramin
Adriamycin	Idamycin		(desipramine)
albuterol	atenolol	clonidine	Klonopin
allopurinol	Apresoline		(clonazepam)
alprazolam	lorazepam	Cordarone	Inocor
Altace	alteplase	Corgard	Cognex
Ambien	Amen	Coumadin	Compazine
Amikin	Amicar	Cozaar	Zocor
amiodarone	amrinone	cyclobenzaprine	cyproheptadine
amitriptyline	nortriptyline	cyclophosphamide	cyclosporine
amoxapine	amoxicillin	cyclosporine	cycloserine
amoxapine	Amoxil	Cytovene	Cytosar
amoxicillin	Amoxil	Cytoxan	Cytosar
Artane	Altace		(cytarabine)
Asacol	Ansaid	Cytoxan	Cytotec
Asacol	Os-Cal	Dantrium	danazol
Atrovent	Alupent	daunorubicin	doxorubicin
Bactocil	Pathocil	Decadron	Percodan
Bentyl	Aventyl	Depo-Medrol	Solu-Medrol
Betalin	Benylin	Diabeta	Zebeta
Brethine	Banthine	Dialose Plus	Dialose Plus
Brevital	Brevibloc	(docusate	(docusate
Bumex	Buprenex	potassium/	sodium/
Cafergot	Carafate	casanthranol)	phenolphthalein)
calcitriol	Calciferol	diazepam	Ditropan
carboplatin	cisplatin	Diflucan	Diprivan
Cardene	Cardizem	Dilaudid	Demerol
Cardene SR	Cardizem SR	Diphenatol	diphenidol
Cardizem CD	Cardizem SR	diphenhydramine	dicyclomine
Cardura	Coumadin	Diupres	Daypro
Cataflam	Catapres	Dobutrex	Diamox
cefaclor	cephalexin	dopamine	dobutamine
Cefotan	Ceftin	doxorubicin	idarubicin
cefprozil	cefuroxime	Edecrin	Eulexin
ceftazidime	ceftizoxime	Elavil	Mellaril
cefuroxime	cefotaxime	Eldepryl	enalapril
cefuroxime	deferoxamine	enalapril	ramipril
Cefzil	Ceftin	Estratest	Estratab
Cefzil	Kefzol	etidronate	etretinate
cephapirin	cephradine	etomidate	etidronate
chlorpromazine	chlorpropamide	Fioricet	Fiorinal
chlorpromazine	prochlorperazine	Flumadine	fludarabine
Clinoril	Clozaril	fluorouracil	flucytosine
Clinoril	Oruvail	FUDR	Fludara

Gamulin Rh	MICRhoGAM
Garamycin	kanamycin
Glucotrol	glyburide
Halotestin	haloperidol
Hycodan	Vicodin
hydrocodone	hydrocortisone
hydromorphone	meperidine
hydromorphone	morphine
Imferon	Roferon-A
imipenem	Omnipen
imipramine	Desipramine
Imuran	Imferon
Inderal LA	IMDUR
Klonopin	clonidine
Lamictal	Lomotil
Lanoxin Lasix	Lomotil
leucovorin Leukine	Leukeran
Levsin	Levoxine
Librium	Librax
Lodine	codeine
Lortab	Lorabid
Lotensin	Lioresal
Lotensin	Loniten
Lotrimin	Otrivin
Lupron	Lopurin
Luvox	Lasix
Mazicon	Mivacron
Mepron	Mepron
(atovaquone	(meprobamate
in U.S.)	in Australia)
methyldopa	L-Dopa (levodopa)
methylphenidate	methadone
methylprednisolone	medroxypro-
	gesterone
metolazone	methotrexate
metolazone	metoclopramide
metoprolol	misoprostol
Monopril	minoxidil
Mylanta Gas	Mylicon
Narcan	Norcuron
Nasalide	Nasalcrom
Nicobid	Nitro-Bid
Norflex	Noroxin
	(norfloxacin)
Norpramin	nortriptyline
Norvasc	Navane
Novolin 70/30	Novolin 70/30
Penfill Prefilled	
Nuprin	Lupron
Ocufen	Ocuflox
	(ofloxacin)
Ocufen	Ocupress
Oruvail	Elavil
paroxetine	paclitaxel

Paxil	paclitaxel
Paxil	Taxol
pentobarbital	phenobarbital
Phenergan	Theragran
phenobarbital	pentobarbital
pindolol	Parlodel
Plendil	pindolol
Plendil	Prinivil
Pravachol	Prevacid
prednisone	methylprednisolone
prednisone	prednisolone
Premarin	Primaxin
Prepidil	bepridil
Prilosec	prednisone
Prilosec	Prozac
Prinivil	Prilosec
Prinivil	Proventil
Prokine	Proleukin
Provera	Premarin
Prozac Proscar	Prosom
Psorion	Psorcon
quinidine	quinine
ranitidine	amantadine
Reglan	Megace
Regroton	Hygroton
reserpine	Risperdal
	(risperidone)
Ridaura	Cardura
rifampin	rifabutin
rimantadine	amantadine
Roxanol	Roxicet
Sinequan	Serentil
Soma	Soma Compound
Stadol	Haldol
sulfasalazine	sulfisoxazole
Symmetrel	Synthroid
Taxol	Paxil
Tegretol	Toradol
Temaril	Demerol
thiamine	Tenormin
Thyrar	Thyrolar
Timoptic	Viroptic
Tobrex	TobraDex
Toradol	Inderal
Toradol	Torecan
Toradol	tramadol
torsemide	furosemide
trifluoperazine	trihexyphenidyl
Trimox	Diamox
Trimox	Tylox
Tronothane	Tronolane
Uridon	Vicodin
Urispas	Urised
Vantin	Ventolin

Versed	Vistaril	Xanax	Zantac
Versed	Vepesid	Zantac	Xanax
vincristine	vinblastine	Zinacef	Zithromax
Viroptic	Timoptic	Zocor	Zoloft
Wymox	Tylox	Zofran	Zantac
Xanax	Lanoxin	Zosyn	Zofran
Xanax	Tylox		

Appendix i

Herbal products

agrimony

Uses: Mild diarrhea, gastroenteritis, intestinal mucous secretion, inflammation of the mouth and throat, cuts and scrapes, amenorrhea

alfalfa

Uses: Poor appetite, hay fever and asthma, high cholesterol, nutrient source

aloe

Uses of aloe vera gel:
• *External:* Minor burns, skin irritations, minor wounds, frostbite, radiation-caused injuries
• *Internal:* To heal intestinal inflammation and ulcers, as a digestive aid to stimulate bile secretion

angelica

Uses: Heartburn, indigestion, gas, colic, poor blood flow to the extremities, bronchitis, poor appetite, psoriasis, vitiligo, as an antiseptic

arnica

Uses: Topical application for muscle and joint inflammation and swelling; in homeopathic preparations as a remedy for shock, injury, pain

astragalus

Uses: Immune stimulant, viral infections, HIV/AIDS, cancer, vascular disorders, improve circulation, lower blood pressure, possible efficacy in myasthenia gravis

bilberry

Uses: Diabetic retinopathy, macular degeneration, glaucoma, cataract, capillary fragility, varicose veins, hemorrhoids, mild diarrhea

black cohosh

Uses:
• *Menopause:* Hot flashes, nervous conditions associated with menopause
• *Dysmenorrhea:* Menstrual cramps, pain, inflammation

Adapted from: Debusk, Ruth, and Treadwell, Phillip. *Serious Drug/Herb Interactions.* Skidmore-Roth Publishing, Inc. 1999.

black haw (cramp bark)

Uses: Dysmenorrhea, menstrual cramps and pain, menopausal metrorrhagia, hysteria, asthma, lower blood pressure, heart palpitations

blessed thistle

Uses: Loss of appetite, indigestion, intestinal gas

blue cohosh

Uses: Menopausal symptoms, uterine and ovarian pain, improve flow of menstrual blood, antiinflammatory, antirheumatic, popular remedy in black ethnic medicine

borage

Uses: Antiinflammatory for premenstrual syndrome, rheumatoid arthritis, Raynaud's disease, other inflammatory conditions, atopic dermatitis, infant cradle cap, cystic fibrosis, high blood pressure, diabetes

burdock root

Uses: Skin diseases, inflammation, rashes, cold and fever, cancer, gout, arthritis

calendula

Uses:
• *External:* Minor skin ailments
• *Internal:* Inflammation throughout the gastrointestinal tract, toxic liver and gallbladder, menstrual bleeding and pain, yeast infections

capsicum (cayenne)

Uses: Muscle spasms, pain of inflammation, neuromas, psoriasis, dry mouth, as an antioxidant food, as a food seasoning

cascara

Uses: Chronic constipation, hepatitis, gallstones

cat's claw

Uses: Cancer, herpes, HIV/AIDS, rheumatoid arthritis, gastritis, gout, wounds, gastric ulcers

chamomile

Uses:
• *External:* As an antiseptic and soothing agent for inflamed skin and minor wounds
• *Internal:* As an antispasmodic, gas-relieving, and antiinflammatory agent for the treatment of digestive problems; light sleep aid and sedative for adults and children; possible anticancer agent

chaparral

Uses: Not recommended—potentially toxic to the liver and kidneys

chicory

Uses: Coffee substitute, source of fructo-oligosaccharides, mild laxative for children, gout, rheumatism, loss of appetite, digestive distress

comfrey

Uses: Bruises, sprains, broken bones, acne, boils

cranberry

Uses: Urinary tract infections (UTIs); susceptibility to kidney stones

dong quai

Uses: To restore vitality to tired women; for a variety of gynecologic, menstrual, and menopausal symptoms; cirrhosis of the liver

echinacea

Uses: Low immune status, hard-to-heal superficial wounds, sun protection

elder (elderberry)

Uses: Susceptibility to colds, flu, yeast infections; nasal and chest congestion; earache associated with chronic congestion; hay fever

eleuthero (See siberian ginseng)

ephedra (ma huang)

Uses: Seasonal and chronic asthma, nasal congestion, cough

evening primrose

Uses: Premenstrual syndrome, arthritis and inflammatory disorders in general, dry skin, eczema, asthma, diabetes, migraines, chronic fatigue syndrome, heart disease and stroke, circulatory disorders, Raynaud's disease, NSAID use, multiple sclerosis

fenugreek

Uses: Loss of appetite, inflamed areas of the skin, water retention, cancer, constipation, diarrhea, high cholesterol, high blood sugar, calcium oxalate stones

---

feverfew

Uses: Migraines, cluster headaches, fever, psoriasis, inflammation

flaxseed

Uses: Constipation, as a source of omega-3 fatty acids

fo-ti

Uses: Tiredness, constipation, elevated cholesterol

garcinia cambogia

Uses: Appetite control, weight loss, high cholesterol

garlic

Uses: Vascular disease, elevated LDL, elevated triglycerides, low HDL, high blood pressure, poor circulation, risk of cancer, inflammatory disorders, childhood ear infection, yeast infection

ginger

Uses: Nausea, motion sickness, indigestion, inflammation

ginkgo

Uses: Poor circulation; age-related decline in cognition, memory; diabetes; vascular disease; cancer; inflammatory disorders; impotence; degenerative nerve conditions

ginseng

Uses: Physical and mental exhaustion, stress, viral infections, diabetes, sluggishness, fatigue, weak immunity, convalescence

goldenseal

Uses: High blood pressure, poor appetite, infections, menstrual problems, minor sciatic pain, muscle spasms, eye washes

gotu kola

Uses: Chronic wounds, psoriasis

grape seed

Uses: Antioxidant, chronic disease prevention, inflammation

green tea

Uses: Cancer prevention, heart disease prevention, hypercholesterolemia, diarrhea

guggul

Uses: High LDL cholesterol, elevated triglycerides, weight loss

---

 = Nursing alert = Herb-drug interaction = Do not crush

gymnema sylvestre

Uses: High blood sugar levels

hawthorn

Uses: Poor circulation, chest pain, irregular heartbeat, high blood fats, high blood pressure

hops

Uses: Mild sedative, diuretic, weak antibiotic, insomnia, hyperactivity, pain, fever, jaundice, improve appetite

horse chestnut

Uses: Fever, fluid retention, frostbite, hemorrhoids, inflammation, lower extremity swelling, phlebitis, varicose veins, wounds

horsetail

Uses: Diuretic, genitourinary astringent, anti-hemorrhagic, Bell's Palsy, healing broken bones

kava

Uses: Nervous anxiety, restlessness, sleep disturbances, stress

khat

Uses: Obesity, gastric ulcers, stimulant

kombucha

Uses: Numerous claims for a wide variety of ills; none has been substantiated to date

konjac

Uses: Blood sugar control, constipation, high blood fats, high blood pressure, excessive appetite

kudzu

Uses: Alcohol cravings, menopausal symptoms

lapacho (pau d'arco)

Uses: Cancer, inflammation, infection

lemon balm (melissa)

Uses: Abdominal gas and cramping, cold sores

licorice

Uses: Allergies, arthritis, asthma, constipation, esophagitis, gastritis, hepatitis, inflammatory conditions, peptic ulcers, poor adrenal function, poor appetite

---

* = Canada only   Side effects: *italics* = common; ***bold italics*** = life-threatening

maitake

Uses: Immunostimulant activity, diabetes, hypertension, high cholesterol, obesity

maté

Uses: Diuretic, depurative

melatonin

Uses: Jet lag, insomnia, cancer protection, oral contraceptive

milk thistle

Uses: Protection for alcoholic cirrhosis and hepatitis, antiinflammatory

monascus

Uses: Maintaining acceptable cholesterol levels

morinda

Uses: Headache, digestive, heart and liver conditions, arthritis

nettle

Uses: Diuretic, hay fever

octacosanol

Uses: Herpes, inflammation of the skin, physical endurance

passionflower

Uses: Antifungal, hypertension, sedative, group A hemolytic streptococcus

peppermint

Uses: GI disorders

pygeum

Uses: Benign prostate hypertrophy, antiinflammatory

raspberry leaves

Uses: Facilitation of childbirth, dysmenorrhea, uterine tonic, fever, vomiting

red clover

Uses: Antispasmodic, expectorant, sedative, psoriasis, eczema, amenorrhea

rose hips

Uses: Source of vit C, cold, fever, mild infections

st. john's wort

Uses: Depression, antiviral

sarsaparilla

Uses: Antiinflammatory, antiseptic, syphilis, skin diseases, rheumatism, necrosis, mercury poisoning

sassafras

Uses: Banned in the United States

saw palmetto

Uses: Benign prostatic hypertrophy

schisandra

Uses: GI disorders, liver protection, tonic

scull cap

Uses: Antibacterial, sedative

senna

Uses: Laxative

siberian ginseng (eleuthero)

Uses: Improve appetite, memory loss, hypertension, insomnia, rheumatism, improve circulation, heart ailments, diabetes, headache

tea tree oil

Uses: Topical use for infections; inhaled for respiratory disorders

uva ursi

Uses: Diuretic, urinary tract infections, contact dermatitis, arthritis

valerian

Uses: Sedative

vitex

Uses: Premenstrual and menstrual disorders, spasms, estrogen gestagen imbalance

yarrow

Uses: To decrease bleeding, Gi disorders, hypertension, thrombi, to improve circulation

yohimbine

Uses: Male organic impotence

Appendix j

FDA pregnancy categories

A   No risk demonstrated to the fetus in any trimester

B   No adverse effects in animals, no human studies available

C   Only given after risks to the fetus are considered; animal studies have shown adverse reactions, no human studies available

D   Definite fetal risks, may be given in spite of risks if needed in life-threatening conditions

X   Absolute fetal abnormalities; not to be used anytime during pregnancy

Note: **UK** = Unknown fetal risk (used in this text but not an official FDA pregnancy category).

Appendix k

Controlled substance chart

Drugs	United States	Canada
Heroin, LSD, peyote, marijuana, mescaline	Schedule I • High abuse potential • No currently accepted medical use	Schedule H
Opium (morphine), meperidine, amphetamines, cocaine, short-acting barbiturates (secobarbital)	Schedule II • High abuse potential; potentially severe psychologic or physical dependence • Currently accepted medical use but may be severely restricted • Telephone orders only in emergencies if written Rx follows promptly • No refills	Schedule G
Glutethimide, paregoric, phendimetrazine	Schedule III • Abuse potential less than the drugs/substances in Schedules I and II; potentially moderate or low physical dependence or high psychologic dependence • Currently accepted medical use • Telephone orders permitted • Prescriber may authorize limited refills	Schedule F

Drugs	United States	Canada
Chloral hydrate, chlordiazepoxide, diazepam, mazindol, meprobamate, phenobarbital (Canada—G)	Schedule IV • Low abuse potential relative to drugs/substances in Schedule III; potentially limited physical or psychological dependence • Currently accepted medical use • Telephone orders permitted • Prescriber may authorize limited refills	Schedule F
Antidiarrheals with opium (Canada—G), antitussives	Schedule V • Lowest abuse potential; potentially very limited physical or psychological dependence • Currently accepted medical use • Prescriber determines refills • Some products containing limited amounts of Schedule V substances (e.g., cough suppressants) available OTC to patients >18 yr	Schedule F

Appendix I

Abbreviations

AAS argininosuccinic acid synthetase
abd abdomen
ABG arterial blood gas
ac before meals
ACE angiotensin-converting enzyme
ADA American Diabetes Association
ADH antidiuretic hormone
ALT alanine aminotransferase
ANA antinuclear antibody
AP anteroposterior
APTT activated partial thromboplastin time
ASA acetylsalicylic acid, aspirin
ASHD arteriosclerotic heart disease
AST aspartate aminotransferase (SGOT)
AV atrioventricular
bid twice a day
BM bowel movement
BMR basal metabolic rate
B/P blood pressure
BPH benign prostatic hypertrophy
BPM beats per minute
BS blood sugar
BUN blood urea nitrogen
C Celsius (centigrade)
Ca cancer
CAD coronary artery disease
cap capsule
Cath catheterization or catheterize
CBC complete blood cell count
CC chief complaint
cc cubic centimeter
CHF congestive heart failure
cm centimeter
CNS central nervous system
CO₂ carbon dioxide
CONT continuous

COPD chronic obstructive pulmonary disease
CPAP continuous positive airway pressure
CPK creatine phosphokinase
CPR cardiopulmonary resuscitation
CPS carbamoyl phosphate synthetase
CrCl creatinine clearance
C&S culture and sensitivity
C sect cesarean section
CSF cerebrospinal fluid
CV cardiovascular
CVA cerebrovascular accident
CVP central venous pressure
D&C dilatation and curettage
DIC diffuse intravascular coagulation
DIR INF direct infusion
dr dram
D₅W 5% glucose in distilled water
ECG electrocardiogram (EKG)
EDTA ethylenediamine tetraacetic acid
EEG electroencephalogram
EENT ear, eye, nose, and throat
EPS extrapyramidal symptom
ESR erythrocyte sedimentation rate
EXT
REL extended release
EXTRA
STREN
SUSP extra strength suspension
FBS fasting blood sugar
FHT fetal heart tones
FSH follicle-stimulating hormone
g gram
GABA γ-aminobutyric acid
GI gastrointestinal

gr	grain	**MAC**	monitored anesthesia care
GT	glucose tolerance test	**MAOI**	monoamine oxidase inhibitor
gtt	drops	**mEq**	milliequivalent
GU	genitourinary	**mg**	milligram
H₂	histamine₂	**μg**	microgram
HCG	human chorionic gonado-tropin	**μm**	micron
		MI	myocardial infarction
Hct	hematocrit	**min**	minute
HDCV	human diploid cell rabies vaccine	**ml**	milliliter
		mm	millimeter
Hgb	hemoglobin	**mo**	month
H & H	hematocrit and hemoglobin	**Na**	sodium
5-HIAA	5-hydroxyindoleacetic acid	**neg**	negative
HIV	human immunodeficiency virus (AIDS)	**ng**	nanogram
		NOS	not otherwise specified
H₂O	water	**NPO**	nothing by mouth (Lat. *nulla per os*)
HOB	head of bed		
HR	heart rate	**NS**	normal saline
hr	hour	**O₂**	oxygen
hs	at bedtime	**OBS**	organic brain syndrome
IgG	immunolobulin G	**od**	right eye
IM	intramuscular	**OR**	operating room
INF	infusion	**os**	left eye
INH	inhalation	**OTC**	over-the-counter
inj	injection	**OU**	each eye
I&O	intake and output	**oz**	ounce
INT	intermittent	**p̄**	after
IPPB	intermittent positive-pressure breathing	**P56**	plasma-lyte 56
		PaCO₂	arterial carbon dioxide ten-sion (pressure)
ITP	idiopathic thrombocytopenic purpura		
		PaO₂	arterial oxygen tension (pressure)
IUD	intrauterine device		
IV	intravenous	**PAT**	paroxysmal atrial tachy-cardia
IVP	intravenous pyelogram		
K	potassium	**PBI**	protein-bound iodine
kg	kilogram	**pc**	after meals
L	liter	**PCWP**	pulmonary capillary wedge pressure
lb	pound		
LDH	lactic dehydrogenase	**PEEP**	positive end-expiratory pressure
LE	lupus erythematosus		
LFT	liver function test	**PERRLA**	pupils equal, round, react to light and accommodation
LH	luteinizing hormone		
LLQ	left lower quadrant		
LMP	last menstrual period	**pH**	hydrogen ion concentration
LOC	level of consciousness	**PO**	by mouth
LR	lactated Ringer's solution	**postop**	postoperative
LT	leukotriene	**PP**	postprandial
LUQ	left upper quadrant	**preop**	preoperative
M	meter	**prn**	as required
m	minim	**PT**	prothrombin time
m²	square meter	**PTT**	partial thromboplastin time

PVC premature ventricular contraction
pwd powder
qAM every morning
qd every day
qh every hour
q2h every 2 hours
q3h every 3 hours
q4h every 4 hours
q6h every 6 hours
q12h every 12 hours
qid four times daily
qod every other day
qPM every night
qs sufficient quantity
qt quart
R right
RAIU radioactive iodine uptake
RBC red blood cell count or red blood cell
RECT rectal
RLQ right lower quadrant
ROM range of motion
RUQ right upper quadrant
SC subcutaneous
SIMV synchronous intermittent mandatory ventilation
SL sublingual
SLE systemic lupus erythematosus
SOB shortness of breath
sol solution
ss one half
suppos suppository

SUS REL sustained release
syr syrup
T&A tonsillectomy and adenoidectomy
tab tablet
tbsp tablespoon
temp temperature
tid three times daily
tinc tincture
TPN total parenteral nutrition
top topical
TRANS transdermal
TSH thyroid-stimulating hormone
tsp teaspoon
TT thrombin time
U unit
UA urinalysis
UTI urinary tract infection
UV ultraviolet
vag vaginal
VMA vanillylmandelic acid
vol volume
VS vital sign
WBC white blood cell count
wk week
wt weight
yr year
> greater than
< less than
= equal
° degree
% percent
γ gamma
β beta

Appendix m

Weights and equivalents

METRIC SYSTEM
Weight

kilogram	= kg	= 1000 grams
gram	= g	= 1 gram
milligram	= mg =	0.001 gram
microgram	= μg =	0.001 milligram

Volume

liter	= L	= 1 L
milliliter	= ml =	0.001 L

AVOIRDUPOIS WEIGHT

1 ounce (oz)= 437.5 grains
1 pound (lb)= 16 ounces = 7000 grains

METRIC AND APOTHECARY EQUIVALENTS
Exact weight equivalents

Metric	Apothecary
1 mg	1/64.8 grain
64.8 mg	1 grain
324 mg	5 grains
1 g	15.432 grains
31.103 g	1 ounce = 480 grains

Exact volume equivalents

Metric	Apothecary		
1.00 ml	16.23 minims		
3.69 ml	1 fluidram	=	60 minims
29.57 ml	1 fluid ounce	=	480 minims
473.16 ml	1 pint	=	7680 minims
946.33 ml	1 quart	=	15,360 minims

Appendix n

Formulas for drug calculations

Surface area rule:

$$\text{Child dose} = \frac{\text{Surface area (m}^2)}{1.73 \text{m}^2} \times \text{Adult dose}$$

Calculating strength of a solution:

Solution Strength: *Desired Solution:*

$$\frac{x}{100} = \frac{\text{Amount of drug desired}}{\text{Amount of finished solution}}$$

Calculating flow rate for IV:

$$\text{Rate of flow} = \frac{\text{Amount of fluid} \times \text{Administration set calibration}}{\text{Running time}}$$

$$\frac{x}{1} = \frac{(\text{ml}) \ (\text{gtt/min})}{\text{min}}$$

Calculation of medication dosages:

Formula method:

$$\frac{\text{Amount ordered}}{\text{Amount on hand}} \times \text{Vehicle} = \text{Number of tablets, capsules, or amount of liquid}$$

Vehicle is the drug form or amount of liquid containing the dosage. Amounts used in calculation by formula must be in same system.

Ratio—proportion method:

1 tablet:tablet in mg on hand::x tablet order in mg

Know or have::Want to know or order

Multiply means and extremes, divide both sides by known amount to get X. Amounts used in equation must be in same system.

Dimensional analysis method:

$$\text{Order in mg} \times \frac{1 \text{ tablet or capsule}}{\text{What 1 tablet or capsule is in mg}}$$
$$= \text{Tablets or capsules to be given}$$

If amounts are in different systems:

$$\text{Order in mg} \times \frac{1 \text{ tablet or capsule}}{\text{What 1 tablet or capsule is in g}} \times \frac{1}{1000 \text{ mg}}$$
$$= \text{Tablets or capsules to be given}$$

Appendix o

Nomogram for calculation of body surface area

Place a straight edge from the patient's height in the left column to the patient's weight in the right column. The point of intersection on the body surface area column indicates the body surface area (BSA). (Reproduced from Behrman RE, and Vaughn VC (editors): *Nelson's textbook of pediatrics,* ed 12, Philadelphia, 1983, WB Saunders.)

Appendix p

Bibliography

Blumenthal M: *The complete German Commission E monographs: Therapeutic guide to herbal medicines,* Austin, 1998, American Botanical Council.

Clark JB, Queener SF, Karb VB: *Pharmacological basis of nursing practice,* ed 5, St Louis, 1998, Mosby.

Drug Information: Bethesda, American Hospital Formulary Service.

Facts and Comparisons: St Louis, updated monthly.

Gahart BL: *Intravenous medications,* ed 14, St Louis, 2000, Mosby.

Goodman A and others: *Goodman and Gilman's The pharmacological basis of therapeutics,* ed 10, New York, 1998, Pergamon Press.

McKenry LM, Salerno E: *Mosby's pharmacology in nursing,* ed 18, St Louis, 1996, Mosby.

Mediphor Editorial Group: *Drug interaction facts,* Philadelphia, updated quarterly, JB Lippincott.

Review of natural products: Philadelphia, updated monthly, *Facts and Comparisons.*

Entries can be identified as follows: generic name, Trade Name, DRUG CATEGORY, *Combination Product, DISEASE/DISORDER,* DISCONTINUED, **Four-Color Illustration.**

Entries can be identified as follows: generic name, Trade Name, DRUG CATEGORY, *Combination Product, DISEASE/DISORDER,* DISCONTINUED, **Four-Color Illustration.**

Entries can be identified as follows: generic name, Trade Name, DRUG CATEGORY, *Combination Product, DISEASE/DISORDER,* DISCONTINUED, **Four-Color Illustration.**

Entries can be identified as follows: generic name, Trade Name, DRUG CATEGORY, *Combination Product, DISEASE/DISORDER,* DISCONTINUED, **Four-Color Illustration.**

Entries can be identified as follows: generic name, Trade Name, DRUG CATEGORY, *Combination Product, DISEASE/DISORDER,* DISCONTINUED, **Four-Color Illustration.**

Entries can be identified as follows: generic name, Trade Name, DRUG CATEGORY, *Combination Product, DISEASE/DISORDER,* DISCONTINUED, **Four-Color Illustration.**

Entries can be identified as follows: generic name, Trade Name, DRUG CATEGORY, *Combination Product, DISEASE/DISORDER,* DISCONTINUED, **Four-Color Illustration.**

Entries can be identified as follows: generic name, Trade Name, DRUG CATEGORY,
Combination Product, DISEASE/DISORDER, DISCONTINUED, **Four-Color Illustration.**

Entries can be identified as follows: generic name, Trade Name, DRUG CATEGORY, *Combination Product, DISEASE/DISORDER,* DISCONTINUED, **Four-Color Illustration.**

Entries can be identified as follows: generic name, Trade Name, DRUG CATEGORY,
Combination Product, DISEASE/DISORDER, DISCONTINUED, **Four-Color Illustration.**

Entries can be identified as follows: generic name, Trade Name, DRUG CATEGORY, *Combination Product*, *DISEASE/DISORDER*, DISCONTINUED, **Four-Color Illustration.**

Entries can be identified as follows: generic name, Trade Name, DRUG CATEGORY, *Combination Product, DISEASE/DISORDER,* DISCONTINUED, **Four-Color Illustration.**

Entries can be identified as follows: generic name, Trade Name, DRUG CATEGORY, *Combination Product, DISEASE/DISORDER,* DISCONTINUED, **Four-Color Illustration.**

Entries can be identified as follows: generic name, Trade Name, DRUG CATEGORY,
Combination Product, DISEASE/DISORDER, DISCONTINUED, **Four-Color Illustration.**

Entries can be identified as follows: generic name, Trade Name, DRUG CATEGORY, *Combination Product, DISEASE/DISORDER,* DISCONTINUED, **Four-Color Illustration.**

Entries can be identified as follows: generic name, Trade Name, DRUG CATEGORY, *Combination Product*, *DISEASE/DISORDER*, DISCONTINUED, **Four-Color Illustration.**

Entries can be identified as follows: generic name, Trade Name, DRUG CATEGORY, *Combination Product, DISEASE/DISORDER,* DISCONTINUED, **Four-Color Illustration.**

Entries can be identified as follows: generic name, Trade Name, DRUG CATEGORY, *Combination Product, DISEASE/DISORDER,* DISCONTINUED, **Four-Color Illustration.**

Entries can be identified as follows: generic name, Trade Name, DRUG CATEGORY, *Combination Product, DISEASE/DISORDER,* DISCONTINUED, **Four-Color Illustration.**

Entries can be identified as follows: generic name, Trade Name, DRUG CATEGORY, *Combination Product, DISEASE/DISORDER,* DISCONTINUED, **Four-Color Illustration.**

Entries can be identified as follows: generic name, Trade Name, DRUG CATEGORY, *Combination Product*, *DISEASE/DISORDER*, DISCONTINUED, **Four-Color Illustration**.

Entries can be identified as follows: generic name, Trade Name, DRUG CATEGORY, *Combination Product, DISEASE/DISORDER,* DISCONTINUED, **Four-Color Illustration.**

Entries can be identified as follows: generic name, Trade Name, DRUG CATEGORY, *Combination Product, DISEASE/DISORDER,* DISCONTINUED, **Four-Color Illustration.**

Entries can be identified as follows: generic name, Trade Name, DRUG CATEGORY, *Combination Product, DISEASE/DISORDER,* DISCONTINUED, **Four-Color Illustration.**

Entries can be identified as follows: generic name, Trade Name, DRUG CATEGORY, *Combination Product, DISEASE/DISORDER,* DISCONTINUED, **Four-Color Illustration.**

Entries can be identified as follows: generic name, Trade Name, DRUG CATEGORY, *Combination Product, DISEASE/DISORDER,* DISCONTINUED, **Four-Color Illustration.**

Entries can be identified as follows: generic name, Trade Name, DRUG CATEGORY,
Combination Product, DISEASE/DISORDER, DISCONTINUED, **Four-Color Illustration.**

Entries can be identified as follows: generic name, Trade Name, DRUG CATEGORY, *Combination Product, DISEASE/DISORDER,* discontinued, **Four-Color Illustration.**

Entries can be identified as follows: generic name, Trade Name, DRUG CATEGORY, *Combination Product, DISEASE/DISORDER,* DISCONTINUED, **Four-Color Illustration.**

Entries can be identified as follows: generic name, Trade Name, DRUG CATEGORY, *Combination Product, DISEASE/DISORDER,* discontinued, **Four-Color Illustration.**

Entries can be identified as follows: generic name, Trade Name, DRUG CATEGORY,
Combination Product, DISEASE/DISORDER, DISCONTINUED, **Four-Color Illustration.**

Entries can be identified as follows: generic name, Trade Name, DRUG CATEGORY, *Combination Product, DISEASE/DISORDER,* DISCONTINUED, **Four-Color Illustration.**

Entries can be identified as follows: generic name, Trade Name, DRUG CATEGORY, *Combination Product, DISEASE/DISORDER,* DISCONTINUED, **Four-Color Illustration.**

Entries can be identified as follows: generic name, Trade Name, DRUG CATEGORY, *Combination Product, DISEASE/DISORDER,* DISCONTINUED, **Four-Color Illustration.**

Entries can be identified as follows: generic name, Trade Name, DRUG CATEGORY, *Combination Product, DISEASE/DISORDER,* DISCONTINUED, **Four-Color Illustration.**

Entries can be identified as follows: generic name, Trade Name, DRUG CATEGORY, *Combination Product, DISEASE/DISORDER,* discontinued, **Four-Color Illustration.**

Entries can be identified as follows: generic name, Trade Name, DRUG CATEGORY, *Combination Product, DISEASE/DISORDER,* DISCONTINUED, **Four-Color Illustration.**

Entries can be identified as follows: generic name, Trade Name, DRUG CATEGORY, *Combination Product, DISEASE/DISORDER,* DISCONTINUED, **Four-Color Illustration.**

Entries can be identified as follows: generic name, Trade Name, DRUG CATEGORY, *Combination Product, DISEASE/DISORDER,* DISCONTINUED, **Four-Color Illustration.**

Entries can be identified as follows: generic name, Trade Name, DRUG CATEGORY, *Combination Product, DISEASE/DISORDER,* DISCONTINUED, **Four-Color Illustration.**

Entries can be identified as follows: generic name, Trade Name, DRUG CATEGORY, *Combination Product, DISEASE/DISORDER,* DISCONTINUED, **Four-Color Illustration.**

Entries can be identified as follows: generic name, Trade Name, DRUG CATEGORY, *Combination Product, DISEASE/DISORDER,* DISCONTINUED, **Four-Color Illustration.**

Entries can be identified as follows: generic name, Trade Name, DRUG CATEGORY, *Combination Product, DISEASE/DISORDER,* DISCONTINUED, **Four-Color Illustration.**

Entries can be identified as follows: generic name, Trade Name, DRUG CATEGORY, *Combination Product*, *DISEASE/DISORDER*, DISCONTINUED, **Four-Color Illustration**.

Entries can be identified as follows: generic name, Trade Name, DRUG CATEGORY,
Combination Product, DISEASE/DISORDER, DISCONTINUED, **Four-Color Illustration.**

Entries can be identified as follows: generic name, Trade Name, DRUG CATEGORY, *Combination Product, DISEASE/DISORDER,* DISCONTINUED, **Four-Color Illustration.**

Entries can be identified as follows: generic name, Trade Name, DRUG CATEGORY, *Combination Product, DISEASE/DISORDER,* DISCONTINUED, **Four-Color Illustration.**

Entries can be identified as follows: generic name, Trade Name, DRUG CATEGORY, *Combination Product, DISEASE/DISORDER,* DISCONTINUED, **Four-Color Illustration.**

Entries can be identified as follows: generic name, Trade Name, DRUG CATEGORY, *Combination Product, DISEASE/DISORDER,* DISCONTINUED, **Four-Color Illustration.**

Entries can be identified as follows: generic name, Trade Name, DRUG CATEGORY, *Combination Product, DISEASE/DISORDER,* DISCONTINUED, **Four-Color Illustration.**

Entries can be identified as follows: generic name, Trade Name, DRUG CATEGORY,
Combination Product, DISEASE/DISORDER, DISCONTINUED, **Four-Color Illustration.**

Entries can be identified as follows: generic name, Trade Name, DRUG CATEGORY, *Combination Product, DISEASE/DISORDER,* DISCONTINUED, **Four-Color Illustration.**

Entries can be identified as follows: generic name, Trade Name, DRUG CATEGORY, *Combination Product, DISEASE/DISORDER,* DISCONTINUED, **Four-Color Illustration.**

Entries can be identified as follows: generic name, Trade Name, DRUG CATEGORY,
Combination Product, DISEASE/DISORDER, DISCONTINUED, **Four-Color Illustration.**

Entries can be identified as follows: generic name, Trade Name, DRUG CATEGORY, *Combination Product, DISEASE/DISORDER,* DISCONTINUED, **Four-Color Illustration.**

Entries can be identified as follows: generic name, Trade Name, DRUG CATEGORY, *Combination Product, DISEASE/DISORDER,* DISCONTINUED, **Four-Color Illustration.**

Entries can be identified as follows: generic name, Trade Name, DRUG CATEGORY, *Combination Product, DISEASE/DISORDER,* DISCONTINUED, **Four-Color Illustration.**

Entries can be identified as follows: generic name, Trade Name, DRUG CATEGORY, *Combination Product, DISEASE/DISORDER,* DISCONTINUED, **Four-Color Illustration.**

Entries can be identified as follows: generic name, Trade Name, DRUG CATEGORY, *Combination Product*, *DISEASE/DISORDER*, DISCONTINUED, **Four-Color Illustration.**

Entries can be identified as follows: generic name, Trade Name, DRUG CATEGORY, *Combination Product, DISEASE/DISORDER,* DISCONTINUED, **Four-Color Illustration.**

Entries can be identified as follows: generic name, Trade Name, DRUG CATEGORY, *Combination Product, DISEASE/DISORDER,* DISCONTINUED, **Four-Color Illustration.**

Entries can be identified as follows: generic name, Trade Name, DRUG CATEGORY,
Combination Product, DISEASE/DISORDER, DISCONTINUED, **Four-Color Illustration.**

Entries can be identified as follows: generic name, Trade Name, DRUG CATEGORY, *Combination Product, DISEASE/DISORDER,* DISCONTINUED, **Four-Color Illustration.**

Entries can be identified as follows: generic name, Trade Name, DRUG CATEGORY,
Combination Product, DISEASE/DISORDER, DISCONTINUED, **Four-Color Illustration.**

Entries can be identified as follows: generic name, Trade Name, DRUG CATEGORY,
Combination Product, DISEASE/DISORDER, DISCONTINUED, **Four-Color Illustration.**

Entries can be identified as follows: generic name, Trade Name, DRUG CATEGORY,
Combination Product, DISEASE/DISORDER, DISCONTINUED, **Four-Color Illustration.**

Entries can be identified as follows: generic name, Trade Name, DRUG CATEGORY, *Combination Product, DISEASE/DISORDER,* DISCONTINUED, **Four-Color Illustration.**

Entries can be identified as follows: generic name, Trade Name, DRUG CATEGORY, *Combination Product*, *DISEASE/DISORDER*, DISCONTINUED, **Four-Color Illustration.**

Entries can be identified as follows: generic name, Trade Name, DRUG CATEGORY,
Combination Product, DISEASE/DISORDER, DISCONTINUED, **Four-Color Illustration.**

Entries can be identified as follows: generic name, Trade Name, DRUG CATEGORY, *Combination Product, DISEASE/DISORDER,* DISCONTINUED, **Four-Color Illustration.**

Entries can be identified as follows: generic name, Trade Name, DRUG CATEGORY, *Combination Product, DISEASE/DISORDER,* DISCONTINUED, **Four-Color Illustration.**

Entries can be identified as follows: generic name, Trade Name, DRUG CATEGORY, *Combination Product, DISEASE/DISORDER,* DISCONTINUED, **Four-Color Illustration.**

Entries can be identified as follows: generic name, Trade Name, DRUG CATEGORY, *Combination Product, DISEASE/DISORDER,* DISCONTINUED, **Four-Color Illustration.**

Herbal Remedies CD-ROM to accompany
Mosby's 2001 Nursing Drug Reference

Herbal Remedies by Steve Blake, ND, MH, DSc, MT, provides you with up-to-date, accurate information on more than 30 of the most commonly used herbal remedies!

Herbal Remedies provides:

• A user-friendly interface that allows you to search for herbs by common name, alternate names, patient health conditions, body systems or organs affected, and actions or constituents of the herb
• A high-quality photograph of every herb
• Detailed information on constituents and actions of each herb
• Warnings, where appropriate, for herbs that may have side effects or contraindications
• Cross-references that link herbs to the appropriate conditions, actions, organs or constituents
• A handy print feature and the ability to save individual herb monographs to a unique file

This mini-CD-ROM *will* work in your CD-ROM drive. Place it on the inner ring of the tray, as shown below, and follow the installation instructions on the facing page.

This mini-CD does not work in:
Floppy Drives
Slot Drives
Zip Drives
Stereos
Insert this mini-CD into your CD-ROM drive as shown at left.

Information on the full spectrum of natural remedies, including herbs, Chinese herbs, Ayurvedic herbs, homeopathic remedies, vitamins, minerals, supplements, aromatherapy oils, and many popular natural formulas, can be found on *Alternative Remedies CD-ROM* by Steve Blake. For more information, or to order, call Mosby toll-free at 1-800-426-4545.